Veterinary Reproduction
and Obstetrics

Veterinary Reproduction and Obstetrics

Seventh Edition

GEOFFREY H. ARTHUR DVSc, FRCVS

Professor Emeritus of Veterinary Surgery, University of Bristol; formerly Clinical Professor, College of Veterinary Medicine and Animal Resources, King Faisal University, Saudi Arabia, and Professor of Veterinary Obstetrics and Diseases of Reproduction, Royal Veterinary College, University of London, UK

DAVID E. NOAKES BVetMed, PhD, FRCVS, DVReprod

Professor of Veterinary Obstetrics and Diseases of Reproduction, Royal Veterinary College, University of London, UK

HAROLD PEARSON BVSc, PhD, FRCVS

Professor of Veterinary Surgery, University of Bristol, UK

TIMOTHY J. PARKINSON BVSc, PhD, DBR, MRCVS

Senior Lecturer in Veterinary Obstetrics and Diseases of Reproduction, University of Bristol, UK

WB Saunders Company Limited
London   Philadelphia   Toronto   Sydney   Tokyo

W. B. Saunders Company Limited   24–28 Oval Road
London NW1 7DX

The Curtis Center
Independence Square West
Philadelphia, PA 19106–3399, USA

Harcourt Brace & Company
55 Horner Avenue
Toronto, Ontario M8Z 4X6, Canada

Harcourt Brace & Company, Australia
30–52 Smidmore Street
Marrickville, NSW 2204, Australia

Harcourt Brace & Company, Japan
Ichibancho Central Building, 22–1 Ichibancho
Chiyoda-ku, Tokyo 102, Japan

First published 1938 as Veterinary Obstetrics by F. Benesch
Second edition 1951 as Veterinary Obstetrics by F. Benesch and J. G. Wright
Third edition 1964 as Wright's Veterinary Obstetrics by G. H. Arthur
Fourth edition 1975 as Veterinary Reproduction and Obstetrics by G. H. Arthur
Fifth edition 1982 as Veterinary Reproduction and Obstetrics by G. H. Arthur, D. E. Noakes and H. Pearson
Sixth edition 1989 as Veterinary Reproduction and Obstetrics by G. H. Arthur, D. E. Noakes and H. Pearson
Reprinted 1992

A catalogue record for this book is available from the British Library

ISBN 0–7020–1785–X

Typeset by J&L Composition, Filey, North Yorkshire
Printed in Great Britain by The Bath Press, Avon

CONTENTS

CONTRIBUTORS

GEOFFREY H. ARTHUR   Professor Emeritus of Veterinary Surgery, University of Bristol. Formerly Professor of Veterinary Obstetrics and Diseases of Reproduction, Royal Veterinary College, University of London, U.K.

DAVID BEE   Practitioner, Petersfield, Hampshire, U.K.

WILLIAM B. CHRISTIE   Embryo Transfer Practitioner, Paragon ET, Hexham, Northumberland, U.K.

GARY ENGLAND   Lecturer in Veterinary Reproduction, Department of Farm Animal and Equine Medicine and Surgery, Royal Veterinary College, University of London, U.K.

CHRISTIANNE E. GLOSSOP   Pig Veterinary Consultant, Malmesbury, Wiltshire, U.K.

M. R. JAINUDEEN   Professor, Faculty of Veterinary Medicine and Animal Science, Universiti Pertanian, Malaysia.

SUSAN E. LONG   Senior Lecturer, Department of Clinical Veterinary Science, School of Veterinary Science, University of Bristol, U.K.

DAVID E. NOAKES   Professor of Veterinary Obstetrics and Diseases of Reproduction, Department of Farm Animal and Equine Medicine and Surgery, Royal Veterinary College, University of London, U.K.

TIMOTHY J. PARKINSON   Senior Lecturer in Veterinary Obstetrics and Diseases of Reproduction, University of Bristol, U.K.

HAROLD PEARSON   Professor of Veterinary Surgery, Department of Veterinary Medicine, University of Bristol, U.K.

JONATHAN F. PYCOCK   Associate Professor of Equine Reproduction, Department of Herd Health and Reproduction, Faculty of Veterinary Medicine, University of Utrecht, Netherlands.

PREFACE

The popularity of this book over the past 30 years has encouraged us to adhere to the objectives of earlier editions, namely to cater for the needs of undergraduate veterinary students and to provide a ready reference for readers in allied disciplines and those in veterinary practice who wish to keep abreast of developments in animal reproductive science. Hence the format of this edition is unchanged.

However, the substantial advances of recent years in basic science have led to a corresponding requirement for specialization in the application of that knowledge to vocational needs. Thus, it is now conceded that a single veterinarian can no longer be expected to provide expert advice and particular skills for the whole range of domestic species. This concept is now well established in veterinary practice and is reflected in the clinics and departments of veterinary schools. Therefore, in producing this Seventh Edition, it seemed reasonable to invite several additional authors to assist with the task, and it is pleasing to welcome Drs England, Glossop and Pycock to cover reproduction in the bitch and queen, pigs, and horses, respectively.

All the chapters have been revised; Dr Parkinson undertook the updating of the whole section on the male animal, while Mr Bee bore the brunt of the revision of the bovine obstetrics chapters. Dr Long kindly undertook the rewriting of the text on abnormal development, including cytogenetics.

The main authors are again indebted to Dr W. B. Christie and Professor Jainudeen for their revisions of the chapters on embryo transfer and buffalo reproduction, respectively.

In the preparation of this Seventh Edition, we are particularly indebted to John Conibear for the generation of much new photographic material. We wish to record our thanks to Rosemary Forster for secretarial support. Katharine Hinton, initially, and Catriona Byres from Saunders subsequently, gave expert advice and showed great tolerance at missed deadlines; thanks are also due to Fran Kingston for supervising the production of a new edition.

Finally, we would like to thank those friends and colleagues who provided constructive criticisms and helpful suggestions, and also illustrative material which is duly acknowledged in the appropriate figure legends.

G. H. ARTHUR
D. E. NOAKES
H. PEARSON
T. J. PARKINSON

1

Part One

Normal Oestrous Cycles

Endogenous and Exogenous Control of Ovarian Cyclicity

In nature it is the general rule that animals breed once annually and parturition occurs in the spring, the time most favourable to the progeny in that they grow up during the period of increasing light and warmth and also at the time when food for the mother is most abundant and adequate lactation is ensured. Under the conditions of feeding and housing provided by domestication the breeding season tends to be lengthened, and some of our species, particularly the cattle, may breed at any time during the year; all domesticated animals, however, show a constant tendency to revert to the natural breeding season.

For an animal to breed it must be mated and hence must attract the male and be sexually receptive, 'in heat' or oestrus. All domestic species show recurring periods of sexual receptivity, or oestrous cycles, which are associated with the ripening in the ovaries of one or more Graafian follicles and culminating in the shedding of one or more ova. If a fertile mating occurs then pregnancy may ensue.

PUBERTY AND THE ONSET OF CYCLIC ACTIVITY

The young female animal shows no evidence of recurring or cyclical periods of sexual receptivity. The onset of such changes when the female becomes sexually mature and able to reproduce is referred to as puberty. Amongst females of the domestic species, puberty precedes the development of physical maturity and, although they become capable of reproducing, their efficiency, particularly with respect to their fecundity, has not reached its maximum.

The initiation of puberty is largely a function of the animal's age and maturity since the female is born with a genetic potential for cyclic reproductive activity. Provided the environmental influences are favourable at this time, then once the 'biological clock' is started it will continue for as long as the environment remains favourable. In none of our domestic species is there a physiological change comparable with the menopause of women.

Amongst polycyclic animals, such as the cow and sow, the recurring cyclical activity is interrupted by pregnancy, lactation and pathological conditions. In those species which are seasonally polycyclic, the mare, ewe and cat, or monocyclic like the bitch, there are periods of sexual quiescence or anoestrus.

When the female reaches puberty the genital organs increase in size. During the prepubertal period the growth of the genital organs is very similar to that of other organ systems, but at puberty their growth rate is accelerated, a point well illustrated in the gilt, where the mean length of the uterine horns is increased by 58%, the mean weight of the uterus by 72% and the mean weight of the ovaries by 32% between 169 and 186 days of age (Lasley, 1968). Females of domestic species reach the age of puberty at the following times:

Mare	1–2 years
Cow	7–18 months
Ewe	6–15 months
Doe or nanny goat	4–8 months
Sow	6–8 months
Bitch	6–20 months
Queen cat	7–12 months

The changes that occur at puberty depend directly upon the activity of the ovaries, which have two functions: the production of the female gametes and the synthesis of hormones. Let us consider the changes that occur in the ovary of the young heifer calf. At birth each ovary may contain up to 150 000 primary or primordial follicles; each consists of an oocyte surrounded by a single layer of epithelial cells, but there are no thecal cells. Soon after birth the ovaries start to develop and produce growing follicles which consist of an oocyte with two or more layers of granulosa cells and a basement membrane. The stimulus for the development of these follicles is intra-ovarian, and until the heifer reaches the age of puberty they will develop only to the stage where they have a theca interna and then start to undergo atresia. Further development of these follicles to produce mature Graafian or antral follicles, of which there are about 200 growing follicles at puberty in the heifer, is dependent upon the stimulus of gonadotrophic hormones.

The sheep has been used extensively for studying many of the mechanisms involved in the initiation of puberty; however, it must be stressed that seasonality will exert an overriding influence in this species (see below). The onset of puberty is signalled by either the occurrence of the first oestrous or the first ovulation; in the ewe lamb these do not occur simultaneously because the first ovulation is not preceded by behavioural oestrus. A similar response is seen in sexually mature ewes at the onset of the normal breeding season (see p. 27).

The hormone that is primarily responsible for the onset of ovarian activity, and hence puberty, is luteinizing hormone (LH). In adult ewes during the normal breeding season, basal LH concentrations increase together with the LH pulse frequency to one per hour during the period of maximum follicular growth. This results in the development of follicles to the preovulatory stage, and their secretion of oestradiol which activates the LH surge causing ovulation and corpus luteum formation. In the prepubertal ewe lamb, LH pulses occur at similar amplitudes but much lower frequencies (one every 2–3 hours). As a consequence, follicular growth is insufficient to activate the LH surge necessary for final follicular maturation and ovulation.

Experimental evidence in prepubertal ewe lambs has shown that ovarian follicles are capable of responding to exogenous gonadotrophin stimulation, and the pituitary is capable of secreting LH at a frequency to stimulate ovulation. The failure of the prepubertal ewe lamb to undergo ovulation and exhibit oestrus is due to the high threshold for the positive-feedback effect of oestradiol, and thus there is no LH surge. At puberty, the threshold is lowered, thus allowing the pituitary to respond. This is sometimes referred to as the 'gonadostat' theory.

Other factors are also involved. The frequency of LH secretion is dependent upon gonadotrophin-releasing-hormone (GnRH) from the hypothalamus, which is controlled by an area in the hypothalamus referred to as the neural GnRH pulse generator. Age-related changes in brain morphology and neuronal cytoarchitecture may also be important, since extrapolation from studies performed in rats, for example, have shown an increase in the number of GnRH cells with spine-like processes on the soma and dendrites. In addition, the inhibitory effect of opioid peptides on LH secretion is reduced with age, which may provide a neurochemical explanation for the changes in pituitary sensitivity to oestradiol feedback which occurs at puberty (Bhanot and Wilkinson, 1983; Wray and Hoffman-Small, 1984).

The reason for the 'silent' first oestrous of the pubertal animal is believed to be because the central nervous system requires to be primed with progesterone before it will respond and the animal show behavioural signs of heat.

External factors influencing the time of onset of puberty

The time of onset of puberty is determined by the individual's genotype, smaller breeds of animals tending to be slightly more precocious. However, this inherent timing is influenced by a number of external factors.

Nutrition. There is good evidence that in most domestic species the age of puberty is closely related to body weight; therefore, it is not surprising that nutrition is an important factor. Animals that are well fed with good growth rates reach puberty before those that are poorly fed with slow growth rates. However, unless the animal is severely malnourished, the onset of cyclical activity will eventually occur.

Season of the Year. In those species which are seasonal breeders, such as the ewe and mare, the age at which puberty occurs will be influenced by the effect of season of the year. For instance, a filly born early in the year, i.e. January or February, may have her first oestrus in the May or June of the following year, i.e. when she is 16 or 17 months old, while a filly foal born late in the year, July or August, may not have her first oestrus until she is 21 or 22 months old. The same is true of ewes which, depending upon the time of year at which they are born, may reach puberty as early as 6 months or as late as 18 months old.

Proximity of the Male. Studies in sheep and pigs have shown that exposure to the male of the species will advance the timing of the onset of puberty. This so-called 'ram or boar effect' is probably mediated by pheromonal and other sensory cues influencing hypothalamic GnRH secretion.

Climate. Anthropomorphic extrapolation has assumed that animals living in the tropics reach puberty at an earlier age than those in temperate climates. Studies carried out in Zambia have shown that in cattle this is not true.

Disease. Any disease which can influence the growth rate, either directly or because of interference with feeding and utilization of nutrients, will delay the onset of puberty.

THE OESTROUS CYCLE AND ITS PHASES

Traditionally, the oestrous cycle is divided into a number of phases.

Pro-oestrus. The phase immediately preceding oestrus. It is characterized by a marked increase in activity of the reproductive system. There is follicular growth and regression of the corpus luteum of the previous cycle (in polycyclic species). The uterus enlarges; the endometrium becomes congested and oedematous, and its glands show evidence of increased secretory activity. The vaginal mucosa becomes hyperaemic; the number of cell layers of the epithelium starts to increase, and the superficial layers become cornified. The bitch shows external evidence of pro-oestrus with vulval oedema, hyperaemia and a sanguineous vulval discharge.

Oestrus. The period of acceptance of the male. The onset and end of the phase are the only accurately measurable points in the oestrous cycle and hence are used as the baseline for determining cycle length. The animal usually seeks out the male and 'stands' for him to mate her. The uterine, cervical and vaginal glands secrete increased amounts of mucus, the vaginal epithelium and endometrium become hyperaemic and congested; the cervix is relaxed.

Ovulation occurs during this phase of the cycle in all domestic species with the exception of the cow, where it occurs about 12 hours after the end of oestrus. Ovulation is a spontaneous process in all domestic species with the exception of the cat, rabbit and camel, in which it is induced by the act of coitus.

During pro-oestrus and oestrus there is follicular growth in the absence of functional corpora lutea, the main ovarian hormones produced being oestrogens. Pro-oestrus and oestrus are frequently referred to collectively as the follicular phase of the cycle.

Metoestrus. The phase succeeding oestrus. The granulosa cells of the ovulated follicle give rise to lutein cells which are responsible for the formation of the corpus luteum. There is a reduction in the amount of secretion from the uterine, cervical and vaginal glands.

Dioestrus. The period of the corpus luteum. The uterine glands undergo hyperplasia and hypertrophy, the cervix becomes constricted, the secretions of the genital tract are scant and sticky; the vaginal mucosa becomes pale. The corpus luteum is fully functional during this phase, and is secreting large amounts of progesterone.

The period of the oestrous cycle when there is a functional corpus luteum is sometimes referred to as the luteal phase of the cycle to differentiate it from the follicular phase.

Since in most of our domestic species oestrus is the only readily identifiable phase of the oestrous cycle there is some merit, in polyoestrous species, in dividing the cycle into oestrus and interoestrus, the latter including pro-oestrus, metoestrus and dioestrus.

Anoestrus. The prolonged period of sexual rest during which the genital system is mainly quiescent. Follicular development is minimal; the corpora lutea, although identifiable, have regressed and are non-functional. Secretions are scanty and tenacious, the cervix is constricted, and the vaginal mucosa is pale.

Natural regulation of cyclical activity

Regulation of cyclical acitivity in the female is a complex process. With the development of new techniques, particularly those of hormone assays, there is a continual advance in the knowledge and understanding of the mechanisms involved. Although much of the early work was done on laboratory animals — notably the rat and guinea-pig — there is now much more information about domestic species, although there are still areas, particularly in the bitch, which are not fully understood.

Regulation of cyclical activity is mainly under the control of the hypothalamic–pituitary–ovarian axis. At one end of this axis there is the influence of the extrahypothalamic areas — the cerebral cortex, thalamus and mid-brain — and the influence upon these of stimuli such as light, olfaction and touch (Ellendorff, 1978), whilst at the other end is the influence of the uterus upon the ovary.

The pineal gland appears to have an important role in controlling reproduction in seasonal breeding species and also in the timing of puberty by influencing the release of follicle-stimulating hormone (FSH), LH and prolactin. Although much of the interest has been on the action of the indole-amine melatonin, there is increasing interest in the other pineal peptide hormones, namely arginine vasotocin, gonadotrophin and prolactin-releasing and inhibitory hormones. There is some suggestion that melatonin may not act directly upon the hypothalamus/anterior pituitary but indrectly via the other pineal peptide hormones.

Melatonin drives the reproductive response of the ewe to inductive photoperiods (Bittman et al., 1983). Rhythmic administration of melatonin to adult ewes exerts a similar effect to increased hours of darkness by inducing the onset of the breeding season (Arendt et al., 1983) and causes changes in prolactin concentrations in the plasma that are similar to those following exposure to short days (Kennaway et al., 1983).

In sheep, an intact pineal gland is required for a normal photoperiodic response to altered daylight patterns; however, other seasonal environmental cues are important since pinealectomized ewes still show seasonal breeding (Lincoln, 1985).

The mare is a seasonal breeder, but is 'switched-on' by increasing day length. The pineal gland is involved, since if it is removed the mare does not show a normal response to changes in photoperiod. In intact mares, melatonin levels increase during hours of darkness (Grubaugh et al, 1982). There is some evidence that foals are conditioned

at an early age and develop a pattern of melatonin secretion from about 7 weeks of age (Kilmer et al., 1982).

The *hypothalamus* is responsible for the control of release of gonadotrophins from the anterior pituitary by the action of specific releasing and inhibitory substances. These are secreted by the hypothalamic neurons, and are carried from the median eminence of the hypothalamus by the hypothalamic–hypophyseal portal system. In 1971 the molecular structure of porcine GnRH was determined (Matsuo et al., 1971) as being a deca-peptide, and subsequently synthesized (Geiger et al., 1971). Opinion is divided as to whether GnRH is responsible *in vivo* for the release of both FSH and LH (Lamming et al., 1979), although the injection of GnRH stimulates the release of both FSH and LH in domestic species (Pelletier, 1976). As yet no specific inhibitory factor such as that for prolactin has been identified for gonadotrophins.

Specific neurotransmitter substances are involved in the regulation of the release of pituitary hormones. The role of three monoamines has now been fairly well established (Kordon, 1978). Noradrenaline stimulates the release of FSH and LH; the inhibition of the conversion of dopamine to noradrenaline blocks the 'oestradiol-induced' release of LH, which is responsible for ovulation; whilst serotonin inhibits the basal secretion of LH and regulates other neurosecretory systems. Dopamine also has an important role in the control of prolactin release.

There is good evidence that in domestic species the secretion of FSH and LH is controlled by two functionally separate but superimposable systems. These are the tonic episodic system, which is responsible for the continuous basal secretion of gonadotrophin and stimulates the growth of both germinal and endocrine components of the ovary, and the surge system which controls the short-lived massive secretion of gonadotrophin, particularly LH, responsible for ovulation. There are two hypothalamic centres that are involved in controlling these two systems (Figure 1.1).

With the exception of the cat, rabbit and camel, all domestic species are spontaneous ovulators. However, in these three species ovulation is induced by the stimulation of sensory receptors in the vagina and cervix at coitus. This initiates a neuro-endocrine reflex ultimately resulting in the

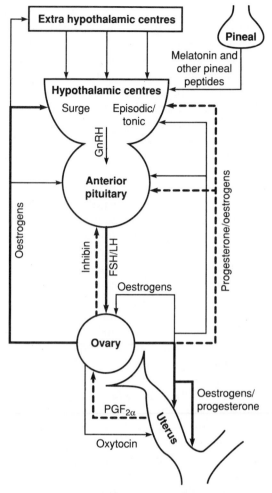

Fig. 1.1 Endocrine control of cyclical reproductive activity; ——, stimulation; - - -, inhibition; PGF$_{2\alpha}$, prostaglandin$_2$. (From Lammin et al., 1979.)

(and probably in other domestic species) FSH secretion is also controlled by a number of ovarian-derived peptide hormones. The first that has been characterized, inhibin, is produced by the granulosa cells of large antral follicles, and can be isolated from follicular fluid. It has also been isolated from the testis and seminal plasma (see Chapter 29). Inhibin and oestradiol act in concert in suppressing FSH secretion. Inhibin, which is produced by all antral follicles, has a longer half-life, and sets the overall level of negative feedback, whereas oestradiol, which is produced only by those antral follicles that have the potential for ovulation, is responsible for the day-to-day fluctuations (Baird et al., 1991). Two other peptide hormones have been isolated from ovarian follicular fluid, these have been designated activin, which stimulates, and follistatin, which suppresss FSH secretion. Their roles in controlling and regulating follicular growth is not known.

The positive-feedback effect of oestradiol on hypothalamic–pituitary function is well demonstrated in farm animals, since the preovulatory surge of oestradiol stimulates the release of LH, which is so necessary for the process of ovulation and corpus luteum formation. The response of the anterior pituitary to GnRH is influenced by the levels of ovarian steroids so that there is increased responsiveness shortly after the level of progesterone declines and that of oestradiol rises (Lamming et al., 1979). There are probably self-regulatory mechanisms controlling gonadotrophin secretion acting locally within the anterior pituitary and hypothalamus.

Tonic release of gonadotrophins, especially LH, does not occur at a steady rate but in a pulsatile fashion in response to a similar release of GnRH from the hypothalamus. The negative feedback of progesterone is mediated via a reduction in pulse frequency of gonadotrophin release, whereas oestradiol exerts its effect via a reduced pulse amplitude. The onset of cyclical activity after parturition (see Chapter 7), at puberty or at the start of the breeding season is associated with increased pulse frequency of tonic gonadotrophin secretion. When the ram is placed in contact with ewes before the start of the breeding season there is increased frequency of pulsatile LH release, which stimulates the onset of cyclical activity (Karsch, 1984).

Progesterone appears to play a critically important role in the inhibition of the tonic mode of LH

activation of GnRH neurons in the surge centre and release of a surge of LH.

Not only does the anterior pituitary have a direct effect upon ovarian functions by stimulating folliculogenesis, follicular maturation, ovulation and corpus luteum formation, but the ovary has an effect upon the hypothalamus and anterior pituitary. This is mediated by oestradiol, produced by the maturing follicle, and by progesterone, produced by the corpus luteum. The episodic/tonic hypothalamic release centre is influenced by the negative-feedback effect of oestradiol and progesterone. Low levels of progesterone also have a modulating influence on this centre, which appears to be particularly important in ruminants (Lamming et al., 1971). In the cow, ewe and sow secretion in the ewe (Karsch et al., 1978). Progesterone is thus the main regulatory hormone which controls the oestrous cycle of the sheep and probably of other species too. Thus when the concentration of progesterone in the circulation falls, associated with the regression of the corpus luteum, there is release of LH from the anterior pituitary. The rise in LH triggers the secretion of oestradiol: this sudden rise stimulates the surge centre for the LH release and, as a result of this sudden increase, ovulation of the mature follicle occurs (Karsh et al., 1978).

In some species, notably the cow (see Figure 1.28), there is also a concomitant surge in FSH; although its significance is unclear it may be part of the 'ovulation-inducing' hormone complex. For this reason it is probably incorrect to assign a separate and specific physiological role for the two pituitary gonadotrophins. Thus although ovulation and steroidogenesis can be initiated by both FSH and LH, it would appear that only FSH can induce early follicular growth, so that when the granulosa cells have matured and are able to respond to endogenous LH, the formation of a fully developed vesicular follicle occurs. Large amounts of a peptide similar to the hormone inhibin, produced by the Sertoli cells of the testis, have been found in bovine and porcine follicular fluid and granulosa cells. This hormone probably selectively inhibits FSH release from the anterior pituitary but it may also have a local role in controlling ovarian function: it has been shown to inhibit the binding of FSH to granulosa cells in the cow (Sato et al., 1982).

The corpus luteum is formed from lutein cells, which are derived from the granulosa cells of the Graafian follicle. Although the corpus luteum develops as a result of ovulation, in some species, notably the bitch, there are early signs of luteinization of the follicle before it has ovulated. The stimulus for the formation and maintenance of the corpus luteum probably varies within species. The hormones which are most likely to be involved are prolactin and LH, but there is some evidence that they are involved together, perhaps in association with FSH. Although all three hormones are probably involved in the induction of luteinization of granulosa cells, the available evidence suggests that FSH is probably not required for the maintenance of luteal function. The difference between species is well illustrated by the

observation that LH will prolong luteal function in the sow but prolactin will not (Denamur et al., 1966; Anderson et al., 1976). However, in the ewe prolactin appears to be more important as a luteotrophic agent since LH will exert an effect only if infused from day 10 to day 12 of the oestrous cycle.

The release of prolactin is largely under the control of a specific prolactin inhibitory factor (PIF), a polypeptide, which is stimulated to be released from the hypothalamus by excess prolactin secretion.

Much interest has been directed towards the role of certain endogenous peptides with opioid activity such as β-endorphin and met-enkephalin. These substances have been found in high concentrations in hypothalamic–hypophyseal portal blood. The administration of exogenous opioid peptides inhibits the secretion of FSH and LH whilst stimulating the secretion of prolactin. If an opiate antagonist such as naloxone is infused, there is an increase in mean concentrations of gonadotrophins in the plasma and the frequency of episodic gonadotrophin secretion. The effect of opioids appears to be influenced by the steroid environment of the animal; for example, in ewes, naloxone increased the mean plasma concentration of LH and the episodic frequency in a high-progesterone environment. However, in ovariectomized ewes or those with oestradiol implants, naloxone had no effect (Brooks et al., 1986). It is possible that the negative feedback of progesterone on LH release (see below) may be mediated via opioids (Brooks et al., 1986).

The prescence of a functional corpus luteum, by virtue of its production of progesterone, inhibits the return to oestrus by exerting a negative-feedback effect upon the anterior pituitary; this is most obvious during pregnancy (see Chapter 3). In the normal, non-pregnant female, oestrus and ovulation occur at fairly regular intervals; the main control of this cyclical activity would appear to be the corpus luteum.

Although it has been known for over 70 years that in certain species of animals the uterus influences ovarian function (Loeb, 1923) the mechanism has been fully understood only in recent years.

It has been demonstrated that in many species, removal of part or all of the uterus will result in the prolongation of the lifespan of the corpus luteum (du Mesnil du Buisson, 1961; Rowson and Moor, 1967); these species include the cow, mare, ewe, goat and sow. In the human, dog and cat the normal lifespan of the corpus luteum is unaltered in the absence of the uterus. In the cow, ewe and goat the 'leutolytic' action of the uterine horn is directed exclusively to the corpus luteum on the adjacent ovary (Ginther, 1974). Thus, if one of the uterine horns is surgically removed on the side adjacent to the ovary with a corpus luteum then the latter will persist. If the contralateral horn is removed, then the corpus luteum will regress at the normal time. It appears that in these species the luteolytic substance is transported directly from the uterus to the ovary. In the ewe it has been shown experimentally that the most likely route for transport of the substance is the middle uterine vein, since when all other structures between the ovary and uterus are severed there is still normal regression of the corpus luteum (Baird and Land, 1973).

In the mare no local effect can be demonstrated, since if the ovary is transplanted outside the pelvic cavity, luteal regression still occurs (Ginther and First, 1971). It is generally assumed that in this species the luteolysin is transported throughout the systemic circulation.

In the pig the luteolytic substance is transported locally (du Mesnil du Buisson, 1961) but not exclusively to the adjacent ovary. It has been shown that, following surgical ablation of parts of the uterine horns, provided at least the cranial quarter of the uterine horn is left, regression of the corpora lutea occurs in both ovaries. If more than three-quarters of the horn are excised, then regression of the corpora lutea occurs only in the ovary adjacent to the intact horn.

Although the importance of the middle uterine vein in the transfer of the luteolytic substance has been demonstrated, the mechanisms whereby the luteolytic substance passes to the ovary have not been conclusively demonstrated in all species, although they have been fairly well evaluated in the ewe and cow. In the former species it appears that the close proximity of the ovarian artery and utero-ovarian vein is important, particularly since at their points of approximation the walls of the two vessels are thinnest; there is no anastomosis (Coudert et al., 1974). This allows the leakage of the luteolytic substance from the uterine vein into the ovarian artery and thus to the ovary, by a form of counter-current exchange through the walls of the vessels. It has been suggested (Ginther, 1974)

that the variation in the response to partial or total hysterectomy in different species is probably due to differences in the relationships between the vasculature of the uterus and ovaries.

It was not until 1969 that the substance responsible for luteolysis was identified, when the duration of pseudo-pregnancy in the rat was shortened by the injection of prostaglandin $F_{2\alpha}$ ($PGF_{2\alpha}$). This same substance has subsequently been shown to have potent luteolytic activity in the ewe, doe, cow, sow and mare. Although it has been proved only in ruminants and the guinea-pig that it is the natural luteolysin, it is likely that it is also true for the other species listed.

$PGF_{2\alpha}$ is a derivative of the unsaturated hydroxy acids lineolenic and arachidonic acids. It derived its name because it was first isolated from fresh semen and it was assumed to be produced in the prostate gland. It is synthesized in the endometrium of a number of species (Horton and Poyser, 1976), and in the ewe it has been demonstrated in increasing amounts at and around the time of luteal regression (Bland et al., 1971).

In ruminants, luteal regression is caused by episodic release of $PGF_{2\alpha}$ from the uterus at intervals of about 6 hours. This is induced by oxytocin secreted by the corpus luteum; thus, each episode of $PGF_{2\alpha}$ release is accompanied by an episode of oxytocin release. Furthermore, $PGF_{2\alpha}$ stimulates further secretion of oxytocin from the ovary.

The sensitivity of the uterus to oxytocin is determined by the concentration of endometrial oxytocin receptors. At the time of luteal regression in sheep they rise approximately 500-fold (Flint et al., 1992). Their concentration is determined by the effects of progesterone and oestradiol. Thus, the high concentrations of progesterone which occur after the formation of the corpus luteum reduce the number of receptors, so that in the normal oestrous cycle of the ewe they start to increase from about day 12. Exogenous oestradiol causes premature induction of oxytocin receptors, resulting in premature luteolysis (Flint et al., 1992).

In non-ruminant species much less is known about the mechanisms of luteolysis.

The corpus luteum becomes more sensitive to the leuteolytic effect of $PGF_{2\alpha}$ as it ages. The early corpus luteum is unresponsive to $PGF_{2\alpha}$.

THE MARE

Cyclical periodicity

Fillies are often seen in oestrus during their second spring and summer (when they are yearlings), but under natural conditions it is unusual for them to foal until they are over 3 years old. The mare is normally a seasonal breeder, with cyclic activity occurring from spring to autumn; during the winter she will normally become anoestrous. However, it has been observed that mares will cycle regularly throughout the year. This tendency can be enhanced if the mares are housed and given supplementary food when the weather is cold and inclement and if additional lighting is provided when the hours of daylight are short.

Horse breeding has been influenced by the demands of thoroughbred racing, because in the northern hemisphere foals are aged from 1 January, irrespective of their actual birth date. As a result the breeding season for mares has been, for over a century, determined by the authorities as running from 15 February to 1 July. Since the natural breeding season does not commence until about the middle of April, and maximum ovarian activity is not reached until July, it is obvious that a large number of thoroughbred mares are bred at a time when their fertility is suboptimal.

The winter anoestrus is followed by a period of transition to regular cyclic activity. During this transition the duration of oestrus may be irregular or very long, sometimes more than a month. The manifestations of heat during the transitional phase are often atypical and make it difficult for the observer to be certain of the mare's reproductive status. Also, before the first ovulation there is poor correlation between sexual behaviour and ovarian activity; it is common for the early heats to be unaccompanied by the presence of palpable follicles, and some long spring heats are anovulatory. However, once ovulation has occurred, regular cycles usually follow.

The average length of the equine cycle is 20–23 days; the cycles are longer in spring and shortest from June to September. Typically, oestrus lasts 6 days and dioestrus 15 days. Ovulation occurs on the penultimate or last day of heat, and this relationship to the end of heat is fairly constant and irrespective of the duration of the cycle or the length of oestrus; Hammond (1938) found that manual rupture of the ripe follicle resulted in termination of oestrus within 24 hours. The diameter of the ripe follicle is 3–7 cm. A few hours before ovulation the tension in the follicle usually subsides, and the palpable presence of a large fluctuating follicle is a sure sign of imminent ovulation.

The onset of heat after foaling occurs on the fifth to 10th day. This foal heat is sometimes rather short, 2–4 days. It is traditional to cover a mare on the ninth day after foaling. The first two post-parturient cycles are a few days longer than subsequent ones.

During oestrus a single egg is usually released, and there is a slight preponderance of ovulations from the left ovary. Assessing the functional activity of the two ovaries on the basis of post-mortem counts of corpora lutea in 792 equine genitalia, Arthur (1958) recorded an incidence of 52.2% of ovulations from the left ovary. Twin ovulation commonly occurs in mares; Burkhardt (1948), in a study of June–July slaughterhouse specimens, saw 27% of double ovulations, and Arthur (1958) found an overall frequency of 18.5%, with a summer peak of 37.5%. However, there is a strong breed influence on twin ovulation: thoroughbreds are prone to it but pony mares

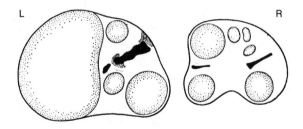

Fig. 1.2 The ovaries of a 5-year-old farm mare in oestrus. Specimens obtained in May. Regressing corpus luteum in left ovary, bright yellow ochre in colour.

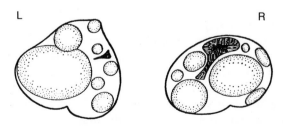

Fig. 1.3 Ovaries of a 9-year-old farm mare in dioestrus. Corpus luteum in right ovary, orange in colour; pleats loose.

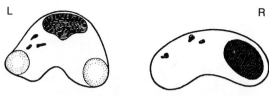

L   R

Fig. 1.4 Ovaries of a 4-year-old shire mare in dioestrus. Corpus luteum in left ovary, brownish-red in colour; pleats distinct; central cavity containing blood clot. Right ovary contains a follicle filled with blood.

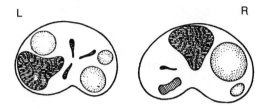

L   R

Fig. 1.5 Ovaries of a 6-year-old farm mare in dioestrus. A corpus luteum in each ovary, orange-yellow in colour; pleats distinct.

rarely show it. A fascinating finding by Van Niekerk and Gernaeke (1966) was that only fertilized eggs pass into the uterus; non-fertilized eggs remain for months in the uterine tubes, where they slowly disintegrate. All equine ovulations occur from the ovulation fossa; only at the ovarian hilus may occasional protrusions of corpora lutea be seen, but because of the curvature of the ovary and the presence of the adjacent substantial fimbriae these protusions cannot be identified by rectal palpation.

Day (1939) has given a clear picture of the changes which occur in the equine ovary during an oestrous cycle. Figures 1.2–1.6 are diagrams of ovaries of the mare, half natural size, at different stages of the oestrous cycle, whereas Figures 1.7–1.12 show examples of whole ovaries, cross-sections and B-mode ultrasound images. Just before the onset of heat, several follicles enlarge

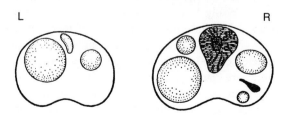

L   R

Fig. 1.6 Ovaries of a 6-year-old hunter mare in dioestrus. Corpus luteum in right ovary, pale yellow in colour; pleats distinct. Central cavity.

to a size of 1–3 cm. By the first day of oestrus one follicle is generally considerably larger than the remainder, having a diameter of 2.5–3.5 cm. During oestrus this follicle matures and ruptures when it has attained a diameter of 3–7 cm. After ovulation the other follicles regress, until, during the first 4–9 days of the ensuing dioestrus, no follicles larger than 1 cm are likely to be present. A few hours before ovulation the ripe follicle becomes much less tense. The collapsed follicle is recognized by an indentation on the ovarian surface; there is usually some haemorrhage into the follicle, and the coagulum hardens within the next 24 hours. Quite frequently the mare shows evidence of discomfort when the ovary is palpated soon after ovulation. Unless sequential rectal examinations are made it is sometimes possible to confuse a mature follicle with the early corpus haemorrhagicum, since before ovulation the follicular antrum is filled with follicular fluid and then soon after ovulation it becomes filled with blood. For this reason mares are sometimes incorrectly diagnosed as having failed to ovulate. For the next 3 days the luteinizing mass can be felt as a resilient focus, but later it tends to have the same texture as the remainder of the ovary. In pony mares, however, of known history from daily examinations Allen (1974) reports that it is possible to follow the growth of the corpus luteum because in ponies it forms a relatively large body in a small ovary. The corpus luteum attains maximum size at 4–5 days, but it does not protrude from the ovarian surface. On section of the ovary it is brown and later yellow and of a triangular or conical shape, with the narrower end impinging on the ovulation fossa. Its centre is commonly occupied by a variable amount of dark-brown fibrin. The cyclical corpus luteum begins to regress at about the 12th day of the cycle, when there is a parallel fall in the blood progesterone concentration. From this day onwards the events previously described recur. Ovulation, with the subsequent formation of a corpus luteum, does not always occur; the follicle may regress or sometimes undergo luteinization (see Figure 1.10(b)).

B-mode ultrasound imaging with a rectal transducer probe has been used to visualize follicles (see Figures 1.8–1.11). This is particularly useful in detecting the possibility of twin ovulations and also in determing the timing of ovulation. Ginther (1986) observed that in the preovulatory period

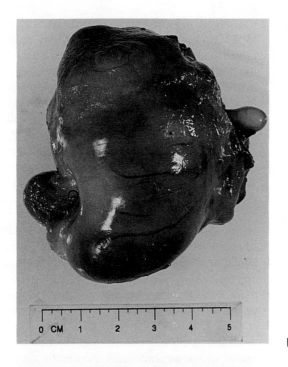

a

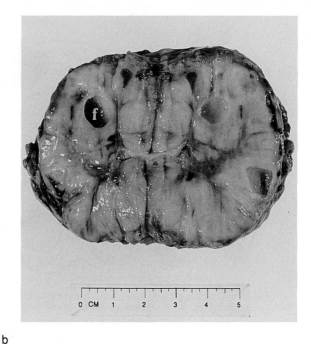

b

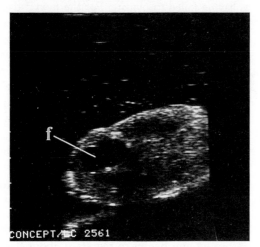

c

Fig. 1.7 Ovary from an acyclical (anoestrus) mare. (a) The ovary was hard on palpation with no evidence of follicular activity. Note the ovulation fossa (o). (b) Cross-section of the ovary. Note that there are a few small follicles (f) <1 cm in diameter which are contained within the ovarian matrix. (c) B-mode ultrasound image of the same ovary showing small anechoic (black) areas <1 cm in diameter which are follicles (f).

there was a change in the shape of the follicle and a thickening of the follicular wall, which, together with the assessment of the size of the follicle, could be used to predict the time of ovulation. The same author has used this technique to assess corpora lutea: he identified differences in the echogenic properties of the corpus luteum depending upon the persistence of the corpus haemorrhagicum — this he identified in about 50%.

During winter anoestrus both ovaries are typically small and bean-shaped, common dimensions being 6 cm from pole to pole, 4 cm from the hilus to the free border and 3 cm from side to side. Not uncommonly, however, in the late autumn or early spring, the anoestrous ovaries are of medium size and knobbly due to the content of numerous follicles of 1–1.5 cm diameter. During the cycle there are large variations in the ovarian size depending on the number and size of the follicles. During oestrus the ovary of the thoroughbred mare may contain two or even three follicles, each of 4–7 cm, and these, with other subsidiary follicles, combine to give it a huge size. During

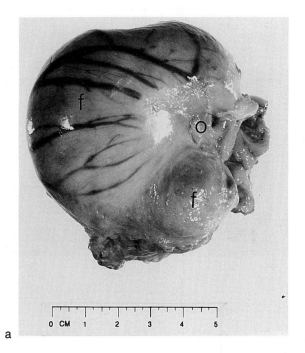

a

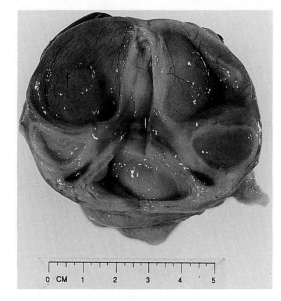

b

c

Fig. 1.8 Ovary from a mare in the early follicular phase. (a) The ovary was soft on palpation with evidence of large follicles near the surface of the ovary (f). Note the ovulation fossa (o). (b) Cross-section of the ovary. Note three follicles are at least 2 cm in diameter. (c) B-mode ultrasound image of the same ovary showing one large anechoic (black) area about 3.5 cm in diameter which is a follicle (f), together with three smaller ones.

dioestrus, however, with an active corpus luteum and only atretic follicles the ovary may be little larger than in anoestrus.

By visual examination of the vagina and the cervix using an illuminated speculum, it is possible to detect the preovulation period. In dioestrus the cervix is small, constricted and firm; it and the vagina are pale pink, while mucus is scanty and sticky. During oestrus there is a gradual increase in the vascularity of the genital tract and relaxation of the cervix with dilatation of the os. As oestrus advances and ovulation time approaches, the cervix becomes very relaxed and its protrusion can be seen lying on the vaginal floor, with its folds oedematous; the vaginal walls are glistening with clear lubricant mucus. After ovulation there is a gradual reversion to the dioestrous appearance.

During anoestrus, as in pregnancy, both the vagina and cervix are blanched; the cervix is constricted and generally turned away from the midline, the external os being filled with tenacious mucus.

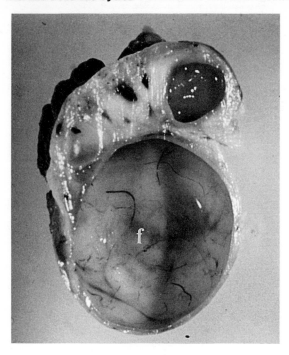

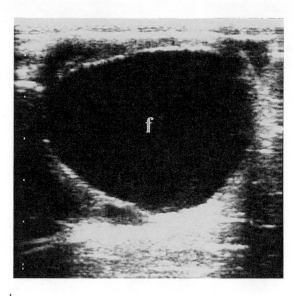

b

a

Fig. 1.9 Ovary of a mare with a single large preovulatory follicle. (a) Section of the ovary showing a 4 cm follicle (f). (b) B-mode ultrasound image of a different ovary showing a 4–5 cm preovulatory follicle (f) as a large anechoic (black) area.

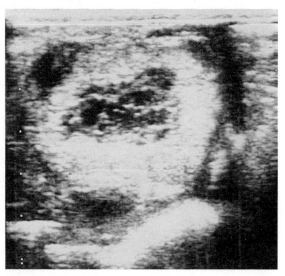

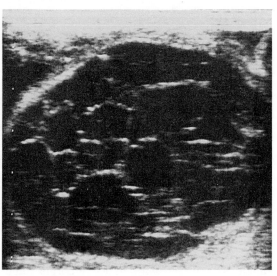

a

b

Fig. 1.10 (a) B-mode ultrasound image of an ovary showing the corpus haemorrhagicum. (b) B-mode ultrasound image of 5 cm anovulatory follicle that is undergoing luteinization.

On palpating the uterus per rectum, cyclic changes can be detected. With the development of the corpus luteum the uterus increases in tone and thickness, but these features diminish when the corpus luteum regresses. At oestrus there is no increase of tone. During anoestrus and for the first few days after ovulation the uterus is flaccid.

During dioestrus, pregnancy and pseudopregnancy the cervix is identified on rectal palpation as a narrow firm tubular structure: at oestrus it is soft

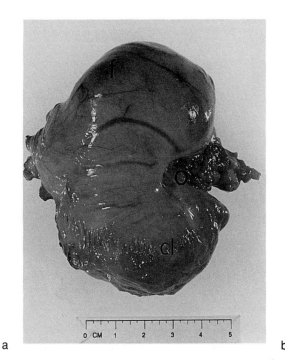

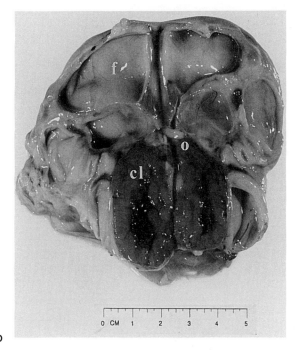

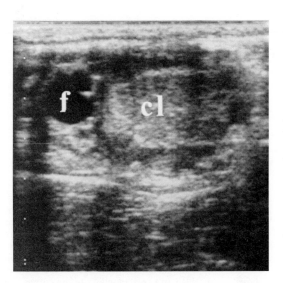

Fig. 1.11 Ovary of a mare in early dioestrus. (a) The corpus luteum (cl), although present, could not be palpated externally, whereas a follicle (f) could be identified. Note the ovulation fossa (o). (b) Section of the same ovary. Note that the corpus luteum (cl), still with a central blood clot, impinges on the ovulation fossa (o) where ovulation occurred. Also, one large follicle (f) and several smaller ones can be identified. (c) B-mode ultrasound image of a different ovary showing the corpus luteum (cl) and follicles (f).

and broad. A temporary pneumovagina assists in this examination (Allen, 1978).

Signs of oestrus

The mare becomes restless and irritable; she frequently adopts the micturition posture and voids urine with repeated exposure of the clitoris (Figure 1.13). When introduced to a stallion or teaser, these postures are accentuated; the mare raises the tail to one side and leans her hindquarters. The vulva is slightly oedematous, and there is a variable amount of mucoid discharge. A mare which is not in heat will usually violently oppose the advances of a stallion, and for this reason when 'trying' mares at stud it should be done over a gate, box-door or stout fence. If the mare is in heat the

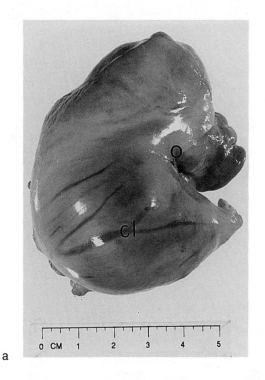

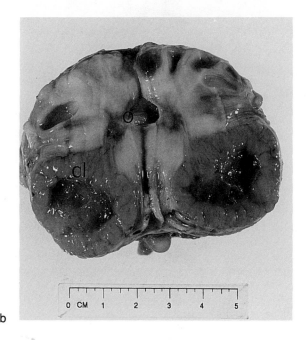

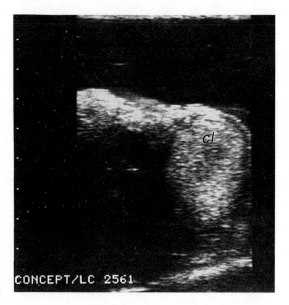

Fig. 1.12 Ovary of a mare in mid-dioestrus. (a) The corpus luteum (cl), although present, could not be palpated externally; there was no evidence of any follicles. Note the ovulation fossa (o). (b) Section of the same ovary. Note the corpus luteum (cl), which impinges upon the ovulation fossa where ovulation has occurred. (c) B-mode ultrasound image of the same ovary showing a speckled area corresponding to the corpus luteum (cl).

stallion usually exhibits 'flehmen'. Good stud management requires that a mare is accustomed to the procedure and that, because of the interval between the end of the last oestrus and the start of the next, she is teased 15–16 days after the end of the last oestrus.

Endocrine changes during the oestrous cycle

The trends in endocrine changes are shown in Figure 1.14. The secretion of FSH is biphasic with surges at approximtely 10–12 day intervals. One surge occurs just after ovulation, with a

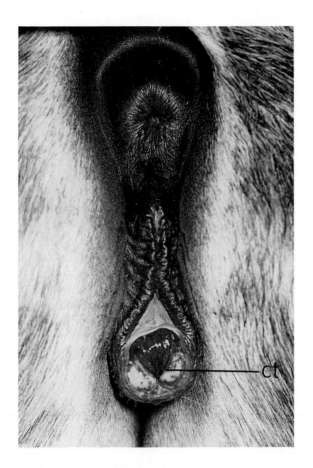

Fig. 1.13 Exposure of the clitoris (ct) in response to teasing.

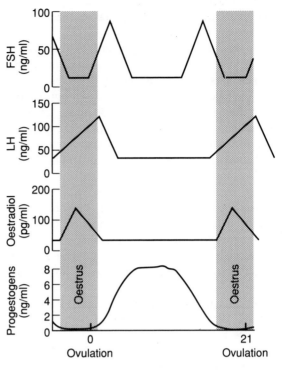

Fig. 1.14 Trends in hormonal concentrations in the peripheral circulation of the mare during the oestrous cycle.

second surge in mid- to late dioestrus approximately 10 days before the next ovulation. It has been suggested that this increase in FSH secretion, which is unique to the mare, is responsible for priming the development of a new generation of follicles, one of which will ovulate at the next oestrous (Evans and Irvine, 1975). The pattern of LH secretion is also unusual in this species since there is no sudden surge of this hormone but a gradual increase and persistence of elevated levels for 5–6 days on either side of ovulation. Oestrogens in the peripheral circulation reach peak values during oestrus whilst concentrations of progesterone and other progestogens follow closely the physical changes of the corpus luteum.

THE COW

Cyclic periodicity

Under conditions of domestication, normal and well-cared-for cattle are polyoestrous throughout the year. The age at first oestrus, or puberty, is affected by nutrition and season of birth, and ranges from 7 to 18 months, with an average of 10 months. A small proportion of heifers do not ovulate at the first heat, and in a majority of young cattle the oestrus associated with the first ovulation is 'silent' (Morrow et al., 1969). Poor feeding and calfhood disease delay puberty. Once puberty has been reached, cyclical activity should persist, except during pregnancy, for 3–6 weeks after calving, during high milk yield, especially if there is some evidence of dietary insufficiency and with a number of pathological conditions (see Chapter 22). Some cows and heifers also fail to show overt signs of oestrus yet have normal cyclical activity, a condition referred to as 'silent heat' or suboestrus.

This may, however, be due to a failure of the herdsman to observe the signs rather than a failure of the cow to show signs.

In heifers the average length of the oestrous cycle is 20 days, and in cows 21 days, the normal ranges being 18–22 and 18–24 days, respectively. The average duration of oestrus is 15 hours; however, there is a wide range of 2–30 hours. There are a number of factors which can influence the duration: breed of animal, season of year, presence of a bull, nutrition, milk yield, lactation number and, perhaps most important, the number of cows that are in oestrus at the same time (Wishart, 1972; Esslemont and Bryant, 1974; Hurnik et al., 1975). There is also good evidence that more signs of oestrus are observed during the hours of night, perhaps when the animals are least disturbed (Williamson et al., 1972; Esslemont and Bryant, 1976).

Ovulation is spontaneous, and occurs on average 12 hours after the end of oestrus.

Signs of oestrus

Where artificial insemination is used, the accurate detection of oestrus by the herdsman is paramount in ensuring optimum fertility. Poor detection is probably the most important reason affecting delayed breeding (Wood, 1976), whilst in the USA Barr (1975) has calculated that in Ohio dairy herds dairymen appeared to be losing twice as many days due to failure to detect heat as to conception failures.

There are great variations amongst individual cattle in the intensity of heat signs; the manifestations tend to be more marked in heifers than in cows. However, it is generally agreed that the most reliable criterion that a cow or heifer is in oestrus is that she will stand to be mounted by another (Williamson et al., 1972; Esslemont and Bryant, 1974; Foote, 1975).

The oestrous animal is restless and more active; Kiddy (1977), using pedometers, found that there was an average increase in activity of 393% at this time. More recently, Lewis and Newman (1984) found that pedometer activity was about twice as great in oestrus compared with the luteal phase of the cycle. In their study, 75% of cows showed peak pedometer readings on the day of onset of oestrus whereas 25% peaked 1 day after oestrus. There tends to be grouping of sexually active individuals; there is a reduction in the time spent eating, resting and ruminating, and frequently a reduction in milk yield. Reduced milk yield has been shown to be a reliable indicator of the onset of oestrus; there is usually a compensatory rebound at the next milking (Horrell et al., 1984). In this study of 73 dairy cows it was found that if a cow produced 75% of her usual yield there was a 50% chance of her being in oestrus. On the rare occasions that it fell to 25%, oestrus was always present. As the cow approaches oestrus she tends to search for other cows in oestrus, and there is licking and sniffing of the perineum. During this period, during oestrus and just afterwards, the cow will attempt to mount other cows; quite often before she does this she will assess the receptivity of the other cows by resting her chin on the rump or loins. If the cow to be mounted is responsive and stands, she will mount and sometimes show evidence of pelvic thrusting (Esselmont and Bryant, 1974). If the cow that is mounted is not in oestrus she will walk away and frequently turn and butt the mounting cow. A positive mounting response lasts about 5 seconds (Hurnik et al., 1975); however, if both cows are in oestrus it will be increased to about 7.5 seconds. In a group of 60 cows, Esslemont and Bryant (1976) observed that 33 cows were mounted on average 56 times.

There is frequent genital discharge of transparent mucus whose elasticity causes it to hang in complete clear strands from the vulva to the ground; it also adheres to the tail and flanks. The vulva is slightly swollen and congested, and there is a small elevation of temperature. The tail may be slightly raised. The hair of the tail-head is often ruffled and the skin sometimes becomes excoriated due to the mounting by other cows. For the same reason the rear of the animal may be soiled with mud. At range the oestrous cow may wander from the herd, and bellowing is a feature of heat. When she is put with a bull the two animals lick each other and the cow often mounts the bull before standing to be mounted by him. For a short time after service the cow stands with raised tail and arched back, and where actual service has not been seen this posture indicates that mating has occurred.

Within 2 days of service there is an occasional yellowish-white vulval discharge of mucus containing neutrophil leucocytes from the uterus. At about 48 hours after heat, irrespective of service, heifers and many cows show a sanguineous discharge, the blood coming mainly from the uterine caruncles.

The body temperature of dairy cows falls about 0.5°C the day before oestrus, increases during oestrus and falls by about 0.3°C at ovulation (Wren et al., 1958). The vaginal temperature, of 37.74°C, was lowest on the day before oestrus, increased by 0.1°C on the day of oestrus, and increased for the next 6 days until a plateau was reached. This was followed by a gradual decline from 7 days before oestrus (Lewis and Newman, 1984). Practical detection of this is tedious; however, the use of microwave telemetry systems may enable such measurements to be made in the future (Bobbett et al., 1977). Automated methods of measuring the related increase in milk temperature in the milking parlour have also been described (Maatje, 1976; Ball, 1977).

Vaginal pH also fluctuates throughout the oestrous cycle but is lowest, namely 7.32, on the day of oestrus (Lewis and Newman, 1984).

Cyclic changes in the vagina
The main variations are in the epithelial cells of the anterior vagina and in the secretory function of the cervical glands (Hammond, 1927; Cole, 1930). During oestrus the anterior vaginal epithelium becomes greatly thickened due to cell division and to the growth of the tall, columnar, mucus-secreting superficial cells. During dioestrus these cells vary from flat to low columnar. Leucocytic invasion of the vaginal mucosa is maximal 2–5 days after oestrus. Copious secretion of mucus by the cervix and anterior vagina begins a day or so before heat, increases during heat and gradually diminishes to the fourth day after heat. The mucus is transparent and flows readily.

Associated with these features of the cervical mucus are variations in its crystallization patterns which can be seen when dried smears of mucus are examined microscopically. During oestrus and for a few days afterwards the crystals are disposed in a distinct aborization pattern, while for the remainder of the cycle this pattern is absent. This phenomenon, together with the character and amount of cervical mucus, are dependent on the concentration of oestrogen. The postoestrous vaginal mucus shows floccules composed of leucocytes, and, as previously mentioned, blood is frequently present. Hyperaemia of the mucosae of the vagina and

cervix is progressive during pro-oestrus and oestrus; the vaginal protrusion of the cervix is tumefied and relaxed so that one or two fingers can be inserted into the cervical os. During metoestrus there is a rapid reduction in vascularity, and from 3 to 5 days after heat the mucosa is pale and quiescent, the external os is constricted while the mucus becomes scanty, sticky and pale yellow or brown. There are also cyclic variations in vaginal thermal conductance and vaginal pH, the former rising just before oestrus (Abrams et al., 1975). When pH electrodes were placed in the cervical end of the vagina the pH fell from 7.0 to 6.72 one day before the first behavioural signs of oestrus, and at the start of oestrus fell again to 6.54 (Schilling and Zust, 1968).

Cyclic changes in the uterus
During oestrus the uterus is congested, and the endometrium is suffused with oedematous fluid; its surface is glistening. The muscularis is physiologically contractile so that when the uterus is palpated per rectum this muscular irritability, coupled with the marked vascularity, conveys a highly characteristic tonic turgidity to the palpating fingers; the horns feel erect and coiled. This tonicity is present the day before and the day after oestrus but is at its maximum during heat, and, with experience, the veterinarian can detect oestrus on this sign alone. Between 24 and 48 hours after oestrus the uterine caruncles show petechial haemorrhages, and these give rise to the postoestrous vaginal discharge of blood. In heifers there are often also associated perimetrial subserous petechiae. During dioestrus the endometrium is covered by a scanty secretion from the uterine glands.

Cyclic changes in the ovaries
Usually one follicle ovulates and one ovum is liberated after each heat, but twin ovulations occur in 4 or 5% of cows, and triplet ovulations more rarely. In dairy cattle about 60% of ovulations are from the right ovary, although in beef cattle the functional disparity between the ovaries is not great.

The size and contour of the ovaries will depend on the phase of the cycle. It is best to begin by studying the organs of a mature unbred heifer. Post-mortem section of such ovaries will reveal the most significant structures in them to be Graafian follicles and corpora lutea.

Follicular growth and development

Follicular growth and atresia throughout the cycle is a feature in the cow (Matton et al., 1983).

In the studies of Bane and Rajakoski (1961) two waves of growth were demonstrated, with the first wave beginning on the third and fourth day and the second starting on the 12th to 14th day of the cycle. Consequently, a normal follicle of 9–13 mm was present from the fifth to the 11th day before becoming atretic. In the second wave the ovulatory follicle developed, and was 9–13 mm between the 15th and 20th days; the ovulatory follicle is selected at about 3 days before ovulation (Pierson and Ginther, 1988). Others have observed three waves of follicular development in most oestrous cycles (Sirois and Fortune, 1988; Savio et al., 1990). The most notable feature was the regularity of the number of waves of follicular growth per oestrous cycle, which probably reflected genetic or environmental influences. Follicular growth is under the influence of FSH, with normally one follicle obtaining dominance and subsequently ovulating. The dominance does not appear to be mediated by the effect of inhibin (see p. 7) but probably by some yet unknown intra-ovarian mechanism which does not involve the suppression of FSH secretion. In addition, other metabolic hormones such as insulin growth factor 1 (IGF1) may also be involved in follicular growth patterns (see review by Webb et al., 1992).

Thus, during dioestrus several large follicles will be found ranging in size up to 0.7–1.5 cm in diameter. These follicles do not alter the general oval contours of the ovaries but do cause some overall variation in gross ovarian size. The ease of palpating them rectally will depend upon the size, degree of protrusion and relationship with the corpus luteum.

During pro-oestrus and oestrus the follicle which is soon to rupture enlarges, and ovulation occurs when it has attained a size of at least 1.9 cm (Hammond, 1927). On rectal palpation of the ovaries during heat it is usually possible to detect the ripening follicle as a slightly bulging, smooth soft area on the surface of one of them. Ovulation may occur from any aspect of the ovarian surface, and the shape of that organ subsequently when the corpus luteum develops will be chiefly influenced

by this site. The point of ovulation is usually in an avascular area of the follicular wall, and consequently haemorrhage is not a feature of bovine ovulation, although there is marked postovulatory congestion around the rupture point, and sometimes a small blood clot is present in the centre of the new corpus lutuem.

The corpus luteum of the oestrous cycle

On rupture, the ovum is expelled through a small breach in the surface of the follicle and, consequent on the escape of the greater part of its fluid, the latter collapses. If the opportunity had arisen for repeatedly carrying out rectal examinations during heat and for the 24 hours succeeding it, this collapse of the follicle would have been detected. The ovary frequently feels flattened and soft. If such an ovary is examined post-mortem it will be seen that the surface from which ovulation has occurred is wrinkled and possibly bloodstained. The corpus luteum develops by hypertrophy and luteinization of the granulosa cells lining the follicle. Enlargement is rapid. By the 48th hour after ovulation it has attained a diameter of about 1.4 cm. At this stage the developing corpus luteum is soft, and yields on palpation. Its colour is dull cream, and the luteinized cells can be seen in the form of loose pleats. The corpus luteum attains its maximum size by the seventh to eighth day of dioestrus (Figure 1.15). The luteinized pleats are now relatively compact, and the body comprises a more or less homogeneous mass, yellow to orange–yellow in colour. Its shape varies; the majority are oval, but some are irregularly square or rectangular. The greatest dimension of the fully developed structure varies from 2.0 to 2.5 cm; the changes in the dimensions of the corpora lutea are shown in Figure 1.16. Its weight also varies; in the authors' series, fully developed corpora lutea have varied from 4.1 to 7.4 g. (Similar variations also occur in the weights of the corpora lutea of pregnancy, ranging from 3.9 to 7.5 g.) Sometimes the centre of the yellow body is occupied by a cavity (Figures 1.17 and 1.27). This has been seen in 25% of those collected by the author. The size of the cavity varies; in the majority it is small, averaging 0.4 cm in diameter, but occasionally it is large, up to 1 cm or more. It is occupied by yellow fluid. In the case just described there is evidence of ovulation by the presence of a pin-head depression in the centre of the projection from the surface of the

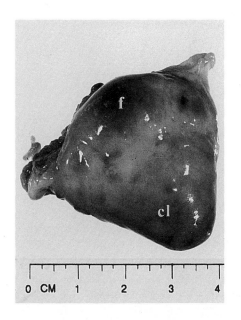

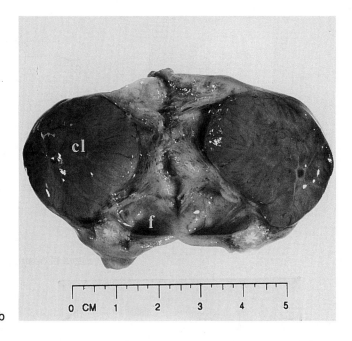

a

b

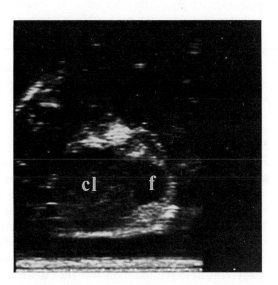

c

Fig. 1.15 Ovary of cow in mid-dioestrus. (a) A mature corpus luteum (cl) with ovulation papilla could be readily palpated together with a mid-cycle follicle (f). (b) Section of the same ovary showing the solid corpus luteum (cl) and mid-cycle follicle (f). (c) B-mode ultrasound image of the same ovary showing a speckled area corresponding to the corpus luteum (cl) and the mid-cycle follicle (f).

ovary. This serves to differentiate them from the abnormality of the cow's ovary: luteinization of the walls of the follicle without ovulation (see p. 367). Nevertheless, it is probable that this is the condition which has been described in the past as cystic corpus luteum and regarded as pathological. The author believes the presence of a cavity to be normal.

Projection of the corpus luteum from the surface of the ovary

As the corpus luteum enlarges, it tends to push itself out of the ovary, stretching the surface of the latter, until by the time it attains maximum development it forms a distinct projection. The degree and type of this projection vary. In the majority it is a distinct bulge about 1 cm in diameter with a clear-cut constriction where it joins the general contour of the ovary. In other cases it is

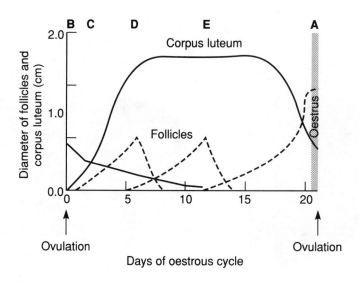

Fig. 1.16 The development of follicles (– – – –) and corpus luteum (————) during the oestrous cycle of the cow.

nipple-like (Figure 1.15). In a third type the projection is indistinct but diffuse and occupying the greater part of the ovary. It would seem that the type of protrusion which develops depends on the extent of the surface of the ovary occupied by the follicle just before ovulation. Figures 1.18–1.26 show bovine ovaries* (natural size) during the oestrous cycle.

Regressing corpus luteum

The corpus luteum maintains its maximum size and remains unaltered in appearance until the onset of pro-oestrus, i.e. 24 hours or so before the onset of heat. From this point it undergoes rapid reduction in size and changes in colour and appearance. By the middle of the heat period its diameter is reduced to 1.5 cm, its protrusion is much smaller and less distinct, while its colour is changing to bright yellow. (This colour contrasts strikingly with that of the active body.) Its consistency is dense, and already scar tissue invasion is commencing. By the second day of dioestrus its size is reduced to about 1 cm and its outline is

* Throughout the book, sketches of bovine ovaries are of a section from the attached to the free border through the poles. In those cases in which this section did not pass through the greatest dimension of the significant corpus luteum or the largest follicle, the sketch has been made as though it did so but without materially altering the size of the ovary.

becoming irregular. By this time its colour is changing to brown. By the middle of dioestrus it has shrunk to a size of about 0.5 cm, and its surface protrusion is little larger than a pin-head. As it gets older its colour tends to change to red or scarlet. Small red remnants of corpora lutea tend to persist for several months.

Size of the ovaries

From the foregoing it will be appreciated that the size of an ovary will depend chiefly on the period in the oestrous cycle at which it is examined and whether or not it contains an active corpus luteum. The presence of follicles does not alter the size of an ovary to anything like the same extent. In the great majority of heifers and young cows examined at any time between the sixth and 18th day of the dioestrous period, one ovary will be distinctly larger than the other. The approximate dimensions of the larger one will be 3.5 cm from pole to pole, 3 cm from the attached to the free border and 2.8 cm from side to side. (All ovarian dimensions given in this book are in this order.) From some part of its surface the corpus luteum will project. The smaller ovary will have approximate dimensions of 2.5 by 1.5 by 1.2 cm, and it will be flat from side to side. During the first 4 or 5 days of the interoestrus phase there will be relatively little

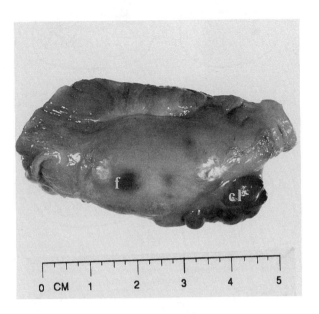

a

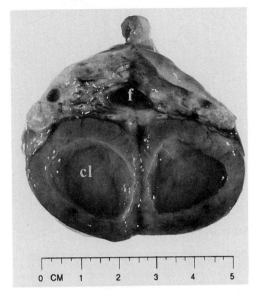

b

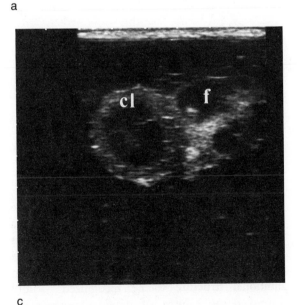

c

Fig. 1.17 Ovary of cow in mid-dioestrus. (a) A mature corpus luteum (cl) with prominent ovulation papilla and mid-cycle follicle (f). (b) Section of the same ovary showing the corpus luteum with a central lacuna which was filled with orange–yellow fluid, and the mid-cycle follicle (f). Note that the 'wall' of the corpus luteum comprises at least 5 mm thickness of luteal tissue. (c) B-mode ultrasound image of the same ovary showing a speckled area corresponding to the 'wall' of the corpus luteum (cl), the central lacuna, and also the mid-cycle follicle (f).

variation in size, for as yet the developing corpus luteum has not attained sufficient bulk significantly to influence the size of the ovary, while the regressing corpus luteum has lost its significant bulk. During the heat period also there will be little difference in size. If the ovary which contains the follicle undergoing preovulation enlargement also contains the regressing corpus luteum (and this is often the case), the ovary containing the two structures will be a little larger than the other, but not strikingly so.

Ovaries of the multiparous cow

The ovaries of the normal multiparous cow do not differ greatly from those of the heifer or first calver. They tend, however, in many cases to be larger. This increase in size is due in part to the progressive deposition of scar tissue resulting from prolonged

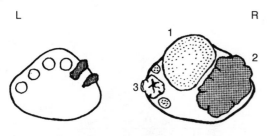

Fig. 1.18 Ovaries of a first-calf heifer in oestrus. 1, ripe follicle; 2, regressing corpus luteum, bright yellow; 3, corpus albicans. Stage A in Figure 1.16.

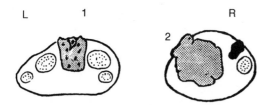

Fig. 1.19 Ovaries of a first-calf heifer in oestrus. 1, ripe follicle; 2, regressing corpus luteum, brick-brown. Stage A in Figure 1.16.

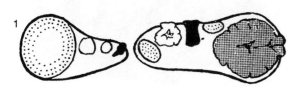

Fig. 1.20 Ovaries of a nulliparous heifer just after ovulation. 1, collapsed follicle, surface wrinkled and blood-stained petechiae in wall; 2, regressing corpus luteum, bright yellow. Stage B in Figure 1.16.

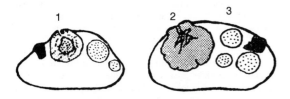

Fig. 1.21 Ovaries of a young cow 1 day after ovulation. 1, developing corpus luteum, pleats loose, colour pale cream, central cavity; 2, regressing corpus luteum, bright orange–yellow; centre filled by connective tissue; 3, corpus albicans. Stage B in Figure 1.16.

function and in some cases also to the presence of large numbers of small but visible follicles. Not infrequently the ovary which does not contain a corpus luteum measures 4 by 3 by 2 cm. Nevertheless, it is generally possible in mid-dioestrus to detect the corpus luteum, for, quite apart from its

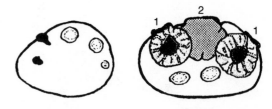

Fig. 1.22 Ovaries of a young cow 2 days after ovulation. 1, twin corpora lutea, some haemorrhage; 2, regressing corpus luteum, bright yellow. Stage C in Figure 1.16.

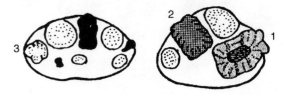

Fig. 1.23 Ovaries of a 4-year-old cow in early dioestrus. 1, active corpus luteum, pleats loose, colour orange–yellow, central cavity; 2, regressing corpus luteum, dense and brown; 3, corpus albicans. Stage C in Figure 1.1.6.

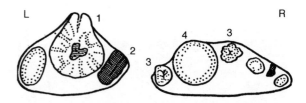

Fig. 1.24 Ovaries of a 6-year-old cow in early dioestrus. 1, active corpus luteum, orange–yellow. Atypical protrusion; 2, regressing corpus luteum, small, shrunken, scarlet; 3, corpus albicans; 4, follicle. Stage D in Figure 1.16.

protrusion, the ovary containing it is plum-like, whereas the other is distinctly flattened from side to side. On section of such ovaries, the corpora lutea, active and regressing, and the follicles approaching maturity are identical with those described for the heifer. There is, however, an additional structure to be recognized — old scarred corpora lutea of previous pregnancies. They generally show as a white, pin-head-sized projection on the surface of the ovary, and on section are found to comprise mainly scar tissue. They are irregular in outline, with a maximum dimension of about 0.5 cm. Their colour is white (corpus albicans) or brownish-white. The corpus luteum of pregnancy does not atrophy after parturition as quickly as does that of the oestrous cycle after it has ceased to function. It is an appreciable structure for several weeks after parturition, brown

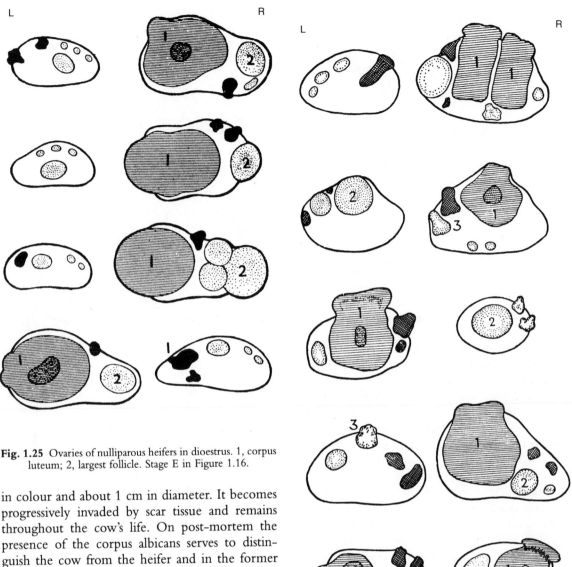

Fig. 1.25 Ovaries of nulliparous heifers in dioestrus. 1, corpus luteum; 2, largest follicle. Stage E in Figure 1.16.

in colour and about 1 cm in diameter. It becomes progressively invaded by scar tissue and remains throughout the cow's life. On post-mortem the presence of the corpus albicans serves to distinguish the cow from the heifer and in the former a count of the corpora albicantia gives the number of calves borne.

The fully developed corpus luteum is present by the seventh day and persists unchanged until the onset of pro-oestrus at the 19th or 20th day. Figure 1.27 shows exceptional corpora lutea.

Ultrasonic appearance of the ovaries

In the previous sections of this chapter there are descriptions of the texture (as determined by palpation) and the appearance (as determined by sectioning after slaughter) of the ovaries and their contents. The advent of transrectal B-mode real-time grey scale ultrasound imaging, particularly using a 7.5 MHz transducer, has enabled detailed,

Fig. 1.26 Ovaries of parous cows in dioestrus. 1, corpus luteum; 2, largest follicle; 3, corpus albicans. Stage E in Figure 1.16.

accurate sequential examination of the ovaries to be made without adversely affecting the cow's health or fertility. The principles of the technique are described on p. 69, and for a detailed description

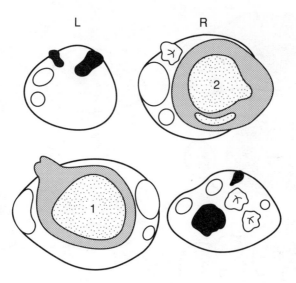

L   R

Fig. 1.27 Examples of vacuolated or cavitated bovine corpora lutea, showing single (1) and sometimes multiple (2) cavities.

of the echogenic appearance of the ovaries, readers are advised to consult Pierson and Ginther (1984) and Boyd and Omran (1990).

The following normal structures can be identified (see Figures 1.15 and 1.17): the ovarian stroma, antral follicles, corpora lutea and ovarian blood vessels. In addition, pathological structures such as ovarian cysts can be seen (see Chapter 22). The ovarian stroma has a mottled echotexture. The antral follicles are readily identifiable as non-echogenic (black) structures of variable size, with a clearly defined line of demarcation between the follicular wall and antrum. Follicles will not always be regular and spherical in shape. Corpora lutea have a well-defined border and a mottled echogenic appearance which is less echogenic than the ovarian stroma; the presence of a fluid-filled lacuna can be readily identified as a dark, non-echogenic area in the centre. Differentiation between developing and regressing corpora lutea can be difficult. Ovarian blood vessels, which can be confused with antral follicles, are black, non-echogenic structures. Movement of the transducer will usually demonstrate their elongated appearance.

Endocrine changes during the oestrous cycle

The trends in concentrations of reproductive hormones in the peripheral circulation are illustrated schematically in Figure 1.28; it is important to

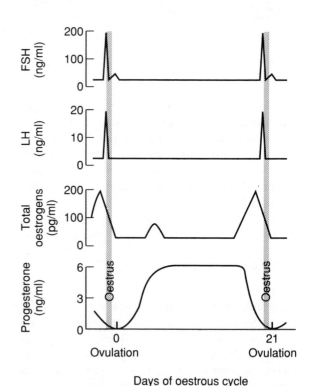

Days of oestrous cycle

Fig. 1.28 Trends in hormone concentrations in the peripheral circulation of the cow during the oestrous cycle.

stress that hormones are secreted in a pulsatile manner and fluctuate considerably. An effective description is given by Peters (1985a,b). Just before the onset of behavioural oestrus there is a sudden rise in plasma oestrogens, particularly oestradiol. Peak values occur at the beginning of oestrus with a subsequent decline to basal levels at the time of ovulation. During the rest of the cycle there are fluctuations in concentrations, although there is a discrete peak around day 6 of the cycle (Glencross et al., 1973) which may be related to the first wave of follicular growth (Ireland and Roche, 1983). The pre-oestrus rise in oestrogens stimulates the surge of LH from the anterior pituitary which is necessary for follicular maturation, ovulation and corpus luteum formation. A secondary less discrete peak has been demonstrated 24 hours after the ovulatory surge of gonadotrophin (Dobson, 1978).

The changes in progesterone concentrations mimic closely the physical changes of the corpus luteum. In a number of cows there is evidence of a delay in progesterone production or secretion by the corpus luteum (Lamming et al., 1979) which does not appear to affect the fertility of the individual adversely. Peak values are reached by days 7 and 8 after ovulation, and decline fairly quickly from day 18. When progesterone values fall to fairly low basal levels the removal of the anterior pituitary block allows the sudden release of gonadotrophins. Prolactin values are frequently difficult to obtain since stress induced by restraint for venepuncture is sufficient to cause a significant rise.

THE EWE

The sexual season of most breeds of sheep in Britain is from October to February, during which time there are eight to 10 recurrent cycles. The stimulus for the annual onset of sexual activity is declining length of daylight. The extent of the breeding season diminishes with increase of latitude; thus at the equator ewes may breed at any time of year, whereas in regions of high latitude — in both northern and southern hemispheres — the breeding season is restricted and distinct, with a prolonged phase of anoestrus after parturition. The breed of ewe also influences the duration of the breeding season; for example, in Dorset Horns it is

distinctly longer than in other breeds — whereby three crops of lambs can be obtained in 2 years — but in hill breeds, like the Welsh Mountain and Scottish Blackface, it is shorter. Local breeds of central Europe and the Merino in Australia may not show an annual anoestrus. Also, in 'ordinary' breeds in Britain, like the Clun Forest, which normally show a distinct seasonal activity, isolated instances of successful mating may occur in every month of the year (Lees, 1969). Ewe-lambs and yearling ewes have shorter breeding seasons than older ewes. The seasonal onset of sexual activity can be advanced by artifical manipulation of the photoperiod and by the use of hormonal agents (described later in this chapter).

The average duration of oestrus in mature ewes of British breeds is about 30 hours, and is at least 10 hours less in immature ewes. In Merinos, heat may last 48 hours. Ovulation occurs towards the end of oestrus, and the length of the oestrous cycle averages 17 days.

Signs of oestrus and mating behaviour

Oestrous ewes are restless. They seek the ram, and together form a following 'harem'. The ram 'tries' members of this group for receptivity by pawing with a forefoot, by rubbing his head along the ewe's side and by nipping her wool. A non-receptive ewe trots away, but when in full heat she stands, waggles her tail and moves it laterally. The vulva is slightly swollen and congested and there is often a slight discharge of clear mucus. The ram mounts and makes a series of probing pelvic thrusts and then dismounts. After variable intervals further mounts occur before intromission is achieved, and this is characterized by a deep pelvic thrust. An essential feature of successful coitus in the Najdi and Awassi breeds of the Middle East is the lateral displacement by the ram of the fat tail of the ewe. Rams of other breeds are unable to move the tail sufficiently to perform intromission.

More ovine matings occur during early morning and evening. When several rams run with a flock a hierarchy is established and the dominant male attracts the largest harem, but, despite this, a majority of ewes mate with more than one ram. Also, ewes show a preference for rams of their own breed or for a ram of their particular group if that group is mixed with other groups of different origin (Lees and Weatherhead, 1970). The number of services received by an oestrous ewe averages a little above four. Rams may serve from eight to 38 ewes in a day.

Changes in the ovaries

The ovaries of the ewe are smaller than those of the cow, and their shape is nearer the spherical. During anoestrus their size is approximately 1.3 by 1.1 by 0.8 cm, and the largest follicles present vary from 0.2 to 0.6 cm. At the onset of heat one or more follicles have attained a size of 1 cm. Their walls are thin and transparent and the liquor folliculi appears purple in colour. Grant (1934) has obseved that rupture of the follicle is preceded by the elevation of a small papilla above the general surface; ovulation occurs through rupture of this papilla about 24 hours after the onset of heat. The development of the corpus luteum is similar to that of the cow; by the fifth day of dioestrus it is 0.6 cm in diameter, and it attains its maximum size, 0.9 cm, by the middle of the dioestrus phase, when it has a central cavity (Roux, 1936). As the dioestrous period advances, its colour changes from blood red to pale pink. Its size remains constant until the onset of the next heat, when atrophy is rapid and the colour changes, first to yellow and later to brownish yellow. In twin ovulations the corpora lutea may occupy the same or opposite ovaries. During pregnancy the corpus luteum remains from 0.7 to 0.9 cm in diameter. Its colour is pale pink, but the central cavity has disappeared, having become filled by white tissue.

Ovulation with corpus luteum formation, but without signs of heat, may occur during the so-called anoestrous period — spurious ovulation (Grant, 1934). As to the number of ova shed at a heat period, genetic and nutritional factors play a part. Hill sheep in this country generally have one lamb, but if they are transferred to lowland pastures where herbage is rich (before the onset of the breeding season), twins become common. With lowland breeds the general expectancy is an average of 1.5 lambs per ewe. Roux (1936) in South Africa has noted that age is also a factor in the incidence of twinning. It attains its maximum when ewes are 5–6 years old, after which it remains constant. Primiparous ewes are very much less likely to have twins than pluriparous

ones. Ewes of the Border Leicester and Lleyn breeds are the most prolific in British sheep, and commonly bear triplets. The Finnish Landrace and Cambridge breeds normally produces two to four lambs per pregnancy.

Endocrine changes during the oestrous cycle

The endocrine changes are shown in Figure 1.29. Just before the onset of oestrus there is a rise in oestrogens in the peripheral circulation, particularly oestradiol-17β. This is followed by a sudden surge of LH which reaches a peak about 14 hours before ovulation; coincidental with this peak is a rise in FSH. There is also a second FSH peak 2 days after ovulation.

Progesterone concentrations follow closely the physical changes of the corpora lutea, but maximum values are lower than those of the cow, i.e. 2.5–4 ng/ml. Prolactin fluctuates throughout the

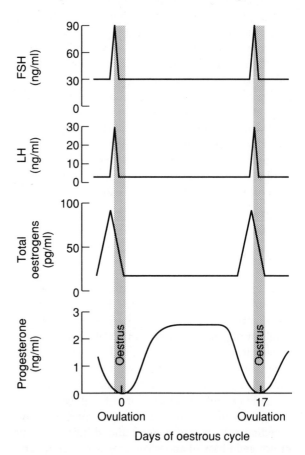

Fig. 1.29 Trends in hormone concentrations in the peripheral circulation of the ewe during the oestrous cycle.

oestrous cycle; however, concentrations rise during oestrus and ovulation, presumably reflecting the role of this hormone in the formation of the corpus luteum.

THE DOE (NANNY) GOAT

The breeding season in Britain is from August to February with the greatest activity in the months of October, November and December. Near the equator there is no evidence of seasonality but continous cyclical activity. The doe is polyoestrous, with an interoestrus interval of 20–21 days, although it is rather irregular at the beginning of the breeding season. The duration of oestrus is 30–40 hours, with ovulation occurring 12–36 hours after the onset.

The detection of heat in a doe is difficult in the absence of a male goat. The vulva shows some evidence of oedema and hyperaemia; the tail is twitched rapidly from side to side and up and down; the doe is restless, more vocal and has a reduced appetite and milk yield. The presence of the pheromones from the male goat, which can be transferred from the scent gland onto a cloth, will often intensify the signs.

The ovaries are of variable shape, depending upon the structures which are present, the longest dimension being about 2.2 cm. The largest follicles reach a maximum size of about 1.2 cm in diameter, and when they protrude from the surface often have a bluish tinge. The corpora lutea are pink.

The endocrine changes measured in the peripheral circulation are very similar to those of the ewe.

THE SOW

Puberty in gilts is reached at about 7 months, but diet, breed (including the degree of in-breeding) and season of birth influence its onset. At the first oestrus the number of ovulations is low, but it increases thereafter so that if mating is delayed until the third heat a larger litter will result. The cross-breeding of in-bred lines increases the ovulation rate, as does the provision of a high-energy diet for 11–14 days before the expected oestrus; continuing such a diet after mating, however, increases

embryonic loss. Fecundity is best from the fourth to seventh gestations.

Although the domestic sow is generally considered to be polyoestrous, the wild pig is a seasonal breeder, the main period being late autumn with a second peak of activity in April (Claus and Weiler, 1985). There is some evidence of the influence of photoperiod on reproduction in the domestic sow; for example, anoestrus is more prevalent in summer, and to a lesser extent February and March, whilst the ovulation rate is lower in summer. Claus and Weiler (1985) found that by reducing the day length artificially from May to August they were able to decrease the interval from weaning to oestrus from 23.6 to 5.7 days. For the most part, the recurrent reproductive cycles of 21 days are interrupted by pregnancy and lactation. The average length of oestrus is 53 hours, with spontaneous ovulation occurring between 38 and 42 hours from the beginning (Signoret, 1971). During lactation the physical stimuli of suckling cause heat to be in abeyance, but many sows show an anovulatory oestrus 2 days after farrowing. Now that satisfactory foods are available for the 'creep feeding' of piglets, the optimum weaning age is probably 5 or 6 weeks, after which oestrus can be expected in 4–6 days. Although early weaning at 3 weeks may be economically desirable, the disadvantages are that thereafter heat will be delayed or not shown so well and that cysts are likely to develop in the ovaries.

Signs of oestrus

Beginning 3 days before heat, the vulva becomes progressively swollen and congested; these features persist throughout heat and gradually subside during the 3 days afterwards. Restlessness is an unfailing sign of the approach of heat, and a peculiar repetitive grunt is emitted. With other sows the pro-oestrous animal sniffs their vulvae and may try to ride them, or will be the recipient of such attentions. The boar is sought, and in his presence the pro-oestrous female noses his testicles and flanks and may mount him but will refuse to be mounted. At the height of oestrus the sow assumes a stationary, rigid attitude with her ears cocked, and she appears to be quite oblivious to her environment. She generally remains still during coitus, which lasts an average of 5–7 minutes, but when mating with heavy boards gilts may become fidgety. Burger (1952) demonstrated that oestrus could readily be determined by firmly pressing the loin of the sow with the palms of both hands; the oestrous sow will stand motionless with cocked ears whereas sows not in heat will object to this approach. The same immobilization response can be elicited if the attendant sits astride the sow, and it can also be obtained in the absence of a boar by reproducing the voice or odour of the boar. The substance responsible for boar odour has been identified as 5α-andost-16-ene-3-one and it is secreted by the salivary glands. In the form of an aerosol it can be sprayed in the vicinity of sows to promote the standing reaction of oestrous.

'Silent heats' occur in about 2% of porcine cycles.

Cyclic changes in ovaries

The ovaries of the mature cycling sow are relatively large and mulberry-like, the surface lobulation being due to the elevations of the large follicles and corpora lutea, which, when mature, attain diameters of 0.8–1 cm and 1–1.3 cm, respectively. Several studies have shown that, except during the follicular phase of the cycle, there is continuous proliferation and atresia of follicles so that there is generally a pool of about 50 between 2 and 5 mm in diameter. Between about day 14 and 16 of the cycle there is recruitment of follicles, under the influence of gonadotrophin stimulation, which are destined for ovulation. The growth of selected preovulatory follicles during the follicular phase is associated with rapid atresia of small follicles and a block to their replacement in the proliferating pool, thus indicating some intraovarian control mechanism (Foxcroft and Hunter, 1985). The ripe follicle is sea-shell pink with a fine network of surface blood vessels and a very transparent focus which indicates the site of imminent ovulation. Haemorrhagic follicles are common. After ovulation there remain a considerable number of follicles of about 0.4 cm, some of which gradually enlarge to 0.9 cm by the succeeding day 18.

Immediately after ovulation the ruptured follicle is represented by a congested depression, but the accumulation of blood clot soon gives it a conical shape. By day 3 its cavity is filled with dark red blood clot, which by day 6 is replaced by a connective tissue plug or by a slightly yellow fluid; clots may persist up to day 12 and fluid up to day 18. The corpora lutea attain their maximum size at 12–15 days, after which they gradually regress to the next oestrus. They are dark red up to day 3 but then change to, and remain, wine red until day 15. As the corpora lutea regress between days 15 and 18 the colour changes rapidly from wine red to yellow, creamy yellow or buff. There is further rapid regression at the next oestrus, but throughout the succeeding dioestrus the corpora lutea remain as distinct entities, after which they regress sharply to grey pin-head foci. When, therefore, a cycling sow is slaughtered in the first half of dioestrus the ovaries may show the wine-coloured corpora lutea of the current cycle, the smaller pale corpora lutea of the previous cycle and the grey specks of the third generation corpora lutea.

Endocrine changes during the oestrous cycle

The endocrine changes are shown in Figure 1.30. Oestrogens in the peripheral circulation start to rise at the time that the corpora lutea begin to regress, reaching a peak about 48 hours before the onset of oestrus. The ovulatory LH peak occurs at the beginning of oestrus and 8–15 hours after the oestrogen peak; values remain low and fluctuate throughout the rest of the cycle. FSH concentrations vary considerably; however, there appears to be some pattern of secretion. Brinkley et al. (1973) demonstrated two surges, one concurrent with the LH peak and a larger one on day 2 or 3 of the cycle; Van de Wiel et al. (1981) found a similar pattern, the peak coinciding with the minimum value of oestradiol. As with other species, the progesterone concentrations follow closely the physical changes of the corpora lutea. For the first 8 days after ovulation there is a good correlation between progesterone levels and the number of corpora lutea; however, by 12 days it is less obvious (Dzuik, 1977).

Two prolactin surges have been identified (Brinkley et al., 1973; Van de Wiel et al., 1981): the first one concomitant with the preovulatory LH and oestrogen surges and a second during oestrus.

THE BITCH

Reproductive activity in the bitch differs from the polycyclic pattern of other species in that there are

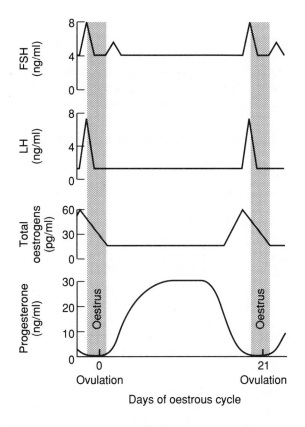

Fig. 1.30 Trends in hormone concentrations in the peripheral circulation of the sow during the oestrous cycle.

no frequent, recurring periods of heat. All bitches have a prolonged period of anoestrus or sexual quiescence between successive heats irrespective of whether they have been pregnant or not; this pattern has been described as monocyclic (Jöchle and Andersen, 1977).

The average interval between successive oestrous periods is 7 months, but it is variable, and there is some evidence that the breed of the bitch can have an effect. For example, for rough collies it is 37 weeks and for the German shepherd 26 weeks (Christie and Bell, 1971): other breeds that were studied had mean intervals between these two figures. Mating does not appear to influence the interval, although pregnancy caused a slight increase (Christie and Bell, 1971). There does not appear to be any seasonal effect on reproductive function since there is a fairly even distribution of the occurrence of oestrus throughout the year (Sokolowski et al., 1977).

The oestrous cycle is traditionally divided into four phases (Heape, 1900).

Pro-oestrus. The bitch has a true pro-oestrus characterized by the presence of vulval oedema, swelling and a sanguinous discharge. Some fastidious bitches show no evidence of discharge as they are continually cleaning the perineum. The bitch is attractive to males but will not accept the male.

Oestrus. The bitch will accept the male and adopts the breeding stance. The vulva becomes less oedematous and the vulval discharge becomes clearer, less sanguinous and less copious.

The duration of pro-oestrus and oestrus combined is about 18 days, i.e. 9 days each. However, this can be very variable, some bitches showing very little sign of pro-oestrus before they will accept and stand for the dog and others producing a copious sanguinous discharge during true oestrus. Some bitches also show evidence of sire preference, which can affect the timing. Ovulation usually occurs 1 or 2 days after the onset of oestrus, although, using laparoscopy, it has been observed that some follicles continue to ovulate up to 14 days later (Wildt et al., 1977).

Metoestrus. This stage starts when the bitch ceases to accept the dog; however, there is dispute about its duration. Some consider that it ends when the corpora lutea have regressed at 70–80 days whilst others measure it in relation to the time taken for repair of the endometrium, 130–140 days.

Anoestrus. At the end of metoestrus the bitch passes into a period of anoestrus without any external signs. The same is also true after parturition following a normal pregnancy. This phase lasts about 3 months before the bitch returns to pro-oestrus.

Signs of oestrus

The first indication that heat is approaching is the onset of slight swelling of the vulval lips. This indication generally precedes the commencement of bleeding by several days. Labial swelling is progressive during the pro-oestrus period. Bleeding attains its maximum early in pro-oestrus and continues at this level into the early part of the true heat phase. During the greater part of pro-oestrus the bitch, although attractive to the dog, takes no interest in his attentions. She will not stand for him and generally attacks him if he attempts to mount her. A day or so before the end of pro–oestrus her attitude changes, and she shows signs of courtship towards the male. These comprise sudden darting movements which end in a crouching attitude with her limbs tense and her face alert. She barks invitingly, but as the dog approaches she moves suddenly again. She will not yet allow him to mount. With the onset of oestrus the invitation to coitus is obvious. She stands in the mating position with her tail slightly raised or held to one side. She remains still while the male mounts and copulates. In the later stages of the copulatory tie, which occupies from 15 to 25 minutes, she becomes restless and irritable and her attempt to free herself may cause the male considerable physical embarrassment. After the first 2 days of heat, sexual desire gradually recedes, but with the continued persuasion of the male she will accept coitus until the end of the period. Bleeding, although reduced in amount, generally continues well into the heat period and may persist until the end. More often, however, the

discharge becomes yellow as heat proceeds. Vulval swelling and tumefaction are greatest at the onset of the stage of acceptance. During the course of oestrous the enlarged labia become softer in consistency. Some labial swelling continues into the first part of the metoestrous phase.

Changes in the vagina and uterus

Vaginal smear
The cyclical changes which occur in vaginal cytology have been described in detail (Griffiths and Amoroso, 1939; Hancock and Rowlands, 1949; Schutte, 1967; Rozel, 1975). Vaginal smears stained with either a simple stain such as Leishman's or a trichrome stain such as Shorr's can, with practice, be used to determine the stage of the oestrous cycle. The advent of the 'Diff-Quik' staining method has greatly simplified the procedure. At the onset of pro–oestrus large numbers of erythrocytes are present; however, when true

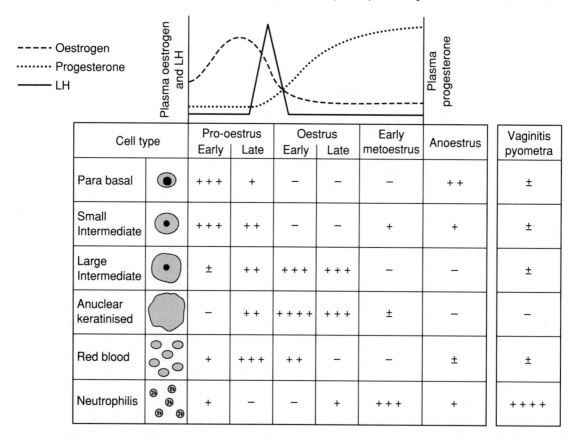

Cell type		Pro-oestrus Early	Pro-oestrus Late	Oestrus Early	Oestrus Late	Early metoestrus	Anoestrus	Vaginitis pyometra
Para basal		+ + +	+	−	−	−	+ +	±
Small Intermediate		+ + +	+ +	−	−	+	+	±
Large Intermediate		±	+ +	+ + +	+ + +	−	−	±
Anuclear keratinised		−	+ +	+ + + +	+ + +	±	−	−
Red blood		+	+ + +	+ +	−	−	±	±
Neutrophilis		+	−	−	+	+ + +	+	+ + + +

Fig. 1.31 Changes in the types of cells, and their relative numbers, in vaginal smears from the bitch during the stages of the oestrous cycle, and changes in oestrogen, progesterone and luteinizing hormone levels in the peripheral plasma.

oestrus occurs the number of erythrocytes is reduced, and the smear consists of superficial cell types from the stratified squamous epithelium, such as anuclear cells, cells with pyknotic nuclei and large intermediate cells. Towards the end of oestrus, numbers of polymorphonuclear neutrophil leucocytes appear in the smear, and these become the dominant cell type during metoestrus. In anoestrus nucleated basal and intermediate cells of the stratified squamous epithelium, together with a few neutrophils, form the characteristic smear.

Figure 1.31 shows the cyclical changes of the cell types.

Vaginal epithelium

The vaginal epithelium during anoestrus is of the low columnar, cuboidal type and comprises two or three layers only. During pro-oestrus the epithelial cells change to the high, squamous, stratified type and persist in this form until the later stages of oestrus. The stratum corneum and the layers immediately beneath it are lost by desquamation during the pro-oestrous and oestrous period, leaving a low, squamous structure which becomes converted to columnar epithelium in from 1 to 3 weeks after the end of heat. During metoestrus (and pregnancy) the epithelium is of a higher columnar type than during anoestrus.

During pro-oestrus, oestrus and early metoestrus the epithelium and lamina propria are infiltrated with large numbers of neutrophils which eventually escape into the vaginal lumen.

Endometrium

The endometrium shows considerable change during the oestrous cycle. The endometrial glands in pro-oestrus and oestrus are loosely coiled with very obvious lumina and deep epithelial lining. During metoestrus the glands become larger, the lumina smaller and the coiled parts in the basal layer of the endometrium more tortuous. As the bitch passes into anoestrus there is a reduction in the amount and degree of coiling of the glands.

At about 98 days after the onset of oestrus, i.e. in metoestrus, there is evidence of desquamation of the endometrial epithelium; however, by about 120–130 days the epithelium has been restored by proliferation of cells from the crypts of the endometrial glands.

Changes in the ovaries

During anoestrus the ovaries are oval and slightly flattened. In a bitch of medium size they measure approximately 1.4 cm from pole to pole and 0.8 cm from the attached to the free border. No appreciable follicles can be seen, although on section the minute remnants of the corpora lutea of the previous cycle may be seen as yellow or brown spots. In the young bitch the surface of the ovaries is smooth and regular, but in the aged animal it is irregular and scarred. At the commencement of pro-oestrus, developing follicles have already attained a diameter of 0.5 cm. They progressively enlarge, until at the time of ovulation their size varies from 0.6 to 1 cm. By this time the ovary is considerably enlarged, its size depending on the number of ripe follicles present, and its shape is irregular due to the projection of the follicles from its surface. Owing to the thickness of the follicle wall it may be difficult to distinguish between follicles and corpora lutea. Prior to ovulation the surface of the follicle shows a slightly raised papule, pin-head sized, and the epithelium covering it is brown, which contrasts with the flesh colour of the remainder of the follicle. A remarkable feature of the ripening follicle of the bitch is the thickness of its wall, due to hypertrophy and folding of the granulosa cells, which can be seen on section with the naked eye as evidence of pre-ovulatory luteinization. Ovulation is spontaneous and normally occurs 1 or 2 days after the onset of the period of acceptance. Most of the follicles rupture over a period of 48 hours (Wildt et al., 1977). The oocyte is capable of being fertilized for up to 108 hours after ovulation (Tsutsui and Shimizu, 1975). The corpus luteum at first contains a central cavity, but becomes filled by compact luteinized cells by the 10th day after ovulation, by which time the body has attained its full size (0.6–1 cm). Corpora lutea now comprise by far the greater mass of the ovary. As a rule an approximately equal number of corpora lutea are found in each ovary, although occasionally there are wide differences. (In this connection it is interesting to note that the numbers of fetuses in the respective cornua in pregnancy frequently differ from those of the corpora lutea in the ovaries on the respective sides.) Embryonic migration into the cornua on the opposite side would appear to be common. On section the corpus luteum is yellowish pink: it

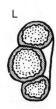
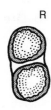

Fig. 1.32 Ovaries of an 8-month-old bitch weighing 6.8 kg after 2–3 days of pro-oestrus. Marked hypertrohy of the granulosa cells lining the follicles.

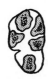

Fig. 1.33 Ovaries of an 8-month-old bitch weighing 6.8 kg just after ovulation. The follicles of the right ovary are collapsed. The left ovary shows remnants of corpora lutea from a previous heat.

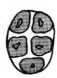

Fig. 1.34 Ovaries of an 8-month-old bitch weighing 6.8 kg late in heat. Corpora lutea are forming; pleats loose and flesh coloured. Central cavities.

Fig. 1.35 Ovaries of a bitch weighing 11 kg. Three fetuses in each cornu. Corpora lutea are flesh coloured. Old remnants still visible.

Fig. 1.36 Ovaries of a bitch weighing 11 kg 4 weeks after parturition (five fetuses). Corpora lutea are shrunken and cream in colour.

remains unchanged in the non-pregnant bitch until about the 30th day after ovulation, after which it slowly atrophies. Visible vestiges may be present throughout anoestrus. During pregnancy the corpora lutea persist at their maximum size throughout, but regress fairly rapidly after parturition. The changes in the ovaries of the bitch are shown diagramatically in figures 1.32 to 1.36.

Ultrasound appearance of the ovaries

Using a transabdominal approach via the flank, with the bitch standing and a 7.5 MHz real-time linear array transducer, England and Allen (1989) were able to identify ovarian structures at the onset of pro-oestrus; these were circular and anechoic and were obviously developing antral follicles. When the bitch was in oestrus they had increased in size, reaching a maximum of 4–13 mm in diameter on day 13 (day 0 being onset of pro-oestrus). The walls of the follicles became thickened from day 10 onwards, due presumably to preovulatory luteinization; there was no evidence

of follicular collapse associated with ovulation. At 25–30 days after the onset of pro-oestrus the ovaries were difficult to identify.

Endocrine changes during the oestrous cycle

The trends in endocrine changes are shown in Figure 1.37. The main feature which distinguishes them from other species previously described is the prolonged luteal phase, illustrated by the persistence of high progesterone levels in the peripheral blood. It is noticeable that progesterone levels start to rise before ovulation has occurred, which confirms the morphological evidence of preovulatory luteinization of the mature follicles 60–70 hours before ovulation (Concannon et al., 1977). This preovulatory rise in progesterone may provide the stimulus for the bitch to accept the male (Concannon et al., 1975). In addition, it can also be used as a method to determine the timing of artificial insemination in that it should not be delayed long after concentrations >2–3 ng/ml are observed in peripheral plasma (Jeffcoate and Lindsay, 1989; see Chapter 28).

Oestrogens rise rapidly just before the onset of standing oestrus, and are rapidly followed by the LH peak, which lasts much longer than that of other species; ovulation occurs 24–96 hours after this (Phemister et al., 1973; Wildt et al., 1977). FSH levels at oestrus reach a peak, coincident with that of LH. Prolactin appears to have a negative correlation with progesterone; thus, as

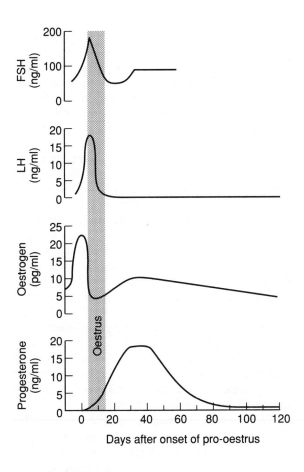

Fig. 1.37 Trends in hormone concentration in the peripheral circulation of the bitch during the oestrous cycle.

progesterone levels fall towards the end of metoestrus or pregnancy, prolactin increases.

Pseudopregnancy

Most, if not all, bitches show some evidence of pseudopregnancy during metoestrus, the intensity and signs being very variable; for this reason it is preferable to refer to *covert* pseudopregnancy, where the bitch will be in metoestrus but will show little or no signs, and *overt* pseudopregnancy. In the latter, the clinical signs will range from slight mammary development and lactogenesis whilst at the opposite extreme the bitch will show all the external signs of pregnancy and will ultimately undergo a mock parturition, with nesting, loss of appetite, straining, emotional attachment to inanimate objects and heavy lactation.

Pseudopregnancy was originally believed to be due to an intensification and prolongation of metoestrus; however, a number of workers have demonstrated that there is no difference in the progesterone concentrations in the peripheral blood of bitches with or without signs of pseudopregnancy. It is likely that the prolactin may well be responsible for initiating the changes. The negative correlation between progesterone and prolactin levels is shown in Figure 1.37, the decline in progesterone appearing to coincide with the rise in prolactin. If bitches undergo ovarohysterectomy when they are pseudopregnant the condition can be intensified and prolonged. Furthermore, antiprolactin drugs such as 2-Brα-ergocryptine have been successfully used to cause remission of the signs of pseudopregnancy (Arbeiter and Winding, 1977).

THE CAT

Body weight is the most important factor in determining puberty in non-pedigree cats (Scott, 1970). Females will usually show their first oestrus once a weight of 2.3–2.5 kg has been attained at an approximate age of 7 months. Puberty occurs a month or two later in males at a weight of approximately 3.5 kg. Puberty is also influenced by the season of birth; females born very early in the year may mature in the autumn of the same year, whilst those born later will not normally show oestrus until the following spring (Gruffydd-Jones, 1982). Puberty is much more variable in pedigree cats (Jemmett and Evans, 1977). Oriental queens (such as Siamese and Burmese) may show their first oestrus before 5 months of age, whilst pedigree longhair cats may not mature until over a year of age.

Free-living non-pedigree and feral cats are seasonally polyoestrus, with a period of anoestrus beginning in the late autumn. Increasing daylight length is the most important factor in inducing the resumption of reproductive activity and the first oestrus will usually be seen soon after the shortest day of the year. If a constant 14 hours of lighting is provided daily, sexual activity will continue throughout the year, and this manipulation of photoperiod will alter the circadian rhythm of melatonin production (Leyva et al., 1985). If the lighting regimen is changed from 14 to 8 hours then cyclical activity will cease immediately (Leyva et al., 1989). There may be a period of apparent lack of oestrous activity in the early summer, but this corresponds with the pregnancy or lactation following mating earlier in the year, rather than true anoestrus.

Some non-pedigree cats have regular oestrous cycles lasting approximately 3 weeks, but others may show no regular pattern (Shille et al., 1979). The duration of oestrus is 7–10 days, and is not significantly shortened by mating (Shille et al., 1979; Gruffydd-Jones, 1982). Oestrous cycle patterns show considerably more variation in pedigree cats. Long-hairs may have only one or two oestrous cycles each year, whilst the period of oestrus may be longer in Oriental queens with a reduced interoestrual interval. Oestrogen concentrations increase dramatically at the time of oestrus from the baseline of 60 pmol/l, and may double within 24 hours, reaching a peak of up to 300 pmol/l (Shille et al., 1979). The principal oestrogen produced by the ovary is oestradiol-17β. The rapid rise in oestrogen concentrations corresponds to an abrupt appearance of behavioural changes indicative of oestrus, and queens do not usually show a distinctive pro-oestrous phase. The oestrual display is characterized by increased vocalization, rubbing and rolling. The queen becomes generally more active, and she will solicit the attention of a tom. The queen may adopt the mating posture either in response to the tom or occasionally spontaneously. She lowers her front quarters with the hind legs extended, resulting in lordosis. The tail is held erect and slightly to one side. There may occasionally be a slight serous vaginal discharge, but there are usually no changes in the appearance of the external genitalia. The extent of the oestrual display varies considerably between queens but is generally more prominent in the Oriental breeds.

Mating and ovulation

During mating, the tom mounts the queen and grasps her neck with his teeth. The queen's hind legs paddle as he adjusts his position, and this becomes more rapid during coitus, which lasts up to 10 seconds. The queen cries out during copulation, and as the tom dismounts, she may strike out at him, displaying the typical 'rage reaction'. This is followed by a period of frantic rolling and licking at the vulva. As soon as this postcoital reaction has ceased, the tom will usually attempt to mate the queen again, and there may be several matings within the first 30–60 minutes.

The cat is an induced ovulator, and thus mating is important in triggering ovulation. Receptors are present within the queen's vulva which are stimulated during copulation, ultimately resulting in release of LH from the posterior pituitary. Only about 50% of queens will ovulate after a single mating, and multiple matings may be required to ensure adequate release of LH to induce ovulation (Concannon et al., 1980). The ovulatory surge of LH begins within minutes of coitus, peaks within 2 hours and returns to basal values within about 8 hours; peak LH concentrations of over 90 ng/ml have been reported (Tsutsui and Stabenfeldt, 1993). Further matings before the peak of LH concentrations has been reached will lead to additional increments. However, after multiple matings over a period of 4 hours or more, further matings may fail to induce any additional increase in LH concentrations, and this is thought to result from depletion of the pituitary pool of the hormone or development of refractoriness to GnRH (Johnson and Gay, 1981).

Ovulation is an 'all or nothing' phenomenon, and once significant concentrations of LH have been achieved all ripe follicles will rupture (Wildt et al., 1980). The mean ovulatory rate for non-pedigree cats is approximately four but is more variable in pedigree animals.

Occasionally, ovulation will occur in the absence of any contact with entire toms. Receptors similar to those found in the vulva are also located in the lumbar area (Rose, 1978), and these may be stimulated if the queen is mounted by other females or castrated male cats, or by stroking over this area. Neutered toms may mate queens in oestrous even if they have been castrated prepubertally. However, in a study involving a colony of American short-haired cats in which the queens were housed individually, and where tactile stimulation of the hindquarters and perineal regions by handlers was avoided, ovulation was detected; this was defined if progesterone concentrations ≥4.8 nmol/l in the peripheral circulation. The queens had sight and sound of other cats, including males. It is noteworthy that six of the seven cats that ovulated were older than 7 years of age (Lawler et al., 1993).

Pseudopregnancy

Sterile matings which successfully induce ovulation lead to pseudopregnancy. Concentrations of progesterone are very similar to those of pregnancy for the first 3 weeks, after which levels gradually fall, reaching baseline by approximately 7 weeks (Paape

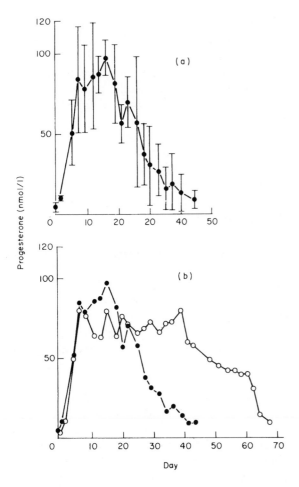

Fig. 1.38 *(a) Mean* ±SD) plasma concentrations of progesterone throughout pseudopregnancy (four cats). (b) Mean plasma concentrations of progesterone throughout pregnancy (o——o) and pseudopregnancy (●——●). Day 0 represents the day of mating. (Figure reproduced courtesy of Dr T. J. Gruffydd Jones.)

et al., 1975; Shille and Stabenfeldt, 1979) (Figure 1.38). Oestrus will usually occur shortly afterwards.

Nesting behaviour and milk production are rarely seen in pseudopregnant queens, but hyperaemia of the nipples will usually be evident as in pregnancy. The queen's appetite may increase, with some redistribution of fat leading to an increase in abdominal size.

ARTIFICIAL CONTROL OF CYCLIC REPRODUCTIVE ACTIVITY

In the management of livestock, or in dealing with companion animals, there are many times when the manipulation of normal cyclic activity ensures optimum production or is convenient for the owner. In the case of seasonal breeders the ability to produce offspring out of season or to advance the time of onset of cyclical activity has advantages. In these and in other species, the ability to ensure that an individual or group of animals does not come into oestrus, or is in oestrus at the same time, has attractions. The methods that are available can be divided into two main groups, first, those which do not involve the use of hormones and, second, those that do.

Non-hormonal methods

Light
The onset of cyclical activity in the mare, ewe, goat and cat is dependent upon changes in the hours of daylight. The mare and queen are stimulated to activity by a lengthening photoperiod, whilst in the ewe and goat it is the effect of a decreasing photoperiod which is the stimulus.

In ewes, the provision of housing with controlled lighting enables the breeding season to change from the autumn and winter to spring and summer. Furthermore, by subjecting the ewes to a lighting regimen which does not have any change in duration it is possible to ensure breeding throughout the year, as is the case in equatorial climates.

If mares are stabled at the end of December in the northern hemisphere and are subjected to artificial light, preferably of increasing duration, then it is possible to advance the onset of normal cyclical activity so that there is oestrus and ovulation.

Both tungsten and fluorescent lights have been used, although the former would appear to be better. The provision of a 200 watt incandescent bulb in each loose-box is adequate, and if it is controlled by an automatic timing device, so that the duration of lighting is increased by 25–30 minutes each week, reproductive activity will be initiated when the mare is receiving 15–16 hours of light each day (Kenney et al., 1975).

Nutrition
The effect of nutrition in initiating reproductive activity in seasonally breeding species is not clear. There is some evidence that the stabling of mares and the provision of good feeding assists in stimulating the onset of cyclical activity in early spring.

There is also evidence for the converse, since Allen (1978) has reported that when yarded mares are turned out to fresh spring grass about 80% of them have come into oestrus and ovulated within 14 days. Furthermore, he has found that barren and maiden mares maintained in yards on adequate but mainly dried feedstuffs during the winter and spring remain in anoestrus longer than those which are kept out at grass. An explanation for this is difficult to find, although it may be related to the β-carotene content of the diet: fresh spring grass containing large amounts of this substance.

Improved nutrition can exert a profound effect on ovarian function by increasing the number of follicles which mature and ovulate. This effect is described as 'flushing', a practice which has been used in lowland flocks of sheep for many years. By increasing the dietary intake, particularly that of energy, before ewes are tupped it is possible to increase the number of lambs that are born. A similar technique can also be used in the sow to increase litter size. There is no evidence, however, that, provided the ewes are adequately fed, it is possible to advance the onset of the breeding season by this means.

The opinions on the effect of nutrition on reproduction in the sow are conflicting. It is generally assumed that flushing gilts and sows 4–6 days before oestrus increased prolificacy by increasing the ovulation rate (Dailey et al., 1972). Whether this effect occurs in adequately fed individuals is difficult to determine (Aherne and Kirkwood, 1985).

Other methods

The presence of a male animal can exert its effect upon the cyclical activity of the female. This is well demonstrated in sheep, where the introduction of a vasectomized tup at the start of the breeding season will stimulate the onset of oestrous cycles in the majority of ewes and can also bring about some degree of synchronization of cyclical patterns (see Chapter 24).

In sows and gilts the weaning of piglets hastens the return of cyclical ovarian activity postpartum. If litters from a number of sows are weaned at the same time this will result in some degree of synchrony of oestrus.

It has also been shown in gilts and sows that stress associated with a change in environment or transportation can stimulate the onset of oestrus postpartum.

Hormonal methods

A large number of different hormones have been used to manipulate cyclic activity in domestic species. Some of the methods have been based upon attempts to mimic closely the normal endocrine changes that occur; however, some have been rather more empirical.

They can be considered in various groups: (1) preparations which stimulate the release of anterior pituitary hormones; (2) preparations which replace or supplement anterior pituitary gonadotrophins; (3) oestrogens; (4) progestogens; (5) prostaglandins; and (6) melatonin.

Preparations which stimulate the release of anterior pituitary hormones

Ovarian steroid hormones, paticularly oestrogens, have been shown to exert a positive-feedback effect upon the anterior pituitary and hypothalamus (see Figure 1.1). A large number of oestrogens, both naturally occurring and synthetic, have been used to stimulate oestrus. It is likely that their effect is purely a direct one in stimulating oestrous behaviour and changes in the genital tract, but it is possible that they may also stimulate the release of pituitary gonadotrophins. However, with the synthesis of GnRH, a substance is now commercially available which can be used to stimulate the release of endogenous gonadotrophins, GnRH has been used to induce premature puberty in gilts following equine chorionic gonadotrophin (eCG) stimulation (Webel, 1978). The results of its use in controlling the time of ovulation in the cow have not been very satisfactory (Cooper, 1978) although it can be used to stimulate the onset of oestrus in the postpartum cow (Lamming et al., 1979). It has not proved to be effective in inducing oestrus in mares during the seasonal anoestrus (Allen and Alexiev, 1979).

Preparations which supplement or replace pituitary gonadotrophins

It is possible to extract purified FSH and LH from pituitary glands obtained at abattoirs. However, it is expensive and time-consuming to obtain sufficient quantities for routine commercial use. Furthermore, there is a danger of transmitting diseases such as BSE. Fortunately, two readily available substitutes are available: (1) eCG, obtained from the serum of pregnant mares, has mainly an

'FSH-like' effect but with some 'LH-like' activity and (2) human chorionic gonadotrophin (hCG), obtained from the urine of pregnant women, has mainly an 'LH-like' effect but with some 'FSH-like' activity.

Pseudopregnancy can be achieved by mating queen cats with a vasectomized tom or through simulating coitus by swabbing the vagina. Administration of hCG can also be used to induce ovulation. Pseudopregnant queens may not show a return to oestrus for 4–8 weeks.

As has been previously described, premature puberty has been initiated in most domestic species by the administration of eCG. However, both gonadotrophins have also been successfully used to manipulate cyclic activity. In anoestrous gilts and sows, eCG alone or in combination with hCG will promote follicular growth and oestrus, but a second injection of hCG 72 hours later will ensure that ovulation occurs. The same technique can be used to synchronize cyclic activity, particularly if used in combination with a progestogen or other pituitary-blocking substance (see below).

The use of eCG alone to induce oestrus in seasonally anoestrous ewes is not very successful; but if progesterone is administered to the ewes before the injection of eCG then there is synchronized oestrus and ovulation in such ewes. However, attempts to stimulate an early return to cyclical activity in lactating ewes have proved to be difficult, particularly in those that are lactating heavily, presumably owing to the effect of prolactin release (Kann et al., 1975).

In the anoestrous cow it is possible to stimulate follicular growth and ovulation with eCG treatment. However, the dose response is variable, and it can frequently result in multiple ovulations. Thus, it is necessary to withhold insemination at this induced oestrus. Unfortunately, in many cases, the cow will then return to the anoestrous state.

Combinations of eCG/hCG have been used to induce oestrus in the anoestrous bitch, sometimes in combination with oestrogens. The induction of a behavioural response has usually been good but the numbers of bitches which ovulated and subsequently conceived has usually been poor.

Surprisingly, eCG does not appear to stimulate ovarian activity when given to mares in winter anoestrus. The reasons for this are probably twofold: firstly, it may be that the dose required to stimulate follicular development is large and,

secondly, it is likely that eCG alone is not responsible for stimulating the wave of accessory follicles during early pregnancy. Human menopausal gonadotrophin (hMG) is extracted from the urine of menopausal women; this has a high FSH-like action. It is used to superovulate cows for embryo transfer, but the author is not aware of it being used elsewhere.

Oestrogens

The administration of oestrogens, either synthetic or naturally occurring, has been used to induce oestrus in animals that are anoestrous. In most cases they have a direct effect on the tubular genital tract and on behaviour; however, it is doubtful if they initiate ovarian activity and ovulation, in fact in large doses they could result in pituitary inhibition.

Progestogens

Progesterone and progestational compounds have been used extensively in most domestic species as a method of controlling the oestrous cycle, particularly synchronization within groups of females. In general, the principle behind their use is that the exogenous progestogens act in the same way as a corpus luteum, resulting in a negative-feedback effect upon the anterior pituitary and a suppression of cyclic activity initiated by the release of gonadotrophins. When the source of progestogen is withdrawn, or its effect declines, there is a return to cyclic activity.

Uses in the Mare. In some racehorses and show-jumpers it is desirable to prevent the mare from coming into oestrus at an inopportune time; in some cases it may be desirable to synchronize a group of animals. A daily injection of progesterone at a dose rate of 0.3 mg/kg is effective in preventing oestrous, with a return to a normal fertile heat 3–7 days after treatment ceases (Van Niekerk, 1973). Potent oral progestogens are now also available for suppressing oestrus and synchronizing groups of mares when withdrawn (Webel, 1975). One of these, allyltrenbolone or altrenogest, has been used successfully in a number of ways:

1. To stimulate the onset of cyclical activity. The hormone, which is incorporated into a clear, yellow, vegetable oil, is administered at a dose rate of 0.044 mg/kg bodyweight mixed in the feed for 10 days and then stopped. A good response will be obtained when given in the late transitional phase

from anoestrus to cyclical activity when follicles are present. The results are better if increased lighting is used.

2. To suppress oestrus, for example for shows or other functions. It should be fed for 15 days at a dose rate of 0.044 mg/kg.

3. To suppress oestrus in mares with prolonged oestrus or other aberrant sexual behaviour.

4. To control the time of oestrus so that effective use can be made of a stallion. The hormone should be fed for 15 days and then stopped, so that the mare should come into oestrus 2–3 days later.

Uses in the Cow. Progestogens can be used to suppress oestrus as described in the mare but there are few practical indications for this purpose. However, there is ample indication for their use to synchronize groups of cows and heifers for artificial insemination and to overcome the problems of oestrus detection.

Progesterone was first used by daily injection to synchronize oestrous cycles in groups of cows in 1948 (Christian and Casida, 1948). A large number of synthetic substances have since been used and it is generally accepted that following treatment of randomly cycling animals with these compounds for 18–21 days, there is fairly good synchronization of oestrus 4–6 days after the cessation of treatment (Cooper, 1978). Unfortunately, as with other species, the fertility at the first oestrus is lower than normal, the most likely reason for this being impaired sperm transport as a result of the atypical hormone balance after withdrawal of the progestogen.

Good synchronization and fertility, following double fixed-time artificial insemination, was reported by Wishart and Young (1974) using a synthetic progestogen (Norgestamet). The hormone was given as a subcutaneous implant at the same time as an injection of oestradiol valerate. The implant was removed after 9 days, and following two inseminations at 48 and 60 hours afterwards, conception rates were 65%.

The main disadvantage of such a scheme is the need to handle the cattle a second time to remove the implant.

Another method of administering progestogens is in the form of a progesterone-releasing intravaginal device (PRID) (Figure 1.39), or controlled internal drug release device (CIDR-type B) containing 1.9 g of progesterone. The PRID, which is a stainless steel coil covered with an inert elastomer incorporating 1.55 g of progesterone, is placed in the vagina, using a special speculum, and whilst it is in position progesterone is absorbed, producing concentrations in the peripheral blood comparable with the maximum levels of dioestrus. When the coil is removed after 12 days the cow will come into oestrus in 2 to 3 days. Good conception rates have been obtained following two fixed-time inseminations at 57 and 74 hours after the removal of the device. Some of the coils also contain a small capsule of oestradiol benzoate. The CIDR, which is a hinged, 't'-shaped device impregnated with progesterone, functions in a similar manner.

In the case of PRID and Norgestamet (see above) the oestradiol benzoate or oestradiol valerate is used as an antiluteotrophic and luteolytic agent. However, there is good evidence that oestrogens are only weakly luteolytic, especially when used in the early luteal phase (Smith and Vincent, 1973). This is probably the reason why in an earlier study on the use of Norgestamet to synchronize heifers only 75% were observed in oestrus within 4.5 days of implantation (Drew et al., 1979). In a study using Norgestamet, Peters (1984) found that, of eight cows treated with oestradiol valerate during the first six days of the oestrous cycle, in only one was there prevention of luteal function. Thus in those cows where this occurred the corpus luteum would have persisted beyond the time that the implant was *in situ*, and hence they would have returned to oestrus only when the corpus luteum had regressed spontaneously. By using $PGF_{2\alpha}$ at the time of removal of the implant, synchronization approaching 100% should be achieved. Better results are obtained if the prostaglandin is injected 24 hours before removal. Norgestamet is available commercially as a 3 mg implant: on insertion, 3 mg of Norgestamet and 5 mg of oestradiol valerate are injected as a 2 ml dose intramuscularly.

In a study comparing the effect of the stage of the oestrous cycle when PRIDs are inserted, and the degree of synchronization, it was found that it was much better when they were inserted on days 13 or 14 compared with days 2–4 (Cumming et al., 1982). When PRIDs were inserted for 12 days and $PGF_{2\alpha}$ injected 24 hours before removal, very good synchronization was achieved (Roche and Ireland, 1981; Folman et al., 1983), with a pregnancy rate of 67% following fixed-time artificial insemination at 56 hours.

The same PRID has also been used successfully

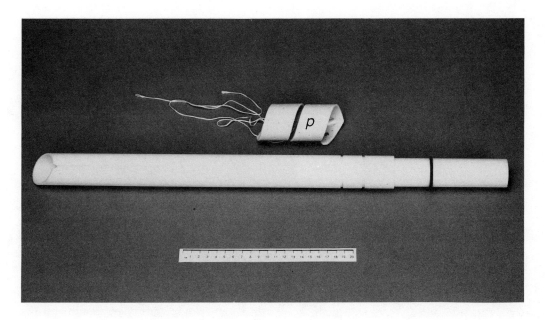

Fig. 1.39 Progesterone-releasing intravaginal device (PRID) (p) with speculum/applicator.

to induce oestrus in dairy cows and beef suckler cows that are anoestrus (Lamming and Bulman, 1976), as has Norgestamet and CIDR. This will be discussed further in Chapter 22.

Uses in the Ewe. Progestogens have been widely used in controlling reproduction in the ewe, either on their own or in conjunction with other hormones. They have been used to induce oestrus in the anoestrous ewe during the non-breeding season and also for synchronization of groups of ewes that are already showing cyclical activity. Most of the progestational substances are administered via the intravaginal route in the form of impregnated sponges or tampons (Figure 1.40). Provided that the progestogen is correctly incorporated into the sponge, it is readily absorbed at a sufficient rate to ensure a full negative-feedback effect on pituitary function. Although progesterone was used initially in the sponges the potent short-acting analogues, notably fluorogestone acetate (FGA) and medroxyprogesterone acetate (MAP), have superseded it.

When intravaginal sponges are used outside the normal breeding season it is necessary to use eCG as a source of gonadotrophin at the end of the progesterone priming period. The onset of normal cyclical activity can be determined by running vasectomized rams with a harness several weeks before. However, it is possible to use a simple rule-of-thumb calculation to determine if eCG is necessary: from the lambing records of the non-synchronized flock, calculate the date when 50% of the ewes had lambed, then, if the sponges are not to be inserted earlier than 150 days before the same date for the current year, eCG will not be required (Henderson, 1985).

The dose of eCG required is such that it should stimulate oestrus and ovulation without causing superovulation. Some approximate dose rates are listed below in Table 1.1.

Opinions vary on the time of injection of eCG. Whilst it is claimed that better results are obtained if it is injected 48 hours before sponge removal, the advantage is so small that the additional handling of the ewes does not make it cost-effective.

Fertility may be reduced when ewes are mated at the first synchronized oestrous; this may be due to poor absorption of the progestogen from the sponge or to an effect of the abnormal steroid balance on sperm transport and survival. However, if ewes fail to conceive at the first oestrus there is usually good synchrony at the second, when better conception rates are likely.

Attempts to induce oestrus in the early post-partum and lactating ewe have been unsuccessful, probably due to the influence of prolactin (Kann et al., 1979).

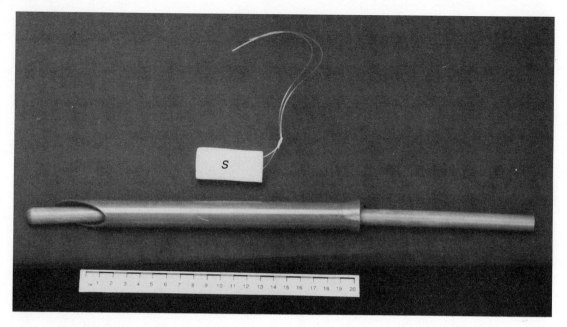

Fig. 1.40 Progestogen-impregnated intravaginal sponge or tampon (s) with speculum and introducer.

Table 1.1. Dose of eCG (IU) required to induce 'out-of-season' oestrus in ewes following withdrawal of progestogen sponges

Month	Dorset Horn, Finn/Dorset	Suffolk, Suffolk cross	Scottish half breeds, Mules, Greyfaces
July	600–500	750–600	Poor results
August	400–300	500–400	750–600
September	0	300–0	500–300
October	0	0	0

From Henderson (1985)

Use in Goats. The same type of sponges used in sheep are quite successful for synchronization of oestrus and, in conjunction with eCG, for the initiation of oestrus during the normal period of anoestrus. Some manufacturers produce a specific sponge for use in goats with a higher dose rate of progestogen. Goats object to the insertion of the sponges, particularly the applicator, much more than ewes, and in maiden goats it is preferable to insert a lubricated sponge with the use of a finger only (Henderson, 1985). Goats show intense oestrus 36–48 hours after sponge removal.

When eCG is used to stimulate oestrus, dose rates of 600–500 IU should be used in July, 500–400 IU in August, and 300–0 IU in September; from October onwards eCG is not required (Henderson, 1985).

Uses in Sows and Gilts. A number of different progestogens have been tried unsuccessfully to synchronize oestrus in sows and gilts. Altrenogest/allyltrenbolone is now sold in many countries for this purpose. This progestogen effectively suppresses follicular maturation when fed daily at a dose rate of 15–20 mg, with no apparent effect upon the life span of the corpora lutea. When fed at lower dose rates, i.e. 2.5–5 mg daily, follicular growth was not inhibited and cystic follicles developed by 10 days after the start of treatment (Martinat-Botte et al., 1985). Similar problems have been encountered with other progestogens.

Allyltrenbolone or altrenogest is sold as an oily solution within a pressurized container and calibrated so that a single 5 ml volume (0.4 w/v) contains the required dose. In an extensive trial involving 1223 gilts of various breeds, Martinat-Botte et al. (1985) found that after feeding the compound for 18 days there was good synchronization of oestrus 5–7 days after withdrawal. There were breed differences in the degree of synchronization. In cross-bred gilts good farrowing rates (average 64–73%) were obtained following fixed-time artificial insemination on days 6 and 7 after withdrawal of the progestogen; litter sizes ranged on average from 9.5 to 9.8. When pure-bred and cross-bred gilts were inseminated at observed oestrus the overall farrowing rates were improved.

A similar study, involving 2215 gilts and sows, was undertaken to see if synchronization after weaning could be improved following feeding of altrenogest/allyltrenbolone. It was found that there was some improvement following short-term feeding at a dose of 20 mg from 3 days before the weaning date. It was improved by boar proximity.

Much of the interest in developing suitable progestational compounds was inhibited when a non-progestational, pituitary-inhibiting substance was developed. This substance, Methallibure, was effective in regulating cyclic activity, and sows and gilts which had been on treatment had good fertility. Unfortunately, it was withdrawn for safety reasons because if fed to pregnant animals it had a severe teratogenic effect on the developing fetuses.

Uses in Bitches and Queen Cats. A number of different progestogens, such as megoestrol acetate, proligestone and medroxyprogesterone acetate, have been used to suppress oestrus in the bitch; these are available for oral administration as tablets or by injection. They can be used to postpone the onset of oestrus when administered during anoestrus or to prevent oestrus from occurring at the first signs of pro-oestrus. The latter is not too difficult to achieve in the bitch. Postponement can be maintained for over a year by injections of progestogens at intervals of 3–5 months or, after a 40-day course of daily oral administration, by tablets twice per week. Prevention of oestrus can be achieved by a singe injection of the progestogen or by the administration of oral progestogen at a higher dose rate than for postponement, but for a shorter duration.

Unfortunately, following the administration of progestogens, the time interval before the onset of the next oestrus is rather unpredictable if treatment is not continued. Furthermore, there is good evidence that continued and frequent use of such preparations can predispose to reproductive disorders, particularly cystic glandular hyperplasia of the endometrium (see p. 527). Because of this problem owners should be warned of the possible dangers, particularly if they wish to use the bitch subsequently for breeding.

In the cat, suppression of oestrus may be desirable for a number of reasons, but, particularly, for planning of litters throughout the year and to allow the queen a period of rest from sexual activity after a litter and to enable her to regain condition before being bred again. If a queen is allowed to call repeatedly without mating this may lead to considerable loss of condition due to relative inappetance during oestrus, particularly in Oriental breeds, which have short interoestrual intervals and long periods of oestrus. In addition, breeders report that difficulties are sometimes encountered in breeding from queens that have been allowed to call incessantly and have been unmated for long periods.

The most widely used method of oestrous suppression is by administration of progestogens. Injectable depot forms are available of proligesterone and medroxyprogesterone acetate which will suppress oestrus for up to 7 months or more following a single injection and can be repeated every 5 months to achieve permanent oestroussuppression. Loss of pigmentation in the area overlying injection sites is occasionally encountered. Oral progestogens have the advantage of greater flexibility, and the most commonly used of these is megoestrol acetate. This can be used to prevent an individual oestrous period by administering 5 mg as soon as signs of oestrus are observed. However, this approach is less suitable in cats than in dogs in view of the very rapid and sudden onset of oestrous behaviour. Postponement is achieved by administering 2.5 mg daily or weekly dependent on whether treatment is begun during the breeding season or anoestrus, although, in some queens, lower dosages may prove effective.

Many queens treated with progestogens will show behavioural changes, most commonly lethargy and weight gain (Øen, 1977). A proportion of treated queens may also develop endometritis. A more serious side-effect which has occasionally been reported, and may not be reversible in some cats, is the development of diabetes mellitus (Moise and Reimers, 1983).

Prostaglandins

Since the length of the interoestrus interval in most domesticated species is controlled by the duration of the lifespan of the corpus luteum, premature lysis, induced by the administration of $PGF_{2\alpha}$ or its analogues, can be used to manipulate the normal pattern of cyclic activity.

The corpora lutea of the cow, mare, sow, ewe and goat normally respond to the administration of exogenous prostaglandins; but in the bitch and the queen the corpora lutea are generally unresponsive

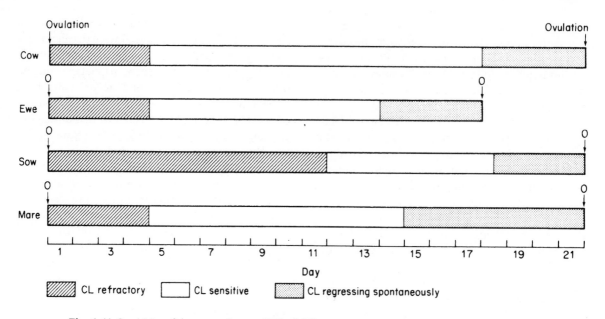

Fig. 1.41 Sensitivity of the corpus luteum (CL) of different species to $PGF_{2\alpha}$ during the oestrous cycle.

unless subjected to repeated doses. It is important to examine, in the first five species mentioned, when the corpora lutea are responsive or are refractory; this is summarized in Figure 1.41. In the cow, mare, ewe and goat the pattern is fairly similar, the new developing corpus luteum being refractory for 3–5 days after ovulation. At the other end of the oestrous cycle the corpus luteum is unaffected by exogenous prostaglandin, since it is already regressing under the influence of its own endogenous luteolysin; there is no evidence that this can be accelerated. Therefore in the cycles of the cow, goat, mare and ewe the corpus luteum is responsive for 13, 13, 10 and 9 days, respectively. The sow, however, is different since the corpus luteum is refractory for up to 11 days after ovulation, and thus is responsive for a much shorter period of only 7 or 8 days.

Since prostaglandins are abortifacients, they must not be used in animals that might be pregnant. If there is any doubt, pregnancy diagnosis must be performed.

Uses in the Cow. Prostaglandins have been used successfully to synchronize oestrus in groups of cows and heifers. This technique has applications in beef cows and heifers, and in dairy heifers where oestrous detection is frequently difficult, thus enabling the routine use of artificial insemination at a predetermined time. The availability of artificial insemination in such situations allows the

use of semen from genetically superior sires and thus can result in the improved genetic potential of the offspring.

It has been found that if two injections of $PGF_{2\alpha}$ or one of its synthetic analogues, e.g. cloprostenol, are given at an interval of 11 days to a group of cows or heifers at randomly different stages of the oestrous cycle, then 3–5 days after the second injection all the animals treated will come into oestrus and ovulate at about the same time. It has also been shown that if they are inseminated twice at a fixed time of 72 and 96 hours or 72 and 90 hours after the second injection, conception rates are comparable with those following artificial insemination or natural service at a spontaneous oestrus. A single fixed-time injection results in a reduction in conception rates. Figure 1.42 shows how three cows at different stages of the oestrous cycle can have their heats synchronized with the double-injection technique. Those animals which have a sensitive corpus luteum at the time of the first injection, as in cow B, will have an induced oestrus 3–5 days later, and if this is observed it is possible to save an additional injection of $PGF_{2\alpha}$ by inseminating them at this stage.

The efficiency of synchronization following the double-injection regimen is usually much better in heifers than in cows. It is not known precisely why this should be so, but one possible explanation is that frequently in cows (as opposed to heifers) the

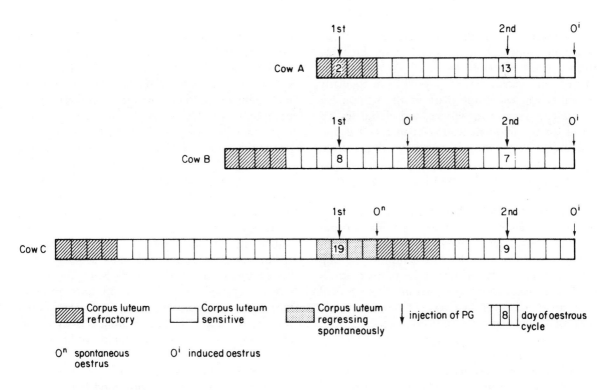

Fig. 1.42 Synchronization of oestrus in cows by the administration of two injections of $PGF_{2\alpha}$ or an analogue at an 11 day interval.

progesterone concentrations remain low for a much longer period of time after ovulation than normal (see Figure 1.28). This phenomenon, referred to as long-low progesterone, has been recorded as occurring in up to 15% of cows in some herds. Presumably the delay in the corpus luteum reaching a sensitive stage interferes with the synchronization scheme outlined in Figure 1.42.

Largely to reduce cost and to improve the pregnancy rates, a compromise regimen has been used. All animals are injected with $PGF_{2\alpha}$ on the same day and observed for oestrus during the following 5 days. Any identified in oestrus are inseminated as normal, and those not identified receive a second injection of prostaglandin followed by fixed-time artificial insemination. Any individuals exhibiting oestrus a few days after fixed-time artificial insemination should be reinseminated.

There is some suggestion that pregnancy rates are improved after a prostaglandin-induced oestrus where cows are inseminated in relation to an observed oestrus. In a review of 17 trials using cloprostenol, McIntosh et al. (1984) found that there was evidence of improved pregnancy rates in 13 of the trials. There is no physiological explanation for this response, but the authors suggest

that it might be a management phenomenon: oestrus can be anticipated over a restricted period of time and there is the opportunity for interaction between several animals in oestrus which may improve the timing of artificial insemination.

Two points are worthy of further consideration. First, it is important to liaise with the local artificial insemination organization before starting the regimen since they will be able to ensure the availability of inseminations when they are required. Second, particularly in heifers, it is important to ensure that they are receiving adequate nutrition since disappointing conception rates have been obtained when feeding has been inadequate. The use of prostaglandins to overcome oestrous detection problems and to treat pathological conditions will be described later (see Chapter 22).

Uses in the Mare. There are a few practical indications for synchronizing groups of mares or fillies. When it is used, the onset of oestrus is generally well synchronized 3 days after treatment, although the subsequent ovulation has a time spread of 7–12 days (Allen, 1978). Some improvement has been achieved by the injection of hCG or GnRH on the second or third day of the induced oestrus (Allen and Rowson, 1973).

Prostaglandins, both $PGF_{2\alpha}$ and the synthetic analogue cloprostenol, are useful in the breeding management of mares. By enabling mares to be mated on predetermined days it is particularly useful where either the mare or the stallion has to travel a distance for service, and eliminates the need for the frequent teasing of mares. It is also useful if a heat is missed, especially the foal heat, since it enables oestrus to be induced prematurely and obviates the need to wait for the next spontaneous heat.

Uses in the Ewe. When $PGF_{2\alpha}$ or an analogue is given to ewes with a sensitive corpus luteum, oestrus occurs 36–46 hours after injection (Haresign, 1979). In order to synchronize a group of ewes at randomly different stages of the oestrous cycle it is necessary to give two injections 8 or 9 days apart. Conception rates and prolificacy following natural matings have been comparable with unsynchronized ewes (Haresign, 1979). There are obvious advantages of using such a technique in conjunction with artificial insemination since it could enable the use of genetically superior sires in many flocks.

Uses in the Sow. Reliable synchronization of oestrus in groups of sows and gilts would have many applications, particularly in conjunction with the use of artificial insemination and to enable batch farrowing to occur. Unfortunately, prostaglandins and their analogues are not luteolytic until the 11th or 12th day of the oestrous cycle; thus, it is not possible to devise a regimen of injections which will synchronize groups of animals with randomly distributed cyclic activity.

However, it is possible to prolong the lifespan of the corpora lutea in the pig with injection of oestrogens on days 10–14 of the oestrous cycle; having done this, prostaglandins can be injected after 5–20 days to induce oestrus 4–6 days later (Guthrie and Polge, 1976). Another approach that has been used is to induce luteolysis, by prostaglandin administration, of accessory corpora lutea produced by the injection of eCG and hCG at any stage of the oestrous cycle (Caldwell et al., 1969).

Uses in the Dog and Cat. Prostaglandins do not readily cause luteolysis in these species.

Melatonin

The pineal gland controls reproductive activity in seasonal breeding species such as sheep, goats, horses and cats by the secretion of melatonin as the daylight hours are reduced (see p. 6). Perhaps not surprisingly, it has not been used successfully to modify seasonal activity in the mare because it would be necessary to inhibit the secretion of melatonin or neutralize its effect to advance the time of onset. However, in the ewe and doe, which are long-day breeders, it has been developed and exploited successfully commercially to advance the timing of the onset of the breeding season. The hormone is administered as an implant containing 18 mg of melatonin which is inserted subcutaneously at the base of the ear.

It is critical that rams (and bucks) should be sufficiently separated from the ewes so that they are out of sight, sound and smell at least 7 days before the insertion of the implant. They must remain separated for at least 30 days and not more than 40 days, when rams (or bucks) should then be reintroduced. Peak mating activity occurs 25–35 days later. Melatonin should not be used in ewe lambs.

The breeding season can be successfully advanced by 2–3 months with good fertility.

Immunization procedures

Increased lambing rates have been obtained by the use of an immunogen, produced by conjugating a derivative of the natural ovarian hormone androstenedione with human serum albumen. When injected into ewes the conjugate stimulates the production of antibodies to androstenedione, which binds free, naturally occurring androstenedione in the blood. This results in an increase in the ovulation rate and the number of lambs born; the precise mode of action is not fully understood (Scaramuzzi et al., 1983; Harding et al., 1984).

The conjugant is injected twice, 8 weeks before tupping and 4 weeks before tupping, although if ewes have been treated in the previous season one injection only is required (4 weeks before tupping). The effect of immunization is to increase the lambing percentage by about 25%.

It is important that only those ewes which are likely to be fed adequately during pregnancy should be treated because of the dangers of pregnancy toxaemia; for this reason, mountain and hill breeds should not be treated.

Immunization against inhibin, which has been used experimentally to increase the ovulation rate in cattle and sheep, may well become available for commercial use.

REFERENCES

Abrams, R. M., Thatcher, W. W., Chenault, J. F. and Wilcox, C. J. (1975) *J. Dairy Sci.*, **58**, 1528.

Aherne, F. X. and Kirkwood, R. N. (1985) *J. Reprod. Fertil. Suppl.*, **33**, 169.

Allen, W. E. (1974) *Equine Vet. J.*, **6**, 25.

Allen, W. E. and Alexiev, M. (1979) *Equine Vet. J.*, **12**, 27.

Allen, W. R. (1978) In: *Control of Ovulation*, ed. D. B. Crighton *et al.*, p. 453, London: Butterworth.

Allen, W. R. and Rowson, L. E. A. (1973) *J. Reprod. Fert.*, **33**, 539.

Anderson, L. L., Dyck, C. W., Mori, H., Hendricks, D. M. and Melampy, R. M. (1967) *Amer. J. Physiol.*, **212**, 1188.

Arbeiter, K. and Winding, W. (1977) *Kleintier Praxis*, **22**, 271.

Arendt, J., Symons, A. M., Laud, C. A. and Pryde, S. J. (1983) *J. Endocrinol.*, **97**, 395.

Arthur, G. H. (1958) *Vet. Rec.*, **70**, 682.

Baird, D. T. and Land, R. B. (1973) *J. Reprod. Fertil.*, **33**, 393.

Baird, D. T., Campbell, B. K., Mann, G. E. and McNeilly, A. S. (1991) *J. Reprod. Fertil. Suppl.*, **43**, 125.

Ball, C. (1977) Personal communication.

Bane, A. and Rajakoski, E. (1961) *Cornell Vet.*, **51**, 77.

Barr, H. L. (1975) *J. Dairy Sci.*, **58**, 246.

Bhanot, R. and Wilkinson, M. (1983) *Endocrinology*, **113**, 596.

Bittman, E. L., Dempsey, R. J. and Karsch, F. J. (1983) *Endocrinology*, **113**, 2275.

Bland, K. P., Horton, E. W. and Poyser, N. L. (1971) *Life Sci.*, **10**, 509.

Bobbett, R. E., Koelle, A. R., Landt, J. A. and Depp, S. W. (1977) *Progress Report LA 6812 PR*. Los Alamos Scientific Laboratory, University of California.

Boyd, J. S. and Omram, S. N. (1991) *In Practice*, 109.

Brinkley, H. J., Willfinger, W. W. and Young, E. O. (1973) *J. Anim. Sci.*, **37**, 333.

Brooks, A. N., Lamming, G. E., Lees, P. D. and Hayes, N. B. (1986) *J. Reprod. Fertil.*, **76**, 693.

Burger, J. F. (1952) *Onderstepoort J. Vet. Sci. Anim. Indust.*, **6**, 465.

Burkhardt, J. (1948) *Vet. Rec.*, **60**, 243.

Caldwell, A. K., Moor, R. M., Wilmut, I., Polge, C. and Rowson, L. E. A. (1969) *J. Reprod. Fertil.*, **18**, 107.

Christian, R. E. and Casida, L. E. (1948) *J. Anim. Sci.*, **7**, 540.

Christie, D. W. and Bell, E. T. (1971) *J. Small Anim. Pract.*, **12**, 159.

Claus, R. and Weiler, U. (1985) *J. Reprod. Fertil. Suppl.*, **33**, 185.

Cole, H. H. (1930) *Amer. J. Anat.*, **48**, 261.

Concannon, P. W., Hansel, W. and Visek, W. J. (1975) *Biol. Reprod.*, **13**, 112.

Concannon, P. W., Hansel, W. and McEntee, K. (1977) *Biol. Reprod.*, **17**, 604.

Concannon, P. W., Hodgson, B. and Lein, D. (1980) *Biol. Reprod.*, **23**, 111.

Cooper, M. J. (1978) In: *Control of Ovulation*, ed. D. B. Crighton, p. 412. London: Butterworth.

Coudert, S. P., Phillips, G. D., Faimin, C., Chernecki, W. and Palmer, M. (1974) *J. Reprod. Fertil.*, **36**, 319.

Cumming, I. A., McPhee, S. R., Chamley, W. A., Folman, Y. and Davis, I. F. (1982) *Aust. Vet. J.*, **59**, 14.

Dailey, R. A., Clark, J. R., First, N. L., Chapman, A. B. and Casida, L. E. (1972) *J. Anim. Sci.*, **35**, 1210.

Day, F. T. (1939) *Vet. Rec.*, **51**, 581.

Denamur, R., Martinet, J. and Short, R. V. (1966) *Acta Endocrinol., Copenh.*, **52**, 72.

Dobson, H. (1978) *J. Reprod. Fertil.*, **52**, 51.

Drew, S. B., Wishart, D. F. and Young, I. M. (1979) *Vet. Rec.*, **104**, 523.

Dzuik, P. J. (1977) In: *Reproduction in Domestic Animals*, 3rd edn, ed. H. H. Cole and P. T. Cupps, p. 456. London: Academic Press.

Ellendorff, F. (1978) In: *Control of Ovulation*, ed. D. B. Crighton, p. 7. London: Butterworth.

England, G. C. W. and Allen, W. E. (1989) *J. Reprod. Fertil. Suppl.*, **39**, 91.

Esslemont, R. J. and Bryant, M. J. (1974) *ADAS Q. Rev.*, **12**, 175.

Esslemont, R. J. and Bryant, M. J. (1976) *Vet. Rec.*, **99**, 47.

Evans, M. J. and Irvine, G. H. G. (1975) *J. Reprod. Fertil. Suppl.*, **23**, 193.

Flint, A. P. F., Stewart, H. J., Lamming, G. E. and Payne, J. H. (1992) *J. Reprod. Fertil. Suppl.*, **45**, 53.

Folman, Y., McPhee, S. R., Cummings, I. A., Davis, I. F. and Chamley, W. A. (1983) *Aust. Vet. J.*, **60**, 44.

Foote, R. H. (1975) *J. Dairy Sci.*, **58**, 248.

Foxcroft, G. R. and Hunter, M. G. (1985) *J. Reprod. Fertil. Suppl.*, **33**, 3.

Geiger, R., Konig, W., Wissman, H., Geisan, K. and Enzmann, F. (1971) *Biochem. Biophys. Res. Comm.*, **45**, 767.

Ginther, O. J. (1974) *J. Anim. Sci.*, **39**, 550.

Ginther, O. J. (1986) *Ultrasonic Imaging and Reproductive Events in the Mare*, pp. 142–145, 158–163. Cross Plains: Equiservices.

Ginther, O. J. and First, N. L. (1971) *Amer. J. Vet. Res.*, **32**, 1687.

Glencross, R. G., Munro, I. B., Senior, B. E. and Pope, G. S. (1973) *Acta Endocrinol.*, **3**, 374.

Grant, R. (1934) *Trans. R. Soc. Edinb.*, **58**, 1.

Griffiths, W. F. B. and Amoroso, E. C. (1939) *Vet. Rec.*, **51**, 1279.

Grubaugh, W., Sharp, D. C., Berglund, L. A., McDowell, K., Kilmer, D. M., Peck, L. and Seamans, K. W. (1982) *J. Reprod. Fertil. Suppl.*, **32**, 293.

Gruffydd-Jones, T. (1982) Ph.D. Thesis, University of Bristol.

Guthrie, H. D. and Polge, C. (1976) *J. Reprod. Fertil.*, **48**, 423.

Hammond, J. (1927) *Physiology of Reproduction in the Cow*. Cambridge: Cambridge University Press.

Hammond, J. (1938) *York Agric. Soc. J.*, **95**, 11.

Hancock, J. L. and Rowlands, I. W. (1949) *Vet. Rec.*, **61**, 771.

Harding, R. B., Hardy, P. R. D. and Joby, R. (1984) *Vet. Rec.*, **115**, 601.

Haresign, W. and Acritopolou, S. A. (1978) *Livestock Production Science*, **5**, 313.

Heape, W. (1900) *Q. J. Microsc. Soc.*, **44**, 1.

Henderson, D. (1985) *In Practice*, **7**, 118–123.

Horrell, R. I., Kilgour, R., Macmillan, K. L. and Bremner, K. (1984) *Vet. Rec.*, **114**, 36.

Horton, E. W. and Poyser, N. L. (1976) *Physiol. Rev.*, **56**, 595.

Hurnick, J. F., King, C. J. and Robertson, H. A. (1975) *Appl. Anim. Ethol.*, **2**, 55.

Ireland, J. J. and Roche, J. F. (1983) *Endocrinology*, **112**, 150.

Jeffcoate, I. A. and Lindsay, F. E. F. (1989) *J. Reprod. Fertil. Suppl.*, **39**, 277.

Jemmett, J. E. and Evans, J. M. (1977) *J. Small Anim. Pract.*, **18**, 21.

Jöchle, W. and Andersen, A. C. (1977) *Theriogenology*, **7**, 113.

Johnson, L. M. and Gay, V. L. (1981) *Endocrinology*, **109**, 240.

Kahn, G., Carpentier, M. C., Meusnier, C., Schirar, A. and Martiner, J. (1975) *J. Res. Ovine. Caprine Fr.*, 272.

Karsch, F. J. (1984) *The Hormonal Control of Reproduction*, pp. 10–19, Cambridge: Cambridge University Press.

Karsch, F. J., Legan, S. J., Ryan, D. and Fostre, D. L. (1978) In: *Control of Ovulation*, ed. D. B. Crighton, p. 29. London: Butterworth.

Kennaway, D. J., Dunstan, E. A., Gilmore, T. A. and Seamark, R. F. (1983) *Anim. Reprod. Sci.*, **5**, 587.

Kenney, R. M., Gamjam, V. K. and Bergman, S. J. (1975) *Vet. Scope*, **19**.

Kiddy, C. A. (1977) *J. Dairy Sci.*, **60**, 235.

Kilmer, D. M., Sharp, D. C., Berglund, L. A., Grubaugh, W., McDowell, K. J. and Peck, L. (1982) *J. Reprod. Fertil. Suppl.*, **32**, 303.

Kordon, C. (1978) In: *Control of Ovulation*, ed. D. B. Crighton, p. 21. London: Butterworth.

Lamming, G. E. and Bulman, D. C. (1976) *Brit. Vet. J.*, **132**, 507.

Lamming, G. E., Foster, J. P. and Bulman, D. C. (1979) *Vet. Rec.*, **104**, 156.

Lasley, J. F. (1968) In: *Reproduction in Farm Animals*, ed. E. S. E. Hafez, p. 81. Philadephia: Lea and Febiger.

Lawler, D. F., Johnston, S. D., Hegstad, R. L., Keltner, D. G. and Owens, S. F. (1993) *J. Reprod. Fertil. Suppl.*, **47**, 57.

Lees, J. L. (1969) *Outlook Agric.*, **6**, 82.

Lees, J. L. and Weatherhead, M. (1970) *Anim. Prod.*, **12**, 173.

Leyva, H., Addiego, L. and Stabenfeldt, G. (1985) *Endocrinology*, **115**, 1729.

Leyva, H., Madley, T. and Stabenfeldt, G. H. (1989) *J. Reprod. Fertil. Suppl.*, **39**, 125.

Lewis, G. S. and Newman, S. K. (1984) *J. Dairy Sci.*, **67**, 146.

Lincoln, G. A. (1985) In: *Hormonal Control of Reproduction*, ed. C. R. Austin and R. V. Short, pp. 52–75. Cambridge: Cambridge University Press.

Loeb, L. (1923) *Proc. Soc. Exp. Biol. Med.*, **20**, 441.

Maatje, R. (1976) *Livestock Prod. Sci.*, **3**, 85.

McIntosh, D. A. D., Lewis, J. A. and Hammond, D. (1984) *Vet. Rec.*, **115**, 129.

Matsuo, H., Baba, Y., Nair, R. M. G. and Schally, A. V. (1971) *Biochem. Biophys. Res. Comm.*, **43**, 1334.

Matton, P., Adelakoun, V., Couture, Y. and Dufour, J. J. (1983) *J. Anim. Sci.*, **52**, 813.

du Mesnil du Buisson, F. (1961) *Ann. Biol. Anim. Biochem. Biophys.*, **1**, 105.

Moise, N. S. and Reimers, T. J. (1983) *J. Amer. Vet. Med. Assn*, **182**, 158.

Morrow, D. A., Roberts, S. J. and McEntee, K. (1969) *Cornell Vet.*, **59**, 134.

Øen, E. O. (1977) *Nord. Vet. Med.*, **29**, 287.

Paape, S. R., Schille, V. M., Seto, H. and Stabenfeldt, G. H. (1975) *Biol. Reprod.*, **13**, 470.

Peters, A. R. (1984) *Vet. Rec.*, **115**, 164.

Peters, A. R. (1985a) *Brit. Vet. J.*, **141**, 564.

Peters, A. R. (1985b) *Vet. Rec.*, **115**, 164.

Phemister, R. D., Holst, P. A., Spano, J. S. and Hopwood, M. L. (1973) *Biol. Reprod.*, **8**, 74.

Pierson, R. A. and Ginther, O. J. (1984) *Theriogenology*, **21**, 495.

Pierson, R. A. and Ginther, O. J. (1988) *Anim. Reprod. Sci.*, **16**, 81.

Roche, J. F. and Ireland, J. J. (1981) *J. Anim. Sci.*, **52**, 580.

Rose, J. D. (1978) *Exp. Neurol.*, **61**, 231.

Roux, L. L. (1936) *Onderstepoort J. Vet. Sci. Anim. Indust.*, **6**, 465.

Rowson, L. E. A. and Moor, R. M. (1967) *J. Reprod. Fertil.*, **13**, 511.

Rozel, J. F. (1975) *Vet. Scope*, **19**, 3.

Sato, E., Ishibashi, T. and Iritani, A. (1982) *J. Anim. Sci.*, **55**, 873.

Savio, J. D., Boland, M. P. and Roche, J. F. (1990) *J. Reprod. Fertil.*, **88**, 581.

Scaramuzzi, R. J., Geldard, H., Beels, C. M., Hoskinson, R. M. and Cox, R. I. (1983) *Wool Technol. Sheep Breeding*, **31**, 87.

Schutte, A. P. (1967) *J. Small Anim. Pract.*, **8**, 301.

Schilling, E. and Zust, J. (1968) *J. Reprod. Fertil.*, **15**, 307.

Scott, P. P. (1970) In: *Reproduction and Breeding Techniques for Laboratory Animals*, ed. E. S. E. Hafez, p. 192. Philadelphia: Lea and Febiger.

Shille, V. M. and Stabenfeldt, G. H. (1979) *Biol. Reprod.*, **21**, 1217.

Shille, V. M., Lundström, K. and Stabenfeldt, G. H. (1979) *Biol. Reprod.*, **21**, 953.

Signoret, J. P. (1971) *Vet. Rec.*, **88**, 34.

Sirois, J. and Fortune, J. E. (1988) *Biol. Reprod.*, **39**, 308.

Smith, L. E. and Vincent, C. K. (1973) *J. Anim. Sci.*, **36**, 216.

Sokolowski, J. H., Stover, D. G. and Van Ravenswaay, F. (1977) *J. Amer. Vet. Med. Assn*, **171**, 271.

Tsutsui, T. and Shimizu, T. (1975) *Jpn. J. Anim. Reprod.*, **21**, 65.

Tsutsui, T. and Stabenfeldt, G. H. (1993) *J. Reprod. Fertil. Suppl.*, **47**, 29.

Van de Wiel, D. F. H., Erkens, J., Koops, W., Vos, E. and Van Lendegheim, A. A. J. (1981) *Biol. Reprod.*, **24**, 223.

Van Niekerk, C. H. (1973) Cited by Allen (1978).

Van Niekerk, C. H. and Gernaeke, W. H. (1966) *Onderstepoort J. Vet. Res.*, **25**(Suppl. 2).

Webb, R., Gong, J. G., Law, A. S. and Rusbridge, S. M. (1992) *J. Reprod. Fertil. Suppl.*, **45**, 141.

Webel, S. K. (1975) *J. Anim. Sci.*, **44**, 385.

Webel, S. K. (1978) In: *Control of Ovulation*, ed. D. B. Crighton, p. 421. London: Butterworth.

Wildt, D. E., Chakraborty, P. K., Banks, W. B. and Seager, S. W. J. (1977) *Proc. Xth Ann. Meet. Soc. Study Reprod.*, Abstr. 110.

Wildt, D. E., Seager, S. W. J. and Chakraborty, P. K. (1980) *Endocrinology*, **107**, 1212.

Williamson, N. B., Morris, R. S., Blood, D. C. and Cannon, C. M. (1972) *Vet. Rec.*, **91**, 50.

Wishart, D. F. (1972) *Vet. Rec.*, **90**, 595.

Wishart, D. F. and Young, I. M. (1974) *Vet. Rec.*, **95**, 503.

Wood, P. D. P. (1976) *Anim. Prod.*, **22**, 275.

Wray, S. and Hoffman-Small, G. E. (1984) *J. Steroid. Biochem.*, **20**, 1420.

2

Part Two

Pregnancy and Parturition

The Development of the Conceptus

As the ripe follicle is about to rupture, the fimbriated end of the uterine tube is applied to it and, at ovulation, the follicular fluid and egg are discharged into the oviduct. If the female had been mated at the current oestrus, spermatozoa will be waiting in the ampulla of the uterine tube for the arrival of the oocyte. Although the nucleus of only one sperm is required to fuse with that of the ovum, it has been estimated that approximately a million sperms are necessary to create a suitable environment for fertilization. Following fertilization, cleavage of the zygote begins and, as a result of peristaltic contractions and ciliary currents in the uterine tube, it is propelled towards the uterus. When it reaches the uterus, at 3–4 days in cattle and at 5–8 days in the dog and cat, the zygote consists of 16–32 cells in the form of a morula. With further cell division and cell orientation the morula becomes hollowed out to form a blastocyst. Up to the time of shedding of the zona pellucida at the ninth day there is little absolute growth of the mammalian egg from its original dimension of 0.14 mm. The fertilized egg of the ewe reaches the uterus at the eight cell stage on day 3, while in the sow it passes down the uterine tube within 2 days of ovulation and arrives in the uterus at the four to eight cell stage. Tubal transport of the fertilized eggs of the mare probably takes 5–6 days, by which time they are at the blastocyst stage, but van Niekerk and Gernaeke (1966) have shown that unfertilized equine eggs remain in the tubes for several months, where they slowly degenerate. The variable duration of travel by the fertilized egg in the oviduct of the domestic species appears to be determined positively by the degrees of activity of the tubal muscle and cilia and negatively by the muscular constriction either at the tubal isthmus or at the uterotubal junction; both positive and negative factors are probably influenced by variable concentration of ovarian steroids and possibly by locally produced prostaglandins. From the time of its arrival in the uterus until attachment, the zygote is propelled or aspirated in the uterine lumen, where it is nourished by the uterine milk. In the polytocous species, the blastocysts are arranged throughout the uterus so as to utilize effectively the uterine space; thus there occurs free migration of embryos between the cornua, regardless of the side of ovulation. In the monotocous cow such migration hardly ever occurs, but in the ewe it is not uncommon.

After the ninth day the blastocyst elongates rapidly. For example, the sheep embryo is 1 cm long at 12 days, 3 cm at 13 days and 10 cm at 14 days, while by day 13 in the sow the apparent length of each blastocyst is about 33 cm, but its real length when disconnected from the much corrugated endometrium is 55–191 cm; by day 21 in the mare the blastocyst measures 7 × 6.5 cm, but in the cow it extends almost throughout the pregnant horn. Embryonic attachment to the uterus occurs at the following times: 12 days, cow; 14 days, sow; 15 days, ewe; 13–17 days, dog and cat; and 25–30 days, mare.

Interesting facts about the intrauterine mobility and location of the equine embryo have been obtained by means of ultrasonic echography by Leith and Ginther (1984). The location of the vesicle was observed in seven mares over a 2-hour period daily from days 9 to 17. There was increasing mobility from day 9 to day 12, when a plateau of high mobility persisted until day 14, after which there were few location changes on day 15 and none on days 16 and 17, indicating that fixation had occurred. On days 9 and 10 the vesicle was at least twice as likely to be in the uterine body as in a uterine horn; on days 11–14 this proportion was reversed, and beyond day 15 the embryo was always cornually disposed.

The bovine embryo itself, although differentiating fast, elongates slowly as compared with the chorion, and at a month after mating it is only just over 1 cm long. The chorionic vesicle, which is at first string-like with a central distended sphere of amnion containing the embryo, is progressively filled by allantoic fluid to form an extensive allantochorionic sac, which first begins to distend the gravid cornu at about 35 days in the cow (Figure 2.1). At this time the chorion already extends into the non-gravid horn; its length is about 40 cm and at its widest part in the dependent portion of the gravid horn it is 4–5 cm in diameter. The early development of the sheep is very similar to that of the cow, but the equine conceptus does not show the initial rapid elongation of the blastocyst-chorion. For example, at 35 days the equine chorion is oval rather than cylindrical and is more distended by the allantoic fluid. This causes an earlier, more discrete uterine enlargement than in the cow, and this is helpful in early clinical pregnancy diagnosis (Figure 2.2).

The allantois, which is an outgrowth of the embryonic hindgut, spreads out into the chorionic vesicle and, as a protruding sac, it makes contact outwardly with the chorion to form the vascular allantochorion, and inwardly it fuses with the amnion, to give rise to the allanto-amnion. The allantochorion, which eventually surrounds the allanto-amnion, is separated from it by allantoic fluid. When the vascularization of the chorion by the allantois is complete (at 40–60 days in the cow) the allantochorion is ready to participate in pla-

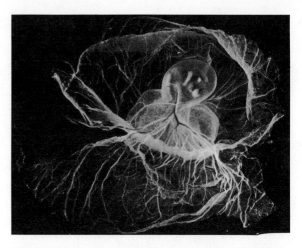

Fig. 2.2 Equine conceptus at 7 weeks. The allantochorion has been opened to show the yolk sac and early fetus within the amnion.

cental function. (Figures 2.1 and 2.2). Prior to this time the embryo has been nourished through its chorion and amnion by diffusion from the uterine milk. In the ruminant uterus, where the allantochorion contacts the uterine caruncles, finger-like processes or villi, containing capillary tufts, grow out from the allantochorion into the crypts of the maternal caruncles, which also are surrounded by capillary plexuses. Thus is formed the characteristic ruminant cotyledon, or placentome, through which takes place nutrient and gaseous exchange between the mother and fetus. On an average there are some 120 functioning cotyledons in the cow (Figure 2.3) and about 80 in the sheep, arranged in four rows along each of the uterine horns. It will be recalled that the chorion, and following it the allantois, extends into the non-gravid horn, and thus it is normal in the ruminant for there to be numerous functioning cotyledons in the non-pregnant horn. The pregnant uterus of the mare, sow, bitch and cat show no cotyledons, for in these species the villi are dispersed over the placental area.

During early development of the ruminant embryo there occurs an extensive fusion between the allanto-amnion and the allantochorion, thus largely obliterating the cavity of the allantois. As a result, where it lies over the amnion, the allantois is reduced to a narrow channel. Here its shape resembles the letter 'T' with the stem coming out of the urachus, along the umbilical cord and then diverging as the two cross-pieces over the

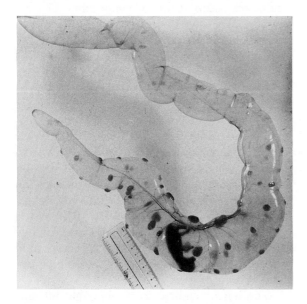

Fig. 2.1 Bovine conceptus at 60 days. Note the fetus contained within the discrete — almost spherical — amniotic sac, with an elongated allantochorion and evidence of the formation of cotyledons.

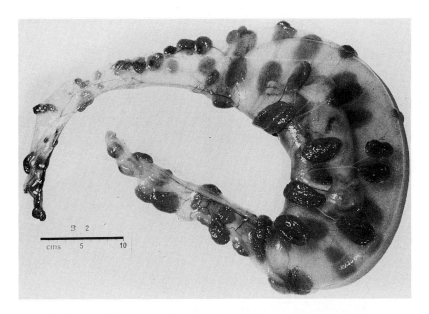

Fig. 2.3 Bovine conceptus at 90 days. Note the relatively larger amniotic sac compared with Figure 2.1, and obvious cotyledons which are larger towards the centre of the allantochorion.

lateral face of the amnion. Consequently there is little allantoic fluid over the amniotic area; most of it lies in the extremities of the allantois, one of which lies in the non-gravid horn (Figures 2.3–2.5). A similar fusion takes place between the amnion and allantois of the pig. However, studies of bovine uteri in late gestation (Arthur, 1959) have shown that, with the increasing pressure of accumulating allantoic fluid, the allantochorion tends to become separated again from the allanto-amnion so that at term the allantois may almost surround the amnion. Thus the final

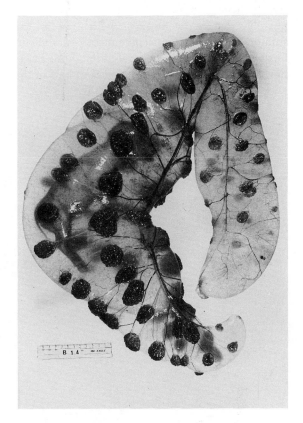

Fig. 2.5 Bovine conceptus at 115 days. Note the blood supply to and from the developing cotyledons.

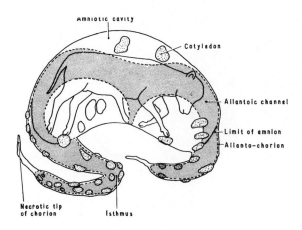

Fig. 2.4 Drawing of a bovine conceptus to show the allantochorion of early pregnancy. (After Zeitzschmann (1924).)

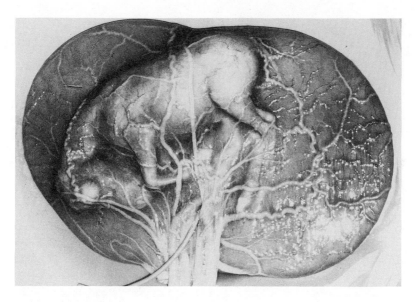

Fig. 2.6 Equine fetus of approximately 3 months of age. The allantochorion has been incised to expose the fetus enclosed within the almost transparent amnion. Note the umbilical cord at the bottom of the picture and the tortuous blood vessels on the surface of the amnion.

arrangement of the two fetal sacs may closely resemble that of the horse, in which species the amnion, except for its attachment at the umbilicus, floats freely in the allantoic fluid throughout gestation (Figures 2.6 and 2.7). The relationships of the

fetal sacs at birth will be referred to again in Chapter 6 on parturition.

In carnivora, as in the domestic herbivora, the allantois also grows out into the cylindrical chorion, but only the central part of it becomes vascu-

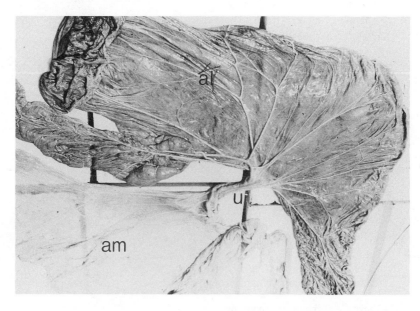

Fig. 2.7 Equine fetal membranes at term. Not the denser allantochorion (al), which is red in colour with its smooth inner surface exposed, the amnion (am), which at term is almost transparent, and the umbilicus (u).

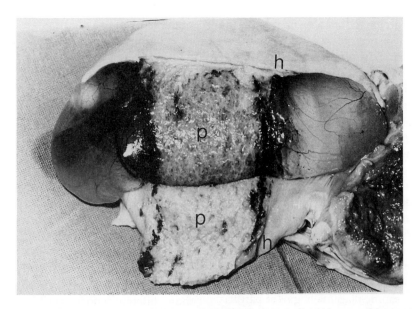

Fig. 2.8 Canine conceptus at approximately 8 weeks of gestation, partially contained within part of the uterine horn, showing marginal haematomata on the allantochorionic sac (h), and the areas of placentation (p).

larized and serves as a placenta. The amnion is surrounded by allantoic fluid, as in the horse (Figures 2.8 and 2.9). A 35-day Beagle embryo is 35mm in crown–rump length and it increases by 6 mm per day between the 35th and 40th days (Evans, 1983).

TYPES OF PLACENTA

Placentae may be classified according to the way the villi are distributed on the fetal chorion. Thus,

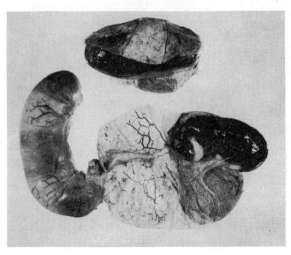

Fig. 2.9 Uterus from a pregnant cat near term dissected to show the placental areas and zonal placenta.

where they are uniformly dispersed, as in the mare and sow, the placenta is said to be *diffuse*. Where they are grouped into multiple circumscribed areas, as in the ruminant, the placental arrangement is called *cotyledonary*, while in the bitch and cat the villi are disposed in the form of a broad encircling belt forming a *zonary* placenta.

Formerly, the placentae were differentiated according to whether or not maternal tissue separated off with the fetal tissue at birth. Thus, of the domestic mammals, the placentae of the bitch and cat were said to be deciduate and those of the remainder non-deciduate.

More recently, embryologists have favoured Grosser's (1909) division of placental types in which the degree of proximity of the maternal and fetal blood circulations is the criterion of classification. Such a concept recognizes the phagocytic property of the trophoblast, or chorionic epithelium, that may be exerted on tissues with which it comes in contact. In the simplest, or *epitheliochorial*, type of placenta, seen in the horse and pig, the chorion is everywhere in contact with the endometrium, and there is no loss of maternal tissue. In the cow, the placenta is described as being *synepithelialchorial* (Wooding, 1992). Soon after embryonic attachment a syncytium is formed on the maternal side of the placentome by the fusion of binucleate cells derived from the trophectoderm and the endometrium. Unlike the sheep and goat the syncytium is only temporary, as fairly soon the syncytial plaques are overgrown by the rapid division of the remaining maternal epithelium (King et al., 1979). In the third, *endotheliochorial* type, there is further invasion of the endometrium by the trophoblast, which is now apposed to the maternal capillaries. Such a type is typical of the carnivora. In the *haemochorial* placenta of primates only the tissues of the chorionic villi separate the fetal and maternal blood. The placenta of the dog and cat is partly haemochorial in that the main zonary placenta of endotheliochorial type is flanked by marginal haematomata — 'the green border' in the dog and 'brown border' in the cat — in which an accumulation of maternal blood between the uterine epithelium and the chorion directly bathes the chorionic villi that project into it. When separation of the canine placenta begins at parturition it is the escape of this altered blood from the marginal haematoma which gives the characteristic green colour to the normal parturient discharges. A simple diagrammatic representation of the types of placenta based on Grosser's (1909) original classification is shown in Figure 2.10.

The degree of intimacy of the maternal and fetal placental blood vessels is the basis for the variable function of the 'placental barrier' of different species. This is of interest in certain diseases

of the fetus and newborn, for example the haemolytic disease of foals in which antigens from the fetus pass across the placenta to the mother but the resultant antibodies can return to the foal only via the colostrum, whereas in women similar antibodies may traverse the placenta and cause an antigen–antibody reaction in the unborn fetus.

FETAL FLUIDS

Sheep

The studies of Malan and Curson (1937) and Cloete (1939) have revealed that the total volume of fetal fluid increases with advancing age of the conceptus but that the separate fetal fluid volumes show different tendencies. Thus, during the first 3 months, apart from an initial preponderance, the allantoic fluid accumulates slowly, e.g. 131 ml at 3 months, whereas the increase in amniotic fluid occurs largely during this time and at 3 months reaches 604 ml. In the fourth month the increase in allantoic fluid is greatly accelerated to 485 ml, while the amniotic fluid increases only slightly. During the last (fifth) month of gestation the allantoic fluid almost doubles its volume to 834 ml but the volume of amniotic fluid dimini-

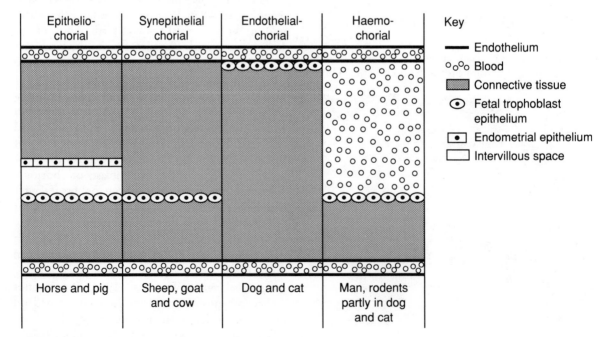

Fig. 2.10 Diagrammatic representation of types of placenta found in domestic species based on Grosser's original classification.

Table 2.1. Volume of fetal fluids in the sheep (ml)

Month of gestation	Amniotic	Allantoic	Total
1	3	38	41
2	169	89	258
3	604	131	735
4	686	485	1171
5	369	834	1203

Data from Malan and Curson (1937) and Cloete (1939).

shes to 369 ml (Table 2.1). When twins are present the totals of fluid are approximately doubled (Arthur, 1956).

Cattle

The total quantity of fetal fluid of cattle increases progressively throughout pregnancy; it averages about 5 litres at 5 months and 20 litres at term. Sharp rises in the total quantity occur between 40 and 65 days, between 3 and 4 months and again between $6\frac{1}{2}$ and $7\frac{1}{2}$ months. The first and last of these are due to allantoic and the second to amniotic increases. For nearly the whole of the first third of pregnancy when the conceptus consists of an elongated allantochorion with a central spheroidal amnion — closely investing the relatively small embryo — there is more allantoic fluid; during most of the second third of pregnancy amniotic fluid predominates but for the greater part of the final third allantoic fluid is again clearly in excess (Figure 2.11).

Throughout gestation the allantoic fluid is watery or urine-like. In the first two-thirds of pregnancy the amniotic fluid is similar but for the remainder of gestation it is a mucoid fluid. The latter change gives it the lubricant property which is so helpful at parturition. At birth the allantoic sac forms the first and the amnion the second 'water-bag'. The allantochorion is thicker and tougher than the transparent amnion.

Horses

Ranges of weights of the total fetal fluid for each month of pregnancy in the mare as given by Richter and Götze (1960) are shown in Table 2.2.

Serial values for the separate amounts of amniotic and allantoic fluids are not available, but the author's observations (Table 2.3), together with

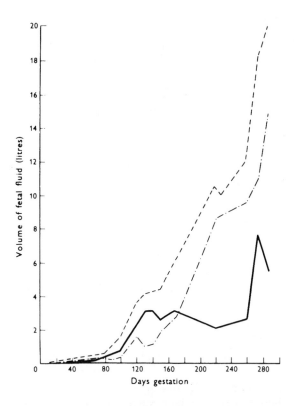

Fig. 2.11 Volume of fetal fluids at successive stages of pregnancy in the cow. – – – –, total; –·—·–, allantoic; ⸺, amniotic. (From Arthur (1969).)

Table 2.2. Weight of fetal fluids in the horse

Month of gestation	Weight of total fluid (kg)
1	0.03–0.04
2	0.3– 0.5
3	1.2– 3.0
4	3.0– 4.0
5	5.0– 8.0
6	6.0–10.0
7	6.0–10.0
8	6.0–12.0
9	8.0–12.0
10	10.0–20.0
11	10.0–20.0

data provided by Amoroso (1952) and Zietzschmann (1924), suggest that the trends are similar to those of cattle. Thus, allantoic fluid predominates in early as well as late pregnancy and measures 8–15 litres at term. The amniotic fluid volume differs from that of cattle: it is low during the first 3 months, for example only 27 ml at 74 days; thereafter it increases more rapidly and at midpregnancy

Table 2.3. Volume of fetal fluids in the horse

Estimated gestation (months)	Fetal body length (cm)	Amniotic (ml)	Allantoic (ml)
3	10	30[a]	2300
4½	20	100	4090
6	44	6200	4090
	77	3700	4800[b]
9	80	9200	—
	81.5	1670	5210

[a] Estimated volume in a preserved specimen.
[b] Some allantoic fluid lost in transit.

equals the volume of allantoic fluid, while at term it is 3–5 litres.

Pigs

The volume of allantoic fluid shows an early rise to about 130 ml at 1 month. Thereafter it increases gradually to nearly 200 ml, although a terminal decrease to 100 ml is sometimes seen. During the first 2 months the amount of amniotic fluid does not exceed 20 ml; in the next months it rises to a maximum which may vary from 75 to 200 ml; thereafter there is wide variation with a tendency to decline.

Carnivora

In kittens of fetal body length up to 9 cm the amniotic fluid rises gradually to 10–15 ml, after which there is some decrease followed by a slight rise just before term. The allantoic fluid starts with a more rapid rise, and at mid-term is higher than the amniotic (20 ml), but towards the end of gestation declines to about 6 ml.

FORM AND FEATURES OF THE FETAL SACS

Ruminants

Throughout the gestation the amnion enclosing the fetus, together with the larger portion of the allantochorion, remains in the uterine horn corresponding to the ovary with the corpus luteum; a smaller 'limb' of allantochorion projects across the uterine body into the other horn. Most of the allantoic fluid gravitates to the poles of the allantochorion, which lie in the dependent parts of the uterine horns, and the uterine distension thus

caused in cattle is the chief clinical sign of early pregnancy. By the third month, considerable fluid (up to 0.75 litres) has accumulated in the spherical amnion, and it now gives rise to the main palpable mass in the pregnant horn (see Figure 2.3).

On the inner face of the amnion of ruminants, particularly near the umbilicus, are numerous raised, rough, discrete, round foci called amniotic plaques. They are rich in glycogen but of unknown function and disappear after 6 months of gestation. Towards the end of pregnancy smooth, discoid, rubber-like masses float in the amniotic and occasionally in the allantoic fluids. They probably comprise aggregations of fetal hair and meconium around which salts are deposited from the fetal fluids. They are called 'hippomanes', and are of no functional significance.

Mare

Much of the allantochorion and the greater part of the amnion are contained within the gravid horn with a direct continuation of similar width into the uterine body. The part of the allantochorion which projects into the non-gravid horn is much narrower and is about two-thirds the length of the gravid horn segment, but in the rare bicornual pregnancy the allantochorion occupies both cornua to a similar extent.

Projecting into the allantoic fluid are peculiar invaginations of the allantochorion. They are first found at a fetal body length (FBL) of about 11 cm and occur in juxtaposition with the endometrial cups whose secretion accumulates in them. Their size corresponds with the secretory activity of the endometrial cups, being largest at FBL 15–20 cm, and regressing after FBL 30 cm. When distended with secretion they are appropriately called allantochorionic pouches. They are few in number, not more than six, and are sometimes absent. The endometrial cups are crateriform structures which are disposed in a concentric manner at the base of the pregnant horn. They are present from the sixth to the 20th weeks of gestation, and in them the equine chorionic gonadotrophin (eCG) is produced. The endometrial cups are formed from cells which invade the endometrium from the trophoblastic girdle of the embryo (Allen and Moor, 1972); this invasion provokes a reaction by the maternal tissue and leads to the dehiscence of the endometrial cups at about day 140.

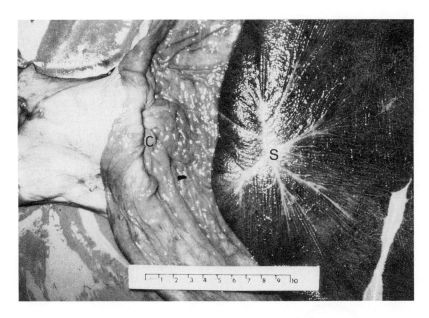

Fig. 2.12 Outer surface of the allantochorion showing the 'star' (s) which is adjacent to the internal opening of the cervix (c) and is devoid of placental villi.

The immunological importance of the endometrial cups in protecting the 'foreign' conceptus has been demonstrated by Allen (1982). In interspecies transfers of fertilized eggs between horses and donkeys no endometrial cups were formed, and the donkey fetuses died at 80–90 days.

The surface of the allantochorion adherent to the endometrium is red in colour and has a 'velvety' appearance and texture. The area adjacent to the internal opening of the cervix is devoid of placental villi, giving rise to the so-called 'star' (Figure 2.12). The inner surface of the allantochorion which is outermost when the placenta is shed has a smooth surface (see Figure 2.7).

Sow

The uterine surface of the sow's allantochorion is studded with small, round, grey foci called 'areolae' in which villi are absent. They occur opposite focal aggregations of uterine glands.

RELATIONSHIP BETWEEN FETAL MEMBRANES OF TWINS AND MULTIPLE FETUSES

The relationship of the membranes of contiguous fetuses is simplest in carnivora, in which, although the extremities of the allantochorionic sacs impinge on each other, they remain separate. The next gradation is in the mare pregnant with twins; here, apparently owing to the lack of uterine length, the distal pole of one allantochorion invaginates the proximal extremity of the other. According to Williams (1939) this results in an unequal sharing of the uterine space and is the reason for the commonly observed disparity of twin foals. Adjacent membranes of porcine fetuses tend to become 'glued' together by a gelatinous substance but the junction is not a strong one. In 66% of cases the adjacent chorions grow together and the intervening tissue breaks down with the formation of a common chorion, and occasionally with a common allantoic cavity. In the rare case of anastomosis of allantoic blood vessels of porcine fetuses of unlike sex, a basis for the 'freemartin' condition exists, as in cattle (see Chapter 4).

In the majority of twin or triplet pregnancies of sheep and cattle, contiguous chorionic sacs coalesce (Figures 2.13 and 2.14) and in many cases the allantoic cavities are confluent, while in cattle — but only in about 0.8% of sheep — allantoic vascular intercommunication is the rule. Such anastomosis, according to Lillie (1917), is present between bovine fetuses from the 40th day, and it forms the main premise of his theory of origin of the bovine freemartin (see Chapter 4).

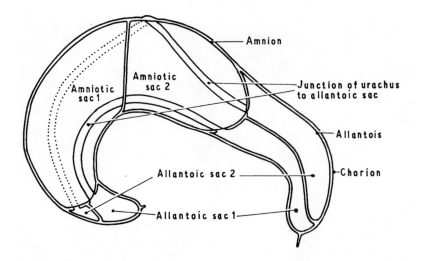

Fig. 2.13 Fetal membranes of bovine twins in unicornual gestation. (Courtesy of M. J. Edwards.)

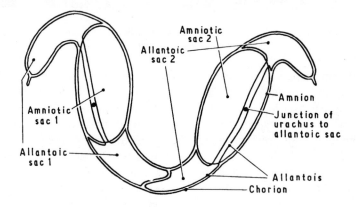

Fig. 2.14 Fetal membranes of bovine twins in bicornual gestation. (Courtesy of M. J. Edwards.)

Of 25 sets of equine twins, 11 were found by Vandeplassche et al. (1970) to have blood chimerism, thus indicating vascular anastomosis between the twin placentae. However, on dissection, the genital organs of the female members of four heterosexual chimerical pairs were found to be normal while five other mares of heterosexual chimerical pairs were found clinically to have normal genitalia, and they had normal oestrous cycles and became pregnant. The fact that blood chimerism has been found in adjacent fetuses of horse, sheep and pig — as well as cattle — gestations indicates that there is a basis for the freemartin condition in these species also. But the observed incidence of freemartinism is very low in pigs and sheep and is nil in horses, and this may be due, according to Vandeplassche et al. (1970), to late allantoic vascular anastomosis in these three species as compared with the early (30-day) fusion in cattle.

FETAL MOBILITY DURING PREGNANCY

While discussing placental relationships it is instructive to consider the subject of fetal mobility within the uterus. Obviously in all species, within the amnion, fetal movement around both longitudinal and transverse axes is possible. Rotation about the first is limited by the length of amniotic umbilical cord and about the second when the length of the fetus exceeds the width of the amnion. In cattle, not more than a three-fourths revolution around the long axis is possible and,

Table 2.4 Pregnant equine uteri: disposition of fetus

Months of gestation	No. of cases	Anterior presentation	Posterior presentation	Right horn pregnant	Left horn pregnant
2–$3\frac{1}{2}$	4	2	2	2	2
$3\frac{1}{2}$–$4\frac{1}{2}$	12	7	5	6	6
$4\frac{1}{2}$–$5\frac{1}{2}$	9	4	5	6	3
$5\frac{1}{2}$–$6\frac{1}{2}$	16	9	7	11	5
$6\frac{1}{2}$–$7\frac{1}{2}$	12	8	4	7	5
$7\frac{1}{2}$–$8\frac{1}{2}$	11	9	2	8	3
$8\frac{1}{2}$–10	4	4	0	3	1
$10\frac{1}{2}$–11	4	4	0	3	1
11–12	3	3	0	2	1
Total	75	50	25	48	27
				64%	36%
10	1	Transverse presentation		Bicornual pregnancy	
5	1			Twin pregnancy	

although several turns around the transverse axis may occur, a complete revolution of the bovine umbilical cord is not normal and has been seen only in mummified fetuses. In equine and porcine fetuses, however, complete revolutions of the amniotic portion of the umbilical cord are common.

Another possibility of intrauterine fetal movement is the potential mobility of the amniotic sac (with contained fetus) within the allantochorion. Owing to the extensive fusion of the allantochorion to the allanto-amnion in the cow, ewe and sow, such mobility is impossible (except perhaps near term) whereas in the mare, bitch and cat such movement does take place and leads to twisting of the allantoic portion of the umbilical cord.

Data collected from pregnant bovine uteri by the present author and from equine specimens by Vandeplassche (1957) (Table 2.4) indicate that initially anterior and posterior presentations occur in equal numbers. At between 5 and 6 months of pregnancy the body length of the fetal calf exceeds the width of the amnion and thus at this stage the final polarity of 95% of fetuses in anterior presentation is adopted. In the mare, however, at $6\frac{1}{2}$ months, 40% of the fetuses are still in posterior presentation; the final gestational presentation of 99% of foals anteriorly disposed is not taken up until the ninth month. Messervy (1958), from observations made during laparotomy of pregnant mares, has also concluded that the presentation of a foal may alter after the eighth month. It would seem likely that these changes of longitudinal presentation that occur during late gestation in the mare are due to movements of the amnion within the allantochorion. The reason for the final overwhelming proportion of anterior presentations in the mare and cow is not known.

The size of the bovine fetus at the various stages of pregnancy is given on p. 78 and the fetal growth curve is shown in Figure 2.15.

Richardson et al. (1976) have shown that long bone length (conveniently radius and tibia) is a reliable indicator of fetal age from 50 days of gestation to term in the sheep, and may be obtained radiographically in the living fetus or by post-mortem measurement. Mean values for the respective ages are shown in Table 2.5.

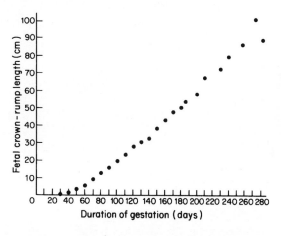

Fig. 2.15 The growth curve of the bovine fetus.

Table 2.5. Length of ovine fetal long bones at various stages of conception

Days after conception	Length of radius (mm)	Length of tibia (mm)
50	4.8	5.0
60	10	12
70	16	19
85	25	32
100	36	47
110	47	63
120	56	76
130	67	91
140	74	100
150	79	107

Richardson (1980) has provided the following formulae for calculating the age of the fetus from its crown–anus length:

Pig $X = 3 (Y + 21)$
Calf $X = 2.5 (Y + 21)$
Lamb $X = 2.1 (Y + 17)$

where X is the developmental age in days and Y is the crown–anus length in centimetres.

REFERENCES

Allen, W. R. (1982) *J. Reprod. Fertil. Suppl.*, **31**, 57.
Allen, W. R. and Moor, R. M. (1972) *J. Reprod. Fertil.*, **29**, 313.

Amoroso, E. C. (1952) Placentation. In: *Marshall's Physiology of Reproduction*, ed. A. S. Parkes, Vol. 2. London: Longmans, Green.
Arthur, G. H. (1956) *J. Comp. Pathol.*, **66**, 345.
Arthur, G. H. (1959) *Vet. Rec.*, **71**, 345.
Arthur, G. H. (1969) *J. Reprod. Fertil. Suppl.*, **9**, 45.
Cloete, J. H. L. (1939) *Onderstepoort J. Vet. Sci. Anim. Indust.*, **13**, 418.
Evans, H. E. (1983) *Proc. XIIth World Vet. Congr., Perth*, p.27.
Grosser, O. (1909) *Eihaute und der Placenta*. Wien and Leipzig.
King, G. J., Atkinson, B. A. and Robertson, H. A. (1979) *J. Reprod. Fertil.*, **55**, 173.
Leith, G. S. and Ginther, O. J. (1984) *Proc. 10th Int. Congr. Anim. Reprod. AI*, **1**, 118.
Lillie, F. R. (1917) *J. Exp. Zool.*, **23**, 371.
Malan, A. P. and Curson, H. H. (1937) *Onderstepoort J. Vet. Sci. Anim. Indust.*, **8**, 417.
Messervy, A. (1958) Personal communication.
Richardson, C. (1980) Personal communication.
Richardson, C., Herbert, C. N. and Terlecki, S. (1976) *Vet. Rec.*, **99**, 22.
Richter, J. and Götze, R. (1960) *Tiergeburtschilfe*. Berlin and Hamburg: Paul Parey.
Vandeplassche, M. (1957) *Vlaams Diergeneesk. Tijdschr.*, **26**, 60.
Vandeplassche, M., Podliachouk, L. and Beaud, R. (1970) *Can. J. Comp. Med.*, **34**, 318.
van Niekerk, C. H. and Gernaeke, W. H. (1966) *Onderstepoort J. Vet. Res.*, **23**(Suppl. 2), 3.
Williams, W. L. (1939) *Diseases of the Genital Organs of Domestic Animals*. Baltimore: Williams and Wilkins.
Wooding, F. B. P. (1992) *Placenta*, **13**, 101.
Zietzschmann, O. (1924) *Lehrbuch der Entwicklungsgeschichte der Haustiere*. Berlin and Hamburg: Paul Parey.

3

Pregnancy and its Diagnosis

MATERNAL RECOGNITION OF PREGNANCY

In most domestic species the establishment and maintenance of pregnancy requires that the luteal phase of the oestrous cycle is prolonged by the persistence of a single corpus luteum or a number of corpora lutea. As a result of the persistence of the luteal tissue, progesterone concentrations remain elevated. This results in a negative feed-back on the anterior pituitary with a resultant inhibition of follicular development and ovulation and, in polyoestrous species, a prevention of return to oestrus. In many species the placenta subsequently replaces or supplements the luteal source of progesterone.

In Chapter 1 the importance of the corpus luteum in regulating the periodicity of the oestrous cycle was discussed, and the role of prostaglandin $F_{2\alpha}$ ($PGF_{2\alpha}$), produced by the endometrium, in causing regression of the corpus luteum and the consequent return to oestrus was described. The presence of a viable, developing embryo, however, prevents the corpus luteum from regressing and thus, in polyoestrous species, inhibits the return to oestrus. This phenomenon was described by Short (1969) as the 'maternal recognition of pregnancy'. It is particularly interesting because a maternal endocrine response is detectable before the blastocyst is attached to the endometrium by microvilli, which either directly or indirectly prevents regression of the corpus luteum. In five of the domestic species the time of maternal recognition of pregnancy has been determined (Table 3.1).

It is likely that the developing embryo exerts its effect in one of two ways: either it has an anti-luteolytic action, preventing the synthesis, release or action of $PGF_{2\alpha}$, or it exerts a luteotrophic effect and thus over-rides the effect of the luteolysin. In most species studied there is some evidence

Table 3.1. Time of maternal recognition of pregnancy

Species	Day of maternal recognition of pregnancy	Day of definite attachment
Sow	12	18
Ewe	12–13	16
Cow	16–17	18–22
Mare	14–16	36–38
Goat	17	

After Findlay (1981).

for both (Heap et al., 1978), although their relative importance probably varies between species.

In *sheep*, early work by Moor (1968) and Martal et al. (1979) demonstrated that the ovine conceptus produces a protein. In recent years it has been characterized as existing in three or four isoforms of molecular weight about 18000; it has been named ovine trophoblast protein or oTP-1. It is produced by the trophectoderm from about day 10, when the blastocyst starts to elongate, until about day 23; its molecular configuration is similar to interferon-α (IFN-α), although since it has been shown that recombinant bovine IFN-α is not as effective as oTP-1 in extending the interoestrus intervals of sheep it is possible that it may have unique biological properties which distinguish it from other IFN-α molecules (Bazer et al., 1991; Roberts et al., 1991).

Details of the mechanism of luteolysis have been described earlier (see p. 9). Although oTP-1 probably exerts its effect in a number of different ways, the result is the reduction in the pulsatile release of $PGF_{2\alpha}$ that occurs between days 15 and 17 in non-pregnant ewes. IFN or oTP-1 act by inhibiting the expression of uterine oxytocin receptors during the period following the inhibitory effect of circulating progesterone on oxytocin receptor concentration. In addition, it may indirectly inhibit the synthesis of $PGF_{2\alpha}$ (Bazer et al.,

1991). It has been suggested that luteal protective mechanisms may be involved in the maternal recognition of pregnancy. Watson et al. (1979) suggested that the trophoblast protein may act directly on the synthetic pathways of prostaglandin by increasing the production of PGE_2 rather than PGF_2; alternatively, it may cause the conversion of $PGF_{2\alpha}$ to PGE_2. More recently, it has been shown that concentrations of PGE in utero-ovarian vein plasma of pregnant ewes increases on days 13 and 14 (Silvia et al., 1984).

In the *cow*, the importance of the blastocyst in prolonging the lifespan of the corpus luteum was shown by the studies of Northey and French (1980). They found that if the blastocyst was removed at day 17 or day 19, the interoestrus intervals were extended to 25 and 26 days, respectively, compared with those in which the embryo was removed at day 13, or were not mated; in the latter cases the intervals were 20–21 days. The antiluteolytic signal produced by the bovine conceptus is bovine trophoblast protein-1 (bTP-1). It cross-reacts immunologically with oTP-1, has high amino acid sequence homology with both oTP-1 and IFN-α and possesses antiviral activity (Bazer et al., 1991). The molecular weight is around 24 000. The maximum secretion of bTP-1 is between days 16 and 19. It commences at the time of elongation of the blastocyst and, unlike oTP-1, continues to be secreted until day 38 of gestation (Bartol et al., 1985; Godkin et al., 1988). When bTP-1 is infused into the uterine lumen of non-pregnant cyclical cows between days 14 and 17, the lifespan of the corpus luteum is extended. Similar results have been obtained following the administration of recombinant bovine INF-α_1 (rBO IFN-α_1) using the same route of administration and also intramuscularly (Plante et al., 1989).

As in the ewe, it is likely that bTP-1 exerts its antiluteolytic effect by modifying endometrial oxytocin receptors, thereby inhibiting the release of $PGF_{2\alpha}$.

In the *goat*, the removal of conceptuses from the uterine lumen between days 13 and 15 does not prolong the lifespan of the corpus luteum, but on day 17 it increases the interoestrus interval by 7–10 days. The caprine conceptus secretes a protein, designated cTP-1, which together with other proteins probably exerts an antiluteolytic effect similar to that described above for sheep and cattle (Gnatek et al., 1989).

In the *sow*, maternal recognition of pregnancy is not controlled by a single event but rather a series of complex biochemical and cellular interactions. The porcine conceptus has been shown to convert progesterone to oestrone and oestradiol-17β as well as another isomer of 16α,17-oestradiol (Fischer et al., 1985). The production of oestrogens increases with the rapid elongation of the blastocyst so that the conceptus is able to stimulate locally a large surface of endometrium. Oestrogen production by the conceptus plays a vital role in the maternal recognition of pregnancy and the extension of the lifespan of the corpora lutea. The administration of exogenous oestrogens parenterally after day 9 of the oestrous cycle was shown to extend the interoestrus interval in gilts by Kidder et al. (1955). The secretion of oestrogens by the blastocyst at the time of elongation also stimulates the release of calcium, specific polypeptides and proteins. These may play a role in the establishment of pregnancy. In addition to the initial secretion of oestrogens at day 11, it is necessary for the second sustained release of oestrogens between days 14 and 18 for luteal persistence beyond day 25 (Geisert et al., 1990). Several mechanisms by which the conceptus-secreted oestrogens prevent luteal regression have been proposed. These include a direct luteotrophic effect, a reduction in the endometrial synthesis, and release of $PGF_{2\alpha}$. However, there is evidence that they probably exert their effect by altering the transport of $PGF_{2\alpha}$ from an endocrine (towards the uterine vasculature) to an exocrine (into the uterine lumen) direction, thereby preventing $PGF_{2\alpha}$ reaching the corpora lutea (Bazer et al., 1984). The fate of the intrauterine $PGF_{2\alpha}$ is not known; however, fetal membranes readily metabolize it to PGFM, which is inactive. The oestrogen stimulation of calcium secretion into the uterine lumen appears to be involved in the process.

As in ruminant species, the pig conceptus produces interferons at the time of elongation (11–17 days of gestation) (Cross and Roberts, 1989); to date two IFNs have been identified, namely IFN-γ and a type 1 IFN. Since the infusion of total conceptus-derived secretory proteins into the uterine lumen failed to prolong the lifespan of the corpora lutea in cyclical sows (Harney and Bazer, 1989), their precise functions are not known. It has been postulated that they may have a specific protective antiviral role or that they may act in conjunction with conceptus-derived oestrogens in prolonging the lifespan of the corpora lutea (La Bonnardière, 1993).

In the *mare*, the mechanisms responsible for the recognition of pregnancy are less well understood than in some other species. However, evidence of the importance of the developing conceptus has been shown by its removal at varying stages of gestation: if it was removed at 10, 15 and 20 days then the return to oestrus was 22.3, 38.0 and 47 days respectively (Hershman and Douglas, 1979). A low molecular weight protein has been identified in the uterine flushings of mares in dioestrus; this persists during pregnancy (McDowell et al., 1982). The equine conceptus also produces oestradiol and oestrone (Berg and Ginther, 1978; Zavy et al., 1979), which enhance the production of a glycoprotein, uteroferrin, by the uterus. PGF secretion from the pregnant uterus is apparently blocked, since lower levels of PGF have been identified in the uterine venous blood of pregnant mares compared with non pregnant mares (Douglas and Ginther, 1976) and similarly lower levels of PGFM in the peripheral circulation (Kindahl et al., 1982). There does not appear to be any sequestration of PGF in the uterine lumen during early pregnancy but when endometrial tissue is incubated *in vitro* with material of conceptus origin there was a reduction in PGF synthesis/ or secretion (Berglund et al., 1982). The importance of the migration of the conceptus within the uterine lumen until it becomes 'fixed' at 16–18 days of gestation at the base of the uterine horn, has been demonstrated in some elegant experiments by McDowell et al. (1988). By restricting the mobility of the conceptus using ligatures at various parts of the uterus, the maternal recognition was compromised so that the corpus luteum regressed spontaneously. It is likely that the stimulus elicited by the migratory conceptus in its contact with the endometrium is compared with the stimulus associated with the rapid elongation of the blastocyst in ruminants and the pig.

The *bitch* is atypical in that the luteal phase (metoestrus) is prolonged in the absence of pregnancy, there being very little difference in the interoestrus intervals of bitches that have been pregnant or non-pregnant. Until more is known about the mechanisms which control the lifespan of the corpus luteum, maternal recognition of pregnancy in this species will not be fully understood.

Possible mechanisms involved in the endocrine recognition of pregnancy, resulting in failure of luteolysis have already been discussed. However, there is some evidence that a maternal response can be identified within hours of fertilization and may well be involved in protecting the embryo, and subsequently the fetus, from being rejected by the dam as a semi-allograft. In 1974, Morton and her co-workers discovered that in pregnant mice it was possible to identify a substance in the peripheral blood from 4 to 6 hours after mating and for 2 weeks of gestation. This substance called early pregnancy factor (EPF) has been identified in sheep, cattle and pigs as well as man and several other species. The method by which it exerts a protective role for the early embryo is not known, but it has been suggested that it binds to the T lymphocytes, thus preventing recognition of the embryonic antigen (Koch, 1985). It can be identified using the rosette inhibition test (Morton et al., 1976).

PREGNANCY AND ITS DETECTION IN THE MARE

Endocrinology

The endocrine changes in the mare during pregnancy are particularly unusual when compared with other domestic species because of the development of temporary hormone-producing structures, the endometrial cups.

After ovulation and the formation of the corpus haemorrhagicum and the corpus luteum, plasma progesterone concentrations in the peripheral plasma rise to 7–8 ng/ml by 6 days. They persist at about these levels for the first 4 weeks of gestation, but there is frequently a transient fall at about 28 days after ovulation to 5 ng/ml. (Holtan et al., 1975), followed by a later rise. Published values for progesterone in the blood and plasma vary considerably between laboratories. This is because there are other progesterone-like substances which cross-react with the antisera during the assay; for this reason several authors refer to 'total progestogen' levels.

In the early part of the second month of pregnancy the endometrial cups are formed. These are

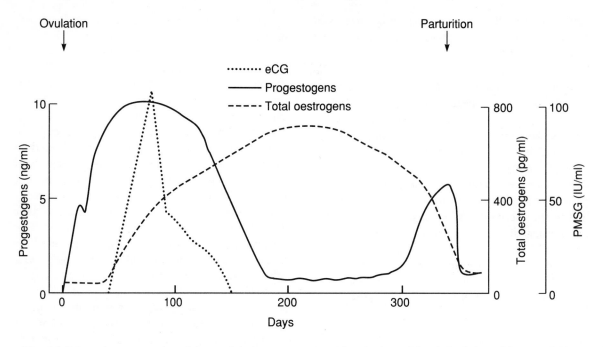

Fig. 3.1 Schematic representation of the trends in hormone concentrations in the peripheral circulation of the mare during pregnancy and at parturition.

discrete outgrowths of densely packed tissue within the gravid horn, derived as a result of the invasion of fetal trophoblast cells into endometrium where they subsequently give rise to the endometrial cup cells (Moor et al., 1975). Usually there are about 12 cups present at the junction of the gravid horn and body as a circumferential band. The endometrial cups produce pregnant mare serum gonadotrophin (PMSG), which is now referred to as equine chorionic gonadotrophin or eCG. It is first demonstrable in the blood 38–42 days after ovulation, reaches a maximum at 60–65 days, declines thereafter and disappears by 150 days of gestation (Figure 3.1). eCG has both follicle-stimulating hormone (FSH)-like and luteinizing hormone (LH)-like activity, and it is generally assumed that, in association with pituitary gonadotrophins, it provides the stimulus for the formation of accessory corpora lutea (Allen, W. R. 1975). These structures start to form between 40 and 60 days of gestation, either as a result of ovulation, in the same way that the corpus luteum of dioestrus is formed (32%), or as a result of luteinization of anovulatory follicles (68%) (Squire et al., 1974). Because of the presence of the accessory corpora lutea the progestogen concentrations in the peripheral circulation increase, to reach and maintain a

plateau from about 50 to 140 days and then decline (Figure 3.1). By 180–200 days the concentrations are below 1 ng/ml and they remain so until about 300 days of gestation, when they increase rapidly to reach a peak just before foaling and subsequently decline rapidly to very low levels immediately after parturition.

Concentrations of total oestrogens in the peripheral circulation during the first 35 days of pregnancy are similar to those of dioestrus, although there is a temporary production of oestrogen by the embryo at 12–20 days (Mayer et al., 1977). After this time they increase to reach a plateau between 40 and 60 days, at values slightly above those that occur before ovulation, about 3 ng/ml; the rise is probably due to the increased follicular development associated with eCG production. After day 60 it is likely that the increase is due to the activity of the fetus or placenta (Terqui and Palmer, 1979). Maximum values are observed at about 210 days, the main source being the fetal gonads (Cox, 1975), with a gradual decline towards the time of foaling and a precipitous fall post-partum. The main oestrogens in the mare are oestrone and a ketonic steroid equilin; oestradiol-17β, oestradiol-17α and equilenine are also present.

Prolactin levels show no distinct pattern, there being considerable variation within and between mares, but there is some evidence of a slight increase towards the end of gestation (Nett et al., 1975).

The main source of progesterone in early pregnancy is the true corpus luteum and the accessory corpora lutea. The true corpus luteum is active for the first 3 months of gestation, and regresses at the same time as the accesssory corpora lutea (Squire and Ginther, 1975).

The placenta must take over the production of progesterone after the regression of the accessory corpora lutea, and although concentrations fall in the peripheral circulation they remain high in the placental tissue and must maintain pregnancy by virtue of a localized effect (Short, 1957). When ovariectomy is performed at 25–45 days of gestation, mares will abort or resorb the fetus; when it is performed after 50 days the response is variable; between 140 and 210 days the pregnancy is continued uninterrupted to term. Thus after 50 days there is evidence of a non-ovarian source of progesterone, and by 140 days the ovaries are no longer necessary for the maintenance of pregnancy (Holtan et al., 1979).

Changes in the genital organs

Conception to 40 days

Ovaries. The corpus luteum verum can only be palpated per rectum for 2 to 3 days after its formation. Thereafter, although it persists for 5 or 6 months, it cannot be identified. In pony mares (Allen, W. E., 1975) there is some palpable follicular development at about 15 days whilst during the next 14 days there is quite a marked increase in folliculogenesis with a large number of follicles less than 3 cm diameter giving the ovaries a 'bunch of grapes' appearance. Ovulations during this period are rare.

Uterus. During late dioestrus and oestrus the uterus is soft and the endometrium thin. After ovulation, tone increases and the uterus becomes more tubular; these textural changes are not marked in the non-pregnant animal, in which they subside after the corpus luteum begins to regress at 10–14 days, but in the pregnant mare the corpus luteum persists, and the tone of the uterus increases to a maximum at 19–21 days, when the conceptus causes a soft, thin-walled

cornual swelling close to the uterine body. The horn involved is not necessarily on the same side as the ovary which produced the ovum because there is extensive mobility of the conceptus within the horns and uterine body before fixation occurs between days 12 and 14 (see p. 65). Most clinicians have reported more equine pregnancies in the right horn, e.g. Vandeplassche (1957) noted 64%, although in ponies there is only a small majority of right horn pregnancies. The excess of right-side pregnancies, coupled with the slightly greater incidence of left-side ovulations, indicates a major embryonic migration from left to right in horses generally. There is, however, good evidence that other factors can influence the horn in which pregnancy occurs. In a survey of 937 thoroughbred mares, Butterfield and Mathews (1979) found that there was no significant difference between the numbers of right or left horn pregnancies: 469 left and 468 right. However, when they examined the results for mares that conceived when they were not lactating there was a significantly greater number of right horn pregnancies. There is also good evidence that implantation usually occurs on the opposite side to that of the previous pregnancy. Feo (1980) found that 19 of 22 mares which conceived at the foal heat were pregnant in the opposite horn to that of the previous gestation. Allen and Newcombe (1981) found that in 82.5% of cases the conceptus was present in the opposite horn.

The conceptual swelling of the uterine horn protrudes ventrally and anteroposteriorly and grows slowly during the phase of organogenesis, i.e. until about 30 days. Thereafter, growth is faster and the swelling progressively extends to the tip of the pregnant horn. Twins are usually disposed at the base of each horn, and in this situation there will be two groups of endometrial cups. If both twins are present in the same horn only one set of cups will be present.

Vagina and Cervix. The vagina becomes progressively paler and dryer and is covered by thin, tacky mucus. The cervix is small and tightly closed; the external os is gradually filled by a plug of mucus and points eccentrically.

40–120 days

Ovaries. This period is characterized by marked ovarian activity, with multiple follicular development causing one or both ovaries to become temporarily larger than during heat, in some cases very much larger. Ovulations, forming accessory corpora lutea, and luteinization of unruptured follicles occur. Follicular activity has usually subsided by 100 days, and the corpora lutea begin to regress. In pony mares, Allen (1971) found ovulations in pregnancy between 21 and 112 days, with the highest incidences between days 40–42, 54–56 and 63–66.

Uterus. The conceptus completely occupies the pregnant horn by about 60 days, after which the body and then the non-pregnant horn are invaded by the allantochorionic membrane. The pregnant horn now changes from a transverse to a longitudinal disposition in the mare's abdomen. By 100 days the fluid-filled uterus is a somewhat tense swelling on the pelvic brim. At this time the small fetus, closely enveloped in the amnion, is floating in a relatively large volume of allantoic fluid.

120 days to term

Ovaries. With the gradual regression of all luteal elements and follicles the ovaries become progressively smaller and harder and are drawn forwards and downwards by the gravid uterus. Except in very large mares they can usually be palpated throughout pregnancy.

Uterus. Gradual distension of the uterus by the fetus and fluids causes increased tension on the utero-ovarian ligament, and the anterior border of the uterus sinks downwards and forwards. After the eighth month the fetus normally assumes an anterior longitudinal presentation. Except in very large mares the fetus can be palpated throughout this period. Fremitus can be detected in the uterine arteries although it is less obvious than in the cow.

Methods of pregnancy diagnosis

The methods available are of four types, managemental, clinical, ultrasonic and laboratory.

Managemental methods

Failure to return to oestrus is a good sign that a mare is pregnant. The demonstration of the signs of oestrus (see Chapter 1) usually requires the presence of a teaser stallion, although some mares will respond to geldings and to androgenized geldings. It is preferable that mares should be accustomed to the teasing routine, which should

commence 16 days after service and continue for a further 6 days.

False positives will occur:

1. If the mare has a silent heat, a common problem when the foal is at foot.

2. If the mare becomes anoestrus as a result of lactation or environmental factors.

3. If the mare has a prolonged dioestrus yet has not conceived (see Chapter 26).

4. If the mare has a prolonged luteal phase associated with embryonic death; this is referred to as 'pseudopregnancy' (see Chapter 26).

False negatives will occur in a few mares which will show oestrus at this time although they are pregnant.

Clinical methods

Vaginal Examination. This is best done using a speculum; however, manual exploration can be used. The vaginal mucosa is pale pink, the mucus is scant and sticky, and the cervix small and tightly closed; the external os is gradually filled with thick tacky mucus, although it is not really apparent as a plug, and points eccentrically.

False positives can occur in early pregnancy because the vagina is indistinguishable from that seen in dioestrus. Errors can also be made as a result of prolonged dioestrus and pseudopregnancy.

Rectal Palpation. The presence of *follicles* during the third week after service does not necessarily indicate that the mare is returning to heat. Follicles are normally present during the first 3 months of gestation, and give considerable size to the ovaries.

Uterine tone is marked at 17–21 days of pregnancy, when the uterine cornua can be palpated as resilient tubular organs. If no conceptual swelling is palpable, then this tone should only be interpreted as suggestive of pregnancy. The uterine body and non-pregnant horn remain tonic until at least day 50 of gestation. Marked uterine tone may also be found in: (1) the puerperal mare covered at the foal heat; (2) acute endometritis; and (3) pseudopregnancy, i.e. when early embryonic death is followed by autolysis or expulsion of the conceptus but the uterus retains the texture of pregnancy because of the persistent corpus luteum.

Palpation of the conceptus is first possible at 17–21 days when it is a small soft swelling of 2.4–2.8 cm or as an apparent 'gap' in the otherwise tonic horn.

It is more easily felt between 21 and 30 days, but still only the anteroventral portion of the distension can be appreciated. At 25 days the conceptual swelling is 3–3.4 cm. At 30 days its dorsoventral diameter is 3–4 cm. At 35 days it is 4.5–6 cm and at 40 days 6–7 cm in diameter — about the size of a tennis ball. Thereafter, it is not possible for the conceptual swelling to be completely cupped within the palm of the hand. By 60 days it is becoming oval in shape and measures approximately 13 × 9 cm, whilst by 90 days it has increased to approximately 23 × 14 cm.

There is a natural variation in the size of the conceptual swelling in mares of similar size and ovulation dates owing to the variation in the volumes of fetal fluids present. However, swellings that appear small for the given stage of pregnancy should be checked later to exclude the possibility of resorption (hence the clinician should keep written records of the findings for later comparisons). Twin conceptuses can be identified up to 60 days. After this a single conceptus is likely to involve both horns, and the swelling becomes more diffuse. Care must be taken not to confuse a partially filled urinary bladder with the pregnant uterus during the 70–100 day period or with an inflated large colon during days 90–120; when in doubt a search should be made for the ovaries in order to establish an anatomical link between them and the uterus via the utero-ovarian ligament.

At about 100 days it is often possible to *ballotte the fetus* as it floats in the fetal fluid of the uterine body. Growth of the fetus and reduction in tension of the fetal sacs enable the examiner to palpate parts of the fetus in the uterine body from the end of the fourth month onwards. It may be difficult to locate between the fifth and seventh months in large pluriparous mares and very occasionally in mares near term. The palpable absence of a non-pregnant uterus and tension in the mesovarium are reassuring features.

False positive results by rectal palpation can be obtained when: (1) in rare instances it is confused with pyometra (see Chapter 26) or (2) in the very early stages, when the uterine tone due to incomplete involution might be assumed to be due to pregnancy in mares which have been served at the foal heat and in those that have developed a pseudopregnancy. It should also be remembered that mares may suffer embryonic or fetal death with resorption or abortion after they have been confirmed pregnant.

False-negative results can be obtained if there is confusion over the service date, i.e. later than the one recorded, or if the uterus is not palpated completely.

Ultrasonic methods

Three types of ultrasound have been used for pregnancy diagnosis. The ultrasonic fetal pulse detector was the first type that was used. This is based upon the Doppler phenomenon in which high-frequency (ultrasonic) sound waves emitted from a probe, placed on the exterior of an animal or in the rectum, are reflected at an altered frequency when they strike a moving object or particles, e.g. the fetal heart or blood flowing in arteries. The reflected waves are received by the same probe; the difference in frequencies are converted into audible sounds and amplified. This has had limited application in the mare.

The ultrasonic amplitude depth analyser (A mode) relies upon a transducer head that emits the high-frequency sound waves and receives the reflected sound, which is shown as a one-dimensional display of echo amplitudes for various depths, usually on an oscilloscope but also on the newer light-emitting diodes. This has been used successfully in many species, notably the sow, but was largely oversold as a method of diagnosing pregnancy in mares in the late 1970s (Ginther, 1986).

The most recent development is that of the B (brightness) mode, which has become a very versatile tool in studying reproductive events in many species, in particular the mare (see Chapter 26). Readers who wish to extend their knowledge of this technique are recommended to consult Ginther (1986).

It is worthwhile outlining briefly the principles behind the technique. The probe or transducer, as it should properly be called, is applied to the skin surface or inserted into the rectum. The transducer contains numbers of piezoelectric crystals which, when subjected to an electric current, expand or contract and produce high-frequency sound waves. When these sound waves are transmitted through tissues a proportion will be reflected back to the transducer, depending upon the characteristic of the tissue, where the returning echoes will compress the same piezocrystals, resulting in the

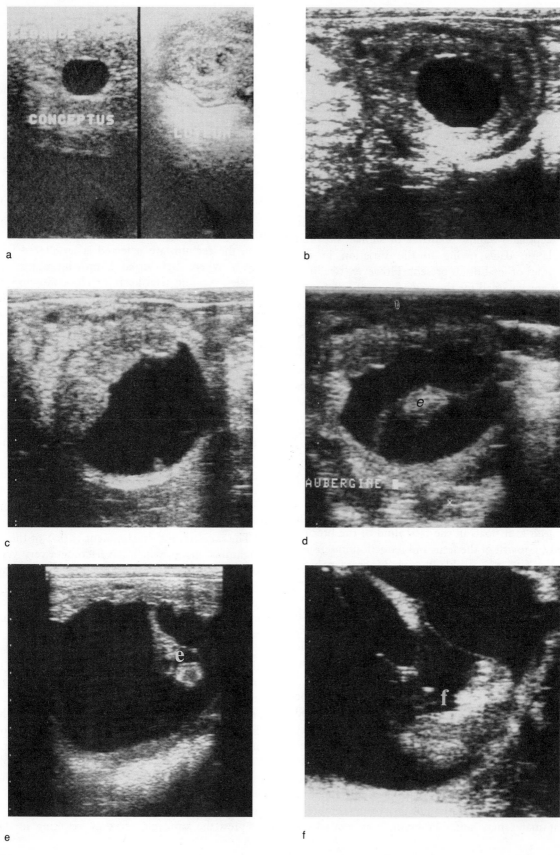

production of electric impulses, which are displayed as a two-dimensional display of dots on a screen. The brightness of the dots will be proportional to the amplitude of the returning echoes and hence will provide an image ranging from black, through various shades of grey, to white.

Liquids do not reflect ultrasound, and thus are depicted as black on the screen, i.e. non-echogenic, whereas solid tissues such as bone or cartilage reflect a high proportion of sound waves, i.e. they are echogenic and appear white on the screen. Since a tissue-gas interface can result in up to 99% of the sound waves being reflected, it is important that air should not be trapped between the transducer face and the tissues to be examined. For this reason a coupling medium or gel (usually methyl cellulose) is applied to the transducer face before it is placed on the skin or rectal mucosa so that air is eliminated. It is also important to select an area that is relatively hairless, or alternatively it may be necessary to clip the hair.

The technique is frequently referred to as real-time ultrasound or imaging. This just implies that there are live or moving displays in which the echoes are recorded continuously. The transducers may have the piezocrystals or elements arranged side by side in lines (hence they are referred to as linear array transducers); the field under examination and the two-dimensional image are in the shape of a rectangle. Sector transducers contain a single crystal which oscillates or rotates to produce a fan-shaped beam. They allow ready access to most of the thoracic viscera, although very superficial structures may not be readily identified because of the shape of the beam. Sector scanners require less skin surface contact, which can reduce the time required to examine each animal, hence they are used for the transabdominal approach, especially in sheep. Linear transducers are usually cheaper to buy, more robust and they produce a rectangular image which is easier to interpret. Straight linear arrays are quite adequate. The transducer should be small enough to be cupped in the hand, smooth in contour,

waterproof and easy to clean (Boyd and Omran, 1991).

Each transducer produces ultrasonic waves at frequencies of between 1 and 10 MHz. The most frequently used frequencies are 3.5, 5, and, more recently, 7.5 MHz. The lower-frequency transducers give better tissue penetration but poorer resolution. Since using the transrectal approach the structures requiring imaging are within a few centimetres of the transducer head; high-frequency equipment is the most effective. Thus, in the case of the mare, using a linear array transducer transrectally to diagnose pregnancy, it is possible to identify a 3–4 mm conceptual vesicle with a 5.0 MHz transducer whereas a 3.5 MHz transducer will only identify a vesicle of 6–7 mm diameter.

Using a 5.0 MHz transducer, the earliest gestational age that pregnancy has been confirmed in 9 days, when the conceptual vesicle appears as a black sphere of about 3 mm in diameter. By 11 days the vesicle has been identified in 98% of ponies and horses examined (Ginther, 1986). The conceptus at this stage moves freely within the uterus, and has been identified in all parts of the uterine horns and in the uterine body just cranial to the cervix; in fact it is found more frequently in the body at this stage. Rapid growth of the conceptual vesicle occurs from 9 to 16 days, with evidence of some reduction in growth rate from 16 to 28 days, before it increases. This plateau in growth may be an artefact because, with a reduced turgidity of the vesicle, it is capable of being compressed by the uterine walls. This is also associated with an apparent change in the shape of the vesicle from spherical, to oval, to triangular; it then becomes irregular in outline. Fixation at the base of the horn occurs between 14 and 16 days, when the conceptual vesicle is about 19–24 mm in diameter (Ginther, 1986).

Twin ovulations are very common in mares, especially in Thoroughbred and draught mares where they can occur in up to 25% of ovulations. The birth of live twins is relatively uncommon, ranging between 0.8 and 3% depending

Fig. 3.2 Transrectal B-mode ultrasound images of the pregnant uterus of the mare, and its content, using a 7.5 MHz linear transducer. Scale in cm. (a) Conceptus at 13 days (left) which is 9 mm in diameter with a dorsal and ventral specular echo. Adjacent ovary (right) showing corpus luteum verum. (b) Conceptus at 16 days; note that it is starting to lose its spherical shape. (c) Conceptus at 21 days; note embryo at 5 o'clock and thickening of uterine wall extending from 8 o'clock to 10 o'clock. (d) Conceptus at 30 days; note embryo (e) which is starting to move towards the dorsal pole of the vesicle. (e) Conceptus at 35 days; note embryo (e) and that the yolk sac has now regressed leaving only the anechoic allontoic sac. (f) Conceptus at 50 days; note fetus (f).

upon the breed. The reasons for the discrepancy are: (1) fertilization failure; (2) death of one or both embryos before or after fixation; (3) death of one fetus, which is relatively uncommon; and (4) abortion of both fetuses (see p. 483). The last event is the most common sequel and is obviously the most costly. Whilst the detection of double ovulations by B-mode ultrasound has enabled better management, and hence the presention of the problem, it is still possible for double ovulations to go undetected. Thus, early identification of twin embryos, preferably between days 12 and 14 before fixation occurs, can enable more effective management of the problem (see p. 479). For this reason it is important to scan the whole of the uterine body and uterine horns.

Laboratory methods

Milk or Blood Progesterone.   As can be seen in Figure 3.1, in the pregnant mare plasma progesterone concentrations remain elevated just before or during the time when the mare would have returned to oestrus. Blood or milk samples collected 16–22 days after service should have elevated progestogen levels in pregnant mares whilst in non-pregnant mares the levels would be low and typical of those obtained at oestrus. Although Hunt et al. (1978) have quoted 100% accuracy in diagnosing pregnancy using this method, false-positive results occur with prolonged dioestrus, and, in general, the method is not very reliable.

Identification of eCG.   Blood samples should be collected, preferably between 50 and 90 days after service, although it is possible to identify the hormone between 40 and 120 days. The test is performed on serum, and thus no anticoagulant is required.

Originally biological methods were used to identify the presence of the gonadotrophin. The most frequently used method was the injection of serum into $3\frac{1}{2}$-week-old immature mice, a positive result being the production of ripe follicles in the ovaries and the presence of a swollen enlarged uterus. The method has been described in detail by Miller and Day (1938).

Immunological methods are now used, either gel diffusion or the haemagglutination inhibition technique. The latter method is available commercially in a simple kit form; all of the reagents are provided, and it is possible for the procedure to be done in any veterinary practice laboratory (MIP

Test, Intervet Ltd, Cambridge, UK). The method is about 95% accurate.

False-negative results are obtained if the blood sample is taken either too early or too late, and for this reason it is important to sample at the optimum times stated above. Some mares produce low levels of eCG that are briefly sustained and which cannot be detected using the method.

False-positive results are obtained as a result of embryonic or fetal death, either after the blood sample was collected or in some cases before. Once the endometrial cups have formed they will persist and still secrete eCG, even if the fetus has died. They regress at the time that they would have done if the pregnancy had continued normally. For this reason owners should always be warned of the problems, to save subsequent disappointment, and certificates should indicate that a positive result has been obtained with an explanation of the significance of such a result.

Blood Oestrogens.   A method of detecting pregnancy by determining the concentration of total oestrogens in the peripheral blood has been suggested by Terqui and Palmer (1979). By 85 days of gestation the concentration should exceed the maximum values obtained in non-pregnant mares.

Urinary Oestrogens.   Oestrogens (oestrone and oestradiol-17β) are present in the urine of pregnant mares in sufficient amounts for accurate detection by a chemical method (Cuboni, 1937) between 150 and 300 days of gestation. A modification of this test (Cox and Galina, 1970) can be carried out easily by the practitioner. Very little equipment is required and the results are easy to interpret.

Because the presence of blood oestrogens depends on a functional placenta, false positives, as seen with the eCG test, do not arise. This chemical test is not sensitive enough to identify the urinary oestrogens of oestrus. It is nearly 100% accurate between 150 and 300 days.

Optimum time for diagnosing pregnancy

The optimum time, as with all species, is as early and as accurately as possible. The use of B-mode ultrasonic imaging has enabled early identification to be made; however, it is important to stress that good results depend upon good equipment and knowledgeable interpretation of the images. Similarly, many of the earlier changes in uterine tone can be identified only by an expert using sequential palpation. Termination of prenancy in the case of twins must be done before the endometrial cups develop, and the mare will become pseudopregnant.

If the mare is not pregnant and has not been observed in oestrus, or if she is in prolonged dioestrus or anoestrus, the necessary action can be taken (see Chapter 26).

Hazards of pregnancy diagnosis

There is no evidence that careful palpation of the genital tract will cause failure of the pregnancy. In those mares where fetal death occurs after a normal rectal examination has been performed the pregnancy would have failed in the absence of the examination.

PREGNANCY AND ITS DIAGNOSIS IN THE COW

Endocrinology

The main source of progesterone for the maintenance of pregnancy in the cow is the corpus luteum, the placenta producing only small amounts. The results of ovariectomy and removal of the corpus luteum are controversial. Up to about 200 days of gestation, removal of the ovary containing the corpus luteum, or ablation of the corpus luteum either surgically or with the use of

$PGF_{2\alpha}$, usually results in abortion. However, after this stage, until just before term, pregnancy usually continues. Some difference has been noted between the effects of ovariectomy and corpus luteum removal, which would suggest that the ovarian stroma may produce some progesterone, whilst the localized effect of placental hormones upon uterine function must also be considered.

The hormonal changes during pregnancy are illustrated in Figure 3.3. Progesterone concentrations in the peripheral circulation during the first 14 days of gestation are similar to those of dioestrus; thereafter, those of the non-pregnant cow decline sharply from about the 18th day after ovulation (see Figure 1.28). In the pregnant cow there is normally only a slight fall at this stage with a rapid recovery. Thereafter the concentration increases slightly during pregnancy until it starts to decline at about 20–30 days prepartum. Oestrogen concentrations during early and mid-gestation are low, less than 100 pg/ml; however, towards the end of gestation, in particular after day 250, oestrogen concentrations increase to reach peak values 2–5 days prepartum of 7 ng/ml oestrone sulfate and 1.2 ng/ml oestrone (Thatcher et al., 1980). These rapidly decline about 8 hours prepartum to low levels immediately postpartum.

Both FSH and LH concentrations remain low during gestation and show no significant fluctuations. Prolactin is low during pregnancy until just before calving when it increases from basal levels of 50–60 ng/ml to peak values of 320 ng/ml 20

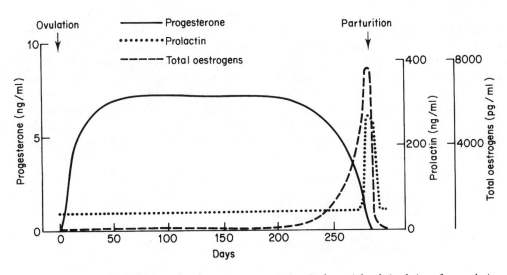

Fig. 3.3 Schematic representation of the trends in hormone concentrations in the peripheral circulation of a cow during pregnancy and at parturition.

L R

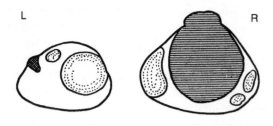

Fig. 3.4 Ovaries of the cow at 35 days of pregnancy. Fetal body length (FBL) 1.6 cm; corpus luteum verum (CLV) yellow.

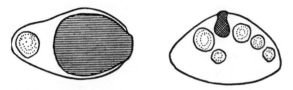

Fig. 3.5 Ovaries of the cow at 48 days of pregnancy. FBL 3.4 cm; CLV orange.

L R

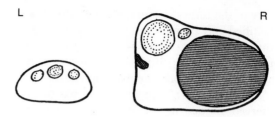

Fig. 3.6 Ovaries of the cow at 70 days of pregnancy. FBL 6.3 cm; CLV yellow–orange.

hours prepartum, until a subsequent decline to basal levels by 30 hours postpartum (Hoffmann et al., 1973). Bovine placental lactogen is present in the peripheral circulation of the dam at about 160 days of gestation, increasing dramatically to maximum concentrations of 1000 ng/ml between 200 days and term (Bolander et al., 1976). The role of this hormone is still unclear but it appears to have prolactin and growth hormone-like activities.

Anatomical changes

Ovaries

In the cow the corpus luteum of pregnancy (corpus luteum verum) persists at its maximum size throughout the whole of the period of gestation. Fundamentally it is indistinguishable from the fully developed corpus luteum of dioestrus, but there are certain features by which its persistence can be recognized when examined post-mortem. The chief is that the protrusion of the structure from

the surface of the ovary is less marked and the epithelium over it is white and scarred. The corpus luteum of oestrus often contains a central lacuna, whereas during pregnancy this becomes filled. It is considered by some that the corpus luteum verum is larger than that of oestrus. The author's series indicates that if this is the case it is too slight to be of significance, and moreover that there are considerable variations in the weights of pregnancy corpora lutea in individuals (3.9–7.5 g) which bear no relationship to the duration of pregnancy. The colour of the corpus luteum of pregnancy, however, differs somewhat from that of dioestrus. There is a wider range from yellow through orange to light brown, and the appearance of the luteal tissue is duller. Figures 3.4–3.9 show drawings of examples of bovine ovaries (natural size) obtained from gravid genital tracts recovered after slaughter. Note the variations in the shape of the ovaries and the position of the corpus luteum verum. In addition, these sagittal sections also show that folliculogenesis and regression continue throughout pregnancy.

As pregnancy advances, the position of the ovaries changes. Their location, however, in non-gravid animals is not constant. In heifers and young cows they are generally situated on each side of, and slightly below, the conjoined cornua at the level of the pelvic brim. They may lie in the pelvic cavity. In multiparous animals they are often situated in the abdominal cavity 5–8 cm in

L R

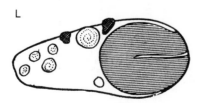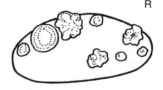

Fig. 3.7 Ovaries of the cow at 100 days of pregnancy. FBL 16 cm; CLV yellow–brown.

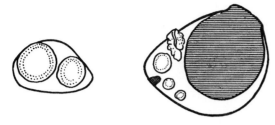

Fig. 3.8 Ovaries of the cow at 120 days of pregnancy. FBL 25 cm; CLV orange.

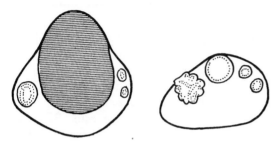

Fig. 3.9 Ovaries of the cow at 190 days of pregnancy. CLV orange.

front of the pelvis, where their detection is more difficult. Consequent on the increase in the weight of the uterus and hypertrophy of the ovarian and uterine ligaments, the ovaries pass deeper and deeper in the abdominal cavity as pregnancy advances. From the fifth month onwards the weight and size of the uterus is such that it sinks down into the abdomen to rest on the abdominal floor. Hammond (1927) found the weight of the uterus and its contents in primigravidae at 5 months to be 48.4 kg. Provided that the animal is comparatively easy to examine, it is generally possible to palpate the ovaries with reasonable certainty up to day 100, by which time in heifers the one on the gravid side is about 8–10 cm in front of, and slightly below, the pelvic brim, and that on the non-gravid side a little nearer the pelvis. In occasional cases both ovaries may be detected as late as day 150, although by this time there is a risk that they will be confused with cotyledons. In the later stages of pregnancy it is not so much that they are beyond the reach of the hand as that one is unable to depress the rectum sufficiently deeply into the abdomen to locate them.

Uterus

During the early stages, detection of an increase in size of the uterus affords strong evidence of pregnancy, but the recognition of these changes necessitates an appreciation of the size of the quiescent uterus in subjects of varying ages and parity (Figure 3.10 and Table 3.2), the quantities of fluid present in the respective fetal sacs and the disposition of those sacs in the uterus (see Figure 2.11).

At 28 days of pregnancy the amniotic sac is spherical in outline and about 2 cm in diameter.

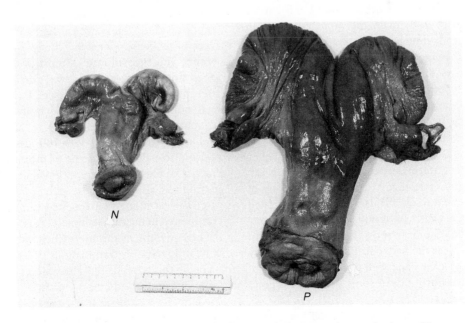

Fig. 3.10 Genital tracts of a nulliparous heifer (N) and pluriparous (seven calves) cow (P).

Table 3.2. Uterine dimensions (non-gravid organ) (cm)

	Unbred nulliparous heifer	Pluriparous cow
Width of conjoined cornua immediately anterior to cervix	2.5	4.0
Width of each cornu at external bifurcation	2.0	3.5
Length of externally connected parts of cornua	9.0	14.0
Length of free portions of cornua	15.0	20.0
Thickness of wall or cornua	0.5	1.2
Length of cervix	5.0	10.0
Width of cervix	3.0	5.0

It occupies the free portion of the gravid horn. The allantoic sac is about 18 cm long, but the amount of contained fluid is insufficient to distend it, and its width is negligible. It occupies almost the whole of the gravid cornu. At this stage the embryo is 0.8 cm long, a quite inappreciable size.

At 35 days, fetal body length is 1.8 cm and the diameter of the spherical amniotic sac 3 cm. They still occupy the free part of the cornua. The conjoined portions of the cornua and the free portion of the non-gravid cornua are not appreciably changed. It is possible, particularly in a heifer easy of examination, that the distension in the free part of the gravid cornua will be detected.

At 60 days the fetal crown–rump length is approximately 6 cm. The amniotic sac is oval and tense, having a transverse measurement of about 5 cm. This causes the free part of the gravid horn to be distended to a width of about 6.5 cm, as compared with 2–3 cm in the quiescent stage in the heifer and young cow. In such subjects this distension may be recognized.

At 80 days the fetus measures 12 cm and the total quantity of fluid is about 1 litre. Distention of the free part of the gravid horn varies from 7 to 10 cm, while that of the conjoined part is but little greater than normal. The greater length of the gravid horn can often be detected.

By 90 days uterine distension is such that it can be detected with accuracy in the great majority of cases. The conjoined cornua are tense, the gravid one having a width of about 9 cm and the non-gravid about 4.5 cm. In most individuals the organ is still high up at the pelvic brim and it is generally possible to pass the hand well over the curvature of the distended horn, but in some multigravid cows the uterus lies in the abdomen, and to palpate it effectively it is necessary to retract the organ by the application of vulsellum forceps to the cervix. Sometimes it is possible to detect the fetus at this stage. Tapping of the distended cornua with the fingers may reveal the fetus rather like a piece of wood floating in the fluid beneath. By gently squeezing the uterus one may be able to pick up the fetus. Its body length is about 15 cm.

By the fourth month the uterus sinks below the pelvic brim, and distension is less easy to recognize as the fluid gravitates towards the extremities of the cornua. The cervix lies on the pelvic brim.

Changes in the size and shape of the gravid uterus during the first 4 months of gestation are shown in Figure 3.11.

Fetus

Several workers (Hammond, 1927; Winters et al., 1942) have recorded fetal body lengths (crown–rump) during the various stages of pregnancy. Data have been collected chiefly from pregnant heifers, and thus allowance must be made for the greater size of the fetus in cows, particularly in the later periods of pregnancy (see Table 3.3). The fetal bulk in relation to these body lengths will be appreciated.

During the period 120–160 days it will be possible to palpate the fetus in more than 50% of cases. The presented extremity will lie within reach in front of and below the pelvic brim. In some cases the fetus may be touched transiently at the commencement of examination and then sinks into the depths of the uterus beyond reach. Similarly, if a series of examinations of an individual is made at this period, the fetus may be detected at some and not at others.

Fig. 3.11 Gravid genital tracts from cows at different stages of gestation. (a) Right horn at 6 weeks. (b) Right horn at 12 weeks. (c) Left horn at 16 weeks. (d) Right horn at 19 weeks.

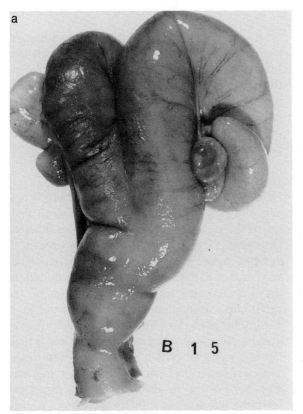

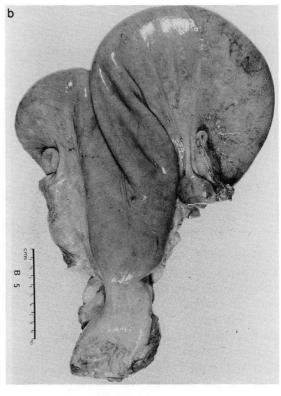

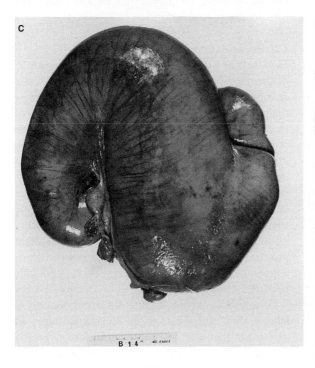

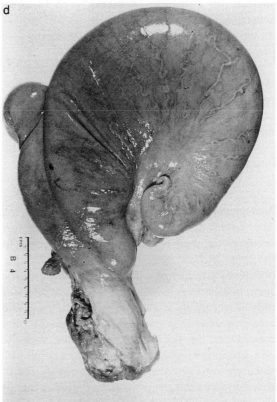

Table 3.3. Fetal body length in cows at various stages of pregnancy

Pregnancy (months)	Fetal body length (cm)
1	0.8
2	6
3	15
4	28
5	40
6	52
7	70
8	80
9	90

Between $5\frac{1}{2}$ and $7\frac{1}{2}$ months the fetus is detected less often than during the previous period. The author would put it at 40–50%. In favourable cases the fetal head and/or flexed limbs are palpated just anterior to the pelvic brim. Touching the fetus often provokes reflex movement.

From $7\frac{1}{2}$ months to the end of gestation the fetus will in the majority of cases be detected readily. Again, however, cases will be encountered, especially in deep-bellied, multiparous cows in which the fetus cannot be detected, at any rate on a single examination, even to term. Several authors (Rüsse, 1968; Dufty, 1973) have shown variations in myometrial tone during late pregnancy.

The latter author found that in a large number of Hereford heifers, which were examined daily by rectal palpation near term, it was frequently impossible to palpate the fetal calf. The reason for this finding was the considerable relaxation of the myometrium, which allowed the calf to descend into the abdomen.

Non-gravid cornu

The extent to which the allantochorionic sac occupies the non-gravid horn varies greatly. In the great majority of bovine pregnancies the sac occupies some part of it, in some it extends to the apex, in others the posterior two-thirds or one-half only is occupied, while in exceptional cases the non-gravid horn is entirely unoccupied by fetal membranes. In the majority of cases also the non-gravid horn plays its part in placentation and its cotyledons hypertrophy, although the degree of cotyledonary enlargement is not as great as that of the pregnant horn. Occasionally the non-gravid horn, although occupied by the allantochorion, plays no part in placentation and its cotyledons remain undeveloped. In such cases, and also in those in which the non-gravid horn is unoccupied, the cotyledons in the gravid horn, particularly those in the region of the fetal trunk, become grossly hypertrophied and may at the time of parturition be as large as 8×12 cm.

Caruncles

Detection of the hypertrophied cotyledons is evidence of pregnancy, but variations occur in their size at the various stages of pregnancy in different individuals. This is probably due to differences in number. Again there is variation throughout the same uterus. Those situated about the middle of the gravid cornu are larger than those of the extremities, while those in the non-gravid horn are smaller than those in the gravid one. (Occasionally there is no placentation in the non-gravid horn.) As pregnancy continues they become progressively larger, until in the terminal stages they may be 5–6 cm in diameter, but because the pregnant uterus sinks into the abdomen, it may not be possible to palpate cotyledons from the fifth to the seventh month.

Uterine arteries

Evidence of pregnancy is afforded by hypertrophy of the middle uterine arteries and a characteristic change in their pulse wave. The latter ceases to be the usual pulse and instead becomes a 'thrill' or tremor. There is considerable variation in the time at which the change can first be felt and also when it becomes continuous. The earliest the author has been able to detect it is at 86 days. During the period 100–175 days cases will frequently be met which 'thrill' at first but later pulsate. It is probable that the degree of pressure applied to the artery infuences the feeling imparted to the fingers; light pressure detects a 'thrill', whereas a pulse wave is apparent to heavy pressure. The 'thrill' generally becomes continous after day 175, although cases will be met in which there is distinct pulsation as late as day 200. During the terminal stages of gestation the uterine arteries become greatly hypertrophied and tortuous; they can be distinctly felt, the thickness of a pencil, with a continuous, tremor-like pulse, laterally situated 2 cm or so in front of the anterior border of the iliac shaft. A difference in size of the two uterine arteries is usually recognizable from about day 100, and this indicates the side of the pregnant cornu.

Fremitus in the posterior uterine arteries was detected between 200 and 248 days on the gravid side and between 235 and 279 days on the non-gravid side (Tsolov, 1978). He also found that the onset of fremitus was later the greater the number of times the cow had been pregnant.

Pregnant side

It is generally accepted that dairy cows are more often pregnant in the right uterine cornua, and that the corpus luteum is in the ovary on the side of the pregnant horn. In a large series of pregnant bovine uteri examined by the author the proportion has been 60 right-side pregnancies to 40 left-side; in only one case was the fetus present in the cornua opposite to the ovary containing the corpus luteum; another case showed a corpus luteum of normal size in each ovary with a single fetus in the right horn. In a series of 1506 uteri of dairy cattle examined in the USA, Erdheim (1942) found the fetus in the right horn in 1015 (67.4%) and in the left in 474 (31.4%). In a series of 2318 uteri of beef cattle, however, the side incidence of pregnancy was approximately equal: right, 1178 (50.8%), and left, 1121 (48.3%). Among all Erdheim's specimens there was one exceptional single pregnancy in which he found the corpus luteum in the left ovary and fetus in the right horn. Of 133 pregnant uteri from Swedish Highland cattle, Setterg-

ren and Galloway (1965) found 59.4% pregnant on the right side and 40.6% on the left. This series also included one specimen in which the corpus luteum was in the left ovary and the fetus in the right horn.

Twinning

World statistics show incidences of 1.04% of twins in dairy cattle and 0.5% in beef cattle (Gilmore, 1952) but carefully kept individual breed records show higher figures: 2.7–8.85% for Brown Swiss, 3.08–3.3% for Holsteins, 2.8% for Ayrshires, 1.95% for Guernseys and 1% for Jerseys (Meadows and Lush, 1957; Johansson, 1968). The rate increases with age, and figures for Holsteins show 1.3% for heifers rising to 7% in 10-year-old cows.

In the majority of cases one corpus luteum is present in each ovary and a fetus in each horn. Not infrequently, however, two corpora lutea are found in a single ovary with gestation bicornual. In 25 pairs of twins in Erdheim's series five were unilateral. This observed natural preponderance of bilaterally disposed twins conforms with the experimental results of Rowson et al. (1971) which showed that induced twin pregnancies were more stable when an embryo was transplanted into each horn than when two embryos were placed in one horn. Arthur (1956) and Erdheim (1942) each encountered only one case of identical twinning — a single corpus luteum with two developing fetuses — and the aggregate

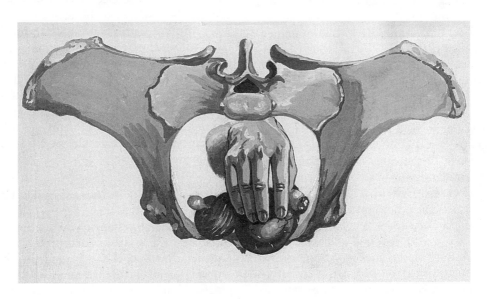

Fig. 3.12 Detection of pregnancy in the cow by rectal examination. Uterus gravid 70 days.

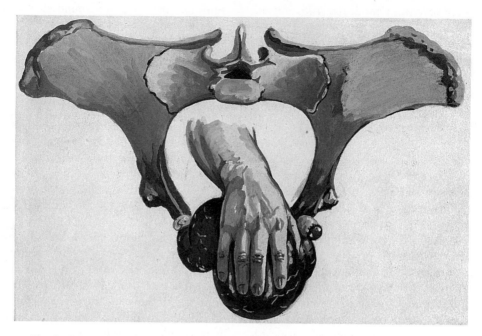

Fig. 3.13 Detection of pregnancy in the cow by rectal examination. Uterus gravid 90 days.

recorded statistics for identical twinning is 4–6% of all twins. The incidence of bovine triplets is 1 in about 7500 single births.

Methods of pregnancy diagnosis

Rectal palpation (Figures 3.12–3.15) has been used for pregnancy diagnosis in the cow during the last 50 years and is still generally accepted as the simplest and most reliable method. However, it is surprising how few farmers have cows examined. In the UK, figures produced by the Milk Marketing Board in 1969 showed that in 767 herds which used the artificial insemination service, 67% had no pregnancy diagnosis performed at all and only 6.5% had all of their cows examined. A more recent survey performed in 1979 (Newton et al., 1982) reported some improvement of use of pregnancy diagnosis. In this study of 1692 dairy herds using Milk Marketing Board artificial insemination services, 42% had no veterinary pregnancy diagnosis done, 14.2% had more than half, and 43.8% had less than half their cows examined. There was greater use in pedigree than non-pedigreee herds. Failure to return to oestrus after service or artificial insemination is used by the herdsman as an indication of pregnancy. However, it should be remembered that cows and heifers sometimes show signs of oestrus during pregnancy, some individuals showing signs on three separate occasions (Donald, 1943). Thus, if this is used as the sole method of diagnosis, a number of cows will be incorrectly assumed to be non-pregnant.

Conversely, how reliable is the detection of oestrus? In a large group of cows it can be expected that about 65% will not return to oestrus after natural service or artificial insemination and can be assumed to be pregnant, whilst 35% will return to oestrus and can be assumed to have failed to conceive. However, assuming the average oestrous detection rate in the UK is 60% (see Chapter 1) therefore 14% of cows will be incorrectly assumed to be in calf. This constitutes a large error and fully justifies the use of diagnostic procedures. Table 3.4 gives a list of the methods of pregnancy diagnosis available and the earliest time that they can be made.

Failure to return to oestrus and persistence of the corpus luteum

Failure of the regression of the corpus luteum at about 21 days, as determined by rectal palpation, provides a method of anticipating that the cow is probably pregnant. It is seldom used as a practical procedure and there are reasons (see Chapter 23) for the corpus luteum persisting in the absence of

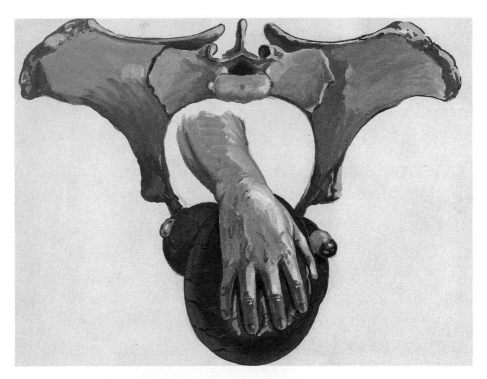

Fig. 3.14 Detection of pregnancy in the cow by rectal examination. Uterus gravid 110 days.

pregnancy. Rectal examination at about this time in an individual which was close to or at oestrus would demonstrate the presence of a turgid, coiled uterus and a mucous vaginal discharge.

Progesterone concentration in plasma and milk

In 1971, Robertson and Sarda described a method of diagnosing pregnancy by the determination of the progesterone concentration in the plasma of cows. Since the corpus luteum persists as a result of the pregnancy, if a blood sample is taken at about 21 days after the previous oestrus progesterone levels remain elevated. If the cow is not pregnant and is close to or at oestrus then the progesterone levels will be low; this can be seen if the progesterone curves in Figures 1.28 and 3.3 are studied. Although this is a perfectly valid and reliable laboratory method, it has the one disadvantage that it requires the collection of a blood sample by a veterinary surgeon.

In 1969, Heap et al. showed that progesterone crossed the mammary gland and appeared in milk. Laing and Heap (1971) confirmed that the changes in progesterone concentrations in the milk closely followed those in the blood or plasma. Further-

more, since progesterone is very soluble in milk fat there were higher concentrations per unit volume in milk than in the blood or plasma. Heap et al. (1973) described the use of the technique to diagnose pregnancy, and since then a large number of different workers in many different countries of the world have described similar methods. The technique depends upon the herdsman collecting about 20 ml of milk, usually at the afternoon milking because the fat content is higher, into a glass or plastic bottle. Then a tablet of potassium dichromate and mercuric chloride as a preservative is added; provided that the sample is not exposed to high temperature or excessive ultraviolet light there is very little loss of progesterone activity.

Initially, progesterone concentrations in the milk were assayed using the method of radioimmunoassay, it is an effective method of measurement but requires the use of radio-isotopes and the equipment to measure radioactive emissions. It can only be performed in a specialist laboratory and hence has the big disadvantage of taking several days before a result is known.

A number of qualitative 'cow-side' tests have been developed which can be used on the farm

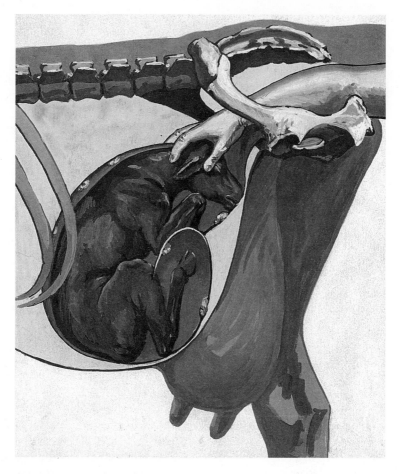

Fig. 3.15 Detection of pregnancy in the cow by rectal examination. Pregnancy approaching term.

Table 3.4. Methods of pregnancy diagnosis in the cow

Method	Earliest time
Real-time ultrasound (direct imaging)	13 days
Failure to return to oestrus and persistence of corpus luteum	21 days
Progesterone concentration in plasma and milk	21–24 days
Assay of pregnancy-specific protein B (PSPB)	24 days
Palpation of the allantochorion (membrane slip)	33 days
Unilateral cornual enlargement and disparity in size, thinning of the uterine wall, fluid-filled fluctuation of enlarged horns	35 days
Palpation of the early fetus when the amnion loses its turgidity	45–60 days
Palpation of the caruncles/cotyledons	80 days
Hypertrophy of the middle uterine artery until presence of fremitus	85 days
Oestrone sulfate in blood or milk	105 days
Palpation of the fetus	120 days

and hence enable the herdsman to obtain a result within 1 hour of collecting the milk sample. All the necessary reagents and equipment are provided in kit form. Semiquantitative or fully quantitative tests are also available but these are designed for use in a veterinary practice laboratory, since they require a minimum amount of equipment and some expertise. Both tests are

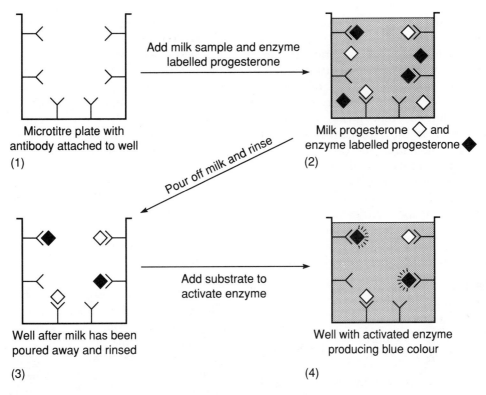

Add milk sample and enzyme labelled progesterone

Microtitre plate with antibody attached to well
(1)

Milk progesterone ◇ and enzyme labelled progesterone ◆
(2)

Pour off milk and rinse

Well after milk has been poured away and rinsed

(3)

Add substrate to activate enzyme

Well with activated enzyme producing blue colour

(4)

Fig. 3.16 ELISA using a microtitre plate.

based on the enzyme-linked immunosorbent assay (ELISA).

The basic principle of the assay is as follows: the plastic wells of the microtitre plates are precoated with a specific progesterone antibody; a milk sample, containing unlabelled progesterone if the cow is pregnant or in dioestrus, is added to each well, together with a fixed quantity of progesterone labelled with an enzyme (usually alkaline phosphatase). After a period of incubation all the contents of the wells are washed away; however, progesterone will remain bound to the antibody and hence the well. A substrate reagent is then added to each of the wells, which, after the second incubation period, reacts with the enzyme-labelled progesterone to produce a colour reaction. The colour can be assessed visually or by a spectrophotometer by comparison with those produced by known standard solutions of progesterone. The amount of labelled progesterone that remains bound to the antibody on the wells is inversely proportional to the amount of unlabelled progesterone in the milk sample. Thus, the higher the concentration of progesterone in the unknown milk sample, the less labelled progesterone will adhere to the wells

and hence the lighter the colour reaction. Zero progesterone in the milk sample will result in the most intense colour reaction. The procedure is outlined and illustrated in Figure 3.16. Rapid, solid phase, dip-stick methods are likely to become available.

The laboratory-based quantitative tests have a series of progesterone standards that enable a standard curve to be drawn: it is usually recommended that duplicate assays are done for each sample, at least until the operator becomes conversant with the procedure.

There are a few problems in using the assay on the farm. These can be summarized as follows: (1) instructions are not always readily understood by persons not used to laboratory procedures; (2) simple equipment requires a fair degree of manual dexterity; (3) instructions should be closely adhered to, particularly with regard to timing of incubation and quantities of reagents; (4) the kits should be kept in a refrigerator at 4°C and should be allowed to warm to room temperature before use, they should not be heated; (5) interpretation of the colour differences can be difficult for some persons; (6) milk samples should be kept at 2–8°C until assayed, and the recommended preservative tablets must be used.

The optimum time for collecting the milk sample is 24 days after service or artificial insemination (Heap et al., 1976). This time interval prevents those cows with a longer than average interoestrus interval from giving false-positive results; however, in those animals with a shorter than average interoestrus interval, false positives will occur. The accuracy of the method in the diagnosis of pregnancy is between 80 and 88% (Heap et al., 1976; Hoffmann et al., 1976; Koegood-Johnsen and Christiansen, 1977); the accuracy of the method for detecting the absence of pregnancy is nearly 100%.

The reasons for false-negative results are:

1. Mistaken identity of the animal either on the farm or in the laboratory.
2. Milk storage problems due to excessive heat or ultraviolet light.
3. Low progesterone production by the corpus luteum.
4. Inadequate mixing of milk so that a low fat sample is obtained.

The reasons for false-positive results are:

1. Cows with shorter than average interoestrus intervals. When milk samples are taken 24 days after service or artificial insemination, if the cow is not pregnant she will already be in the luteal phase of the next cycle.
2. Embryonic death, if it occurs after the day when the milk was collected (see Chapter 24).
3. Luteal cysts which produce progesterone (see Chapter 22).
4. Incorrect timing of insemination. Several reports (Hoffmann et al., 1976) have shown that up to 15% of cows are presented for artificial insemination when they are not in oestrus. Thus if a milk sample is taken 24 days after the cow was incorrectly inseminated in early or mid-dioestrus, then she will be in the subsequent dioestrus, with a functional corpus luteum and elevated milk progesterone concentrations.
5. Pathological prolongation of the lifespan of the corpus luteum; this will be discussed in Chapter 23.

The main advantage of the milk progesterone test is that, with the exception of transrectal B-mode ultrasound imaging, it identifies those cows that are not pregnant before it is possible to do so by other methods, such as rectal palpation. A 24 day sample will enable the herdsman to anticipate the return to oestrus 42 days after the service if she is not pregnant, or enable the veterinarian to examine the animal, if she is a problem, before she returns again. Cows which are found to be pregnant at 24 days should be checked at a later date by rectal palpations. The on-farm tests can be used as early as 19 days after service since a low progesterone concentration at this time is highly indicative of non-pregnancy and thus the first return to oestrus can be anticipated (see p. 449). Daily sequential samples can be taken at or around this time, but it is expensive and time-consuming for the herdsman.

Assay of pregnancy-specific protein B (PSPB)

This protein has been identified in the maternal serum of cows from 24 days of gestation; the concentration is measured by radio-immunoassay (Sasser and Ruder, 1987). It is secreted from the binucleate cells of the trophoblastic ectoderm (Reimers et al., 1985), and thus its presence can be used to confirm pregnancy. However, since it has a long biological half-life it can also be identified in serum for many weeks postpartum.

At present, it can only be measured by radio-immunoassay but, with the development of suitable ELISA methods, it could well become an 'on-farm' diagnostic test (Sasser and Ruder, 1987).

Palpation of the amniotic vesicle

The method was first described in 1923 by two German veterinarians Pissl and Rüther (see Cowie, 1948) who reported that they were able to identify the amnion towards the end of the first month of pregnancy. Several others (Schmidt, 1932; Wisnicky and Casida, 1948; Studer, 1969; Abbitt et al., 1978) have described the technique and commented upon its safety and accuracy. The method is briefly as follows. The bifurcation of the uterine horns is located, the horns uncoiled and gently palpated along their entire length between the thumb and middle two fingers. The amniotic sac can be felt as a distinct, round turgid object 1–2 cm in diameter floating in the allantoic fluid. The vesicle should not be compressed directly but gently pushed backwards and forwards.

Others (Rowson and Dott, 1963; Ball and Carroll, 1963; Zemjanis, 1971) consider that this technique is dangerous because of the possibility of rupture of the amniotic sac or of the embryonic heart. As with all rectal techniques care is the rule, and excessive pressure and rough handling should be avoided.

Palpation of the allantochorion (membrane slip)

The method is dependent upon the fact that in the cow, attachment of the allantochorion to the endometrium occurs only between the cotyledons and the caruncles and that the intercotyledonary part of the fetal membrane is free.

The method was first described by Abelein (1928) (see Cowie, 1948) who reported that it could be used from the fifth week of gestation. It was subsequently popularized by Euler (1930) (see Cowie, 1948), Götze (1940) and Fincher (1943). The method is as follows. Identify the bifurcation of the uterine horns, pick up the enlarged, gravid horn between thumb and either index or middle finger just cranial to the bifurcation and gently squeeze the whole thickness of the horn. The allantochorion will be eventually identified as a very fine structure as it slips between the thumb and finger before the uterine and rectal walls are lost from grasp. It is important in the early stages of pregnancy to grasp the whole width of the horn because as the allantochorion is very thin at this stage the structure which can be more readily identified is the connective tissue band which contains the blood vessels supplying the allantochorion (see Figure 2.1). Fincher (1943) recommended that it should not be used before 40 days of gestation and that it was infallible up to 95 days. The advantage of the method is that it enables the differential diagnosis of pregnancy from mucometra or pyometra. In some cases, particularly after 60 days of gestation, it can be more readily elicited in the non-gravid horn since the tension on the wall is less and this allows it to be grasped more readily.

For the beginner it is a worthwhile exercise to practise it on a fresh gravid genital tract from the abattoir.

Unilateral cornual enlargement

Unless there are twin conceptuses, one in each horn, it is possible to detect a difference in the size of the two horns. This is largely due to the presence of fetal fluids, in particular allantoic fluid, which gives the uterine horn a fluctuating feel with good tone. It can be likened to the feel of a toy balloon which has been filled with water to a point when the wall just starts to stretch. At the same time, if the wall of the horn is squeezed it is noticeable that it is much thinner than that of a non-gravid tract.

In many cases a definite diagnosis of pregnancy can be made on these signs alone. The presence of a corpus luteum in the ovary adjacent to the enlarged horn is a useful confirmatory sign; however, a false diagnosis of pregnancy may be made in cases of pyometra, mucometra or incomplete uterine involution (see Chapter 7).

Palpation of the early fetus

At about 45–50 days of gestation the amniotic sac becomes less turgid, and it is sometimes possible to palpate directly the small devloping fetus. This should be done with care.

Palpation of caruncles/cotyledons

Caruncles/cotyledons first become recognizable by rectal palpation at about 90–100 days. They are first felt in the midline, about 8–10 cm in front of and over the pelvic brim, by pressing down upon the uterine body and base of the horns. In the early stages it is difficult to identify them as distinct, individual structures. The uterus feels as if it has an irregular corrugated surface; it has been likened to palpating a sackful of small potatoes. As pregnancy proceeds, the cotyledons become larger, but once the uterus has sunk into the abdomen between 5 and 7 months, it is frequently impossible to palpate them.

Identification of cotyledons is virtually diagnostic of pregnancy, but in the immediate postpartum uterus they can also be felt.

Hypertrophy and fremitus of the middle uterine arteries

In a non-gravid or early pregnant cow, identification of the middle uterine artery is impossible by rectal palpation. The artery runs in the broad ligament, along a tortuous course, passing downwards and forwards over the pelvic brim. Usually, it is identified 5–10 cm lateral to the cervix. Inexperienced persons sometimes confuse it with the iliac and obturator arteries, but the middle uterine artery is very mobile and can be encircled with thumb and finger.

Identification of hypertrophy and fremitus of the middle uterine artery is usually regarded as

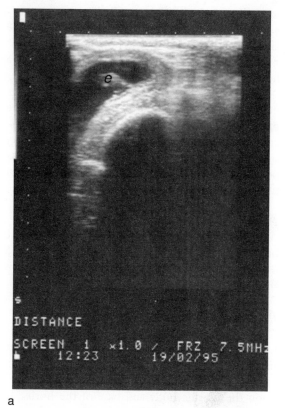

a

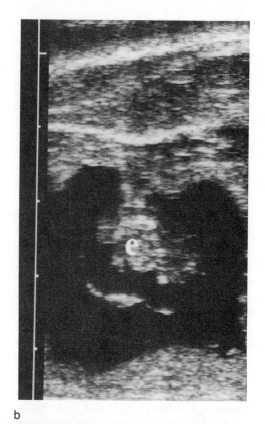

b

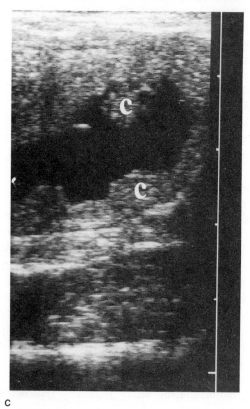

c

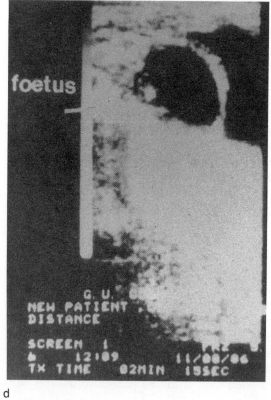

d

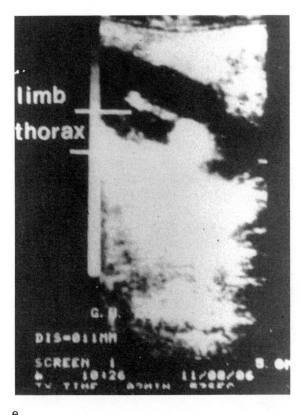

limb

thorax

e

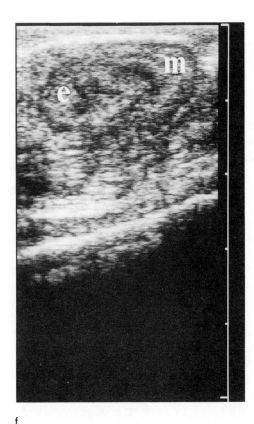

m

e

f

Fig. 3.17 Transrectal B-mode ultrasound images of the gravid uterus of a cow using 7.5 MH$_Z$ transducer. (a) At 32 days of gestation. Note embryo (e) surrounded by anechoic (black) area of amniotic fluid. (b) At 38 days of gestation. Note embryo (e). (c) At 38 days of gestation. Note rudimentary caruncles (c). (d) At 41 days of gestation. Note fetus. (e) At 59 days of gestation. (f) Cross-section of non-gravid uterine horn. Note endometrium (e) and muscularis (m).

diagnostic of pregnancy, but it also persists for a few days postpatum, and is present in established cases of pyometra.

Palpation of the fetus

Palpation of the fetus, either per rectum or by abdominal ballottement, is diagnostic of pregnancy. The ease of palpation depends upon the size of the cow, the degree of stretching of the suspension of the uterus and the degree of relaxation of the rectum and uterine wall.

Other methods

Abdominal Ballottement. This is often possible as early as 7 months of gestation in some small breeds such as the Jersey. However, in some fat cows of large breeds it is sometimes impossible even at term.

The method involves fairly vigorous pummel-ling of the ventral abdomen and flank with clenched fists. The object is to push the fetus, which is floating in the fetal fluids, away from the body wall and then identify it as it swings back against the fist which is kept pressed against the abdominal wall.

Vaginal Examination. Examination may be manual or visual. In the latter case, an illuminated speculum is used. The condition of the vaginal mucous membrane does not afford definite clinical evidence of pregnancy, for the degree of 'dryness' and blanching which occur during the dioestrous period are very similar to those of pregnancy. It is to the external os of the cervix that attention is directed. During pregnancy the secretion of the cervical glands becomes gelatinous and tough, forming a plug for sealing the canal. In many cases the seal covers or protrudes from the external os. It has developed by day 60.

On manual examination the finger should be pressed gently into the os. The detection of an adhesive, tenacious secretion rather than a slimy, moist one is strong evidence of pregnancy. With a speculum the seal can sometimes be seen, light brown in colour, covering the os. In many cases, however, the seal occupies the canal only and cannot be detected with certainty.

Mammary Glands. Mammary changes during pregnancy are best observed in primigravida. The teats of the pregnant heifer commence to enlarge about the fourth month and with a little experience it is an easy matter to distinguish them from those of the non-pregnant or early pregnant animal. From the sixth month the mammary glands become more firm to the touch and their enlargement can be seen. Hypertrophy is progressive and is particularly marked during the terminal month. As parturition approaches the glands become grossly enlarged and oedematous and the teats take on a waxy, tumefied appearance. The abdominal wall, particularly in the region of the umbilicus, may also become swollen by oedema. In the dry, milch cow, mammary enlargement occurs during the last 14 or so days of pregnancy. After the fourth month a honey-like secretion may be withdrawn from the teats of pregnant heifers.

Cervix. Evidence of pregnancy can be assumed when there is tension on the cervix. In the nonpregnant or early pregnant cow or heifer the cervix is freely moveable from side to side. However, as pregnancy advances the cervix becomes less mobile and it is pulled forwards and downwards over the pelvic brim.

Ultrasonic Techniques. Using the ultrasonic fetal pulse detector which employs the Doppler principle it is possible to identify the fetal heart from 6–7 weeks using a rectal probe. Ultrasonic depth analysers (A mode) have been used to detect pregnancy as early as 40 days. Although a level of accuracy of 85–95% has been achieved in positively identifying pregnant cows, a large percentage of non-pregnant cows (57–87%) were incorrectly diagnosed as being pregnant (Tierney, 1983). Neither of these two ultrasonic methods would appear to have any advantage over rectal palpation with regard to time of examination or accuracy of the diagnosis. Real-time B-mode grey scale ultrasound scanning is rapidly becoming the method of choice for the early diagnosis of pregnancy in the cow. The limiting factors are the price of the

equipment and its comparative lack of mobility for on-farm use; both are likely to change in the future. Details of the principle of the technique and the equipment available have been described earlier (see p. 69). For an excellent description, the reader is advised to consult Boyd and Omran (1991).

The uterus is imaged transrectally; for early pregnancies a 7.5 MHz linear transducer is required, whereas a 3.5 MHz transducer is preferable for late pregnancies. After insertion of the transducer both ovaries should be examined to determine the presence of a corpus luteum (see p. 21), followed by the right and left horns. Because of the shape of the probe, the diameter of the rectum and the coiled nature of the horns, it is impossible to scan each horn along its length at the same time, thus cross-sectional images of the horns are frequently identified (Figure 3.17 (f)). Diagnosis of an early pregnancy is dependent upon the identification of a non-echogenic (black) area within the lumen of the uterine horn due to the presence of fetal fluids. Since this occurs first in the horn ipsilateral to the corpus luteum of pregnancy, ovarian imaging for the presence of this structure is important.

Using a 7.5 MHz transducer, Boyd et al. (1988) were able to confirm pregnancy as early as 9 days, whilst Pierson and Ginther (1984) using a 5 MHz transducer were able to do so at 12 and 14 days in heifers before the blastocyst had elongated (see Chapter 2). By 17 days the blastocyst will have elongated and extended into the contralateral horn; this can usually be easily identified by 26 days.

Experienced persons can accurately diagnose pregnancy, either at the time of, or before, the expected date of return to oestrus in the non-pregnant cyclical animal. This is also true up to 30 days; however, after this stage an accurate and rapid diagnosis can be made relatively easily.

Figure 3.17 shows images at various stages of pregnancy.

The technique can be used to estimate fetal age up to 140 days of gestation (White et al., 1985) following the measurement of a number of different fetal dimensions; of these, the crown–rump length was least frequently capable of being measured, whereas the trunk diameter was the most readily assessed.

Fetal Electrocardiography. Fetal electrocardiography has been noted as a method of pregnancy diagnosis (Larks et al., 1960; Lindahl et al., 1968).

It is not applicable before 5 months of gestation, but it might have application for the diagnosis of multiple pregnancies.

Oestrone Sulfate in Milk. Oestrone sulfate is quantitatively one of the major oestrogens in the milk of pregnant, lactating cows. During gestation the concentration increases gradually so that after day 105 it is present in the milk of all pregnant animals, whereas in non-pregnant individuals it is low or undetectable; the source of the hormone is the fetoplacental unit. The identification of oestrone sulfate in the milk of a cow of 105 days of gestation, or later, is a very reliable method of pregnancy diagnosis (Hamon et al., 1981). Furthermore, unlike progesterone assays the precise date of sampling is not required. However, it has limited applications because of the lateness of the time that a positive diagnosis is obtained.

The optimum time of pregnancy diagnosis

The aim of pregnancy tests is to identify, as early and as accurately as possible, the absence of pregnancy so that steps can be taken to ensure that she is served again and thus ensure an optimum calving pattern (see Chapter 24). However, it is important that inexperienced veterinarians should select a time when they are confident of their accuracy in making the diagnosis, irrespective of the method used.

Accuracy of pregnancy diagnosis by rectal palpation

It is difficult to obtain reliable information on the accuracy of rectal palpation. However, Hancock (1962) and Meacham et al. (1976) report between 94.9 and 99.1% of positive and negative diagnoses.

The most likely reason for making a false-positive diagnosis is subsequent embryonic or fetal death, which is impossible to exclude. Other reasons for false positives are incomplete uterine involution (see Chapter 7), pyometra, mucometra and hydrometra (see Chapter 23) and failure to retract the uterus. The reasons for false negatives are incorrect recording of the date of service or artificial insemination, so that when the cow is examined she is pregnant but a cycle length earlier than expected, and incomplete retraction of the uterus. The latter reason is worthy of further consideration and can be a particular problem in

large pluriparous cows with deep abdomens. In order to make a complete examination of the uterus by palpation full retraction is necessary. The inexperienced person may well make a diagnosis of pregnancy because the uterus is out of reach and cannot be palpated. It is important that the diagnosis should be made on the identification of positive signs. It is perfectly permissible to admit uncertainty, to note in writing the changes that can be identified and re-examine the animal in 2 or 3 weeks time.

Induced prenatal death due to rectal palpation

Concern is sometimes expressed that rectal palpation can induce embryonic or fetal death. There have been several studies to evaluate the risks, either by recording if a cow failed to calve having previously been diagnosed as being pregnant by rectal palpation or, more recently, in association with milk progesterone assays.

The results have been equivocal, but although it is possible that certain methods and certain individuals may increase the incidence of prenatal death, it is likely that the rectal palpation of cows at 41–45 days of gestation is a safe and reliable method when performed carefully and skilfully. In those cows where the pregnancy failed, it would probably have occurred irrespective of the procedure used. Furthermore, in experiments where attempts have been made to induce abortion by damaging the fetus at rectal palpation, extensive trauma has frequently been necessary (Paisley et al., 1978).

PREGNANCY AND ITS DIAGNOSIS IN THE SOW

Endocrinology

In the non-pregnant sow the plasma progesterone concentration falls rapidly 15–16 days after the previous oestrus, but if conception occurs the corpora lutea persist and the peripheral progesterone level remains elevated at between 30 and 35 ng/ml. Although there is a slight fall to 17–18 ng/ml on day 24, the elevated level persists for most of the gestation, decreasing rapidly just before farrowing. The ovaries and corpora lutea are always necessary for the maintenance of pregnancy. The number of embryos present in utero does not influence the progesterone concentration (Monk and Erb, 1974). The minimum concentration of progesterone in the peripheral circulation for the maintenance of pregnancy is about 6 ng/ml (Ellicott and Dzuik, 1973); at lower levels the pregnancy is lost but higher levels do not appear to increase embryonic survival.

Total oestrogen concentrations remain fairly constant during pregnancy but about 2–3 weeks prepartum they begin to increase to about 100 pg/ml, with a sudden surge to values about 500 pg/ml a few days before farrowing. This is followed by a rapid decline after parturition. Oestrone sulfate rises to a peak at 20–30 days of gestation, which is used as a method of diagnosing pregnancy (see later).

Methods of pregnancy diagnosis

Traditionally, failure to return to oestrus at 18–22 days after service or artificial insemination has been regarded as a sign of pregnancy. However, the detection of oestrus can be difficult, and it is time-consuming; even the back pressure or riding test, which is generally accepted to be the most reliable (Reed, 1969), is inconsistent. Failure to return to oestrus may be due to a reluctance to show signs, anoestrus or ovarian cysts. It is important to know as soon as possible if a sow or gilt is not pregnant so that she can be served again, treated or culled. A reliable method is also necessary so that breeders can certify that an animal is pregnant before sale. Any technique must be accurate, capable of being used early in gestation and fairly inexpensive.

Rectal palpation

The method was first described by Huchzermeyer and Plonait (1960) and Keel-Diffey (1963), and more recently by Meredith (1976) and Cameron (1977). It is dependent upon palpation per rectum of the cervix, uterus and middle uterine arteries. The details of the method according to Cameron (1977) are as follows.

0–21 Days of Gestation. The cervix and uterus feel very similar to their state at dioestrus (see Chapter 1). However, during this period the bifurcation of the cornua becomes less distinct and the uterus becomes slightly enlarged, with soft walls. The middle uterine artery increases to approximately 5 mm in diameter towards the third week. It is located as it passes across the external iliac artery (the latter can be identified as it runs along the anteromedial border of the ilium towards the hindleg, ventrally and slightly posteriorly; it is about 1 cm in diameter in the adult sow) running forwards towards the abdominal cavity.

21–30 Days of Gestation. The bifurcation of the cornua is less distinct, the cervix and uterine walls are flaccid and thin. The middle uterine artery is 5–8 mm in diameter and more easily identified.

31–60 Days of Gestation. The cervix feels like a soft-walled tubular structure; the uterus is ill defined and thin walled. The middle uterine artery has enlarged to about the same size as the external iliac. Fremitus can be first identified at 35 days to 37 days (Meredith, 1976); the pulse pattern can be compared with that of the external iliac artery.

60 Days to Term. The middle uterine artery is greater in diameter than the external iliac and it has strong fremitus; it now crosses the external iliac artery more dorsally than before. Only towards the end of gestation is it possible to palpate piglets at the level of the cornual bifurcation.

The technique can be performed without the need of much restraint, preferably when the animal is feeding. Unfortunately, it is not possible to perform the technique in gilts because they are too small, and even in large sows a slender arm is advantageous. Cameron (1977) found that between 30 and 60 days of gestation he was 94% accurate in making a diagnosis of pregnancy and 97% accurate in diagnosing non-pregnancy, whilst Meredith (1976) reported an accuracy of 99% and 86%, respectively. The accuracy improves with experience and advancing pregnancy.

Ultrasonic methods

The use of the fetal pulse detector (Doppler) to diagnose pregnancy in the sow was first described by Fraser and Robertson (1967). The earliest diagnosis made using a rectal probe is about 25 days of gestation. The accuracy of the method is reasonable for the diagnosis of pregnant sows (92–100%) but it is less reliable for non-pregnant sows (25–100%) (McCaughey, 1979).

Ultrasonic amplitude–depth analysis (A-mode ultrasound) has proved to be more reliable. In a

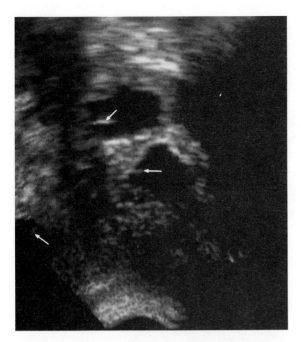

Fig. 3.18 Transabdominal B-mode (5 MHz transducer) ultrasound image of a pregnant sow 25 days after service. Note embryos (arrows) surrounded by amniotic fluid (black). (By courtesy of M. J. Meredith.)

study involving 1001 sows using a 2 MHz external transducer probe, Lindahl et al. (1975) reported a 99% accuracy in identifying pregnant sows and a 98% accuracy for non-pregnant sows. These results were obtained between 30 and 90 days of gestation; unreliable results were obtained before 30 days. Similar results were obtained in a smaller sample of 84 sows which were examined between 30 and 64 days after service.

B-mode direct imaging has proved to be very successful in the sow. The transducer probe is applied to the abdominal wall of the standing sow about 5 cm posterior to the umbilicus, to the right of the mid-line and just lateral to the teats, and is directed towards the posterior abdomen; a coupling medium is always required. In a study of 145 sows, Inabe et al. (1983) reported a 100% accuracy for the diagnosis of pregnancy from 22 days of gestation. Similarly Jackson (1980) reported a 100% accuracy for identifying non-pregnant sows and a 99% accuracy for diagnosing pregnancy from 24 to 37 days of gestation. The small number of errors in this study of 285 sows was due to prenatal death. Using a simple 5 MHz rectal probe a correct diagnosis of pregnancy was made in 10 sows between 12 and 20 days (mean

15.4 days) (Thayer et al., 1985). Figure 3.18 is a computer-enhanced transabdominal ultrasound image of a gravid sow at 25 days of gestation.

Vaginal biopsy

Histological assessment of the number of layers of the stratified squamous epithelium of the vaginal mucosa obtained by biopsy (Figure 3.19) can be used as a method of diagnosing pregnancy in the sow (Done and Heard, 1968; Morton and Rankin, 1969).

The accuracy of this method between 30 and 90 days of pregnancy is over 90%. Between 18 and 22 days after service it is 97 and 94% for the diagnosis of pregnancy and non-pregnancy, respectively (McCaughey, 1979). There is no doubt that the difference in the histological picture is greater between oestrus and pregnancy than between dioestrus and pregnancy. The diagnosis depends on the number of layers of vaginal epithelial cells, which, in turn, relates to the endocrine state; thus during pro-oestrus, when oestrogen is dominant, a rapid proliferation of the stratum germinativum occurs so that at oestrus there are up to 20 layers (Figure 3.19(a)). From the end of oestrus and throughout the luteal phase, when progesterone is dominant, the depth of vaginal epithelium falls so that by day 11 or 12 there are only three or four irregularly arranged layers (Figure 3.19(b)) and only two or three layers in late dioestrus. With the onset of pregnancy progesterone domination continues, and by day 26 the typical histological picture is two parallel rows of epithelial cells with condensed darkly staining nuclei (Figure 3.19(c) and (d)). This pattern persists until the final 3 weeks of gestation. In deciding when to apply this test one should remember that if return to oestrus has inadvertently occurred and the sow is tested at, say, 32–35 days after service, she may then actually be between days 11 and 14 of the second dioestrus when the histology is not markedly different from pregnancy. The best time to test is from 18 to 25 days after mating.

Sections taken erroneously from the cervix or posterior vagina are unsatisfactory for diagnosis.

False-negative results are probably due to errors in the processing of the tissue or mistaken identification of the animal or sample. The same reasons can also account for the false-positive results, although sows which are sampled during the luteal phase of the oestrous cycle or which

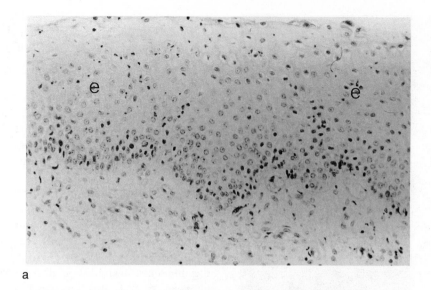

a

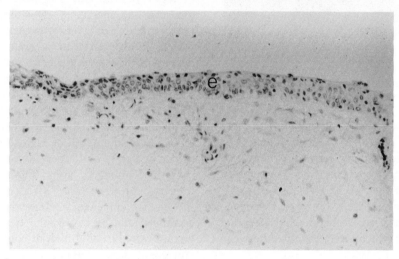

b

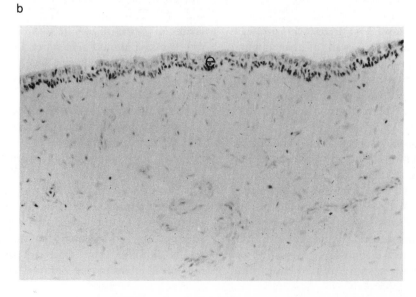

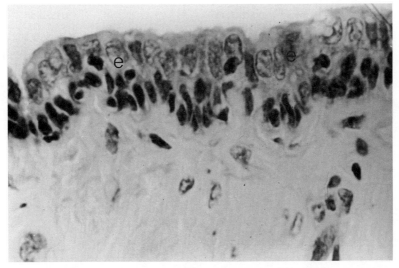

d

Fig. 3.19 Photomicrographs of sections of sow's vaginal wall biopsies. (a) At oestrus with multilayered epithelium (× 350). (b) During dioestrus (day 10) (× 350). (c) At 32 days of gestation (× 350). (d) At 32 days of gestation (× 1000). Note epithelium (e).

subsequently resorb or abort can be causes of error. However, the technique is a satisfactory one, the big disadvantages being the cost of the procedure and the delay in knowing the result of the test.

Estimation of plasma progesterone

Since there is a decline in progesterone concentrations in the peripheral blood from about day 16 in non-pregnant cyclical animals (see Figure 1.30) estimation of progesterone levels from this time after service would be worthwhile. Meding and Koegood-Johnsen (1978) reported that when sows were bled 16–24 days after service a 96% accuracy of pregnancy diagnosis was achieved; they assumed that values in the plasma ≥ 7.5 ng/ml were indicative of pregnancy. Because of the irregularity of the interoestrus interval it was more reliable in identifying those sows which were not pregnant. The biggest problem with technique was the difficulty of obtaining blood samples.

Plasma oestrogen assay

Robertson et al. (1978) were unable to detect oestrone sulfate in the blood of non-pregnant cyclic sows and yet in pregnant animals it was detectable from day 20 of gestation. This can therefore be used as a method of diagnosing pregnancy. A small volume of blood sufficient for the assay can be collected from the ear vein; the optimum time for diagnosis, when maximum con-

centrations of oestrone sulfate are present, is at about 24–28 days.

PREGNANCY AND ITS DETECTION IN THE EWE AND GOAT

Endocrinology

Ewe (Figure 3.20)

In the non-pregnant cyclical ewe, progesterone concentrations in the peripheral blood fall rapidly just before the onset of oestrus (see Figure 1.29). Following conception the corpus luteum persists and peak dioestrous values are maintained and gradually increase to about 60 days of gestation, when there is a considerable increase, this rise being due to the placental contribution to progesterone production. Levels remain high until the last week of pregnancy when they decline rapidly to 1 ng/ml at parturition. The concentration of progesterone is significantly higher in multiple pregnancies (Basset et al., 1969) since it has been calculated that in late pregnancy the placenta produces five times as much progesterone as the ovary (Linzell and Heap, 1968). Maximum progesterone concentrations in the peripheral blood of ewes with a single lamb was 3.78 ng/ml between days 105 and 110, with twins 5.09 ng/ml between days

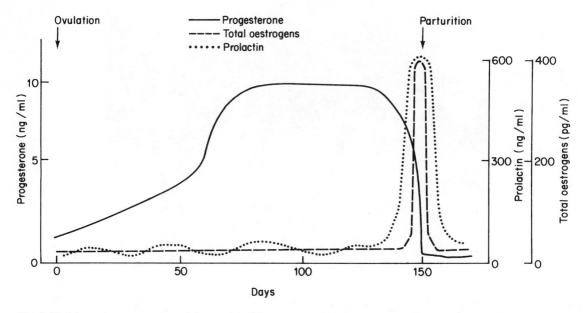

Fig. 3.20 Schematic representation of the trends in hormone concentrations in the peripheral circulation of the ewe during pregnancy and parturition.

125 and 130 and with triplets 9.18 ng/ml between days 125 and 130 (Emady et al., 1974).

Oestrogen concentrations in the peripheral circulation remain low throughout gestation. A few days before parturition they start to rise then suddenly increase to about 400 pg/ml at the time of lambing, followed by a rapid fall (Challis, 1971).

Prolactin concentrations fluctuate during pregnancy between 20 and 80 ng/ml; towards the end, however, they start to increase and reach a peak of between 400 and 700 ng/ml on the day of lambing (Davies and Reichert, 1971; Kann and Denamur, 1974).

Placental lactogen has been detected in maternal plasma from 48 days of gestation; it reaches a maximum by about 140 days, gradually decreasing until lambing. It has been identified in trophoblast tissue from 16 to 17 day blastocysts (Martal and Djiane, 1977). The role of this hormone is still unclear, it may have a role in the luteotrophic complex of the pregnant ewe and also in controlling fetal growth and mammary development.

Bilateral ovariectomy after 55 days will not result in abortion because by this stage of gestation the placenta has taken over the major role of progesterone production. However, it should be remembered that the corpora lutea persist for the duration of the pregnancy and regress only at the time of parturition (see Chapter 6).

Goat

As in the ewe, progesterone concentrations in the peripheral blood and milk decline around the time of oestrus, thus sampling approximately 21 days after service or artificial insemination will enable a distinction to be made between non-pregnancy and pregnancy. In the latter, they increase until a plateau is reached, and then decline rapidly a few days before parturition. Total oestrogens in the peripheral circulation are much higher than those recorded in the ewe. They increase gradually from 30 to 40 days of gestation, reaching a peak value of over 600 pg/ml just before parturition (Challis and Linzell, 1971). Prolactin remains low during pregnancy but rises rapidly just before parturition.

Bilateral ovariectomy at any stage of gestation will result in loss of the pregnancy; thus, extra-ovarian sources would appear to be unable to produce sufficient progesterone for the maintenance of pregnancy.

Methods of diagnosing pregnancy in the ewe

There are a large number of published methods of diagnosing pregnancy in the ewe, these have been reviewed in detail (Richardson, 1972). The number and variety of methods point to the fact that there was not a simple, accurate and inexpensive clinical method of diagnosing pregnancy in the ewe until the advent of B-mode ultrasonography, which is without doubt the method of choice.

Management methods

Traditionally the method used by shepherds is the observation that ewes, which have been marked by a 'keeled' or 'raddled' ram, fail to be marked again within 16–19 days. This is a sufficiently reliable sign of pregnancy for most purposes, but subsequent embryonic death will reduce its accuracy, and 20–30% of pregnant ewes will show oestrous during early pregnancy. It is important to ensure that the raddle crayon is changed regularly every 16 days, that it is sufficiently soft to produce a mark and that the colour sequence allows easy colour identification.

Beyond 100 days of gestation the fetus may be palpated through the abdominal wall, and development of the udder is then obvious in primipara. The best way to ballotte the fetus is to have the ewe standing normally and to lift the abdomen repeatedly immediately in front of the udder; the fetus can be felt to drop on to the palpating hand.

Ultrasonic methods

The fetal pulse detector (Doppler) has been used to diagnose pregnancy in ewes, and two types of probe are available. The external probe is applied to the skin surface of the abdomen just cranial to the udder. The fleece in this region is sparse and with transmission gel applied to the end of the probe it is slowly moved over the surface. The ewe can be restrained either standing or sitting on her haunches. Characteristic sounds indicate the presence of the fetal heart ('tack, tack, tack') or vessels ('swish, swish, swish'); the frequency greatly exceeds that of the mother's heart rate, except in late gestation when the fetal heart rate is reduced and can be less than the maternal. Between 40 and 80 days of gestation the accuracy of detection is no better than 60% (Hulet, 1968; Richardson, 1972). However, after 80 days, with a reasonable amount of practice, it is over 90% accurate and it takes an average three or four minutes per ewe to make a diagnosis.

Using a rectal probe Lindahl (1970) reported an accuracy of 97% between 35 and 55 days after mating. There are a large number of reports giving similar results from as early as 20–25 days. The rectal probe is safe and easy to use and requires limited restraint of the ewe.

With the fetal pulse detector the diagnosis of false positives should be virtually nil, the only source of error being the confusion of the maternal pulse sounds with those of the fetus. However, false negatives are always a possibility, since there is a limit to the amount of time that the search for confirmatory sounds can be made.

The external probe can also be used between 80 and 100 days to differentiate between single and multiple pregnancies, although the accuracy in identifying the precise number of fetal lambs is poor. Fukui et al. (1984) used an external probe together with the fetal pulse detector to determine the number of fetuses between 60 and 140 days of gestation. The results were rather disappointing with an accuracy of 76.9% for the correct diagnosis of no pregnancy and 74.4% for the identification of twins. The stage of gestation did not appear to influence the accuracy of the procedure.

The use of A-mode ultrasound has been described by Madel (1983) using an external probe. He obtained an overall accuracy of differentiating between pregnant and non-pregnant ewes of 80.1%, with poorer results obtained for the correct diagnosis of non-pregnant ewes. The average time to examine each ewe was about 2 minutes.

A B-mode ultrasound sector transducer probe, using the transabdominal approach, has proved to be an accurate and rapid method of not only differentiating pregnant from non-pregnant ewes but also accurately determining fetal numbers (Figure 3.21). The cost-effectiveness of such a procedure is obvious since it is possible not only to eliminate barren ewes but also to adjust feeding levels to accommodate the number of lambs. Not only does this save on feed cost but also reduces the chances of pregnancy toxaemia occurring. Pregnancy can be detected as early as 30 days, although the optimum time to differentiate fetal numbers is 45–50 days. White et al. (1984) using a 2.25, 3 or 3.5 MHz transducer examined a total of 1120 ewes 36–90 days after tupping. The fleece was shorn on the abdomen of each ewe extending some 20 cm cranial to the udder and across the whole width. The ewe was restrained on her back and, using vegetable oil as a coupling medium, the abdomen was scanned. A positive diagnosis of pregnancy based upon the imaging of a fluid-filled uterus and placental material, especially caruncles/cotyledons, could be made quite quickly. Care was taken

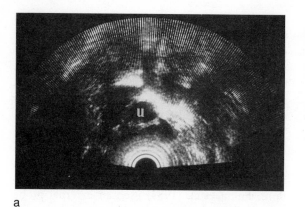

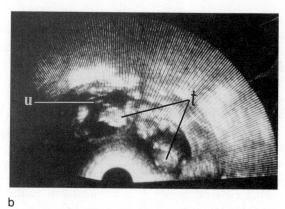

a

b

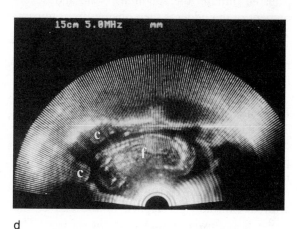

c

d

e

Fig. 3.21 Transabdominal B-mode ultrasound images of the ewe's pregnant uterus and its contents using 3.0 or 5.0 MHz sector transducer. (a) At approximately 35 days of gestation. At this stage it is possible to identify fluid-filled sections of the uterine horns (u). In the absence of an embryo or fetus it is only indicative of a possible pregnancy. (b) At approximately 55 days of gestation. Note twin fetuses (t) surrounded by non-echogenic (black) amniotic fluid. The umbilical cord can be seen attached to the left fetus (u). (c) At approximately 70 days of gestation. Note twin fetuses (t) and cotyledons (c). (d) At approximately 80 days of gestation. Note the large single fetus (f) in which the spine can be identified; also cotyledons (c). (e) At approximately 81 days of gestation. Note the single fetus (f) with ribs (r) and heart (h). (Courtesy Dr P. J. Goddard.)

to examine the limits of the uterus so that fetal numbers could be detected accurately. An experienced person could examine on average 75 ewes per hour. It is possible to examine the ewe in a sitting position with the transducer applied to the hairless area just cranial to the udder and to one side of the midline, thus obviating the need to shear the fleece. An experienced person was over 99% correct in differentiating pregnant from non-pregnant ewes and 98.9% in identifying fetal numbers. The commonest source of error was failing to identify the third fetus in ewes with triplets. Inexperienced persons soon developed a high level of accuracy.

Vaginal biopsy

The method is similar to that reported for the sow where the stratified squamous epithelium of the vaginal mucosa is sensitive to the hormonal changes that occur during the oestrous cycle and pregnancy (Radev et al., 1960).

Richardson (1972) found that it was 81% accurate in detecting barren ewes; after 40 days it was 91% accurate in detecting pregnancy, and accuracy increased to 100% after 80 days of gestation. Doubtful interpretations in some ewes are likely in late dioestrus and late anoestrus since the histological appearance of the sections is then similar to that of pregnancy.

Radiography

Both dorsoventral and lateral radiographs can be taken. Richardson (1972) recommends the use of a 12 × 15 medium-speed film with a grid voltage of 80–90 kV and maximum current of 100 mA. Using an exposure time of 0.3–0.5 seconds and depending on the dorsoventral dimension of the ewe, fetuses were detectable from 70 days of gestation. The overall accuracy of the method in detecting pregnancy increases with advancing gestation: 52% between 66 and 95 days to 100% after 96 days (Richardson, 1972).

The accuracy in detecting fetal numbers is not so great. Ardran and Brown (1964) quote 22% between 51 and 70 days, 79% between 71 and 90 days and 87% between 91 and 110 days. The method is also useful for estimating the gestational length from 110 days by the measurement of the fetal long bones.

Although the technique is reliable, it is expensive and time-consuming and hence is not practicable for normal farming enterprises.

Milk and plasma progesterone

Pregnancy can be diagnosed on the fact that in the pregnant ewe the corpora lutea persist and hence peripheral progesterone concentrations will remain elevated at 15–18 days after mating. In lactating ewes it is also possible to determine the progesterone levels in milk. Plasma and milk progesterone values in pregnant sheep 18–22 days after mating were similar (3.7 ng/ml), whereas in non-pregnant ewes they were 1 ng/ml. Lambing results showed a similar accuracy of 82 and 84% (Shemesh et al., 1979).

Rosette inhibition titre (RIT) test

This is an established test for determining the immunosuppressive potential of anti-lymphocyte serum which has been applied to determining the presence of an 'early pregnancy factor' (EPF) in ewes. In ewes which were subsequently found to be pregnant, the factor could be demonstrated as early as 24 hours after mating (Morton et al., 1979). The RIT test is time-consuming and difficult to maintain; according to Sasser and Ruder (1987), the development of a radio-immunoassay or ELISA for EPF should provide a more reliable method.

Palpation of caudal uterine artery

Identification of enlargement of the caudal uterine artery has been reported as a fairly reliable method of diagnosing pregnancy; the technique requires patience and skill. The arteries can be palpated per vaginum as they run outside the arterior vaginal wall at the 10 o'clock and 2 o'clock positions (Richardson, 1972). Quite often it is necessary to displace a pad of fat ventrally to enable identification of the vessel. In the non-pregnant ewe the artery is very small or cannot be palpated at all. After about 50 days of gestation there is some enlargement. The accuracy of the method after 60 days of gestation was 62%, but a large number of barren ewes were incorrectly diagnosed as being pregnant (Richardson, 1972).

Peritoneoscopy

Phillipo et al. (1971) obtained 91% accuracy of pregnancy detection between 17 and 28 days by means of direct inspection of the uterus and ovaries with a laparoscope, using general anaesthesia.

Methods of diagnosing pregnancy in the goat

Many of the methods which have been described above for the ewe are also applicable to the goat. Using the fetal pulse detector a reliable diagnosis of pregnancy is possible at 50 days with an abdominal probe and 25 days with a rectal probe. Excellent results have also been obtained with B-mode direct imaging from about 30 days of gestation.

The milk progesterone test has been used extensively since most parous goats are lactating at the time of mating. Whole milk samples are collected from the bucket after thorough mixing on or about the day of mating and, in the absence of return to oestrous, 22 and 26 days later (Holdsworth and Davies, 1979). The accuracy for identifying goats that were not pregnant was 100%; however, some false-positive results were obtained due to pseudopregnancy, ovarian cysts and elevated progesterone values at oestrus. It is likely, however, that the method will become routine in goat husbandry.

Oestrone sulfate is produced by the fetoplacental unit; its presence in plasma or in milk is a positive indication of pregnancy, thus enabling differentiation from pseudopregnancy. Although it has been shown that oestrone sulfate concentrations from 30 days of gestation exceed those in non-pregnant individuals (Heap et al., 1981) the earliest optimum time is 50 days or later after service (Chaplin and Holdsworth, 1982).

PREGNANCY AND ITS DIAGNOSIS IN THE DOG AND CAT

Endocrinology

Dog

The bitch has a prolonged luteal phase with persistence of the corpora lutea for 70–80 days in the non-pregnant animal. Progesterone concentrations in the peripheral circulation of pregnant bitches are similar to those of non-pregnant individuals and for this reason, unlike other species, cannot be used to diagnose pregnancy. Concannon et al. (1975) obtained mean maximum values of 29 ng/ml for pregnant and 27 ng/ml for non-pregnant bitches. However, there was a lot of individual variation,

with peak values obtained between 8 and 29 days after the LH peak in pregnant bitches and between 12 and 28 days in non-pregnant bitches. There is some evidence that at the time of implantation (17–21 days), or just after implantation, progesterone concentrations increase, due possibly to the effect of a placental gonadotrophin (Jones et al., 1973). From about 30 days of gestation there is a gradual decrease in progesterone so that by about day 60 values of 5 ng/ml are obtained, followed by a sudden decline just before parturition, to zero just afterwards. In the non-pregnant bitch there is no rapid fall; low levels of progesterone persist. The number of days in which values $\geqslant 1$ ng/ml were obtained were 68 days in non-pregnant compared with 63.8 days in pregnant bitches (Concannon et al., 1975).

Total oestrogen values are slightly higher in the pregnant bitch than in the non-pregnant bitch, with some evidence of an increase at the time of implantation (Concannon et al., 1975). They remain fairly constant during the rest of gestation (20–27 pg/ml), before declining 2 days prepartum to non-pregnant values by the day of parturition (Figure 3.22).

Although prolactin concentrations increase during the first half of the luteal phase in both pregnant and non-pregnant bitches, there is a much greater rise in the second half of the former. The gradual rise during pregnancy ends with a sudden surge during the rapid decline in progesterone which occurs 1–2 days before whelping (De Coster et al., 1983; McCann et al., 1988).

Relaxin can be detected in the peripheral circulation of pregnant Labrador and Beagle bitches at 20–30 days of gestation, where it was absent in non-pregnant bitches at all stages of the reproductive cycle in non-pregnant animals (Steinetz et al., 1989).

The ovaries of the bitch are necessary for the maintenance of pregnancy; even their removal as late as 56 days resulted in abortion (Sokolowski, 1971).

The average gestation length in the bitch is normally quoted as 63–64 days, but the interval from first mating to whelping can vary from 56 to 71 days. However, if gestation length is measured from the time of the pre-ovulatory LH peak it is very constant at between 64 and 66 days (Concannon et al., 1983).

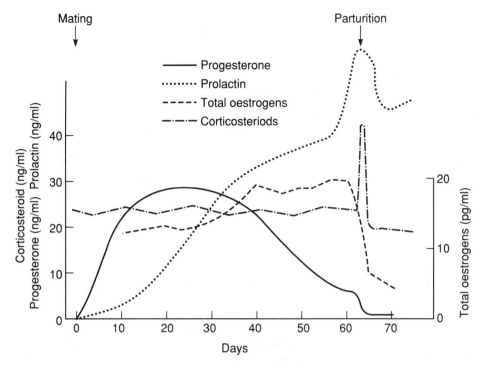

Fig. 3.22. Schematic representation of the trends in hormone concentrations in the peripheral circulation of the bitch during pregnancy and parturition.

Cat

Ovulation occurs 23–30 hours after mating (Schille et al., 1983), and serum progesterone concentrations rapidly increase from the baseline of under 10 nmol/l to reach peak values of around 100 nmol/l between the first and fourth week of pregnancy (Verhage et al., 1976) (Figures 3.23 and 3.24).

Cats are unusual in that queens may continue to display oestrous behaviour and accept mating, even though ovulation may have occurred and there is significant production of progesterone (Stabenfeldt, 1974).

At 3–4 weeks of pregnancy, hyperaemia of the teats occurs. This is particularly prominent in maiden queens. It is a progesterone-dependent phenomenon and is also seen in pseudopregnancy. There is conflicting evidence concerning the relative roles of the corpora lutea and fetoplacental units in the synthesis of progesterone during pregnancy. Whereas Scott (1970) and Gruffydd-Jones (1982) have reported the maintenance of pregnancy following ovariectomy after 45–50 and 49 days, respectively, Verstegan et al. (1993a) have reported abortion following ovariectomy at 45 days of gestation. Progesterone concentrations

gradually fall from their peak values during the first month of pregnancy, the fall becoming precipitous during the last 2 days prior to parturition. There may be a slight pre-parturient increase in oestrogen concentrations but this declines just before parturition.

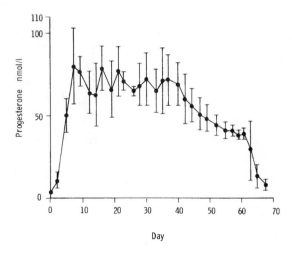

Fig. 3.23 Mean (± SD) plasma concentrations of progesterone throughout pregnancy (four cats). Day 0 represents the day of mating. (By courtesy of T. J. Gruffydd-Jones.)

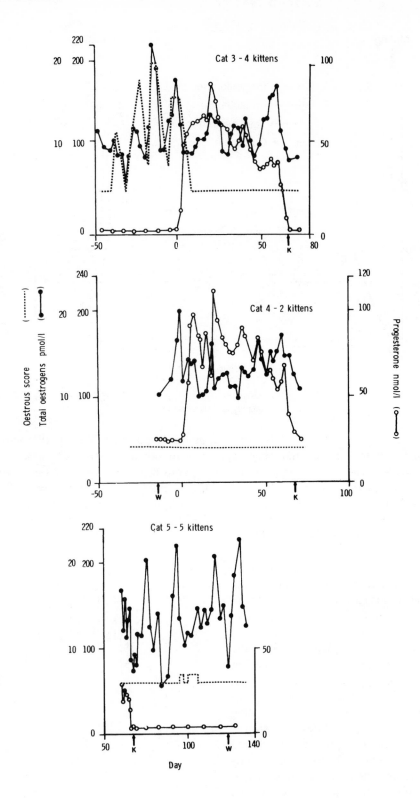

Fig. 3.24 Plasma concentrations of total oestrogens (●——●) and progesterone (○——○), and oestrous scores (- - - - -) throughout oestrus, pregnancy and lactation in individual queens. Day 0 represents the day of mating; K, the day of kittening; W, the day of weaning. (By courtesy of T. J. Gruffydd-Jones.)

Relaxin is produced by the placenta during pregnancy and is thought to contribute to its maintenance by inhibiting uterine activity. It appears during the third week of pregnancy, with concentrations declining just before parturition (Stewart and Stabenfeldt, 1985). Prolactin is produced during the last third of pregnancy and concentrations decline as weaning takes place (Banks et al., 1983).

The average gestation length is 63–65 days but is reported to vary between 59 and 70 days. The fact that ovulation may not necessarily occur after the first mating may partly explain this considerable variation.

The modal litter size for non-pedigree cats is four with a range of three to seven but there is variation in litter size between pedigree breeds. Oriental breeds tend to have larger litters, sometimes in excess of 10 kittens, whilst pedigree Longhair queens tend to have smaller litters, often of only two or three kittens. Singleton litters are unusual and this may reflect fetal resorption due to inadequate fetoplacental endocrine contribution to the maintenance of pregnancy.

A proportion of queens will display oestrous behaviour whilst pregnant. Some of these cats will mate, and this may lead to superfetation. Free-living queens may mate with several competing toms during oestrus and hence superfecundity is common.

Methods of pregnancy diagnosis in the bitch

Since the bitch is not polycyclic, pregnancy cannot be anticipated by a failure to return to oestrus. There is some evidence that pregnancy does increase the interoestrus interval and causes greater regularity of oestrus (Anderson and Wooten, 1959). It is also generally accepted that the period of oestrus ends more quickly after conception.

The main problem in diagnosing pregnancy in the bitch is that overt pseudopregnancy is very common, the degree varying from individual to individual.

The deposition of abdominal and subcutaneous fat during pregnancy is often marked. It is a storing of fat for the subsequent lactation, for it is generally lost again during the period of nursing. The gravid uterus and its contents cause no appreciable increase in body weight during the first 5 weeks. From this point body weight rapidly increases

according to the number of fetuses. The increase will vary from 1 kg in a 5 kg bitch to 7 kg or more in one of 27 kg, but by the time body weight has become a guide there are other very definite signs of pregnancy (Figure 3.25). In multiple pregnancy, abdominal distension becomes progressive and obvious from the fifth week onwards, but in animals gravid with one or two fetuses only, particularly when the bitch is large or very fat, distension may not be noticeable.

There are several causes of abdominal distension in the bitch which must be differentiated from pregnancy. The most important is pyometra, which occurs during pseudopregnancy; others are ascites, peritonitis with effusion, splenic enlargement and neoplasia of the liver, abdominal lymphatic glands or uterus.

Mammary glands
Characteristic changes occur in the mammary glands. Unfortunately, similar, but less definite, changes may occur during pseudopregnancy.

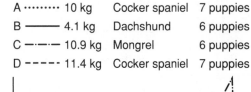

A ········ 10 kg	Cocker spaniel	7 puppies
B ——— 4.1 kg	Dachshund	6 puppies
C —·—·— 10.9 kg	Mongrel	6 puppies
D − − − − 11.4 kg	Cocker spaniel	7 puppies

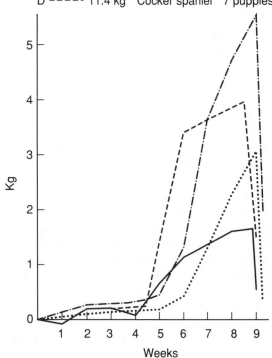

Fig. 3.25 Increase in body weight in bitches during pregnancy.

These changes are more easily recognized in primigravida. At about day 35, in unpigmented skins, the teats become bright pink, enlarged and turgid; they protrude. This condition persists until about day 45, when the teats become larger still but softer and tumefied. They may become pigmented. Appreciable hypertrophy of the glands commences at day 50. It progresses until at term the mammary glands comprise two parallel, enlarged and oedematous areas with a depression between them, extending from the pelvic brim to the anterior part of the chest. A watery secretion can generally be expressed from the teats two to three days before parturition. The onset of milk secretion coincides with parturition. In multigravida, mammary hypertrophy commences about seven days before term and in some cases milk can be expressed from the teats several days before parturition.

Abdominal palpation

The ease and accuracy of abdominal palpation will depend upon the following factors:

1. The size of the animal: the smaller the easier.
2. Its temperament: whether palpation is resisted.
3. The period in gestation at which examination is made.
4. The number of fetuses *in utero*.
5. Whether the bitch is of normal size or grossly fat.

Days 18–21. At this stage the embryos represent a series of tense, oval distensions in the cornua, about 12 mm long by 9 mm broad. In small bitches which can be readily manipulated it may be possible to state approximately the number present. Those situated in the posterior parts of the cornua are most easily felt; if only one or two, situated anteriorly, are present they may be missed. In large or fat bitches it is improbable that embryos will be detected at this stage. Care must be taken not to confuse faeces in the colon with fetuses.

Days 24–30. This is the optimum period for the early diagnosis of pregnancy. By day 24 these distensions have become spherical in outline, from 6 to 30 mm in diameter. They remain tense and are easily recognized (Figure 3.26). Sometimes there is variation in size, the posterior ones being rather smaller than those in front. The embryonic units maintain this spherical form until about day 33.

Days 35–44. The constricted portions of the cornua between the embryonic units progressively dilate, the distensions become elongated and much of their tenseness is lost. At this period the uterus comes into contact with the abdominal wall, and in the animal pregnant with multiple fetuses abdominal distension is commencing to be visible. Nevertheless, palpation of the fetuses themselves is not yet possible and as the uterus itself has lost much of its tension positive diagnosis may be difficult, particularly in those pregnant with one or two only.

Days 45–55. During this stage increase in the size of the fetuses is rapid. At day 45 it may be possible to detect the posteriorly situated ones between the fingers; in a 9 kg bitch they are approximately 63 mm long and 12 mm broad. It is during this stage that the disposition of the uterus in the abdominal cavity changes. In animals pregnant with multiple fetuses, each cornua represents an elongated cylinder, 38–51 mm in diameter and 228–300 mm long. Posteriorly they extend into the uterine body, which has by this time become dilated. Each horn is in two segments: the posterior, which lies on the abdominal floor and passes forwards to the margins of the liver, and the anterior, which lies dorsal and lateral to it, with its long axis directed backwards towards the pelvis. In the last stages the uterus almost entirely fills the abdomen.

Days 55–63. During this period there should be no difficulty in diagnosing pregnancy provided the bitch allows manipulation of the abdomen. The size of the fetuses is such that they can readily be detected. High in the flank the one occupying the apex of the cornua will be felt, while in the midline just in front of the pelvic brim is the one with its extremity in the uterine body. If manipulation is resisted, digital examination per rectum is helpful. The bitch's foreparts should be raised and the uterus pressed backwards towards the pelvic inlet by pressure on the abdomen. The presented part of the posterior fetus will be detected beneath the finger. In big or fat bitches pregnant with one or two only, doubt may still exist, although by this time the mammary glands afford valuable confirmatory evidence.

Accuracy. The accuracy of abdominal palpa-

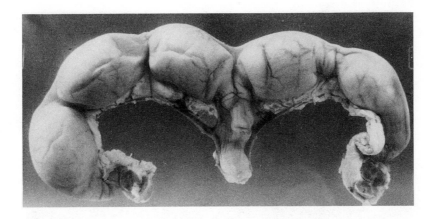

Fig. 3.26 Uterus and ovaries of a bitch, pregnancy of about 30 days. Note five conceptual swellings.

tion is sometimes questioned, particularly in differentiating pregnancy from overt pseudopregnancy (see p. 35). Apart from Hancock and Rowlands (1949), and more recently Allen and Meredith (1981), there have been no reports on the assessment of the accuracy of this method. The latter authors found that although pregnancy was detected at 21–25 days of gestation, the accuracy was only 52% compared with 87% from 26 to 35 days. However, in the case of the correct diagnosis of bitches that did not subsequently whelp, the accuracies were 92 and 73%, respectively, for the same gestational ages. The optimum time for accuracy is between 26 and 35 days of gestation. It is important for a high level of accuracy that the interval from mating to examination is known, since assessment of whether a bitch is pregnant or not is dependent upon the identification of conceptual swellings of a size comparable with the gestational age of the bitch.

Radiography

Radiography is a particularly useful diagnostic aid in the terminal stages of pregnancy, especially in the obese dog where a differential diagnosis from pseudopregnancy is required or in bitches with a single puppy that may have suffered prolonged gestation. It is also very valuable in dystocia cases to disclose the presence of retained puppies and the disposition of a presenting puppy.

In most cases a single radiograph with the bitch in lateral recumbency will suffice, although in an attempt to identify more accurately fetal numbers and fetal presentation a dorsoventral view may be useful. An intensity of less than 100 mA, voltage between 65 and 90 kV and a speed of 0.15–0.03 seconds should be adequate, depending on the size of the bitch and the amount of body fat (Royal et al., 1979). In interpreting radiographs, three points require identification: firstly, displacement of the intestinal mass by the early gravid uterus; secondly, identification of the uterus; and, thirdly, the presence of fetal skeletons. It is possible to see fetal sacs as early as 23–25 days of gestation (Royal et al., 1979). At the end of 6 weeks there may be evidence of fetal skeletons, with the skulls identifiable by 45 days. At the end of 7 weeks it is normally possible to identify the whole fetal skeleton. The technique is not reliable in the identification of fetal numbers. The accuracy of radiographic diagnosis is very much dependent upon the quality of the radiograph that is obtained (Figure 3.27).

Ultrasonic methods

Using the Doppler method (see p. 69) with an external transducer probe placed on the abdominal wall adjacent to the mammary glands, fetal heart sounds were detected as early as 29 days of gestation (Helper, 1970), although in all the 25 bitches confirmed to be pregnant the fetal hearts were heard by 32 days; they were consistently twice the maternal heart rate. Sounds associated with placental blood flow were heard in some bitches as early as 25 days, although it was sometimes difficult to distinguish them from maternal sounds. Helper reported an accuracy of 100%. Riznar and Makek (1978) found that the earliest time a positive diagnosis could be made was at 44 days. They stressed its value in late gestation, 61–70 days after mating, especially as a method of confirming the presence

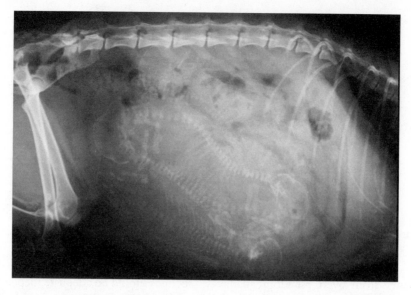

Fig. 3.27 Radiograph of the abdomen of a pregnant bitch near term. Note the fetal skeletons.

of live or dead puppies. Using two different instruments, Allen and Meredith (1981) found a low level of accuracy between 25 and 35 days of gestation, which improved with advancing gestational age to reach 100% with one instrument between 43 and 64 days.

A-mode ultrasound depth analysers have been used to diagnose pregnancy using an external transducer probe. Smith and Kirk (1975) were able to detect pregnancy as early as 18 days after mating; these authors stressed the importance of not scanning too far caudally because of the chance of reflections from a full urinary bladder. Using a similar instrument with a 2.25 MHz transducer probe, the earliest correct positive diagnosis of pregnancy was made at 26 days (Allen and Meredith, 1981). From 32 days to term a level of accuracy of about 90% was obtained for the correct diagnosis of pregnant and non-pregnant bitches.

As with other species, B-mode ultrasound has been clearly demonstrated to be the most accurate method of diagnosing pregnancy in the bitch (Figure 3.28). Furthermore, with the development of improved transducers it is likely to become more accurate and become a widely used diagnostic tool. Using a 2.4 MHz linear array transducer probe placed on the abdominal wall, positive identification of pregnancy at a high level of accuracy was achieved 28 days after natural mating or artificial insemination (Bondestam et al., 1984). Of 77 bitches that whelped, only

one was incorrectly diagnosed as being non-pregnant, an accuracy of 99.3%, and she expelled a macerated fetus, whilst all 58 that were diagnosed non-pregnant failed to give birth to puppies. Earlier identification of the conceptus has been reported at 14 days (Tainturier and Moysan, 1984) and 21 days (Taverne, 1984). However, the former workers suggested that it was preferable to wait until 20 days.

The accurate estimation of litter size has proved to be difficult, especially in larger breeds of dogs. A figure of 40% accuracy at 29 days after mating and 83.3% accuracy from 50 days to term has been reported (Bondestam et al., 1984).

It is generally unnecessary to clip the hair of dogs, even those breeds with long coats, provided that the hair is parted and plenty of coupling gel is used.

Measurement of serum proteins

Gentry and Liptrap (1981) observed a three-fold rise in serum fibrinogen concentrations during pregnancy, with peak values occurring 4–5 weeks after mating. Since this phenomenon did not occur at the corresponding stage of metoestrus in non-pregnant bitches, it can be used as a method of detecting pregnancy.

Recent studies (Eckersall et al., 1993) have reported an acute phase response in pregnant bitches as demonstrated by the rise in serum C-reactive protein (CRP) in mid-gestation. This is

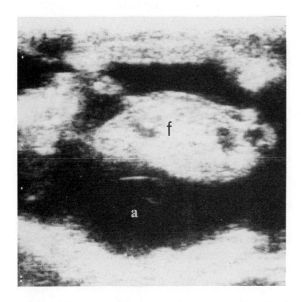

Fig. 3.28 Ultrasound image of the abdomen of a gravid bitch 32 days after plasma LH surge. Note the fetal puppy in transverse section (f) surrounded by amniotic fluid (a).

likely to be produced in response to the implantation of the embryo causing tissue damage.

Methods of pregnancy diagnosis in the cat

Cats lend themselves particularly well to pregnancy diagnosis by abdominal palpation. This is most satisfactorily performed 16–26 days after mating when conceptuses are readily identifiable as individual turgid spherical swellings. Pregnancy may be confirmed as early as 13 days after mating, but, at this stage, the conceptuses may be confused with faecal boluses. After six weeks, the conceptual swellings increase markedly in size, elongating and merging, thus making palpation more difficult. However, by this stage, there will usually be significant abdominal enlargement.

B-Mode ultrasound enables pregnancy diagnosis to be confirmed by demonstration of an enlarged uterus as early as the first week of pregnancy and, more reliably, by identifying the gestational sacs from the second week (Davidson et al., 1986) (Figure 3.29). Fetal cardiac activity can be detected from the third week onwards to assess fetal viability.

PREVENTION AND TERMINATION OF PREGNANCY

In all domestic species there will be occasions when it will be desirable to either prevent pregnancy occurring or terminate it prematurely. Such occasions may follow an unintended mating (misalliance), where pregnancy and parturition may

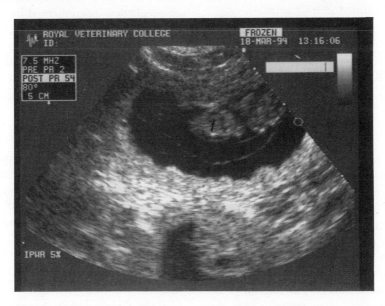

Fig. 3.29 Ultrasound image of the abdomen of a gravid queen approximately 35 days after mating (7.5 MHz sector transducer). Note the fetus (f).

present a severe risk to the dam's health, or where the owners of the animal do not want the pregnancy to continue.

Mare

The management and treatment of twinning is discussed in detail in Chapter 26. If the pregnancy needs to be curtailed for this and other reasons, such as mismating, the treatment of choice is $PGF_{2\alpha}$ or an analogue administered after the corpus luteum has become responsive to the hormone, i.e. 4 days after ovulation (see Chapter 1) and before the formation of the endometrial cups, i.e. about 35 days (see p. 58). Therefore, it is preferable to treat approximately 10–15 days after mating. Alternatively, intrauterine infusion of 250–500 ml of physiological saline during the same period will also be effective, since as well as a physical effect in flushing out the conceptus, it also stimulates the release of endogenous $PGF_{2\alpha}$.

Cow

Pregnancy can be terminated from 4–5 to 100 days after ovulation with $PGF_{2\alpha}$ or an analogue, and even up to 150 days many cows will respond. After 150 days, the placenta is the major source of progesterone for the maintenance of pregnancy, until about 270 days of gestation, $PGF_{2\alpha}$ alone is not effective. During this period, either long-acting corticosteroids alone, or in combination with $PGF_{2\alpha}$, are required (see Chapter 4).

Large doses of oestradiol benzoate can terminate pregnancy up to about 150 days by stimulating endogenous $PGF_{2\alpha}$ release; however, it is not as effective as using the hormone directly.

Doe

Pregnancy can be terminated at any stage with $PGF_{2\alpha}$.

Ewe

$PGF_{2\alpha}$ is effective in terminating pregnancy after day 4 and before day 12. During the day 12–21 period, there will be no response because of the protective effect of oTP–1 ensuring the survival of the corpus luteum. There is also some suggestion of another refractory period between days 25 and 40. After 45–55 days, the corpus luteum is no longer the main source of progesterone for the maintenance of pregnancy, and at this stage corti-

costeroids will be necessary to terminate pregnancy (see p. 151).

Sow

Pregnancy can be terminated at any stage with $PGF_{2\alpha}$.

Bitch

Pregnancy can be prevented in the bitch by the strategic use of oestrogens during the first 5 days after mating. They exert their effect by interfering with the transport of the zygotes from the uterine tube to the uterine horns, probably by causing oedema of the endosalpinx and thus a temporary tubal occlusion. Oestradiol benzoate can be administered by intramuscular or subcutaneous injection at a dose rate of 5–10 mg. Signs of oestrus will be prolonged, and it is not advisable to repeat treatment if a mismating occurs again. Oral diethylstilboestrol and ethinyl oestradiol treatment has also been used. Oestrogen therapy, particularly repeated use, can predispose to cystic endometrial hyperplasia (pyometra) and bone marrow suppression.

Attention has also focused on the termination of pregnancy at a later stage. Natural $PGF_{2\alpha}$ rather than analogues has been found to be effective when administered at a dose rate of 150–270 μg/kg subcutaneously twice daily consecutively on days 10–14 after the bitch has entered metoestrus or pregnancy, as confirmed by exfoliative vaginal cytology (see Chapter 1) (Romagnoli et al., 1993). Earlier reports in which pregnancy was terminated at a later stage, namely 25–30 days, resulted in unacceptable side-effects (Lein et al., 1989). At present, it is doubtful if $PGF_{2\alpha}$ should be used for this purpose.

Recently a dopamine agonist, cabergoline, which also inhibits prolactin secretion and hence indirectly withdraws the luteotrophic support for the corpora lutea, has been used to terminate pregnancy in bitches. It has been used at a dose rate of 1.65 μg/kg subcutaneously for 5 days at 25–40 days of gestation (Onclin et al., 1993). Unlike the prolactin inhibitor, bromocryptine, it does not have unpleasant side-effects.

Cat

Oestradiol cypionate by intramuscular injection at a dose rate of 125–250 μg within 40 hours of mating has been shown to be effective in preventing pregnancy, probably by interfering with the normal transport of the zygotes within the uterine tubes (Herron and Sis, 1974). Similarly, injections of diethylstilboestrol have been used. However, there is little data on possible side-effects, and such treatments should only be used in exceptional circumstances.

Recently, both $PGF_{2\alpha}$ and the dopamine agonist cabergoline have been shown to be fairly effective in causing abortion; however, the former has unpleasant side-effects (Verstegen et al., 1993b).

REFERENCES

Abbitt, B., Ball, L., Kitto, G. P., Sitzman, C. G., Wilgenburg, B., Raim, L. W. and Seidel, G. E. (1978) *J. Amer. Vet. Med. Assn*, **173**, 973.

Allen, W. E. (1971) *Vet. Rec.*, **88**, 508.

Allen, W. E. (1975) *J. Reprod. Fertil. Suppl.*, **23**, 425.

Allen, W. E. and Newcombe, J. R. (1981) *Equine Vet. J.*, **13**, 51.

Allen, W. E. and Meredith, M. J. (1981) *J. Small Anim. Pract.*, **22**, 609.

Allen, W. R. (1975) *J. Reprod. Fertil. Suppl.*, **23**, 405.

Andersen, A. C. and Wooten, E. (1959) In: *Reproduction in Domestic Animals*, ed. H. H. Cole and P. T. Cupps. New York: Academic Press.

Ardran, G. M. and Brown, T. H. (1964) *J. Agr. Sci. Camb.*, **63**, 205.

Arthur, G. H. (1956) *J. Comp. Pathol.*, **66**, 345.

Ball, L. and Carroll, E. J. (1963) *J. Amer. Vet. Med. Assn*, **143**, 373.

Banks, D. R., Paape, S. R. and Stabenfeldt, G. H. (1983) *Biol. Reprod.*, **28**, 923.

Bartol, F. F., Roberts, R. M., Bazer, F. W., Lewis, G. S., Godwin, J. D. and Thatcher, W. W. (1985) *Biol. Reprod.*, **32**, 681.

Bassett, J. M., Oxborrow, T. J., Smith, I. D. and Thorburn, G. D. (1969) *J. Endocrinol.*, **45**, 449.

Bazer, F. W., Marengo, S. R., Geisert, R. D. and Thatcher, W. W. (1984) *Anim, Reprod. Sci.*, **7**, 115.

Bazer, F. W., Thatcher, W. W., Hansen, P. J., Mirando, M. A., Ott, T. J. and Plante, C. (1991) *J. Reprod. Fertil. Suppl.*, **43**, 39.

Berg, S. L. and Ginther, O. J. (1978) *J. Anim. Sci.*, **47**, 203.

Berglund, L. A., Sharp, D. C., Vernon, M. W. and Thatcher, W. W. (1982) *J. Reprod. Fertil. Suppl.*, **32**, 335.

Bolander, F. F., Ulberg, L. C. and Fellows, R. E. (1976) *Endocrinology*, **99**, 1273.

Bondestom, S., Karkkainen, M., Alitalo, T. and Forss, M. (1984) *Acta Vet. Scand.*, **25**, 327.

Boyd, J. S. and Omran, S. N. (1991) *In Practice*, **13**, 109.

Boyd, J. S., Omran, S. W. and Ayliffe, T. R. (1988) *Vet. Rec.*, **123**, 8.

Butterfield, R. M. and Mathews, R. G. (1979) *J. Reprod. Fertil.*, **27**, 447.

Cameron, R. D. A. (1977) *Aust. Vet. J.*, **53**, 432.

Challis, J. R. G. (1971) *Nature, Lond.*, **229**, 208.

Challis, J. R. G. and Linzell, J. L. (1971) *J. Reprod. Fertil.*, **26**, 401.

Chaplin, V. M. and Holdsworth, R. J. (1982) *Vet. Rec.*, **111**, 224.

Concannon, P. W., Hansel, W. and Visek, W. J. (1975) *Biol. Reprod.*, **13**, 112.

Concannon, P. W., Whaley, S., Lein, D. and Wissler, R. (1983) *Amer. J. Vet. Res.*, **44**, 1819.

Cowie, A. T. (1948) *Pregnancy Diagnosis Tests: A Review,* No. 13. Edinburgh: Commonwealth Agricultural Bureau.

Cox, J. E. (1975) *J. Reprod. Fertil.*, **23**, 463.

Cox, J. E. and Galina, C. S. (1970) *Vet. Rec.*, **86**, 97.

Cross, J. C. and Roberts, R. M. (1989) *Biol. Reprod.*, **40**, 1109.

Cuboni, E. (1937) *Clin. Vet. Milano*, **60**, 375 (Abstr. *Vet. Rec.* (1938), **50**, 791).

Davidson, A. P., Nyland, T. G. and Tsutsui, T. (1986) *Vet. Radiol.*, **27**, 109.

Davis, S. L. and Reichert, L. E. (1971) *Biol. Reprod.*, **4**, 145.

De Coster, R., Beckers, J. F., Beerens, D. and De May, J. (1983) *Acta Endocrinol. Copenh.*, **103**, 473.

Donald, H. P. (1943) *Vet. Rec.*, **55**, 297.

Done, J. T. and Heard, T. W. (1968) *Vet. Rec.*, **82**, 64.

Douglas, R. H. and Ginther, O. J. (1976) *Prostaglandins*, **11**, 251.

Dufty, J. H. (1973) *Aust. Vet. J.*, **49**, 177.

Eckersall, P. D., Harvey, M. J. A., Ferguson, J. M., Renton, J. P., Nickson, D. A. and Boyd, J. S. (1993) *J. Reprod. Fertil. Suppl.*, **47**, 159.

Ellicott, A. R. and Dzuik, P. J. (1973) *Biol. Reprod.*, **9**, 300.

Emady, M., Hadley, J. C., Noakes, D. E. and Arthur, G. H. (1974) *Vet. Rec.*, **95**, 168.

Erdheim, M. (1942) *J. Amer. Vet. Med. Assn*, **100**, 343.

Feo, J. C. S. A. (1980) *Vet. Rec.*, **106**, 368.

Fincher, M. G. (1943) *Cornell Vet.*, **33**, 257.

Fischer, H. E., Bazer, F. W. and Fields, M. J. (1985) *J. Reprod. Fertil.*, **75**, 69.

Findlay, J. K. (1981) *J. Reprod. Fertil. Suppl.*, **30**, 171.

Fukui, Y., Kimura, T. and Ono, H. (1984) *Vet. Rec.*, **114**, 145.

Geisert, R. D., Zavy, M. T., Moffatt, R. J., Blair, R. M. and Yellin, T. (1990) *J. Reprod. Fertil. Suppl.*, **40**, 293.

Gentry, P. A. and Liptrap, R. M. (1981) *J. Small Anim. Pract.*, **22**, 185.

Gilmore, L. O. (1952) *Genetics and Animal Breeding.* New York: Lippincott.

Ginther, O. J. (1986) *Ultrasonic Imaging and Reproductive Events in the Mare.* Cross Plains: Equiservices.

Gnatek, G. G., Smith, L. D., Duby, R. T. and Godkin, J. D. (1989) *Biol. Reprod.*, **41**, 655.

Godkin, J. D., Lifsey, G. J. and Gillespie, B. E. (1988) *Biol. Reprod.*, **38**, 703.

Götze, R. (1940) *Dt. Tierärztl. Wschr.*, **48**, 183.

Gruffydd-Jones, T. J. (1982) Ph.D. Thesis, University of Bristol.

Hamon, M., Fleet, I. R., Holdsworth, R. J. and Heap, R. B. (1981) *Brit. Vet. J.*, **137**, 71.

Hancock, J. L. (1962) *Vet. Rec.*, **74**, 646.

Hancock, J. L. and Rowlands, I. W. (1949) *Vet. Rec.*, **61**, 771.

Hammond, J. (1927) *Physiology of Reproduction in the Cow.* Cambridge: Cambridge University Press.

Harney, J. P. and Bazer, F. W. (1989) *Biol. Reprod.*, **41**, 277.

Heap, R. B.., Linzell, J. L. and Slotin, C. R. (1969) *J. Physiol. Lond.*, **200**, 38.

Heap, R. B., Gwyn, M., Laing, J. A. and Walters, D. E. (1973) *J. Agr. Sci. Camb.*, **81**, 151.

Heap, R. B., Holdsworth, R. J., Gadsby, J. E., Laing, J. A. and Walters, D. E. (1976) *Brit. Vet. J.*, **132**, 445.

Heap, R. B., Flint, A. P. F. and Jenkin, G. (1978) In: *Control of Ovulation*, ed. D. B. Crighton *et al.*, p. 295. London: Butterworth.

Heap, R. B., Flint, A. P. F., Hartmann, P. E., Gadsby, J. E., Stables, L. D., Ackland, N. and Harman, M. (1981) *J. Endocrinol.*, **89**, 77.

Helper, L. C. (1970) *J. Amer. Vet. Med. Assn.*, **156**, 60.

Herron, M. A. and Sis, R. F. (1974) *Amer. J. Vet. Res.*, **35**, 1277.

Hershman, L. and Douglas, R. H. (1979) *J. Reprod. Fertil. Suppl.*, **27**, 395.

Hoffmann, B., Günzler, O., Hamburger, R. and Schmidt, W. (1976) *Brit. Vet. J.*, **132**, 469.

Hoffmann, B., Schams, D., Giminez, T., Ender, M. L., Hermann, C. and Karg, H. (1973) *Acta Endocrinol.*, **73**, 385.

Holdsworth, R. J. and Davies, J. (1979) *Vet. Rec.*, **105**, 535.

Holtan, D. W., Nett, T. M. and Estergreen, V. L. (1975) *J. Reprod. Fertil. Suppl.*, **23**, 419.

Holtan, D. W., Squire, E. L., Lapin, D. R. and Ginther, O. J. (1979) *J. Reprod. Fertil. Suppl.*, **27**, 457.

Huchzermeyer, F. and Plonait, H. (1960) *Tierärztl. Umsch.*, **15**, 399.

Hulet, C. V. (1968) *J. Amin. Sci.*, **27**, 1104.

Hunt, B., Lein, D. H. and Foote, R. H. (1978) *J. Amer. Vet. Med. Assn*, **172**, 1298.

Inabe, T., Nakazima, Y. and Matsui, N. (1983) *Theriogenology*, **20**, 97.

Jackson, G. H. (1980) *Vet. Rec.*, **119**, 90.

Johansson, I. (1968) *Genetics and Animal Breeding.* San Francisco: Freeman.

Jones, G. E., Boyns, A. R., Bell, E. T., Christie, D. W. and Parkes, M. F. (1973) *Acta Endocrinol.*, **72**, 573.

Kann, G. and Denamur, R. (1974) *J. Reprod. Fertil.*, **39**, 473.

Keel-Diffey, S. J. (1963) *Vet. Rec.*, **75**, 464.

Kidder, H. E., Casida, L. E. and Grummer, R. H. (1955) *J. Anim. Sci.*, **14**, 470.

Kindahl, H., Knudsen, O., Madej, A. and Edquist, L. E. (1982) *J. Reprod. Fertil. Suppl.*, **32**, 353.

Koch, E. (1985) *J. Reprod. Fertil. Suppl.*, **33**, 65.

Koegood-Johnsen, H. H. and Christiansen, J. (1977) *Ann. Rep. R. Vet. Agric. Univ. (Copenhagen)*, **67**.

La Bonnardiere, C. (1993) *J. Reprod. Fertil. Suppl.*, **48**, 157.

Laing, J. A. and Heap, R. B. (1971) *Brit. Vet. J.*, **127**, XIX.

Larks, S. D., Holm, L. W. and Parker, H. R. (1960) *Cornell Vet.*, **50**, 459.

Lein, D. H., Concannon, P. W., Hornbuckle, W. E., Gilbert, R. O., Glendening, J. R. and Dunlop, H. L. (1989) *J. Reprod. Fertil. Suppl.*, **39**, 231.

Lindahl, I. L. (1970) *J. Anim. Sci.*, **31**, 225.

Lindahl, I. L., Reynolds, P. J. and Allman, K. E. (1968) *J. Anim. Sci.*, **27**, 1412.

Lindahl, I. L., Totsch, J. P., Martin, P. A. and Dzuik, P. (1985) *J. Anim. Sci.*, **40**, 220.

Linzell, J. L. and Heap, R. B. (1968) *J. Endocrinol.*, **41**, 433.

McCann, J. P., Temple, M. and Concannon, P. W. (1988) Cited by Concannon, P. W., McCann, J. P. and Temple, M. (1989) *J. Reprod. Fertil. Suppl.*, **39**, 3.

McCaughey, W. J. (1979) *Vet. Rec.*, **104**, 255.

McDowell, K. J., Sharp, D. C., Fazleabas, A., Roberts, R. M. and Bazer, F. W. (1982) *J. Reprod. Fertil. Suppl.*, **32**, 329.

McDowell, K. J., Sharp, D. C., Grubaugh, W., Thatcher, W. W. and Wilcox, C. J. (1988) *Biol. Reprod.*, **39**, 340.

Madel, A. J. (1983) *Vet. Rec.*, **112**, 11.

Martal, J. and Djiane, J. (1977) *Cell Tissue Res.*, **184**, 427.

Mayer, R. E., Vernon, M. M., Zavy, M. T., Bazer, F. W. and Sharp, D. C. (1977) *Proc. 69th Ann. Meet. Soc. Anim. Sci., University of Wisconsin*, No. 466.

Meacham, T. N., Bovard, K, P. and Bond, J. (1976) *J. Anim. Sci.*, **42**, 274.

Meadows, C. E. and Lush, J. L. (1957) *J. Dairy Sci.*, **40**, 11.

Meding, J. H. and Koegood-Johnsen, H. H. (1978) *Dansk. Vettidsskr.*, **61**, 530.

Meredith, M. J. (1976) *Proc. IV Int. Pig Vet. Soc. Congr., Ames*, D3.

Miller, W. C. and Day, F. T. (1938) *J. R. Army Vet. Corps*, **10**, 101.

Monk, E. L. and Erb, R. E. (1974) *J. Anim. Sci.*, **39**, 366.

Moor, R. M., Allen, W. R. and Hamilton, D. W. (1975) *J. Reprod. Fertil. Suppl.*, **23**, 391.

Morton, D. B. and Rankin, J. E. F. (1969) *Vet. Rec.*, **84**, 658.

Morton, H., Hegh, V. and Clunie, G. J. A. (1974) *Nature*, **249**, 459.

Morton, H., Nancarrow, C. D., Scaramuzzi, R. J., Evison, B. N. and Clunie, G. J. A. (1979) *J. Reprod. Fertil.*, **56**, 75.

Nett, T. M., Holtan, D. W. and Estergreen, V. L. (1975) *J. Reprod. Fertil. Suppl.*, **23**, 457.

Newton, J. M., Shaw, R. C. and Booth, J. M. (1982) *Vet. Rec.*, **110**, 123.

Northey, D. L. and French, L. R. (1978) *Proc. Am. Soc. Anim. Sci.*, East Lansing, 0380.

Northey, D. L. and French, L. R. (1980) *J. Anim. Sci.*, **50**, 298.

Onclin, K., Silva, L. D. M. M., Donnay, I. and Verstegen, J. P. (1993) *J. Reprod. Fertil. Suppl.*, **47**, 403.

Paisley, L. G., Mickelsen, W. D., Frost, O. L. (1978) *Theriogenology*, **9**, 481.

Phillipo, M., Swapp, G. H., Robinson, J. J. and Gill, J. C. (1971) *J. Reprod. Fertil.*, **27**, 129.

Pierson, R. A. and Ginther, O. J. (1984) *Theriogenology*, **22**, 225.

Plante, C., Hansen, P. J., Martinod, S., Siegenthalev, B., Thatcher, W. W., Pollard, J. W. and Leslie, M. V. (1989) *J. Dairy Sci.*, **72**, 1859.

Radev, G., Todorov, A. and Danov, D. (1960) *Proc. IV Int. Congr. Anim. Reprod., The Hague.*

Reed, H. C. B. (1969) *Brit. Vet. J.*, **125**, 272.

Reimers, T. J., Sasser, R. G. and Ruder, C. A. (1985) *Biol. Reprod.*, **32**(Suppl. 65), Abstr.

Richardson, C. (1972) *Vet. Rec.*, **90**, 264.

Riznar, S. and Mahek, Z. (1978) *Anim. Breeding Abstr.*, **46**, Abstr. 5183.

Roberts, R. M., Klemann, S. W., Leaman, D.W., Bixby, J. A.,

Cross, J. C., Farin, C. E., Imakawa, K. and Hansen, T. R. (1991) *J. Reprod. Fertil. Suppl.*, **43**, 3.

Robertson, H. A. and Sarda, I. R. (1971) *J. Endocrinol.*, **49**, 407.

Romagnoli, S. E., Camillo, F., Cela, M., Johnston, S. D., Grassi, F., Ferdeghini, M. and Avia, G. (1993) *J. Reprod. Fertil. Suppl.*, **47**, 425.

Robertson, H. A., King, G. J. and Dyck, G. W. (1978) *J. Reprod. Fertil.*, **52**, 337.

Rowson, L. E. A. and Dott, H. M. (1963) *Vet. Rec.*, **75**, 865.

Rowson, L. E. A., Lawson, R. A. S. and Moor, R. M. (1971) *J. Reprod. Fertil.*, **25**, 261.

Royal, L., Ferneg, J. and Tainturier, D. (1979) *Rev. Med. Vet.*, **130**, 859.

Rüsse, M. (1968) *Arch. Exp. Vet. Med.*, **19**, 963.

Sasser, R. G. and Ruder, C. A. (1987) *J. Reprod. Fertil. Suppl.*, **34**, 261.

Schille, V. M., Munro, C., Walker-Farmer, S., Papkoff, H. and Stabenfeldt, G. H. (1983) *J. Reprod. Fertil.*, **68**, 29.

Schmidt, W. (1932) *Tierärzl. Rdsch.*, **38**, 825, 845.

Scott, P. P. (1970) In: *Techniques for Laboratory Animals*, ed. E. S. E. Hafez, pp. 192–208. Philadelphia: Lea and Febiger.

Settergren, I. and Galloway, D. B. (1965) *Nord. Vet. Med.*, **17**, 9.

Shemesh, M., Ayalon, N. and Mazor, T. (1979) *J. Reprod. Fertil.*, **56**, 301.

Short, R. V. (1957) *J. Endocrinol.*, **15**, 1.

Short, R. V. (1969) *Implantation and the Maternal Recognition of Pregnancy in Foetal Autonomy*. London: Churchill.

Silvia, W. J., Ottolove, J. S. and Inskeep, E. K. (1984) *Biol. Reprod.*, **30**, 936.

Smith, D. H. and Kirk, G. R. (1975) *J. Amer. Anim. Hosp. Assn*, **11**, 201.

Sokolowski, J. H. (1971) *J. Anim. Sci.*, **21**, 696.

Squire, E. L. and Ginther, O. J. (1975) *J. Reprod. Fertil. Suppl.*, **23**, 429.

Squire, E. L., Douglas, R. H., Steffenhager, W. P. and Ginther, O. J. (1974) *J. Anim. Sci.*, **38**, 330.

Stabenfeldt, G. H. (1974) *J. Amer. Vet. Med. Assn*, **164**, 311.

Steinetz, B. G., Goldsmith, L. T., Harvey, H. J. and Lust, G. (1989) *Amer. J. Vet. Res.*, **50**, 68.

Stewart, D. R. and Stabenfeldt, G. H. (1985) *Biol. Reprod.*, **32**, 848.

Studer, E. (1969) *Vet. Med. Small Anim. Clin.*, **59**, 613.

Tainturier, D. and Moysan, F. (1984) *Rev. Med. Vet.*, **135**, 525.

Taverne, M. A. M. (1984) *Tidjschr. Diergeneesk.*, **109**, 494.

Terqui, M. and Palmer, E. (1979) *J. Reprod. Fertil. Suppl.*, **27**, 441.

Thatcher, W. W., Lewis, G. S., Eley, R. M., Bazer, F. W., Fields, M. J., Williams, W. F. and Wilcox, C. J. (1980) *Proc. IX Int. Congr. Anim. Reprod. Artific. Insem., Madrid.*

Thayer, K. M., Zalesky, D., Knabe, D. A. and Forrest, D. W. (1985) *J. Ultrasound Med., Suppl.*, **4**, 186.

Tierney, T. J. (1983) *Aust. Vet. J.*, **60**, 250.

Tsolov, T. (1978) *Vet. Bull.*, Abstr. 5718.

Vandeplassche, M. (1975) *Vlaams Diergeneesk. Tijdschr.*, **26**, 60.

Verhage, H. G., Beamer, N. B. and Brenner, R. M. (1976) *Biol. Reprod.*, **14**, 579.

Verstegen, J. P., Onclin, K., Silva, L. D. M., Wouters-Ballman, P. and Ectors, F. (1993a) *J. Reprod. Fertil. Suppl.*, **47**, 165.

Verstegen, J. P., Onclin, K., Silva, L. D. M. and Donnay, I. (1993b) *J. Reprod. Fertil. Suppl.*, **47**, 411.

Watson, J., Shepherd, T. S. and Dodson, K. S. (1979) *J. Reprod. Fertil.*, **57**, 489.

White, I. R., Russel, A. J. F. and Fowler, O. G. (1984) *Vet. Rec.*, **115**, 140.

White, I. R., Russel, A. J. F., Wright, I. A. and Whyte, T. K. (1985) *Vet. Rec.*, **117**, 5.

Winters, L. M., Green, W. W. and Comstock, R. E. (1942) *Univ. Minn. Tech. Bull.*, 151.

Wisnicky, W. and Casida, L. E. (1948) *J. Amer. Vet. Med. Assn*, **133**, 451.

Zavy, M. T., Mayer, R., Vernon, M. W., Bazer, F. W. and Sharp, D. C. (1979) *J. Reprod. Fertil. Suppl.*, **27**, 403.

Zemjanis, R. (1971) *Diagnostic and Therapeutic Techniques in Animal Reproduction*. Baltimore: Williams and Wilkins.

4

Abnormal Development of the Conceptus and its Consequences

The early development of the conceptus has been described in connection with the development of the fetal membranes (see Chapter 2). However, a number of factors can influence this. The conceptus may be exposed to harmful agents during the pre-attachment, embryonic or fetal stages of development, and the vulnerability to these agents varies with these different stages. For example, during the pre-attachment stage the embryo is very resistant to teratogens and the zona pellucida is an efficient barrier to many viruses. By contrast, the embryonic stage, with rapid cell growth and differentiation, is most susceptible to teratogens. Furthermore, each organ has a critical period of development. For example, the palate, cerebellum and urogenital systems develop relatively late in the fetal period. It should also be remembered that the membranes are part of the conceptus and so any impairment to their development will affect the foetus.

Embryonic or fetal death together with the birth of abnormal offspring represent a considerable biological waste as well as being of economic significance to humans.

FERTILIZATION FAILURE AND EMBRYONIC/FETAL LOSS

Fertilization rates in domestic animals are very high. Under normal circumstances one would expect approximately 90% of ova shed to be fertilized. However, a high proportion of ova fail to develop to full-term offspring. In some instances as many as 65% are lost during embryonic and fetal development (Table 4.1). Commercially, this loss is of great economic importance.

Table 4.1 Embryonic wastage in domestic animals

Species	Wastage (%)	Reference
Cattle	45–65	Ayalon (1981)
Pig	30–50	Scofield (1976)
Sheep	20–30	Edey (1969)
Horse	15–24	Ball (1993)

DETECTION OF EMBRYONIC/ FETAL LOSS

Embryonic loss can be suspected when there is an irregular extension of the interoestrus-period. However, this will be an underestimate of total loss because it will not detect that which is occurring early on, before the maternal recognition of pregnancy and the resultant extension of the life of the corpus luteum (see Chapter 3). Furthermore, in polytocous species, like the pig, embryos may be lost without termination of pregnancy.

More accurate estimations of embryonic loss can be made by slaughtering at different times during gestation and correlating the number of embryos with the number of corpora lutea. However, this method requires the sacrifice of the animal and hence the loss of the pregnancy. A non-invasive method is preferable, but one, such as the per rectum examination of the fetus, has the disadvantage that it can be carried out only in the larger domestic animals. Furthermore, since the pregnancy can be palpated only relatively late, early embryonic loss goes undetected. More recently, ultrasonic scanning, such as Doppler, A mode and real B-mode time techniques, has allowed the very early detection of pregnancy and embryonic loss in a non-invasive manner.

TIME OF EMBRYONIC LOSS

The various techniques for estimating embryonic loss have shown that most occurs very early in gestation. For example, in mares, it is between days 10 and 14 post-service, in beef cattle it is before day 15 post-service, and in dairy heifers losses plateau after about day 19 post-service. In sheep most losses occur between days 15 and 18 post-service. In the pig, there appears to be two critical stages of embryonic loss, i.e. when the blastocyst begins to expand on day 9 and around implantation at day 13 post-service.

CAUSES OF EMBRYONIC/ FETAL LOSS

Prenatal development is a continuous process of tissue differentiation, organogenesis and maturation. The process is complex, and critical periods of development occur at different times in the different species. Agents causing embryonic loss are therefore highly variable.

Broadly speaking, embryonic loss may be due to either genetic or environmental factors or a combination of the two. The exact effect of each factor depends upon when, during gestation, it is encountered and how it exerts its influence.

ENVIRONMENTAL FACTORS CAUSING EMBRYONIC/FETAL LOSS

Environmental factors include climate, nutrition, stress, ovulation rate, failure of the normal fetomaternal recognition factors, uterine conditions, hormones, infectious agents, and teratogens. Some infectious agents causing embryonic or fetal loss in the different species are described in Chapters 23, 25, 26, 27 and 28. Teratogenic agents are discussed below, and some are shown in Table 4.2. The remaining environmental causes of embryonic or fetal loss are discussed under separate species headings.

Table 4.2 Some teratogenic agents in ruminants

	Cattle	Sheep	Goats
Viruses			
Akabane virus	+	+	+
Bluetongue virus	+	+	+
Border disease virus	−	+	−
Bovine viral diarrhoea virus	+	+	−
Cache valley virus	−	+	−
Rift valley fever virus	+	+	+
Wesselbron virus	+	+	−
Plants			
Veratrum californicum		+	
Lupins	+	+	
Others			
Hyperthermia	+	+	
Iodine deficiency	+	+	

GENETIC CAUSES OF EMBRYONIC/FETAL LOSS

Genetic factors causing embryonic loss include single-gene defects, polygenic abnormalities and chromosomal anomalies. A few single gene mutations are lethal and result in the death of the conceptus. If the gene is dominant, a single copy may be sufficient to cause death, whilst in other instances it is only the homozygous state that is

Table 4.3 Genetic abnormalities in cattle (recessive conditions)

Abnormality	Breed
Achondroplasia	Holstein Freisian
Amputates	Holstein Friesian
Oedematous calves	Ayrshire
Tibial hemimelia	Galloway
Arthrogryposis	Charolais (linked to production characteristics?)
Hip dysplasia	Charolais
Familial ataxia	Charolais
Hairless condition	Many
Factor XI deficiency	Holstein Friesian
Syndactyly	Holstein Friesian
DUMS[a]	Holstein Friesian
Weaver	Brown Swiss
Arachnomelia	Brown Swiss
Spinal muscular atrophy	Brown Swiss
α-Mannosidosis	Aberdeen Angus
BLAD[b]	Holstein Friesian

[a] DUMS, deficiency of uridine monophosphate synthesis.
[b] BLAD, bovine leukocyte adhesion deficiency.

Table 4.4 Common hereditary defects in pigs

Abnormality	Progeny with defect (%)		Probable genetic basis
	Large White	Landrace	
Congenital tremors	0.02	0.05	Possibly sex linked or recessive
Congenital splay leg	0.14	1.43	Recessive, may be sex linked
Porcine stress sydrome (malignant hyperthermia)	—	—	Recessive genes linked to genes for lean carcass. Mainly in Pietrain
Inguinal (scrotal) hernia	0.44	0.71	Recessive gene
Atresia ani	0.25	0.32	Recessive, 50% penetrance
Cryptorchidism	0.09	0.23	Recessive, incomplete penetrance
Cleft palate	—	—	Recessive
Pityriasis roseae	0.09	0.42	Unknown
Umbilical hernia	0.13	0.07	Recessive
Intersex	0.06	0.08	Unknown
Dermatosis vegetans	—	—	Recessive
Inherited thick forelegs	—	—	Recessive
Crooked tails	—	—	Dominant
Microphthalmia	—	—	Dominant, with low penetrance
Epitheliogenesis imperfecta	—	—	Recessive
Arthrogryposis	—	—	Recessive (dominant in Large White)
Cerebrospinal lipodystrophy	—	—	Recessive
Bilateral renal hypoplasia	—	—	Recessive
Renal cysts	—	—	Dominant

Table 4.5 Some inherited defects in sheep

Abnormality	Probable genetic cause
Agnathia	Lethal recessive
Brachygnathia	Recessive (also teratogens)
Arthrogryposis	Recessive (also teratogens)
Inguinal hernia	Recessive
Atresia ani	Recessive
Cryptorchidism	Recessive
Bilateral cystic renal dysplasia	Dominant
Neuraxonal dystrophy	Recessive
Entropian	Unknown
Cataracts	Dominant in New Zealand Romney
Split eyelid	Unknown
Photosensitivity (hyperbilirubinaemia)	Recessive
Micropthalmia/ anopthalmia	Recessive
Cerebellar ataxia	Recessive
Muscular dystrophy	Recessive
Goitre	Recessive (also nutitional)
Dwarfism	Recessive

Table 4.6 Some inherited defects in goats

Abnormality	Probable genetic cause
Myotonia congenita	Unknown
β-Mannosidosis	Recessive
Intersexuality (associated with the polling gene which is dominant)	Recessive
Afibrinogenaemia	Incompletely dominant
Anotia/microtia	Incompletely dominant
Udder hypoplasia	Polygenic
Extra teats (polythelia)	Polygenic
Achondroplasia	Incompletely dominant

lethal (e.g. the dominant Manx gene (M) in the cat). Recessive genes only exert their effect in the homozygous state.

Not all genetic defects are lethal. Some abnor-

mal fetuses survive to term, but these represent an economic loss. For this reason carrier animals should be eliminated from the breeding programme wherever possible. Some genetic and congenital abnormalities in domestic animals are shown in Tables 4.3–4.9 (for reviews, see: pig — Woollen, 1993; sheep — Dennis, 1993; dog — Stockman, 1982, 1983a, b; Robinson, 1990; cat — Robinson, 1991).

It was once thought that chromosomal abnormalities might be an important cause of loss of the conceptus because, in humans, it was found that approximately 50% of spontaneously aborted

Table 4.7 Some genetic defects in dogs

Abnormality	Breed	Possible cause
General		
Elbow displasia (ununited anconeal process)	Many breeds	Polygenic?
Hip dysplasia	German shepherd dogs, Labrador retrievers and others	Polygenic, multifactorial
Von Perthes's disease	West Highland white Miniature and toy poodles	Autosomal recessive but possibly polygenic
Giant axonal neuropathy	German Shepherd	Autosomal recessive
Progressive axonopathy	Boxer dogs	Autosomal recessive
Scottie cramp	Scottish terrier	Autosomal recessive
Cryptorchidism	Many	?
High uric acid secretion	Dalmations	Autosomal recessive
Dermoid sinus	Rhodesian Ridgeback	Autosomal recessive?
Deafness	Dalmations	Polygenic?
Clotting factor deficiencies		
Factor VII deficiency	Beagles	Autosomal recessive
Haemophilia A (factor VIII deficiency=classic haemophilia)	Many	X-linked recessive
Haemophilia B (factor IX deficiency=Christmas disease)	Cairn terrier, St Bernard, America cocker spaniel, French bulldog, Scottish terrier, Old English sheepdog, Shetland sheepdog, Alaskan malamute, Black and tan coonhound	X-linked recessive
Von Willebrand's disease	Scottish terrier, Chesapeake Bay retriever	Autosomal recessive
	Many other breeds	Autosomal dominant
Ocular defects		
Progressive retinal atrophy	Many breeds	Dominant or recessive depending upon type and breed
Hereditary cataract (HC)	Many breeds	?
Collie eye anomaly (CEA)	Collies	?
Cataract	Many	Many different types and genetic causes
Entropian/ectropian	Many	Polygenic
Merle eye	Many	Dominant gene affecting coat colour and tapetum formation. The homozygote is more seriously affected

fetuses had a chromosomal abnormality (Lauritsen et al., 1972). However, investigations in domestic animals have shown that probably less than 10% of pre-implantation losses are caused by gross chromosomal abnormalities (Table 4.10).

Certain specific chromosomal abnormalities, for example reciprocal translocations, do result in reduced litter sizes because of embryonic death. These are discussed separately below.

CHROMOSOME ABNORMALITIES AS A CAUSE OF INFERTILITY AND EMBRYONIC DEATH IN DOMESTIC ANIMALS

It is now well recognized that chromosomal abnormalities play an important role in infertility in some species. The chromosome complement can be determined from any dividing cell. The most common cell type used is peripheral blood lymphocytes. A *heparinized* blood sample is

Table 4.8 Some hereditary defects in cats

Abnormality	Probable genetic cause
Oesophageal stenosis	Recessive (?)
Cataract	Recessive (?)
Chediak–Higashi syndrome	Recessive
Cutaneous asthenia	Dominant
Deafness in white cats	Dominant ?
Episodic weakness	Recessive
Flat-chested kitten syndrome	Recessive
Four ears	Recessive (semilethal?)
Gangliodosis GM$_1$	Recessive
Gangliodosis GM$_2$	Recessive
Haemophilia A	Sex-linked recessive
Haemophilia B	Sex-linked recessive
Hageman factor deficiency	Incomplete dominant
Hairlessness (hypotrichosis)	Recessive
Hydrocephalus	Recessive
Hyperoxaluria	Recessive
Hyperchylomicronaemia	Recessive
Mannosidosis	Recessive
Manx tailessness	Dominant (lethal in homozygous state)
Meningoencephalocoele	Recessive
Mucopolysaccharidosis I	Recessive
Mucopolysaccharidosis VI	Recessive
Neuroaxonal dystrophy	Recessive
Polydactyly	Dominant
Porphoryria	Dominant
Progressive retinal atrophy	Two forms, one recessive, one dominant
Spheroid lysosomal disease	Recessive
Sphingomyelinosis	Recessive
Umbilical hernia	Unknown

Table 4.9 Some inherited defects of horses

Abnormality	Probable genetic cause
Cryptorchidism	Recessive (?)
Haemophilia	Sex-linked recessive
Combined immunodeficiency (CID)	Recessive
Primary agammaglobulinaemia	Sex-linked recessive (?)
Aniridia	Dominant
Hereditary ataxia	Recessive
Occipito-atlanto-axial malformation (OAAM)	Recessive
Torticollis	Recessive
Atresia coli	Recessive
Overshot/undershot jaw	Unknown
White foal syndrome	Recessive
Epitheliogenesis imperfecta	Recessive
Umbilical/inguinal hernia	Unknown
Lethal dominant white	Dominant
Cerebellar abiotropy	Recessive (?)
Hereditary multiple exostosis	Dominant
Ulnar/tibial malformation	Recessive

Table 4.10 Incidence of chromosomal abnormalities in pre-implantation embryos of domestic animals

Species	Abnormalities (%)
Sheep	6.6
Cattle	10.4
Pig	5.0
Horse	0

Data from King (1990).

required, and this should be sent for analysis as soon as possible after collection. The process depends upon obtaining dividing cells after a 2 or 3 day culture in a simple tissue culture medium with suitable supplements. After this short-term culture, the cells are inhibited from completing their division by the addition of a spindle blocker to the medium. The effect of this is to accumulate cells at mitotic metaphase. The cells are then fixed and dropped on to slides, which makes the chromosomes spread out so that they can be analysed.

Whilst blood is the most convenient source of dividing cells, longer-term fibroblast cultures can be established from almost any tissue, e.g. skin and peritoneum. Direct preparations (i.e. without any culture) can be made from tissue that is normally rapidly dividing, such as bone marrow, but this is difficult and often painful to obtain and the preparations tend to be of a poorer quality.

Various differential staining techniques enable chromosomes to be individually identified and small abnormalities to be detected. The simplest staining technique (conventional staining) reveals the chromosomal number and morphology, whilst differential staining techniques either identify areas of highly repetitive DNA sequences (C banding) or bands of euchromatin and heterochromatin (G banding and R banding). The chromosome spreads can be photographed, cut out and arranged in an agreed order to construct a *karyotype* (Figure 4.1). The normal diploid chromosome number in our domestic species is shown in Table 4.11.

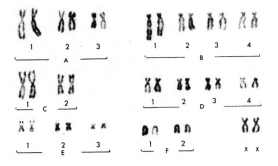

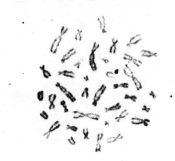

Fig. 4.1 Karyotype and spread from a female domestic cat, *Felis cattus. 2n = 38.*

Chromosome abnormalities may be numerical (e.g. aneuploidy or polyploidy) or structural and may occur in the sex chromosomes (X or Y) or the non-sex chromosomes, which are called the autosomes. Furthermore, an individual may have more than one cell line and therefore be a mixaploid.

Table 4.11 Chromosome number in domestic animals

Species	Chromosome number
Cattle	60
Sheep	54
Goat	60
Horse	64
Donkey	62
Pig	38
Swamp buffalo	48
River buffalo	50
Bactrian camel	74
Cat	38
Dog	78

Aneuploidy

Aneuploidy is when the chromosome number is almost diploid but there are one or two chromosomes too many or too few. Aneuploidy arises if there is non-disjunction during meiosis so that the chromosomes do not separate in a balanced fashion. X chromosome aneuploidy in females (XO, Turner's syndrome, and XXX, triple-X syndrome) results in infertility because two X chromosomes are required for normal meiosis in the embryo. Deviation from the normal number results in oocyte atresia during embryonic development.

Extra X chromosomes in the male (XXY, i.e. Klinefelter's syndrome) results in infertility because the extra X interferes with spermatogenesis at puberty. Animals with Klinefelter's syndrome are phenotypic males but with small testes and are azoospermic and sterile.

Aneuploidy of the autosomes results in either too many (trisomy) or too few (monosomy) copies of a particular chromosome and its associated genes. The outcome of this depends upon the genes involved. Either the individual has developmental abnormalities or, if these are not compatible with life, there is embryonic death.

Polyploidy

This is when there are whole multiples of the haploid (i.e. half the diploid) chromosome number in excess, e.g. triploidy is three times the haploid number, and tetraploidy is four times the haploid number. Polyploidy arises when there is a failure of the block to polyspermy or if there is retention of the first or second (or both) polar bodies during oogenesis.

Structural abnormalities

Problems caused by structural chromosomal abnormalities will depend upon whether genetic material has been lost (deletions) or just rearranged (insertions, inversions and translocations). In the case of deletions, carriers of the anomaly may have developmental abnormalities, depending upon which genes have been lost, which may cause embryonic death. In the latter case, balanced carriers of the anomaly are phenotypically normal, but problems arise during meiotic prophase because the chromosomes have problems at pairing. This often results in non-disjunction and the production of chromosomally unbalanced gametes, which, if they participate in fertilization events, produce unbalanced zygotes (trisomies or monosomies). Such unbalanced embryos are usually not viable.

Different abnormalities are found at different frequencies in the different species. The more common anomalies in each species are discussed below, but for a more comprehensive description the reader should consult McFeely (1990).

Horse

Chromosomal anomalies are an important cause of infertility in mares. Between 50 and 60% of mares with gonadal dysgenesis have an abnormal chromosome complement. The commonest chromosomal abnormality in mares is X chromosome aneuploidy, e.g. XO or XXX. Another common anomaly is XY sex reversal, i.e. the animal presents as a phenotypic mare but is, in fact, a genetic male.

XO mares are usually small for their age and some have poor body conformation. They usually fail to show any signs of oestrus, and the ovaries are small, fibrous and underdeveloped. The uterus is small and often described as infantile. All XO mares to date have been infertile. In women, the infertility is due to accelerated oocyte loss during fetal development and ovarian atresia in the pre-pubertal period. A similar mechanism is believed to be involved in the horse.

XXX mares often present with the same clinical history as XO mares. Others have shown irregular cyclic activity, but all have been infertile. In humans, some XXX women have been fertile, although with a reduced fertility. Since it is only infertile mares that are usually examined, it may be that some XXX horses are fertile and so are never presented for examination.

XY sex reversal is not uncommon in the horse. Most cases have been seen in Arabs and Thoroughbreds, but this may merely reflect the common breeds examined. All are phenotypically female but are genetic males. The clinical signs are variable. Some animals fail to show signs of oestrus at all whilst others have irregular but strong oestrous behaviour. Some animals have had small, undifferentiated gonads whilst others have had apparently normal ovaries with follicular activity. Most are infertile, but a very few have been fertile and at least one has produced an XY 'filly'.

In some cases the mare may be a *mixaploid* and have normal as well as abnormal cells, e.g. XO/XX, XX/XXX, XO/XX/XXX or XO/XY. In animals with a very low incidence of abnormal cells in an otherwise normal XX population, diagnosis of the condition can be difficult.

The fertility in mixaploid animals with a normal XX cell line is difficult to predict because, although most have been infertile, some have produced a foal. If the animal is actually showing oestrus and follicles are palpable on the ovary it is probably advisable not to declare the animal infertile.

Diagnosis of a chromosomal cause of a fertility problem cannot be made on the basis of the clinical history alone because animals with a normal karyotype present with the same history and clinical findings.

Few studies have been carried out on *stallions* with a fertility problem. Two colts have been reported with autosomal trisomies (Power, 1990). One was a cryptorchid (Power, 1987) and the other had small testes (Klunder et al., 1989). Structural abnormalities have also been found in chromosome 1 in a stallion with a history of early embryonic death in mares which he covered (Long, unpublished data).

Cattle

The commonest chromosomal abnormality in cattle is a structural anomaly known as a centric fusion translocation. Two chromosomes fuse together near the centromere, resulting in a reduction in the chromosome number but little or no loss in genetic material (Figure 4.2). Over 30 different centric fusion translocations have been reported in cattle, and the commonest of these is the 1/29 translocation which is found in a large number of breeds throughout the world (Table 4.12). Heterozygosity (i.e. carrying one copy) for a centric fusion translocation results in a drop in fertility, the extent of which depends upon which translocation is being carried. Animals heterozygous for the 1/29 translocation have a reduced fertility of the order of 5%. The drop in fertility is due to non-disjunction at meiosis and the production of chromosomally unbalanced gametes. The resultant unbalanced embryos undergo early embryonic death. The reduced fertility is manifested as a small increase in services per conception in the female and a lower non-return rate in the male.

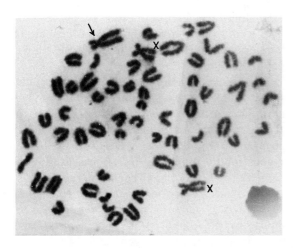

Fig. 4.2 Chromosome spread from a cow, heterozygous for the 1/29 centric fusion translocation. $2n = 59$. The arrow indicates the translocation chromosome.

Carriers of some of the other centric fusion translocations have an even greater reduction in fertility, e.g. 46% with the 25/27 translocation in the Alpine Grey.

Artificial insemination organizations in many European countries now screen their bull population, and animals carrying translocations are not used. Many countries will not allow the importation of animals carrying such translocations.

A number of other chromosomal anomalies have been reported in cattle but these are much less common. Some phenotypically abnormal calves have been born with autosomal trisomies, a few cases of infertility in the bull have been due to the XXY Klinefelter syndrome, and XXX infertile cows have been found.

Chromosomal analysis is used in the diagnosis of *freemartins* because, in this condition, the fusion of the placental blood vessels not only allows the Mullerian inhibition substance (MIS) and testosterone from the male to affect the female development, but also allows the mixing of haemopoetic precursor cells and so leads to the establishment of male and female cells in the blood of each twin. This can be detected by a simple chromosome analysis at any time after birth, and therefore freemartinism can be predicted (Long, 1990). Diagnosis is easier if blood samples from both the suspect freemartin and the male twin are analysed. This is because sometimes there is a very low number of male cells in the

Table 4.12 Cattle breeds carrying the 1/29 centric fusion translocation

Breed	Incidence (%)
Barrosa	65.1
Bauole	
Blonde d'Aquitaine	14.2–21.6
British White	65.6–78.8
Brown Mountain	
Brown Atlas	
Brown Swiss	0.2
Charolais	1.9
Chianina	13.6
Corsican	40.0
Czechoslovakian Red Pied	
De Lida	8.2
Fleckvieh	3.1
Galicia	11.8
Gascons	
German Red Pied	
Grauviel	
Hungarian Grey	3.8
Japanese Black	
Kuri	
Limousin	6.0
Maremmana	
Maronesa	49.5
Marchigiana	18.9
Modicana	6.5
Montebeliard	2.2
Nguni	10.2
Norwegian Red	
Ottenese	
Pisa	
Podolian	
Red Poll	19.0
Romagnola	22.5
Russian Black Pied	
Santa Gertrudis	
Siamese	
Simmental	3.0
Swedish Red and White	13.4
Vosgienne	
Zamora	24.0

female, but if that is so, there will be an equally low number of male cells in the male, if placental anastomosis has taken place. Examination of the male saves considerable time in these cases. However, diagnosis is possible using samples from the female alone. No samples are required from the sire or dam.

There is some debate as to the fertility of males, born twin to females. Some surveys have shown reduced non-return rates (Cribiu and Popescu, 1982), poor sperm freezability (Switonski et al.,

1991) or poor sperm concentration and motility in the ejaculate (Dunn et al., 1979) in chimeric bulls. However, other surveys have shown no reduced fertility (Gustavsson, 1977), and a normal semen picture (Gustavsson, 1977; Jaszczak et al., 1988) in such animals. There is no obvious reason for the contradictions in these findings.

Pigs

In the pig, reciprocal translocations are the most common chromosome anomalies. These are structural abnormalities where parts of chromosomes are exchanged with little or no loss of genetic material. Carriers of reciprocal translocations are phenotypically normal but have problems at meiosis, and produce unbalanced gametes. This leads to a reduced litter size or even infertility. In Sweden, 50% of boars culled for small litter sizes were found to be heterozygous for a reciprocal translocation. Of some concern is the fact that most of these translocations appear to have arisen *de novo* and were not inherited. This implies that there is something in the pig's environment that is inducing new translocations. Approximately 45 different reciprocal translocations have been identified in the pig to date.

Sheep

Cases of infertility in the ram have been due to the XXY Klinefelter syndrome. Centric fusion translocations are found in New Zealand Romney, Perendale and Drysdale sheep in New Zealand and in the Romney Marsh breed in Britain. However, unlike in cattle, centric fusion translocations have not been associated with a reduction in fertility in sheep. Reciprocal translocations have been reported in sheep with reduced fertility but these are rare (Glahn-Luft and Wassmuth, 1980; Anamthawat-Jonsson et al., 1992).

In a recent survey of barren ewes, XX/XY (freemartinism) was the commonest finding (Smith et al., unpublished data). The XO (Turner's syndrome) may be another cause of barren ewes, since one or two cases have been reported.

Goat

Centric fusion translocations have been found in Saanen and Toggenburg goats, but the effect on fertility is difficult to assess because of the con-

founding factor of the intersex gene associated with polledness in this species. Nevertheless, it does seem that heterozygosity for a centric fusion translocation is associated with reduced fertility in the Saanen breed.

The intersex gene is an autosomal recessive which is linked to the dominant gene for polledness. Thus, females that are homozygous for the polling gene are also homozygous for the intersex gene and are intersexes. Males that are homozygous for the polling gene are usually normal. However, 10–30% have been infertile due to tubular blockage in the head of the epididymis. This intersex gene in goats is thought to be similar to the *Sxr* gene in mice which causes testicular development in genetic females.

Cat

Chromosomal abnormalities are not common in the cat except in association with the tortoiseshell coat colour in the male. Many of these are XXY Klinefelter cats, and they are always sterile. However, the mixaploid animals which have a normal XY male cell line may be fertile. Fertility presumably depends upon whether the normal XY cell line is found in the testis. Fertile male tortoiseshell cats will breed as if they were normal XY toms, and will pass on the coat colour genes in a normal Mendelian fashion.

Since there is no reason to suppose that these chromosomal anomalies are only found in tortoiseshell cats they are probably responsible for fertility failure in other cats but have gone undiagnosed because very few cats are examined cytogenetically.

The XO condition has been reported and is therefore a possible cause of infertility in the female.

Dog

Chromosomal abnormalities have not been associated with infertility in the dog except in one case of Klinefelter's syndrome. Centric fusion translocations have been reported, but there have been no consistent clinical findings. Their influence on fertility has not been investigated.

Mules and hinnies

The mule is a cross between a female horse and a male donkey, and the hinnie is a cross between a female donkey and a male horse. The males of

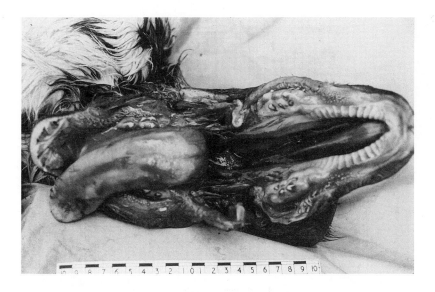

Fig. 4.3 Extreme example of cleft palate in a calf.

both crosses show abnormalities of chromosome pairing at the pachytene stage of meiotic prophase, and little or no mature spermatozoa are produced. Thus the males are infertile. Females are also affected during the fetal development of the germ cells, and most oogonia die as they are entering meiosis. However, sometimes a mature follicle is present in the adult, and, rarely, confirmed foalings have been reported in both mules and hinnies.

CONGENITAL ABNORMALITIES AND TERATOGENS

Congenital abnormalities are abnormalities that are present at birth (Figure 4.3). They may be caused by genetic factors or some other agent. A teratogen is an agent that can induce abnormalities in a developing conceptus. Teratogenic agents may not kill the developing conceptus, but many of the abnormalities they induce are incompatible with life.

Teratogens have their major effect during the embryonic stages. Before this, during pregastrulation, the conceptus is relatively resistant to the effects of teratogens, and after this, at the fetal stage, it is only the late-developing systems such as the palate, cerebellum and parts of the cardio-

vascular and urogenital system that are affected. A teratogen may be a drug, hormone, chemical, gamma irradiation, trace element, variations of temperature, or an infectious agent (particularly viruses — see Oberst (1993) for a review). For example, in the pig, Swine fever (hog cholera) virus will produce neurological abnormalities such as demyelination, cerebellar and spinal hypoplasia, hydrocephalus and arthrogryposis. Table 4.2 shows some of the known teratogenic agents in ruminants. In the dog, some common pharmacological agents such as corticosteroids and griseofulvin are known teratogens, and care must be exercised in their use in pregnant bitches. In the cat, the panleucopenia virus will cause teratogenic effects in pregnant queens.

Congenital abnormalities may cause obstetrical problems. For example, *perosomus elumbis*, which occurs in ruminants and swine, is characterized by hypoplasia or aplasia of the spinal cord which ends in the thoracic region. The regions of the body, including the hind limbs, which are normally supplied by the lumbar and sacral nerves, exhibit muscular atrophy, and joint movement does not develop. The rigidity of the posterior limbs may then cause dystocia.

Schistosoma reflexus, another abnormality common in ruminants and swine, has as the main defect, acute angulation of the vertebral column such that the tail lies close to the head (Figure 4.4). The chest and abdominal cavities are incomplete

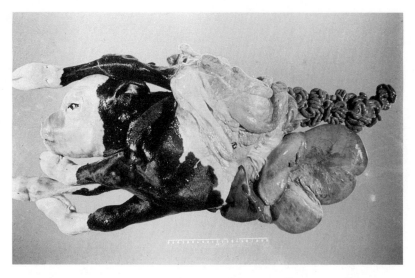

Fig. 4.4 *Schistosoma reflexus* in a calf.

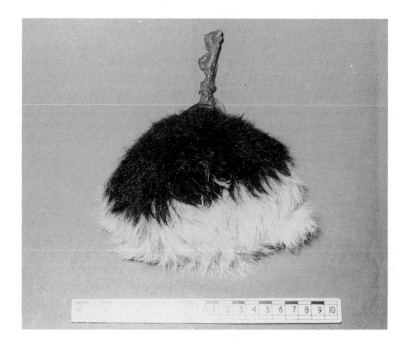

Fig. 4.5 *Amorphous globosus* in the cow.

ventrally so that the viscera are exposed. Again such cases may cause dystocia (see Chapter 16).

Another strange entity is that known as *amorphous globosus*, acardiac monster or fetal mole (Figure 4.5). These are spherical bodies, attached to the fetal membranes of a normal fetus. They are formed from connective tissue surrounded by skin and may be of a different sex to that of the normal twin. Since there is not usually any gonadal devel-

opment they do not pose a threat of freemartin development.

Double monsters (Figures 4.6 and 4.7), which are found in a number of species, will present as absolute fetal oversize. Other examples of causes of fetal oversize are hydrocephalus (Figures 4.8 and 4.9) and accessory limbs (Figure 4.10)

Some of the congenital anomalies that are of importance in veterinary obstetrics have a genetic

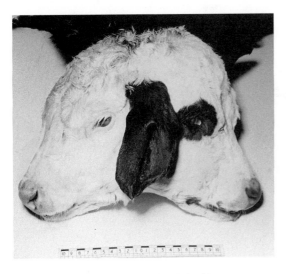

Fig. 4.6 Double-headed calf.

EMBRYONIC/FETAL LOSS IN THE DIFFERENT SPECIES

Pig

Ovulation rate is not usually a limiting factor in productivity in the pig but, in general, as ovulation rates increase, the embryo survival rate decreases. This can be demonstrated in gilts, where the ovulation rate can be artificially increased but embryo survival rate decreases.

Even if early embryonic death does not occur with high ovulation rates, a problem may arise later in pregnancy with competition for uterine space. It has been suggested that a higher fetal death rate exists when there are more than five fetuses *per* horn, with those embryos in the middle of the horn being smaller (Perry and Rowell, 1969).

Apart from the above intrinsic factors, extrinsic factors such as nutrition and stress play an important part in embryonic loss in the pig. For example, it is well documented that high energy levels after service result in reduced embryo survival. Stress, associated with extremes of temperature, or certain management systems such as sow stalls or tethers, is also known to result in increased embryo mortality. Other husbandry policies, such as lactation length, also affect embryonic death rates, and lactation lengths of less than 3 weeks produce a marked rise in embryonic mortality (Varley and Cole,

cause. For example, achondroplasia (dwalf calves) (Figure 4.11) and amputates (otter calves) (Figure 4.12) in Friesians, double muscling and arthrogryposis (Figure 4.13) in the Charolais, and oedematous calves in the Ayrshire breed (Figure 4.14) (see Table 4.3). Leipold and Dennis (1986) described rectovaginal constriction in Jersey cattle, due to a simple autosomal recessive, as an important cause of severe dystocia. Affected animals required episiotomy or Caesarian section at parturition.

Some congenital abnormalities, such as spastic paresis (Figure 4.15), resolve in time.

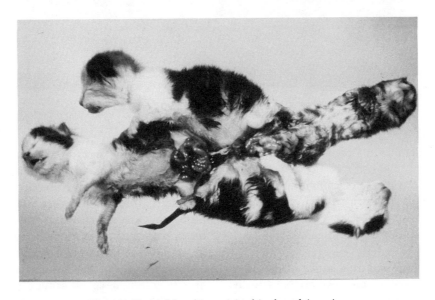

Fig. 4.7 Litter of four kittens joined in the pelvic region.

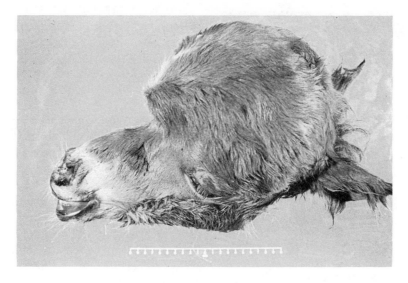

Fig. 4.8 Hydrocephalus in a foal fetus.

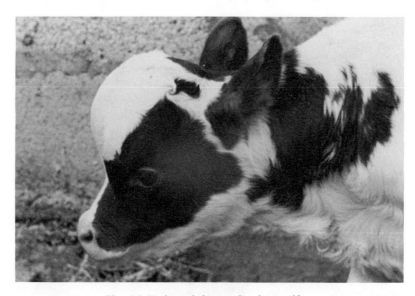

Fig. 4.9 Hydrocephalus in a live-born calf.

1976), presumably due to a poor uterine environment.

Some infectious causes of embryonic loss and abortion in the pig are discussed in Chapter 27.

Cattle

Considering the size and importance of the dairy industry in Western countries there is actually relative little hard experimental data on the causes of embryonic loss in cattle. The timing of insemination is important. Insemination too late in the oestrous period leads to ovum ageing and embryonic death. (In laboratory species, ovum ageing has been shown to result in chromosomal abnormalities.) Artificial insemination during pregnancy will induce loss, either through mechanical trauma to fetal membranes or the introduction of infection. Specific infectious agents causing loss are described in Chapter 23. Cows conceiving too soon after

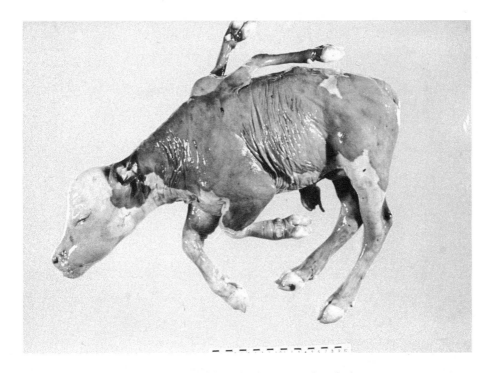

Fig. 4.10 Calf embryo with accessory front limbs.

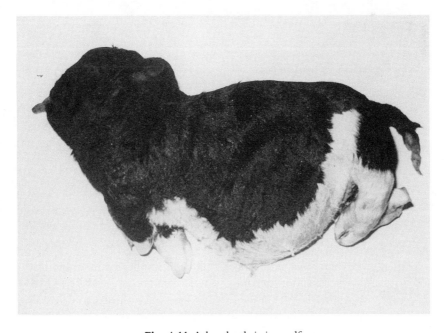

Fig. 4.11 Achondroplasia in a calf.

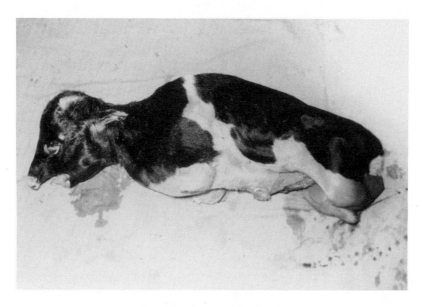

Fig. 4.12 Amputate (otter) calf.

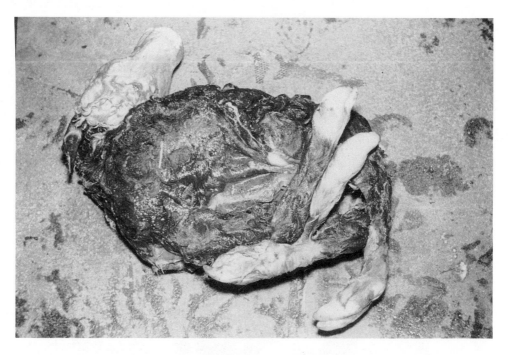

Fig. 4.13 Arthrogryposis in a calf.

calving have a higher embryonic loss rate, and this is presumed to be due to a poor uterine environment.

Nutritional causes such as β-carotene, selenium, phosphorus and copper deficiencies have all been implicated in embryonic loss, but unequivical data are not available.

Stress, e.g. heat stress, has also been shown to result in embryonic loss (Thatcher and Collier, 1986).

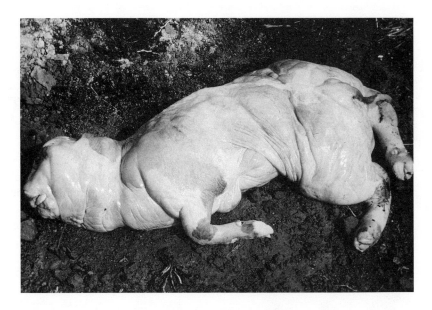

Fig. 4.14 Oedematous Ayrshire calf.

Horse

The commonest cause of embryonic loss in mares is twin conceptions (see Chapter 26). Competition for placental space usually results in one fetus growing more slowly than the other, and the smaller fetus, with a smaller placenta, dies. Death of one fetus often results in the loss of the second. Other intrinsic factors which are thought to be related to embryonic loss in the mare include oviductal secretions, embryonic vesicle mobility and uterine environment. Since the mare's embryo is at a more advanced stage whilst still in the uterine tube, the environment may be relatively more important in this species than others. In addition, the embryonic vesicle remains free in the lumen of the uterine horn much longer in the mare than in other species, and the degree of mobility of this vesicle is thought to be important in maternal recognition of pregnancy (Ginther, 1985; McDowell et al., 1985). Greater mobility enhances the suppression of luteolysis and results in higher levels of progesterone (Ginther et al., 1985). As regards the uterine environment, recurrent endometritis and post-service infection leads to perivascular fibrosis, and this is a common cause of embryonic and fetal death between 40 and 90 days of gestation (see Chapter 26). Increased maternal age has also been associated with increased embryonic loss, but this may merely reflect increased chronic uterine pathology.

Other factors such as lactation and service at the foal heat also result in higher embryonic death rates, although the latter may be due to lactational stress. Stress, due to transportation, is thought to cause embryonic losses in the mare. However, recent studies failed to confirm this even though transport did result in raised plasma ascorbic acid levels, which has been associated with prolonged stress (Baucus et al., 1990). Nutritional stress, in the form of restricted energy intake, does increase embryonic loss.

Infectious causes of loss are discussed in Chapter 26.

Sheep

Nutrition, specifically energy level, is known to affect embryonic survival in sheep in a complex manner. Low body condition at mating is detrimental to embryo survival, irrespective of post-mating nutrition. However, in ewes that lose weight post-service, embryo mortality is increased. Prolonged, moderate, undernutrition has more effect on ewe lambs than adult ewes. Nutritional energy may exert its effect via peripheral blood progesterone levels since there is an inverse relationship between food intake and progesterone levels. Other nutrients important in embryo survival are vitamin E and selenium.

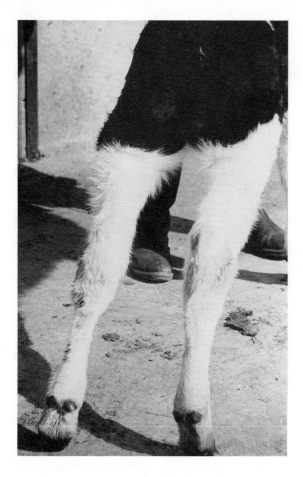

Fig. 4.15 Spastic paresis in a calf.

Certain plants, such as kale and *Veratrum californicum*, will cause embryonic death. The latter is also a teratogenic agent (see Table 4.2).

The effects of nutrition may be exaggerated or confounded by differences in ovulation rate since losses have often been reported to be disproportionately high in twin ovulations. In breeds with very high ovulation rates (i.e. litter bearers), the embryonic death rate rises proportionately, but this is probably due to limitations of uterine space.

High environmental temperature, particularly in the first week after mating, has been shown experimentally to increase dramatically the embryonic death rate. This could be important in climatic heat waves. However, if there is diurnal variation, as would occur naturally, the loss is much less.

Physiological stress, such as that produced by overcrowding or handling of sheep, also increases embryonic loss. This may be due to excess secre-

tion of progesterone by the adrenals and/or raised corticosteroid levels (Wilmut et al., 1986).

The age of the ewe is also important, since there is some evidence that ewe lambs have a higher incidence of embryonic loss than mature ewes (Quirke and Hanrahan, 1977). Infectious causes of fetal loss are discussed in Chapter 25.

Goat

Goats are particularly susceptible to non-infectious fetal loss, and this is particularly true of the Angora breed. Losses are also common in poorly fed animals of any breed. Another reported cause of fetal loss is dosing with anthelmintics such as carbon tetrachloride and phenothiazine.

Infectious causes of abortion in goats are discussed in Chapter 25.

Dog

Very little information is available on the non-infectious causes of embryonic loss in the dog. In some instances whole litters are resorbed. It used to be thought that this was due to progesterone insufficiency, but there is no real evidence for this proposition. Furthermore, high levels of exogenous progesterone may cause abnormal sex differation in the male puppies.

The commonest infectious cause of fetal loss is *Brucella canis*. This organism is not, however, found in Britain. Canine herpes virus can also cause fetal death and mummification. In this condition, infection of the fetus can be transplacental in pregnant bitches, but more commonly the neonate is infected during passage through the birth canal at parturition (see Chapter 28).

Cat

Very little information is available on the non-infectious causes of embryonic loss in the cat. Cats are susceptible to the loss of embryos due to stress, and care should be taken not to distress a pregnant queen. The infectious causes of embryonic loss include feline viral rhinotracheitis (FVR) and feline panleucopenia virus (FPV), which cause abortion, fetal mummification and stillborn kittens, and feline leukaemia virus (FELV), which causes fetal resorption and abortion and is also responsible for producing the fading kitten syndrome (see Chapter 28).

SEQUELAE TO EMBRYONIC OR FETAL DEATH

Following early embryonic death the embryonic tissues are usually *resorbed*, and the animal returns to oestrus if there is no other conceptus in the uterus. If death occurs before there has been maternal recognition of pregnancy the oestrous cycle is not prolonged. If it occurs after recognition has taken place, the oestrous cycle will be prolonged (see pp. 63–65).

If death of the embryo is due to an infection then, even although the embryonic material may be absorbed, a *pyometra* may follow. In cattle this condition is characterized by persistance of the corpus luteum, closed cervix and pus accumulation in the uterine body and horns. It is a particular characteristic of infection with *Tritrichomonas fetus* (see Chapter 23).

If fetal death occurs after ossification of the bones has begun, complete resorption of fetal material cannot take place. Instead, *fetal mummification* occurs. The commonest form of mummification is *papyraceous mummification*, where the fetal fluids are resorbed and the fetal membranes become shrivelled and dried so that they resemble parchment (hence the name). The uterus contracts on to the fetus, which becomes twisted and contorted. In polytocous species, if mummification occurs in only some embryos, this does not interfere with the continuation of the pregnancy of the live fetuses. The mummified fetus is simply expelled at parturition.

Mummification is very common in the pig, and is a particular characteristic of infection with the SMEDI viruses (see p. 510). It is also seen in large litters as a consequence of uterine overcrowding and placental insufficiency. In the cat, fetal mummification is not uncommon in large litters, and is again assumed to be due to uterine overcrowding. In the dog, fetal mummification is a characteristic of canine herpes virus (CHV) infection. In the ewe, fetal mummification may be seen with twins and/or triplets when one of the embryos has died. In the mare, mummification is rare and is always associated with twin pregnancies (see p. 478). If twinning does occur, one of the fetuses usually develops more slowly than the other and is smaller. The small fetus usually dies, and if the other fetus survives and the pregnancy is maintained, the

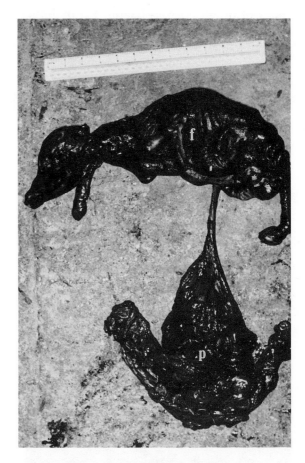

Fig. 4.16 Mummified foal (f) with attached placenta. (p), twin to a normal foal.

dead fetus will mummify and be delivered at term with the live foal (Figure 4.16).

In cattle, fetal mummification occurs with an incidence of 0.13–1.8% (Barth, 1986). Although papyraceous mummification does occur, *haematic mummification* is more common. In this condition the fetal fluids are resorbed but the fetus and membranes are surrounded by a viscous, chocolate-coloured material. It was once thought that the colour was due to pigments from the blood and that the condition was due to caruncular haemorrhage (hence the name) which resulted in fetal death. However, the haemorrhage is thought now to be an effect of fetal death, rather than the cause. Various theories have been put forward as to the aetiology of the condition. It has been suggested that there is a genetic cause, particularly since the condition appeared to be more common in Channel Island breeds (Jersey and Guernsey) and occurred with a high frequency in a particular family of British Friesians (Logan, 1973). Torsion of the umbilical cord has been suggested as the primary cause of fetal death, but this has not been a consistent finding in haematic mummies. On the other hand, the condition has been induced hormonally using oestradiol and trembolone acetate (Gorse, 1979), which suggests that a hormonal anomaly may be the cause.

Haematic mummification can occur following fetal death at ages ranging from 3 to 8 months of gestation. Since there is no fetal signal for the onset of parturition the *corpus luteum* is retained and the 'pregnancy' will be maintained for an unpredictable time. The condition is often only diagnosed when the cow is examined because of a *prolonged gestation* period. Treatment of choice is the induction of abortion by luteolysis using prostaglandins. The fetus is normally expelled in 2–4 days. The prognosis for further breeding is good since there has been no intrinsic damage to the reproductive tract. However, care needs to be taken that the mummified fetus is indeed expelled, otherwise a possible sequel is *fetal maceration*. Fetal maceration

can occur in any species, but it is described most frequently in cattle. It occurs as a consequence of the failure of an aborting fetus to be expelled, due perhaps to uterine inertia. Bacteria enter the uterus through the dilated cervix, and by a combination of putrefaction and autolysis the soft tissues are digested, leaving a mass of fetal bones within the uterus. Sometimes these become embedded in the uterine wall and are difficult to remove other than by hysterotomy (Figure 4.17). Under these circumstances a chronic endometritis ensues and there is severe damage to the endometrium. The animal should therefore be sent for slaughter.

Prolonged gestation need not be always related to fetal death. It is, for example, a characteristic of anencephalic pregnancies (Figure 4.18), in which, due to the absence of the fetal pituitary, normal parturition cannot be initiated (see Chapter 6). If the fetus is alive it continues to grow, and so the result of prolonged gestation is absolute fetal oversize, which leads to *dystocia*.

Other sequelae to fetal death are *abortion* and *stillbirth*. Abortions are often caused by infectious

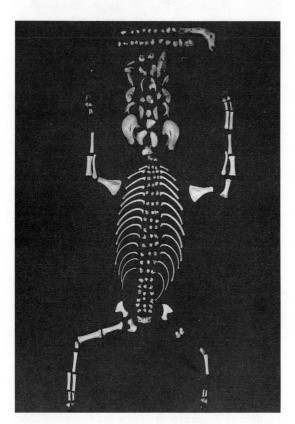
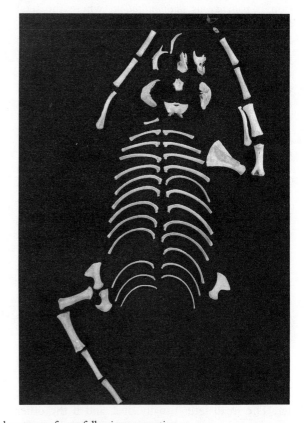

Fig. 4.17 Fetal bones removed from the uterus of cow following maceration.

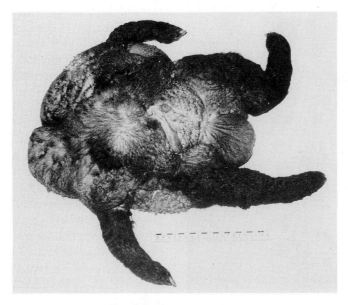

Fig. 4.18 Anencephalic lamb.

agents, and these are dealt with elsewhere (see Chapters 23 and 25–28). Stillbirths may occur because of developmental anomalies incompatible with life.

DROPSY OF THE FETAL MEMBRANES AND FETUS

Three dropsical conditions of the conceptus may be seen in veterinary obstetrics: oedema of the placenta, dropsy of the fetal sacs and dropsy of the fetus. They may occur separately or in combination.

Oedema of the placenta

This frequently accompanies a placentitis, for example *Brucella abortus* infection in cattle. It does not cause dystocia but is frequently associated with abortion or stillbirth.

Dropsy of the fetal sacs

Both the amniotic and allantoic sacs can contain excessive quantities of fetal fluid (see Chapter 2); when this occurs it is referred to as hydramnios or hydrallantois, depending on which sac is involved. Hydrallantois is much more common than hydramnios, although the latter is always seen in

association with specific fetal abnormalities such as the 'bulldog' calf in the Dexter. Although dropsy of the fetal sacs is essentially a bovine condition, Vandeplassche (1973) has seen 48 equine cases in which pluriparous mares of 10–20 years of age showed very rapid onset of the condition between $7\frac{1}{2}$ and $9\frac{1}{2}$ months of gestation. A few cases have been recorded in sheep, associated with either twins or triplets, in which the excess of fluid — amounting to about 18.5 litres — was in the amniotic sac. It has also been reported in the dog involving all fetuses in a litter.

Apart from the hereditary cases of hydramnios which accompany the Dexter 'bulldog' calf, and which may occur as early as the third or fourth month, most instances of dropsy of the fetal sacs of cattle are seen in the last 3 months of gestation. The cause is not known. Arthur (1957) found the number of functioning cotyledons was abnormally low — the non-pregnant horn usually was not participating in placental formation — and there was a compensatory accessory caruncular development in the pregnant horn. Histologically, there was a non-infectious degeneration and necrosis of the endometrium and, as already observed, the fetus was undersized. Normally, in cattle, there is a markedly accelerated production of allantoic fluid at 6–7 months of gestation, and it is suggested that, where placental dysfunction exists,

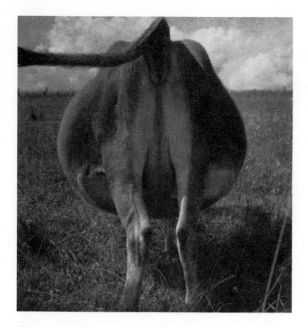

Fig. 4.19 Jersey cow with the distended 'pear-shaped' abdomen typical of hydrops allantois.

gression. The essential symptom is distension of the abdomen by the excess of fetal fluid (Figure 4.19). The later in gestation the condition occurs, the more likely it is that the cow will survive to term, whereas if the abdomen is obviously distended at 6 or 7 months, the cow will become extremely ill long before term. The volume of allantoic fluid varies up to 273 litres, and such large amounts impose a serious strain on the cow and greatly hamper respiration and reduce appetite. There is gradual loss of condition, eventually causing recumbency and death (Figure 4.20). Occasionally, the animal becomes relieved by aborting. The less severely affected reach term in poor condition and, because of uterine inertia (often accompanied by incomplete dilation of the cervix), frequently require help at parturition.

The diagnosis of bovine hydrallantois is based on the easily appreciable fluid distension of the abdomen, with its associated symptoms, in the last third of pregnancy. Confirmation may be obtained by the rectal palpation of the markedly swollen uterus and by the failure to palpate the fetus either per rectum or externally.

The *treatment* of hydrallantois calls for a realistic approach and a nicety of judgement. Cases that have become recumbent should be slaughtered. Where the animal is near term, a one- or two-stage caesarian operation is indicated. With both

this increase may become uncontrolled and lead to massive accumulation. It is also frequently associated with twins.

All cases of hydrallantois are progressive, but they vary in time of clinical onset (within the last 3 months of pregnancy) and in their rate of pro-

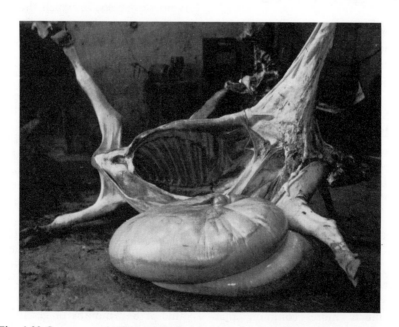

Fig. 4.20 Same cow as in Figure 4.19 after slaughter showing the greatly enlarged uterus.

methods it is imperative that the fluid is allowed to escape slowly, so as to prevent the occurrence of hypovolaemic shock associated with splanchnic pooling of blood. Since hydrallantois is frequently seen in twin pregnancies in cows, it is particularly important to search the grossly distended uterus for the second calf.

Cases of hydrallantois which calve, or are delivered by caesarian operation, frequently retain the placenta and, owing to tardy uterine involution, often develop metritis. This may lead to a protracted convalescence and delayed conception.

By using a synthetic corticosteroid (dexamethazone or flumethazone) in conjunction with oxytocin, Vandeplassche (1973) reported improved therapy for hydrallantois. About 4 or 5 days after an injection of 20 mg of dexamethazone or 5–10 mg of flumethazone the cervix relaxes and the cow is given oxytocin by means of intravenous drip for 30 minutes. Of 20 cows so treated, 17 recovered. In respect of the management of equine hydrallantois, the same writer advises that affected mares enter a spontaneous abortion phase but fail to expel the fetus because of uterine atony. Vandeplassche breaks the allantochorion to release its fluid (commonly amounting to 100 litres). The mare is then given oxytocin by intravenous drip, and when the cervix has relaxed sufficiently the fetus is manually withdrawn. The placental itself is markedly oedematous, and retention is prevented by further administration of oxytocin.

DROPSY OF THE FETUS

There are several types of fetal dropsy, and those of obstetric importance are hydrocephalus (see Figure 4.8 and 4.9), ascites and anasarca. The form of the fetus and the degree of obstetric hazard are determined by the location and amount of the excess of fluid. Dystocia is due to the increased diameter of the fetus.

Hydrocephalus

Hydrocephalus involves a swelling of the cranium due to an accumulation of fluid which may be in the ventricular system or between the brain and the dura. It affects all species of animals and is seen most commonly by veterinary obstetricians in pigs, puppies and calves (see Figures 4.8 and 4.9).

In the more severe forms of hydrocephalus there is marked thinning of the cranial bones. This facilitates trocarization and compression of the skull so as to allow vaginal delivery. Where this cannot be done, the dome of the cranium may be sawn off with fetotomy wire or chain saw. If the fetus is decapitated there is still the difficulty of delivering the head. Caesarian section may be performed, but there is no merit in obtaining a live hydrocephalic calf; however, this operation may be necessary in severe cases affecting pigs and dogs, and in cattle when the calf is presented posteriorly or when hydrocephalus is accompanied by ankylosis of the limb joints.

Fetal ascites

Dropsy of the peritoneum is a common accompaniment of infectious disease of the fetus and of developmental defects, such as achondroplasia (see Figure 4.11). Occasionally, it occurs as the only defect. Aborted fetuses are often dropsical; when the fetus is full term, ascites may cause dystocia. This can usually be relieved by incising the fetal abdomen with a fetotomy knife.

Fetal anasarca

The affected fetus is usually carried to term, and concern is caused by the lack of progress in second-stage labour. This is due to the great increase in fetal volume caused by the excess of fluid in the subcutaneous tissues, particularly of the head and hindlimbs. In the case of the head, there is so much swelling that the normal features are masked and the resultant appearance is quite grotesque. It is an interesting point that an undue proportion of these anasarcous fetuses are presented posteriorly, in which case the enormous swelling of the presenting limbs is very conspicuous. There is frequently an excess of fluid in the peritoneal and pleural cavities with dilatation of the umbilical and inguinal rings as well as hydrocele. The substance of the fetal membranes is also oedematous and occasionally there is a degree of hydrallantois.

SUPERFECUNDATION

Superfecundation is the condition in which offspring from two sires are conceived contemporaneously. Owing to the number of ova shed and their longevity, as well as to the length of oestrus and the promiscuous mating behaviour of the species, superfecundation is most likely in the bitch. The phenomenon is suspected when mating to two dogs of different breeds is known to have occurred, and the suspicion is heightened when the litter shows marked dual variation in colour pattern, conformation and size. Corroboration of superfecundation by inspection of the progeny is valid only when pure-bred partners are involved. It is likely that the majority of alleged cases are due simply to genetic variation in the offspring of impure parents.

Superfecundation has been reported when a mare gave birth to twin horse and mule foals, and when a Friesian cow delivered twin Friesian and Hereford calves.

SUPERFETATION

Superfetation is the condition that arises when an animal already pregnant mates, ovulates and conceives a second fetus or second litter. It is not uncommon for a cow to be mated when pregnant, but no evidence is available that ovulation occurs in a cow carrying a live fetus. Ovulation does occur in pregnant mares, and in this species superfetation is theoretically possible. Superfetation is suspected when fetuses of very different size are born together or when two fetuses, or two litters, are born at widely separated times. Apparently authentic cases have been described in which two normally mature fetuses, or litters, have been delivered at times corresponding in gestation length to two widely separated and observed matings.

In general there is considerable doubt about superfetation; however, Vandeplassche et al. (1968) have produced convincing proof that this is so in the double parturitions of sows. They investigated 12 cases of double porcine parturition following a single mating, and in two of them they explored the uterus and ovaries by laparotomy after the second farrowing. They concluded that double parturition followed a single mating at which an excessively large number of eggs were fertilized and which later distributed themselves normally throughout both uterine horns. Instead of the more usual subsequent reduction of the litter size

by embryonic death, the embryos in the cranial halves of both cornua remained unimplanted in a state of 'embryonic diapause' for periods varying from 4 to 98 days, after which they were reactivated and implanted, thus constituting a spontaneous superfetation in the cranial parts of the horns. The embryos which implanted in the caudal parts of the horns underwent a normal gestation and parturition; a second parturition at variable intervals occurred when the piglets from the delayed implantation reached maturity. Vandeplassche and his co-workers believe that the cases of double parturition in pigs and in other species which follow mating at separate oestrous periods are also due to embryonic diapause rather than to superfetation; also that occasional cases of prolonged gestation may be due to the same cause.

REFERENCES

Anamthawat-Jonsson, K., Lang, S. E., Basrur, P. K. and Adalsteinsson, S. (1992) *Res. Vet. Sci.*, **52**, 367–370.

Arthur, G. H. (1957) *Brit. Vet. J.*, **113**, 17.

Ayalon, N. (1981) *Zuchthygiene*, **16**, 97.

Ball, B. A. (1993) Embryonic death in mares. In: *Equine Reproduction*, ed. A. O. McKinnon and J. L. Voss, p. 517. Philadelphia: Lea and Febiger.

Barth, A. D. (1986) Induced abortion in cattle. In: *Current Therapy in Theriogenology 2*, ed. D. A. Morrow, p. 205. Philadelphia: W. B. Saunders.

Baucus, K. L., Ralston, S. L., Nockels, C. F., McKinnon, A. O. and Squires, E. L. (1990) *J. Anim. Sci.*, **68**, 345.

Cribiu, E. P. and Popescu, C. P. (1982) Sur la frequence du chimerisms leucocytaire XX/XY parmi les taureaux d'insemination. *Proc. 5th Eur. Colloq. Cytogenet. Domestic Anim.*, *Milano-Gargnano*, p. 215.

Dennis, S. M. (1993) *Vet. Clin. N. Amer. Food Anim. Pract.*, **9**, 203.

Dunn, H. O., McEntee, K., Hall, C. E., Johnson, R. M. and Stone, W. H. (1979) *J. Reprod. Fertil.*, **57**, 21.

Edey, T. N. (1969) *Anim. Breeding Abstr.*, **37**, 43.

Ginther, O. J. (1985) *Equine Vet. J. (Suppl.)*, **3**, 41.

Ginther, O. J., Garcia, M. C. and Bergfeldt, D. R. (1985) *Theriogenerology*, **24**, 409.

Glahn-Luft and Wassmuth, R. (1980) *Proc. 31st Ann. Meeting Europ. Assn Anim. Prod.*

Gorse, M. (1979) *Vet. Bull.*, **49**, 349 (Abstr. 2729).

Gustavsson, I. (1977) *Ann. Genet. Selection Anim.*, **9**, 531.

Jaszczak, K., Parada, R., Boryczko, Z., Romanowicz, K. and Wijas, B. (1988) *Genet. Polonica*, **29**, 369.

King, W. A. (1990) *Advan. Vet. Sci. Comp. Med.*, **34**, 229.

Klunder, L. R., McFeely, R. A., Beech, J. and McClune, W. (1989) *Equine Vet. J.*, **21**, 69.

Lauritsen, J. G., Jonasson, J., Therkelsen, A. J., Lass, F., Lindsten, J. and Petersen, G. B. (1972) *Hereditas*, **71**, 160.

Leiopold, H. N. and Dennis, S. M. (1986) *14th World Congr. Dis. Cattle, Dublin*, p. 63.

Logan, E. F. (1973) *Vet. Rec.*, **93**, 252.

Long, S. E. (1990) *In Practice*, **12**, 208.

McDowell, K. J., Sharp, D. C. and Peck, L. S. (1985) *Equine Vet. J. (Suppl.)*, **3**, 23.

McFeely, R. A. (1990) *Advan. Vet. Sci. Comp. Med.*, **34**.

Oberst, R. D. (1993) *Vet. Clin. N. Amer. Food Anim. Pract.*, **9**, 23.

Perry, J. S. and Rowell, J. C. (1969) *J. Reprod. Fertil.*, **19**, 527.

Power, M. M. (1987) *Cytogenet. Cell Genet.*, **45**, 163.

Power, M. M. (1990) *Advan. Vet. Sci. Comp. Med.*, **34**, 131–167.

Quirke, J. F. and Hanrahan, J. P. (1977) *J. Reprod. Fertil.*, **51**, 487.

Robinson, R. (1990) *Genetics for Dog Breeders*. Oxford: Pergamon Press.

Robinson, R. (1991) *Genetics for Cat Breeders*. Oxford: Pergamon Press.

Scofield, A. M. (1976) *Vet. Annual.*, **15**, 91.

Stockman, M. (1982) *In Practice*, **4**, 170.

Stockman, M. (1983a) *In Practice*, **5**, 103.

Stockman, M. (1983b) *In Practice*, **5**, 202.

Switonski, M., Lechniak, D. and Landzwojczak, D. (1991) *Genet. Polonica*, **32**, 227.

Thatcher, W. W. and Collier, R. J. (1986) Effects of climate on bovine reproduction. In: *Current Therapy in Theriogenology 2*, ed. D. A. Morrow, p. 301. Philadelphia: W. B. Saunders.

Vandeplassche, M. (1973) Personal communication.

Vandeplassche, M., Vandevelde, A., Delanote, M. and Ghekiere, P. (1968) *Tijdschr. Diergeneesk.*, **93**, 19.

Varley, M. A. and Cole, D. J. A. (1976) *Anim. Prod.*, **22**, 79.

Wilmut, I., Sales, D. I. and Ashworth, C. J. (1986) *J. Reprod. Fertil.*, **76**, 851.

Woollen, N. E. (1993) *Vet. Clin. N. Amer. Food Anim. Pract.*, **9**, 163.

5

Typically, prolapse of the vagina is a condition of ruminants in late gestation. Occasionally it is seen after parturition and rarely it occurs unconnected with pregnancy or parturition.

Its exact cause has not been ascertained but several factors are generally believed to play a part. Cattle of the beef breeds, particularly Herefords, are most commonly affected. Woodward and Queensberry (1956) recorded 1.1% of vaginal prolapses in 7859 pregnancies in Hereford cattle in the USA, and it has been suggested that in them the anatomical anchorage of the genital tract is less efficient than in other animals. An excessive deposition of fat in the perivaginal connective tissue, and ligamentous relaxation, may increase the mobility of the vagina. Both these effects might be due to a state of endocrine imbalance, in which oestrogenic hormones predominate. The administration of stilboestrol is known to soften the genital ligaments and to increase the bulk of the genital tract. Where oestrogenic substances are present in inordinate amounts in the diet, as in subterranean clover pastures of Western Australia (Bennetts, 1944), or when they are purposedly fed for fattening purposes, vaginal prolapse may frequently occur. Mouldy maize and barley are considered to have a high oestrogen content, and when young gilts and heifers are fed on them they may show vulvovaginitis with oedema of the vulva, relaxation of the pelvic ligaments, tenesmus and vaginal prolapse (Koen and Smith, 1945; McErlean, 1952). Vaginal prolapse in gilts may be seen at oestrus.

It is postulated that the endocrine predisposition to vaginal prolapse is inherited. Mechanical factors such as the increasing intra-abdominal pressure of late pregnancy and gravity, acting through the medium of a sloping byre floor, are of probable aetiological significance (McLean and Claxton, 1960).

In so far as sheep are concerned, and in this species the affection may be of real economic importance with an average incidence of 0.53 which may rise to 20% in some flocks (Edgar, 1952), close confinement undoubtedly predisposes to vaginal prolapse. Similarly, hill sheep, brought down to unnaturally lush lowland pastures, with consequent restriction of exercise, are especially prone. In this connection, ewes of the Kerry Hill and Clun Forest breeds seem to be particularly susceptible. It is not yet known whether sex hormones present in herbage play a part in the causation of vaginal prolapse in British sheep, but it appears that the disease occurs more frequently as pastures are improved and that it is more troublesome in twin-bearing ewes in seasons when there is plentiful herbage. The feeding of high-roughage diets such as silage, poor-quality hay or root crops can also predispose to the condition. There is a similarity of incidence, and probably an aetiological relationship, between vaginal prolapse and 'ringwomb' in sheep; not uncommonly the same ewe is consecutively affected by the two conditions. In both sheep and cattle vaginal prolapse is commoner in pluripara than primipara.

Whatever the cause of prolapse of the vagina, parturiton or abortion relieves the condition.

In some bitches, hyperplasia of the vaginal mucosa occurs at oestrous and may protrude through the vulva. This is sometimes referred to as vaginal prolapse, although such a description is incorrect and is not comparable with the condition in other species (see Chapter 28). Recently, chronic prolapse during pregnancy requiring hysteropexy has been described (Memon *et al.*, 1993).

Symptoms and course
Initially the lesion involves a protrusion of the mucous membrane — more particularly of the floor — of that part of the vagina which lies just in front of the urethral opening. In severe cases the whole of the anterior vagina and cervix may

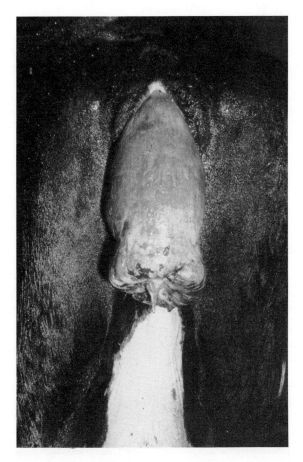

Fig. 5.1 Prolapse of vagina in a Friesian cow.

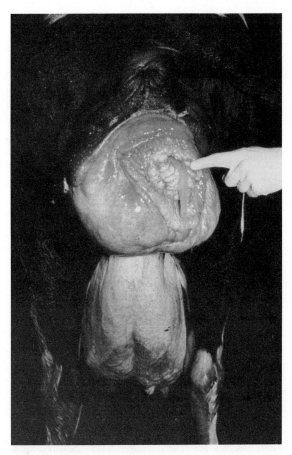

Fig. 5.2 Prolapse of vagina and cervix (as indicated by the finger).

protrude. The further from parturition that the disease begins the more serious it is likely to become because advancing pregnancy tends to accentuate the condition. Most bovine cases are seen in the last 2 months of gestation, and the majority of affected sheep are within a fortnight of lambing. In the mildest cases the lesion appears only when the cow is recumbent; when the animal rises the prolapse recedes. The tendency is, however, to a progressive degree of prolapse and, in time, a larger bulk protrudes and does not disappear in the standing position. Now the dependent tissue, with its circulation impeded, is prone to injury and infection. The resultant irritation causes expulsive straining efforts. This increases the degree of prolapse, and a vicious circle is established. Eventually the whole of the vagina, cervix and even the rectum may become everted (Figures 5.1–5.5). Thrombosis, ulceration and necrosis of the prolapsed organ, accompanied by toxaemia and severe straining, lead to anorexia,

rapid deterioration in bodily condition and occasionally death. In sheep a severe prolapse with heavy straining is not well tolerated, and fatalities from shock, exhaustion and anaerobic infection are common. Abortion, or premature delivery, often of a dead fetus, may be followed by a quick maternal recovery.

Postparturient prolapse of the vagina of cattle is usually due to severe straining in response to vaginal trauma, or infection, following a serious dystocia. Vaginal contusion at parturition, followed by *Fusiformis necrophorus* infection, exerts a high degree of irritation with frequent exhausting expulsive efforts.

Treatment

If prompt attention is given, simple measures often succeed. The aim is to arrest the process by early replacement and retention of the prolapsed portion. Epidural anaesthesia is indicated both to

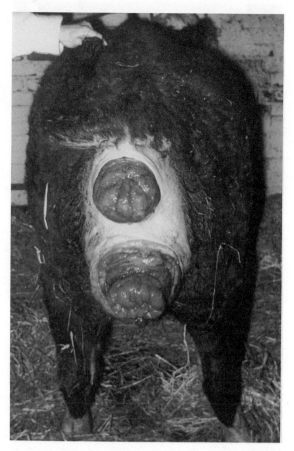

Fig. 5.3 Prolapse of vagina, cervix and, because of persistent straining, the rectum.

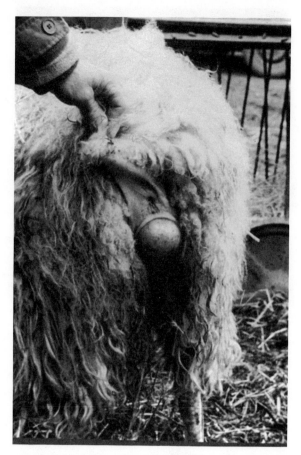

Fig. 5.4 Moderate, early prolapse of the vagina in a ewe.

obviate straining and to desensitize the perineum for suturing. The everted mass is washed clean, dressed with an antiseptic — and preferably anaesthetic — lubricant and replaced. It is retained by tape or stout nylon sutures which cross the vulva and are inserted in the perineal skin. Quill sutures tied over rubber tubing are best. Alternatively, special vulval clamps or metal sutures may be used. In sheep, the perineal wool, or string fastened to it, may be tied across the vulva; large safety-pins are often used. In cases where the vagina has suffered little damage and especially where parturition is imminent, such measures are usually sufficient, particularly when, as is possible with dairy cows, the patient can be stalled on a forward slope. But where there is much irritation from trauma and infection with consequent vigorous straining, the retaining sutures may be dislodged and prolapse recur. Straining may be controlled by epidural anaesthesia but it is not practicable to provide continuous anaesthesia by this means. Perineural injection of the pudic nerves has the same effect, and disadvantage. Tenesmus can be prevented for several days to a week or more by the induction of artificial pneumoperitoneum: a sterile 10 cm hypodermic needle is passed through the abdominal wall at the sublumbar fossa and connected to an udder inflation pump with which filtered air is pumped into the peritoneal cavity until the flanks are distended above the thorax. In contemplating adoption of this device in the case of a cow near parturition it must be understood that pneumoperitoneum will prevent second-stage labour (Espersen, 1962; Svendsen, 1967). For cows showing recurrent prolapse and which are remote from parturition, and also for postpartum cases, Roberts (1949) has suggested a method of almost complete surgical occlusion of the vulva by a technique which is really an extension of Caslick's plastic operation for preventing vaginal aspiration (Figure 5.6).

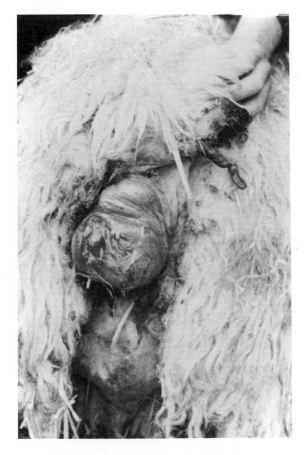

Fig. 5.5 Severe prolapse of the vagina in a ewe.

approximated by means of fine nylon sutures and a few mattress sutures of tape or stout nylon are deeply placed across the vulva to protect the coapted lips from the effects of straining. First-intention healing should occur, and the suture line must be incised when parturition is imminent.

Farquharson (1949), who saw hundreds of cases of vaginal prolapse in Hereford range cattle in Colorado, successfully applied a technique of submucous resection, or 'reefing' operation, on the prolapsed organ. The object of the operation, which should not be performed later than 3–4 weeks from term, is to excise the protruding mucosa — which forms the bulk of the everted mass — and then approximate the cut edges. Proximal and distal encircling incisions through the mucous membrane are made near the urethral opening and the cervix respectively, and the intervening mucosa, in the form of a crescent, is removed by blunt dissection through the oedematous submucosa. In order to control haemorrhage and to facilitate suturing, it is best to perform the circumferential dissections in separate segments and, as the resection of each segment is completed, so the cut edges are coapted with continuous catgut or other absorbable sutures. The operation is performed under posterior epidural anaesthesia. Subsequent parturition and conception are not affected, and the cure is permanent.

In the author's experience the best means of retaining the replaced vagina is the technique described by Bühner (1958). (Figure 5.7) It entails the placing, by use of a special needle, of a

Under posterior epidural or local infiltration anaesthesia, strips of mucous membrane, 1.2 cm wide, are dissected from the upper three-fourths of each vulval lip. The denuded areas are then

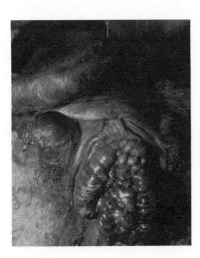
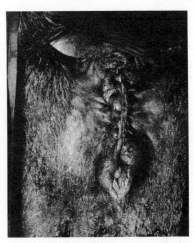

Fig. 5.6 Chronic prolapse of the cervix. This was treated by using Robert's modification of Caslick's operation.

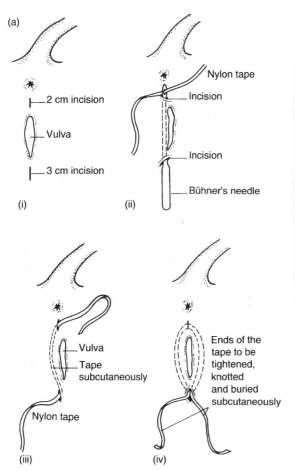

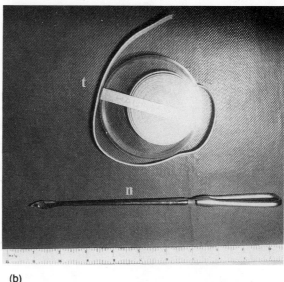

(b)

Fig. 5.7 (a) Bühner's method for the retention of vaginal prolapse. (b) Bühner's needle (n) and nylon tape (t)

subcutaneous suture of nylon tape around the vulva. To facilitate introduction of the large needle two 'stab' incisions are made (under epidural anaesthesia previously induced to aid replacement of the vagina) in the midline; the upper one is midway between the dorsal commissure of the vulva and the anus, while the lower one is immediately beneath the ventral vulval commissure. The needle is inserted into the lower incision and gradually passed subcutaneously up the right side of the vulva until its point emerges through the upper incision whereupon the needle is threaded with a double length of nylon tape. While one end of the tape is firmly held, the loaded needle is pulled downwards until free of the lower incision when it is unthreaded, thus leaving a length of tape protruding from each incision. The needle is now inserted again into the lower incision and passed subcutaneously up the left vulval labium. When its point emerges the needle is threaded, then pulled backwards and

outwards from the lower aperture and unthreaded. The tape now encircles the vulva subcutaneously and its two ends hang from the lower incision. These ends are tied with a simple knot with such a degree of tightness that four fingers can be inserted flatwise up to their second joints into the vulva. The upper incision is closed with a couple of sutures of fine monofilament nylon while the lower incision can be either left open or sutured according to the cow's proximity to parturition. The suture causes practically no tissue reaction: the vulval labiae are not damaged by it, and it can remain *in situ* for months, until the cow is on the point of calving, when the knot should be cut so as to release the thread and allow the vulva to dilate for the birth of the calf.

Bühner's method is equally applicable to ewes with prolapsed vaginas, a suture of monofilament nylon being laid by means of a large half-curved, cutting suture needle.

Another method of retaining the replaced

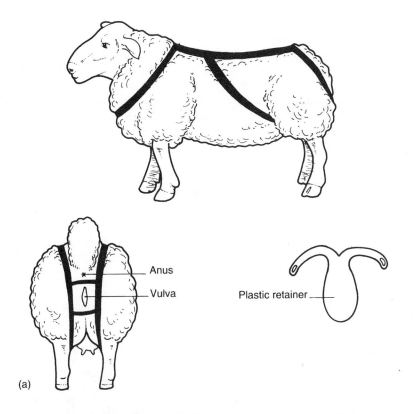

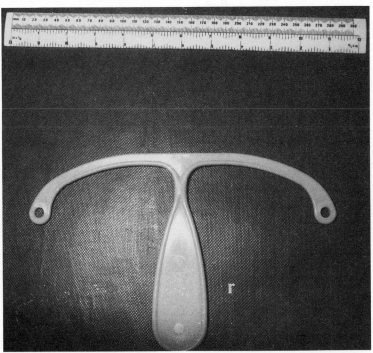

Fig. 5.8 (a) Diagram to show positioning of a harness (constructed of baling twine or nylon strapping) in a ewe together with the plastic retainer. The latter is not always used if pressure from the harness on the perineum is sufficient to retain the prolapse. (b) The plastic retainer (r). This can be used without the harness, and can be attached to the wool using tapes.

vagina, devised in the USA by Winkler (1966), entails fixation of the cervix to the prepubic tendon with a suture of monofilament nylon which is placed from the anterior vagina by means of a 10 cm 'U'-shaped cutting needle loaded with a long 0.9–1.2 m strand of nylon. Before inserting the suture (under epidural anaesthesia) the bladder is pushed to one side.

For retaining the prolapsed vagina of ewes, Fowler and Evans (1957) and Jones (1958) first described the use of a stainless steel stay which, in the form of the letter 'U', is placed in the vagina. The emerging ends are bent at right angles and fitted with 'eyes' which are securely fastened with string on either side to the wool of the gluteal region. This type of prolapse retainer has been improved by the development of a plastic spoon which is fastened in the same way as the 'U'-shaped device, or in association with a harness made from baling twine or nylon strapping (Figure 5.8). The early replacement and retention of the prolapse is very important to prevent trauma and to ensure that the ewe maintains pregnancy to term.

White (1961) first described a fatal condition of heavily pregnant ewes in which the intestines become prolapsed through a spontaneous rupture of the dorsal or lateral wall of the vagina. This has been shown to be associated with vaginal prolapse, although why it should occur is not entirely clear.

In so far as genetic aspects are concerned, it would seem unwise to breed from animals which have shown vaginal prolapse. There is little doubt that by adopting this culling policy over the years, stock owners have exerted a large measure of control over the condition.

REFERENCES

Bennetts, H. W. (1944) *J. Agr. West Aust.*, **21**, 104.
Bühner, F. (1958) *Tierärztl. Umsch.*, **13**, 183.
Edgar, D. G. (1952) *Vet. Rec.*, **64**, 852.
Espersen, G. (1962) *Wien. Tierärztl. Mschr.*, **49**, 825.
Farquharson, J. (1949) *Rep. 14th Int. Vet. Congr.*, **3**, 264.
Fowler, N. G. and Evans, D. A. (1957) *Vet. Rec.*, **69**, 501.
Jones, B. V. (1958) *Vet. Rec.*, **70**, 362.
Koen, J. S. and Smith, H. C. (1945) *Vet. Med.*, **40**, 131.
McErlean, B. A. (1952) *Vet. Rec.*, **64**, 539.
McLean, J. W. and Claxton, J. H. (1960) *N.Z. Vet. J.*, **8**, 51.
Memon, M. A., Pavletic, M. M. and Kumar, M. S. A. (1993) *J. Amer. Vet. Med. Assn*, **202**, 295.
Roberts, S. J. (1949) *Cornell Vet.*, **39**, 434.
Svendsen, P. (1967) *Nord. VetMed.*, **19**, 163.
White, J. B. (1961) *Vet. Rec.*, **73**, 281.
Winkler, J. K. (1966) *J. Amer. Vet. Med. Assn*, **149**, 768.
Woodward, R. R. and Queensberry, J. R. (1956) *J. Anim. Sci.*, **15**, 119.

PARTURITION

It is essential that the veterinarian shall be perfectly familiar with the normal course of parturition in domestic species in order to be able to differentiate between physiological and pathological birth. The appropriate intervention at the correct time can increase the likelihood of a successful outcome by ensuring that both mother and offspring survive.

Initiation of parturition

Parturition is one of the most fascinating of biological processes, for although its physiology is explicable and its associated endocrine changes have been fairly well established, the factors which initiate birth and thereby terminate pregnancy after a constant length of gestation for a given species are still imperfectly understood. The modern concept, which is firmly based on experimental studies and clinical observations, is that the fetus exerts an overriding control of the length of gestation and that the mother can influence the time of birth only within narrow limits.

The uterine musculature is the key component of labour, and the essential physiological change between gestation and birth is a liberation of the contractile potential of the myometrium; the factors involved in this transformation are neural, humoral and mechanical.

Of the humoral factors the most important is the reversal of those mechanisms which are necessary for the maintenance of pregnancy, in particular the removal of the progesterone block, which ensures that, during this phase of the animal's reproductive life, the myometrium is largely quiescent.

The mechanisms that are responsible for the initiation of parturition vary slightly between species. Initially much of the experimental work to determine the mechanisms involved was done in the ewe. This, together with circumstantial evidence obtained from cattle, sheep, goats and humans, in which it was observed that prolonged gestation was usually associated with abnormalities of the fetal brain and adrenal, supported the hypothesis first advocated by Hippocrates that the fetus is responsible for controlling the time when parturition occurs.

The mechanisms are fairly well defined in sheep, cattle, goats and pigs, but in the horse there are a number of important areas which are not well understood, whilst in the dog and cat little information is currently available. Since much of the work has been reported in sheep it is proposed to describe in detail the mechanisms in this species and subsequently to indicate those differences which have been identified in other species.

Ewe

Before 120 days of gestation, much of the cortisol present in the circulation of the fetal lamb is derived from the ewe via transplacental transfer. During the last 20–25 days of gestation there is a dramatic rise in fetal cortisol concentrations, which reach a peak 2–3 days before birth, thereafter declining 7–10 days postpartum. The source of the increase in fetal cortisol is the fetal adrenal; in fact, maternal cortisol concentrations only rise around the time of parturition. At the same time, the binding capacity of the fetal plasma increases, thus reducing the amount of free cortisol in the fetal circulation and thereby reducing the negative-feedback effect on the secretion of adrenocorticotrophic hormone (ACTH) by the fetal pituitary.

Although it has been known for some time that the rise in fetal cortisol is critical for the initiation of parturition in this species, the mechanisms are not fully understood. It is likely that it is due both to a change in trophic hormone stimulation from the fetal pituitary and also enhanced responsiveness of the fetal adrenal to a given level of trophic stimulation.

In sheep fetal pituitaries, the 'fetal' corticotrophs are replaced by smaller stellate cells, the so-called 'adult' corticotrophs, around 125 days of gestation, which might reflect an increased potential for ACTH secretion (Antolovich et al., 1988). There is an increase in corticotrophin-releasing hormone (CRH) in the fetal hypothalamus during the last 10 days of gestation, and, in addition, it has been suggested that the placenta of the sheep can also secrete CRH (Jones et al., 1989). Endogenous opioids may also play a role in stimulating ACTH secretion via their effect upon the fetal hypothalamus rather than the pituitary. It has been shown experimentally that when exogenous opioids are infused into the fetal lamb, there is an increase in ACTH which can be abolished by the administration of the opioid antagonist naloxone (Brooks and Challis, 1988). Pro-opiomelanocortin (POMC) peptides and arginine vasopressin may also be involved in ACTH secretion since both increase towards the end of gestation.

It has been known for some time that the fetal adrenal becomes more responsive to ACTH stimulation with advancing age (Glickman and Challis, 1980). Maturation is induced by ACTH, particularly the pulse pattern of its secretion. Recent work has shown that insulin-like growth factors (IGFs) may have an autocrine and/or paracrine role in regulating ovine fetal adrenal function (Hann et al., 1992). Fetal growth hormone, which is elevated from 50–70 days of gestation then falls to 100 days before increasing to term, may also modify the response of the fetal adrenal to ACTH (Devaskar et al., 1981).

The rise in fetal cortisol stimulates the conversion of placentally-derived progesterone to oestrogen by activating the placental enzyme 17α-hydroxylase; this hydroxylates progesterone via androstenedione to oestrogen (Figure 6.1). The consequences of the rise in oestrogens in the peripheral circulation are threefold. First, oestrogens have a direct effect upon the myometrium, increasing its responsiveness to oxytocin; second, they produce softening of the cervix by altering the structure of collagen fibres; third, they act upon the cotyledon–caruncle complex to stimulate the production and release of prostaglandin $F_{2\alpha}$ ($PGF_{2\alpha}$). The latter change is induced by the activation of the enzyme phospholipase A_2 stimulated by the decline in progesterone and rise in

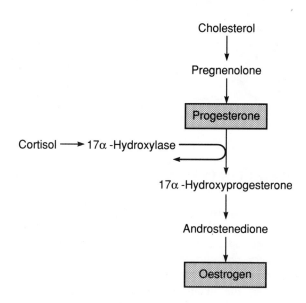

Fig. 6.1 Diagrammatic representation of the conversion of placentally derived progesterone to oestrogen. (After Liggins (1982).)

oestrogen. This enzyme stimulates the release of arachidonic acid from phospholipids, so that under the influence of the enzyme prostaglandin synthetase, $PGF_{2\alpha}$ is formed (Figure 6.2).

Further stimulation of synthesis and release of the latter hormone from the myometrium can also be induced by the action of oxytocin and mechanical stimulation of the vagina.

Prostaglandins play a key role in initiating parturition; because of their molecular structure they are soluble in fat and water so that they readily pass

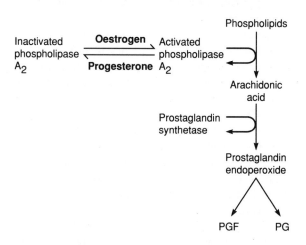

Fig. 6.2 Diagrammatic representation of the induction of PGE PGF release. (After Liggins (1982).)

from cell to cell via cell membranes or between cells in the extracellular fluid (Liggins, 1982). Two prostaglandins are produced by the uterus — $PGF_{2\alpha}$ in the endometrium and, during expulsion of the fetus in the myometrium, prostacyclin (PGI_2). Prostaglandins have a wide range of actions; they cause smooth muscle contraction, luteolysis, softening of cervical collagen and stimulate smooth muscle cells to develop special areas of contact called gap junctions, thereby allowing the passage of electrical pulses and ensuring coordinated contractions.

$PGF_{2\alpha}$ is considered to be the intrinsic stimulating factor of smooth muscle cells (Csapo, 1977) and thus its release is important in initiating myometrial contractions. The effect of these contractions is to force the fetal lamb towards the cervix and vagina where it will stimulate sensory receptors and initiate Ferguson's reflex, with the release of large amounts of oxytocin from the posterior pituitary. Oxytocin will stimulate further myometrial contractions and the release of $PGF_{2\alpha}$ from the myometrium. Hence both these

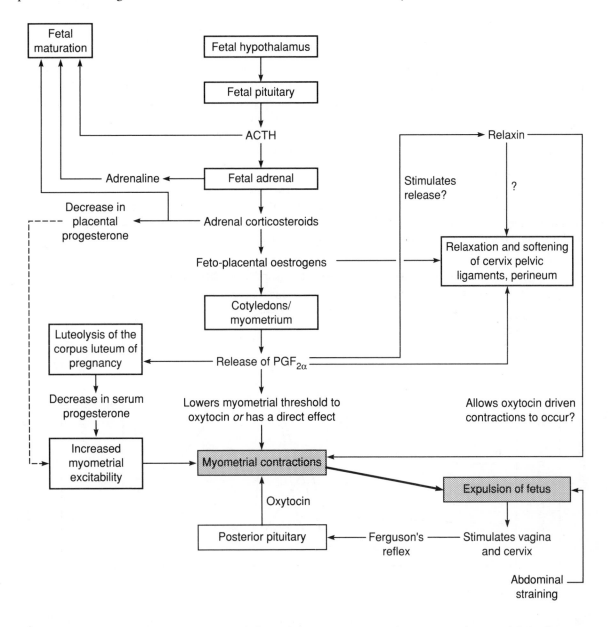

Fig. 6.3 The endocrine changes that occur before and during parturition in the sow, ewe and cow, and their effects.

hormones, together with uterine contraction, seem to work as a positive-feedback system of increasing magnitude, thus stimulating further uterine contractions and consequent expulsion of the fetus (First, 1980).

Other important changes which are brought about by the endocrine events of parturition have been observed. For instance, maturation of the fetal lamb's lungs, especially the production of alveolar surfactant, is stimulated by cortisol, as are many other changes in fetal function and structure that enable the lamb to survive after birth. A schematic representation of the endocrine changes that are involved in the initiation of parturition in the ewe and some other species is shown in Figure 6.3, whilst overall trends in reproductive and other hormones occurring in the peripheral circulation of the ewe around the time of parturition are shown in Figure 6.4.

Cow

As stated in Chapter 3, the placenta assumes the main role of progesterone production at between 150 and 200 days of gestation, so that if the ovary containing the corpus luteum, or the corpus luteum itself is removed after this stage, pregnancy

will continue (McDonald et al., 1953). However, it has been observed that in cows that have been ovariectomized parturition is frequently abnormal (McDonald et al., 1953). For although the corpus luteum is not required to maintain pregnancy after this time it has been shown that its regression plays an important role in the endocrine changes which are necessary for the initiation of parturition.

Other mechanisms, such as the direct effect of glucocorticoids or the direct effect of placental oestrogen, may be responsible for luteal regression, but it is most likely that it is initiated by the action of $PGF_{2\alpha}$. The latter is released as a result of the effect of placental oestrogens acting upon the fetal cotyledons (see Figures 6.1 and 6.2). The endocrine changes responsible for initiating parturition are very similar to those described in the sheep (see Figure 6.3). Overall trends in reproductive and other hormones occurring in the peripheral circulation of the cow around the time of parturition are shown in Figure 6.5.

Doe (nanny) goat

In this species the corpora lutea provide the essential source of progesterone necessary for the maintenance of gestation, since ovariectomy

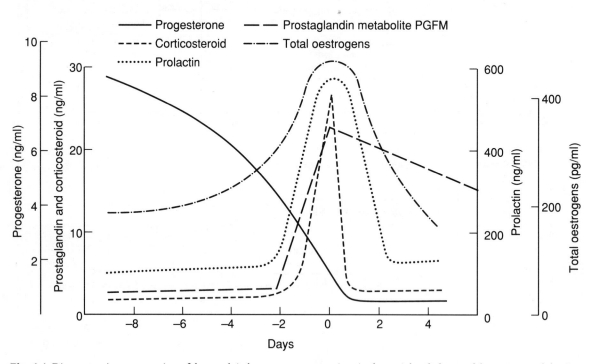

Fig. 6.4 Diagrammatic representation of the trends in hormone concentrations in the peripheral plasma of the ewe around the time of parturition. Day 0 at parturition.

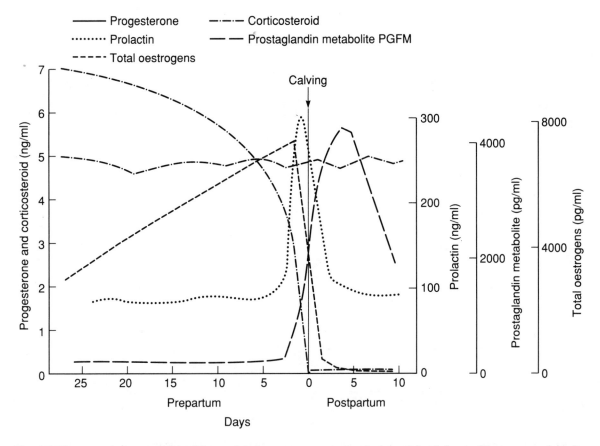

Fig. 6.5 Diagrammatic representation of the trends in hormone concentrations in the peripheral plasma of the cow around the time of parturition. Day 0 at parturition.

or extirpation of the corpora lutea will terminate pregnancy. Placental 17_α-hydroxylase, which is stimulated by the rise in fetal cortisol, diverts the synthesis of progesterone by the corpora lutea into oestrogen. The change in the oestrogen:progesterone ratio stimulates $PGF_{2\alpha}$ synthesis as in the ewe (see Figures 6.1 and 6.2), resulting in luteolysis with a further decline in progesterone. Progesterone disappears from the circulation before parturition can occur. The endocrine changes are very similar to those in the sheep and cow.

Sow
Progesterone from the corpora lutea is necessary for the maintenance of pregnancy throughout its entire duration. Parturition is preceded initially by increased levels of cortisol in the fetal plasma which results in a rise in the maternal blood cortisol, oestradiol and $PGF_{2\alpha}$ metabolites and a decrease in progesterone. It is unlikely that oestrogens are

responsible for stimulating the release of $PGF_{2\alpha}$ as occurs in the other species (First, 1979). Otherwise the scheme for the initiation of parturition is similar to that illustrated for the ewe. The hormonal changes in the peripheral circulation are illustrated in Figure 6.6.

Mare
The mechanisms responsible for the initiation of parturition are not as well understood as those of the previous four species; there is less circumstantial and experimental evidence. However, it is likely that the fetal foal is responsible for the initial trigger mechanism, since the fetal adrenal undergoes rapid hypertrophy immediately before parturition (Comline and Silver, 1971) and fetal plasma cortisol concentrations have been shown to increase nearly 10-fold during the last 8 days before foaling (Card and Hillman, 1993). Since it has been shown that in the peripheral circulation of the newborn foal, β-endorphin concentrations

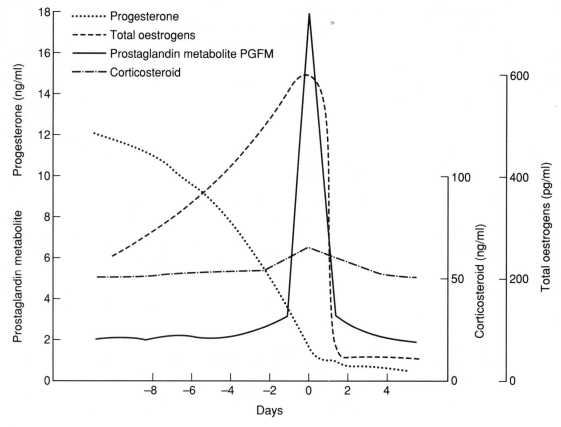

Fig. 6.6 Trends in hormone concentrations in the peripheral circulation of the sow around the time of parturition. Farrowing at day 0.

are raised, it has been suggested that they may be involved in triggering parturition. However, it is also possible that they are produced in response to the act of parturition (Dudan et al., 1988).

The main difference relates to the endocrine changes that occur in the maternal circulation (see Figure 3.1). Progestogens (progesterone and progestins) remain low from the middle of pregnancy until the last 2–3 months of gestation; they then increase, especially during the last 20 days, to reach a peak about 48 hours before parturition. They then decrease rapidly to low levels at the time of parturition. Plasma oestrogen concentrations decline during the last 100 days of gestation, rather than increase as in other species, reaching relatively low levels at parturition, although this is largely a reflection of the decline in oestrone and the species-specific oestrogens, equilin and equilenin, since concentrations of oestradiol-17β remain fairly constant.

Bitch and queen cat

Far less is known about the mechanisms that are responsible for initiating parturition in either of these two species.

In the bitch a prepartum rise of cortisol has been detected in the peripheral circulation with peaks obtained 8–24 hours prepartum (Concannon et al., 1975). Progesterone concentrations start to decline gradually from about the 30th day of gestation, and there is a precipitous fall between 12 and 40 hours before the birth of the first puppy (Concannon et al., 1975). This latter change is probably due to the release of luteolytic amounts of $PGF_{2\alpha}$ since, during the 48 hours before whelping, there is a rise in the metabolite PGFM. As the latter increased from a mean of 395 to 2100 pg/ml, progesterone decreased from a mean of 2.8 to 0.7 ng/ml (Concannon et al., 1989). Oestrogens remain at a fairly constant level throughout pregnancy and start to decline about 2 days prepartum, reaching non-pregnant values at the time of parturition (see Figure 3.22). Prolactin increases as progesterone concentrations decrease 1–2 days before whelping (Concannon et al., 1977); it is not known if this hormone plays any role in parturition.

In the queen cat progesterone remains between 20 and 50 ng/ml for the first two-thirds of gestation before starting to decline gradually towards term. Just before parturition it declines more rapidly to almost zero at the time of parturition (Verhage et al., 1976). Oestradiol concentrations increase slightly just before parturition.

Relaxin

Sources of relaxin

Relaxin, a polypeptide hormone, was shown to be responsible for causing relaxation of the pubic symphysis of guinea-pigs by Hisaw in 1926. The most potent sources of this hormone are the corpora lutea of the pregnant sow, however it is now known to be produced by a number of other tissues such that it has a wide diversity of chemical structure and physiological effects between species.

In the pig, as well as the corpora lutea of the pregnant sow, it is also produced by preovulatory follicles. In the cow, the corpus luteum appears to be the main source of the hormone, with values increasing just before calving; however, because a reliable assay is not available in this species, some of the results are equivocal. There is conflicting evidence in the ewe concerning the secretion of the hormone as well as its likely source of production.

In the horse, dog and cat, the main or sole source of the hormone is the placenta. In the mare, concentrations start to rise from about 80 days of gestation, although there is considerable breed variation (Stewart et al., 1992). In the bitch, relaxin increases from about 4 weeks of gestation, and remains elevated until term, whereas in the cat there is a sudden rise from 23 days of gestation with a peak at 36 days and a dramatic decline just before parturition (Stewart and Stabenfeldt, 1985).

Actions of relaxin

Crude extracts and purified forms of the hormone have a wide range of actions on a variety of target tissues including the pubic symphysis, pelvic ligaments, cervix, myometrium and the mammary gland.

In the sow, relaxin stimulates the growth of the cervix during late pregnancy as well as causing relaxation before parturition. The latter changes, which are also influenced by the oestrogen:progesterone ratio, involve changes at a biochemical level by influencing the glycosaminoglycans:collagen ratio (O'Day-Bowman et al., 1991) and histological structure (Winn et al., 1993).

Despite the fact that there is not a reliable assay for relaxin in the cow, there is long-standing circumstantial evidence that it plays an important role in cervical relaxation at term. Studies have shown that when highly purified porcine relaxin was placed directly on the external os of the cervix at 276–278 days of gestation, cervical relaxation occurred 8–12 hours later (Musah et al., 1986). Similar results have been obtained when parturition has been induced with dexamethasone (Musah et al., 1987). The reports on the effect of porcine relaxin on the cervix of the sheep are equivocal. Recent work (Roche et al., 1993) has shown that a relaxin-like mRNA cannot encode a functional relaxin molecule, which suggests that sheep may not produce relaxin and thus, in this species, cervical relaxation may not be relaxin-dependent.

Relaxin also exerts an influence on myometrial activity, with several studies reported in domestic species, in particular the pig. In general, relaxin reduces both the frequency and amplitude of uterine contractions, particularly the former. It appears to act in concert with progesterone, oestrogens, oxytocin and prostaglandins. Thus in the sow, although the progesterone concentrations have fallen significantly 10–24 hours before farrowing, with the removal of the progesterone block (see below), myometrial activity is low. At this time, relaxin concentrations increase significantly. Furthermore, in sows there is a relationship between relaxin concentrations and the duration of farrowing (Wathes et al., 1989).

Fetal maturation

As has already been described, the fetal endocrine changes that occur in late pregnancy not only initiate parturition but also stimulate a variety of maturational changes which enable the newborn animal to survive. In the absence of these changes, sometimes referred to as 'preparation for birth'

(Liggins et al., 1979), neonatal death may occur because of malfunction of immature organs.

If the premature induction with the exogenous hormones bypasses some of the endocrine changes that normally occur, the newborn may be unprepared. This has been demonstrated when goat kids which were born following the injection of $PGF_{2\alpha}$ were compared with those which were born after induction with ACTH (Currie and Thorburn, 1973). The link between parturition and maturation of the fetus appears to be related to the adrenal cortex and the prepartum surge of fetal cortisol (Liggins, 1976).

During its intrauterine life the fetus is in a thermally neutral environment, but at birth it has to be able to maintain its own body temperature. The mechanisms which enable this are the accumulation of brown fat and glycogen in late gestation and maturation of the thyroid gland. The latter process occurs as a result of the prepartum rise in fetal cortisol which stimulates the monodeiodination of the thyroid hormones, thus enhancing their biological activity (Liggins et al., 1979).

The maintenance of glucose homeostasis immediately after birth, when the newborn loses its placental source of glucose, is dependent on adequate stores of liver glycogen. There is strong evidence that in sheep the stimulus for the accumulation of glycogen stores in late gestation is the rise in fetal cortisol (Jost et al., 1966). The glycogen stores are just sufficient to provide energy before sources of glucose become available from food. A similar stimulus to the production of insulin by the pancreas has also been attributed to the effect of elevated fetal cortisol, which enables the newborn to respond quickly to maintain glucose homeostasis.

The fetal adrenal medulla also shows evidence of maturational changes in that its ability to produce catecholamines, especially adrenaline, is increased in response to asphyxia (Comline and Silver, 1971). There is some evidence that adrenaline, together with fetal ACTH and cortisol, stimulates lung maturation, thus enabling normal respiratory function to occur.

Premature induction of parturition

Although it is usually possible to predict approximately when parturition will occur in domestic species there are obvious advantages in being able to predetermine when the event will occur. Many of the methods that are used have originated from studies of the endocrine changes responsible for the initiation of normal parturition. Since the first published reports of premature induction by Van Rensberg (1967) in the ewe, and Adams (1969) in the cow, a large number of successful reports have been published in these two species as well as in the doe, sow and mare; little success has been achieved in the bitch and the cat.

Mare

The indications for the premature induction of foaling are few, the main one being to ensure that it occurs in the presence of skilled assistance; then if dystocia occurs it is possible quickly to correct the difficulty so as to ensure survival of the foal and reduce the danger to the mare. There are also a few occasions when, because of disease or illness in the mare, it may be advantageous for foaling to be induced.

A number of different hormone preparations have been used. Britton (1972) and Purvis (1972) described the successful induction of over 1500 foaling with an intramuscular injection of oxytocin, either with or without priming with stilboestrol dipropionate. If the cervix showed evidence of 'ripening', i.e. was soft on palpation and able to allow the insertion of one or two fingers in the external os, and the foal was in normal presentation, position and posture, oxytocin was given at a dose of 120 IU to mares between 360 and 600 kg live weight. Foaling occurred 15–60 minutes later. If the cervix was 'unripe', 30 mg of stilboestrol dipropionate in oil was given intramuscularly, followed by oxytocin 12–24 hours later, provided that the cervix had responded. Both authors recommend that a second vaginal examination is made 10–15 minutes after the oxytocin to determine the foal's position and posture so that if it is abnormal correction can be made. Purvis (1972) also recommended that the allantochorion is ruptured manually if it has not ruptured naturally by the time that the foal is well advanced into the vagina.

Purvis (1972) recorded no difficulty with placental retention although this was a problem in the cases described by Rossdale and Jeffcoat (1975). A relationship between the dose of oxytocin and placental separation has been demonstrated (Hillman, 1975), doses of less than 60 IU resulting in retention.

In the author's experience, dystocia has sometimes occurred owing to the lateral position of the foal, as a result of incomplete rotation before the onset of the second stage of parturition. Furthermore, foal viability has often been poor due to anoxia during expulsion because of premature placental separation. It is important to know the precise gestational age since induction should not be attempted before 320 days.

Dexamethasone, a quick-release synthetic corticosteroid, has been used successfully to induce foaling in ponies (First and Alm, 1977) and large 'saddle-type' mares (Alm et al., 1975). A dose rate of 100 mg every day for 4 days resulted in parturition 6–7 days after the start of treatment in the latter type, whilst the ponies responded more rapidly. The regimen was started at 321 days of gestation, with satisfactory foal survival and subsequent growth rate.

$PGF_{2\alpha}$ and its analogue fluprostenol have also been used to induce foaling. A single dose of $PGF_{2\alpha}$ is not always effective; quite often it is necessary to use repeated injections of 1.5–2.5 mg every 12 hours. In some cases these prostaglandins can cause discomfort and can result in a high incidence of dystocia due to abnormalities in the position of the foal (Allen, 1980). Fluprostenol will successfully induce foaling between 322 and 367 days of gestation when given as a single dose of 250 µg to ponies and 1000 µg to thoroughbred mares (Rossdale et al., 1976). The time from injection to the onset of second-stage labour ranged from 33 to 183 minutes; second stage lasted 5–33 minutes, and the placenta was shed by 112 minutes. The viability of the foals was generally good, although a number suffered rib damage.

It is also possible to induce foaling by the administration of progesterone; the interval from injection to effect is very similar to that following dexamethasone (Alm et al., 1975). It is possible that, as in other species, progesterone is metabolized by the adrenal or placenta to corticosteroid (First, 1980).

Cow

The indications for the induction of calving are as follows:

1. Advancing the time of calving to coincide with the availability of suitable pasture for milk production. This is used in New Zealnd and parts of Ireland. In the latter country it is important that the cows calve over a period of 3 months as close to 23 March as possible (O'Farrell, 1979). O'Farrell has calculated that for every day that a cow calves after this date the yield is reduced by an average of 6.4 litres per day; he found that over 40% of the cows were in this category.

2. Ensuring that cows calve at a predetermined time when skilled assistance is available so that prompt attention can be given. This should reduce calf mortality and injury to the cow.

3. Reducing the birth weight of the calf by shortening the length of gestation. During the last weeks of gestation the growth rate of the calf is rapid; in some of the exotic breeds, such as the Charolais, the live weight of the calf can increase by between 0.25 and 0.5 kg per day. Thus if the dam is immature, with a small pelvis, or pregnancy is prolonged beyond 280 days, as occurs in some exotic breeds, the calf may be too large to traverse the birth canal. Premature induction can thus reduce the likelihood of dystocia due to fetomaternal disproportion (see Chapter 11).

The stage at which calving is induced must be a compromise between the birth of the calf which is small enough to be born unaided and yet is large enough to be viable and subsequently to have an adequate growth rate. This threshold weight will vary from breed to breed. In the pluriparous Aberdeen Angus and Hereford cow it is 40 kg, for the pluriparous Friesian 42–45 kg, for the 2-year-old Charollais 35 kg and for the 3-year-old Charollais 40–45 kg (Meniscier and Foulley, 1979).

4. In diseased or injured cows where the termination of pregnancy will alleviate the condition, or where a live calf can be obtained before slaughter, premature induction may be used. Cows suffering from hydrallantois will frequently respond.

A number of different hormones have been used successfully to induce calving so that a live calf is born. Since induction before 270 days will usually result in the birth of a small, weakly calf with poor prospects of survival it is important that the date of service or insemination is accurately known.

Although ACTH has been used to induce calving, since it exerts its effect by stimulating endogenous corticosteroid production, it is best replaced by the direct administration of corticosteroids. A number of potent synthetic ones are available. There are three main categories: these are referred to as long-acting, medium-acting and short-acting, their classification being based upon the duration of the latent period (time interval from treatment to effect). Thus, when given at a normal therapeutic dose rate, the long-, medium- and short-acting corticosteroids have latent periods of 11–18, 5–11 and 1–6 days, respectively (Parkinson, 1993). It is important to give large breeds of cows an adequate dose; in the case of betamethasone up to 35 mg is necessary in the Charollais. Corticosteroids are also immunosuppressive and thus they should not be given without broad-spectrum antibiotics if infection is present; the lungs and udder should be carefully examined beforehand.

PGE_1, PGE_2 and $PGF_{2\alpha}$ and analogues of the latter have been used. In the first reported use of prostaglandins (Zerobin et al., 1973), a minority of calvings were described as being associated with 'explosive expulsions', a 42% incidence of dystocia due to poor cervical dilatation was also reported by Hendricks et al. (1977). However, both $PGF_{2\alpha}$ and the analogues have been successfully used from about 275 days of gestation with a latent period of 2–3 days (Kordts and Jöchle, 1975; Day, 1977).

Good results have been obtained by using a combination of corticosteroid and prostaglandin. Beal et al. (1976) injected $PGF_{2\alpha}$ if no effect had occurred 40 hours after treatment with dexamethasone. Day (1978) obtained good results using a prostaglandin analogue, cloprostenol, administered 8 or 12 days after pretreatment with dexamethasone trimethylacetate; all the cows calved within 72 hours. In a similar trial, involving 26 adult Friesian cows ranging in gestation from 237 to 270 days, 20 mg of dexamethasone phenylproprionate was given, and induced calving in 13 cows on average 5.6 days later. Those that failed to respond received 500 µg of cloprostenol after 10 days, and all calved within 3 days; all liveborn calves survived (Murray et al., 1982). In summary, for early induction (250–275 days of gestation) a long-acting corticosteroid is administered followed by a short-acting corticosteroid, or $PGF_{2\alpha}$ after 8 days if calving has not occurred; the latent period is about 48 hours. After 275 days, a medium-acting corticosteroid, with either a short-acting corticosteroid or $PGF_{2\alpha}$ after 8 days if the cow has failed to calve, is used. After 282 days,

$PGF_{2\alpha}$ or short- or medium-acting corticosteroids are effective on their own.

There are, however, some disadvantages of premature induction of calving. It is not always effective. The birth weight of the calf is lower than it would have been at term, and thus the subsequent growth rate is reduced. There is also a high incidence of placental retention, up to 53% when 'short-acting' preparations are used (Wagner et al., 1971), although it is less common following the use of slow-release preparations (Welch et al., 1973; O'Farrell and Crowley, 1974). Milk yield is initially affected, with a delay in reaching peak lactation, although there appears to be very little influence on the overall yield (Bailey et al., 1973; Welch et al., 1977; O'Farrell, 1979). Subsequent fertility is fairly normal although the calving to conception interval and the number of services per conception are slightly increased in those cows that retain their placentae. There is a reduction in the quality and quantity of colostral immunoglobulins, especially following the use of slow-release corticosteroid preparations, but it is unlikely that the calf will not acquire an adequate passive immunity.

Sow

On average, 5–7% of all piglets are stillborn, and it is estimated that 75% of stillbirths occur during parturition. The time interval between the birth of the first and last piglets influences the stillbirth rate so that prolonged farrowing results in an increase. Probably 80% of the stillbirths occur in the last third of the litter to be born.

It has been shown that the time interval between the birth of two live piglets is generally shorter than the time interval whch precedes the birth of a stillborn piglet. The death of the piglet may have been due to a delay in expulsion, although there is good evidence that dead piglets are expelled more slowly. One of the causes of stillbirth is the premature rupture of the umbilicus; surveys have shown the 94% of stillborn piglets had ruptured umbilical cords at birth compared with 39% when all piglets were included (Randall, 1972).

The stillbirth rate could be reduced by greater care and attention during farrowing; however, the time of farrowing can be difficult to predict. For this reason the induction of farrowing of groups of sows at predetermined times has many attractions because this can enable a skilled person to be in attendance to a group of sows during normal working hours.

Since there is also evidence that delayed or prolonged parturition can increase the stillbirth rate then methods which accelerate the process, or at the very least prevent delays, have obvious attractions.

There are also a number of other management requirements which have stimulated a need to plan and regulate the timing of farrowing:

1. Group farrowing facilitates multiple suckling and allows cross fostering to take place. Thus the piglets from sows with large litters or agalactia have a greater chance of surviving and being reared.

2. Groups of sows and litters can be managed on an 'all in, all out' principle, thus enabling disinfection and cleaning to be performed more efficiently.

3. Group farrowing facilitates group weaning.

4. Farrowing can take place on certain days of the week and during normal working hours, as well as reducing the stillbirth rate it can reduce the death rate due to overlaying of newborn piglets.

5. It increases the reproductive efficiency by reducing the farrowing interval by a few days.

Synthetic corticosteroids have been used successfully to induce parturition in sows by injecting them on days 101–104 with a single daily dose, 75–100 mg; farrowing occurs on day 109. The procedure is expensive, and piglets born on day 109 have a poor survival rate.

Since the first reports of successful induction of farrowing using $PGF_{2\alpha}$ (Diehl et al., 1974; Robertson et al., 1974) or a synthetic analogue (Ash and Heap, 1973) a large number of reports have been published worldwide. It is now an accepted procedure in the pig industry. More recently, attempts have been made to improve its efficiency by combining prostaglandins with other hormones.

The basic procedure with prostaglandin treatment is that either 10 mg of $PGF_{2\alpha}$ or 175 µg cloprostenol is injected intramuscularly on days 112–113 of gestation, and farrowing will occur on average 28 hours later. Thus, if the timing of injection is between 08.00 and 10.00 hours, the majority of sows will farrow during normal working hours. Adjustments have to be made for herd variations in the average gestational length.

In general, the earlier the time of induction the lower the birth weights; however, if attempts are made to delay the time of induction in order to obtain large birth weight the degree of synchronization is not as good.

In an interesting study involving the use of dinoprost to induce farrowing on 229 occasions (Young and Harvey, 1984), it was found that 95% of farrowings occurred within 48 hours of injecting dinoprost, the majority (76%) within 24–36 hours, which corresponded with normal working hours on the farm. Those sows which did not farrow within 48 hours were deemed not to have responded to the injection of prostaglandin. Apart from very small litters (up to five piglets), litter size had no effect upon the response to prostaglandin; however, the duration of farrowing was directly related to litter size.

There is apparently no difference in the efficiency of $PGF_{2\alpha}$ (dinoprost) or the analogue cloprostenol, although it is generally recognized that side-effects such as biting cage bars and increased respiration rate are greater following $PGF_{2\alpha}$ (Einarsson et al., 1981).

Improved expulsion of the piglets was observed when cloprostenol was combined with oestradiol benzoate. Bonte et al. (1981) reported that the best expulsion occurred when 10 mg of oestradiol benzoate was given 24 hours before cloprostenol although there was some improvement when 1 mg of oestradiol benzoate was given 5–6 hours after cloprostenol. Oxytocin has also been used routinely after induction (see below).

Ewe

Parturition can be induced in the ewe by means of ACTH, corticosteroids and oestrogens. The indications for induction are limited since dystocia due to fetomaternal disproportion is not common. However, a system which can guarantee that lambing will occur only during the hours of daylight when skilled assistance is available might reduce any problems due to dystocia and increase lamb survival rates. However, it is not possible to shorten gestation length appreciably without increasing lamb mortality.

As with other species, an accurately known gestational age is important. When corticosteroids such as dexamethasone, flumethasone and betamethasone are given by a single intramuscular injection within 5 days of term, normal parturition occurs in 2–3 days. Induction is also possible with two intramuscular injections of 1–2 mg of oestradiol benzoate 5–6 days before term or with a single injection of 15 mg of oestradiol benzoate 5 days before term (Bosc et al., 1977). Cahill et al. (1976), using similar methods, had a. higher than normal incidence of dystocia with poorer lamb survival.

Unfortunately, attempts to concentrate lambing to the hours of daylight by premature induction with corticosteroids have not been very successful (Bosc, 1972). Induction of lambing in groups of ewes that have been synchronized with progestogens (see p. 41) can ensure that ewes lamb over a relatively short period of time in a single batch.

Doe (nanny) goat
Parturition has been successfully induced with ACTH, corticosteroids, $PGF_{2\alpha}$ and analogues, and oestrogens; however, lactation sometimes occurs prematurely (Currie and Thorburn, 1977).

Bitch and queen cat
Except for the induction of abortion using $PGF_{2\alpha}$, epostane and a prolactin inhibitor cabergoline, attempts to induce parturition in these species have been unsuccessful.

Accelerating parturition
Oxytocin, administered as a bolus injection, has long been used to treat sows which appeared to be suffering from uterine inertia as shown by prolonged farrowing times.

Routine use of oxytocin 1–2 IU used repeatedly in delayed farrowing was effective in accelerating the process. Doses in excess of 10 IU induce uterine spasm and are contraindicated (Zerobin, 1981). Depot or slow-release oxytocin preparations are not effective.

Studies by Pejsak and Tereszczuk (1981), in which 10 IU of oxytocin was given to 836 primiparous and pluriparous gilts and sows by the intramuscular or intranasal route as a routine procedure, demonstrated some favourable results. In their regimen, oxytocin was given immediately after the birth of the first piglet and was repeated if there was a delay of more than 1 hour before the birth of the next piglet. If no response was

observed in 10–20 minutes, a vaginal examination was performed. All the oxytocin treated sows farrowed within 10 hours whilst some in the control group exceeded this duration.

A β-blocking agent, carazolol, has been used to shorten the duration of farrowing with encouraging results. The rationale behind its use is that during pregnancy, because β receptors in the uterus become dominant, the stress resulting in adrenaline release will cause relaxation of the uterus. If these receptors are blocked with carazolol then in stressed animals (especially gilts) the adrenaline will have little or no effect upon the myometrium, the uterus will retain its tone and parturition will not be delayed. In a double-blind trial, involving 1000 sows using a dose rate of 0.5 mg/50 kg given at the beginning of labour, there was a significant reduction in the duration of farrowing ($P < 0.05$), a reduction in the stillbirth rate and in the incidence of obstetrical complications, especially in gilts (Bostedt and Rudolf, 1983). There may also be some effect upon milk let down.

Delaying parturition
β-Adrenergic agents
β-Adrenergic agents which stimulate the β_2 receptors of uterine muscle cells can abolish uterine contractions and delay parturition for a short time. One such substance, clenbuterol, has been used successfully in cows, sows and ewes (Balarini et al., 1980; Collins et al., 1980; Jotch et al., 1981). In cows, provided that the cervix is not fully dilated and second stage has not commenced, an injection of 0.3 mg of clenbuterol hydrochloride (10 ml) followed by a second injection of 0.21 mg (7 ml) 4 hours later will inhibit calving for 8 hours after the second injection. As well as being used as a management tool it can be effective in ensuring improved relaxation of the vulva and perineum in heifers.

In sows, it causes relaxation of the myometrium and hence interrupts expulsion of the piglets. After several hours there is a return of spontaneous myometrial contractions without any adverse effects upon the viability of piglets. Zerobin (1981) obtained good responses with a dose rate of 150 μg. He also recommends the use of oxytocin 20–40 IU to reverse the effect of the clenbuterol; this is said to produce strong myometrial contractions without spasm of the smooth muscle. He recommends the combination of both drugs to manage farrowing.

Course of parturition: physiology and maternal behaviour

The essential components of the birth process are the expulsive forces, the fetus(es) and the birth canal. Normal birth will result when these forces are sufficient to expel a normal, correctly disposed fetus (and fetal membranes) through a birth canal of adequate dimensions.

The expulsive forces consist of the contractions of the myometrium and the abdominal musculature; the relative importance of these two components varies from species to species. During pregnancy the fetus occupies as small a space as possible; in order to do this it flexes its limbs and neck and, particularly in the monotocous species, assumes a position so that its dorsum is adjacent to the greatest curvature of the uterus. In order to negotiate the birth canal the fetus must be correctly disposed so that its body conformation is as 'streamlined' as possible to match the shape and direction of the birth canal, this being particularly important in monotocous species. Finally, the birth canal must allow the passage of the correctly disposed fetus. Changes occur in the maternal structures which allow this to occur. The cervix must dilate, the bony pelvis and its related ligaments must relax, and the vagina, vulva and perineum must soften.

Myometrial contractions

The hormones which bring about some of these changes have already been discussed. The mechanisms involved in the myometrial contractions have not. The myometrium is formed from two main types of muscle protein, namely myosin and actin. The contractions of the myofibrils occur because of the formation of covalent cross-linked bonds between the actin and myosin filaments. Contractions are initiated when the ATPase of myosin light chain (MLC), which is one of the myosin components, is phosphorylated by the action of MLC kinase (MLCK). This enzyme, MLCK, is activated by a calcium-binding protein — calmodulin. Myometrial relaxation occurs because of dephosphorylation of MLC by the action of MLC phosphatase or cAMP-dependent protein kinase which inhibits MLCkinase and hence phosphorylation of MLC.

It is important to consider the structural arrangement of the smooth muscle bundles. In domestic species with a bicornuate uterus the myometrium comprises two layers. In the outer layer the bundles are arranged parallel to the long axis of the uterus so that when these contract the uterus is shortened cephalocaudally. The myometrium is continuous with the cervix which is fairly well secured within the pelvic cavity; thus when the longitudinal bundles contract the uterine horns will be pulled caudally. When the uterus contains a full-term fetus the ability of the uterus to shorten is reduced and, as a result, the contractions may cause some dilatation of the cervix. The inner layer of the myometrium is formed by bundles of fibres arranged concentrically around the longitudinal axis, thus these contractions will constrict the uterine lumen (Porter, 1975).

During pregnancy, as a result of the stimulus of oestrogens on protein synthesis and the localized influence of distention by the developing conceptus, there is hypertrophy of the myometrium. In early pregnancy there is also some evidence of hyperplasia. As a result of this the length of the myofibrils is increased 10-fold and the width twofold. Since the myometrial mass is increased its work capacity is increased.

As well as the physical changes in the myometrium there are also changes in the electrophysiology of the smooth muscle. It has been demonstrated that in many species during pregnancy there is an increase in the resting membrane potential. With the prepartum rise in oestrogens and the removal of the progesterone block there is discharge of action potentials and the initiation of myometrial contractions. The resting membrane potential of the oestrogen-dominated myometrial cell is also close to the threshold level for the spontaneous firing of action potentials. Thus, if the myometrium is stretched there is slight depolarization and discharge of action potentials. However, in the case of the rat myometrium there is no triggering of action potentials in response to stretch when it is under the dominance of progesterone; at present there is no report of a similar effect in domestic species.

Effects of progesterone and oestrogens on myometrial activity

Progesterone dominance during pregnancy ensures that the myometrium remains relatively quiescent, although there is some evidence in some species that relaxin and PGI_2 may also play a role (see below). Oestrogens have the reverse effect. Although the mechanisms involved are not fully understood, it has been suggested that oestrogens might exert their effect by: (1) increasing contractile protein synthesis; (2) increasing the number of agonist receptors for oxytocin and prostaglandins; (3) increasing calmodulin synthesis; (4) increasing MLCK activity; and (5) increasing the number of gap junctions, which are low-resistance pathways for the transmission of electrical and molecular information between smooth muscle cells. Oestrogens, in this way, increase the effectiveness of the myometrium as a contractile unit. Progesterone has the opposite effects: (1) reduces the number of gap junctions; (2) reduces the number of agonist receptors; (3) inhibits the synthesis of prostaglandins and the release of oxytocin; and (4) increases calcium binding.

Role of prostaglandins and oxytocin

Prostaglandins play a critical role in parturition, not only in the initiation of the process but in the control of myometrial contractions. These actions are facilitated because their molecular structure enables them to move freely through extracellular fluids and lipid cell membranes. Whereas $PFG_{2\alpha}$ and PGE are responsible for stimulating uterine contractions, it has been shown that PGI_2 inhibits uterine contractions (Omini et al., 1979). Prostaglandin action is mediated through specific receptors, and as a consequence they influence the number of gap junctions and also the movement of Ca^{2+} between the myofibrils; $PGF_{2\alpha}$ and PGE enhance and PGI_2 inhibits these changes.

The pattern of oxytocin release during late pregnancy and parturition has been studied in the ewe (Fitzpatrick, 1961), goat (Chard et al., 1970), mare (Allen et al., 1973), cow (Schams and Prokopp, 1979) and sow (Forsling et al., 1979). It is interesting that in all these species the oxytocin levels during late pregnancy and the early stages of parturition remain fairly low and increase to reach peak values at the time when the fetal head emerges from the vulva and when the fetal membranes are expelled. Therefore, it is likely that oxytocin plays only a minor role in the initiation of uterine contractions. The main release of this hormone occurs as a result of the stimulation of sensory receptors in the anterior vagina and cervix (Ferguson's reflex). There is certainly a good correlation between electromyographic activity and oxytocin release in the sow (Ellendorff et al., 1979) which is suggestive of a local positive-feedback mechanism operating in the uterus of this species.

Oxytocin receptors increase during late gestation and with the onset of parturition; this is dependent mainly on the decline in progesterone and increase in oestrogens. Little is known in domestic species about their distribution in the circular and longitudinal muscle layers. Oxytocin stimulates uterine contractions in two ways: firstly, by increasing prostaglandin release, with which there is a synergistic effect; secondly, by increasing Ca^{2+} release which increases MLC phosphorylation (MacKenzie et al., 1990).

Stages of labour

Traditionally the process of parturition has been divided into three separate stages referred to as the stages of labour. Whilst it is convenient to consider the process in this way, it is important to remember that the stages do not start and end abruptly but pass gradually from one to the other.

First stage of labour

The changes that occur during this phase of parturition are not visible externally but are important because they prepare the birth canal and the fetus for expulsion. A number of important changes occur. Firstly the structure of the cervix changes so that it can dilate; secondly there is the onset of myometrial contractions; and finally the fetus assumes the disposition for expulsion, which involves rotation about its longitudinal axis and extension of the extremities.

The change in the structure of the cervix has been studied by Fitzpatrick (1977b), who has described a loosening of the ground substance of its structure due to changes in the composition of collagen components. There is also increased incorporation of water, which permits the collagen fibres to separate from each other particularly under the extension forces, and possibly also allows ready access of previously inactive proteases to susceptible sites for the breakdown of the collagen molecules (Fitzpatrick and Dobson, 1979).

The cervix of the cow dilates, with the external os opening before the internal os (Abusineina, 1963); the same has also been reported in the ewe (Fitzpatrick, 1977b).The time taken for cervical dilatation varies. In the sow, using sequential vaginal exploration, it was found that it takes between 1 hour and 2 days, with 50% taking 6–12 hours (Schmidt, 1937). The mechanism responsible for dilatation is still not fully understood. For many years it was assumed to be a passive process brought about by the passage of the fetus and the fluid-filled fetal membranes through the ripened cervix. It has also been suggested that it is mainly an active process caused by the contraction of the longitudinal muscle bundles. However, it has been found that in some ewes only weak myometrial contractions precede dilatation (Hindson et al., 1968) and in some women the cervix can dilate in the absence of uterine contractions (Liggins, 1978). More recently, Ledger et al. (1985) demonstrated that in ewes, even when the cervix and uterus were isolated surgically, cervical softening still occurred. Thus the biochemical changes, previously described, are more important than the contributions from the smooth muscle of the cervix or myometrium. These changes are probably not just the degradation of collagen but rather a remodelling of the cervical matrix with new collagen and proteoglycan synthesis (Challis and Lye, 1994). It is likely that in normal parturition it is a combination of active and passive mechanisms.

In the cow there is initially wide dilatation of the external os, whose perimeter is palpable as a frill at the cranial end of the vagina. The cone-shaped cervix then undergoes a simultaneous shortening before the internal os dilates and when this has occurred the vagina and uterus form a continuous canal which becomes tightly engaged by the distended allantochorion.

The first stage of labour is also characterized by the onset of regular myometrial contractions, which frequently produce signs of discomfort and mild colic, the degree of response varying from species to species and individual to individual. However, in most cases there is restlessness with elevated pulse and respiratory rates; the body temperature usually falls a degree or so. In the sheep and goat during late gestation, in some cases as early as two months before parturition, uterine contractions occur once every 30–60 minutes; they are of low amplitude but of five to ten minutes duration. This pattern continues until at least the last four days prepartum when the frequency and amplitude increase. It is only in the last 12 hours, and in some ewes in the last 2 hours, that clearly coordinated contractions occur at a regular frequency (30 per hour), of short duration (1 minute) and substantial amplitude (20–25 mmHg) (Fitzpatrick and Dobson, 1979). Ward (1968) found that there is a significant increase in myometrial activity during the last 4 hours before the expulsion of the lamb.

In the cow, the myometrial contractions show a transition from isolated, uncoordinated waves during late pregnancy, 'contractures', to a regular co-ordinated peristaltic type nearer to expulsion of the calf. The frequency also increases from 12 to 24 per hour in the last 2 hours, and 48 per hour just before expulsion (Gillette and Holm, 1963).

Myoelectrical activity increases during the last 24 hours before birth in association with pressure changes, but strong progressive changes occur only just before expulsion (Taverne et al., 1976). One feature identified in the cow by Gillette and Holm (1963), which will also be discussed below in the sow, was the presence of cervicotubular and tubular–cervical contractions. The function of the former type is not known in this species. The myometrial contractions in the sow are more complex. However, as in other species, there is a tendency for their duration, frequency and amplitude to increase and for them to become more regular 12–72 hours before the onset of second stage (Zerobin and Spörri, 1972; Ngiam, 1979). Contraction frequencies of eight to 24 per hour, durations of 0.5–3.5 minutes, at amplitudes up to 60 mmHg, have been recorded from about 24 hours prepartum. A change in the pattern of the contractions was observed by Zerobin and Spörri (1972) at the time that milk appeared in the teats. The same authors, using pressure recordings, and Taverne et al. (1979), using myoelectrical techniques, identified the presence of cervicotubular and tubular–cervical contractions. The latter authors observed that once one of the horns was empty cervicotubular contractions decreased or disappeared, yet tubular–cervical contractions were present in the opposite horn. Since it has been known for some time that uterine volume is important in regulating myometrial activity by altering myo-electrical activity (Csapo et al., 1963), it has been postulated that the cervicotubular contractions prevent the premature displacement of piglets, thus ensuring orderly expulsion from the horns (Taverne et al., 1979).

The contractions of the uterine musculature cause other changes in the uterus and probably also in the fetus. In the placenta, the attachments to the endometrium become less intimate and the superficial cells undergo fatty degeneration, while in those species with a deciduate placenta, separation of the margins, with haemorrhage, is beginning. The increased resistance to blood circulation in the maternal side of the placenta causes a correspondingly greater flow of blood to the fetus. On the maternal side this impediment to circulation may aid diversion of blood to the mammary glands.

As regards the fetus in first-stage labour, it becomes more active and disposes itself in a manner which will allow it to negotiate the birth canal. Thus, in the foal and puppy there is a progressive rotation from the ventral to the dorsal position, while the forelimbs, head and neck become extended. In the case of the calf and lamb extension only is necessary to change the fetus from its gestational posture to that of parturition. The nature of the mechanism whereby the forelimbs become straightened in front of the body is unknown. In the bovine species this is a unique attitude which is never repeated after birth. In his studies of the first stage of labour, Abusineina (1963) noticed that the flexed knees of the calf first occupied the dilating cervix; 30 minutes later the digits were in the cervix. The author suggests that at this time the fetus is practising righting reflexes and that it extends the carpal joints in its efforts to 'stand up in utero'. It is likely also that these spontaneous fetal movements occur in response to increased uterine pressure caused by the myometrial contractions of the first stage. If this view is correct then the mother, through the medium of an indifferent myometrial function, could be partly responsible for fetal dystocia due to postural errors. With further reference to the importance of myometrial function, it is significant that when birth is premature cervical dilatation is often incomplete and fetal postural defects are then common; also retention of the afterbirth is likely: all these clinical effects are due to uterine inertia which may result from a disordered sequence of preparturient endocrine events.

Second stage of labour

In the monotocous species this refers to the expulsion of the fetus; however, in polytocous species the fetal membranes are sometimes voided together with fetuses and hence this stage cannot be separated from the third stage.

The sign of the onset of second stage is the appearance of abdominal contractions. In the cow it has been shown that eight to 10 of these are superimposed upon the onset of each myometrial contraction whose frequency at this stage is 24–48 per hour, so that one contraction is almost immediately followed by another (Gillette and Holm, 1963; Zerobin and Spörri, 1972). Similar observations were made in the ewe where the frequency of contractions increased to 40 per hour, with only very short periods of rest, and intrauterine pressure is increased to 30–40 mmHg with each contraction (Fitzpatrick and Dobson, 1979). In the cow the disappearance of waves of cervicotubular contractions during second stage has been observed (Zerobin and Spörri, 1972).

In many species the superimposition of abdominal contractions upon myometrial contractions has been demonstrated; this is shown in an intrauterine pressure recording obtained from a sow (Figure 6.7). It should be remembered that these abdominal contractions which cause straining are not related directly to the release of oxytocin and should not be confused with Ferguson's reflex. The coordination between the two is due to the fact that the myometrial contractions force the fetus into the pelvic inlet, which activates the pelvic reflex and stimulates straining; this is a similar response to the one that stimulates defaecation. The straining forces the fetus against the cervix and anterior vagina, thus initiating Ferguson's reflex, so that the oxytocin which is released causes further contractions of the myometrium.

The allantochorionic sac, as a consequence of its backward movement being restricted by its placental attachments, ruptures, and a gush of urine-like fluid escapes from the vulva. The distended amnion, together with parts of the fetus, is forced into the pelvic inlet, thus stimulating the pelvic reflex, which induces powerful contractions of the abdominal muscle. Similar, substantial straining occurs later when first the fetal shoulders and later the fetal hips engage the pelvis. These distensions of the maternal birth canal cause great

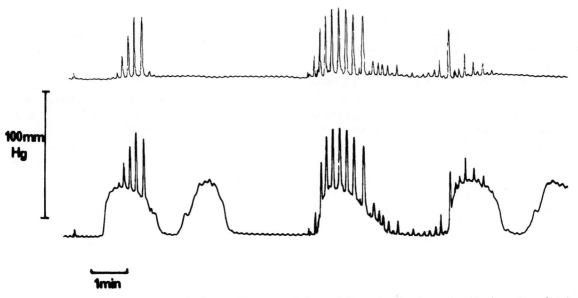

100mm
Hg

1min

Fig. 6.7 Pressure changes at parturition in the sow. Upper trace is from a balloon-tipped catheter placed in the peritoneal cavity. Lower trace is from an intrauterine balloon-tipped catheter.

increases in the release of oxytocin from the posterior pituitary and this, in turn, accentuates the myometrial contractions; thus there is a conjunction of uterine and abdominal expulsive efforts. As the intermittent straining continues the amnion traverses the vagina and appears at the vulva as the 'water-bag'. With further straining fetal limbs appear in the water-bag; in the case of the monotocous species one limb slightly precedes the other. The amnion is progressively expelled and may, or may not, become ruptured by a fetal foot, with escape of some of the lubricant amniotic fluid. The fetal head next occupies the vulva, and at this time the contractions of the uterine and abdominal muscles reach a climax of expulsive effort, maximum effort coinciding with the birth of the fetal occiput. When the head is born the mother may rest for a while but soon a further bout of straining causes the fetal thorax to pass through the vulva. Usually, birth of the hips quickly follows and the hindlimbs may be expelled at the same time; in many cases in the monotocous species, however, no further expulsive effort occurs after the birth of the hips, the hindlimbs remaining in the vagina until they are freed either by movement of the young one or by the mother rising from the ground.

Attempts have been made to quantify the importance of the two components involved in the expulsion of the fetus. In the ewe the com-

bined effect of the myometrial and abdominal contractions is about two-and-a-half times the effect of the uterus on its own (Ward, 1968; Hindson et al., 1965, 1968). Similar observations have been made in the cow (Gillette and Holm, 1963), although since the myometrium is involved alone during the first stage of labour it probably contributes to about 90% of the total work done in the expulsion of the calf. The abdominal effort is of high intensity at certain critical stages of delivery.

If the fetus is born in the amnion, or if the partially ruptured amnion covers the face of the offspring, fetal movement quickly causes it to be ruptured or drawn away; respirations, often accompanied by a cry, then begin. There seems to be very little risk of a healthy fetus being suffocated by an enveloping amnion. The stimulus to breathing is apparently the impact of air at the nostrils, for occasionally during the expulsive phase of equine and bovine births when the protruding face has become uncovered, breathing has begun some time before delivery was completed.

When the mother gives birth in lateral recumbency the offspring is often born with an intact umbilical cord, and some minutes may elapse before the cord is ruptured by movement of the young animal or mother. It is important to allow this to happen naturally, for artificial and premature rupture, or ligation, of the cord may deprive the newborn of a large volume of blood which would normally pass to it from the placenta. When rupture occurs, the two umbilical arteries and urachus retract towards, or into, the abdomen, and this prevents haemorrhage.

In physiological birth the fetus does not come in direct contact with the genital tract, for the surrounding amnion has served as a glistening and well-lubricated sheath through which the fetus has passed.

The second stage of labour is complete when all fetuses have been delivered; it lasts from an average of 17 minutes in the mare to an average of 4 hours in the sow. Its duration and the degree of effort associated with it are usually greater in primigravida than in multigravida.

In the mare, cow and ewe (when monotocous) the fetus is usually delivered in anterior presentation, dorsal position and extended posture, although a small proportion of normal deliveries may occur in posterior presentation, dorsal position and extended posture. In the polytocous bitch and sow up to 40–45% of fetuses may be normally delivered in posterior presentation (see p. 223).

During its passage from the uterus to the exterior the fetus of the monotocous species follows an arched route. This tends to reduce the dorsoventral diameter of the fetal pelvis and also tends to keep the fetal pelvis high in the birth canal where the maternal bisiliac diameter is widest.

Third stage of labour

After birth of the young, regular abdominal contractions largely cease. Although a temporary lull has been recorded in the cow (Gillette and Holm, 1963), myometrial contractions persist; in general, they decrease in amplitude but become more frequent and less regular. These contractions are important for dehiscence and expulsion of the fetal membranes. Not only do the waves of contractions passing from uterine tube to cervix persist, but in both the cow and sow there is the re-appearance of contractions in the reverse direction (Zerobin and Spörri, 1972; Ngiam, 1978); the former authors noted their return in the cow within 10 minutes of the expulsion of the calf. Taverne et al. (1976a) reported in the sow the presence of regular contractions of a frequency of 15–27 per hour which frequently progressed in a peristaltic fashion over the entire length of the uterus.

During the last 5 days of gestation, maturational changes occur in the placenta; these are likely to be related to the changes in the endocrine environment that triggers parturition (see pp. 141–144). Grunert (1984) has identified collagenization of the placentome and flattening of the maternal crypt epithelium in the cow. In the same species he also observed significant cellular changes, such as leucocyte migration and increased activity, and a reduction in the number of binucleate cells in the trophectoderm. However, these changes may occur as a result of the maturational changes rather than causing them.

A weakening of the acellular layer of adhesive protein, the 'so-called' glue line that has been demonstrated in the cow between the cotyledonary and caruncular epithelium, is probably important in ensuring placental separation (Bjorkmann and Sollen, 1960).

The effect of the contractions is to open up the endometrial crypts which in the case of those species with cotyledons resemble the openings of a succession of fans. The fetal villi have shrunk, owing mainly to the sudden loss of turgidity related to the loss of blood from the fetal side of the placenta when the umbilical cord ruptures. Exsanguination of the placenta is also aided by the squeezing effect of myometrial contractions. These actions, together with some of the early degenerative or maturational changes which are seen in the caruncles of the ewe and cow, cause separation of the fetal membrane. As a result, the apex of the allantochorionic sac becomes inverted and as the sac is 'rolled' down the cornua the fetal villi are drawn out of the crypts. When a large portion of the afterbirth becomes detached and inverted it forms a mass within the maternal pelvis which stimulates reflex contractions of the abdominal muscles; this straining completes the expulsion of the allantochorionic sac, which is seen to have its smooth, shining allantoic surface outermost. In the polytocous species the dehiscence and expulsion of the fetal membranes are interspersed with the fetal births; but only the expulsion of the last afterbirth simulates the third stage of the monotocous species. The third stage lasts from an average of 1 hour in the mare to 6 hours in the cow. With the exception of the mare, domestic animals normally eat the afterbirth.

The nature of the third-stage uterine contractions can be easily appreciated with the exercise of a little patience by direct palpation of the cow's uterus per rectum. At intervals of a few minutes, profound waves of contraction are generated, during which the texture of the uterus is transformed from a flaccid state into a condition of intense tone.

With the exception of the sow, the females of the other domestic species indulge in intensive licking of the newborn offspring. Within an hour of birth it is normal for the young of all species to be suckling, and it is known that the stimulus of suckling causes release of oxytocin, which promotes the 'let down' of milk as well as an augmentation of myometrial contractions. This has been clearly demonstrated in the sow, where suckling resulted in greater synchrony of the contractions and an increase in the number of tubocervical contractions (Ngiam, 1979). Hence suckling exerts a favourable influence on expulsion of the afterbirth. In the mare the resumption of substantial contractions of the uterine musculature in the third stage causes abdominal pain, and it is quite common for expulsion of the membranes to be preceded by mild symptoms of colic.

CARE OF PARTURIENT ANIMALS

Mares approaching term should be put in a handy paddock during the day and brought in at night. As soon as the udder and teats become distended, or waxing occurs, the mare should be put in a foaling box at night and kept under continuous, but unobtrusive observation. The majority of mares foal between 18.00 hours and midnight, so that by daybreak in natural conditions the foal has suckled and can gallop away. It is still uncertain to what extent foaling may be delayed as a result of some (to the mare) untoward environmental influence. Where continuous vigil is kept by relays of students who, being curious, may be rather obtrusive, the mare seems as likely to foal by day as during the night. The cervix does not apparently require the same degree of preparatory dilatation as in the cow. The author has seen a mare foal with ease immediately after a gynaecological examination at which the cervix seemed relaxed but not at all dilated.

If the presentation is seen to be normal, i.e. two feet and muzzle at the vulva, then the mare is almost certain to deliver the foal; an exception is 'dog-sitting position' where, with forelimbs and head showing, the presentation *looks* normal. As soon as an irregular presentation, position or posture is recognized, or if no progress occurs within 10 minutes of the onset of straining, a veterinary examination should be called for (see p. 223). In these ideal circumstances the obstetrician will have little more than an hour in which to arrive and deliver a live foal — often an impossibility because he cannot be located or cannot cover the distance in time. The early dehiscence of the allantochorion in equine dystocia makes stillbirth the rule rather than the exception. Even if the foal is dead on arrival, however, the veterinary surgeon's prompt attention will make a much more favourable prognosis for the mare.

As soon as a cow shows complete relaxation of the posterior border of the sacrosciatic ligament she should be put in a clean, well-bedded box and kept under frequent observation. If after 12 hours of restlessness there is no straining a veterinary examination should be made to exclude primary uterine inertia, failure of the cervix to dilate and uterine torsion. If a cow comes into a normal second stage and there is no progress after an hour's straining she should be examined to ascertain the cause of the obstructive birth.

Heavily pregnant ewes should be kept in a handy paddock or in a lambing yard or pen whose location can be frequently changed during the lambing season.

Sows should be well washed and introduced to a farrowing crate several days before the expected farrowing. The majority of sows farrow at night, and there is a substantial loss of piglets due to overlying by the sow; in fact more than half the piglet deaths up to weaning occur within 48 hours of farrowing. By using a $PGF_{2\alpha}$ analogue to control the time of farrowing, Hammond and Matty (1980) were able to reduce both the number of stillbirths and the mortality due to crushing by the sow and thus significantly increase the number of piglets weaned (at 3 weeks) (see p. 150).

It is clear that the mother, by reacting to environmental influences, can exert some control over the time of parturition. For example, most mares and sows, and probably other domestic species kept in more natural conditions, produce their offspring at night in quiet, undisturbed surroundings. However, constant obtrusive interference can override this natural tendency. For example, in five beagle bitches it was observed that electromyographic activity of the uterus during late gestation was influenced significantly by external stimuli (Van der Weyden et al., 1989). Parturient bitches which are transferred for whelping to a strange environment may suffer from nervous voluntary inhibition of labour. The maternal stress occasioned by the adverse surroundings is considered to inhibit the release of oxytocin, or the resultant adrenaline secretion stimulates the β receptors of the myometrium causing relaxation.

Studies of 1151 calvings of beef cattle in Canada (Yarney et al., 1979) and of 522 parturitions in Friesian cows in Britain (Edwards, 1979) showed that the distribution of calvings was fairly uniform throughout the 24 hour period, but that the disturbances caused by farm staff at feeding and milking times exerted significant inhibiting effects, particularly in milking cows of third and later parities. There was also evidence from the beef cattle study and from data on lambing times collected by George (1969) that there is a genetic effect on the time of parturition: thus of the several beef breeds studied, 55.9–59% of cows with a Hereford grandparent calved during the day (between 07.00 and 19.00 hours), and under uniform husbandry more Merino ewes lambed at night and more Dorset Horn ewes during the day.

Mare

The imminence of labour can be recognized by the degree of mammary hypertrophy, waxing of the teats and possibly the escape of milk from the glands (Figure 6.8).

The best indication that the first stage has begun is the onset of patchy sweating behind the elbows and about the flanks. Although it occurs in the majority of mares, it is by no means invariable. It commences about 4 hours before the birth of the foal and increases as the stage progresses.

Initially the mare yawns, there are no obvious indications of pain and food is generally taken readily. Respirations are normal and the pulse is about 60. (This increase in pulse rate is not significant of the onset of labour, for it develops during the terminal stages of pregnancy.) There is evidence that body temperature may become slightly subnormal during the first stage (36.5–37°C).

As the stage advances the mare becomes restless and tends to wander aimlessly around the loose-

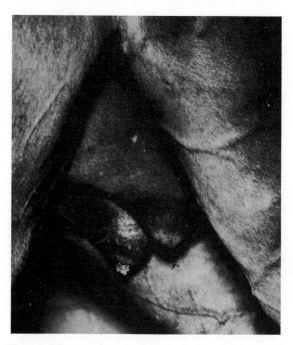

Fig. 6.8 Mammary hypertrophy, tumefaction of the teats and waxing in a Thoroughbred mare 4 hours before the birth of the foal.

box. The tail is frequently raised or held to one side. There may be swishing of the tail or slapping of it against the anus and kicking at the abdomen. As the end of the stage approaches the mare becomes very restless. This is indicated by crouching, straddling of the hindlimbs, going down on the knees or sternum and rising again, glancing at the flank. The stage terminates with rupture of the allantochorionic membrane and the escape of urine-like, allantoic fluid from the vulva. Its quantity is not copious. It will be noticed that there is no reference to visible straining during this period in the mare.

The onset of the second stage occurs abruptly. It is characterized by the appearance of the amnion or the commencement of forcible straining. There is never very much delay between them, and they often coincide. Very soon after straining begins, the mare goes down. She passes on to her side with limbs extended, and generally remains in this position until the foal is born. The presence of the transparent bluish-white water-bag (amnion) at the vulva is quickly followed by the appearance in it of a digit. Straining efforts recur at fairly regular intervals; each bout comprises three or four powerful expulsive efforts followed by a period of rest, generally of about 3 minutes. One forelimb precedes the other by a distance of about 7–8 cm and this position is maintained until the head is born. The point is a significant one, for it indicates that one elbow passes through the bony pelvic inlet before the other and in this way nature has provided that the foal shall present the minimum obstruction at the pelvic inlet. During its delivery, the head is generally in the oblique position, it may even be transverse — the cheek lying on the limbs — but this is probably due to rotation of the cervical joints within the pelvis and should not be taken as evidence that the presentation was oblique. (The second stage is illustrated in Figure 6.9.)

The greatest and longest effort is associated with birth of the head; the chest presents less difficulty, and following this the hips slip out easily. Although equine delivery is comparatively rapid it constitutes a tremendous effort, and after expulsion of the foal the mare may remain lying on her side exhausted for anything up to 30 minutes.

The umbilical cord is intact when the foal is born. It subsequently ruptures, 5–8 cm beneath the belly, as the result of movement by either the mare or the foal. Usually also the foal is born within the amnion, the membrane being ruptured by the movements of the foreparts of the fetus. Respiratory movements may be seen within the intact amnion.

The lower portions of the foal's hindlimbs often remain within the mare's vagina for some minutes after the rest of the foal is born. Their final emergence is due to movement of the foal rather than to the expulsive efforts of the mare.

The duration of the second stage in the mare is about 17 minutes; it may be as short as 10 minutes. The longest the writer has observed within normality was 70 minutes, and in this case it was seen that the greater part of the placenta came away with the fetus. It is probable that this is near the limit of the time available if parturition is to remain normal, for in the mare separation of the placenta tends to proceed rapidly once the second stage begins, and if delivery occupies too long a time it is likely the fetus will succumb from this cause.

In the majority of mares the membranes are expelled quickly after the birth of the foal, generally within 3 hours; in fact they may fall away in about 30 minutes. The average duration of the third stage is about 1 hour. Occasionally, however, cases are met in which periods up to 24 hours elapse before the membranes fall away, yet the animal suffers no ill-effect. Straining is not a feature of the third stage, the afterbirth being expelled by the myometrial contractions. The recognition of the exact time at which a case becomes pathological and interference is necessary is a difficult problem. As has already been pointed out, the membranes are passed with the allantoic surface (smooth and shiny) of the allantochorion outermost. This statement holds for those cases in which expulsion occurs early after parturition, but it has been noticed that in those in which there is delay, the placental surface (roughened and red) is outermost, indicating that separation was complete before expulsion began.

Cow

The immediate approach of labour has been recognized by slackening of the pelvic ligaments and the change of the mammary secretion from a relatively transparent, honey-like secretion to an opaque cellular secretion — colostrum. About 54 hours before birth of the calf, Ewbank (1963) noticed a fall in the cow's body temperature of 0.6°C. He observed that a cow showing signs of imminent labour would be unlikely to calve during the succeeding 12 hours if its temperature was 39°C or more. Parturition will usually begin within 12 hours of the appreciation of complete relaxation of the posterior borders of the sacrosciatic ligaments. The first stage of labour can easily be recognized by direct palpation of the cervix.

There is great variation in the intensity of the symptoms of the first stage; in fact, many subjects, particularly multigravida, show none. Others, usually heifers, may show signs of abdominal pain for periods up to 24 hours before the cervix is completely dilated. The first stage usually lasts about 6 hours. Another feature of the cow is that occasional straining may occur during the first stage. Food is only 'picked'; rumination is irregular; there may be 'lowing' or kicking at the belly. The animal is obviously restless; she may stand with her back arched and tail raised; she may go down and rise again frequently. The line of demarcation between the first and second stages is not clear-cut, as in the mare. Body temperature is generally normal, but the pulse rate is often increased to between 80 and 90.

In 40% of normal calvings observed by the

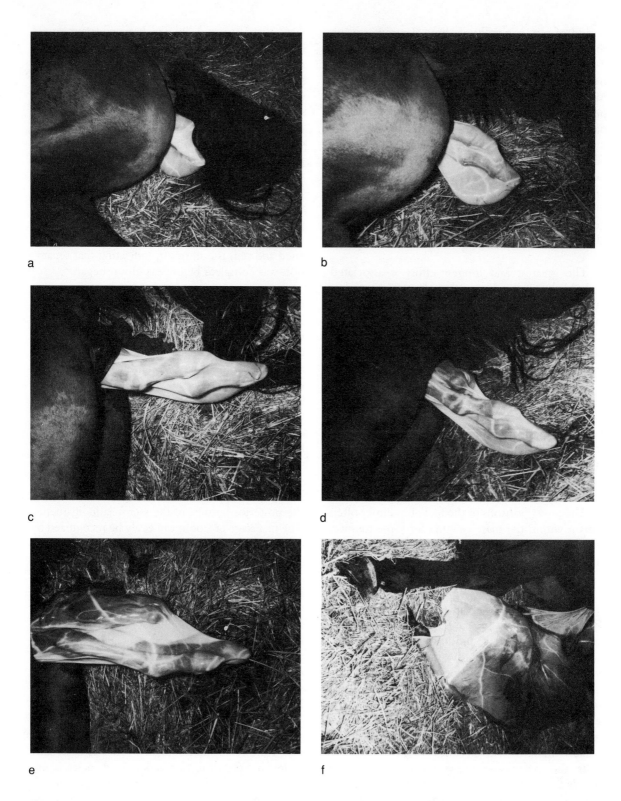

Fig. 6.9 The second stage of labour in the mare. Note the relative positions of the forelimbs and head. The foal is born in the amnion but breaks out of the sac without difficulty. In the final photograph much of the allantochorion has been passed but the umbilical cord is still intact.

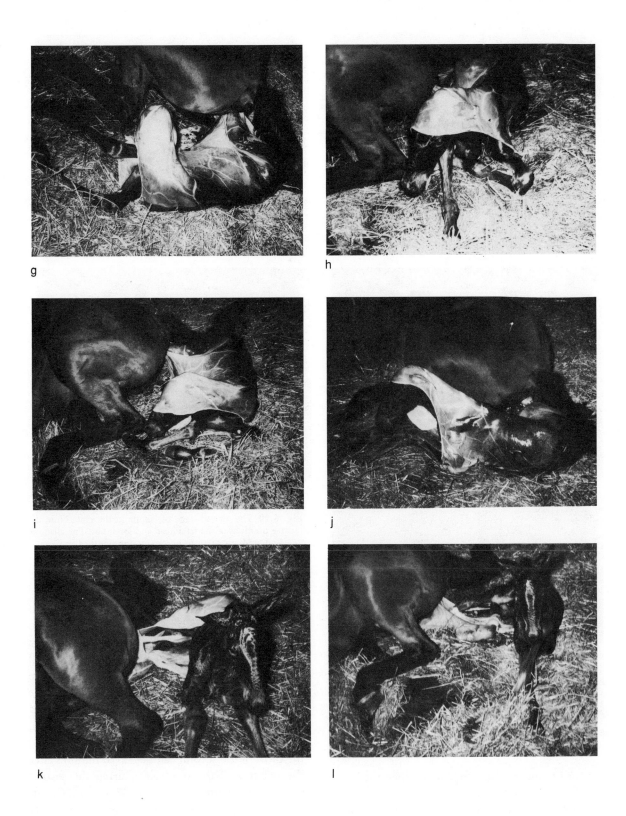

g

h

i

j

k

l

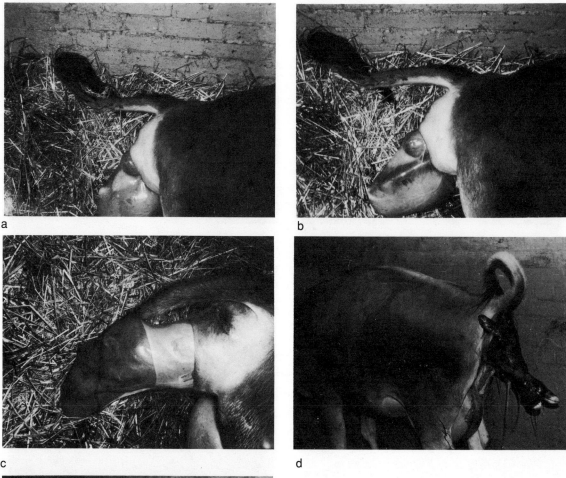

a

b

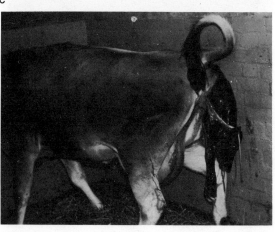

c

d

e

Fig. 6.10 The second stage of labour in the cow. Note the relative positions of the fetal head and forelimbs. The allantoic and amniotic sacs can be clearly distinguished in C.

(Figure 6.10). During the passage of the head through the vulva, however, the cow generally goes down and remains recumbent until the calf is born. She may lie on her side, but more often adopts breast recumbency. Taking the appearance of the water-bag as the time of its onset, the second stage may occupy from 30 minutes to 4 hours, the average duration being about 70 minutes. The second stage is longer in heifers than cows, and male calves take longer to be born. In twin births, Owens et al. (1984) noted that intense straining for the birth of the second calf began 10 minutes after the delivery of the first calf. During the second stage, temperature may rise to 39.5 or 40°C, but this is by no means constant and is probably dependent on the degree of effort required. The pulse rate may increase to 100 or more. About 20%

author the intact allantochorion reached the vulva as a 'first water-bag'.

The second stage is less intense but of longer duration than in the mare. Straining is less frequent and the animal often remains standing at first of calves are born almost completely enclosed in the amnion.

Placental separation occurs more slowly in the cow than in the mare and thus the stage of expulsion may occupy considerably longer without jeopardizing the life of the young one. The process of expulsion is similar to that described for the mare. The umbilical cord is shorter in the calf than in the foal and its rupture generally occurs as it falls from the vulva.

Expulsion of the fetal membranes usually takes place about 6 hours later; occasionally it may be delayed to 12 hours, but when 24 hours elapses and the membranes are still in the uterus it is probable that the cause is pathological retention. Unless prevented from doing so, it is customary for the cow to eat the fetal membranes. It will also be noticed during the first and second stages that there is a tendency to lick up vulval discharges.

Bitch

The imminence of parturition has been indicated by the animal preparing her bed. In primigravida the onset of lactation coincides with parturition, but in multigravida milk may be expressed from the teats for several days prior to its onset. There is a transient drop in body temperature of at least 1.2°C within the 24 hours before the onset of labour.

There is nothing characteristic about the first stage, but it is generally noticed that the bitch is restless, indifferent to food and inclined to pant. It is most obvious in primigravida and occupies about 12 hours.

Electromyographic (EMG) pattern during late pregnancy comprises episodes of myoelectrical activity (EMEAs) lasting 3–10 minutes and recurring at a low frequency (maximum 2.5/hour). During the last 7 days before whelping and especially during the last 48 hours, more short bursts (< 3 minutes) appeared between the EMEAs; this was closely correlated with the decline in progesterone concentrations. The total duration of EMG and the burst frequency increased dramatically as the progesterone concentration and body temperature fall 12–24 hours before whelping (Van der Weyden, 1989).

The onset of the second stage is indicated by straining. In the majority of cases the animal remains in her bed in sternum recumbency, although sometimes she may stand and move about during straining efforts. The water-bag of the first fetus appears at the vulva, and following a series of efforts attains the size of a golf-ball. It is generally ruptured by the bitch who licks vigorously at her vulva. As with other species, delivery of the head coincides the the greatest effort; in the majority of instances once this is born the remainder of the fetus follows easily. Expulsion of the first fetus may occupy up to an hour, but seldom longer if the process is normal. It is often quicker; a matter of a quarter of an hour or so. About 40% of puppies are born in posterior presentation.

The umbilical cord is intact at the birth of the puppy, but it is quickly torn by the mother, who bites it away.

As a rule the bitch rests for a time after the birth of her first puppy. She lies licking her young one, which soon begins to suckle. She pays frequent attention to her vulva and licks up any discharges. The fetal membranes are generally voided in 10–15 minutes and are promptly eaten by the bitch.

Straining recommences after a variable delay. This delay maybe 30 minutes only; it may comprise 1–2 hours. (The writer has seen it occupy 7 hours in a bitch pregnant with two fetuses only.) The effort required and time occupied for the delivery of the second fetus is usually less than for the first. This may be followed by a further period of rest, but quite frequently a third puppy quickly follows the second.

The stage of expulsion of the fetuses is most irregular; one bitch may have her first puppy and then rest for several hours, then deliver two or three more in quick succession and then rest again before expelling several more; while another may expel them at fairly regular intervals throughout the period. There is no rule. In an exceptional case a bitch may deliver the whole of her litter in an hour or so. Unlike the sow (see later), there is a tendency for the puppies to be expelled from alternate horns. In addition, reversal of the presentation or 'leapfrogging' of puppies is very uncommon (Van der Weyden, 1989).

Expulsion of the fetal membranes is also irregular. They may come individually. In other instances a puppy may be born with the membranes of its predecessor around its neck.

The total time occupied by the second stage will depend chiefly on the number of fetuses, but as a general rule when the litter is within the usual limits (four to eight) it occupies about 6 hours. The question arises of what is the maximum time it may occupy, especially when the number of fetuses is very high (10–14). The writer would put it at 12 hours at the outside. It is very improbable that puppies born after this time, even without assistance, will be alive.

The fetal membranes of the last fetus are generally expelled with it or shortly afterwards. Exceptionally, however, there is a delay up to 24 hours before parturition is finally completed.

A feature of parturition in the bitch is that much of the uterine discharge is dark green in colour. This is due to the breakdown of the marginal haematoma ('green border') and to the escape of the blood pigment, biliverdin.

Cat

During the last week of pregnancy, the queen will seek out a suitable nesting area for kittening. Most cats are secretive about kittening and will select a quiet, undisturbed spot, whilst some socialized pet cats show less interest in selecting a suitable nesting position and become more demanding of human contact.

Mammary development becomes noticeable in the last week of pregnancy, and this may be particularly prominent in maiden queens. Rectal temperature may fall a day or two before parturition, but this is not a consistent feature.

During the first stage of parturition the queen may become restless, frequently visiting the site selected for kittening, whilst other queens hide away quietly in the chosen nesting area, occasionally lying down and straining unproductively. The second stage begins with straining in lateral recumbency. Expulsion of the kittens is usually rapid, with only a short interval between each birth, and parturition is usually completed within a few hours. However, in other cases, the pattern of fetal expulsion may be much more variable and, on some occasions, part of the litter may be born one day and the remainder 24 hours or more later. If the queen is alarmed, this may disrupt the pattern of births and she may move the kittens already born to a new nesting area before resuming parturition. The placentae are usually expelled still attached to the fetuses or shortly afterwards and are quickly consumed by the queen. Breakdown of the marginal haematoma releases the pigment which gives a brown coloration to the parturient

discharge. Soon after birth, the kittens will seek out the nipples and begin to suckle.

Ewe

In the ewe the course of parturition is very similar to that described for the cow, except that the incidence of twinning and even triplets is high in those ewes which have 'been done well' previous to mating time. Wallace (1949) found that 72% of ewes complete second-stage labour in 1 hour and that the majority of ewes pass the afterbirth within 2 or 3 hours of the expulsion of the lamb. Ninety-five per cent of lambs were presented anteriorly. Spontaneous birth may occur despite retention of a forelimb. In their observations of ovine parturition, Hindson and Schofield (1969) noted that in twin births where one fetus occupied each horn, one horn developed contractility before the other. This observation supports the author's contention that dystocia in cattle and sheep due to simultaneous presentation of twins is more likely when both fetuses occupy the same horn.

Sow

From 60 to 75% of sows farrow at night (Bichard et al., 1976; Korensic and Avakumovic, 1978). The fetal membranes of adjacent piglets are usually fused and because individual or aggregated afterbirths may be expelled during the phase of fetal expulsion as well as after the birth of the last fetus, it is unrealistic to speak of separate second and third stages of labour in porcine species. Good accounts of farrowing have been given by Jones (1966) and by Randall (1972).

Sows in late pregnancy are mostly asleep in lateral recumbency but within 24 hours before the birth of the first piglet a marked restlessness develops — apparently caused by the discomfort of the first-stage labour pains — accompanied by bed-making activity. The intensely active period is followed by recumbency and rest but after a variable pause clawing and champing of the bedding is resumed. There are several alternating periods of rest and bed-making and then, in the hour preceding the birth of the first piglet, the sow settles quietly into lateral recumbency.

Conspicuous mammary growth is a feature of late gestation, 1–2 days before farrowing the individual glands are clearly demarcated, turgid, tense and warm, and milk can be expressed from the prominent teats during the final 24 hours.

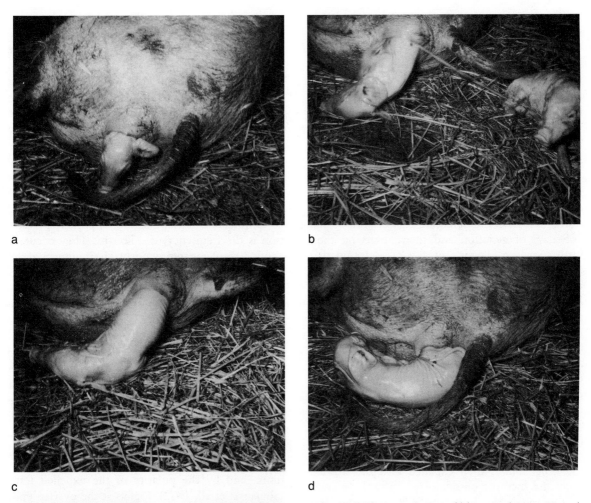

a

b

c

d

e

Fig. 6.11 The second stage of labour in the sow. Note the lack of extension of the forelimbs. the intact umbilical cord can be seen in E.

There is progressive swelling of the vulval labia from about 4 days before parturition and the mucosa becomes reddened.

Prepartum temperature variations of between 37.5 and 38.5°C, but with no constant temperature change, have previously been reported, but Elmore et al. (1979) recorded a 1°C rise at 12–15 hours before the birth of the first piglet.

Parturient sows usually remain in lateral recumbency but gilts more particularly may get up after the birth of the first or second piglet, or change from one side to the other, or from lateral to ventral recumbency. After the prepartum quiet period there is intermittent straining accompanied by paddling leg movements. The birth of the first pig (and subsequent ones) is heralded by the passing of a small quantity of fetal fluid and by marked tail-switching. The greatest parturient effort is expended over the first piglet, succeeding fetuses being expelled with surprising ease and sometimes with projectile force. The allantochorion and amnion usually rupture as the conceptus traverses the birth canal but occasionally piglets are born within the amnion, and not uncommonly, a fetus becomes surrounded by the membranes of another fetus. Only small amounts of fetal fluid are voided.

The expulsive phase of parturition is illustrated in sequence by Figure 6.11. By means of laparotomy and transuterine marking of the uterine location of fetuses of the miniature pig between 80 and 105 days of gestation and then observing their birth sequence, Taverne et al. (1977) found that the offspring were delivered randomly from both uterine horns. As had previously been observed by Perry (1954), there were occasional instances of a piglet apparently overtaking its neighbour in the uterus. In 18 of 95 piglets the observed presentation at birth differed from that previously detected at laparotomy but it was not determined whether these changes of polarity occurred in the uterus during gestation or within the uterine body during delivery. Both explanations would seem valid although Taverne (1981) has postulated that the polarity change is most likely to occur because a piglet passes down from one horn into the base of the other and is then expelled into the uterine body and then the outside.

Observing the birth of 1078 piglets in 103 litters Randall (1972) recorded 55.4% anterior and 44.6% posterior presentations. In both presentations the fetus was usually in dorsal position with the presenting limbs flexed alongside the fetal body; thus the fetal snout or tail were the first parts to protrude. The mean interval between consecutive births was 16 minutes and the mean duration of the expulsive stage was 2 hours 36 minutes. Between 60 and 70% of piglets were born with intact umbilical cords; in the case of the early-born fetuses the elasticity of the cord allowed the newborn piglet to reach the middle of the sow's abdomen without the cord breaking. The later-born piglets were more likely to be expelled with broken cords. Newborn piglets were remarkably active and within two minutes had reached a teat and attempted to suck.

The porcine fetal membranes tend to be expelled as two or three masses of joined allantochorions with the placental stalks of the umbilical cords indicating the number of separate conceptuses in each mass; single afterbirths may also be voided. One or more of the coalesced masses are commonly passed before all the fetuses are born but the largest mass is usually passed about four hours after the last piglet.

When all the piglets have been expelled, the sow usually stands up and micturates profusely. She then lies down again, sometimes very clumsily — with consequent risk of crushing the surrounding piglets — and the feature of the next phase is that the sow lies quietly for a long time and allows the piglets to suck.

A notable economic feature of porcine parturition is the frequency of stillbirths. They occur in about 30% of apparently normal farrowings and the overall stillbirth percentage in unassisted deliveries is 3–6% (Randall and Penny, 1970).

Because piglets are nearly always found alive when premeditated hysterectomies or hysterotomies are performed just before the onset of parturition, it is concluded that stillbirths occur during farrowing. Early-born piglets are more likely to survive than either the middle-born ones, which are of smaller size, or the late-born ones from the tips of the uterine horns (Dzuik and Harmon, 1969; Sprecher et al., 1974; Leman et al., 1979). The stillbirth rate is also influenced by litter size, being greatest in litters of four or less or in those of 14 or more, and by the polarity of the expelled fetus (Sovjanski et al., 1972). Piglets at the ovarian ends of the uterine horns have to traverse the entire length of the respective horn and in the case of small litters they may have to negotiate a previously unoccupied and non-dilated length or horn. Piglets born posteriorly are nearly four times as likely to be born dead as those presented anteriorly. Also, extension of the intervals between successive births up to 20 minutes or more predispose to stillbirth.

High progesterone and/or low oestrogen levels, produced experimentally in the preparturient sow's blood, can delay farrowing and increase the stillbirth rate from 10 to 97% (Wilson et al., 1979); the authors suggest that such hormonal derangements may occur naturally.

REFERENCES

Abusineina, M. E. A. (1963) Thesis, University of London.
Adams, W. M. (1969) *J. Amer. Vet. Med. Assn*, **154**, 261.

Allen, W. E. (1980) Personal communication.

Allen, W. E., Chard, T. and Forsling, M. L. (1973) *J. Endocrinol.*, **57**, 175.

Alm, C. C., Sullivan, J. J. and First, N. L. (1975) *J. Reprod. Fertil.*, **23**, 637.

Antolovich, G. A., McMillen, I. O. and Perry, R. A. (1988) In: *Research in Perinatal Medicine*, ed. C. T. Jones, p. 243. New York: Perinatal Press.

Ash, R. W. and Heap, R. B. (1973) *J. Agr. Sci.*, **81**, 383.

Bailey, L. F., Lennan, H. W., McLean, D. M., Harford, P. R. and Munro, G. (1973) *Aust. Vet. J.*, **49**, 567.

Ballarini, G., Belluzi, G., Brisighella, C., Fanini, G. and Signorini, G. C. (1980) *Tierärztl. Umschau*, **35**, 504.

Beal, W. E., Graves, N. W., Dunn, T. G. and Kaltenbach, C. C. (1976) *J. Anim. Sci.*, **42**, 1564.

Bichard, M., Stork, M. G., Rikatson, S. and Pese, A. H. R. (1976) *Proc. Brit. Soc. Anim. Prod.*, March.

Bjorkman, N. and Sollen, P. (1960) *Acta Vet. Scand.*, **1**, 347.

Bonte, P., Coryn, M. and Vandeplassche, M. (1981) *Proc. Int. Pig Vet. Congr.*

Bosc, M. J. (1972) *J. Reprod. Fertil.*, **28**, 347.

Bosc, M. J., DeLouis, C. and Terqui, M. (1977) *Management of Reproduction in Sheep and Goats*, p. 89. Madison, W.: University of Wisconsin.

Bostedt, H. and Rudolf, P. R. (1983) *Theriogenology*, **20**, 191.

Britton, J. W. (1972) *Proc. 18th Ann. Conv. Amer. Assn Equine Practnrs.*, 116.

Brooks, A. N. and Challis, J. R. G. (1988) *J. Endocrinol.*, **119**, 389.

Cahill, L. P., Knee, B. W. and Lawson, R. A. S. (1976) *Theriogenology*, **5**, 289.

Card, C. E. and Hillman, R. B. (1993) In: *Equine Reproduction*, eds. A. O. McKinnon and J. L. Voss, pp. 567–573. Philadelphia: Lea and Febiger.

Challis, J. R. G. and Lye, S. J. (1994) In: *The Physiology of Reproduction*, 2nd edn, ed. E. Knobil and J. D. Neill, p. 1018. New York: Raven Press.

Chard, T., Boyd, N. R. H., Forsling, M. L., McNeilly, A. S. and Landon, J. (1970) *J. Endocrinol.*, **48**, 223.

Collins, K., Hardebeck, H. and Sommer, H. (1980) *Berl. Münch. Tierärztl. Wschr.*, **93**, 310.

Comline, R. S. and Silver, M. (1971) *J. Physiol., Lond.*, **216**, 659.

Concannon, P. W., Hansel, W. and Visek, W. J. (1975) *Biol. Reprod.*, **13**, 112.

Concannon, P. W., McCann, J. P. and Temple, M. (1989) *J. Reprod. Fertil. Suppl.*, **39**, 3.

Concannon, P. W., Powers, M. E., Holder, W. and Hansel, W. (1977) *Biol. Reprod.*, **16**, 517.

Csapso, A. I. (1977) In: *The Fetus and Birth. Ciba Foundation Symposium 47*, ed. J. Knight and M. O'Connor, p. 159. Amsterdam: Elsevier North Holland.

Csapo, A. I., Takeda, H. and Wood, C. (1963) *Amer. J. Obst. Gynec.*, **85**, 813.

Currie, W. B. and Thorburn, G. D. (1973) *Prostaglandins*, **4**, 201.

Currie, W. B. and Thorburn, G. D. (1977) In: *The Fetus and Birth. Ciba Foundation Symposium 47*, ed. J. Knight and M. O'Connor, p. 49. Amsterdam: Elsevier North Holland.

Day, A. M. (1977) *N.Z. Vet. J.*, **25**, 136.

Day, A. M. (1978) *N.Z. Vet. J.*, **27**, 22.

Devaskar, U. P., Devaskar, S. U., Voina, S., Velayo, N. and Sperling, M. A. (1981) *Nature*, **290**, 404.

Diehl, J. R., Godke, R. A., Killian, D. B. and Day, B. N. (1974) *J. Anim. Sci.*, **38**, 1229.

Dudan, F. E., Little, T. V., Hillman, R. B., Lit, W. I. and Chen, C. L. (1988) *Equine Vet. J. Suppl.*, **5**, 46.

Dzuik, P. J. and Harmon, B. G. (1969) *Amer. J. Vet. Sci.*, **30**, 419.

Edwards, S. A. (1979) *J. Agr. Sci., Camb.*, **93**, 359.

Einarsson, S., Fischier, M. and Karlberg, K. (1981) *Nord. Vet. Med.*, **33**, 354.

Ellendorff, F., Taverne, M., Elsaesser, F., Forsling, M. L., Parvizi, N., Naaktgerboren, C. and Smidt, D. (1979) *Anim. Reprod. Sci.*, **2**, 323.

Elmore, R. G., Martin, C. E., Riley, J. L. and Littledyke, T. (1979) *J. Amer. Vet. Med. Assn*, **174**, 620.

Ewbank, R. (1963) *Vet. Rec.*, **75**, 367.

First, N. L. (1979) *J. Anim. Sci.*, **48**, 1407.

First, N. L. (1980) *Anim. Reprod. Sci.*, **3**, 215.

First, N. L. and Alm, C. C. (1977) *J. Anim. Sci.*, **44**, 1072.

Fitzpatrick, R. J. (1961) *Oxytocin. Proceedings of International Symposium*. Oxford: Pergamon Press.

Fitzpatrick, R. J. (1977) *Ann. Réch. Vet.*, **8**, 438.

Fitzpatrick, R. J. and Dobson, H. (1979) *Anim. Reprod. Sci.*, **2**, 209.

Forsling, M. L., MacDonald, A. A. and Ellendorff, F. (1979) *Anim. Reprod. Sci.*, **2**, 3.

George, J. M. (1969) *J. Agr. Sci., Camb.*, **73**, 295.

Glickman, J. A. and Challis, J. R. G. (1980) *Endocrinology*, **106**, 1371.

Gillette, D. D. and Holm, L. (1963) *Amer. J. Physiol.*, **204**, 115.

Grunert, E. (1984) *Proc. 10th Int. Conf. Anim. Reprod. AI*, **XI**, 17.

Hammond, D. and Matty, G. (1980) *Vet. Rec.*, **106**, 72.

Hann, V. K. M., Lu, F. and Bassett, N. (1992) *Endocrinology*, **131**, 3100.

Hendricks, D. M., Dawlings, N. C., Ellicott, A. R., Dickey, J. F. and Hill, J. R. (1977) *J. Anim. Sci.*, **44**, 438.

Hillman, R. B. (1975) *J. Reprod. Fertil. Suppl.*, **23**, 641.

Hindson, J. C. and Schofield, B. M. (1969) *H, Reprod. Fertil.*, **18**, 355.

Hindson, J. C., Schofield, B. M. and Turner, C. B. (1968) *J. Physiol., Lond.*, **195**, 19.

Jones, C. T., Gu, W. and Parer, J. T. (1989) *J. Dev. Physiol.*, **260**, R389.

Jones, J. E. T. (1966) *Brit. Vet. J.*, **122**, 47, 420.

Jost, A., Dupouy, J. P. and Monchamp, A. (1966) *C. R.Hebd. Séanc. Acad. Sci., Paris, Set D*, **262**, 147.

Jotsch, O., Flach, D. and Finger, K. H. (1981) *Tierärztl. Umschau*, **36**, 118.

Kordts, E. and Jöchle, W. (1975) *Theriogenology*, **3**, 171.

Kovenic, I. and Avakumovic, D. J. (1978) *Proc. 5th Wld. Congr. Hyology Hyoiatrics, Zabgreb*.

Ledger, W. L., Webster, M., Harrison, C. P., Anderson, A. B. M. and Turnbull, A. C. (1985) *Amer. J. Obstet. Gynaecol.*, **151**, 397.

Liggins, G. C. (1978) *Seminars Perin.*, **2**, 261.

Liggins, G. C. (1982) In: *Reproduction in Mammals 2*, ed. C. R. Austin and R. V. Short, pp. 126–141. Cambridge: Cambridge University Press.

Liggins, G. C., Kitterman, J. A. and Forster, C. S. (1979) *Anim. Reprod. Sci.*, **2**, 193.

MacKenzie, L. W., Word, R. A., Casey, M. L. and Stull, J. T. (1990) *Amer. J. Physiol.*, **258**, 92.

McDonald, L. E., McNutt, S. H. and Nichols, L. E. (1953) *Amer. J. Vet. Res.*, **14**, 539.

Meniscier, F. and Foulley, J. L. (1979) In: *Calving Problems and Early Viability of the Calf*, ed. B. Hoffman, I. C. Mason and J. Schmidt, p. 30. The Hague: Martinus Nijhoft.

Murray, R. D., Nutter, W. T., Wilman, S. and Harker, D. B. (1982) *Vet. Rec.*, **111**, 363.

Musah, A. I., Schwabe, C., Willham, R. L. and Anderson, L. L. (1986) *Endocrinology*, **118**, 1476.

Musah, A. I., Schwabe, C., Willham, R. L. and Anderson, L. L. (1987) *Biol. Reprod.*, **37**, 797.

Ngiam, T. T. (1979) *Singapore Vet. J.*, **1**, 13.

O'Day-Bowman, M. B., Winn, R. J., Djuik, P. J., Lindley, E. R. and Sherwood, O. D. (1991) *Endocrinology*, **129**, 1967.

O'Farrell, K. J. (1979) In: *Calving Problems and Early Viability of the Calf*, ed. B. Hoffman, I. C. Mason and J. Schmidt, p. 325. The Hague: Martinus Nijhoft.

O'Farrell, K. J. and Crowley, J. P. (1974) *Vet. Rec.*, **94**, 364.

Omini, V., Folco, G. C., Pasargiklian, R., Fano, M. and Berti, F. (1979) *Prostaglandins*, **17**, 113.

Owens, J. L., Edey, T. N., Bindon, B. M. and Piper, L. N. (1984) *App. Anim. Biol. Sci.*, **13**, 32.

Parkinson, T. J. (1993) *In Practice*, 135.

Pejsack, S. and Tereszczuk, S. (1981) *Proc. Int. Pig Vet. Congr.*

Perry, J. S. (1954) *Vet. Rec.*, **66**, 706.

Porter, D. G. (1975) In: *The Uterus*, ed. C. A. Finn, p. 133. London: Elek.

Purvis, A. D. (1972) *Proc. 18th Ann. Conv. Amer. Ass. Equine Practnrs*, p. 116.

Randall, G. C. B. (1972) *Vet. Rec.*, **84**, 178.

Randall, G. C. B. and Penny, R. H. C. (1970) *Brit. Vet. J.*, **126**, 593.

Robertson, H. A., King, G. J. and Elliott, J. I. (1974). *Can. J. Comp. Med.*, **42**, 32.

Roche, P. J., Crawford, R. J. and Tregear, G. W. (1993) *Mol. Cell. Endocrinol.*, **91**, 21.

Rossdale, P. D. and Jeffcoat, L. B. (1975) *Vet. Rec.*, **97**, 371.

Rossdale, P. D., Jeffcoat, L. B. and Allen, W. R. (1976) *Vet. Rec.*, **99**, 26.

Schams, D. and Prokopp, S. (1979) *Anim. Reprod. Sci.*, **2**, 267.

Schmidt, R. (1937) cited by Taverne, M. A. M. (1979) Thesis, University of Utrecht.

Sovjanski, B., Milosovljevic, S., Miljkovic, V., Stankov, M., Trbojevic, G. and Radovic, B. (1972) *Acta Vet. Belgrade*, **22**, 77.

Sprecher, D. J., Leman, A. D., Dzuik, P. J., Cropper, M. and Dedecker, M. (1974) *J. Amer. Vet. Med. Assn*, **165**, 698.

Stewart, D. R. and Stabenfeldt, G. H. (1985) *Biol. Reprod.*, **32**, 848.

Stewart, D. R., Addiego, L. A., Pascoe, D. R., Haluska, G. F. and Pashen, R. (1992) *Biol. Reprod.*, **46**, 648.

Taverne, M. A. M. (1981) Personal communication.

Taverne, M. A. M., Naaktgeboren, C. and Van der Weyden, G. C. (1979) *Anim. Reprod. Sci.*, **2**, 117.

Taverne, M. A. M., Van der Weyden, C. C., Ellendorff, F., Elsaessen, F., Fontijne, P. and Smidt, D. (1976) *Proc. VIIIth Ann. Congr. Anim. Reprod. Artific. Insem., Cracow.*

Taverne, M. A. M., Van der Weyden, G. C., Fontijne, P., Ellendorff, F., Naaktigeboren, C. and Smidt, D. (1977) *Amer. J. Vet. Res.*, **38**, 1761.

Van der Weyden, G. C., Taverne, M. A. M., Dieleman, S. J., Wurth, Y., Bevers, M. M. and van Oord, H. A. (1989) *J. Reprod. Fertil. Suppl.*, **39**, 211.

Van Rensburg, S. J. (1967) *J. Endocrinol.*, **38**, 83.

Verhage, H. G., Beamer, N. B. and Brenner, R. M. (1976) *Biol. Reprod.*, **14**, 570.

Wagner, W. C., Willham, R. L. and Evans, L. E. (1971) *Proc. Amer. Soc. Anim. Sci.*, **33**, 1164.

Ward, W. R. (1968) Ph.D. Thesis, University of Liverpool.

Wathes, D. C., King, G. J., Porter, D. G. and Wathes, C. M. (1989) *J. Reprod. Fertil.*, **87**, 383.

Welch, R. A. S., Newling, P. and Anderson, D. (1973) *N.Z. Vet. J.*, **21**, 103.

Welch, R. A. S., Crawford, J. E. and Duganzich, D. M. (1977) *N.Z. Vet. J.*, **25**, 111.

Wilson, M. E., Edgerton, L. A., Cromwell, G. L. and Stahly, T. S. (1979) *J. Anim. Sci.*, **49**(Suppl. 1), 24.

Winn, R. J., O'Day-Bowman, M. B. and Sherwood, O. D. (1993) *Endocrinology*, **133**, 121.

Yarney, T. A., Rahnefield, G. W., Konetal, G., Boston, A. C., McCannel, B., Sigurdson, M., Parker, K. J. and Palmer, W. M. (1979) *Rep. Can. Soc. Anim. Sci., Alberta*, 836.

Young, I. M. and Harvey, M. J. A. (1984) *Vet. Rec.*, **115**, 539.

Zerobin, K. (1981) *Proc. Int. Pig Vet. Congr.*

Zerobin, K. and Spörri, H. (1972) *Adv. Vet. Sci. Comp. Sci.*, **16**, 303.

Zerobin, K., Jöchle, W. and Steingruber, C. H. (1973) *Prostaglandins*, **4**, 891.

7

The Puerperium and the Care of the Newborn

THE PUERPERIUM

The puerperium is that period after the completion of parturition, including the third stage of labour, when the genital system is returning to its normal non-pregnant state. In the polyoestrous species (the cow, mare and sow) it is important that there should be a normal puerperium since it is the practice under most systems of husbandry to breed from individuals of these species fairly soon after they have given birth. Thus any extension of the puerperium may have a detrimental effect on the reproductive performance of the individual animal concerned. The genital system does not completely return to the original pregravid state since, particularly after the first gestation, certain changes are not completely reversible.

There are four main areas of activity:

1. The tubular genital tract, especially the uterus, is shrinking and atrophying, thus reversing the hypertrophy that occurs in response to the stimulus of pregnancy. Myometrial contractions, which continue for several days after parturition, aid this process and help in the voiding of fluids and tissue debris; this is normally referred to as involution.
2. The structure of the endometrium and deeper layers of the uterine wall is restored.
3. There is a resumption of ovarian function in polyoestrous species and a return to cyclical activity.
4. Bacterial contamination of the uterine lumen is eliminated.

Cow

Although the stimulus for the changes that occur during the puerperium is primarily due to the removal of the fetus, oxytocin and prostaglandin $F_{2\alpha}$ ($PGF_{2\alpha}$) are also probably involved. The latter hormone increases after the end of parturition to reach peak values 3 days postpartum and does not return to basal levels until 15 days (Edquist et al., 1978, 1980).

The puerperium has been studied in detail by Rasbech (1950), Gier and Marion (1968) and Morrow et al. (1969).

Involution

The reduction in the size of the genital tract is called involution; it occurs in a decreasing logarithmic scale, the greatest change occurring during the first few days after calving. Uterine contractions continue for several days, although decreasing in regularity, frequency, amplitude and duration. The atrophy of the myofibrils is shown by their reduction in size from 750 to 400 μm on the first day to less than 200 μm over the next few days.

Gier and Marion (1968) found that the diameter of the previously gravid horn was halved by 5 days and its length halved by 15 days. The results of their study are summarized in Figure 7.1 and show that after the initial rapid phase of involution the subsequent changes proceed more slowly. Others (Morrow et al., 1969) recorded a reduction in the rate of involution between 4 and 9 days postpartum, with a period of accelerated change from days 10 to 14 and a gradual decrease thereafter. Associated with this phase of rapid involution is uterine discharge. The whole of the uterus is usually palpable per rectum by 8 and 10 days postpartum in primipara and pluripara, respectively. The speed of involution of the non-gravid horn is more variable than that of the previously gravid horn, which depends upon its degree of involvement in placentation.

There is some dispute about when uterine involution is complete; the differences are probably only subjective. In six studies reported in dairy cattle the time taken for complete involution ranged from 26.0 to 52.0 days whilst in three studies in beef cattle it was 37.7–56.0 days. The changes after 20–25 days are generally almost imperceptible.

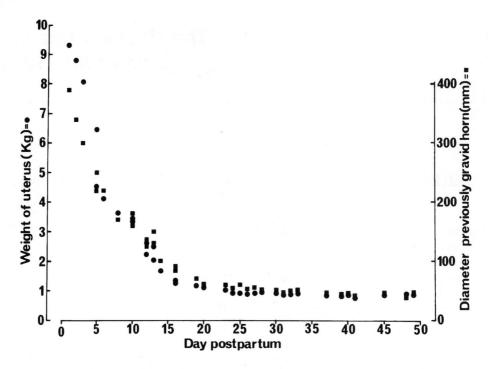

Fig. 7.1 Gross changes in the uterus of the cow during the puerperium. (Drawn from the data of Gier and Marion (1968).)

The cervix constricts rapidly postpartum; within 10–12 hours of a normal calving it becomes almost impossible to insert a hand through it into the uterus, and by 96 hours it will admit just two fingers. The cervix also undergoes atrophy and shrinkage due to the elimination of fluid and the reduction in muscle tissue. Gier and Marion (1968) found that the mean external diameter was 15 cm at 2 days postpartum, 9–11 cm at 10 days, 7–8 cm at 30 days and 5–6 cm at 60 days. A useful guide that involution is occurring normally is to compare the diameter of the previously gravid horn with that of the cervix, since at about 25 days postpartum the latter starts to exceed the former.

Prostaglandins must have a role in controlling uterine involution. Eley et al. (1981) have shown a positive correlation between PGFM concentrations in the peripheral circulation and the diameter of the uterine horn. Using exogenous $PGF_{2\alpha}$, twice daily for 10 days starting from 3 days postpartum, uterine involution has been accelerated by 6–13 days (Kindahl et al., 1982).

Restoration of the endometrium
Although placentation in the cow is considered to be of a non-deciduous type it is well recognized that during the first 7–10 days after calving there is usually a noticeable loss of fluid and tissue debris. This is sometimes referred to by the herdsman as the 'second cleansing' or 'secundus'. In human gynaecology the postpartum vaginal discharge is referred to as lochia. The presence of such a discharge is normal, although sometimes herdsmen will mistake it for an abnormal discharge due to uterine infection and request treatment.

The lochial discharge is usually yellowish brown or reddish brown; the volume voided varies greatly from individual to individual. Pluripara can void up to a total of 2000 ml, although it is more usually about 1000 ml. In primipara it is rarely more than 500 ml and in some animals it is occasionally nil, owing to the complete absorption of the lochia. The greatest flow of lochia occurs during the first 2–3 days; by 8 days it is reduced and by 14–18 days postpartum it has virtually disappeared. At about 9 days it is frequently bloodstained, whilst before it ceases it becomes lighter in colour and almost 'lymph-like'. Normal lochial discharge does not have an unpleasant odour.

The lochia is derived from the remains of fetal fluids, blood from the ruptured umbilical vessels and shreds of fetal membranes, but mainly from the

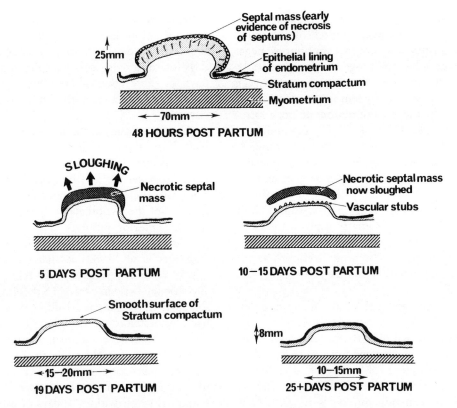

Fig. 7.2 The changes that occur in the caruncles of the cow during the puerperium. (Drawn from the data of Gier and Marion (1968).)

sloughed surfaces of the uterine caruncles. The slough occurs following degenerative changes and necrosis of the superficial layers, first described by Rasbech (1950). The changes that occur are illustrated diagrammatically in Figure 7.2.

After the shedding of the allantochorion the caruncle is about 70 mm long, 35 mm wide and 25 mm thick. The endometrial crypts frequently contain remnants of the chorionic villi which were detached from the rest of the allantochorion at the time of placental separation. Within the first 48 hours postpartum there is evidence of early necrotic changes in the septal mass of the caruncle; the caruncular blood vessels become rapidly constricted and are nearly occluded. At 5 days the necrosis has proceeded rapidly so that the stratum compactum is now covered by a leucocyte-laden necrotic layer. Some of this necrotic material starts to slough and contributes to the lochia. Small blood vessels, mainly arterioles, then protrude from the surface of the caruncle, from which there is oozing of blood, causing a red coloration of the lochia. By 10 days, most of the necrotic

caruncular tissue has sloughed and undergone some degree of liquefaction and by 15 days postpartum sloughing is complete, leaving only stubs of blood vessels protruding from the exposed stratum compactum. This eventually becomes smooth by 19 days, owing to the disappearance of the vessels.

Regeneration of the epithelium of the endometrium occurs immediately after parturition in those areas which were not seriously damaged and is complete in the inter-caruncular areas by 8 days. Complete re-epithelialization of the caruncle, which is largely derived from centripetal growth of cells from the surrounding uterine glands, is complete from 25 days onwards, although the stage at which complete healing occurs is variable.

Whilst these changes are taking place the caruncles are becoming smaller (Figure 7.2), so that at 40–60 days they consist of small protrusions 4–8 mm in diameter and 4–6 mm high. They also differ from those of nullipara because they are larger and have melanin pigmentation and a more vascular base.

Return of cyclical activity (ovarian rebound)

Because of the prolonged period of inhibition during pregnancy, due to the continuous negative-feedback effect of progesterone secreted by the corpus luteum and placenta, the pituitary is refractory postpartum, as demonstrated by a lack of response to the administration of gonadotrophin-releasing hormone (GnRH) (Lamming et al., 1979). This eventually recovers with time. As a result of the absence or low output of gonadotrophins the ovary is relatively quiescent and the cow is in the anoestrous phase which may be prolonged in suckler and high-yielding cows. However, during this postpartum phase the ovaries frequently contain numerous large anovulatory follicles which quickly become atretic, these are sometimes incorrectly diagnosed as cysts (see Chapter 22).

Opinions vary about the time of the first oestrus postpartum. In a survey of 14 publications on this subject (Garcia, 1982), the mean interval from calving to first oestrus ranged from 33 to 85.5 days. In a similar review by Morrow et al. (1966) a difference in the time of onset of first oestrus was identified between different types of cattle, 30–76.3 days for dairy cows and 52.2–80.2 days for beef cows. However, it is now accepted that the first sign of oestrus is not always a true reflection of the onset of cyclical activity (Moller, 1970; King et al., 1976). Using continuous time-lapse video recording of herds, 50, 94 and 100% of cows were identified in oestrus at the first, second and third postpartum ovulations (King et al., 1976); however, with daily observations the frequencies of detected oestrus were 16, 43 and 57%, respectively.

The availability of the milk progesterone assay has enabled the onset of cyclical activity to be determined by the presence of elevated progesterone concentrations. In a survey of 533 dairy cows in four herds (Bulman and Wood, 1980) nearly half (47.8%) of the cows had resumed normal cyclical ovarian activity within 20 days of calving and by 40 days this had increased to 92.4%. In this study only 4.9% appeared to have a delayed return to cyclical activity, i.e. had not returned by 50 days postpartum and 5.1% of the cows subsequently ceased normal cyclical activity having initially returned. A small number, 1.9%, had prolonged luteal activity, presumably due to a persistent corpus luteum or luteal cyst (see p. 364). These ovarian abnormalities depressed fertility, as measured by the calving to conception interval, which was 98 days for those with a delayed start to ovarian activity, 102 days for those with persistent luteal function, 124 days for those cows where there was cessation of cyclical activity compared with 85 days for normal cows.

Details of the endocrine changes postpartum have been discussed in detail (Lamming et al., 1982; Peters and Lamming, 1986). At calving both progesterone and oestradiol-17β concentrations fall, the latter precipitously so that there is removal of the hypothalamic/pituitary block.

The anterior pituitary is capable of releasing FSH during the first few days postpartum (Schallenberger et al., 1982) so that with the sporadic release of endogenous GnRH there is a gradual and sustained rise in plasma FSH. This causes some follicular development resulting in negative feedback by oestradiol and inhibin. The ability of the pituitary to release luteinizing hormone (LH) is much slower, for although the early release of GnRH causes some rise in LH, it quickly returns to basal levels. If a very large dose of endogenous GnRH is given within 10 days of calving there is no release of LH (Foster et al., 1980). If standard doses of GnRH are given at 10 and 16 days postpartum in milked cows then LH rises; however, in autumn calved suckler beef cows 20 days had to elapse and in spring calved suckler beef cows 30 days had to elapse (Lamming et al., 1982). Further evidence of the refractory state of the hypothalamus and pituitary gland has been demonstrated by the failure of a 1 mg dose of oestradiol benzoate to elicit a surge of LH at 0–5 days postpartum; a response was obtained by 10 days which was increased by 25 days. This is probably related to the delay in the restoration of oestrogen receptors in both hypothalamus and pituitary so that the positive-feedback mechanism necessary for the preovulatory LH surge cannot occur. The same dose rate of oestradiol stimulated an FSH surge as early as five days postpartum (Schallenberger et al., 1982).

The endocrine changes can be summarized thus: immediately postpartum there are no clearly defined episodes of follicle-stimulating hormone (FSH) or LH activity irrespective of suckling, milking or other function; thereafter, the levels of FSH rise first in the plasma followed by LH. In normal milked cows, due to increased GnRH release, there are increases in basal levels of LH together with increased frequency and amplitude of LH pulses culminating in an ovulatory surge. After ovulation there is a luteal phase which may be of normal length with a return to oestrus after 18–24 days or it may be much shorter. These short luteal phases probably arise because of inadequate preovulatory development of the follicle so that it either becomes luteinized in the absence of ovulation (see p. 361) or luteinization is inadequate. These short luteal phases are more prevalent the earlier the return of normal ovarian activity, i.e. 100% at 0–5 days, 60% at 10–15 days and 10% at 25–30 days postpartum (Terqui et al., 1982).

Other endocrine organs are involved in controlling ovarian function postpartum (Peters and Lamming, 1990). The uterus exerts an influence since it has been known for some time that the majority of ovulations postpartum occur in the ovary contralateral to the previously gravid horn (Gier and Marion, 1968); the effect is less, the later ovulation occurs. It has also been shown that prostaglandin metabolite (PGFM) usually returns to normal levels before the first postpartum ovulation (Thatcher, 1986). Similarly, the ovario-uterine axis exerts an inhibitory effect on pituitary LH secretion during the early postpartum period; experimental hysterectomy results in a rapid increase in plasma gonadotrophin concentrations (Schallenberger et al., 1982).

The adrenal cortex plays an important role in influencing the return to oestrus postpartum. Adrenocorticotrophic hormone (ACTH) (Liptrap and McNally, 1976) and corticosteroid administration (da Rosa and Wagner, 1981) suppress the secretion of LH. Stimulation of the teat, and milk removal cause a rise in glucocorticoids (Wagner and Oxenreider, 1972; Schams, 1976). Suckling, which is known to delay the return of cyclical ovarian activity, may exert its effect by modifying the tonic release of GnRH and LH by the release of opioid peptides. The role of prolactin is equivocal, for although bromocriptine treatment during lactation had little or no effect on LH release in cows, there appears to be a reciprocal relationship between the hypothalamic control of LH release and prolactin release. Opioid antagonists increase LH and decrease prolactin secretion; the effects of the agonists are the reverse. The mammary gland has also been shown to have an endocrine role (Peters and Lamming, 1990).

Elimination of bacterial contamination

At calving, and immediately postpartum, the vulva is relaxed and the cervix is dilated thus allowing bacteria to gain entry into the vagina, and thereafter the uterus. A wide range of bacteria are isolated from the uterine lumen; Elliott et al. (1968) identified 33 different species, those most frequently isolated being *Actinomyces* (*Corynebacterium*) *pyogenes*, *Escherichia coli*, streptococci and staphylococci (Johanns et al., 1967; Elliott et al., 1968; Griffin et al., 1974). The last authors stressed that the flora fluctuated as a result of spontaneous contamination, clearance and recontamination during the first seven weeks postpartum. In all studies there is a decrease with time in the percentage of uteri from which bacteria are isolated. This is exemplified in the study of Elliott et al. (1968) in which 93% of uteri examined within 15 days of calving were contaminated, compared with 78% between 16 and 30 days, 50% between 31 and 45 days and only 9% between 46 and 60 days.

Blood, cell debris and sloughed caruncular tissue provide an ideal medium for bacterial growth; however, in most cases the bacteria do not colonize the uterus to produce a metritis/endometritis (see Chapter 23). The main mechanism involved in the elimination of the bacteria is phagocytosis by migrating leucocytes; however, persistence of uterine contractions, sloughing of caruncular tissue and uterine secretions all assist in the physical expulsion of the bacteria. Early return to cyclical activity is probably important since the oestrogen-dominated uterus is more resistant to infection. However there is evidence that in some cases early return to oestrus may be disadvantageous (Olson, 1984; and see Chapter 23).

Factors influencing the puerperium

Uterine involution. Many of the methods used to measure the rate of involution have been largely subjective and thus inaccurate; however, with the advent of transrectal ultrasound imaging, accurate measurements of uterine and cervical dimensions are now possible (Tian and Noakes, 1991). Some of the factors are:

1. *Age.* Most observers have found that involution is more rapid in primipara than pluripara.

2. *Season of year.* If there is any influence,

involution is probably most rapid in spring and summer.

3. *Suckling vs milking.* Results are contradictory, it may be a breed influence on the effect of time to return of cyclical ovarian activity.

4. *Climate.* There is evidence that heat stress can accelerate and inhibit the speed of involution.

5. *Periparturient abnormalities.* Dystocia, retained placenta, hypocalcaemia, ketosis, twin calves and metritis delay involution. Periparturient problems cause an overall delay in the completion of this process of 5–8 days (Buch et al., 1955; Tennant and Peddicord, 1968).

6. *Delayed return to cyclical ovarian activity.* Inhibits involution.

Restoration of the Endometrium. There is little related documented evidence; however, retained placenta and metritis inhibit healing, whilst ovarian rebound to cyclical activity may have an influence.

Return of cyclical ovarian activity (ovarian rebound).

1. *Periparturient abnormalities.* A number of authors have shown that a whole range of periparturient problems delay ovarian rebound.

2. *Milk yield.* There is much contradictory evidence on the influence of current milk yield; some authors have demonstrated an effect of the lactation preceding calving. It is frequently difficult to differentiate the influence of nutrition and milk yield.

3. *Nutrition.* In both beef suckler and dairy cows, inadequate feeding, especially of energy, during the dry period and after calving inhibits ovarian rebound. This is likely to be mediated by modification of GnRH and LH secretion from the hypothalamus and pituitary, respectively. Recent work has implicated insulin-like growth factor 1 (IGF-1) (see review by Peters and Lamming, 1990).

4. *Breed.* Whilst it has been known for some time that there is a longer delay in beef compared with dairy cows there is evidence of a breed effect within the two groups especially in the former.

5. *Parity.* Most observers have recorded a delay in primipara compared with pluripara — up to the fourth lactation. Conflicting opinions have probably arisen because of the problems of separating

the influences of nutritional status, milk yield and weight loss.

6. *Season of the year.* There is good evidence that photoperiod has an effect. This has been shown by experimentally subjecting heifers to continuous darkness which inhibited the return of cyclical activity (Terqui et al., 1982). Peters and Riley (1982) showed that suckler cows that calved between February and April were acyclic significantly longer than those that calved between August and December. By stimulating the effects of short day length using exogenous melatonin it has been possible to delay the return to oestrous and ovulation in postpartum beef cows (Sharp et al., 1986).

7. *Climate.* Cows in tropical climates show a delay compared with those in temperate zones.

8. *Suckling intensity and milking frequency.* The greater the frequency of milking and the intensity of suckling (number of calves) the longer the period of acyclicity.

Elimination of Bacterial Contamination. This problem is associated with the development of metritis and endometritis (see Chapter 23).

1. *Magnitude of bacterial contamination.* A massive bacterial flora may overwhelm natural defence mechanisms.

2. *Nature of bacterial flora.* Many obligate Gram-negative anaerobes, such as *Fusobacterium necrophorum* and *Bacteroides* spp., exhibit synergy with Gram-positive aerobic contaminants.

3. *Delayed uterine involution.*

4. *Retained placenta.*

5. *Calving trauma to the uterus.*

6. *Return of cyclical ovarian activity.* There is contradictory evidence since, with an early return to oestrous there is an early oestrogen peak which should assist in the elimination of the bacteria. However, if the level of contamination is such that a significant bacterial flora persists after the first oestrus the subsequent luteal phase may allow the bacteria to proliferate (Olson et al., 1984).

Mare

The puerperium is shorter in the mare than in the cow, with rapid involution and relatively good conception rates at the first postpartum oestrus.

For the reader who wishes to study the subject in greater detail than outlined below there are two excellent papers (Andrews and McKenzie, 1941; Gygax et al., 1979).

In pony mares it is usually possible to identify the outline of the uterine body and horns by rectal palpation at about 12 hours postpartum; in Thoroughbreds it is longer. Lochial discharge is relatively slight in most mares and usually ceases by 24–48 hours after foaling, although in a few cases it can persist for up to a week. The uterine horns shrink rapidly, reaching their pregravid size by day 32. Although the previously non-gravid horn was initially smaller, it shrinks at a slower rate. The cervix remains slightly dilated until after the first oestrus.

Ovarian rebound is rapid, the foal heat occurring five to 12 days postpartum. Evidence of follicular activity can be determined as early as the second day. Although conception rates at this first oestrus are lower than at other times, a large number of mares are fertile, which proves that the endometrium is capable of sustaining a pregnancy. Andrews and McKenzie (1941) found that the endometrium was fully restored by 13–25 days postpartum.

There is nothing comparable with the degeneration and sloughing of the endometrium that occurs in the cow; small amounts of villous debris are frequently attached to the maternal crypts but are removed by autolysis. The maternal crypts disappear as a result of lysis and shrinkage of the epithelial cells of the endometrium, condensation of their contents and collapse of the lumen of the crypt. By 14 days the endometrium is usually quite normal, apart from some pleomorphism of the luminal epithelium, but in some mares inflammatory changes may persist for several weeks (Gygax et al., 1979).

As in the cow, bacterial contamination of the uterus from the environment is a frequent occurrence, the species most frequently isolated being β-haemolytic streptococci and coliforms. These organisms are usually eliminated at the foal heat; if not, although they may increase during the subsequent dioestrus, they usually disappear at the second postpartum oestrus.

Placental retention delays involution, whilst exercise is said to hasten it. The process is more rapid in primipara than in pluripara.

Ewe and doe (nanny goat)

The puerperium in both these species is very similar to that in the cow, being typical of ruminants in general. The main difference is that, since they are both seasonal breeders, parturition is followed by a period of anoestrus. There is little information available for the doe so that the changes that are described relate only to the ewe, although it is unlikely that there will be major differences.

Involution

There is rapid shrinkage and contraction of the uterus, particularly during the third to 10th day postpartum, as determined by measurements of uterine weight and length, diameter of uterine body and previously gravid horn. According to these measurements, involution is complete by 20–25 days (Uren, 1935; Hunter et al., 1968; Foote and Call, 1969).

Restoration of the endometrium

As in the cow there are profound changes in the structure of the caruncles with degeneration of the surface, necrosis, sloughing and subsequent regeneration of the superficial layers of the endometrium. There is evidence, determined by the slaughter of animals three days before the expected date of lambing, of prepartum hyaline degenerative changes. This occurs in the connective tissue at the base of, and adjacent to, the endometrial crypts and also involves both directly and indirectly the walls of the arteries and veins, thus reducing their lumens; the fetal villi are unaffected (Van Wyk et al., 1972).

After dehiscence and separation of the placenta there is further hyaline degeneration of caruncular tissue, which results in constriction of the blood vessels at the base of the maternal crypts. There is necrosis of the surface layer of the caruncle so that at about 4 days postpartum the most superficial layers are undergoing autolysis and liquefaction, which is responsible for the dark reddish brown or black coloration of the lochial discharge at this time. By 16 days postpartum, necrosis of the whole superficial part of the caruncle has occurred with, in most cases, separation of the brown necrotic plaque so that it is lying free in the uterine lumen. The caruncles now have a clean, glistening surface, and the process of regeneration is completed by the re-epithelialization of the caruncles by about 28 days.

The quantity of lochia voided is variable. Initially it arises from blood, fetal fluids and placental debris but as the puerperium proceeds it is contributed to by the liquefied, sloughed caruncular tissue.

Return of cyclical activity (ovarian rebound)
Although in temperate climates ewes normally become anoestrous after lambing there are numerous reports of ovarian activity occurring within a few days to two weeks postpartum. Follicular growth is common but ovulation is unusual and when it does occur it is usually associated with a silent heat. Failure of follicular maturation and ovulation is probably due to inadequate release of LH as a result of a deficiency in GnRH synthesis and secretion. As a result, basal LH levels and the pulse frequency of episodic LH secretion are inadequate to stimulate normal ovarian function (Wright et al., 1981). It is possible that the time of the year when the ewes lamb has a profound effect, with those that lamb early and within the normal breeding season being more likely to have normal ovarian rebound. Hafez (1952) has suggested that it is most likely to occur in those breeds which have a longer-than-average breeding season.

Elimination of bacterial contamination
Although it would have been expected that similar events to those previously described for the cow and mare would occur, the author was unable to isolate bacteria from uterine swabs obtained from 10 ewes, 1–14 days postpartum.

Sow
There are a number of studies which describe the changes that take place during the puerperium of the sow (Palmer et al., 1965; Graves et al., 1967; Svajgr et al., 1974). It is important that the changes should occur rapidly, with a return to a normal pregravid state, so that pregnancy can be established as quickly as possible after weaning.

Involution
Apart from the rapid initial uterine weight loss which occurs in the first 5 days postpartum, involution is fairly uniform and is complete by 28 days.

After day 6 most of the loss of weight is due to changes in the myometrium, notably a reduction in cell numbers, cell size and amounts of connective tissue. The decrease in the thickness of the endometrium and myometrium is completed by 28 days.

Restoration of the endometrium
The uterine epithelium one day after farrowing is a low columnar or cuboidal type and there is evidence of the extensive folding that is present during pregnancy. The epithelial cells at seven days are very low and flattened and show signs of degenerative changes; however, there are also signs of active cell division which is subsequently responsible for regeneration of the epithelium. This latter process is complete by 21 days and is capable of sustaining pregnancy.

Return of cyclical activity (ovarian rebound)
Suckling and subsequent weaning have a profound effect upon ovarian rebound and indirectly on other puerperal changes in the genital tract. In most cases there will be no return to oestrus and ovulation until the piglets are removed. In the study by Palmer et al. (1965) there was no evidence of ovulation during suckling periods of up to 62 days. In general, the later the time of weaning, the shorter the time interval to the first oestrus; for example, if the litter is weaned at 2, 13, 24 and 35 days postpartum the mean times to first oestrus were 10.1, 8.2, 7.1 and 6.8 days, respectively (Svajgr et al., 1974). The time to the first ovulation can also be shortened by the temporary removal of the whole litter for varying periods during the day (partial weaning), or the permanent removal of part of the litter (split weaning) (Britt et al., 1985).

There is rapid regression of the corpora lutea of pregnancy, with signs of cellular degeneration by three days postpartum, so that by day 7 they consist mainly of connective tissue. There is considerable follicular activity during suckling, with follicles sometimes reaching a diameter of 6–7 mm. This is sometimes associated with behavioural oestrus shortly after farrowing but in no cases is there ovulation; the follicles become atretic.

In a study of the endocrine changes of the postpartum sow, Edwards and Foxcroft (1983) showed that, irrespective of whether weaning occurred at 3 or 5 weeks, the great majority of sows showed a preovulatory LH surge within 7 days of weaning. At the time of weaning there was a transient rise in basal LH of about 2 days' duration but, unlike the cow, there was no consistent change in the episodic release of LH. Prolactin concentrations are high during lactation but decline rapidly to basal levels a few hours after weaning; mean FSH concentrations rise 2–3 days after weaning. Follicular growth and ovulation are inhibited during lactation because of suppressed LH secretion; this probably occurs as a result of direct neural inhibition of GnRH synthesis and release. Inadequate nutrition, particularly severe weight loss, can delay the onset of cyclical ovarian activity, as can the season of the year (Britt et al., 1985). It is generally accepted that exposure to the boar has the reverse effect.

The time of weaning, and thus the time of first oestrus, also has other effects on reproductive function, owing to the time taken for the completion of the puerperium. Fertilization rates and pregnancy rates are improved the later the time of weaning and hence the later sows are served after farrowing.

Bitch

Since the bitch is monocyclic, parturition is followed by anoestrus, the onset of the next heat being unpredictable. Regression of the corpora lutea of pregnancy is initially rapid, so that by 1 or 2 weeks postpartum they have been reduced in size. However, thereafter it is much slower, so that even after 3 months the corpora lutea measure 2.5 mm in diameter.

The rate of involution is similar to that of other species and the uterine horns are restored to their pregravid size by 4 weeks. The lochial discharge immediately postpartum is very noticeable because of its green colour due to the presence of uteroverdin; unless there are complications this should change to a blood-stained, mucoid discharge within 12 hours.

In the non-pregnant bitch, the surface of the endometrium undergoes desquamation followed by regeneration, with repair completed by 120 days after the onset of oestrus (see Chapter 1). After pregnancy and normal parturition, the time taken for regeneration of the endometrium is about 2 weeks longer. The areas of placental attachment are not readily identifiable immedi-

ately postpartum but by four weeks they are easy to identify. Desquamation of the epithelial lining of the endometrium starts at 6 weeks postpartum, is complete by 7 weeks, and the whole process of regeneration has ended by 12 weeks.

Cat

Lactation will usually suppress oestrus effectively (Schmidt et al., 1983) but if the queen has no kittens to suckle or only one or two, she may show a postpartum oestrus 7–10 days after parturition.

THE NEWBORN AND ITS CARE

The sudden change at birth from the constant, controlled, cosseted environment of the uterus to the variable and frequently stressful free-living environment demands great adaptability from the newborn. In domestic species, provided that parturition is normal, most survive this transition without assistance. It should also be remembered that during the latter part of gestation the fetus is already undergoing a number of maturational changes, probably stimulated by the hormonal changes that occur in the initiation of parturition, in preparation for the free-living state (see Chapter 6). However, at birth, and for a variable period of time afterwards, a number of important events must occur.

Onset of spontaneous respiration

During fetal life episodes of muscular movements similar to those of respiration have been observed in a number of species; whether these are truly the precursors of the continuous respiratory movements of the newborn is debatable. However, if parturition occurs normally then spontaneous respiratory movements will occur within 60 seconds of expulsion; if there is a delay then respiratory movements can sometimes occur before the offspring has been completely expelled.

There are probably a number of factors that are responsible for the initiation of spontaneous respiration. During the birth process P_{O_2} and blood pH are falling and P_{CO_2} is rising due to the start of placental separation and occlusion of the umbilicus, thus restricting gaseous exchange.

These changes have been shown in the lamb to stimulate chemoreceptors in the carotid sinus (Chernick et al., 1969). Tactile and thermal stimuli are also important, for it has been shown that if the face of the fetal lamb is cooled there is stimulation of respiratory movements (Dawes, 1968), whilst the licking and nuzzling of the dam probably provides some stimulus.

The first respiratory movement is usually a deep, forceful inspiration which is necessary to force air into the lungs. It has been demonstrated in the fetal lamb that a pressure of 18 cm of water is necessary to force air into the lungs at the first inflation; once this has occurred only a small pressure is needed to cause full inflation thereafter (Reynolds and Strang, 1966). The importance of pulmonary surfactant which occurs with maturation of the fetus has been demonstrated by the same authors. Although the initial work done in the first breath is greater in mature than in immature fetal lungs, for the second and subsequent breaths it is much less.

Survival of the newborn is dependent upon the rapid onset of normal, spontaneous respiration. Once birth is complete it is important first to ensure that the upper respiratory tract is cleared of fluid, mucus and attached fetal membrane. This can be done with the aid of fingers or, preferably, with a simple suction device. Elevation of the rear of the calf, particularly by suspension from the hindlimbs, results in the escape of copious quantities of fluid. Some of this comes from the stomach and it may not necessarily be beneficial since it has been shown that one-third of this fluid can be absorbed from the lungs of the newborn via the lymphatic system (Humphreys et al., 1967). Brisk rubbing of the chest with straw or towels frequently provides the necessary tactile stimulus to stimulate respiration, whilst a portable oxygen cylinder and resuscitator are useful equipment to have available. This comprises a small portable cylinder of oxygen, a reducing valve, rebreathing bag and either a face mask or intranasal tube. Respiratory stimulants such as coramine and adrenaline are not particularly useful; however, a mixture of solutions of crotethamide and corpropamide placed on the tongue can stimulate respiratory activity in some cases. Over enthusiastic compression of the chest can sometimes cause injury to the ribs and the thoracic organs.

In most cases, if resuscitation does not result in spontaneous respiration in 2 or 3 minutes it is unlikely that the newborn will survive, even though there is a good strong pulse and heart beat.

Most perinatal deaths are associated with dystocia and subsequent assistance. In a study involving the post-mortem examination of 327 calves that died during the perinatal period (within 48 hours of birth), 13.2% had fractured ribs, 4.3% diaphragmatic tears and 2.8% fracture of the spine in the thoracolumbar region (Mee, 1993). In a study involving the perinatal death of 22 calves born after an unassisted calving there was some evidence that deficiencies of selenium, iodine and other trace elements were involved (Mee, 1991). In addition, premature separation and expulsion of the placenta can also result in perinatal death in all species.

Thermoregulation

In the period immediately following birth the newborn has to adjust to an environment whose temperature may fluctuate widely and which is also usually below that of the uterus.

Following birth the body temperature of the newborn falls quickly from that of the dam before it eventually recovers; the degree of fall and speed of recovery vary from species to species and with the environmental temperature. In the foal and calf the fall is transient; in the lamb recovery occurs within a few hours; the piglet takes up to 24 hours or even longer in cold conditions; whilst in the kitten and puppy the period before the temperature recovers to approximately that of birth is 7–9 days.

In the newborn, thermoregulation is controlled in two ways. Firstly the metabolic rate is increased to three times the fetal rate soon after birth. The increased rate is dependent upon adequate substrate and since glycogen and adipose tissue reserves are low in the newborn it is very important that immediate and adequate food is available. However, the metabolic rate can increase only to a certain level, known as summit metabolism; if this is insufficient to maintain body temperature then hypothermia occurs (Alexander, 1970). The second method of thermoregulation is to reduce heat loss. The newborn has little subcutaneous fat and hence insulation is poor. The body surface is wet and thus heat is lost due to evaporation, whilst in species such as the pig the coat provides little protection. Heat loss is greatest in smaller individuals because they have a greater surface area per unit of body weight.

Thermoregulation in the newborn can be improved in a number of ways:

1. Ensure that there is adequate food intake.

2. Arrange for birth to occur in at least a thermally neutral environment and in those species where thermoregulation is delayed this environment should be maintained. The new-born puppy should be placed in an environmental temperature of 30–33° C for the first 24 hours, which can be reduced to 26–30° C by three days. Puppies born at a normal room temperature of 18–22° C can suffer a fall in rectal temperature of 5° C.

3. Reduce heat loss by ensuring that the coat is adequately and quickly dried. A proper nest area should be provided with good insulation and supplementary heating in polytocous species which will also encourage the huddling together of the litter, thus reducing the overall surface area. In the case of lambs, simple plastic jackets can be an effective way of reducing heat loss.

Umbilicus

At birth the umbilicus usually ruptures passively or in some species, such as the dog, the dam bites through the structure; there are few indications for ligation. Premature severance, especially in the foal, should be prevented, since it has been shown that in the foal the pulse can persist for up to nine minutes after expulsion of the foal, thereby ensuring an adequate blood volume (Rossdale, 1967).

Provided that birth occurs in a clean environment with adequate hygiene it should not be necessary to handle the umbilicus. However, if there is an outbreak of 'navel ill' it may be necessary to introduce some prophylactic measures. The navel should be carefully cleansed with an antiseptic solution, dried and treated with an antibiotic spray or dressing.

Protection from an excitable or vicious dam

Occasionally the dam will attack or savage the newborn, in which case it may be necessary to provide some physical protection and resort to the use of tranquillizer drugs.

REFERENCES

Alexander, G. (1970) In: *Physiology of Digestion and Metabolism in the Ruminant*, ed. A. T. Phillipson, p. 199. Newcastle: Oriel Press.

Andrews, F. N. and McKenzie, F. F. (1941) *Res. Bull. Univ. Mo.*, 329.

Britt, J. H., Armstrong, J. D., Cox, N. M. and Esbenshade, K. L. (1985) *J. Reprod. Fertil. Suppl.*, **33**, 37.

Bulman, D. C. and Wood, P. D. P. (1980) *Anim. Proc.*, **30**, 177.

Chernick, V., Faridy, E. E. and Pagtakhan, R. D. (1969) *Proc. Amer. Soc. Exp. Biol. Med.*, **28**, 439.

da Rosa, G. O. and Wagner, W. C. (1981) *J. Anim. Sci.*, **52**, 1098.

Dawes, G. S. (1968) *Foetal and Neonatal Physiology*. Chicago, Ill.: Year Book.

Edquist, L. E., Kindahl, H. and Stabenfelt, G. (1978) *Prostaglandins*, **16**, 111.

Edquist, L. E., Lindell, J. O. and Kindahl, H. (1980) *Proc. 9th Int. Cong. Anim. Reprod. Artific. Insem., Madrid*.

Edwards, S. and Foxcroft, G. R. (1983) *J. Reprod. Fertil.*, **67**, 163.

Eley, D. S., Thatcher, W. W., Head, H. H., Collier, R. J., Wilcox, C. J. and Call, E. P. (1981) *J. Dairy Sci.*, **64**, 312.

Elliott, K., McMahon, K. J., Gier, H. T. and Marion, G. B. (1968) *Amer. J. Vet. Res.*, **29**, 77.

Foote, W. C. and Call, J. W. (1969) *J. Anim. Sci.*, **29**, 190.

Foster, J. P., Lamming, G. E. and Peters, A. R. (1980) *J. Reprod. Fertil.*, **59**, 321.

Garcia, M. (1982) *Nordisk Vet. Med.*, **34**, 255.

Gier, W. C. and Marion, G. B. (1968) *Amer. J. Vet. Res.*, **29**, 83.

Graves, W. E., Lauderdale, J. W., Kirkpatrick, R. L., First, N. L. and Casida, L. E. (1967) *J. Anim. Sci.*, 26, 365.

Griffin, J. F. T., Hartigan, P. J. and Nunn, W. R. (1974) *Theriogenology*, **1**, 91.

Gygax, A. P., Ganjam, V. K. and Kennedy, R. M. (1979) *J. Reprod. Fertil. Suppl.*, **27**, 571.

Hafez, E. S. E. (1952) *J. Agr. Sci., Camb.*, **42**, 189.

Humphreys, P. W., Normand, I. C. S., Reynolds, E. O. R. and Strang, L. B. (1967) *J. Physiol., Lond.*, **193**, 1.

Hunter, D. L., Erb, R. E., Randel, R. D., Gaverick, H. A., Callahan, C. J. and Harrington, R. B. (1968) *J. Dairy Sci.*, **52**, 904.

Johanns, C. J., Clark, T. L. and Herrick, J. B. (1967) *J. Amer. Vet. Med. Assn*, **151**, 1692.

King, G. J., Hurnik, J. F. and Robertson, H. A. (1976) *J. Anim. Sci.*, **42**, 688.

Lamming, G. E., Foster, J. P. and Bulman, D. C. (1979) *Vet. Rec.*, **104**, 156.

Lamming, G. E., Peters, A. R., Riley, G. M. and Fisher, M. W. (1982) In: *Factors Influencing Fertility in the Postpartum Cow*, ed. H. Karg and E. Schallenberger, pp. 173–186. The Hague: Martinus Nijhoff.

Liptrap, R. M. and McNally, P. J. (1976) *Amer. J. Vet. Res.*, **37**, 369.

Mee, J. F. (1991) *Irish Vet. J.*, **44**, 80.

Mee, J. F. (1993) *Vet. Rec.*, **133**, 555.

Moller, K. (1970) *N.Z. Vet. J.*, **18**, 83.

Morrow, D. A., Roberts, S. I. and McEntee, K. (1969) *Cornell Vet.*, **59**, 134, 190.

Olson, J. D., Ball, L., Mortimer, R. G., Farin, P. W., Adney, W. S. and Huffman, E. M. (1984) *Amer. J. Vet. Res.*, **45**, 2251.

Palmer, W. M. H., Teague, H. S. and Venzke, W. G. (1965) *J. Anim. Sci.*, **24**, 541.

Peters, A. R. and Lamming, G. E. (1990) In: *Oxford Reviews of Reproductive Biology*, ed. S. R. Milligan, Vol. 12, pp. 245–288. Oxford: Oxford University Press.

Peters, A. R. and Riley, G. M. (1982) *Anim. Prod.*, **34**, 145.

Rasbech, N. O. (1950) *Nord. VetMed.*, **2**, 655.

Reynolds, E. O. R. and Strang, L. B. (1966) *Brit. Med. Bull.*, **22**, 79.

Rossdale, P. D. (1967) *Brit. Vet. J.*, **123**, 470.

Schallenberger, E., Oerterer, U. and Hutterer, G. (1982) In: *Factors Influencing Fertility in the Postpartum Cow*, ed. H. Karg and E. Schallenberger, pp. 123–146. The Hague: Martinus Nijhoff.

Sharpe, P. H., Gifford, D. R., Flavel, P. F., Nottle, M. B. and Armgtrong, D. T. (1986) *Theriogenology*, **26**, 621.

Svajgr, A. J., Hays, V. W., Cromwell, G. L. L. and Dutt, R. H. (1974) *J. Anim. Sci.*, **38**, 100.

Tennant, B. and Peddicord, R. G. (1968) *Cornell Vet.*, **58**, 185.

Terqui, M., Chupin, D., Gauthier, D., Perez, B., Pelot, J. and Mauleon, P. (1982) In: *Factors Influencing Fertility in the Postpartum Cow*, ed. H. Karg and E. Schallenberger, pp. 384–408. The Hague: Martinus Nijhoff.

Thatcher, W. W. (1986) Cited by Peters, A. R. and Lamming, G. E. (1986) *Vet. Rec.*, **118**, 236.

Tian, W. and Noakes, D. E. (1991) *Vet. Rec.*, **128**, 566.

Uren, A. W. (1935) *Mich. State Coll. Agric. Exp. Stn. Tech. Bull.*, 144.

Van Wyk, L. C., Van Niekerk, C. H. and Belonje, P. C. (1972) *J. S. Afr. Vet. Assn*, **43**, 13, 29.

Wagner, W. C. and Oxenreider, S. L. (1972) *J. Anim. Sci.*, **34**, 360.

Wright, P. J., Geytenbeek, P. E., Clarke, I. J. and Findlay, J. K. (1981) *J. Reprod. Fertil.*, **61**, 97.

3

Part Three

Dystocia and Other Disorders Associated with Parturition

8

AETIOLOGY

Dystocia means difficult birth. Its diagnosis and treatment constitute a large and important part of the science of obstetrics. The economic importance of bovine dystocia is emphasized in published figures collected by Sloss and Duffy (1980). They show that about a third of the total of 17% of fetal and calf losses occur at the time of parturition and that most of these arise from calving difficulties. Similarly, Greene (1984) in a 7 year study in Ireland found a stillbirth rate of 5.2% of all calves on dairy farms. The major cause of these losses was dystocia due to fetopelvic disproportion. To this loss of offspring must be added maternal deaths and subsequent infertility which derive from dystocia in all species as well as the cost of treatment and the diminished productive capacity of the dam. In a survey of the effects of dystocia on fertility in 1889 cows, Laster et al. (1973) found that cows which had had calving difficulties experienced delay in resuming oestrous and showed 15.9% reduction in conception rate compared with cows which had calved normally.

Obstetricians have usually regarded dystocia as being either maternal or fetal in origin. More realistically, however, it should be considered in relation to defects in the three components of the birth process — the expulsive forces, the birth canal and the fetus. Difficult birth will occur when the expulsive forces are insufficient, when the birth canal is constricted or when the presenting diameter of the fetus is inordinately large. The types and causes of animal dystocia can be set out as in Figure 8.1.

The immediate causes of difficult birth are, in general, readily recognized and easily understood and thus permit the application of rational treatment. But modern veterinary obstetricians should be as much, or more, concerned to prevent dystocia as to treat it and this standpoint requires a more profound consideration of its fundamental causes. In particular, there should be a constant awareness of the possibility of underlying hereditary causes. For example, if it is accepted that primary inertia has a high incidence in a particular breed, then it is a reasonable supposition that occasional bulls will sire daughters which have a predisposition to uterine inertia. Indeed, records from artificial insemination stations show that this is so. Similarly, bitches of brachycephalic breeds show high incidences of dystocia which is partly due to a relatively short depth of the pelvic inlet. In addition, certain bulls beget heifer progeny whose pelves appear too small to admit calves of normal size. Environmental influences can also be of fundamental importance. For instance, when litter numbers are low in the polytocous species the individual offspring grow to unusually large size — presumably due to more favourable uterine nutrition — and cause dystocia. As might be expected, therefore, if ewes pregnant with singletons are overfed in the last weeks of gestation the mean birth weight may be increased from 3.7 to 4.6 kg (Underwood and Shier, 1942) and the incidence of dystocia correspondingly raised. Incomplete dilatation of the cervix in the same flock of ewes may vary from year to year, and peak incidences occur in years when prolapse of the vagina is common; this would seem to indicate an environmental cause acting through the endocrine system. With respect to bovine fetal dystocia it is now clear that difficult birth due to fetal oversize is very largely of hereditary origin and capable of being partially controlled by rigorous selection of artificial insemination bulls. Drew (1986–1987) studied the factors affecting dystocia in Friesian dairy heifers, based on a field trial involving 2973 calvings on 58 farms. She concluded that the following advice should be given to farmers and veterinary surgeons:

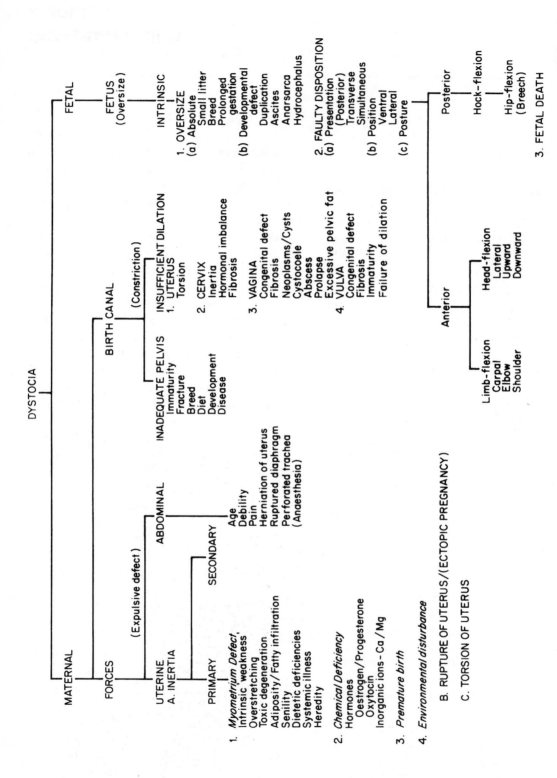

Fig. 8.1 The causes of dystocia.

Management at service
- Ensure service weight is more than 260 kg.
- Take care when selecting the service sire:
  – Artificial insemination bulls:
  Select a well-proven bull of high genetic merit. Select a bull which has been used successfully on heifers on several farms or, if this is not possible, one with a below average incidence of calving difficulties and gestation length when used on cows.
  – Natural service bulls:
  Avoid bulls of large breeds. Select a bull with a record of easy calvings or, if this is not possible, one with a sire with a good record.

Management pre-calving
- Adjust feed levels to avoid calving in an over-fat condition.
- Restrict energy intake in the last 3 weeks of pregnancy.
- Check iodine and selenium levels if calf mortality has been high in previous years.
- Ensure supplementary magnesium is provided.
- Ensure that an adequate exercise area is available.
- Observe the heifers at least four or five times daily during the last 3 weeks of pregnancy, especially if short-gestation length bulls are used.
- If possible, run as a heifer group or with dry cows. If fed with the milking cows ensure 'parlour feed' is restricted to the amount required to acquaint the heifer with her post-calving diet.

Management at calving
- Calve grazed heifers in their field or paddock if possible. Housed heifers should calve in familiar surroundings. Avoid moving them to a calving box unless essential for adequate assistance.
- Ensure the field is well fenced to avoid the possibility of heifers rolling into positions from where it is difficult to assist.
- Observe hourly (approximately) when calving starts. Too frequent observations (more frequently than $\frac{1}{2}$ hourly) can delay calving.
- Be a good stockman. Watch for signs of fear, abnormal pain or distress and be ready to assist if these are noted or if calving is prolonged.
- Ensure that the stockmen are trained to identify potential problems and know when to call professional help. If calving aids are used,

instruction should be given as to the correct method of application.
- Call professional advice if an unusually high percentage of the first heifers to calve require assistance — there may be a herd *problem* which will affect the whole group.

Little attention has been paid to the study of the basic causes of that other large category of dystocia which is due to faulty disposition of the fetus. It is unlikely that its aetiology will be clarified until the normal birth mechanism for parturient extension of the limbs from the flexed gestational position is understood. It seems likely to the author that the uterus, through its myometrial activity, plays a part in this limb extension: postural defects are more common with twins and with premature births, in both of which instances a degree of uterine inertia is commonly present. Hormone ratios and hormone concentrations (particularly that of progesterone) are probably important in determining limb posture, for Jöchle et al. (1972) have found that when progesterone was given to cows in which labour had been induced by flumethasone there was a high incidence of dystocia due to postural deviation. Similarly, Hendricks et al. (1977) found that five of 12 pregnant Hereford heifers in which premature parturition was induced with prostaglandin $F_{2\alpha}$ given at day 267, and which calved 90 hours later, had dystocia due to flexion of either the head or a forelimb. Moreover, 10 of the 12 prematurely induced heifers retained the afterbirth beyond 72 hours of calving. Also, Chew et al. (1979) found that four of eight cows from which the ovaries were removed on day 218 and which calved prematurely between days 269 and 278 had dystocia. The authors attributed this dystocia to the chronically low levels of progesterone during the several weeks prepartum in the ovariectomized cows. The type of dystocia was not maldisposition but appeared to be due either to a lack of expulsive effort or to a measure of fetopelvic disproportion. Prepartum hormone measurements in a group of intact control heifers, some of which, incidentally, had dystocia, showed that the dystocia was associated with progesterone levels which were higher and oestrogen levels which were lower than normal. In some animals with high progesterone the level dropped suddenly and in others very gradually before parturition. Crenshaw et al. (1966) had previously demonstrated that high concentrations of progesterone, artificially induced in ewes at term, reduced the myometrial activity of the mother as well as the muscular reactivity of the fetus.

O'Brien and Stott (1977) made daily blood hormone assays from day 260 until term on 12 Holstein heifers from a herd with a high incidence of dystocia. Six heifers developed dystocia and, as compared with others, they showed lower concentrations of oestradiol-17β and higher concentrations of progesterone from day 23 to day 12 before calving. These authors concluded, and their conclusion may be applied to the preceding reports, that dystocia may be due to a delay in the development of the hormone changes which precede normal parturition, or to the changes being less pronounced than in normal animals or, one may add, to the ratio between plasma levels of certain hormones — particularly oestradiol-17β and progesterone — being abnormal at a crucial prepartum period. At any rate, these reports on the association of hormone concentrations with dystocia tend to bridge the aetiological gap between maternal expulsive deficiency and fetal maldisposition.

When a certain type of dystocia has a high incidence in a particular breed it is probably due to genetic factors. Hence one is not surprised to find that when in-breeding has been intentionally practised over several generations the dystocia incidence rises. For example, records of in-bred and non-in-bred herds of Hereford cattle in Montana, USA, studied by Woodward and Clark (1959), showed that of 8857 births, 3.6% of calves were stillborn; for the in-bred population the stillborn birth rate was 4.3% as compared with 2.8% for the non-in-bred cattle; posterior presentation accounted for 25% of the still-births and the posterior presentation rate in calves born to one sire was high enough to suggest that a hereditary factor was involved.

INCIDENCE

The overall incidence of dystocia varies with the species and with breeds within the species, as also does the incidence of particular types of dystocia. The bovine species is most often affected but ewes, particularly when carrying twins, can show a high incidence. Mares and sows are much less commonly affected. In the bitch the incidence varies with the breed: it is comparatively common in the Scottish, Boston and Sealyham terriers and in the miniature varieties of corgi, poodle and dachshund, but is less common in the more natural breeds and in mongrels. In the cat the incidence is higher than in the normal breeds of dog but lower than in the special canine breeds mentioned.

Published incidence of bovine dystocia per 100 births varies from 2.1 and 2.3 in Denmark (Rasbech et al., 1967; Ellerby et al., 1969), through 10.8 in Holland (Grommers et al., 1965) to 12.2 in Sweden (Ekesbo, 1966). Most of the figures apply to dairy cattle and will vary with the breeds surveyed. An extreme figure would be obtained in districts of the Low Countries, where muscular hypertrophy of calves of the Belgian White and Blue and the Charolais breeds is favoured by farmers. Also, in some surveys, only cases requiring veterinary aid are included, while in others all calvings requiring assistance, lay or professional, are reckoned. Vandeplassche (1993) gave an incidence of 4% for Thoroughbred horses and about 10% for Belgian draught horses, while for pigs Jones (1966) gave a figure of 0.25% and Randall (1972) 2.9%. No figures are available for the other species.

Maternal dystocia occurs less frequently than fetal dystocia in the mare, cow and ewe, but in the sow and bitch it predominates.

In cattle, Tutt (1944) has recorded 85.5% of fetal dystocia and 14.5% maternal. Only about 5% of the more serious equine dystocias are of maternal origin (mainly uterine torsion) (Vendeplassche, 1972). Jackson (1972) found that two-thirds of 202 cases of porcine dystocia were due to maternal causes.

Dystocia is commoner in primipara than in multipara. As regards the effect of parity in cattle, Edwards (1979) recorded 66.5, 23.1 and 14.3% of assisted deliveries in the first, second and third calvings in a Friesian herd. In cattle the heavier male calves are more frequently associated with difficult births than are female calves. Twin births increase the incidence of dystocia, while in the multiparous species an abnormally low litter size predisposes to large fetuses and difficult births. Pregnancies that terminate early are conducive to dystocia through the medium of uterine inertia and fetal malposture, while one type of prolonged gestation increases difficult birth by leading to fetal oversize. Close confinement and overfeeding of the mother militate against normal birth, while gross underfeeding or too early breeding of primipara are deleterious factors causing retarded skeletal developments in the dam.

Accepting the importance of the foregoing basic aetiological factors, it is obvious to the veterinarian that the incidence of serious clinical dystocia depends largely on the degree and quality of the supervision that parturient animals are given. All forms of dystocia worsen with the passage of time.

TYPES OF DYSTOCIA WITHIN THE SPECIES

Cow

Both relative and absolute fetal oversize are common, especially in the Friesian breed. Disproportion due to emphysema of a dead fetus is frequently encountered but it is an outcome, rather than a primary cause, of dystocia. Local or general oedema of the fetus is a relatively rare cause of oversize and is seen particularly in the Ayrshire breed. The incidence of monsters is relatively high in the cow; they are generally of the distorted and celosomian types, *schistosoma reflexus* and *perosomus elumbis* being commonest. Achondroplastic calves, typified by the 'bulldog' calf of the Dexter–Kerry breed, are encountered.

Departures from longitudinal presentation are uncommon because the anatomical arrangement of the uterine cornua and the absence of a distinct uterine body do not favour transverse presentation. Postural irregularities of the head and limbs are common, particularly carpal flexion, lateral deviation of the head and 'breech presentation'. Simultaneous presentation of twins is a well-recognized cause of bovine dystocia, and one of the first duties of the obstetrician when proceeding to manipulative delivery is to ensure that the presenting limbs belong to the same fetus. Uterine inertia, often associated with hypocalcaemia, is well known, particularly in pluriparous Jersey cows; uterine torsion has its highest incidence in cattle, while instances of incomplete dilatation of the cervix are occasionally seen.

In 200 dystocia cases in dairy practice in Cheshire, Morton and Cox (1968) found the three most important causes of dystocia to be fetal

Table 8.1. Causes of dystocia in 635 beef cattle

Cause	Percentage of all dystocias
Fetal oversize	46
Fetal displacement	26
Cervical and vaginal incomplete dilatation	9
Uterine inertia	5
Uterine torsion	3

After Sloss and Johnston (1967).

malpresentation 44.5%, fetomaternal disproportion 21.8% and uterine inertia 18%. In a Hampshire general practice, Tutt (1944) recorded 97 cases of bovine dystocia, 85.5% of which were due to fetal causes and 14.5% to maternal factors. Of the maternal factors uterine torsion headed the list, followed by immature pelvis with smallness of the vagina and vulva, incomplete dilatation of the cervix and fibrous hymen. In the fetal group, postural abnormalities were by far the commonest; others were oversize of the fetus and monstrosities. In a review of 200 bovine dystocias in Kent, Williams (1968) found more difficult births in heifers than cows, due to the higher frequency in heifers of disproportion. Fetal maldisposition and uterine inertia were much commoner in cows. In 635 dystocias in beef cattle (cows and heifers) in the USA, Sloss and Johnston (1967) found the main causes of dystocia as set out in Table 8.1.

There are important breed differences in cattle dystocia: for example, in two Friesian and two Ayrshire herds Wright (1958) recorded incidences of 8.25 and 11.7% as against 2.7 and 3.0%. The most common forms of dystocia in these four herds were fetal oversize (55%), uterine inertia (17%) and postural abnormalities (16%). When heifers (or cows) of one breed are crossed with sires of other breeds the importance of the breed factor in bovine dystocia is well shown, as in Table 8.2.

Mare

According to Vandeplassche (1972) only about 5% of the more serious equine dystocias are of maternal origin, and they are mainly uterine torsions. Most cases result from irregularity of presentation, position and posture of the fetus, of which the commonest single cause is lateral deviation of the

Table 8.2. Difficult calvings and stillborn calves resulting from crossing Swedish red and white heifers with six breeds of sire

Breed of sire	Completed pregnancies	Calving difficulty (%)	Stillborn calves (%)
SRB Swedish	218	8.72	2.75
Friesian	267	13.11	3.00
Red Danish milk breed	131	12.21	3.82
Aberdeen Angus	218	4.13	1.83
Hereford	257	12.84	3.11
Charolais	164	17.30	4.70

After Lindhé (1966).

head. Fetomaternal disproportion and uterine inertia are rare, except in some draught breeds. Transverse presentation of the foal across the uterine body (either dorsotransverse or ventrotransverse) is well known, and another form of transverse disposition in which the extemities of the fetus occupy the uterine horns is notorious and peculiar to the equine species. In respect of the influence of presentation of the fetus on dystocia, Vandeplassche (1993) summarizes the presentations in 170 000 normal equine births in Belgium, compared with the presentations diagnosed in 601 dystocia cases brought to his clinic in Gent (Table 8.3). Whereas posterior and transverse presentations occurred in only 1.0% and 0.1%, respectively, of normal births, they were present in 16% and 16% of dystocia cases. An obliquely vertical or 'dog-sitting' position of the fetus is another well-known dystocia peculiar to horses.

Failure of the fetus to rotate into the dorsal position and its consequent engagement at the maternal pelvis in the ventral or lateral position is often encountered. It may be complicated by laceration of the dorsal wall of the vagina and even of the rectum and anus.

All forms of postural irregularity occur in the mare. The head and neck may be displaced laterally or downwards between the forelegs. Such displacements may be further complicated by rotation of the cervical joints. The limbs are frequently presented abnormally; one, several or all of the joints of the limbs may be flexed, and the irregularities are classified according to their clinical significance as carpal flexion, shoulder flexion, hock

Table 8.3 Influence of fetal presentation on dystocia in the mare (Vandeplassche, 1993)

Presentation	Normal foalings	Dystocia cases
Anterior	168 130 (98.9%)	408 (68%)
Posterior	1 700 (1.0%)	95 (16%)
Transverse	170 (0.1%)	98 (16%)

flexion and hip flexion. Bilateral hip flexion is known as breech presentation. An exceptional equine postural abnormality which occurs in anterior presentation is displacement of one or both extended forelimbs above the fetal neck (foot–nape posture).

Gross fetal monstrosities are rare, but occasional developmental anomalies which cause dystocia are wryneck (fixed lateral deviation) and hydrocephalus. Wryneck is likely to occur with transverse bicornual pregnancy.

Ewe

Wallace (1949) provided a useful basis for sheep dystocia considerations by observing all parturitions (275) in a flock (Table 8.4). He found 94.5% anterior presentations and 3.6% posterior, strikingly similar figures to those for bovine parturitions. Gunn (1968) collected data from 15 584 births in Scottish hill flocks and reported a dystocia incidence of 3.1% (3.5% with singles and 1.3% with twins) but McSporran et al. (1977) recorded 20–31% of difficult lambings in a particular flock of Romney sheep in which fetopelvic disproportion was prevalent.

It is uniformly believed that in the generality of sheep populations fetopelvic disproportion is the commonest type of dystocia, that its incidence varies with breeds and that it frequently occurs where there is crossing of disparate breeds for commercial lamb production. Also, assistance at lambing for this type of dystocia is more frequently required in primipara; male lambs, being larger, predispose to it. Where pelvic size of the ewe is the major factor in the disproportion there is likely to be repeated dystocia. McSporran et al. (1977) have demonstrated that its incidence can be markedly reduced (from 31 to 3.3% in a period of 4 years) — to the level in Gunn's survey for Scottish hill sheep — by culling ewes that had required assistance at consecutive parturitions and

Table 8.4 Classification of ovine births according to the type of presentation

Presentation	Number
Anterior, with head and both forefeet extended	191 (69.5%)
Anterior, with head and one foreleg normal, other leg retained	49 (17.8%)
Anterior, with head presented and both forelegs retained	18 (6.5%)
Anterior, with forefeet presented and head retained	2 (0.7%)
Breech presentation — both hind legs retained	7 (2.5%)
Posterior — lamb being right way up and both hind legs presented	2 (0.7%)
Posterior — lamb upside down, i.e. ventrosacral position	1 (0.4%)
Other miscellaneous types	5 (1.8%)
Total	275

Data from Wallace (1949).

by breeding to rams that had sired lambs of lower birth weight.

In certain breeds and flocks the incidence of dystocia due to maldisposition exceeds that due to fetopelvic disproportion, e.g. in Gunn's survey it was more than 60%. It is more common in pluripara than primipara and is more frequent with twins than with single births. Among maldisposition dystocias, shoulder flexion is commonest, followed by carpal flexion, breech presentation, lateral deviation of the head and transverse presentation. Ewes with unilateral shoulder flexion often lamb spontaneously.

Only the more difficult dystocias are referred for treatment to veterinary surgeons, and in veterinary lists of assisted lambings the incidence of particular types of dystocia varies with the prevalent breed and with flock management techniques in the practice area. In Ellis's (1958) series of 1200 cases of sheep dystocia attended in a North Wales practice over a 10 year period, lateral deviation of the head was the commonest type, whereas in Wallace's (1949) and Blackmore's (1960) reports it was cervical non-dilatation (32 and 15%, respectively). Next after these two types in the veterinary surveys came shoulder flexion, carpal flexion, simultaneous presentation of twins, breech presentation and fetal oversize. Other occasional causes of severe sheep dystocia are uterine torsion, monstrosities (including schistosoma reflexus), fetal duplication, fetal oedema and perosomus elumbis.

It appeared from Gunn's data and from other reports that twinning does not significantly increase sheep dystocia overall. The explanation for this is that whereas twins increase maldisposition dystocia they reduce the incidence of feto-

pelvic disproportion dystocia because of their smaller individual size.

There is no doubt from all published work that posterior presentation markedly predisposes to difficult births.

Sow

The types of dystocia encountered in the sow resemble more closely those of the bitch than those of the uniparous species, maternal forms being almost twice as common as fetal forms. In Jackson's (1972) series of 202 dystocias, 37% were caused by uterine inertia, 13% by obstruction of the birth canal and 9% by downward deviation of the uterus; whereas 14.5% were caused by breech presentation, 10% by simultaneous presentation, 3.5% by downward deviation of head and 4% by fetal oversize. The incidence of fetal dystocia increases when the litter is small, for in these the size of the individual tends to be large and obstruction may result. Irregularities of limb posture and even uncomplicated posterior presentation often cause dystocia when the litter is small whereas had the litter been large and its individuals small, these irregularities would not have interfered with normal expulsion. Monstrosities are not uncommon; they are generally of the double type but schistosomes, perosomes and hydrocephalic specimens also occur.

Among litters of sows attended for dystocia there is a collective stillbirth rate of about 20% as compared with 6% in sows which farrow unaided.

Bitch

The two principal causes of canine dystocia are primary uterine inertia and fetopelvic

Table 8.5 Details of parturition in the bitch

Animal Age Parity	Weight before and after parturition (kg)	Gestation length (days)	Sex and weight (g) of puppies									Remarks
			1st	2nd	3rd	4th	5th	6th	7th	8th	9th	
Toy dachshund 6½ years Multipara	B5.6 A4.9	60	F169	M141	M169	F169	M169	6th puppy fetal death at week 8				Normal parturition, 9 hours
Mongrel 2 years Primipara	B6.3 A4.5		M275	M261	M219							Dystocia, big fetus and breech
Pekingese 4 years Multipara	B6.4 A5.5	64	M141	F155								Normal parturition, 4½ hours
Terrier 1½ years Primipara	B6.3 A4.9		M148	M212	M191	F191						Metrectomy at day 60, fracture of pelvis
West Highland 1½ years Primipara	B7.7 A7.0	60	M219	F198								Dystocia, uterine inertia. Forceps delivery
Shetland collie 8 years Multipara	B9.5 A8.6		F247	F191	3rd puppy fetal death at week 6							Dystocia, butt presentation. In labour 3 days. Metrectomy
Mongrel/pom 4½ years Primipara	B9.5 A7.7	59	M254	F240	F212	F169						Normal parturition. Pelvic inlet narrow, old fracture
Sealyham 5 years Multipara	B13.1 A11.3		M254	M240	M226	F198	F183					Dystocia, cervical stricture. Metrectomy
Spaniel 1 year Primipara	B13.1 A10.1	66	aF226	M226	M254	F283	F254	F226	M198			Normal parturition, 4 hours
Spaniel 3 years Primipara	B15.0 A12.7	62	F254	F311	F268	M254	M254	F191	M191			Normal parturition, 6½ hours
Mongrel 9 months Primipara	B16.5 A13.1	63	M339	F297	F240	F268	F290	F155				Normal parturition, 4½ hours
Spaniel	B A12.2	58	F311	M283	M339	M311	M283	M283	F311	F283		Normal parturition, 8 hours

a Order of puppies not known.

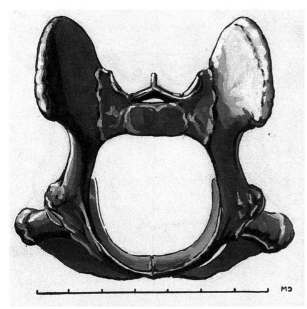

Fig. 8.2 The pelvic inlet of the bitch. The specimen was obtained from a 9 kg animal.

disproportion. The dachshund and Aberdeen terrier are particularly prone to primary uterine inertia. The corgi shows extreme variation in the size of its puppies and hence absolute and relative oversize may occur (Table 8.5). Brachycephalic breeds, together with the Sealyham and Scottish terrier, are prone to obstructive dystocia due to the fetuses having comparatively large heads and the dams having narrow pelves. Absolute fetal oversize is commonly encountered in bitches gravid with only one or two young; it may also result from a pathological fetus. A primigravid bitch of the small breeds often has trouble from relative fetal oversize with her first puppy but provided timely assistance is forthcoming she usually expels the remainder of her litter normally; if, however, assistance is delayed the onset of secondary inertia may make the outcome serious. Irregularities of limb posture are generally of little importance provided the puppy is of normal size. In fact many puppies are born with their fore- or hindlimbs flexed. When, however, the fetus is relatively large these postural deviations are often the factor that causes dystocia. Not infrequently a bitch or cat, in attempting to expel a fetus with its forelimbs retained, partially succeeds in that the head is born but the thorax with the limbs becomes obstructed in the maternal pelvic inlet. Similarly a puppy or kitten may have

its hindparts born while its distended thorax is obstructed.

Irregularities of head posture are common, and vertex ('butt') presentation and lateral deviation of the head are frequently encountered. An interesting feature of the latter abnormality is that it often involves the last puppy to be born.

Fetal hydrocephalus and anasarca are occasionally met, but other forms of monster are rare. In the achondroplastic types and in the kitten, gross umbilical hernia (schistocormus) is seen, but it is seldom a cause of dystocia.

Abnormalities of position are common in both anterior and posterior presentation and are themselves a cause of obstruction. Failure of the fetus to rotate prior to presentation results in its engaging in the pelvic inlet in the ventral or lateral position (Figure 8.2).

Traverse presentation is rare. When it occurs the bitch is generally gravid with a single fetus only and gestation is of the bicornual type. It is generally accompanied by uterine inertia.

Further information on the incidence and types of canine dystocia may be obtained from Wright (1939), Freak (1948, 1962), Kirk et al. (1968), Bennett (1974), Hall and Swenberg (1977) and Donovan (1980).

REFERENCES

Bennett, D. (1974) *J. Small Anim. Pract.*, **15**, 101.

Blackmore, D. K. (1960) *Vet. Rec.*, **72**, 631.

Chew, B. P., Erb, R., Fessler, J. F., Callahan, C. J. and Malvern, P. V. (1979) *J. Dairy Sci.*, **62**, 557.

Crenshaw, M. C., Meschia, G. and Barron, D. H. (1966) *Nature, Lond.*, **212**, 842.

Donovan, E. F. (1980) In: *Current Veterinary Therapy VIII. Small Animal Practice*, ed. R. W. Kirk, p. 1212. Philadelphia: W. B. Saunders.

Drew, B. (1986–1987) *Proc. BCVA*, 143.

Edwards, S. A. (1979) *J. Agr. Sci., Camb.*, **93**, 359.

Ellerby, J., Jochumsen, P. and Veirup, H. (1969) *Kgl. Vetoglandbohogst. Sterilitsfoskn. Aarsberetn.*, **77**.

Ellis, T. H. (1958) *Vet. Rec.*, **70**, 952.

Ekesbo, I. (1966) *Acta Agr. Scand. Suppl.*, 15.

Freak, M. J. (1948) *Vet. Rec.*, **60**, 295.

Freak, M. J. (1962) *Vet. Rec.*, **74**, 1323.

Greene, H. J. (1984) *Proc. 13th World Congr. Diseases of Cattle, London*, p. 859.

Grommers, F. J., Brands, F. A. and Shoenmakers, A. (1965) *Tijdschr. Diergeneesk.*, **90**, 231.

Gunn, R. G. (1968) *Anim. Prod.*, **10**, 213.

Hall, M. A. and Swenberg, L. N. (1977) In: *Current Veterinary*

Therapy VII. Small Animal Practice, ed. R. W. Kirk, p. 1216. Philadelphia: W. B. Saunders.

Hendricks, D. M., Rawlings, N. C., Ellicott, A. R., Dickey, J. F. and Hill, J. R. (1977) *J. Anim. Sci.*, **44**, 438.

Jackson, P. G. G. (1972) Personal communication.

Jöchle, W., Esparza, P., Gimenez, T. and Hidalgo, M. A. (1972) *J. Reprod. Fertil.*, **28**, 407.

Jones, J. E. T. (1966) *Brit. Vet. J.*, **122**, 420.

Kirk, R. W., McEntee, K. and Bentink-Smith, J. (1968) In: *Canine Medicine*, ed. E. J. Catcott, p. 470. Wheaton, Ill.: American Veterinary Publications.

Laster, D. B., Glimp, H. A., Cundiff, L. V. and Gregory, K. E. (1973) *J. Anim. Sci.*, **36**, 695.

Lindhé, B. (1966) *Wld Rev. Anim. Prod.*, **2**, 53.

McSporran, K. D., Buchanan, R. and Fielden, E. D. (1977) *N.Z. Vet. J.*, **25**, 247.

Morton, D. H. and Cox, J. E. (1968) Vet. Rec., **82**, 530.

O'Brien, T. and Stott, G. H. (1977) *J. Dairy Sci.*, **60**, 249.

Randall, G. C. B. (1972) *Vet. Rec.*, **90**, 178.

Rasbech, N. O., Jochumsen, P. and Christiansen, I. J. (1967) *Kgl. Vetoglandbohogst. Sterilitsfoskn. Aarsberetn.*, **265**.

Sloss, V. and Dufty, J. H. (1980) *Handbook of Bovine Obstetrics*. Baltimore: Williams and Wilkins.

Sloss, V. and Johnston, D. E. (1967) *Aust. Vet. J.*, **43**, 13.

Tutt, J. B. (1944) *Vet. J.*, **100**, 154, 182.

Underwood, E. J. and Shier, F. L. (1942) *J. Dep. Agric. West. Aust.*, **19**, 37.

Vandeplassche, M. (1972) Personal communication.

Vandeplassche, M. (1993) *Equine Reproduction*. Philadelphia: Lea and Febiger.

Wallace, L. R. (1949) *Proc. N.Z. Soc. Anim. Prod.*, 85.

Williams, K. R. (1968) *Vet. Rec.*, **83**, 87.

Woodward, R. R. and Clark, R. I. (1959) *J. Anim. Sci.*, **18**, 85.

Wright, J. G. (1939) *Vet. Rec.*, **51**, 1331.

Wright, J. G. (1958) *Vet. Rec.*, **70**, 347.

Each case of dystocia constitutes a clinical problem which may be solved if a correct procedure is followed. The veterinary surgeon arrives with a knowledge of the various types of abnormalities that may occur in that particular species and then, by a careful consideration of the facts elicited from the attendant and the information obtained from his or her own methodical examination of the patient, the nature of the abnormality with which he or she is confronted must be ascertained. A correct diagnosis is the basis of sound obstetric practice.

HISTORY OF THE CASE

Before proceeding to interfere with the animal, therefore, a comprehensive history of the case should, whenever possible be obtained. Much of it will be the outcome of questioning of the attendant, but many points also will be elicited from personal observation of the animal.

- Has full term arrived or is delivery premature?
- Is the animal a primigravida or multigravida?
- What is her previous breeding history?
- What has been the general management during pregnancy?
- When did straining begin; what was its nature — slight and intermittent or frequent and forceful?
- Has straining ceased?
- Has a water-bag appeared and, if so, when was it first seen?
- Has there been any escape of fluid?
- Have any parts of the fetus appeared at the vulva?
- Has an examination been made and has assistance been attempted; if so, what was its nature?
- In the case of the multiparous species, have any

young been born, naturally or otherwise, and, if so, when? Were they alive at birth?
- Is the animal still taking food?
- In the case of the bitch and cat, has there been vomiting?

By a consideration of the answers to these and similar questions it is possible to form a fairly accurate idea of the case to be dealt with. The inference to be drawn from many of them is obvious, but there are several points associated with them which merit discussion. The greatest attention will be paid to the duration of labour. If the animal, particularly a heifer, has been exhibiting slight and occasional efforts only and there has been no appearance of the water-bag, it is probable that the second stage of labour has not begun and that parturition will proceed normally. The onset, however, of vigorous and frequent straining, together with the appearance of the amniotic sac, indicates that the second stage of delivery has commenced; if several hours have elapsed since its onset, it is reasonably certain that obstructive dystocia exists. Nevertheless it is probable in all species except the mare that the fetus or fetuses are still living. In the primigravida, particularly the heifer and the bitch, it is often found that the cause of the dystocia is relatively simple, such as slight oversize of the fetus, and the application of a little assistance is all that is required. In the mare, the normal course of delivery is so rapid, and separation of the placenta occurs so quickly once the second stage has commenced, that any delay generally results in the death of the young one.

When, however, the call for assistance has been delayed 24 or more hours and it is noticed that straining efforts have ceased, it may be taken that the fetus is dead, much of the fluid has been lost, the uterus is exhausted and putrefaction of the fetus has begun. These facts in themselves, quite apart from the more detailed features of the case, indicate that the prognosis must be guarded. This is especially the case in the multiparous species, for it is probable that there are several fetuses in utero.

If the history is that efforts to deliver the animal have already been made, or when such evidence is absent but one suspects it to be the case, a search for injury of the genital canal will be the first feature of the detailed examination of the animal.

GENERAL EXAMINATION OF THE ANIMAL

The animal's physical and general condition should be noted. If recumbent, is she merely resting or is she exhausted? Body temperature and pulse rate should be noted and the significance of abnormalities considered. Particular attention should be paid to the vulva. Parts of a fetus may be protruding and it may be possible to assess the nature of the dystocia from these. Are exposed fetal parts moist or dry? Such evidence serves not only as a guide to the duration of the condition but also to the effort that will be necessary to correct it. Should parts of the amnion protrude, what is their condition? Are they moist and glistening and is fluid caught up in their folds? If so, their exposure is recent and the case is an early one. If, however, the membranes are dry and dark in colour, it may be taken that the case is protracted. Maybe nothing protrudes from the vulva. Particular attention should be paid to the nature of the discharge. Blood, especially if profuse, generally indicates recent injury to the birth canal. A dark brown fetid discharge indicates a grossly delayed case. In cases in which it is clear from the evidence already adduced that the fetus is dead and the uterus grossly infected, the desirability of inducing epidural anaesthesia before proceeding to a vaginal examination should be considered. In this way the risk of infecting the neural canal should spinal anaesthesia later be found to be necessary is reduced.

When dealing with the bitch and cat, the degree of abdominal distension should be observed, for it is thus possible to make an estimate of the number of fetuses which occupy the uterus. The onset of vomiting together with a great increase in thirst should be regarded as grave signs in the bitch.

DETAILED EXAMINATION OF THE ANIMAL

Large animals

The animal should be effectively restrained with someone at its head and its right side pressed firmly against a partition. In the case of the mare, a twitch should be applied and a forelimb raised until one is satisfied as to the animal's temperament and likely behaviour. Several clean buckets full of hot water with soap should be available, as well as a table, bench or truss of straw covered with a sterile cloth, on which the instruments may be placed. A plentiful supply of clean straw should be placed under and behind the animal; also, since the floor is often wet and slippery, a prior application of sand or grit is a worthwhile precaution.

With an assistant holding the tail to one side, the external genitalia and surrounding parts are thoroughly washed from one bucket. The operator, having washed and lathered his or her hands and arms from another bucket, proceeds to make a vaginal examination. The introduction of the hand through the vulval labiae almost invariably provokes defaecation in the cow and it becomes necessary to wash the vulva and the operator's arms again.

Without the previous induction of epidural anaesthesia and the resultant paralysis of the rectum, it is almost impossible to make a vaginal examination in the cow without introducing some faeces. This statement certainly holds true for animals which have been fed on grass and in which faeces are semi-fluid. Nevertheless, it may be taken that such material is not highly infective and no serious consequence will result from this contamination of the vaginal mucous membrane provided the latter is intact.

To proceed to a consideration of a recent case. If the vagina is found to be empty, attention should be directed to the cervix. Is it completely obliterated? If it is not and is still occupied by some sticky mucus, it may be concluded that the second stage of labour has not yet begun and the animal should be given more time. Maybe the case is one of uterine torsion. Does the vagina end abruptly at the pelvic brim and is the mucosa drawn into tight, spirally arranged folds? In the event of the vagina being occupied by amnion only, the nature of the fetal parts presented at the pelvic inlet must be ascertained. Can a fetal tail and anus be identified? If so it is highly probable that the case is one of breech presentation. Is it the flexed neck which is being palpated? Can the mane be detected? A search on one or other side may reveal the ears and occiput, the case being one of lateral deviation of the head. But what of the forelimbs? Can the flexed carpi be felt beneath the neck or is there complete retention of the forelimbs in addition to the head abnormality? In the mare, complete emptiness of the vagina apart from the membranes may be due to postural defects, as previously outlined, but more often indicates a dorsotransverse presentation. If it is impossible or almost impossible to reach any parts of the fetus in this species, the case is probably one of bicornual gestation.

But in the majority of cases some part of the fetus occupies the vagina — the head, a limb or limbs. Recognition of the head is not difficult: the mouth and tongue, the orbits and the ears are generally obvious. In the case of a limb, the first requirement is to ascertain whether it is a fore or hind. If the plantar aspect of the digit is downwards, it is highly probable that it is a forelimb; the converse is equally true. This statement applies with greater force to the cow than the mare, for in the latter, presentation of the fetus in the ventral position is relatively common. Proof is obtained by noting the direction of flexion of the limb joints. If the joint immediately above the fetlock flexes in the same direction as the latter, the limb is a fore one and the converse holds true. The beginner may experience some difficulty in recognizing the fetal parts he is palpating if they are covered by amnion. To overcome this, he should first pick up and open the torn edges of the amniotic sac and pass his hand into it so that his fingers come into direct contact with the fetus. If two limbs are present, it must be ensured that they belong to the same extremity and to the same fetus.

Not infrequently it is necessary to repel the fetus in the uterus to ascertain the nature and direction of displaced parts. If continued straining makes this difficult, the induction of epidural anaesthesia should be considered at once.

In the protracted case, assessment of the exact nature of the dystocia and methods of correction may be more difficult. Often, particularly in the case of the heifer, the vaginal mucous membrane has become grossly swollen and there is no room in which to carry out manipulations. Loss of fluid has resulted in the mucous membrane and the fetal parts becoming dry. Contraction of the uterus directly on the irregular contour of the fetus makes retropulsion difficult or even impossible, while in many cases the fetus has become impacted in the pelvis.

Bitch

Examination should if possible be carried out in a room where running water and a wash-basin are available. The bitch, unless an exceptionally large one, should be placed standing on a table. It is preferable that a person with whom the animal is familiar should hold its head. This person should be warned that the bitch may resent a vaginal examination.

As a general rule, the operator will proceed to make a digital examination per vaginam, especially in early cases in which it is likely that obstruction is the cause of the delay and also in protracted ones in which it is estimated that a single fetus only remains unborn. Nevertheless, cases will be met in which it is obvious that inertia has supervened and there are several fetuses to be delivered, in which case immediate caesarian section or hysterectomy is indicated.

Whether or not the hair is clipped from the area around the vulva before making a vaginal examination will depend on the length of the coat. In long-coated animals it is a great convenience to do so; although it is impossible to render the area sterile, it should be thoroughly washed with hot water and soap.

Sometimes on raising the tail it is seen that part of a fetus, a head or hind parts, is outside the vulva. Such a finding is more common in the cat than the bitch. The case is a simple one: traction on the exposed parts effect delivery without difficulty and, provided this assistance has been forthcoming early, it is probable that parturition will proceed normally. Occasionally it is found that the vagina is occupied by a fetal head or buttocks which have become impacted. In the majority, however, the pelvic canal is unoccupied and obstruction occurs at the inlet.

What is the presentation? If a head, can one detect the mouth? Or is it the occiput with the ears? If the latter, the case is one of vertex presentation. Maybe a single limb is felt, but there is no sign of the head: the case is probably one of lateral deviation of the head. Is the presentation posterior? Recognition of the tail is generally simple, although it may be directed forwards over the fetal back. Have the hindlimbs entered the pelvis or are they retained? Has the fetus rotated into the dorsal position or is the case one of ventral or lateral position? Is the uterine body unoccupied?

CONSIDERATION OF TREATMENT TO BE ADOPTED

General

The great majority of dystocia cases in the monotocous species are fetal in type and are the outcome of either faulty disposition or oversize. In the former, the first aim of treatment is to convert it to normal, and having done this hasten delivery by relatively gentle traction. Such correction must, if possible, be performed by manipulation, assisted perhaps by the use of simple instruments such as snares and repellers. In cases of oversize of the fetus a decision must be made promptly on whether to attempt delivery by traction or by caesarian section. Various studies in cattle have shown that one of the major factors which determines the outcome for the cow and calf in cases of caesarian section is the degree of traction to which the cow was subjected before the decision to operate was made. The rationale for the obstetrician should always be that if presented with live and viable young, at term, inside a viable dam, then the only measure of success is the delivery of live and viable young, without compromising the health or future fertility of the dam. However, the decision as to whether delivery should be accomplished by traction or caesarian section is one of the most difficult facing the obstetrician.

In the majority of cases of relative oversize, strong but controlled traction will be successful.

In cattle, in general, if the calf's head and legs, or, in cases of posterior presentation, if the calf's hips are within the maternal pelvis, before any external traction has been applied, then successful delivery by traction should be possible. If the calf is clearly too large, or if controlled traction does not result in any progress being made, then the decision to carry out a caesarian section should be made promptly.

In respect of bovine dystocia cases diagnosed as fetopelvic disproportion over which there is frequently an element of doubt as to whether traction will succeed or whether a caesarean operation should be decided on, Hindson (1978) has devised a formula in an attempt to resolve the problem. It involves taking two measurements: the interischial distance of the dam and the diameter of the calf's digit. The formula which is then applied to obtain the traction ratio (TR) is:

$$TR = \frac{\text{Interischial distance}}{\text{Calf digital diameter}} \times \frac{P_1}{P_2} \times \frac{1}{E}$$

where P_1 is the parity factor of 0.95 for heifers, P_2 is the correction factor of 1.05 for posterior presentation, and E is a factor of 1.05 for breeds with muscular hypertrophy.

TRs of 2.5 or more are likely to be resolved by traction; TRs of less than 2.5 require a caesarean operation.

Caesarean section is a common and usually successful operation in the mare, cow, ewe, sow, bitch and cat. In uniparous species, when it is impossible to correct a faulty fetal disposition or when the fetus is deformed or grossly emphysematous, fetotomy should be considered.

Uncontrolled forcible traction may lead to laceration and contusion of maternal soft tissues, pelvic nerve damage and occasionally sacral displacement. If the mother survives, a third-degree perineal laceration, deformity of the perineum, fistula of the vagina and rectum, or paralysis may ensue. The obstetrician should seek to avoid these complications at all costs.

Special

Mare

The first consideration is whether attempts at correction should be made with the animal standing or cast, restrained and narcotized? The decision will be influenced in part by the size and temperament of the mare, but more especially by the type of dystocia. Not infrequently the operator begins manipulative correction with the mare standing, but soon realizes that for success, recumbency with narcosis and possibly anterior epidural anaesthesia will be necessary. It is important in such cases that this decision shall be made early, so that the obstetrician shall not have become exhausted as the result of prolonged but futile efforts. If operation is to be performed with the mare in the standing position, the induction of posterior epidural anaesthesia should be considered, particularly if efforts at correction are negated by the vigorous straining of the mare. It is important, however, that the quantity of anaesthetic solution injected shall not be such as seriously to impair the action of the hind-limbs, for a partial motor paralysis may result in serious injury to the animal. Relatively simple abnormalities, such as carpal flexion or lateral or downwards deviation of the head, can often be corrected using the hand alone, particularly when the mare is comparatively small and straining has been eliminated. When, however, one of the more difficult forms is present, such as transverse presentation or impaction of the fetus in the pelvis, or when there is laceration of the vagina or vulva, it is generally best to cast and narcotize the animal at the outset. One of the advantages of recumbency is that by changing the position of the mare the weight of the fetus can be utilized to facilitate correction. Whenever fetotomy is required, both heavy sedation and epidural anaesthesia should be used. For the former, either detomidine or guaphenesin may be preferred. In veterinary hospitals, general anaesthesia is preferable.

In all severe cases the operator should consider the advisability of seeking the assistance of a colleague, for it is always possible that the combined efforts of two will succeed where those of one alone fail.

The value of *partial* fetotomy as a treatment of equine dystocia where the fetus is dead or deformed has been emphasized by Vandeplassche (1972, 1980), but *total* fetotomy was not recommended because it usually causes severe damage, particularly of the uterus. He pointed out that in the mare, fetotomy was difficult because of heavy straining, long birth canal and early dehiscence of the placenta. A long Thygesen fetotome was the best instrument. The indications for, and results of, partial fetotomy are shown in Table 9.1. Vandeplassche found that 25% of mares retained the afterbirth after fetotomy compared with 5% after normal birth and that the fertility after fetotomy was 42%. From his results he draws the wise conclusion that training in the basic rules of partial fetotomy in both cows and mares should form part of the veterinary curriculum. He goes on to show, however, that the caesarean operation has a definite place in equine obstetrics, particular indications being maternal dystocia due to bicornual gesta-

Table 9.1 Results of fetotomy in mares suffering from dystocia

Cause of dystocia	No. of mares	No. recovered	
Reflection of head and neck	72	67	(93%)
Hydrocephalus of two heads	6	6	(100%)
Breech presentation with ankylosis	17	14	(82%)
Partial transverse presentation	25	21	(84%)
Deformity, ankylosis or reflexion of forelegs	12	11	(92%)
Total	132	119	(90%)

tion, uterine torsion and narrow or deformed pelvis, as well as those cases of fetal dystocia where there is oversize or fetal malposition combined with maternal injury or with uterine involution and emphysema. His maternal recovery rates for fetotomy (132 cases) and caesarean operation (77 cases) were, respectively, 90 and 81%. Because of early dehiscence of the allantochorion in mare dystocia only 30% of foals survived the caesarean operation (as compared with 85% of calves after the bovine operation).

Cow

In the cow also, delivery by the natural route is the foremost consideration. The delay before professional aid is sought varies greatly, and this is a factor which influences the course to be adopted. In protracted cases there is often severe impaction of parts of the fetus in the pelvis; the greater part of the fetal fluids has often been lost and there is insufficient space to repel the fetus; the fetal skin and the vaginal mucosa have lost their natural lubrication, while the vagina and vulva are often swollen and manipulation is rendered difficult. Correction of the faulty disposition in such cases may prove very difficult and may prompt an early decision to undertake fetotomy or caesarean section. If, however, fetal disposition is normal and the case is one of relative oversize, controlled traction will be first attempted, but before this is done it is important that the vagina and those parts of the fetus occupying it shall be lubricated as well as possible. For this purpose, mucilage of linseed or acacia or one of the proprietary brands of cellulose-based obstetric lubricant may be used. Failing these the copious application of soap and water is indicated. Traction, however, must be employed with consideration and discretion, for if it is impossible to extract the fetus by this means its continued application makes for more severe impaction and this renders subsequent fetotomy very difficult or even impossible. In all cases such as these, epidural anaesthesia should be induced at the outset. Under the influence of the anaesthetic it is generally possible to repel the fetus sufficiently for the performance of intra-uterine fetotomy. When applying epidural anaesthesia subsequent to handling a putrid fetus, great care must be taken that infection is not introduced into the neural canal through the medium of either the needle or the anaesthetic solution.

More often, however, the case will be an early one; the calf is living and the uterus healthy. In the heifer it is often found that presentation is normal and that obstruction is due to slight oversize. In these it is a comparatively simple matter to apply snares to the extremities and, following the principles which are described in detail in later chapters, to effect delivery by traction. As a rule the animal remains standing during the application of snares but often goes down during the passage of the calf's head through the vulva. In the multigravid cow, while oversize is often encountered, it is more likely that the cause of obstruction is malpresentation. If it is found that the space required for correction is continually lost due to straining, epidural anaesthesia should be adopted without further waste of effort. It is preferable in all relatively simple cases to employ posterior rather than anterior epidural anaesthesia, for the animal is still able to stand under its influence and, speaking generally, reposition is easier in the standing than in the recumbent position. A further advantage of epidural anaesthesia is that an animal which has become recumbent often rises again after its induction.

If the calf is a monster, e.g. schistosoma reflexus presented viscerally, it is almost certain that fetotomy will be necessary before it can be delivered via the vagina. In many, especially schistosoma reflexus in which the head and limbs are directed towards the pelvic inlet, fetotomy may be extremely difficult, and a better means of removing the fetus is by laparohysterotomy.

In cases of relative fetal oversize of an otherwise normal calf presented normally, the inclination of the operator will be to resort to traction. In many cases this attitude is a proper one, for by this means delivery is often effected without the mother sustaining irreparable injury. However, the amount of traction must be limited to that of three persons, and the progress of the operation must be very closely scrutinized by the veterinary surgeon, who will pay due regard to lubrication and to the method and direction of traction. If no progress is made after 5 minutes, or if the fetus becomes lodged and fails to yield to 5 minutes of further traction, then a caesarian section should be performed.

Here again, the operator should always consider the advisability of seeking the aid of a colleague.

Ewe

In this species the facility with which malpresentations can be corrected will depend in large measure on the operator's ability to pass a hand through the pelvis into the uterus. In the majority of ewes this is possible, but occasionally, especially in primigravid animals of the smaller breeds, it is impossible, and delivery per vaginam may fail. The same difficulty arises in cases of 'ringwomb'. In this troublesome condition, unless patient digital and manual efforts to dilate the cervix soon succeed, caesarean section must be resorted to.

In cases of relative oversize in normal presentation, the application of cords after retropulsion of the head or hips from the pelvic inlet is not difficult, and gentle traction effects delivery. Similarly in malpresentation of the limbs or head, reposition after retropulsion is, as a rule, relatively easy. Retropulsion, replacement of lost fetal fluids and correction of a faulty disposition are made much easier by elevating the hindquarters of the ewe. This can be done by rolling her on to her back and getting an assistant to pull both hind legs upwards and forwards. In cases of lateral deviation of the head and breech presentation in which manipulative reposition fails, fetotomy using the guarded wire-saw is indicated. Owing to the smallness of the lamb, the operation is easier than in the calf.

In the ewe it is especially important to ensure that the presented parts belong to a single fetus. The young, in cases of twins and triplets, are small and retropulsion and reposition are seldom difficult.

In ewes in which it is impossible to pass the hand into the uterus, delivery by forceps traction may be possible. The manner of the application of the forceps is similar to that later to be described for the bitch. Forceps of the Hobday type, of appropriate size and fitted with a ratchet to maintain a secure hold when applied, are best for the purpose. Snare forceps of the Roberts's type are also useful in head presentations.

Great care must be taken during intravaginal manipulations that the mucous membrane at the pelvic inlet is not lacerated. It is an accident which may occur quite simply, particularly when a finger is being used to lever a head or limb upwards. Such lacerations are usually followed by acute infection and death but a fatal outcome may be prevented by the general use of prophylactic vaccination against anaerobic bacterial infections before the breeding season and by the obstetric administration of antibiotic drugs.

Sow

In the sow also, the ease with which obstructive dystocia can be relieved depends almost entirely on the operator's ability to pass a hand through the pelvic inlet. Provided this is possible it is usually a relatively easy matter to grip the head or hind parts and withdraw the fetus. The disposition of the limbs is seldom of much consequence. When such assistance has been forthcoming early, i.e. within an hour or two of the onset of second-stage labour, removal of a fetus is often followed by the normal expulsion of the remainder. But assistance in the sow is frequently delayed, and in these cases the obstetrician will be well advised to remove as many piglets from the uterine body and cornua as are within reach. The subsequent course will depend chiefly on the measure of delay and thus the degree of inertia which has supervened. It may be found in an hour or so that normal expulsion has recommenced or that on further examination more fetuses are accessible to manual extraction and by continued attention to the sow in this manner the whole litter can be removed. Quite often, however, complete inertia has developed and no further progress follows the removal of the accessible fetuses. In these, caesarean hysterotomy is the only means of saving the sow.

Cases will be encountered, however, in which, as the result either of natural smallness or of previous injury, the hand cannot be introduced into the uterus. In these, one's procedure will be influenced by the number of fetuses it is estimated are still unborn and also by the duration of the dystocia. If the case is recent and one or two fetuses only are thought to be present, delivery by forceps will probably be attempted. If, on the other hand, difficulty has occurred with one of the early fetuses and many more remain, or if inertia has supervened and the removal of the presented fetus will not significantly change the situation, immediate caesarean section is indicated. The place of pituitary extract in porcine dystocia has not been evaluated, but for the treatment of agalactia and uterine inertia Straub and Gotte (1959) have successfully used synthetic oxytocin in doses of 5–10 units intravenously and 15–20 units intramuscularly. In a series of 200 porcine dystocias, Jackson (1972) found that an injection of 1 ml of a solution containing 0.5 mg of ergometrine maleate and 5 units of oxytocin gave a better and more prolonged ecbolic effect than 10 units of pituitary extract. The same author observed that the greatest problem in porcine obstetrics was to know when a parturient sow had expelled all her piglets. Good, but not infallible, indications of the end of labour are that the sow rises, passes a large volume of urine and then resumes recumbency in an attitude of contentment. When it is suspected that parturition is incomplete, the clinician should pass a hand as far as possible into the uterus and sweep it gently about the abdomen in the hope of ballotting indirectly a piglet in an adjacent segment of the long uterine horn. Aids to the location of a retained fetus are the detection of the fetal pulse by auscultation or by ultrasonography (see Chapter 3). The possibility of the retention of a portion of placenta is an even greater clinical problem. Where the clinical manifestations suggest that a portion of conceptus is still retained and there has been no response to the administration of ecbolics, an exploratory laparotomy is indicated.

Bitch

The primary consideration in the management of a case of dystocia in the bitch is — shall one proceed with delivery per vaginam or shall one immediately resort to laparotomy? Factors which will influence the decision are:

1. The cause of dystocia, whether obstruction or primary inertia.
2. The duration of second-stage labour and

hence the condition of the fetuses and the uterine muscle.

3. The number of fetuses involved.

When the case is recent, a matter of a few hours only, one will proceed to assist the bitch per vaginam. If the cause is relative oversize in anterior or posterior presentation it is probable that traction, using the finger and vectis or forceps, will succeed in effecting delivery and parturition will then proceed normally. Similarly in cases of malpresentation such as vertex posture or breech, traction may succeed after correction of the posture. If, however, there is gross oversize of the fetus, and this should be suspected in litters of one or two only, early laparotomy is indicated.

In protracted cases of 24 hours or more, laparotomy is the primary consideration, for it is probable that secondary inertia has supervened and removal of the obstructed fetus will not alter the ultimate outcome.

The question arises of whether one should first attempt to remove the presented fetus per vaginam. It is probable that this fetus is grossly infected, and interference with it through an abdominal wound will favour the development of peritonitis. There is also, of course, the possibility that forceps interference will subject the bitch to even graver risk. The author's attitude is that when the presented puppy is impacted in the pelvis, it is best to attempt its removal with forceps prior to commencing abdominal operation, but in all others he removes the presented fetus by laparotomy.

A further question which arises in laparotomy cases, and this has special reference to the anaesthetic to be employed, is how long after the onset of second-stage labour it is likely that the puppies are alive. The author's experience has been that it is very improbable that the presented fetus will live longer than 6–8 hours, for by that time its placenta will have completely separated. The remaining fetuses, however, may be alive for much longer periods; in fact, he has seen cases in which after 36 hours delay the presented fetus was dead and emphysematous yet those occupying the anterior parts of the cornua were alive. He has never encountered living fetuses after a delay of 48 hours.

In all cases in which inertia has supervened, whether it be primary or secondary in nature, and three or more fetuses remain, laparotomy is indicated.

The respective indications for the two operations, hysterotomy and hysterectomy, will be discussed in a later chapter.

REFERENCES

Hindson, J. C. (1978) *Vet. Rec.*, **102**, 327.
Jackson, P. G. G. (1972) Personal communication.
Straub, O. C. and Gotte, J. O. (1959) *J. Amer. Vet. Med. Assn*, **135**, 171.
Vandeplassche, M. (1972) *Equine Vet. J.*, **4**, 105.
Vandeplassche, M. (1980) *Equine Vet. J.*, **12**, 45.

Dystocias which arise in the mother are due either to constriction of the birth canal or to a deficiency of expulsive force; they are set out in Figure 8.1, p. 186. The constrictive forms, of which the most important are pelvic inadequacies, incomplete dilatation of the cervix and uterine torsion, will be considered first.

CONSTRICTION OF THE BIRTH CANAL

Pelvic constriction
Developmental abnormalities of the pelvis are generally rare in animals, but in the achondroplastic types of dog the pelvic inlet is flattened in the sacropubic dimension, and this, together with the large head of the fetus in these types, is a common cause of dystocia. An inadequate pelvis is a very frequent cause of dystocia in bovine primipara (heifers) and is due to immaturity or retarded development: it is discussed in Chapter 13.

Incomplete dilatation of the cervix
Failure of the cervix to dilate completely is a relatively common cause of dystocia in dairy cattle. It may occur in both the heifer and the multiparous cow. In the latter, the condition has generally been ascribed to fibrosis of the cervix resulting from injury at previous parturitions, but the author is doubtful if this explanation is correct. He thinks it more likely to be the outcome of hormonal dysfunction, for generally the course of labour in such cases is atypical. Pains are weak and transient only. Often it is difficult to ascertain accurately how long labour has been in existence for, other than discomfort, little may have been noticed. On examination the cervix is found to comprise a frill about 5 cm broad, separating the vagina from the uterus, and it is clear that delivery by traction must inevitably cause severe tearing.

Often the amniotic sac has passed through the cervix and may be present at the vulva; it may have ruptured with escape of amniotic fluid. Sometimes fetal limbs have passed into the anterior vagina.

In order not to be precipitate in any actions, the obstetrician may decide to wait several hours before interfering in the hope that the case is simply one of delay and that normal dilatation will later occur. (He or she is aware of the relative frequency with which discomfort, particularly in heifers, is a feature of the first stage of labour during which the cervix is dilating normally.) In the condition under review, however, there will be no further dilatation. The author has on occasion waited for a further 12 hours, by which time the calf had died, without any change in the cervix.

In some cases of abortion also the cervix fails to dilate properly and the fetus is retained, subsequently to undergo putrefactive maceration in the uterus. Incomplete dilatation of the cervix is frequently an accompaniment of uterine torsion.

Ringwomb
Incomplete dilatation of the cervix of the ewe is descriptively named ringwomb. It accounts for 15–32% of the ovine dystocia cases referred to veterinary surgeons. The condition is suspected when, after protracted restleness, the ewe does not progress to the second stage of labour. Manual exploration of the birth canal reveals that the cervix is in the form of a tight, unyielding ring which will admit only one or two fingers. Usually the intact allantochorion can be felt beyond the cervix but occasionally this membrane has ruptured and a portion of it may have passed into the vagina; the latter observation distinguishes the condition from a protracted first stage, with which it may easily be confused and thus wrongly diagnosed. If there is a fetid vaginal discharge and necrotic fetal membrane in the vagina, in the

presence of a non-dilated cervix, there is no doubt that the condition is abnormal. When there is doubt over the diagnosis the ewe should be left for 2 hours and then re-examined to ascertain if any further cervical dilatation has occurred, as in normal first-stage labour. Caufield (1960), who reported operating on about 50 cases annually from 1952, found that only about 20% of cases of cervical failure recognized by him opened naturally, but even these required some assistance to lamb. Without treatment, ewes with ringwomb develop toxaemia and die within 48 hours, but if caesarean section is performed within a few hours of diagnosis up to 95% recover. Other veterinary surgeons have found that patient effort to dilate the cervix by digital manipulation is rewarding, and Blackmore (1960) was successful by this means in the treatment of 28 of 32 cases of ringwomb. The method of vaginal hysterotomy, whereby the cervix is retracted with vulsellum forceps and then incised by shallow cuts 'at the points of the compass', has its advocates, but in using it the extreme susceptibility of the ewe to anaerobic infection should be borne in mind and effective antibiotic prophylaxis provided.

Many cases of ringwomb follow preparturient prolapse of the vagina and both conditions occur in similar circumstances of breed and environment. Hindson (1961) has drawn attention to an apparent connection between the incidence of 'ringwomb' at parturition and the prevailing weather conditions during pregnancy. Thus during the seasons 1956–1957 and 1957–1958, when there was abundant grass, he saw in his Devonshire practice 158 and 123 cases of ringwomb, respectively, whereas during the very dry season of 1959–1960 only 62 cases were seen. In the latter season there was a high incidence of single lambs (probably due to a lack of flushing) and the ewes had to range widely to get sufficient keep.

Hindson et al. (1967) were able to produce ringwomb experimentally by the injection of 20 mg of stilboestrol into pregnant ewes as early as 85–105 days of gestation. During this type of dystocia the myometrial contractions were normal, and the authors therefore concluded that natural ringwomb was a cervical rather than a myometrial disorder. Hindson and Turner (1972) suggested that ringwomb might be caused by excessive ingestion of oestrogenic substances by pregnant sheep, as for example by grazing on red clover pasture or by feeding on herbage or grain contaminated with a fungus like *Fusarium graminaerum*. Further elucidation of the probable endocrine aetiology of ringwomb has been provided by Liggins et al. (1977), who found that administration of $PGF_{2\alpha}$ into the substance of the cervix caused local softening and dilatation, and by Mitchell and Flint (1978), who demonstrated that when synthesis of prostaglandin was experimentally reduced cervical ripening did not occur.

Incomplete dilatation of the posterior vagina and vulva

This is a relatively common finding in dairy heifers. It seems to be associated with heifers which are in over-fat body condition, or in herds where the animals have been moved just before calving or where the process of calving has been interrupted by too frequent observations or interventions.

Treatment requires the patient application of gentle traction. If continuous progress is made then delivery can be affected. If the vulva will not dilate properly then episiotomy should be carried out (see Chapter 13). If there is any doubt about the likelihood of success with continuing attempts at vaginal delivery, a caesarean section should be performed.

Vaginal cystocele

This is the name given to a condition occasionally encountered in the parturient mare and cow in which the urinary bladder lies in the vagina or vulva. It is of two types:

1. Eversion of the bladder through the urethra. This is more likely to occur in the mare consequent on the great dilatability of the urethra and the force of straining efforts in this species: the everted organ will occupy the vulva and will be visible between the labiae.
2. Prolapse of the bladder through a rupture of the vaginal floor. In this condition the bladder will lie in the vagina and it will further differ from the previous one in that the serous coat of the organ will be outermost.

In both conditions, the first aim of treatment is to overcome straining; this is best effected by the induction of epidural anaesthesia with or without narcosis. This must be followed by retropulsion of those parts of the fetus which already occupy the vagina. In the case of the first, it is then necessary to invert the organ again by manipulation, and in the second, to replace it in the pelvis and close the vaginal rupture by suture. The fetus should be delivered by traction after the correction of any postural abnormality.

Neoplasms

Neoplasms of the vulva and vagina may occur in all species and thus serve as potential causes of dystocia, although in fact it is seldom that they do so. In the cow, the writer has encountered papillomata, sarcomata and submucous fibromata of the vulva, while in the bitch the vaginal submucous myxofibroma is common.

Neoplasms of the cervix are so rare in animals as to be of no consequence in a consideration of the causes of dystocia.

Pelvic obstruction by the distended urinary bladder

Jackson (1972) has described a type of porcine dystocia in which the birth canal was obstructed by the distended urinary bladder being forced back by straining in the form of a mound under the vaginal floor where it acted like a ball-valve in the birth canal. It was associated with a very relaxed birth canal. Catheterization of the bladder relieved the condition.

Other abnormalities

Remnants of the müllerian ducts often persist in the anterior vagina of cattle. They generally have the form of one or more 'bands' passing from the roof to the floor just behind the cervix and are usually broken during parturition. Sometimes they are laterally situated and the fetus passes to one side of them. Occasionally, however, a remnant is of such size and strength that it forms an effective barrier to the birth of the young one. The forelimbs may pass on either side of it. It is important that the obstetrician shall recognize what he or she is dealing with and not confuse the condition with a partially dilated cervix. To examine the vagina satisfactorily, it is often an advantage to induce posterior epidural anaesthesia and repel the fetus into the uterus. The obstruction can be cut without risk, using a hook-knife or a guarded fetotomy knife of the Colin's or Roberts's type.

Cases of bifid and double cervix are occasionally seen on random post-mortem examination of bovine genitalia and there is generally plentiful evidence that the animal involved has had one or more calves. The condition is unlikely to be a cause of dystocia.

A cord-like dorsoventral band behind the cervix is an occasional cause of dystocia in bulldogs (Smith, 1965).

Torsion of the uterus

Rotation of the uterus on its long axis with twisting of the anterior vagina is a common cause of bovine dystocia. In veterinary practices in Britain it has accounted for 6% (Tutt, 1944) and 5% (Morton and Cox, 1968) of dystocia, while in the New York State Ambulatory Clinic, Roberts (1972) reported an incidence of 7.3% among 1555 dystocias attended over a 10 year period. In veterinary hospitals to which the more severe types of dystocia are referred, irreducible uterine torsion is the indication for the caesarean operation in from 13.8 to 26.5% of cases (see Pearson, 1971).

Aetiology

Uterine torsion is a complication of late first-stage or early second-stage labour. It is probably due to instability of the bovine uterus which results from the greater curvature of the organ being dorsal and from the uterus being disposed anteriorly to its subilial suspension by the broad ligaments. However, there must be some contributory factor additional to instability that operates during first-stage labour; otherwise torsion would be more frequently seen during advanced pregnancy than at parturition, but this is not so. The precipitating parturient factor is probably inordinate fetal movement which is a component of the postural adjustments that occur during first-stage labour in response to the contractions of the myometrium. Excessive fetal weight is also a predisposing factor; Wright (1958) recorded an average calf weight of 48.5 kg in torsion cases, and Pearson (1971) a comparable figure of 49.8 kg. The presence of bicornually disposed bovine twins would appear to stabilize the parturient uterus and this view is supported by the great rarity of torsion in twin pregnancy. However, in ewes the anatomical attachment of the mesometrium is sublumbar rather than subilial as in cattle and bicornual gestation is very common. Yet uterine torsion occurs, and of 10 cases recorded by Pearson (1971) five were in bicornual twin pregnancies. Neither breed nor parity appears to affect the incidence of the condition. Regarding the aetiology of bovine torsion, Vandeplassche (1982) observes that uterine instability can be accepted as a cause of torsions of up to 180° but it cannot account for torsions of 360° or more.

Clinical features

The consensus of veterinary opinion is that torsion in an anticlockwise direction preponderates to an extent of about 75%. Although the uterus rotates about its longitudinal axis the actual twist in the majority of cases involves the anterior vagina; in the minority of cases in which the twist affects the posterior part of the uterus there is minimal distortion of the vaginal walls. Wright (1958) considered the most common degree of torsion to be of the order of 90–180°. However, in a series of 133 cases which were possibly more severe because they were referred by practising veterinary surgeons to a veterinary clinic, Pearson (1971) found that in only 37 was the amount of rotation 180° or less while in the majority (88) the angle of torsion was 360°. Williams (1943) maintained that many dystocias diagnosed as due to lateral and ventral positions of the fetus were actually uterine torsions of low magnitude. The severity of the twist does not directly affect the survival of the fetus, fetal death being caused by loss of fetal fluids or separation of the placenta.

The most constant feature of uterine torsion is its association with parturition. It is generally and correctly believed to occur during the first stage of labour because immediately after it has been corrected the cervix is found to be dilated to a variable degree. However, if after correction the cervix is found to be fully dilated or if before correction the membranes are ruptured and portions of them or the fetus are protruding through the cervix, the inference should be that the torsion occurred during early second-stage labour. Roberts (1972) believes that torsions of less than 180° cause little interference with gestation and that they often arise during advanced pregnancy and may persist for weeks or months, being recognized only when they cause dystocia at term. He further contends that torsions of 45–90° are often detected at pregnancy diagnosis and that they probably undergo spontaneous correction.

Symptoms

Up to the onset of parturition the animal has been normal, and when it enters the first stage of labour the usual signs of restlessness due to subacute abdominal pain associated with myometrial contractions and cervical dilatation are shown. In the typical case the only real symptom is that the period of restlessness is abnormally protracted or that it wanes and does not progress into second-stage labour. If the torsion does not occur until early second-stage labour then a short period of straining will have succeeded the restlessness but will have ceased abruptly. In the severe cases of torsion there may be increasing restlessness, but more probably all parturient behaviour will cease and, unless the animal has been closely observed, there may be no knowledge that parturition has begun. Pearson (1971) has noted slight depression of the lumbosacral spine as a frequent symptom.

If the condition is unrelieved, the placenta will separate and the fetus will die. There will develop persistent low-grade abdominal pain, progressive anorexia and constipation. Because the fetal membranes often remain intact, secondary bacterial infection of the fetus will develop later than with other forms of dystocia.

Diagnosis

Diagnosis is readily made by palpating the stenosed anterior vagina whose walls are usually disposed in oblique spirals which indicate the direction of the uterine rotation. The cervix may not be immediately palpable but by carefully following the folds into the narrowing vagina, the lubricated fingers can usually be pressed gently forwards and through the partially dilated cervix. Where the site of the twist is precervical, the vagina is much less involved, and diagnosis is assisted by palpating the uterus per rectum. In torsions of less than 180° portions of the fetus may enter the vagina and the dystocia may be wrongly ascribed to faulty fetal position (lateral or ventral).

Treatment

There are records of spontaneous recoveries but it is generally believed that unrelieved uterine torsion would progress to fetal death, putrefaction and fatal maternal toxaemia. Fetal maceration with maternal survival is possible. With the adoption of prompt treatment prognosis is favourable for mother and fetus. Delay leads to fetal death and makes treatment more difficult but there is still a high rate of maternal recovery. At the New York State Ambulatory Clinic between 1963 and 1968, Roberts (1972) recorded a 4.3% maternal mortality. In Pearson's series of 168 more severe cases treated in a veterinary hospital only 67 calves were born alive, but it is certain that a better rate of survival would be obtained in the less severe cases treated more promptly on farms. The possible forms of treatment are as follows.

Rotation of the Fetus per Vaginam. The aim of this method is to reach the fetus by insinuation of the hand through the constriction of the anterior vagina and partially dilated cervix and then to apply a rotational force to the uterus through the medium of the fetus. Its likelihood of success depends mainly on two factors: whether the cervix is sufficiently dilated to admit the hand and whether the fetus is alive. Pearson was successful in 64 of 104 cases attempted by this method, 39 live fetuses being obtained from the 64 reducible, and 31 dead fetuses from the cases which were irreducible and subsequently treated surgically. Care must be taken not to rupture the fetal membranes for this markedly reduces the fetal viability. When the fetus is reached, purchase is obtained on its shoulder or elbow region in order to rotate it in the opposite direction to the twist, but the first manoeuvres are designed to generate a gently swinging motion in the fetus before attempting to reduce the torsion. The most difficult part of the procedure is rotation through the first 180°: after this, replacement is spontaneous. It is helpful to have the rear of the cow at a higher level than the front, and epidural anaesthesia should be beneficial. When the head of the live calf is readily accessible, pressing on its eyeballs will cause a convulsive reaction which can be translated into a rotation by applying a sufficient torque. Auld (1947) recommended abdominal ballottement to assist swinging the calf prior to reduction per vaginam. The rotation of the fetus by means of Cämmerer's torsion fork to engage canvas cuffs placed on the extended limbs can be recommended, provided the fetus is sufficiently accessible. Great care must be taken to avoid rupture of the uterus with the instrument or by causing a rotating and flexed fetal limb to pierce the organ.

Torsion of the uterus anterior to the cervix cannot be treated by vaginal manipulation, nor can the rare cases of twists of 720° or more.

Rotation of the Cow's Body: correction by 'rolling'. This was the most popular method of correction, but because it requires the assistance of at least three people it is being replaced by the previous method. The aim is to rotate quickly the cow's body in the direction of the torsion while the uterus remains relatively steady. The mechanics of the method may be questioned but it is often successful. The cow is cast by Reuff's method on the side to which the torsion is directed. One assistant holds down the head while first the two front feet and then the two hindfeet are tied together with separate 2.5–3 m lengths of rope, each of which is held taut, preferably by two assistants on each rope. At a given signal a sudden smart coordinated pull is made on the leg ropes so that the cow is rapidly turned over from one side to the other. A vaginal examination is then made to ascertain whether correction has occurred, in which case there is ready manual access to the cervix and probably to the fetus in the uterus. If there is no relief the cow is slowly restored to her original position or the legs can be flexed under her body and she can be turned 180° over her legs on to the original side. The same procedure of rapid turning is repeated, and to check that the rolling is in the correct direction the operator should try to retain a hand in the vagina during the manoeuvre. If there is no success on this occasion and the spiral folds are felt to tighten, one infers that the rolling is in the wrong direction, and sharp rotation in the contrary manner is carried out. Otherwise, repetition of the original procedure is applied until correction is achieved. If a calf's extremity can be grasped and partially flexed whilst the cow is rolled, this will help to fix the uterus and allow correction of the torsion to occur.

A modification of the foregoing traditional technique described by Schäfer (1946) is recommended by the author and has been favourably received by Roberts (1972). It entails the application of a wide plank of wood, 3–4 m long and 20–30 cm wide, to the flank of the cast cow, the one end resting on the ground. An assistant stands on the plank while the cow is slowly turned over by pulling on the leg ropes. The advantages of this technique are that the plank fixes the uterus while the cow's body is turned and that, because the cow is turned slowly, less assistance is required and it is easier for the veterinary surgeon to check the correct direction of the rolling by vaginal palpation; moreover, the first rolling is usually successful.

Surgical Correction. If the case cannot be corrected by either of the previous methods a laparotomy should be performed on the standing cow through the left or right sublumbar fossa and an attempt made to rotate the uterus by intra-abdominal manipulation. Because a caesarean hysterotomy may also be required before the torsion can be corrected — or after the torsion is corrected when the cervix will not dilate — a left flank approach is preferable, although it should be remembered that in cases of uterine torsion there are often loops of small intestine displaced on the left side of the abdomen. Under paravertebral or field infiltration anaesthesia a 15–20 cm incision is made in the left sublumbar fossa. A hand is inserted, the omentum pushed forwards and the direction of twist confirmed. For a twist to the left, the hand is passed down between the uterus and the left flank and a fetal hand-hold sought whereby an attempt is made first to 'rock' the uterus and then to rotate it by strongly lifting and pushing to the right. For a twist to the right, the hand is passed over and down between the uterus and the right flank and as before a swinging man-oeuvre is followed by pulling upwards and to the left. Owing to oedema of its walls the uterus is unusually friable and there is copious peritoneal transudate.

In some cases it is impossible to rotate the uterus by abdominal taxis, and a caesarean opera-tion must then be carried out before the torsion can be corrected. In other cases, despite abdominal relief of the twist, the cervix will not dilate and a caesarean operation must be performed to deliver the cow. Where the fetus has to be removed before the uterus can be turned it may be found that the uterine wound is relatively inaccessible for suturing.

Whatever method is used to correct uterine torsion a decision has to be made on the subse-quent management of the case. Because some placental separation and a degree of uterine iner-tia will have developed in many cases, and because there is a tendency in other cases for the cervix to close quickly after the uterus is replaced and not to dilate again (Pearson, 1971), it is wise to deliver the cow at once, per vaginam if possible or, if failing that, by caesarean operation. Where the cervix is found to be open after correction of the torsion

and provided there is no inordinate fetopelvic disproportion, delivery of the cow by judicious traction on the calf will present no problem. If the cervix is only partially dilated, rather than resort to immediate caesarean operation, Pearson has recommended vaginal hysterotomy if the following clinical features are present:

1. The birth canal caudal to the cervix is dilated sufficiently to allow delivery.
2. The remaining cervical rim is thin and stretches like a sleeve on the fetus when traction is applied. Section is contraindicated if the cervix is thick and indurated.
3. The fetus does not feel excessively large.

The technique of cervical section is simple and painless: the fetus is pulled backwards so as to engage the cervix fully and the stretched cervical rim is incised deeply at one point. This incision gives immediate relief and allows delivery to proceed.

The caesarean operation is indicated if the torsion is irreducible or if the cervix is insuffi-ciently dilated or fails to dilate further after reduc-tion. In the 168 cases of uterine torsion referred to the Bristol Veterinary School Clinic, Pearson (1971) reported that caesarean section was carried out on 137 animals, with a maternal recovery rate of 95%. It was noted that the placenta was either already detached at the time of operation or was passed soon afterwards and that uterine involution was rapid. Other surgical features related to laparo-hysterotomy for uterine torsion are discussed in Chapter 20.

Species affected

Mare. Torsion of the uterus is a rare condition in riding horses in Britain; Day (1972) recalled seeing only three cases over some 30 years in a practice where approximately 1000 mares foaled annually. It is less rare among draught horses in Europe; Skjerven (1965) discussed 15 cases of surgical correction of uterine torsion and Vande-plassche et al. (1972) reported on 42 cases (four of which were included in Skjerven's previous review). The latter authors found that more than half their cases occurred before the end of gestation but that 5–10% of all serious dystocias in Belgian horses were due to torsion; twisting in an anti-clockwise direction was more common and in the majority the extent of rotation was 360° or more.

The possibility of uterine torsion should be considered in cases of colic during late pregnancy. Diagnosis is readily established by rectal palpation of the uterine ligaments. The circulatory disturbance in the uterus is greater than with the same condition in cattle, with consequent risk to the survival of the fetus and the development of shock and dehydration of the dam.

After trying other methods of treatment for the antepartum case, including rolling the mare, Vandeplassche and his colleagues recommend laparotomy and rotation of the uterus by direct taxis, the mare being tranquillized in stocks and operated on under epidural and field infiltration anaesthesia. A high flank incision is made on the side of the torsion and a hand passed into the abdominal cavity and under the uterus. By carefully grasping the uterus, or the fetus through the uterine wall, and using the minimum of rotational force, the uterus is easily restored to its normal position. In cases where the foal is alive and the uterus not too congested there is a good chance of progression to a normal parturition, especially if isoxsuprine is given for 24 hours after the operation (Vandeplassche, 1980). Skjerven prefers to correct the torsion on the recumbent mare under general anaesthesia. He incises the flank opposite to the direction of twist: a hand is introduced and a suitable part of the fetus recognized in the proximal aspect of the uterus. To this fetal component sufficient pressure is applied in a ventral direction to restore the normal position of the uterus. By pressing ventrally from the proximal side rather than by pulling dorsally from the distal side, there is less risk of rupturing the uterus. In the antepartum case where the foal is dead or the uterus severely congested, hysterotomy should be performed (Figure 10.1).

When dystocia is due to uterine torsion an attempt should be made to pass the hand through the cervix and to rotate the uterus by manipulating the fetus. If this method fails, a caesarean operation must be performed.

In Vandeplassche's series of 42 cases, 60% of the mares and 30% of the foals survived. Skjerven's review indicated a favourable prospect for fertility in mares which recovered after torsion.

Ewe. Before 1963 there were very few recorded cases of uterine torsion in ewes. Since then the question of its incidence has been raised in veterinary correspondence, and the small num-

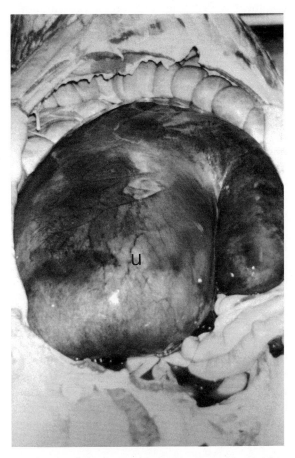

Fig. 10.1 Uterine torsion in a mare, as exposed by mid-line laparotomy. Note the congested uterus (u). Correction by rotating the uterus was impossible, and a dead foal was removed after hysterotomy; thereafter, correction of the torsion was possible.

ber of instances which were subsequently described (Farman, 1965; Moar, 1965; Tallantire, 1965) indicated that its frequency is very low. The condition closely resembles bovine torsion; most cases respond to 'rolling' or to raising and simultaneously rotating the body by means of a twisting grip on the hindlegs. Failing these measures, the caesarean operation must be performed, particularly where the lamb is dead in utero.

Sow. Torsion is rare in sows; there was no case in 200 porcine dystocias attended by Jackson (1972).

Bitch. Uterine torsion is very rare. In describing a successful ovarohysterectomy in a 13-year-old nulliparous bitch for the treatment of a 270° torsion of the left horn around which the right horn was twisted through 1080°, Shutt et al. (1978)

commented that only two other cases in non-pregnant bitches had been recorded and that they had met this one case among 83 000 canine admissions to the Missouri University Small Animal Clinic.

In pregnant bitches a few instances have been discovered on post-mortem examinations of fatal dystocia cases where there were torsions of up to 2160°, while the rare finding of encapsulated fetal bones in a bitch's abdomen may be a legacy of uterine torsion and rupture.

If a uterine torsion arises during whelping and can be promptly diagnosed, a caesarean operation should be successful.

Cat. Torsion of 90–180°, involving either one horn or the uterine body, in near full-term pregnancies (Young and Hiscock, 1963; Farman, 1965) and a cornual torsion of 360° in a 4-month pregnancy (Boswood, 1963) have been described in association with sudden illness in cats. Diagnosis of these conditions can be made only by laparotomy, and the best treatment is a prompt hysterectomy. Occasional instances of extrauterine abdominal fetuses have been recorded (Bark et al., 1980). These probably result from uterine rupture during pregnancy, possibly associated with uterine torsion rather than from ectopic pregnancy.

Displacement of the gravid uterus

Ventral hernia in the mare, cow and ewe

Occasionally in these subjects hernia of the gravid uterus occurs through a rupture of the abdominal floor (Figure 10.2). The accident is one of advanced pregnancy, occurring at the ninth month or later in the mare, from the seventh month onwards in the cow and during the last month in the ewe. It is probable that in the majority of cases a severe blow on the abdominal wall is the exciting cause, although many observers have stated that it may occur without traumatic influence, the abdominal musculature becoming in some way so weakened that it is unable to support the gravid uterus. The site of the original rupture is the ventral aspect of the abdomen, a little to one side of the midline (left in the case of the mare and right in the cow and ewe) behind the umbilicus. It generally commences as a local swelling about the size of a football but rapidly enlarges until it forms an enormous ventral swelling extending from the pelvic brim to the xiphister-

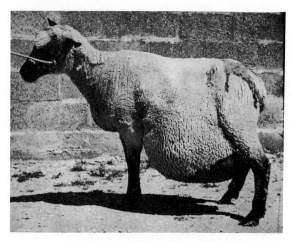

Fig. 10.2 Ventral hernia in the ewe.

num. It is most prominent posteriorly, where it may sink to the level of the hocks. By this time practically the whole of the uterus and its contents have passed out of the abdomen to occupy a subcutaneous focus. In cattle the bulk of the swelling is often situated between the hindlegs, the udder being deflected to one side. Generally, the condition is complicated by gross oedema of the abdominal wall due to pressure on the veins; in fact this oedema may be so great that it is impossible to palpate either the edges of the rupture or the fetus.

As a rule, gestation is uninterrupted but the condition becomes grave for both mother and fetus when parturition commences, particularly in the case of the mare, although there are records of affected cows calving normally. In the mare, if the foal is to be saved, it is essential that aid shall be forthcoming the moment the expulsive forces of labour commence. The writer has encountered a case in which delivery of the foal by traction presented no difficulty despite the downwards deviation of the uterus, but he visualizes cases in which displacement of the uterus places the fetus beyond reach. In these it is advised that the mare be cast, narcotized and turned on to her back and the hernia reduced by pressure. Attempts at delivery should be made with the animal in this position. After parturition and involution of the uterus, the hernia will become occupied by intestine. It is improbable, however, that strangulation will occur and the mare may be able to suckle the foal. At the end of this period she should be destroyed.

Cows and ewes may give birth spontaneously despite severe ventral hernia, but affected animals should be closely watched during labour in case artificial aid is needed.

Downward deviation of the porcine uterus

Downward deviation of the uterus has been described by Jackson (1972) as the cause of 19 of 200 cases of porcine dystocia. Affected animals strained vigorously despite an empty vagina, and at a point about 15–22 cm in front of the pelvic brim the uterus deviated sharply in a downwards and backwards direction. It was very difficult to extract the obstructed piglet manually, and insertion of the arm up to the shoulder was necessary so that the obstetrician's elbow could be flexed within the sow's abdomen. Affected sows were deep-bodied and pregnant with large litters.

Retroflexion of the mare's uterus

During the previous 10 years at the Ghent Veterinary Clinic, Vandeplassche (1980) reported that he and his colleagues saw 18 cases of severe colic in mares near term in which the foal occupied the maternal pelvis. Per rectum, it could be pushed forward into the abdomen, although this manipulation provoked renewed colic, and the fetus soon regained the intrapelvic position. It was found that the injection at intervals of the muscle relaxant isoxsuprine lactate, in doses of 200 mg, relieved the colic and allowed the foal to move forwards in front of the pelvis. Normal parturition followed in due course.

Inguinal hernia in the bitch

Acquired inguinal hernia is common in the bitch and not infrequently the incarcerated uterus becomes the focus of pregnancy. (The author has also seen the condition in the cat, but it is rare in this species). The hernia is generally unilateral and it may contain one or both uterine cornua.

Often the history is that an inguinal swelling the size of an egg has been recognized for months, but that during the last few weeks it has rapidly become larger. In other cases, the recent development of a progressive swelling is the story. There may or may not be a history of recent oestrus and mating.

The lesion is obvious; it is unlikely that it will be confused with a mammary neoplasm or a local abscess if careful examination is made. The condition is painless and there is no systemic disturbance. Although it is tense and irreducible there is little tendency to strangulation provided intestine is not involved in addition. The latter complication is rare. In those cases in which pregnancy is advanced it will probably be possible to detect fetuses on palpation.

The course of the condition depends primarily on the degree of tension in the sac and this will be influenced by its size and the number of fetuses involved. A case has been seen in which the two fetuses involved developed to full term and then underwent partial resorption. Another has been met in which both cornua were involved and each contained two fetal units of about 30 days' development. Death of the embryos with partial resorption of the placentae had occurred. The majority of cases will be presented when pregnancy has advanced about 30 days and each fetal unit is about the size of a golf ball, for by this time the size of the swelling is becoming alarming to the owner (Figure 10.3).

The writer has not seen a case which has been associated with parturition nor one in which fetuses were present in a herniated cornu and an abdominally situated one, but they are cases which must be considered.

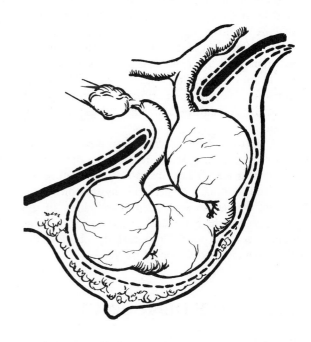

Fig. 10.3 Inguinal cystocele in a bitch gravid with three embryos of about 30 days.

Surgical Interference. The following alternatives present themselves:

1. Reduce the hernia, obliterate the sac and allow pregnancy to take its normal course. In the great majority of cases it will not be possible to reduce the hernia by simple means.

2. Enlarge the hernial ring by incision of the abdominal wall and later close by suture after reduction of the hernia. Obliterate sac; allow pregnancy to continue. From the strictly ethical viewpoint this is the operation to select. Pregnancy is uninterrupted and the animal's full breeding powers are conserved. It presents, however, several technical difficulties: precise incision of the abdominal wall forwards from the inguinal orifice is not easy owing to the presence of the large and tensely filled sac. Moreover, effective closure of the neck of the sac may be difficult after incision of the parietal peritoneum. At the same time cases will be encountered in which, after assessment of all the individual factors, this operation is selected.

3. Dissect out the hernial sac; incise its apex and expose the herniated uterus. Amputate the cornu or cornua involved. Obliterate the hernial sac. If it happens that the animal is also pregnant in an abdominally situated horn this should not be interfered with. If, however, an abdominally situated horn is empty and it is desired that the bitch shall be sterilized, it is an easy matter after location of the bifurcation to draw this horn into the hernia and remove it. As a rule it is not possible to draw the ovaries through the inguinal ring. This is the operation most often performed. It presents no particular difficulties and cure of the hernia is certain.

4. In those cases in which fetal development is at or approaching term, it may be decided to proceed as for (3) but, instead of amputating the involved cornua, to perform hysterotomy and extract the fetuses with their membranes. In the one case in which the author has performed this operation it was possible to return the uterus to the abdomen after extraction of the fetus.

EXPULSIVE DEFICIENCY

The expulsive force of labour comprises the contractions of the uterine and abdominal muscles. Because the abdominal muscles do not come into play until the uterine muscle has lifted the conceptus into the pelvic inlet it is logical to consider first the expulsive deficiencies that may arise in the myometrium; these may occur spontaneously or dependently and are called respectively primary and secondary uterine inertia.

Primary uterine inertia

Primary uterine inertia implies an original deficiency in the contractile potential of the myometrium. It is less common than secondary uterine inertia and is seen most often in the bitch and sow (in which Jackson (1972) found it to account for 37% of dystocia), occasionally in the cow, but rarely in the other species. It varies considerably in degree from cases in which second-stage labour does not begin to others in which parturition is complete, save for the retention of one allantochorion of a polytocous birth. An understanding of the origin of primary uterine inertia is possible from a consideration of the endocrinology and physiology of normal birth, although in veterinary practice the true cause is often obscure. Reference to Figure 8.1 (see p. 186) shows its possible causes. There may be a basic — possibly inherited — 'weakness' in the uterine muscle; this is surmised when there is no other obvious cause and it might be termed 'idiopathic primary uterine' inertia. Examples are seen in the Scottish terrier breed and in Ayrshire cattle; occasionally also within a particular cattle breed a large proportion of the progeny of a certain bull are affected. An individual animal may suffer repeated episodes of inertia at consecutive parturitions. More tangible causes of uterine inertia are:

1. Overstretching of the myometrium by an excessively large fetus, hydrallantois, or an unusually large number of fetuses.
2. Toxic degeneration in bacterial infections.
3. Fatty infiltration of the myometrium.
4. Senility, though this is rare.

The chemical environment of the uterus may be abnormal in respect of the ratio between progesterone and oestrogen concentrations or in respect of a lack of either oxytocin or calcium, as in parturient hypocalcaemia. Such biochemical aberrations may be inherited. In Friesian heifers it has been shown by Drew (1986) that magnesium supplementation before calving will reduce the number of calving difficulties. This is probably because adequate magnesium levels are necessary for the occurrence of normal uterine contractions.

There is no doubt that late abortion or premature birth, irrespective of its aetiology, is an important cause of primary uterine inertia as is also twin parturition in cattle.

An innate 'nervous disposition', as well as environmental disturbances, are considered to interfere with the hypothalamic regulation of oxytocin secretion and release by the pituitary with resultant circulatory deficiency of that hormone. An excessively small litter may fail to supply an adequate fetal pituitary–adrenal endocrine contribution to the termination of pregnancy.

When the uterus is ruptured or when the genital tract becomes twisted on its long axis, myometrial activity ceases. Spontaneous uterine rupture may arise during gestation as a consequence of uterine torsion or it may occur during second-stage labour as a complication of breech presentation (see p. 277).

The *diagnosis* of primary uterine inertia is made from the history and by an examination of the birth canal and presenting fetus. The dam is at or near term, as denoted by mammary changes and ligamentous relaxation in the pelvis, while the psychological manifestations, coupled with restlessness due to abdominal discomfort, will have indicated the first stage has passed. There may have been a few feeble abdominal contractions but no progress has been made; or in the multiparous species, after an adequate beginning of second-stage labour, all further activity has ceased. Examination of the birth canal in the larger animals reveals a patent cervix beyond which can be felt a fetus within its membranes.

It is essential that treatment shall be forthcoming at the appropriate time in order to safeguard the life of the young one as well as that of the mother. It should be instituted as soon as one is satisfied that the second stage is present and that it is not proceeding normally.

In the large, uniparous species, treatment is generally simple. By vaginal manipulation the membranes are ruptured, the posture of the presented extremity corrected if necessary and the fetus delivered by gentle traction. In the bitch, however, the problem is greater, its extent depending on the number of young present in the uterus.

If one only, its delivery by vectis or forceps per vaginam is indicated, although it is probable that if the latter instrument is employed the fetus will be grossly injured. When multiple fetuses are present, however, caesarean hysterotomy should be performed.

Provided that the cervix is dilated, that obstructive dystocia is not present and that the uterus is not abnormally distended, posterior pituitary extract may be injected intra-muscularly in doses of 5–15 IU. The best response to pituitrin is obtained early in second-stage labour, but when, as is often the case, it is used to bring down the last puppy of a litter the result is frequently disappointing. Disadvantages of pituitrin mentioned by Freak (1962) are that it may cause contraction of the cervix, and thus interfere with the expulsion of a puppy or fetal membranes, and that by promoting placental separation of unborn fetuses their survival may be jeopardized; Thus if natural delivery does not ensue within 20 minutes of the injection and live puppies are still to be obtained, the need for assisted delivery has been made much more urgent. Conversely an advantage of pituitrin when given at the close of a caesarean operation for uterine inertia is that by promoting prompt uterine involution it minimizes haemorrhage from the placental zones of the endometrium. Where posterior pituitary has failed to bring down the last fetus, ergometrine maleate may be given orally in doses of 0.25–0.5 mg for the 9–14 kg bitch; it is also useful for causing expulsion of retained afterbirth and for postpartum haemorrhage.

Slow initiation of labour in the bitch may be due to subclinical hypocalcaemia, in which cases Barrett (1949) and Freak (1962) have noted an immediate response to intravenous injection of calcium borogluconate. To prevent possible eclampsia the dose should be repeated subcutaneously after the completion of whelping.

Bulldogs sometimes show dystocia which is apparently due to slack abdominal muscles combined with uterine inertia which gives rise to insufficient force to lift the fetuses into the pelvic cavity (Smith, 1965).

Uterine inertia is the commonest form of porcine dystocia, and Jackson (1972) found it in 37% of 200 cases treated in veterinary practice in England. It is treated as far as possible by consecutive manual extraction of the fetuses, aided by the administration of ecbolics (ergometrine or

Table 10.1. Classification of 272 canine dystocias

Obstructive dystocias, fetal	
Relative oversize of one or more fetuses	77
Absolute oversize	15
Fetal monstrosity or gross abnormality	2
Malpresentation other than posterior	12
Posterior presentation of first fetus	35
Obstructive dystocias, maternal	
Abnormality of maternal soft structures	4
Abnormality of maternal pelvis (addidental)	1
Slackness of abdominal wall	3
Inertias	
Primary inertia	41
Secondary inertia	44
Nervous voluntary inhibition of labour	17
Slow initiation of labour (query hormonal in origin)	1
Slow initiation of labour (due to subclinical eclampsia)	7
Abortion near to term of dead fetuses	2
Death of some fetuses prior to parturition	10
Coincidental illness	1

After Freak (1962).

oxytocin) and, when these measures fail, by caesarean operation.

Nervous voluntary inhibition of labour

In 17 of 272 canine dystocia cases (Table 10.1) recorded by Freak (1962), labour did not begin or, having begun, did not proceed. The factor common to all of the affected bitches was the provision of a special parturition environment. When the bitches were returned to their accustomed quarters they proceeded to whelp. Occasionally, bitches appear to be frightened by labour pains and voluntarily inhibit straining; tranquillizing drugs are helpful in such cases.

Hysteria

In the study of 200 porcine dystocias previously referred to, there were six cases in which the sows were so excitable and aggressive that they were apparently unable to continue normal parturition. The use of the sedative azaperone was followed by a resumption of normal farrowing.

Primary inertia in the bitch pregnant with an abnormally small number of fetuses

It is convenient to refer to this condition here as it is generally regarded as an example of primary uterine inertia. It is probable, however, that the condition results from hormone dysfunction rather than from primary uterine causes.

It is encountered in bitches gravid with one, possibly two and at the most three fetuses. Term arrives and passes without signs of labour. Mammary hypertrophy is absent or slight only and there is no tumefaction of the labiae. The owner has often concluded, in the absence of abdominal distension, that the bitch has failed to conceive. Just how long the fetus or fetuses remain alive is not definitely known, but it is improbable it is beyond day 70, by which time complete separation of the decidua has occurred. From this point the fluids, membranes and soft fetal tissues undergo resorption.

In the majority of the cases the cervix relaxes between days 70 and 80, and a dark green, viscid discharge escapes from the vulva. There is still no evidence of straining. It is improbable that vaginal examination will reveal the fetus for it still occupies its original position in the cornu but it is generally possible to detect it by abdominal manipulation.

In one case recorded by the author, parts of the single fetus occupied both cornua, the head, thorax and forelimbs being in one and the placenta, abdomen and hindlegs in the other. In another, the condition occurred in an inguinal hysterocele.

The writer has met the condition in the chow, retriever, bull terrier and spaniel breeds.

The following exceptional case record illustrates the condition:

Subject: A field spaniel in good health.
   1. At 3 years old, conceived a single fetus which was delivered normally at term.
   2. At 7 years old, again conceived a single fetus, but term arrived and passed without signs of parturition. At 74 days the cervix was still closed and a fully developed but partially resorbed fetus was removed by hysterotomy.
   3. At 8 years old, again pregnant with a single fetus. Again term passed and at day 110, the cervix still being closed, hysterectomy was performed.
   (Fetal membranes and fluids entirely gone and replaced by dark brown, glutinous mucus. Fetus shrunken, eyeballs sunken and shrunken. The abdominal cavity was empty. Pelvis occupied by the terminal rectum and urinary

bladder. Diaphragm complete; heart a small fibrous sac. Unexpanded lungs almost normal.

Factors which will influence the treatment of such cases are the duration of gestation and hence the state of the fetus(es); whether the cervix has opened and if so the degree of infection which may have supervened; and the accessibility of the fetus for forceps traction. Clearly hysterotomy is indicated in the majority, but if infection has supervened, hysterectomy is preferable. In the small proportion of cases in which the cervix is open and the fetus occupies the uterine body, delivery per vaginam will be selected. Such cases are of interest in relation to the factors responsible for the initiation of normal parturition and are comparable to the entity known as *prolonged gestation* of cattle. In the latter there is a complete absence of the parturient mechanism at term and in some of the affected calves an aplasia of the fetal pituitary has been found.

Secondary inertia

This is the inertia of exhaustion and is essentially a result of, rather than a cause of, dystocia. Nevertheless, in multiparous species, prolonged unsuccessful efforts to deliver one fetus may result in dystocia from inertia in regard to the remainder. Secondary inertia is frequently followed by retention of the fetal membranes and retarded involution of the uterus, factors which predispose to puerperal metritis.

Secondary inertia is met with in all species and, speaking generally, is a preventable condition. Its prevention depends on the early recognition that labour has ceased to be normal and the application of the appropriate assistance.

In some breeds of dog, of which the Scottish terrier is the outstanding example, inertia may supervene early and before the expenditure of effort it is reasonable to expect from a healthy bitch. The general history of such a case is as follows.

The bitch is heavily gravid; the gestational period is normal. One or two fetuses have been expelled without exceptional difficulty. From this point all signs of labour cease and the bitch is content to lie suckling the young already born yet it is obvious that the greater part of the litter has still to be expelled. No further progress is made and if appropriate treatment is not forthcoming the fetuses will die, infection of the uterus and toxaemia develop and the bitch succumb.

Sometimes the case conforms with the description given for primary inertia — a short, feeble effort is the sole indication of labour. A similar picture is frequently seen in the toy dachshund.

Treatment

In the uniparous species, correction of the dystocia which provoked the inertia is the essential feature of treatment. In the multiparous species, management of the case will depend on the duration of labour, the number of fetuses still unborn and their condition and the degree of uterine infection. In an early case, delivery of the fetus causing the primary dystocia may be followed after a few hours by a return of uterine contractions and parturition may proceed without further hindrance. Such is often the case in the sow and occasionally in the bitch and cat. When the case is of longer duration and there are still several young to be born it is best to proceed with the delivery of the remainder. In the sow it is often possible to do this with the hand inserted into the uterus per vaginam. In the bitch it may be decided to attempt forceps delivery. But the protracted use of forceps when three or four fetuses remain unborn has very little to commend it. The fetuses occupy the cornua beyond the safe reach of the forceps and 'blind fishing' is likely to result in uterine rupture. Better results attend laparotomy. If the case is not of more than 12 hours' duration since the onset of second-stage labour, hysterotomy is the operation of choice, for not only is the interference of less magnitude than hysterectomy but the animal's breeding function is preserved and the prognosis is good. If, however, the case is of longer duration and the fetuses are dead and putrefaction has commenced, hysterectomy should be resorted to, for in these instances the more simple hysterotomy is attended by a higher risk of postoperative peritonitis. The prognosis after hysterectomy will depend chiefly on the animal's state of health at the time of operation, but if performed up to 24 hours after the onset of labour hysterectomy will be attended by a high recovery rate.

Bostedt and Rudolf (1983) reported a controlled field trial, involving 1066 animals, of a then new method of accelerating porcine parturition and thus reducing the losses that arise from a prolonged expulsive stage. The β blocker, carazolol, was given at the beginning of labour. The duration of parturition was shortened with the result that 3.4% more piglets were reared; moreover, the incidence of the metritis–mastitis–agalactia syndrome was reduced from 20.5 to 9.9%.

REFERENCES

Auld, W. C. (1947) *Vet. Rec.*, **59**, 287.

Bark, H., Sekeles, B. and Marcus, R. (1980) *Feline Practice*, **10**(3), 44.

Barrett, E. P. (1949) *Vet. Rec.*, **61**, 783.

Blackmore, D. K. (1960) *Vet. Rec.*, **72**, 631.

Bostedt, H. and Rudolf, P. (1983) *Proc. XIIth World Vet. Congr., Perth*, p. 180.

Boswood, B. (1963) *Vet. Rec.*, **75**, 1044.

Caufield, W. (1960) *Vet. Rec.*, **72**, 673.

Day, F. T. (1972) *Equine Vet. J.*, **4**, 131.

Drew, B. (1986–1987) *Proc. Brit. Cattle Vet. Assn*, p. 143.

Farman, R. S. (1965) *Vet. Rec.*, **77**, 610.

Freak, M. J. (1962) *Vet. Rec.*, **74**, 1323.

Hindson, J. C. (1961) *Vet. Rec.*, **73**, 85.

Hindson, J. C. and Turner, C. B. (1972) *Vet. Rec.*, **90**, 100.

Hindson, J. C., Schofield, B. M. and Turner, C. B. (1967) *Res. Vet. Sci.*, **8**, 353.

Jackson, P. G. G. (1972) *Personal communication.*

Liggins, G. C., Fairclough, R. J., Grieves, S. A., Foster, C. S. and Knox, R. S. (1977) *The Fetus and Birth. Ciba Foundation Symp. 47*, ed. J. Knight and M. O'Connor, p. 5. Amsterdam: Elsevier.

Mitchell, M. D. and Flint, A. P. F. (1978) *J. Endocrinol.*, **76**, 108.

Moar, J. A. E. (1965) *Vet. Rec.*, **77**, 660.

Morton, D. H. and Cox, J. E. (1968) *Vet Rec.*, **82**, 530.

Pearson, H. (1971) *Vet. Rec.*, **89**, 597.

Roberts, S. J. (1972) *Veterinary Obstetrics and Genital Diseases.* Woodstock, VT.: Roberts.

Schäfer, W. (1946) *Schweizer Arch. Tierheilk.*, **88**, 44.

Shutt, R. M., Johnson, S. D., Johnson, G. R., Caywood, D. and Stevens, J. B. (1978) *J. Amer. Vet. Med. Assn*, **172**, 601.

Skjerven, O. (1965) *Nord. Vet. Med.*, **17**, 377.

Smith, K. W. (1965) *Canine Surgery.* Wheaton, ILL.: American Veterinary Publications.

Tallantire, I. W. (1965) *Vet. Rec.*, **77**, 551.

Tutt, J. B. (1944) *Vet. J.*, **100**, 154, 182.

Vandeplassche, M. (1980) *Equine Vet. J.*, **12**, 45.

Vandeplassche, M. (1982) Personal communication.

Vandeplassche, M., Spincemaille, J., Bouters, R. and Bonte, P. (1972) *Equine Vet. J.*, **4**, 105.

Williams, W. L. (1943) *Veterinary Obstetrics.* New York: Williams and Wilkins.

Wright, J. G. (1958) *Vet. Rec.*, **70**, 347.

Young, R. O. and Hiscock, R. H. (1963) *Vet. Rec.*, **75**, 872.

The two broad divisions of fetal dystocia are fetal oversize and faulty fetal disposition (see Figure 8.1, p. 186. For convenience, inadequacies in the maternal pelvis will be considered with fetal oversize under the joint heading of fetomaternal disproportion: this is quite a practical concept, for in respect of obstetric treatment the delivery of a mother with an inordinately small pelvis and a normally sized calf (relative fetal oversize) is no different from the delivery of a normal cow with an excessively large calf (absolute fetal oversize).

FETOMATERNAL DISPROPORTION

Withers (1953), in a British survey, reported that dystocia was almost three times as common in heifers as in cows. In 6309 pregnancies in cows, difficulty in calving occurred in 1.38%, and in 2814 in heifers difficulty occurred in 3.8%. In a study of 345 bovine dystocias in the USA, 95% of which were in beef cattle, Adams and Bishop (1963) found that 85% of all the dystocias were in heifers, and they were classified as follows: excessive calf size 66%, small maternal pelvis 15% and combination of the two 19%. This preponderance of heifer dystocia is due largely to fetomaternal disproportion. The younger the heifer, the higher is the dystocia rate (Lindhé, 1966). As would be expected, the stillbirth rate is much higher in heifer (6.7%) than in cow parturitions (2.4%).

It has been known for many years that the incidence of fetomaternal disproportion was much higher in the Friesian than in the other dairy breeds and that the Jersey was the least affected. The Friesian is now much the most numerous dairy breed (it accounts for 95% of dairy cattle inseminations in Britain) and the present widespread use of artificial insemination (70%

of cattle in Britain) has enabled artificial insemination officers to collect useful data on the incidence of dystocia for pure-bred and for cross-bred Friesian matings. In America, Boyd and Hafs (1965) recorded an overall dystocia level of 4.7% when 10 Holstein bulls were used on Holstein cows, whereas in matings by four Aberdeen Angus bulls the dystocia rate among Holstein cows was 1.5%. The importation of Charolais bulls into Britain (in 1963) and other countries, and later importations of Simmenthal and Limousin bulls, for crossing with cows of the local breeds has caused many difficult births, and this led to important surveys of cattle dystocia. In Britain, Edwards (1966) showed that the incidence of dystocia in cows bred to Charolais bulls was 14.3%, compared to 1.9% for cows mated to Hereford bulls and 3.5% in matings by bulls of other breeds. There were marked differences in dystocia levels in matings by particular Charolais bulls.

In the USA, Laster et al. (1973) surveyed dystocia rates and subsequent fertility following the mating of 1889 Hereford and Angus cows to bulls of the Angus, Charolais, Hereford, Jersey, Limousin, Simmenthal and South Devon breeds. Calves sired by the Simmenthal, South Devon, Charolais and Limousin bulls caused significantly more dystocia, 32.66, 32.34, 30.9 and 30.78%, respectively, than calves sired by Hereford, Angus and Jersey bulls, 15.78, 9.9 and 6.46%, respectively. Of the other factors influencing dystocia rate, calf birth weight had the greatest effect; each kilogram increase of birth weight increased the rate of dystocia by 2.3%. Hereford cows had more calving difficulty (34.78%) than Angus cows (27.02%). Male calves were heavier at birth (35.12 kg) than females (32.1 kg) and caused more dystocia (28.4% compared with 16.98%). This sex of calf effect was most marked in 2-year-old dams.

In dystocia due to disproportion the important

variables are fetal diameter and the capacity of the maternal pelvis. No single fetal body measurement is as useful a criterion of fetal size as fetal body weight but Wiltbank (1961) found that the maternal pelvic size, i.e. the area of the pelvic inlet (height × width), was a much better parameter for the prediction of dystocia than any fetal measurement. There are variations between the breeds in respect of the ratio of the calf weight at birth to maternal weight as follows: Friesian 1:12.1, Ayrshire 1:12.6 and Jersey 1:14.6. When a Friesian bull was used on Friesian, Ayrshire and Jersey cows the ratios of calf weight to maternal weight were: Friesian 1:12.1, Ayrshire 1:11.3 and Jersey 1:11.1. Although the Friesian–Jersey calves were larger in proportion to their dams than pure-bred Friesian calves, the incidence of dystocia with the pure-bred Friesian calves was about three times the incidence for the Friesian–Jersey calves. These data indicate that the Jersey cow has a more favourable pelvic capacity than the Friesian.

In summary, the literature review reveals that the rate of dystocia is much higher in heifers than cows and that this higher incidence is due mainly to fetopelvic disproportion; also that fetopelvic disproportion is highest in Friesians and in Friesian crosses and that when Charolais bulls are used for crossing on other dairy breeds they cause even higher rates of dystocia than Friesian bulls. Unfortunately, there is an increasing tendency for conformation of beef breeds to change over the years. The modern-day Aberdeen Angus or Hereford is much larger than its counterpart of 15–20 years ago. Furthermore, there is great variation in dystocia rates between individual bulls of the same

breed, and this difference is often greater than that which exists between breeds. The consequence of this is that a farmer may well get less dystocia by using a known 'easy-calving' Charolais bull than would be the case with certain Aberdeen Angus bulls.

Daughters sired by particular bulls may themselves have higher rates of dystocia. Furthermore, published data confirm that the Jersey breed can accommodate a greater degree of fetal weight to maternal weight than other breeds. In seeking to reduce dystocia due to fetopelvic disproportion, therefore, one should study the factors that affect fetal weight and those that affect pelvic capacity.

Factors affecting birth weight

The massive literature on the factors which affect birth weight of calves and lambs has been excellently reviewed by Young (1970).

Heredity, as expressed in different breeds, has the most marked effect, as shown in Table 11.1, which also shows the effects on birth weight of sex of calf and parity of dam. With the increasing use of cross-bred steers out of dairy cows for beef production, there is a growing interest in the effect of parental size on calf birth weight. In general it has been found that when the parents are of disparate size, e.g. Friesian bull and Jersey cow, the birth weight of the cross-bred Friesian–Jersey calf is near the mean of the body weight for the pure-bred Friesian and pure-bred Jersey calves. When the reciprocal crosses are made, however, it can be seen that the dam exerts an influence towards its own birth weight. Hilder and Fohrman (1949) demonstrated this influence on calf birth weight

Table 11.1. Average birth weights of various breeds of cattle

	Average birth weight (kg)				
	Ayrshire	*Brown Swiss*	*Guernsey*	*Holstein*	*Jersey*
Number	213	163	154	587	117
Average	36.4	46.4	32.2	42.9	24.7
Males	38.2	48.4	34.4	44.4	25.7
Females	34.6	44.2	30.6	41.6	23.4
First calving	35.2	44.2	31.7	40.7	22.6
Second calving	36.6	48.3	32.5	44.2	25.7
Third calving	38.1	47.7	31.6	44.6	25.9
Fourth and subsequent calvings	38.1	48.1	33.3	43.2	24.8

After Legault and Touchberry (1962).
Average weights for Aberdeen Angus, Charolais and Hereford calves are 27.1, 47.5 and 32.6 kg respectively.

Table 11.2. Influence of parent on birth weight

Parent	Female calves (kg)	Male calves (kg)
Pure-bred Friesian	43.4	
Pure-bred Jersey	25.0	
Calculated mean birth weight	34.2	
Observed Friesian bull × Jersey cow	33.9	34.5
Observed Jersey bull × Friesian cow	34.7	37.1

After Hilder and Fohrman (1949).

Table 11.3. Influence of parent on birth weight

Parent	Calf weight (kg)
Pure-bred South Devon	45.4
Pure-bred Dexter	23.7
Calculated mean	34.5
Dexter bull × South Devon cow	33.2
South Devon bull × Dexter cow	26.7

After Joubert and Hammond (1958).

for Friesian–Jersey crosses (Table 11.2), and Joubert and Hammond (1958) demonstrated it for South Devon–Dexter crosses (Table 11.3).

The knowledge of the effect of heredity on calf size is applied extensively by farmers who often use an Aberdeen Angus sire or easy calving Friesian on Friesian heifers and thereby reduce the rate of dystocia. Conversely, the use of the larger Charolais bull on Friesian heifers is avoided because it markedly increases the rate of dystocia.

The effect of breed on birth weight has also been shown in sheep by Hunter (1957). The results he obtained by reciprocal crossing between one of the heaviest breeds, the Border Leicester, with one of the lightest breeds, the Welsh Mountain, are shown in Table 11.4.

After heredity, *sex of calf* affects birth weight to an average of about 2 kg in favour of the male calf — regardless of the breed — and several investigations of lamb birth weights have shown that the male is about 5% heavier than the female.

In sheep, *twins* are about 16% lighter at birth than singletons (Starke et al., 1958). In a study of induced twinning in Hereford cows caused by transferring to each uterine horn of each cow an Angus × Hereford embryo, Anderson et al. (1979) found calf birth weights of 35.7 ± 1.8 kg and 27.5 ± 0.5 kg, respectively, for the single and twin calves which resulted. The dams were liberally fed. When one or two Charolais embryos were transplanted to Friesian cows, already inseminated a week earlier with Friesian semen, the resulting Friesian singleton calves weighted 40.97 kg at birth and the Charolais singletons 47.78 kg. In the resulting twin sets, the Friesian calves averaged 37.83 kg and the Charolais 40.53 kg (Kennedy et al., 1984).

In-breeding predisposes to lower birth weights but certain sires may trasmit heavy birth weight which can cancel the effect of homozygosity.

Working with sheep, Hammond (1932) found that birth weight of single lambs increased with the *length of gestation*. There are variations in the gestation lengths of several cattle breeds, and when crosses are made between any two of them the 'cross-bred gestation' length is near the mean for the two breeds, with corresponding variations in the 'cross-bred birth weights' (Tables 11.5 and 11.6).

With pure-bred and cross-bred calves the males tend to be carried a day or two longer than the

Table 11.4. Effect of breed on birth weight

Ewe	Ram	Weight of lambs (kg)	
		Singles	Twins
Border Leicester	Border Leicester	Male 6.6	
		Female 5.9	Female 5.2
	Welsh Mountain		Male 5.2
		Female 5.9	Female 4.3
Welsh Mountain	Border Leicester	Male 4.9	Male 4.3
		Female 4.9	Female 3.8
	Welsh Mountain	Male 3.8	Male 4.0
		Female 3.7	Female 3.4

Table 11.5. Variations in gestation lengths in several cattle breeds

Breed	No. of gestation periods, male and female calves	Average gestation length, male and female calves
Pure-bred Angus	101	276.47
Pure-bred Hereford	100	286.28
Hereford bull × Angus cow	94	281.98
Angus bull × Hereford cow	102	283.30

After Gerlaugh et al. (1951)

Table 11.6. Gestation length and birth weights of calves of pure-bred and reciprocal crosses of Angus and Hereford cattle

Breed	Gestation length (days)	Birth weight (kg)
Calves from Angus cows		
Male pure-bred	277.2	28.3
Male cross-bred	282.7	29.8
Female pure-bred	275.7	25.4
Female cross-bred	281.1	28.4
Calves from Hereford cows		
Male pure-bred	287.5	31.3
Male cross-bred	283.1	30.3
Female pure-bred	285.2	30.7
Female cross-bred	283.5	28.4

After Gerlaugh et al. (1951).

females, and this is reflected in the greater birth weight of the male.

A *sire effect* on gestation length has been noted within a breed, and in a study of five Aberdeen Angus, 10 Hereford and three Shorthorn bulls, Wheat and Riggs (1952) found variations of gestation length of 11, 7 and 7 days, respectively, between bulls within those three breeds.

When Charolais and Hereford bulls were crossed with cows of the Friesian, Ayrshire, Shorthorn, Guernsey and Jersey breeds whose average breed gestation length was 281.7 days, the cross-bred calves to the Charolais and Hereford bulls were carried for 286 and 283 days respectively (Edwards, 1966).

Pathologically prolonged gestation occurs in sheep and cattle; some of the fetuses are grossly oversized but others with pituitary hypoplasia are markedly undersized.

Seasonal effect on fetal weight

In range beef cattle, where calving is planned to begin at the start of the grazing season, there is evidence from several studies that calf birth weights increase in proportion to the extension in calving date; for example Young (1970) found a 0.64 kg increase of birth weight for each 10 day protraction of the calving season.

Intrinsic fetal oversize

The effect of heredity (breed and sire) and prolonged gestation have been mentioned as causes of excessive fetal weight. Pathological conditions are occasional causes of severe oversize, examples being duplication and oedema (including ascites and anasarca); the dystocia with schistosomes is due to excessive fetal diameter rather than to body weight which is decreased (see Chapter 10). A condition of fetal oversize which is in the borderland of normality and pathology and which is of increasing economic importance is *muscular hypertrophy* or *double muscling*. This is a hereditary anomaly of cattle in which there is excessive development of muscles, particularly of the hindquarters but also of the loins and forequarters; the skin is thin and the limb bones tend to be shorter. It is of varying severity, and when mild is favourably regarded by both farmers and butchers because of the greatly increased proportion of meat in the carcass. When marked, however, it is the cause of severe dystocia, particularly in heifers. Muscular hypertrophy has been described in the South Devon breed by MacKellar (1960), and it is well known in the Belgian blue, Charolais and White Flanders breeds. Mason (1963) has described it in the grandsons of a Friesian bull imported into Britain; he ascribed it to a single gene, but there is disagreement over whether it is inherited as a dominant or recessive character (Vandenbussche et al., 1964). Vandeplassche (1973) has stated that 50% of oversized calves in Belgium are due to double muscling and that the condition is a frequent indication for the caesarean operation in Holland, Belgium and France.

The effects of cross-breeding on both calf weight and gestation length have already been mentioned. Within particular cross-breeding programmes and within particular pure-bred herds, *individual sires* have been shown to exert marked effects on the birth weight of their progeny.

Maternal influences on birth weight of progeny

Parity. Parity, which is closely related to *maternal age*, has an effect on calf birth weight, and it is well known that heifers have calves that are 1–4 kg lighter than cows (see Table 11.1). Generally there is an increasing calf birth weight with increasing weight of the dam, but beyond the third parity, by which time the dam is fully grown, there is no increase in calf weight (Braude and Walker, 1949).

Intrauterine Environment. By means of reciprocal transfers of fertilized eggs between sheep breeds of disparate size, Hunter (1957) and Dickenson et al. (1962) have been able to show the relative influence on birth weight of prenatal environment (phenotype) and the genotype of the lamb. In Hunter's work on Border Leicester and Welsh Mountain breeds the mean birth weight of Border Leicester lambs born to Welsh Mountain ewes was 1.13 kg less than that of Border Leicester lambs born to Border Leicester ewes; also, the birth weight of Welsh Mountain lambs born to Border Leicester ewes was 0.56 kg more than that of Welsh Mountain lambs born to Welsh Mountain ewes. Thus the maternal influence can limit the size of a genetically larger lamb as well as increase the size of a genetically smaller lamb. Also, the size limitation imposed on Border Leicester lambs by the Welsh Mountain maternal environment was greater than the size increase produced in Welsh Mountain lambs by the Border Leicester maternal influence.

In reciprocal crossing between the (large) Lincoln and (small) Welsh Mountain breeds, Dickenson et al. (1962) found no lambing difficulties occurred in Lincoln ewes, but in 13 Welsh ewes carrying Lincoln lambs, eight needed assistance at birth. In another experiment, fertilized eggs from pure Lincoln and from pure Welsh donors were transferred to Scottish Blackface ewes. Of 36 Lincoln lambs 16 required obstetric assistance, while only one of 28 Welsh lambs was associated with dystocia. The results of the egg transfer experiments showed that:

1. Lambs of the same breed (genotype) differed in birth weight according to whether their uterine environment (phenotype) was Lincoln or Welsh.

2. Lambs reared in the same uterine environment differed in birth weight according to whether their genotype was Lincoln or Welsh.

3. Both genotype of lamb and maternal environment had significant effects on the birth weight of the lambs.

4. The genotype influence was three or four times as great as the maternal influence on lamb birth weight.

Maternal Nutrition During Pregnancy. There is a vast and varied literature, which is difficult to evaluate succinctly, concerning the effects on fetal weight of variations in the maternal diet. The motivation for this research is mainly economic because birth weight is positively correlated with postnatal weight gain and with the subsequent achievement of commercially desirable slaughter weights of food animals. In the obstetric context the concern over birth weight is two-fold: firstly, large fetuses contribute to dystocia and, secondly, undersized offspring are more prone to neonatal death and disease. Therefore, while it is reasonable to explore how birth weight may be controlled so as to reduce dystocia, any severe reduction in fetal birth weight, achieved by manipulation of the maternal diet, may place the neonate in jeopardy.

In a fundamental consideration of fetal development it must be remembered that the fetus grows by both hyperplasia and hypertrophy of its constituent tissues. Prior and Laster (1979) have shown that in cattle growth by hyperplasia is more important in early gestation but that it decreases rapidly towards the end of pregnancy, whereas growth by hypertrophy continues to increase with advancing gestation. Retardation of growth at any stage of gestation would have a permanent effect on postnatal development but because the relative proportion of growth by hyperplasia gets less as fetal age increases, retardation of growth in late gestation has less effect on subsequent postnatal development. Actually, the growth by hyperplasia that does occur in late gestation is mainly in muscle.

In normal cattle, fetal growth during the final third of gestation accounts for two-thirds of the birth weight. It follows that the nutritional demands of the fetus in early and middle gestation are low and that suboptimum maternal nutrition will exert its maximum influence during the last trimester. Prior and Laster (1979) and Eley et al.

(1978) found that bovine fetal growth was fastest at 232 days of gestation, but the two research groups' findings differed in the amount of the daily increase, 331 and 200 g, respectively. By the end of gestation the increase in fetal weight had declined to 200 g daily. The first group also ascertained that when pregnant heifers were fed varying diets to produce low, medium and high maternal weight gains there was no resultant difference in fetal birth weights between the three categories.

In other nutritional experiments in cattle, sheep and pigs it has been found that only when the maternal diet is severely restricted in late gestation (last 90 days in cattle, last 60 days in sheep and last 45 days in pigs), so that the mother did not maintain her body weight, was fetal birth weight reduced. The reduced fetal birth weight in these instances was due mainly to less fetal muscle. Tudor (1972) fed two groups of cows from 180 days of gestation to term so that one group gained and the other lost weight. Calf birth weights were respectively 30.9 kg from the high-plane dams and 24.1 kg from the low-plane mothers. In another experiment in which cows lost 17.5% of their weight during the last trimester the calves showed a reduction of birth weight of 21.9%. Working with sheep, Wallace (1948) fed groups of ewes on high and low planes of nutrition from day 28 to day 144 of pregnancy, while in other groups the levels of diet were reversed after 91 days. He found that lamb birth weight was markedly affected by nutrition of the ewe in late pregnancy; however, up to 90 days (three-fifths of gestation) the previous level of maternal diet has no effect. Similarly, in varying the diets of pregnant sows, Pike and Boaz (1972) have shown that variable feeding from conception to 70 days gestation exerted no effect and only in the last 45 days did maternal nutrition influence birth weight. The latter finding corresponds with the observation that there is a 10-fold increase in porcine fetal weight during the last 45 days.

Before too rigid general conclusions are made from the foregoing, it should be pointed out that it was the energy content of the maternal diet which was manipulated in the research regimens. It is possible that a maternal diet which is insufficient in protein during early gestation may affect placental development and thus lead to retardation of fetal growth.

Obviously cows and ewes carrying twins will have higher dietary maintenance requirements, which in some circumstances cannot be sustained from the available food supply. By supplementation of the diet of pregnant ewes with 226 g wheat grain per head per day for the last quarter of gestation it was possible to increase the birth weight of single lambs from 3.7 to 4.6 kg and of twins from 2.8 to 3.4 kg (Underwood and Shier, 1942). The lamb survival rates for supplemented ewes as compared with controls were 16:14 for singletons and 23:6 for twins. Similarly, in the case of bovine twin gestation, it is generally believed that better feeding of the pregnant dam would improve the survival rate of the offspring and help to reduce the other deleterious effects of twinning.

Returning to obstetric considerations of birth weight, although effective reduction of birth weight through dietary control is difficult and carries a risk to the newborn, it should be borne in mind that quite small variations in birth weight, as small as 3.21 kg were found between normal calving and dystocia in Aberdeen Angus heifers (Young, 1970). Also, Smith et al. (1976) reported that, on average, over all dam ages calving difficulties increased by 1.63% for each kilogram increase in calf birth weight.

Pelvic capacity in fetomaternal disproportion

Wiltbank (1961), Derivaux et al. (1964), Rice and Wiltbank (1970) and Young (1970) have made valuable observations on maternal pelvic size as a factor in bovine dystocia. The best criterion of pelvic capacity was the 'pelvic area', which is the product of the dorsoventral and (the widest) bisiliac dimensions of the pelvic inlet. These two measurements can be obtained per rectum by employing a pocket calliper. Measurements of pelvic area in Angus heifers, taken at the time of breeding, at 6–7 months of gestation, at 1 week prepartum and at parturition were 147, 184, 227 and 232 cm^2. The rate of pelvic expansion was greatest near parturition. Charolais heifers having a pelvic area less than 300 cm^2 had a high incidence of dystocia. Devon heifers which suffered from dystocia had a mean pelvic area of between 242 and 263 cm^2. Hereford heifers with pelvic area of less than 230 cm^2 showed a 70% incidence of dystocia while those with pelvic areas above 230 cm^2 had a dystocia rate of 12%. These observations suggest that culling of heifers with a small pelvic area would reduce the incidence of dystocia due to fetopelvic disproportion.

In New Zealand, McSporran and Wyburn (1979) and McSporran and Fielden (1979) were able to assess the pelvic area by means of radiographic pelvimetry, and found that variations in the incidence of dystocia between different groups of Romney ewes were related to the pelvic area. Attempts to correlate external bodily measurements with internal pelvic dimensions were not practically useful. Because the particular ovine dystocia studied by these authors was largely due to fetopelvic disproportion they recommended selective breeding of ewes and rams for freedom from dystocia.

Apart from breed, pelvic area within a breed is most influenced by dam body weight and it is noteworthy that the use of growth stimulants in the management of heifer replacements for the dairy herd has caused an increase in pelvic area (Staigmiller, 1983). Also, experimentally, Musah et al. (1986) have shown that in cross-bred beef heifers the intracervical deposition of porcine relaxin on day 278 of gestation caused increases in cervical dilatation, in pelvic expansion and in the rate of pelvic expansion. It also brought forward the time of parturition by 2.1–2.5 days.

In concluding this section on dystocia due to fetopelvic disproportion it is important to consider the preventive aspects, namely the selection of breeding stock for desirable obstetric traits. The suggested guidelines are as follows.

Females
At breeding time select large-for-age heifers with ample pelvic area.

Males

1. In breeding pure-bred replacements for either a dairy or beef enterprise, select sires on their ease-of-calving records and normal (i.e. not unduly long) gestation lengths for the particular breed.

2. In cross-breeding for beef production from dairy herds, avoid sires of the larger breeds such as Simmenthal and Charolais for the heifer inseminations and use instead a known 'easy calving' Aberdeen Angus or Hereford bull. For second and later parities choose a bull of a larger breed on his ease-of-calving record and gestation length.

3. In beef production from beef breeds: for heifer pregnancies use either a sire of a smaller beef breed or a within-breed sire of good ease-of-calving record and gestation length; for later parities use a bull either of the same or larger breed — both on the bases of calving ease and gestation length.

While applying the above principles in the production of offspring for beef, whether purebred, or cross-bred, it should be noted that the weight of the calf at birth assuming equal gestation lengths bears a direct relationship to its weaning weight and to its subsequent slaughter weight, on which the profitability of the enterprise largely depends. On the other hand, unduly large calves at birth predispose to calf deaths and to maternal morbidity, mortality, reduced milk yield and infertility. Thus a breeder must consider how much increase in birth weight can be tolerated in return for increases in growth rate and weaning weight.

Obstetric terminology

In the treatment of animal dystocia by vaginal manipulation the terminology of Benesch will be followed and, at the outset, it is necessary to define the terms *presentation*, *position* and *posture*.

Presentation signifies the relation between the long axis of the fetus and the maternal birth canal. It includes *longitudinal presentation*, which may be anterior or posterior according to which extremity of the fetus is adjacent to the maternal pelvis; *transverse presentation*, ventral or dorsal according to whether the ventral or dorsal aspect of the trunk is presenting; and *vertical presentation*, ventral or dorsal. Vertical presentations are very rare and only the obliquely vertical 'dog-sitting position' of the equine species need be considered.

Position indicates that surface of the maternal birth canal to which the fetal vertebral column is applied. It includes *dorsal*, *ventral* and *right* or *left lateral position*.

Posture refers to the disposition of the movable appendages of the fetus and involves flexion or extension of the cervical and limb joints, for example downward deviation of the head, or hock flexion posture.

FAULTY FETAL DISPOSITION

Presentation

About 99% of foals and 95% of calves are presented anteriorly; when sheep are parturient with singletons they show a similar percentage of anterior presentations to cattle but with twins there is a considerable proportion of posteriorly presented lambs. The polytocous sow and bitch deliver 30–40% of fetuses in posterior presentation. In posterior presentation the hindlimbs may be extended or flexed beneath the fetal body. When the hindlimbs are extended in polytocous births there is little more dystocia than with anterior presentation; however, when the hindlimbs are flexed (breech presentation) in polytocous births the incidence of dystocia is increased. In the monotocous species serious dystocia always occurs with posterior presentation if the hindlimbs are flexed; even when they are extended there is greater likelihood of difficult birth than with anterior presentation. Because of the relatively long limbs of the fetuses of monotocous species and the large space required for hindlimb extension, there is obviously a high probability that a fetus presented posteriorly in late gestation will fail to extend its hindlimbs before second-stage labour begins. In ovine twin births, breech presentation causes dystocia although the twin lamb is smaller than the singleton.

There is a consensus of authoritative veterinary opinion that both dystocia and stillbirth are much more likely to occur if the calf is presented posteriorly rather than anteriorly. Ben-David (1961) found that 47% of posterior presentations in Holsteins were accompanied by dystocia. Also the likelihood of dystocia in equine posterior presentations is exceptionally high. It is therefore important to enquire into the factors that determine fetal polarity. The author and Abusineina (1963) have made post-mortem studies on this problem in cattle, while Vandeplassche (1957) has carried out similar investigations in horses. With respect to cattle, during the first 2 months of gestation no definite polarity was evident but during the third month there were equal numbers of anterior and posterior presentations. Thenceforward to the end of gestation there were only three transverse presentations out of 363 pregnancies. Throughout the fourth, fifth and first half of the 6 months a majority of fetuses were in posterior presentation, but during the sixth month the situation began to change so that at the end of that month anterior and posterior presentation frequencies were equal. By the middle of the seventh month the majority of fetuses were in anterior presentation. Beyond the seventh month only one of 17 fetuses was posteriorly disposed, a situation closely similar to that observed at term. To recapitulate: between $5\frac{1}{2}$ and $6\frac{1}{2}$ months of gestation the polarity of the bovine fetus becomes reversed, and by the end of the seventh month the final birth presentation is adopted. Attempts, using post-mortem pregnant uteri, to alter the presentation beyond the seventh month were unsuccessful because by that time the fetal body length too greatly exceeds the width of the amnion, while successful efforts to change the presentation between $5\frac{1}{2}$ and $6\frac{1}{2}$ months required definite manipulative force. Similar attempts carried out under paravertebral anaesthesia on the standing cow have been successful with a $6\frac{1}{2}$ month fetus but unsuccessful with an 8 month calf.

The natural forces which bring about these changes in polarity are not understood but presumably reflex fetal movements occur in response to changes in the intrauterine pressure due to myometrial contractions, to movements of adjacent abdominal viscera or to contraction of the abdominal musculature. Fetal movements are often felt during rectal palpation of the uterus. The preponderance of posterior presentation in early gestation would be the expected result of suspending an inert body with the same centre of gravity as the fetal calf. With the development of the fetal nervous system and a consequent appreciation of gravity the fetal calf would begin to execute righting reflexes which would tend to bring up the head from the dependent part of the uterus. If these assumptions are true, then posterior presentation, rather than being regarded as an obstetric accident, could be caused either by a subnormally developed fetus or by a uterus deficient in tone. Obviously size of fetus and uterine space must influence the ease with which a fetus can change its polarity in utero; there is a much higher percentage of posterior presentations in bovine twin births, while an above average percentage of posterior presentations occurs with excessively large fetuses, e.g. the hydropic Ayrshire calf in which the anomaly is present as early as 100 days of gestation.

In equine gestation, 98% of foals assume an anterior longitudinal presentation between $6\frac{1}{2}$ and $8\frac{1}{2}$ months (Vandeplassche, 1957). A small proportion of the remaining 2% — possibly about 0.1% — are transverse presentations in which the extremities of the fetus occupy the uterine cornua while the uterine body is largely empty. This presentation causes the most serious of all equine dystocias. It probably arises at about 70 days of gestation when the uterus normally changes from a transverse to a longitudinal direction in front of the maternal pelvis as a result of the allantochorion passing from the pregnant horn into the uterine body. In the abnormal situation either the allantochorion does not intrude into the uterine body or the major, rather than the normally minor, branch of the allantochorion passes into the non-pregnant horn and is followed by the amnion, containing a fetal extremity. Normally neither the amnion nor the fetus passes into the non-pregnant horn. Other, less serious, equine transverse presentations occur across the uterine body; it is uncertain when they occur, but they could occur during birth.

Transverse presentations are very uncommon in cattle and sheep, but in the polytocous species a fetus is not uncommonly found to dispose itself across the entrance to the maternal pelvis; such presentations undoubtedly arise during birth.

The lack of a marked difference in frequency between anterior and posterior presentations in pigs and dogs may be due to the horizontal disposition of the long uterine horns as compared with the sloping uteri of the monotocous species.

Position

As regards position of the fetus, the natural tendency is for the fetus to lie with its dorsum against the greater curvature of the uterus; thus the equine fetus is upside down and the bovine fetus is upright during late gestation. The latter maintains this relationship during birth but in the mare the fetus changes from a ventral to a dorsal position during the course of labour. As might be expected, therefore, ventral, as well as lateral, positions are much commoner in equine than in bovine dystocia; they arise during birth.

Posture

As regards posture, the arrangement of the bovine fetus during the final two months of gestation is one of anterior presentation and dorsal position with flexion of all joints of the movable appendages. The appendages of the equine fetus are similarly flexed on the inverted fetus. This postural disposition of 'universal flexion' achieves the maximum economy of space. The fascinating and unsolved problem is the nature of the parturient mechanism whereby the occipitoatlantal and cervical joints become extended while the forelimbs become straightened in front of the fetus. The extended forelimb posture necessary for normal birth in cattle is the more remarkable because it is a posture which is never repeated postnatally. In his studies of the first stage of labour in cattle Abusineina (1963) noticed that the flexed knees of the calf first occupied the dilating cervix: 30 minutes later the digits were felt in the cervix. The authors believe that the limb extension occurs while the fetus is practising righting reflexes in its attempt to 'stand-up in utero'. No doubt such active fetal movements are provoked by the myometrial contractions of first-stage labour, and presumably the fall in progesterone concentration at this time favours contractions of fetal muscle as well as of the myometrium. In this connection the observation by Jöchle et al. (1972) that progesterone given to parturient cows caused a high incidence of postural dystocia is fascinating. There is also the well-known increased frequency of postural aberrations in premature births and in twin parturitions where, it may be presumed, the usual hormonal ratios do not obtain and in which a degree of uterine inertia is a common accompaniment. If these assumptions are correct then some forms of fetal and maternal dystocia may be due to the same basic causes. For example, calcium deficiency causes uterine inertia: preparturient hypocalcaemia might be a cause of postural defect.

Lateral deviation of the head is a postural abnormality which deserves special mention. It may be due to the same factors as those noted above but lack of uterine space may predispose to it and it may arise during late gestation rather than during birth. A congenital deformity known as *wryneck* in which the head and neck are fixed in flexion arises during the peculiar bicornual gestation of solipeds (Williams, 1940). In 27 difficult equine dystocias treated by Vandeplassche (1957), the majority of which were associated with bicornual gestation, 10 of the foals were affected with a degree of wryneck.

In the monotocous species the dimensions of the non-dilatable maternal pelvis are just sufficient for the normal full-term fetus to negotiate the birth canal; any fetal disposition other than anterior presentation, dorsal position, extended posture is likely to result in dystocia. In the polytocous species the fetomaternal relationship is not so exact, with the result that the disposition of the comparatively small fetal limbs is less important and many piglets and puppies are delivered normally with their limbs in postures which would have caused dystocia in the foal and calf. However, if a female of a polytocous species is parturient with an abnormally low number of fetuses there is likely to be relative fetal oversize and in these circumstances malposture of the limbs may cause dystocia.

Faulty fetal disposition as a cause of difficult births is most frequent in dairy cattle, with a much higher incidence in cows than heifers; it is much less common in the beef breeds. It is not uncommon in sheep parturition and in both cattle and sheep twin births increase its incidence.

From the foregoing account it will be gathered that in the authors' view dystocia due to abnormal presentation of the fetus (posterior and transverse) originates during gestation (between $6\frac{1}{2}$ and $8\frac{1}{2}$ months in the cow and mare), while dystocia due to errors of position and posture arises during the first or early part of the second stage of labour. Furthermore, it is considered that fetal dystocia (with the exception of those forms caused by oversize and gross developmental anomalies) is due mainly to aberrations of neuromuscular function in the fetus and in the myometrium, and that the latter are probably caused by abnormal concentrations of those agents which normally affect neuromuscular activity, such as calcium ions, oestrogens and progesterone. These factors may, in turn, be influenced by hereditary or environmental factors. For example, Woodward and Clark (1959) found that a particular Hereford sire when used on an inbred line of cattle produced a high incidence of posterior presentations while Uwland (1976) reported ranges of between 2 and 9.7% of posterior presentations in the progeny of different bulls; these observations suggest that a hereditary factor may affect the incidence of posterior presentation.

REFERENCES

Abusineina, M. E. A. (1963) Thesis, University of London.

Adams, J. W. E. and Bishop, G. H. R. (1963) *J. S. Afr. Vet. Med. Assn*, **34**, 91.

Anderson, G. B., Cupps, P. T. and Drost, M. (1979) *J. Anim. Sci.*, **49**, 1037.

Ben-David, B. (1961) *Refuah Vet.*, **19**, 152.

Boyd, L. J. and Hafs, H. D. (1965) *J. Dairy Sci.*, **48**, 9, 1236.

Braude, R. and Walker, D. M. (1949) *J. Agr. Sci., Camb.*, **39**, 156.

Dickenson, A. G., Hancock, J. L., Hovell, G. J. R., Taylor, St. C. S. and Wiener, G. (1962) *Anim. Prod.*, **5**, 87.

Edwards, J. (1966) *The Charolais Report*. London: Milk Marketing Board.

Eley, R. M., Thatcher, W. M., Bazer, F. W., Wilcox, C. J., Becker, R. B., Head, H. H. and Atkinson, A. W. (1978) *J. Dairy Sci.*, **61**, 467.

Gerlaugh, P., Kunkle, L. E. and Rife, D. C. (1951) *Ohio Agric. Exp. Stn. Res. Bull.*, 703.

Hammond, J. (1932) *Growth and Development of Sheep*. Edinburgh: Oliver and Boyd.

Hilder, R. A. and Fohrman, M. H. (1949) *J. Agr. Res.*, **78**, 457.

Hunter, G. L. (1957) *J. Agr. Sci., Camb.*, **48**, 36.

Jöchle, W., Esparza, H., Gimenez, T. and Hidalgo, M. A. (1972) *J. Reprod. Fertil.*, **28**, 407.

Joubert, D. M. and Hammond, J. (1958) *J. Agr. Sci., Camb.*, **51**, 325.

Kennedy, L., Boland, M. P. and Gordon, I. (1984) *10th Int. Congr. Anim. Reprod. and AI Urbana-Champaign*, **1**, 232.

Laster, D. B., Glimp, H. A., Cundiff, L. V. and Gregory, K. E. (1973) *J. Anim. Sci.*, **36**, 695.

Legault, C. R. and Touchberry, R. W. (1962) *J. Dairy Sci.*, **45**, 1226.

Lindhé, B. (1966) *Wld Rev. Anim. Prod.*, **2**, 53.

MacKellar, J. C. (1960) *Vet. Rec.*, **72**, 507.

McSporran, K. D. and Fielden, E. D. (1979) *N.Z. Vet. J.*, **27**, 75.

McSporran, K. D. and Wyburn, R. S. (1979) *N.Z. Vet. J.*, **27**, 64.

Mason, I. L. (1963) *Vet. Rec.*, **76**, 28.

Musah, A. I., Schwabe, C., Williams, R. L. and Andersen, L. L. (1986) *Biol. Reprod.*, **34**, 363.

Prior, R. L. and Laster, D. B. (1979) *J. Anim. Sci.*, **48**, 1456.

Pike, I. H. and Boaz, T. G. (1972) *Anim. Prod.*, **15**, 147.

Smith, G. M., Laster, D. B. and Gregory, K. E. (1976) *J. Anim. Sci.*, **43**, 27.

Staigmiller, R. B. (1983) *Proc. Soc. Anim. Breeding, Nottingham*.

Starke, J. S., Smith, J. B. and Joubert, D. M. (1958) *Sci. Bull. Dep. Agric. For. Un. S. Afr.*, **382**.

Tudor, G. D. (1972) *Aust. J. Agr. Res.*, **23**, 389.

Underwood, E. J. and Shier, F. L. (1942) *J. Dep. Agric. W. Aust.*, **19**, 37.

Uwland, J. (1976) *Tijdschr. Diergeneesk.*, **101**, 421.

Vandenbussche, O., Vandenbussche, P. and Vandeplassche, M. (1964) *Vlaams Diergeneesk. Tijdschr.*, **33**, 5.

Vandenplassche, M. (1957) *Bijr. Vlaams Diergeneesk. Tijdschr.*, **26**, 68.

Vandeplassche, M. (1973) Personal communication.

Wallace, L. R. (1948) *J. Agr. Sci., Camb.*, **38**, 367.

Wheat, J. D. and Riggs, J. K. (1952) *J. Hered.*, **43**, 99.

Williams, W. L. (1940) *Veterinary Obstetrics*. New York: Williams and Wilkins.

Wiltbank, J. N. (1961) *Neb. Exp. Stn. Q.*, Summer.

Withers, F. W. (1953) *Brit. Vet. J.*, **109**, 122.

Woodward, R. R. and Clark, R. T. (1959) *J. Anim. Sci.*, **18**, 85.

Young, J. S. (1970) Thesis, University of Sydney.

FARM ANIMALS

General considerations

1. Obstetrics is a branch of surgery and therefore asepsis and gentleness are of prime importance.

2. Whereas the treatment must be humane, it should be carried out under firm discipline so that the available lay help may be used to the best effect.

3. Obstetric cases should always be regarded with urgency but the actual interference requires infinite patience, bearing in mind the duration of normal second-stage labour.

4. The rectification of defects of presentation, position and posture can be achieved only by intrauterine manipulation of the fetus. Thus an essential prerequisite to treatment is retropulsion of the fetus. This is greatly facilitated by posterior epidural anaesthesia. In cases of fetal oversize to be delivered by traction, on the other hand, epidural anaesthesia is not essential or even desirable, except on humane grounds.

5. In cases of delayed dystocia, delivery is expedited by substitution of fluids for the lost fetal fluids. Boiled water, which has been cooled to body temperature, is the best substitute for allantoic fluid. In quantities of up to 14 litres, instilled into the uterus by gravity, it greatly increases the mobility of the fetus in utero. For actual vaginal delivery a lubricant substitute for the amniotic fluid is required, and this may be in the form of a liquid such as Celacol or as a semi-solid substance smeared over the engaging fetus and passage. Lard is a well-tried obstetric lubricant and, in emergency, soap may be used, but there are available many bland proprietary obstetric lubricants which are water-soluble. The value of fetal fluid supplements cannot be too strongly emphasized.

6. The amount of artificial obstetric force used in traction should not be inordinate; in large animals it should not exceed the pulling power of four people. Its application and direction must simulate the physiological as nearly as possible. The veterinarian should be concerned to direct appropriate traction rather than to participate in it. Whereas rectification of postural defects should be performed with the patient standing, in instances where considerable traction is required it is best applied with the cow recumbent.

7. After diagnosing the cause of dystocia and deciding on a plan of action, the obstetrician should consider whether he or she has the necessary facilities, including sufficient lay help, to carry out the treatment successfully. In severe forms of dystocia, more especially in mares, the veterinarian should seek the assistance of a professional colleague.

8. After prolonged vaginal manipulations, or fetotomy, broad-spectrum antibiotics should be given to the dam.

Obstetric equipment

The aim should be to possess the minimum of essential equipment and to be thoroughly conversant with its use. It cannot be stated too often that the best instruments are the *clean and gentle* hands and arms of the obstetrician. Simple instruments which are easy to handle and convenient to sterilize are best. More complex equipment is occasionally required and the important consideration is to know when the use of such complicated instruments is indicated. The following equipment should suffice to deal with all cases:

- Protective clothing (waterproof gown, rubber boots, rubber gloves)
- Obstetric lubricant, funnel and rubber tubing for uterine infusion
- Preparations of oxytocin

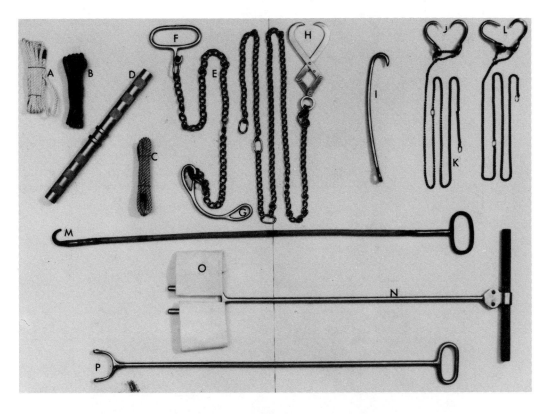

Fig. 12.1 Instruments for manipulative delivery.

- Calcium borogluconate
- Antibiotics
- Xylazine
- Local anaesthetic
- Tetanus antitoxin
- 10 ml syringes with hypodermic and epidural needles
- Intravenous infusion apparatus with intravenous needles
- Drum of sterile gauze swabs
- Cotton wool
- Surgical spirit
- Suture material with needles

Instruments for manipulative delivery (Figure 12.1) include obstetric snares, i.e. 1 m lengths, with loops, of cotton rope (clothes line), nylon cord or webbing (A, B, C) — a finer cord for snaring the mandible is essential — and traction bars (D). As an alternative to snares one may use Moore's obstetric chains (E) with handles (F). A snare introducer (G) is also illustrated. Obstetrical hooks include Krey–Schottler double-jointed hooks (H); Obermeyer's anal hook (I), Harms's

sharp (J) or blunt (L) paired hooks on a fine (farrowing) chain (K), and Blanchard's long, flexible cane hook (M). Additional instruments are Cämmerer's torsion fork (N) with canvas cuffs (O) and Kühn's obstetrical crutch (P). Traction may be applied using a block and tackle or an HK calf puller or Vink calving jack (Figure 12.2).

Instruments for fetotomy (Figure 12.3) include fetotomy knives such as Roberts's (A) or Unsworth's (B), spatula (C), Persson's chain-saw (D), Fetotome (Swedish modification of Thygesen's model) (G), with wire introducer (E), wire (F), hand-grips (H) and Shriever's introducer (J); and Glättli's spiral tubes (K).

Obstetric manoeuvres

The manoeuvres which are practised on the fetus in manipulative obstetrics are as follows.

Retropulsion means pushing the fetus forwards from the birth canal towards the uterus. It is fundamental to all intrauterine measures which may be required to rectify defects of presentation, position and posture. It is effected by pressure with

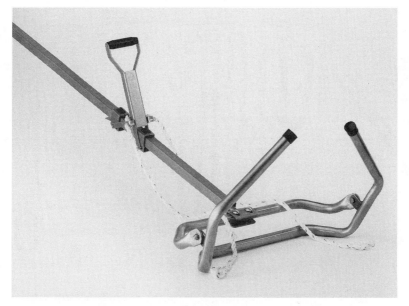

a

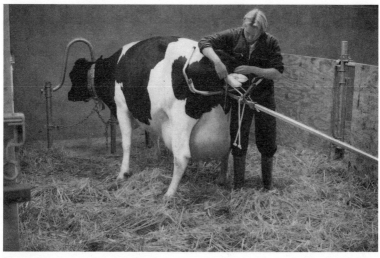

b

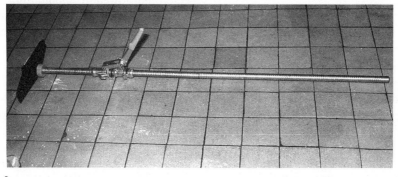

c

Fig. 12.2 (a) Vink calving jack. (b) Vink calving jack in use to apply traction to calf in anterior longitudinal presentation with snare attached to both forelimbs. (c) HK calf puller.

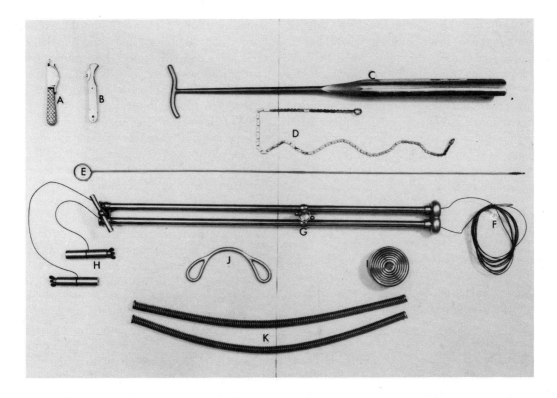

Fig. 12.3 Instruments for fetotomy.

the hand on the presenting bulk of the fetus; in some cases it is convenient for an assistant to repel the fetus while the obstetrician otherwise manipulates it, while in others retropulsion is applied by means of a crutch. As far as possible, the repelling force should be exerted in the intervals between bouts of straining. Alternatively, epidural anaesthesia may be induced, and in many cases this is extremely helpful because it prevents the dam 'straining'.

Extension refers to the extension of flexed joints when postural defects are present. It is carried out by applying tangential force to the extremity of the displaced member so that it is brought through an arc of a circle to the entrance of the pelvis. The force is applied preferably by hand or, failing that, by snare or hook(s).

Traction means the application of force to the presenting parts of the fetus in order to supplement, or in some cases to replace, the maternal forces. Such force is applied by hand or through the medium of snares or hooks. Limb-snares are fixed above the fetlocks, and the head snare may be applied by the Benesch method, in which the loop is placed in the mouth and up over the poll and

behind the ears or, alternatively, the centre of a single rope may be pushed up over the poll and behind both ears, leaving both ends of the rope protruding from the vagina. For replacement of the laterally deviated head where the operator's hand is insufficient a thin rope snare applied to the mandible is essential. A matter often discussed by veterinary obstetricians is the extent to which supplementary force may be used. It is felt that the strength of four average persons should be the limit. Before traction is applied, sand should be sprinkled on the floor so as to improve the foothold of patient and assistants. Mechanical methods of applying traction are deprecated by some, but for the single-handed veterinary surgeon working on remote farms the pulley block and tackle, HK calf puller or Vink calving jack (see Figure 12.2) are invaluable. Nowadays, there is a welcome trend towards caesarean section, or fetotomy, rather than recourse to inordinate and inhumane traction.

Rotation entails alteration of the position of a fetus by moving it around its longitudinal axis, for example from the ventral to dorsal position. It is more often required in horses than in cattle and is much more easily effected on the responsive live fetus, which may be readily rotated by digital pressure on the eyeballs, protected by the lids; this causes a convulsive reaction, and slight rotational force then completes the manoeuvre. If this fails — and in the case of dead fetuses fetal fluid supplements are indicated — rotational force may be exerted on the crossed extended limbs by hand or mechanically through the medium of Cämmerer's torsion fork or Kühn's crutch.

Version means alteration of transverse or vertical to longitudinal presentation.

Obstetric anaesthesia for vaginal delivery

In order to achieve safe, expeditious and humane delivery in some of the more severe types of dystocia the induction of local or general anaesthesia in the dam is essential.

General anaesthesia

Deep narcosis, or general anaesthesia, is better suited to the temperament of mares than local analgesia, although in well-chosen cases epidural anaesthesia may be combined with sedatives. Where a complicated correction, or fetotomy, is required, it is best to cause recumbency by administration of detomidine or guaphenesin. In veterinary hospitals, general anaesthesia is preferable. The application of hobbles will facilitate movement of the mare into dorsal or lateral recumbency; such change of position may greatly expedite obstetric manoeuvres particularly if a pack is placed under the rear of the mare so as to cause the abdominal viscera to move away from the pelvis.

Epidural anaesthesia

In ruminants, epidural anaesthesia is ideal for obstetric purposes. Its merits were first demonstrated to the veterinary profession by Benesch (1927). It is a form of multiple spinal nerve block in which, by means of a single injection of local anaesthetic solution into the epidural space, the coccygeal and posterior sacral nerves are affected, thus producing anaesthesia of the anus, perineum, vulva and vagina. As a result, painless birth is possible, but an outstanding additional advantage of epidural anaesthesia to the veterinary surgeon is that by abolishing pelvic sensation, reflex abdominal contraction ('straining') is prevented. Thus,

intravaginal manipulations are facilitated, retropulsion is made easier, fetal fluid supplements are retained and defaecation is suspended. The patient stands more quietly and, if recumbent initially, often gets up when relieved of painful pelvic sensations; this again makes the obstetrician's task easier and cleaner. This form of anaesthesia is useful whenever straining is troublesome, as in prolapse of the uterus, vagina, rectum or bladder. It is also indicated for episiotomy and for suturing the vulva or perineum.

Provided that the epidural injection is made with due regard to asepsis and that an excessive volume of anaesthetic is not injected (thus causing the animal to fall) the method is free from risk.

The local anaesthetic usually employed is 2% lignocaine, with or without adrenaline. Solutions containing chlorocresol or sodium metabisulphite as preservatives should not be used.

It should be clearly understood that epidural anaesthesia does not affect uterine contractions; the main force of labour is not antagonized and the third stage of labour, as well as uterine involution, are not affected.

Technique of Epidural Injection. The site of injection is the middle of the first intercoccygeal space. This is located by raising the tail 'pump-handle' fashion. The first obvious articulation behind the sacrum is the first intercoccygeal. The area is clipped, thoroughly washed with soap and water and dressed with alcohol. Some inject a small volume of local anaesthetic using a fine needle to desensitize the skin over the injection site, others do not. The epidural needle, which is of 16–18 gauge and 5 cm long, is inserted into the middle of the space at right angles to the normal contour of the tail-head exactly in the mid-line and directed downwards in the mid-sagittal plane. The needle is passed downwards for a distance of 2–4 cm until it strikes the floor of the epidural space; it is then very slightly withdrawn (Figure 12.4 and Plate 1). Confirmation that the needle is correctly placed is obtained by attaching to it the syringe and making a trial injection; if there is no resistance to injection, the needle point is in the epidural space. Alternatively, the hub of the epidural needle can be filled with anaesthetic solution. As the needle is advanced into the epidural space, the anaesthetic solution will be sucked in as a result of the slight negative pressure which exists there. Within 2 minutes of the injection the tail becomes limp. In

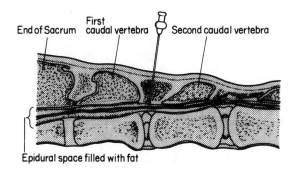

End of Sacrum   First caudal vertebra   Second caudal vertebra

Epidural space filled with fat

Fig. 12.4 Longitudinal section through the caudal vertebrae of the cow.

order to produce obstetric anaesthesia, heifers and small cows require a volume of 5–7 ml of 2% lignocaine solution and large cows will need 7–10 ml. The addition to the local anaesthetic of 2% of adrenaline prolongs the period of anaesthesia from $1\frac{1}{2}$ to 3 hours. Some veterinary surgeons maintain that epidural injections may be made more easily into the sacrococcygeal rather than into the first intercoccygeal space.

The technique of epidural injection in the mare is the same but, because the root of the tail is well covered by muscle and fat, the spines of all coccygeal vertebrae are not so easy to locate (Plate 2). Also, owing to the thickness of the tail, a longer needle must be passed to a depth of 4–8 cm. The dose of local anaesthetic for mares of hunter type should not exceed 15 ml. It is absolutely essential to avoid overdosage in the mare, and most scrupu-lous regard must be paid to the pre-injection preparation of the intercoccygeal space.

Epidural injection is occasionally useful in ovine obstetrics. The method of injection is the same as for the cow, a needle 4 cm long and of 18 gauge and quantities of 2–4 ml of local anaesthetic being used.

Epidural anaesthesia is seldom required for obstetric purposes in swine but may be induced by injecting 5 ml of local anaesthetic solution into the *lumbosacral* space. The wings of the ilia are joined by an imaginary transverse line and where this crosses the mid-dorsal line a 10 cm needle is inserted perpendicularly until it strikes the floor of the vertebral canal. The needle is then withdrawn slightly and the injection made. Injection at this site affects the nerves of the lumbrosacral plexus and produces posterior paralysis. A similar technique is used for the bitch; in this species, epidural anaesthesia should be preceded by a sedative or narcotic; about 1 ml of local anaesthetic solution per 2.25 kg of body weight is required.

BITCH

Before resorting to instrumental assistance the use of the finger should be fully exploited. When parts of the fetus have already passed through the pelvic inlet, for instance, it is often possible by insinuating the finger over the occiput, into the intermaxillary space or in front of the fetal pelvis in posterior

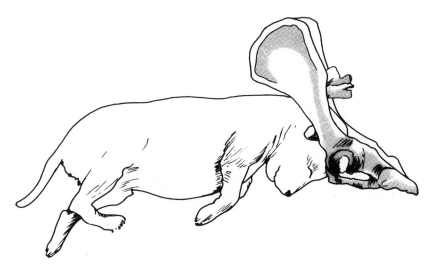

Fig. 12.5 Vertex posture ('butt' presentation) with bilateral shoulder flexion.

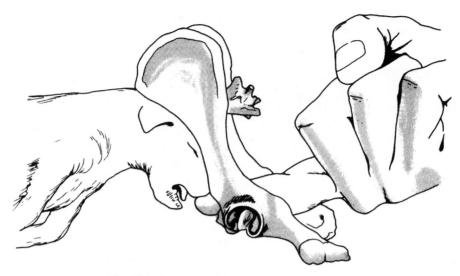

Fig. 12.6 Correction of the vertex posture with the finger.

presentation, to apply sufficient traction to draw these parts into the vulva. Straining on the part of the bitch is of great assistance to one's efforts. Once parts of the fetus are in the vulva, traction delivery is generally simple. In cases of posterior presentation in the ventral position this form of assistance is often effective also. In breech presentation it is generally possible to hook the fingers around the retained limbs and draw them upwards and backwards into the maternal pelvis. In vertex posture it is usually a relatively simple matter to insert the finger beneath the fetal chin and, by drawing it upwards, direct the muzzle into the passage (Figures 12.5 and 12.6). During all these manipulations

it is helpful to fix the position of the fetus in the uterus by gripping it with the left hand through the abdominal wall and to direct the fetus towards the pelvic inlet.

When parts of the fetus have already traversed the pelvic inlet and occupy the vagina, Hobday's vectis is a useful instrument. The vectis is passed into the vagina and, according to the presentation, over the dorsal aspect of the fetal head or pelvis and by pressure downwards engaged behind the occiput or tuber coxae. The index finger is then introduced and pressed upwards into the intermaxillary space or in front of the fetal pelvis and between the opposing grips of the vectis above

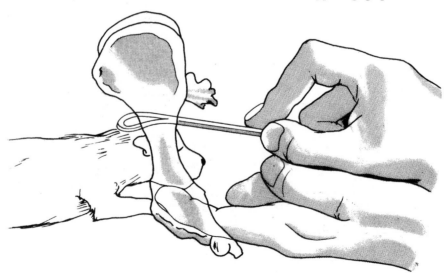

Fig. 12.7 Traction applied to a puppy's head using the vectis and finger.

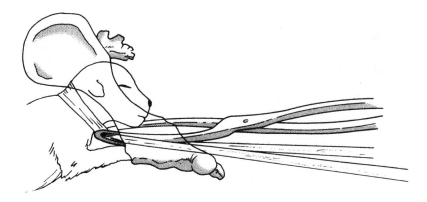

Fig. 12.8 Roberts's snare forceps applied to the fetal neck.

and the finger beneath it is often possible to apply sufficient traction to the fetus to deliver it without injury (Figure 12.7). The method may even be successful in cases in which the forelimbs are retained and the correction of which is difficult because of the presence of the head in the vagina.

In cases of relative oversize in anterior presentation in which the fetus is entirely in the uterus and obstruction is caused by the size of the cranium, Roberts's snare forceps are of value, particularly in small bitches and cats. Such cases may also be associated with retention of the forelimbs. Should the latter be the case it is better to attempt delivery with the posture uncorrected, for the forelegs will cause no greater obstruction lying alongside the chest than they would if extended; moreover, the subsequent traction, applied as it is to the head only, may cause the elbows alongside the head to become impacted at the pelvic inlet. Snare forceps are used as follows: while fixing the fetus at the pelvic brim by holding it through the abdominal wall, the closed forceps carrying the snare are passed into the uterus and over the fetal head until they lie above the neck. The jaws are then opened as widely as possible and depressed downwards until they lie ventral to the neck and then closed. In this way an encircling noose has been applied. By traction on the free ends of the snare the noose is drawn tight and it is held in position by the forceps. Traction is then applied to the forceps and the free ends of the snare (Figure 12.8).

Freak (1948) recommends Rampley's sponge-holding forceps for the application of traction to the living fetus in cases similar to those previously outlined. Using the index finger as a guide to their

application, the forceps are lightly fixed to the upper or lower jaw, or even the whole snout. In the case of posterior presentation they may be applied to a hindlimb until the fetal pelvis is drawn into the maternal inlet and then a more secure hold obtained. Points made by Freak in favour of Rampley's forceps over those of the Hobday type, in relatively simple cases, are: first, they can be applied and fixed by means of the ratchet★ to comparatively small parts of the fetus, and thus they do not increase the total size of the obstructing part when drawing it through the maternal inlet; and, second, consequent on the lightness with which it is possible to apply them, the fetus can be delivered uninjured.

Lateral deviation of the head and nape posture are abnormalities which require special consideration, for the diagnosis may be difficult and attempts to deliver fetuses so presented without correction, even with severe forceps traction, are generally futile, at any rate in the healthy fetus. In lateral deviation, the forelimb on the side opposite to the neck flexion has generally passed through the pelvic inlet (Figure 12.9). Thus, the presence of a single forelimb in the anterior vagina indicates a likelihood of the condition. To verify the diagnosis and also to ascertain the side to which the head is deviated, the fetus must first be repelled forwards. The finger is then directed laterally towards the iliac shaft in order to detect the fetal occiput or ears. In the small bitch this may not be difficult, but in the large one the length of the maternal pelvis and of the fetal neck are often such that it is

★ Care should be exercised in the use of ratchet forceps; there is a great temptation to close the forceps completely. Rampley's forceps without a ratchet are preferable.

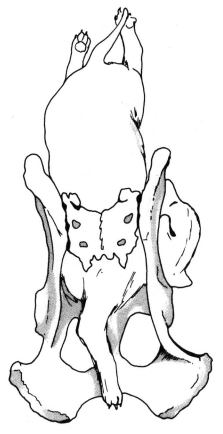

Fig. 12.9 Lateral deviation of the head (shoulder presentation).

impossible to make an accurate diagnosis, let alone correct the condition. In a protracted case it may be impossible to obtain the space in front of the pelvis necessary for exploration with the finger. The fetal fluids have been lost and the uterus has contracted firmly on the fetus, the latter often being enlarged by putrefactive emphysema.

Freak (1948) recommends Rampley's forceps both as an aid to diagnosis and to the correction of downward and lateral deviation of the head. It is proposed to quote her excellent description:

> Breast–head posture: The forceps are of great assistance (to diagnosis) since a light grip may be obtained on one foreleg, if present, or on the neck, raising the fetus sufficiently close into the pelvic inlet for a more complete examination to be made with the finger, when foetal ears may be recognized lying just below the pelvic brim. To correct the posture a light grip should be taken on the skin over the occiput and the foetus slightly repelled. Forceps may be left *in situ*, supported by the finger and thumb, while an attempt

is made with the other hand on the maternal abdominal wall to raise the foetal head above the pelvic brim. Sometimes the forceps grip and repulsion of the foetus are alone sufficient to bring this about, and the finger can then be inserted into the mouth to hold it in position while the forceps are reapplied on the upper jaw. Frequently correction has to be done in stages, obtaining a grip a little lower on the forehead after each repulsion.

Lateral deviation: Forceps are used to assist in the diagnosis of the posture and the side to which the head is deflected. The shoulder of the opposite side may be recognized by the finger, or again, the position of the ears may assist. When this is decided a grip is taken on that side of the head or neck presented and the foetus is repelled diagonally away from the side to which the head is turned. Again the grip and repulsion may need to be replaced, and again, particularly in a small bitch, great assistance is derived from external manipulation assisted by guidance from the finger in the vagina.

Delivery by traction

This method may be employed in cases of oversize when the less drastic methods previously outlined fail. It is used particularly in the case of dead and emphysematous fetuses. The method should always be avoided in the case of a living fetus, for the grip of the forceps generally causes it severe injury. Hobday's forceps are generally employed.

It should always be remembered that caesarean section or, in the case of putrid fetuses, hysterectomy, will carry a better prognosis for the bitch than prolonged attempts at forceps delivery.

In cases requiring traction the whole of the fetus, with the possible exception of limbs, lies in the uterus. Occasionally, in cases of posterior presentation (Figure 12.10) the pelvis and hindlimbs have passed into the pelvic inlet. In these it is best to repel these parts into the uterus before attempting to apply the forceps.

The aim is to obtain a secure grip across the fetal cranium or pelvis so that considerable traction can be applied. The application of the forceps to a limb or the lower or upper jaw is generally futile because the force it is necessary to apply causes either the forceps to slip or the parts to be torn away.

Operation should be carried out under general anaesthesia with the bitch in breast recumbency. The position of the presented fetus is fixed by gripping it through the abdominal wall. The

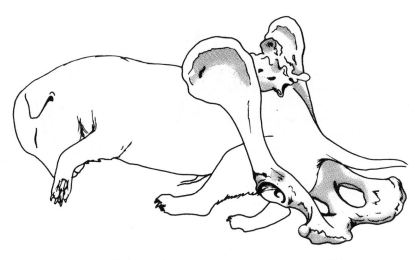

Fig. 12.10 Bilateral hip flexion posture (breech presentation).

closed forceps are introduced into the vulva and directed, at first upwards until they have reached the pelvic floor, then horizontally forwards through the pelvic canal and finally slightly downwards and forwards into the uterus. Here the fetal extremity will be felt beneath. The jaws of the forceps are now opened as widely as possible and again depressed downwards. On closing them it becomes clear from the extent to which the han-

dles are apart that the whole width of a fetal head or pelvis has been gripped. On no account should traction be applied until the operator is satisfied that he or she has a firm grip on the cranium or pelvis (Figure 12.11).

Working in the dark, as the method entails, the operator is always fearful lest the uterine wall has been picked up in addition to the fetus. Fortunately if the forceps are applied within the uterus

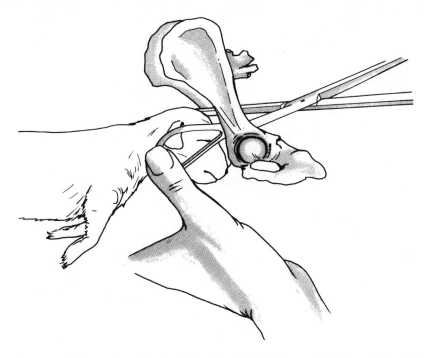

Fig. 12.11 Delivery of a puppy with retention of the forelimbs using Hobday's forceps. While the position of the fetus is fixed through the abdominal wall with the left hand, the forceps are applied to the skull with the right.

in the method described there is little tendency to injury of the maternal soft parts in so doing; nevertheless, as soon as the secured part has been drawn back to a point that can be reached with a finger, the operator will ensure before proceeding that it is the fetus only which is involved.

Steady traction is applied in the upwards and backwards direction until the secured part has passed through the pelvic inlet. From this point delivery is relatively easy. It will be appreciated that there is a limit to the amount of force which can be safely applied, for severe pulling may cause rupture of the vagina at the pelvic brim. Such an accident necessitates immediate laparotomy to remove any fetus(es) and/or to repair the vaginal rent if possible. One author has encountered a case in which such a rupture was followed by progressive passage of the remaining fetuses through it into the abdominal cavity.

In protracted cases in which the fetuses are putrid the application of traction often results in breakage of the fetus, a head or hind parts being torn away. Often in posterior presentation, the fetal trunk is torn away and the head remains in the uterus.

Again in protracted cases in which complete inertia has supervened, attempts must not be made to extract fetuses from the cornua with the forceps, for it is highly probable that by so doing the uterus will be torn. Forceps delivery is only applicable to fetuses the extremity of which has passed into the uterine body.

It cannot be gainsaid that grossly protracted cases should not occur. They are the outcome of ignorance or negligence. It is the duty of the veterinarian to educate the dog-breeding public in the normal course of parturition, to deplore delay, and to carry out the appropriate interference at the proper time.

CAT

Most queens will kitten naturally, with no difficulties and without any need for intervention. If dystocia does occur, it is most likely to be in a queen with only one or two kittens in the litter. Although relative fetal oversize and secondary uterine inertia may contribute to the dystocia, the most important factor may be a failure of fetal endocrine contribution to the initiation of parturition in such cases. Fetal malpresentations do occur but this will not usually prevent their birth.

The decision to intervene during parturition can be very difficult and is compounded by the very variable pattern that parturition can take in cats. Generally, if the queen appears contented, she should be left alone, but the presence of an unpleasant vaginal discharge, which should not be confused with the normal brown pigmented birth fluids, or any signs of illness, may indicate the need for assistance. Oxytocin, at a dosage of up to 5 units, may help, although care is necessary to avoid uterine rupture due to excessive uterine contractions.

REFERENCES

Benesch, F. (1927) *Cornell Vet.*, **14**, 227.
Freak, M. J. (1948) *Vet. Rec.*, **60**, 295.

13

FETAL OVERSIZE IN CATTLE

The clinical diagnosis 'fetal oversize' includes *relative oversize* in which the fetus is of normal dimensions but the maternal pelvis is too small, *absolute oversize* in which the maternal pelvis is normal but the fetus is abnormally large although normal in other respects, and *pathological enlargement* of the fetus; the last may be due to fetal giantism as seen in some forms of prolonged gestation, to fetal dropsy as in the Ayrshire breed and to emphysema of the retained dead fetus. Severe developmental defects such as schistosoma reflexus and double monsters obviously cause serious disproportion at birth but they are usually diagnosed as 'monstrosities'; their delivery will be considered in Chapter 16.

In cases of oversize it may not always be obvious to the obstetrician whether the fetus is too large or the pelvis too small, but the techique of delivery is the same irrespective of the source of the trouble. Fetal oversize may therefore be treated as a single entity. It may be overcome in one of the following ways:

1. The normal expulsive forces may be supplemented by external traction on the fetus. This method is frequently employed by lay attendants and often succeeds. Also in many cases it is resorted to initially by the obstetrician. When this method is used, artificial lubrication of the vagina is often helpful.
2. The diameter of the vulval opening may be increased by episiotomy.
3. The fetus may be removed through an artificial opening made into the dam's abdomen and uterus (laparohysterotomy or caesarean section). In this way, mother and fetus may be saved.
4. The volume of the fetus may be reduced by fetotomy (originally referred to as fetotomy), i.e. dismemberment of its body, and the fetus removed in several parts. Nowadays fetotomy is applied only

when the fetus is already dead, but even then caesarean section may be preferred.

As a guide to deciding which of the foregoing methods to use in a case of oversize the veterinarian should be influenced by the obstetrician's ideal, which is to render the abnormal birth as near to the physiological as possible and to preserve the lives of mother and fetus. In the case of a group of animals where dystocia is being caused by relative fetal oversize, consideration should be given to inducing early parturition in the remainder of the group (see p. 148).

Fetal oversize: anterior presentation

This is probably the commonest type of bovine dystocia. In its simplest form it is often successfully treated by the attendant or stock-owner. It occurs in all breeds but is much more common in Friesians than in other breeds. Heifers are chiefly affected but many cases occur in mature cows; also, gross delay in rendering obstetric aid, with resultant fetal enlargement due to emphysematous decomposition, occurs too frequently in cattle. Often, when the veterinarian arrives, the animal has been in second-stage labour for at least 2 hours and there is a measure of secondary uterine inertia. The allantochorion has ruptured and two forefeet are visible as well as, occasionally, the fetal nose. Difficulty seems to be associated with the birth of the fetal head. In heifers this can be due to a failure of the posterior vagina and vulva to dilate; in adult cows it is often associated with too great a bulk of fetal chest and shoulders at the entrance to the maternal pelvis.

Once the head is expelled the remainder of the calf can usually be delivered, except in the case of calves sired by certain bulls which, at term, have disproportionately large hindquarters. In these cases the head and chest may emerge with relatively little effort, but the calf's hips will not pass into the maternal pelvis. At the initial examination it is difficult to be sure of the degree of oversize. In most cases the disproportion between fetus and birth canal is slight, but gradations of disproportion occur to the most severe form in which the pelvis is so small, or the calf so large, that the fetal head may fail to enter the birth canal. With increasing experience the veterinary surgeon will assess with considerable accuracy the extreme cases which will need fetotomy or caesarean section. In all other cases and, whenever there is any doubt about the possibility of vaginal delivery, the simplest method, namely traction, is tried first. But the plan of action must be tentative, rather than rigid, and when the simple method fails the more complicated procedure is followed, remembering that the outcome in cases of caesarean section will be much worse if the cow and calf have been subjected to prolonged or excessive traction.

Delivery by traction

The vast majority of cases of simple oversize are successfully treated by the application of manual traction to the presenting feet, but birth is greatly expedited by first applying a head snare so that an axial pull may be put on the fetus. For vaginal delivery three sterile snares are required, which should be brought to the case in a sterilizer. The heifer is restrained by tying its head (with a quick-release knot) and by having it held alongside a stall-division, or wall, by an attendant at its flank, who also holds the patient's tail to one side. The vulva, perineum and base of the tail are thoroughly washed from one bucket of water. From a second bucket the obstetrician thoroughly washes his or

her hands and arms and applies to them an obstetric lubricant. A loop is made in the head-snare and this is carried into the vulva where part of the loop is placed in the calf's mouth and the remainder pushed up over the forehead and behind the ears. A simpler alternative which is easier to apply and less stressful to the calf is to push the centre point of a rope snare over the forehead and behind the ears, leaving both ends of the snare outside the vulva. A good axial pull, which also tends to depress the calf's poll ventrally, can be achieved by simultaneous traction on both ends of the snare. Each of the other snares is placed above the fore fetlock of the calf. The head-snare is controlled by one assistant and the foot-snares by another. At first, with the head-rope held taut, traction is applied to one foot-snare with a view to advancing one shoulder at a time through the pelvic entrance (Figure 13.1). Then the other leg is advanced. All three ropes are then pulled on. At all times traction should be synchronous with the expulsive efforts of the cow and, as far as practicable, the initial pulling should be upwards but once the head engages the vulva, the direction of traction should be obliquely downward. After each bout of straining, and with each small advance of the fetus, the veterinarian should ascertain by further examination that delivery is proceeding satisfactorily. Frequent applications of lubricant to the vagina and to the fetal occiput are indicated and the veterinarian should be satisfied with very gradual progress.

Episiotomy. If it is obvious that the vulva is relatively small (as is commonly the case in Friesian heifers) and that further traction on the calf will cause rupture of

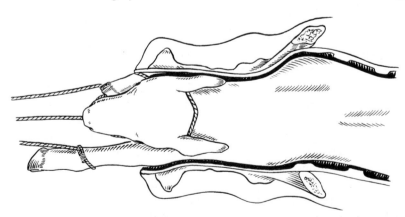

Fig. 13.1 Diagnosis: anterior presentation, dorsal position, extended posture; fetal oversize. Delivery by traction. Alternate traction is first applied to the forelimbs. Note Benesch's head-snare for axial traction.

the vulva and perineum (with subsequent infertility), episiotomy should be performed. Freiermuth (1948) suggested incising, in the shape of an arch and in a dorsolateral direction, the vulval labium in its upper third. Cutting directly upwards into the perineal raphe is contraindicated because, once started, further birth of the calf will cause a traumatic upward extension towards, and sometimes into, the anus. It is preferable to cut both labiae in the manner advised by Freiermuth; the requisite depth of the vulval incisions can be decided only by trial on the basis of the minimum amount to allow delivery. By gentle traction on the fetal head so as to cause firm engagement of the occiput in the vulval orifice, it is easy to ascertain the necessary depth of the incisions. Local infiltration, rather than epidural anaesthesia, should be used so as not to interfere with the maternal expulsive efforts. Immediately after delivery the wounds are repaired by means of mattress sutures, the suture material being passed through all the tissues of the wound except the vulval mucosa.

Birth of the head is facilitated and rupture of the perineum is less likely to occur if, while downward traction is maintained on the head-snare, the obstetrician inserts both hands, 'cups' them over the occiput and presses vigorously downwards. When the fetal head is born, all three ropes may be pulled on as the cow strains and the direction of traction should progressively approach the vertical. Obstruction sometimes occurs as the fetal pelvis engages the pelvic inlet; this is sometimes referred to as 'hip-lock'. At this stage, slight retropulsion and rotation of the calf through an angle of 45° is very helpful. The direction of traction should now be vertically downwards until birth is completed. The calf is attended to so as to free its nostrils of amnion or mucus, and respiration is stimulated. The genital passage of the heifer is explored, first in order to ascertain that another calf is not present and second to make sure that it has sustained no damage. The posterior portion of the allantochorion and attached amnion are left hanging from the vulva. The patient is offered a drink of water and untied and the calf is put towards her head. In the case of impacted hip-lock by a dead fetus where it is found impossible to repel and rotate the calf, Graham (1979) has suggested a method of reducing the fetal diameter so that traction may succeed. He uses a long-handled (75 cm) blunt hook which is passed into the fetal abdomen through an incision made just behind the xiphisternum. The hook is advanced to engage the fetal pelvis and

abrupt traction on it then fractures the pelvic girdle. One or two repetitions of this procedure to cause further fractures and to ensure pelvic collapse may be followed by easy traction delivery. Another method of treating hip-lock in a dead fetus is to make a transverse bisection of the calf in the lumbar region and then to divide the hindquarters by means of a vertical cut, both cuts being made by means of the wire-saw fetotome.

In the case of simple oversize just described, the traction power of two lay attendants, properly directed by the veterinary surgeon, is sufficient. Not infrequently, however, more severe forms of oversize occur in which, following separate advancement of each fetal shoulder into the birth canal, the force of two people pulling on the head and forelegs is found to be insufficient. Where they are available it is now permissible for three attendants to pull on the calf, one pulling on the head-snare and one on each leg-snare. The veterinary surgeon should recheck that the fetus is correctly placed in the birth canal, that the extremities belong to one calf and that there is no developmental abnormality of the fetus apart from oversize. Special attention should be paid to lubrication of the vagina. Traction should coincide with the abdominal contractions of the cow, and the veterinary surgeon should be satisfied with very gradual progress. It is not unusual for a cow to go down when heavy traction is applied; this is not necessarily a disadvantage, provided that she does not fall awkwardly and injure herself. In fact, with the patient in lateral recumbency, traction may be applied to better advantage. In these circumstances also, where adequate lay help is not available, a pulley block and tackle may be used. The pulley block is fastened to a fixed point behind the cow and the rope is attached to the calf's feet. One assistant controls the pulley rope and the other pulls on the head-snare. The employment of pulleys must be very closely supervised. Obviously it is not easy to make the necessary adjustments in the direction of traction when pulleys are employed. Provided, however, that the mechanical advantage is kept in mind and that the sum of the force exerted does not exceed that of four people, then on remote hill farms, where lay help is often scarce, their use is justified. Mechanical calf extractors which have come into general use in several countries are the HK calf puller and the Vink calving jack (see Figures 12.2 and 12.3, pp. 230 and 231).

The mechanical advantage is derived from a lever and ratchet and it is so designed that alternate traction may be applied to the forefeet. Experienced obstetricians regard these appliances as the most useful and humane mechanical aid to bovine delivery that is available.

The HK calf puller is used by attaching snares to the calf's legs and, in anterior presentation, the head. The 'rump bar' of the puller is then placed against the cow's perineum, and the snares are attached to the ratchet. Moving the handle backwards and forwards causes the assembly to move along the pole away from the cow, thus pulling the calf out. Using this device, considerable force, equivalent to the pulling power of six people, can be applied. Its disadvantages are:

1. The amount of force which in unskilled hands can be applied.
2. The fact that the pull is continuous and ungiving, which may lead to damage of maternal soft tissues. (In natural birth the calf would be advanced some way with each contraction, and then go back a little before the next contraction pushes it even further.)
3. The fact that the direction of pull has to be at least slightly down towards the udder. If it is horizontal or away from the udder then the rump bar merely slips down the perineum away from the vulva when traction is applied. This means it is very difficult to apply force in the same direction as the expulsion forces of the cow. Ideally, force should be applied in a slightly upward direction until the calf's head is within the pelvis, then in a horizontal direction until the calf's head and chest have been delivered and, finally, in a progressively more downward direction until the calf's hips have been born.

The third disadvantage has been overcome in a more recent design of the calf puller, the Vink calving jack. This has a rump frame which fits around the tail head and vulva of the cow, allowing traction to be applied in the direction chosen by the obstetrician.

If after 5 minutes of judicious traction by three attendants no progress is made the veterinary surgeon must resort to a caesarean operation or fetotomy. If the calf is alive, caesarean section is indicated; the technique is described in Chapter 20. If, as the result of prolonged second-stage labour, the calf is now dead, the caesarean opera-

tion may still be used and will give a high percentage of maternal recovery, but in occasional cases it may be simpler for the obstetrician and possibly better for the subsequent fertility of the cow if fetotomy is used. There are cases where it is difficult to assess whether a calf is alive or dead. If there is any question, the calf should be given the benefit of the doubt. If certain of success by the employment of limited fetotomy such as the removal of a forelimb, or a forelimb together with the head and neck, this would be the method of choice for the single-handed veterinary surgeon in dealing with an oversized dead fetus. Unfortunately, it not infrequently happens that, having embarked on fetotomy the obstetrician finds that total dismemberment will be necessary to effect delivery. Because of this difficulty in assessing the amount of fetotomy required and the knowledge that total fetotomy is a tedious and arduous task, there is an increasing tendency for veterinary surgeons to resort to caesarean section in cases of disproportion where the fetus cannot be delivered by reasonable traction.

The technique of fetotomy for severe fetal oversize in extended anterior presentation will now be described. The method used involves the removal of one or sometimes two forelimbs, with a view to reducing the circumference of the fetal chest. If the head is likely seriously to impede the proposed manipulations it may be returned to the uterus; failing this, it may first be removed (Figure 13.2) but it must be understood that the head is not itself the cause of trouble in dystocia due to absolute oversize.

Subcutaneous fetotomy: removal of a forelimb

A foreleg may be removed by subcutaneous or percutaneous fetotomy. In either case, posterior epidural anaesthesia is employed. The simpler method, which will now be described, is subcutaneous removal, for which the essential instrument is a fetotomy knife. When both forelegs are equally accessible it is immaterial which is removed, but the right-handed operator will find it easier to perform fetotomy on the left foreleg of the calf. This leg is snared — around the pastern rather than above the fetlock — and sustained traction applied to it by one assistant. The obstetrician makes a small incision with a scalpel into the skin in front of the fetlock joint. Into this 'nick' the beak of Roberts's fetotomy knife is inserted, and a longitudinal

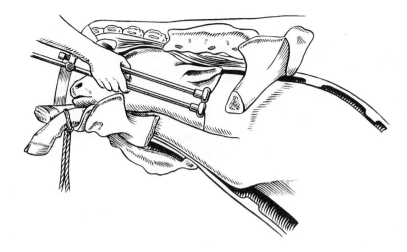

Fig. 13.2 Diagnosis: as in Figure 13.1. Delivery by fetotomy. Amputation of the head using Thygesen's wire-saw fetotome.

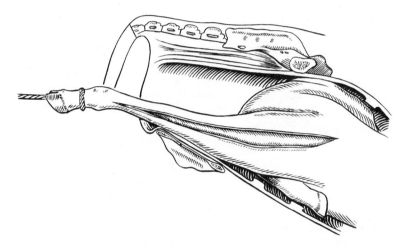

Fig. 13.3 Diagnosis: as in Figure 13.1. The head has been returned to the uterus. Delivery by fetotomy. Subcutaneous removal of the extended forelimb. State 1: the skin has been incised from the fetlock to the scapula, using Roberts's knife.

incision is made up the front of the limb from the pastern to the scapular cartilage (Figure 13.3).

The knife is now laid aside, and the second step in the procedure is literally the 'skinning' of the limb *in situ* (Figure 13.4). This operation requires strong fingers, but with diligent application it may be completed in about 10 minutes. (The separation of the skin from the muscles lying over the scapula completes this second step.)

The third step involves the division of the adductor muscles. This is conveniently done by reintroducing Roberts's knife, and, by vigorous probing with the beak of the instrument, the muscle mass is separated into several 'strings'; then each of these, in turn, is engaged and severed by the knife.

The fourth step (Figure 13.5) is to disarticulate the fetlock joint so that the digit is left connected to the detached skin of the metacarpus. A snare is then attached to the cannon-bone, and, in order to get a more secure hold, an additional half-hitch is put on above the first loop.

The shank of the snare, with traction bars, is then handed to two attendants, and the final step in the operation consists in avulsion of the denuded forelimb by the forcible traction of the two assistants while the operator applies counter-force to the front of the fetus. In this way the remaining muscle attachments to the top of the scapula are broken and the limb comes away.

In many cases the removal of the one forelimb gives a sufficient reduction in fetal diameter to

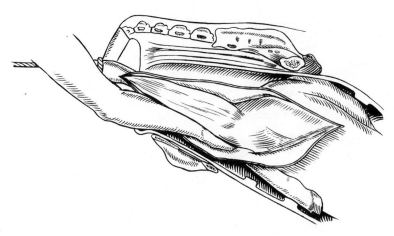

Fig. 13.4 Diagnosis: as in Figure 13.1. Subcutaneous removal of the extended forelimb. Stage 2: finger dissection of the skin around the leg and extending as high as possible in the scapular region.

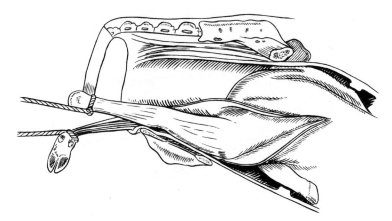

Fig. 13.5 Diagnosis: as in Figure 13.1. Subcutaneous removal of the extended forelimb. Stage 3: after the attachments of the pectoral muscles in the axilla have been broken down and the metacarpophalangeal joint disarticulated, traction is applied to the denuded limb. Note that the foot is still attached to the skin.

allow delivery. The principles of traction previously described are applied and in this case the foot and skin of the amputated limb afford a safe hold for a snare. Should delivery not be possible after this operation, the other foreleg must be removed in the same way, after which moderate traction is usually successful. Occasionally, after removal of one or both forelimbs — and despite partial rotation of the fetus — its hindquarters become locked at the pelvic inlet. Now the calf should be withdrawn as far as possible, and the protruding part of the trunk completely severed. The fetal abdomen is eviscerated, following which one of the hindlegs must be removed. There are two ways of doing this, and the one chosen will depend largely on the mobility of the retained extremity. If it is possible, the posterior part of

the calf should be repelled and one of the hindlimbs brought forward with the aid of a snare; the limb is then removed by subcutaneous fetotomy (presently to be described). If it is not possible to grasp the limb and bring it forward it must be amputated in the following way. Using a direct-cutting fetotomy knife, such as Unsworth's, an incision is made over the hip joint of the leg to be removed. The muscles lateral to the femoral head are also divided and the upper extremity of the femur is isolated. Around this a snare is passed and by vigorous abrupt traction the teres ligament is broken and the articular head freed from the acetabulum. The snare loop is then made secure below the great trochanter and sustained traction applied. This causes the leg to be drawn out from its skin; difficulty occurs over the os calcis but a few strokes of the knife frees this part also. The hind digit should be left attached to the skin and the leg disarticulated at the fetlock joint. After one of the hindlimbs is removed, the remainder of the posterior part of the fetus can be withdrawn by traction through the medium of the double hook — which is attached to the coapted skin of the severed trunk — and the digit and skin of the amputated limb. Amputation of both hindlimbs is rarely needed.

In cases where hip-lock occurs after partial fetotomy of the front extremity, Graham's (1979) method of causing fetal pelvic collapse should be considered as an alternative to further dismemberment of the fetus.

Percutaneous fetotomy

In the opinion of many obstetricians, the delivery of an absolutely oversized calf may be more expeditiously accomplished by percutaneous fetotomy, that is, by means of the wire-saw tubular fetotome. For ease of sterilization the model preferred is the Swedish modification of Thygesen's instrument. Reliable wire, safe handgrips, a wire introducer — such as Schriever's — and a threader are required. Percutaneous fetotomy of an oversized calf in anterior presentation will now be described.

The first operation is the removal, in one piece, of the fetal head, neck and one forelimb (Figure 13.6). To do this the fetotome wire must be looped around the neck and forelimb and pushed back on one side so as to lie behind the posterior angle of the scapula where a deep incision is made with Unsworth's knife to accommodate the wire. The head of the instrument is brought up to the base of

the neck on the side opposite to the foreleg being removed. With the wire loop correctly placed, the section is very easily completed by an assistant who makes long sawing strokes, so as to use the maximum length of available wire. The detached segment of fetus is carefully drawn out of the birth canal. An attempt is now made to deliver the remainder of the calf by traction; a snare is placed on the intact limb and, with the aid of the double hook, another point of traction is available on the exposed lower, cervical vertebral column. If birth is not yet possible, the calf is repelled and the fetotome wire is looped around the trunk of the calf with the head of the instrument laterally, and as far back as possible, in the dorsolumbar region (Figure 13.7). Sawing is continued until the vertebral column is severed, when the anterior part of the calf may be delivered. The remainder of the abdomen is eviscerated, and the next step is to bisect, in the sagittal plane, the hind extremity. To do this, the introducer, with wire attached, is passed over the dorsal aspect of the sacrum and down behind the perineum, where the hand, passed in under the calf, reaches it, pulls it out and completes the loop. The head of the instrument is placed against the fetal spine (Figure 13.8) and the hindquarters divided by direct sawing; then each of the halves can be withdrawn in turn by means of the double hook.

In comparing the facility with which an excessively large calf may be removed by subcutaneous or percutaneous fetotomy, it must be clearly appreciated that the troublesome part of the percutaneous method is the correct placing and retention

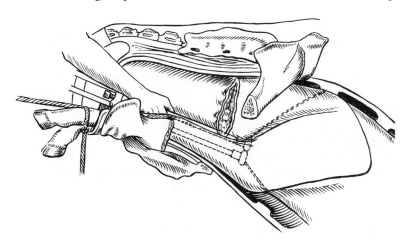

Fig. 13.6 Diagnosis: as in Figure 13.1. Delivery by percutaneous fetotomy. Amputation of the forelimb and neck after removal of the head (as in Figure 13.2). It is sometimes possible to remove the head, neck and forelimb in one operation.

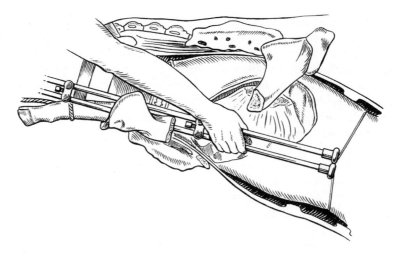

Fig. 13.7 Diagnosis: as in Figure 13.1. Delivery by percutaneous fetotomy. Transverse division through the trunk after removal of the head and forelimb. Note that if the base of the neck had been removed with the forelimb, as in Figure 13.6, the operation would have been simplified.

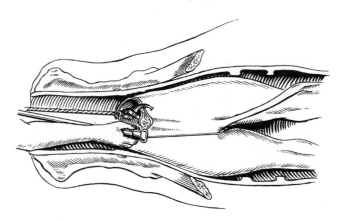

Fig. 13.8 Diagnosis: as in Figure 13.1. Delivery by percutaneous fetotomy. Final stage of total fetotomy: longitudinal division of the hindparts.

of the wire. Given strong wire, the actual sawing presents no difficulty. Occasionally, the two methods may be advantageously combined, e.g. the subcutaneous procedure for the forelimb(s) and the wire-saw fetotome for the head, trunk and hindlimbs. Many veterinary surgeons now prefer caesarean section to total fetotomy. One cannot generalize on which method is preferable, but the subsequent health and fertility of the cow should figure prominently in the reckoning.

Fetal oversize: posterior presentation

The capacity of the fetus to survive obstructive dystocia is diminished by posterior presentation; such cases therefore require prompt attention. Because of the abruptly presenting buttocks and contrary direction of the fetal hair, a posteriorly presented fetus is more difficult to deliver than a comparable one presented anteriorly. The retroverted tail also may be an impediment.

When confronted with such a dystocia the obstetrician should first attempt to assess the degree of disparity between the fetus and birth canal. Where oversize is slight, delivery by traction should first be tried.

Delivery by traction
The hindfeet are usually visible at the vulva, and to them snares are applied above the fetlock joints. It

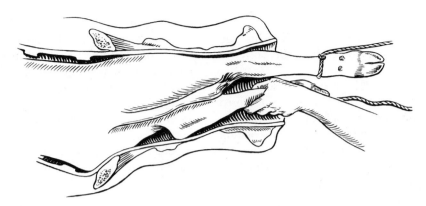

Fig. 13.9 Diagnosis: posterior presentation, dorsal position, extended posture; fetal oversize. Delivery by traction. Alternate traction on the hindlimbs.

should be ascertained that the fetal tail is not retroverted. Epidural anaesthesia is not required, but in delayed cases fetal fluid supplements are essential. With one leg repelled as far as possible (Figure 13.9) the other is pulled on so as to bring its stifle over the pelvic brim. The repelled limb is similarly dealt with. In this way a smaller fetal diameter is presented at the pelvic inlet and, with this simple manoeuvre, traction may succeed. If during traction the fetal pelvis becomes 'jammed' in the birth canal, the calf should be repelled a little, rotated through 45° and again pulled on. This latter manipulation, which brings the greater diameter of the fetus into the largest pelvic dimension, is often successful; it may be accomplished by means of Cämmerer's torsion fork or Kühn's crutch, or by simply bending the protruding metatarsi and using them as levers in a rotary manner. There is a misunderstanding, particularly among farmers, that calves in posterior presentation need to be pulled out very rapidly, otherwise they will die. One must remember that the calf's life will not be compromised until its umbilical cord becomes trapped against the maternal pelvis. In practical terms, therefore, traction should be slow and controlled until such time as the calf's tail head and anus begin to emerge from the cow's vulva. Once this point is reached, delay should be avoided. If the hindquarters can be delivered the forequarters usually follow, but there are exceptions and they will be considered when discussing total fetotomy in posterior presentation.

In cases of posterior presentation where judicious traction by four attendants does not succeed, the fetus must be removed by caesarean section or fetotomy. If the calf is alive, caesarean hysterotomy is indicated. In the case of an immovable, dead fetus there is a choice about which it is difficult to generalize, but if there is obviously gross oversize a laparotomy is preferable. In many instances of medium oversized and dead fetuses, however, it may be easier to remove one limb, for this relatively simple operation often makes birth possible, and this fetotomy will now be described. The presenting legs can be removed by subcutaneous or percutaneous methods, and the former will be described first.

Subcutaneous removal of the hindlimb

Posterior epidural anaesthesia is induced and a 'nick' made just above the fetlock on the posterior aspect of the extended fetal leg. Into this is placed the 'beak' of Roberts's knife, and with it an incision is made from the fetlock up the back of the limb to the anterior gluteal region. The skin is separated all around the leg and the muscles above the hip joint, as well as the adductor muscles, are divided. The femoral head is detached from the acetabulum by introducing a traction bar underneath the Achilles tendon and by forcibly rotating the limb laterally. The skin is then cut sufficiently around the fetlock joint to give scope for disarticulation, and a rope snare is placed over the freed end of the metatarsus. Sustained traction on the snare by two assistants, with retropulsion of the calf by the obstetrician, usually causes avulsion of the denuded limb.

Removal of the one leg followed by traction on its foot — connected to the torso by the skin of the leg — and on the other limb often results in extraction of the calf. If it does not, then the other hindlimb must be similarly removed. This will allow complete delivery or birth of the posterior half of the calf.

Should the forequarters become obstructed at the pelvic inlet, then further fetotomy is required as follows. As much of the calf as possible is withdrawn from the vulva and amputated. Evisceration is now carried out. The remainder is repelled and then, with Unsworth's knife, an incision is made in the skin over the scapula cartilage, and the muscles which connect the scapula to the spine are divided. By blunt dissection the upper end of the shoulder blade is isolated and to it Krey's hooks are fastened and traction applied. In this way the limb is drawn out of its skin as far as the fetlock joint, at which point it is disarticulated and removed. The digit, with skin attached, together with Krey's hooks gripping the thoracic vertebral column, serve as traction points for extraction of the remainder of the calf. In rare cases, before the anterior half can be withdrawn, the other forelimb must be removed.

Percutaneous removal of the hindlimb

Percutaneous fetotomy in posterior presentation is most conveniently performed with the tubular wire-saw Danish fetotome. The instrument is threaded, the wire loop placed over one foot and passed up the limb so that laterally it lies anterior to the external angle of the ilium where a cut in the skin, previously made with Unsworth's knife helps to retain it. The head of the instrument is placed lateral to the anus, and the tail of the calf must be included in the loop, otherwise, during sawing, the wire will slip down the limb and the section will be made through the distal third, instead of through the upper extremity, of the femur. The severed limb is removed. Traction is then applied to the calf by means of the Krey–Schottler hook attached to the perineum or with the aid of Obermayer's anal hook passed over the calf's pubic brim. If delivery is still impossible the other hindleg must be removed and the fetus withdrawn as far as possible. If the calf cannot now be removed completely then its trunk must be bisected by means of the wire loop, the division being made as far forward as possible. One, or if necessary both, forelimbs are afterwards amputated by passing the wire, with the aid of Schriever's introducer, forwards between the neck and foreleg and then

reaching for the introducer underneath the calf; the wire is withdrawn, the threading of the instrument completed and its 'head' passed up the severed end of the vertebral column where the section may be made by sawing. The severed limb may be brought out by attaching to it Krey's hook. An attempt is again made to withdraw the anterior portion of the calf and in most cases this is now possible. In the exceptional case the other foreleg must be removed in like manner.

FETAL OVERSIZE IN OTHER ANIMALS

Mare

Disproportion as a cause of dystocia is uncommon in horses. Apart from being more urgent, the occasional case of relative oversize is treated on similar lines to the bovine case with the exception that because of the late osseous union of the fetal skull, only limited traction should be applied to the fetal head. Although prolonged gestation is not uncommon, excessively large fetuses are rare in horses. When the fetus is alive, the caesarean operation is the first consideration and, with the increasing experience of recent years, it is now preferred to total fetotomy for a dead fetus.

Ewe

Oversize is a common cause of dystocia in ewes carrying single lambs. Ewes of the smaller breeds are often mated to larger rams, and although the fetal size is controlled to a large extent by the dam, bulky body features derived from the ram such as large head and coarseness of shoulders and buttocks often cause trouble. Most cases are successfully overcome by the shepherd applying traction to the forelegs. More severe cases may be brought to the veterinary surgery, where they may be conveniently treated as described for the cow. Where judicious traction — using fine snares, copious lubricants, and with strict regard to asepsis — does not succeed, caesarean section or fetotomy may be employed. Where the fetus is dead, and this is frequently so in cases seen by the veterinary surgeon, fetotomy is often indicated. In this species the subcutaneous methods of limb removal are very easily carried out, but the percutaneous techniques, using the wire-saw protected by Glattli's spinal tubes, or Persson's chain-saw, are quite practicable.

Sow

Although fetal oversize may occur in the multiparous species when pregnant with an abnormally small litter, it cannot be treated by fetotomy; if traction by hand, snare or forceps fails, then hysterotomy is indicated.

REFERENCES

Freiermuth, G. J. (1948) *J. Amer. Vet. Med. Assn,* **113**, 231.
Graham, J. A. (1979) *J. Amer. Vet. Med. Assn,* **174**, 169.

14

POSTURAL DEFECTS OF ANTERIOR PRESENTATION IN CATTLE

Next in frequency to oversize as causes of dystocia in ruminants are the postural defects, of which the commonest are carpal flexion and lateral deviation of the head. All postural defects are readily rectified by manipulation if treatment is forthcoming in early second-stage labour. But in neglected cases associated with secondary uterine inertia, loss of fetal fluids and a dead, emphysematous fetus, tightly enclosed by the uterus, very serious dystocia may occur, for which fetotomy or caesarean section may be required.

The mechanics of postural rectification are extremely simple; the secret of success lies in an appreciation of the value of retropulsion. Except for dystocia of short duration, this means that

epidural anaesthesia is needed. Hence, once the posture has been corrected, the cow must then be delivered by traction, for the accessory expulsive forces are now in abeyance and the uterus may still be inert. The obstetrician with relatively thin arms may have a significant advantage in correcting postural defects, in that it is often possible for both arms to be used inside the cow simultaneously — one to push and the other to pull.

Abnormalities of posture will be considered in series — beginning with the simple and going on to the complicated — in each example.

Carpal flexion posture

One or both forelimbs may be affected. In the unilateral case the flexed carpus is engaged at the pelvic inlet; the other forefoot may be visible at the vulva. The simple recent case requires retropulsion at the fetal head or shoulder: the retained foot is then grasped and, as the carpus is pushed upwards,

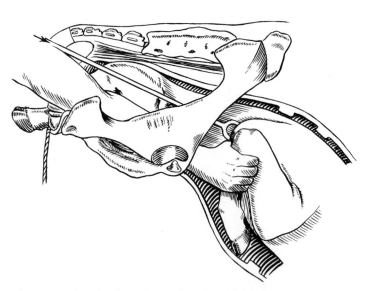

Fig. 14.1 Diagnosis: anterior presentation, dorsal position, unilateral carpal flexion posture. Correction using the hand and a crutch.

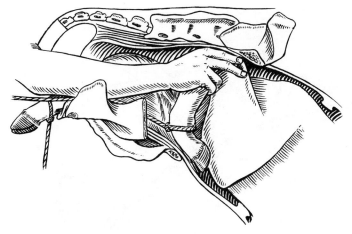

Fig. 14.2 Diagnosis: as in Figure 14.1. Correction using the hand and a digital snare.

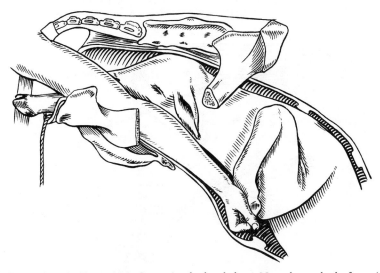

Fig. 14.3 Diagnosis: as in Figure 14.1. Correction by hand alone. Note the method of grasping the foot.

the foot is carried outwards and finally brought forwards in an arc over the pelvic brim and extended alongside the other limb (Figure 14.1). More difficult cases require a snare attached to the retained fetlock to help extend the limb (Figure 14.2). The fetal foot should always be carried over the pelvic brim in the cupped hand of the obstetrician (Figure 14.3). An obstinate case may require the introduction of copious warm water to help mobilize the calf. Rarely, in very protracted dystocia and cases of ankylosis, the limb cannot be extended and then it must be cut through at the carpus by means of the wire-saw fetotome.

Incomplete extension of the elbow(s)

This case is diagnosed on inspection, the digits emerging at the same level as the fetal muzzle instead of being well advanced beyond it. Usually, without the need of epidural anaesthesia, the head is repelled and each limb pulled in turn in an obliquely upward direction so as to lift the olecranon process over the maternal pelvic brim. Delivery is accomplished by traction on the head and both forelimbs as already described in the chapter on fetal oversize.

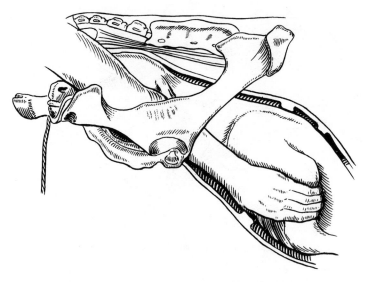

Fig. 14.4 Diagnosis: anterior presentation, dorsal position, unilateral shoulder flexion posture (complete retention of the forelimb). First stage of correction by hand.

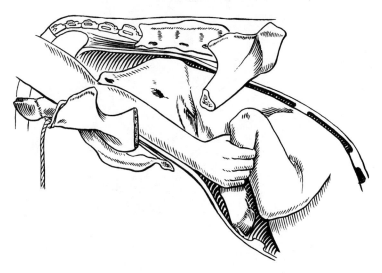

Fig. 14.5 Diagnosis: as in Figure 14.4. Second stage of correction by hand.

Shoulder flexion posture; complete retention of the forelimb(s)

This type of dystocia may be unilateral or bilateral. The diagnosis of bilateral retention is usually obvious by observing that the head is partly or completely born, but there is no sign of the feet. (In bilateral carpal flexion the head cannot be advanced so far.) In a 'roomy' cow with a small full-term or premature calf the dystocia may be overcome by traction in the abnormal posture, but in such cases, unless there has been much delay, postural rectification is usually easy and should be resorted to.

Retropulsion is a very obvious necessity, and if the extruded head is much swollen, the calf being dead, it should be amputated outside the vulva. To this end, Krey's hooks are placed in the orbits and traction applied so as to bring the head beyond the vulva and allow disarticulation at the occipitoatlantal joint. Following this, as the fetus is repelled, the retained forelimbs tend to come forwards; the calf's forearm is then grasped and the defect is easily converted into carpal flexion posture and relieved accordingly (Figures 14.4 and 14.5).

In the more difficult case the limb must be snared, at first proximally, and then the noose passed down until it lies above the fetlock, the shank being placed from before backwards between the claws so as to flex the fetlock and pastern when traction is applied to it. The digits are held in the cupped hand and the carpus forced upwards while an assistant, pulling on the snare, helps the operator to bring the foot over the pelvic brim. In a delayed case such a manoeuvre may be impossible and then fetotomy of the limb is undertaken by the percutaneous or subcutaneous method, of which the percutaneous technique, now to be described, is simpler.

Percutaneous removal of retained forelimb

Epidural anaesthesia is indicated and, if it has not already been done, extravulval decapitation is now essential. At this stage it is wise to employ fetal fluid substitute which is fed into the uterus by gravity flow from an elevated funnel attached to a rubber delivery tube, whose end is controlled by a hand in the uterus. The fetus is now repelled and the fetotomy wire, protruding from one tube of the fetotome and fitted with Schriever's introducer, is passed in dorsally above the neck and down between the thorax and retained limb whence it is sought below by the hand introduced ventrally to the fetal scapula. The introducer and wire are drawn outwards, and the threading of the fetotome completed. The head of the instrument is passed into the birth canal so that finally it rests dorsal to the posterior angle of the scapula. Some force is required to maintain it thus while the muscles which attach the limb to the trunk and the skin at the base of the neck are severed by sawing. The detached portion is extracted by means of Krey's hooks. An attempt should again be made to extend the other retained limb and, this being possible, traction on it, and on the neck — through the medium of Krey's hooks — should result in delivery. Alternatively, the fetus may be withdrawn without extension of the other leg. If both these attempts fail, then the other limb must also be removed, the subsequent procedure being that described for absolute fetal oversize.

Subcutaneous removal of retained forelimb

The operation of subcutaneous detachment of the retained forelimb again requires prior removal of the head so as to allow sufficient space for the hand and arm to carry in Unsworth's knife, which is used to divide the skin and muscles that connect the dorsal border of the scapula to the trunk. Following this division, vigorous blunt dissection is employed in order to expose the upper part of the scapula. To this isolated portion either a snare, or Krey's hook, is attached and traction applied. The operation is expedited by further vigorous incision of the adductor (pectoral) muscles. In this way the limb is pulled out of its skin until the fetlock joint is exposed, at which point disarticulation is performed and the limb removed leaving the foot attached to the skin of the limb. The fetus is now withdrawn by traction on the intact limb and on the foot and skin of the detached limb. If necessary, additional traction may be produced by fastening Krey's hooks to the exposed end of the vertebral column.

Lateral deviation of the head

The head may be displaced to either side, and this constitutes one of the commonest types of ruminant dystocia. When treated in early second-stage labour it is easily rectified by hand, without recourse to epidural anaesthesia. The lubricated hand is introduced and, when the provoked

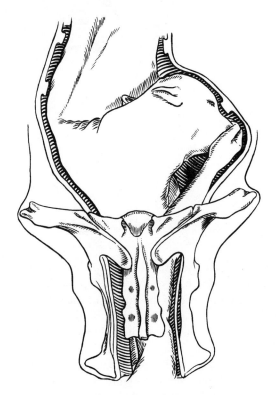

Fig. 14.6 Diagnosis: anterior presentation, dorsal position, lateral deviation of the head. Correction by hand.

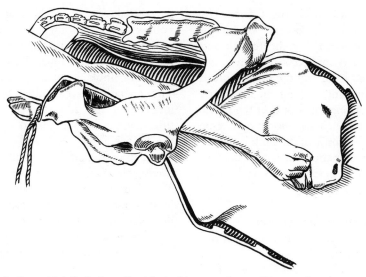

Fig. 14.7 Diagnosis: as in Figure 14.6. Preliminary 'hooking' of the commissure of the mouth, prior to grasping the muzzle of the calf.

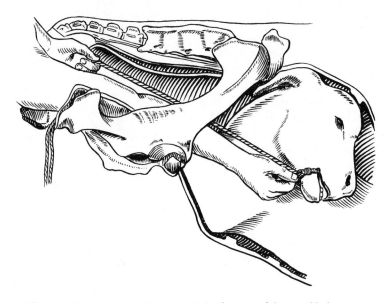

Fig. 14.8 Diagnosis: as in Figure 14.6. Application of the mandibular snare.

straining has ceased, the fetus is repelled by pressing forwards at the base of its neck. The hand is then quickly transferred to the muzzle of the calf, which is firmly grasped and brought round through an arc until the nose is in line with the birth canal (Figure 14.6). In a more inaccessible case the muzzle may be reached after preliminary traction on the commissure of the mouth (Figure 14.7) or on the mandible (Figure 14.8). A head-snare and fore-limb-snares are now affixed, and traction, synchro-nously applied with the cow's expulsive efforts, leads to delivery.

In more protracted cases of head displacement, with greater loss of fetal fluid and with the uterus contracted on the calf, it is more difficult to rectify the posture. Epidural anaesthesia is indicated, followed by the instillation of fetal fluid substitute; this renders the calf more buoyant. A special head cord, of smaller calibre than those used on the limbs, is carried in as a running noose and slipped over the mandible of the calf, where it is tightened, and the shank of the snare is handed to an assistant (Figure 14.8). The operator reintroduces his hand, grasps the calf's muzzle and, as he manipulates it round, directs traction by the assistant. It is obviously important that this head-snare should be passed around the greater curvature of the neck to the mandible. Should the snare inadvertently be passed across the concavity of the neck curvature to the mandible, pulling on it will accentuate, rather than relieve, the displacement.

In very obstinate delayed cases of lateral deviation with a dead fetus and in the occasional congenital rigid curvature of the neck called 'wryneck', correction is impossible and decapitation is required. This is conveniently performed by means of the wire-saw fetotome, the chain or wire being passed in on an introducer around the flexure of the neck. The severed head is first removed, and the remainder of the calf withdrawn by applying traction on the forelimbs by means of snares and to the neck through the medium of Krey's hook.

Downward displacement of the head

This is an uncommon type of dystocia in cattle. It usually takes the form of 'vertex posture' in which the calf's nose abuts on the pubic brim and the brow is directed into the pelvis (Figure 14.9). The more severe varieties of downward deviation of the head, namely 'nape presentation' and 'breast–head'

posture — in which the head is flexed vertically between the forelimbs — are rare in cattle; when present, they have usually been caused by traction on the limbs before the head had extended.

Provided sufficient retropulsion can be achieved, vertex posture is easily overcome. Neglected cases may require epidural anaesthesia and fetal fluid supplement. The obstetrician repels the calf's forehead by means of a thumb while lifting the mandible over the pelvic brim with the fingers.

More severe degrees of downward displacement of the head are treated in a similar way, but if difficulty is experienced one of the forelimbs should be replaced into the uterus. This gives room for the head to be first rotated laterally and then brought upwards and forwards over the pelvic brim. The leg is then extended and the fetus removed by traction. In very difficult cases it may be advantageous to replace both forelimbs into the uterus. Casting the cow and placing her in dorsal recumbency may greatly facilitate extension of the fetal head. Another alternative is to rotate the fetus, by means of Cämmerer's torsion fork applied to its legs, into a temporary ventral position from which the head may be more easily extended. When manipulative correction fails, fetotomy may be practised; either the head is removed in nape presentation or one forelimb is sectioned in breast–head posture.

In difficult cases of downward deviation in which the calf is still alive, caesarean section has much to commend it.

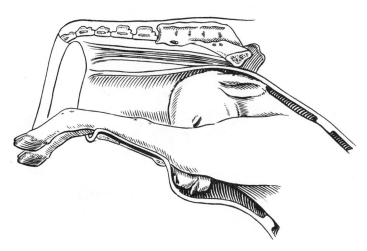

Fig. 14.9 Diagnosis: anterior presentation, dorsal posture, downward displacement of the head ('vertex' posture).

POSTURAL DEFECTS OF ANTERIOR PRESENTATION IN HORSES

Although showing a lower incidence in horses than in cattle, defects of limb posture cause more serious dystocia in mares than in cows. This is due to the severe pelvic impaction that is consequent upon the mare's very strong expulsive efforts and to the longer limbs of foals. In order to prevent rupture of the uterus, or vagina, correction of posture must be done with the utmost care. Where impaction is severe it may be possible to repel the fetus; traction without correction of posture may then be attempted; it has a better chance of success than in the cow. The obstetrician is ever mindful of the urgency of equine dystocia, but if at the outset an impacted fetus is found to be already dead, the advantage of narcotizing the mare and placing her in lateral or dorsal recumbency should be considered.

Carpal flexion posture

The principles of correction are the same as for the cow. Adequate retropulsion of the fetus, in order to make sufficient room for the extension of the longer limbs of the foal, is most essential, and a foot-snare is a great aid to manual extension of the limb. During the final extension of the carpus the birth canal must be protected from injury by holding the fetal foot in the cupped hand.

There is a tendency for a foal in carpal flexion posture to become impacted in the maternal pelvis (Figure 14.10); the procedure required will depend on the degree of impaction, on the relative sizes of the fetus and birth canal and on the duration of second-stage labour. Retropulsion of the fetus, followed by extension of the carpus, should always be attempted. Where there is obviously insufficient room for extension the flexed carpus may be pushed forwards into the uterus so that the retained limb lies under the fetal abdomen. Moderate traction applied to the other limb and to the fetal head then often succeeds without injury to the mare. Where it is found impossible to relieve the impaction there are two alternatives for the veterinary surgeon: either to attempt traction without rectification or to section the leg through the carpal joint. The first alternative will be tried on a live foal and when the flexed carpus is well advanced into the maternal pelvis. In addition to snares on the head and the other extended limb, traction is applied to a snare placed around the flexed carpus. Fetotomy for irreducible carpal flexion is easily effected by means of the wire-saw fetotome, section being made through the carpal joint. A snare is then placed above the carpus, and the fetus is removed by pulling on this as well as on the other limb and head.

In the case of irreducible *bilateral* carpal flexion, affecting a normally developed full-term foal, traction should not be attempted. It is unlikely that the foal will still be alive so that fetotomy is indicated, one or two of the carpal joints being sectioned as required.

Incomplete extension of the elbow
This is uncommon. The treatment is that described for the same condition in cattle.

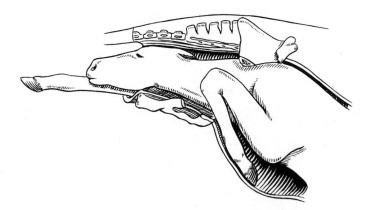

Fig. 14.10 Diagnosis: anterior presentation, dorsal position, unilateral carpal flexion posture in the mare. Note the tendency to impaction in this malposture.

Shoulder flexion posture

One or both forelimbs may be retained. The more slender head and longer neck of the foal give more room in the maternal pelvis for the hand and arm of the obstetrician than is available in the same type of bovine dystocia; but the retained limb is further away and it is consequently more difficult to pass a snare around the forearm. Copious fetal fluid supplement should be infused and vigorous retropulsion applied. If a snare cannot be passed directly around the upper forearm an attempt is made to bring the forearm nearer by engaging it with Blanchard's long flexible hook or by means of Krey's hooks. Once the forearm has been snared it should be possible to advance the limb and to convert the posture into one of carpal flexion and then to proceed accordingly.

When it is found to be impossible to extend the limb, traction may be tried. This often succeeds, but the foal is usually dead. Rather than use inordinate force, it is preferable to remove the retained forelimb by means of the wire-saw fetotome as described for the cow. When both forelimbs are retained and attempts at correction fail, traction may be tried, but it is probably better first to try to remove one limb by means of the wire-saw.

Foot–nape posture

This deviation of posture comprises upward displacement of one or both extended forelimbs so that they come to lie above the extended head in the vagina. It is an equine peculiarity that is made possible by the more slender head and longer limbs of the foal. It is very likely to lead to serious impaction and carries a great danger of penetration of the vaginal roof by the foot of the foal. The uppermost limb is recognized, and as the foal's muzzle is vigorously repelled in a forwards and upwards direction the fetal foot is raised and then pushed, or pulled, to the appropriate side. The other foot is similarly manipulated and, finally, the head is again raised and each foreleg placed underneath it. Traction is then applied to the head and both forelimbs.

If penetration of the vaginal roof has occurred, epidural anaesthesia or deep narcosis should be induced. Reposition is first attempted, and if it is not possible, amputation of the fetal head or the upper limb — whichever is easier — should be performed. The upper limb is sectioned through the radius by means of the wire-saw, and it should then be possible to replace the other limb under the head; the stump of the radius must be carefully controlled during the final delivery.

Where one foot is already protruding from the ruptured perineum, or rectum, it may be necessary to incise the perineum, extract the fetus and then repair both the lacerated and the incised tissue.

Lateral deviation of the head

This is a more serious malposture than in cattle because, owing to the greater length of the neck

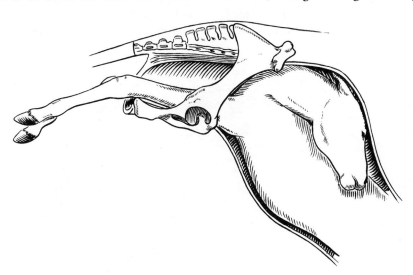

Fig. 14.11 Diagnosis: anterior presentation, dorsal position, lateral deviation of the head in the mare. The fetal nose may lie even further forward on the foal's stifle.

and head, the foal's nose lies further away near the stifle joint instead of on the middle ribs, as in the calf (Figure 14.11). Thus, except in ponies, the displaced head is beyond the reach of the obstetrician's hand. A special instrument is therefore required to help procure the head, and three such are available: Kühn's crutch, Blanchard's long flexible hook and the Krey–Schottler double hook.

Of these the first is the least damaging, and it is used as follows. The mare should be adequately controlled and epidural anaesthesia is indicated. If the mare will not stand quietly it is best to cast her on her side so that the displaced head is uppermost. Narcosis or general anaesthesia may be employed. A snare is fixed to one 'eye' of Kühn's crutch, and the free shank of the snare, to the end of which is tied Schriever's introducer, is carried in dorsal to the neck and pushed ventrally at arm's length down between the neck and thorax where it is sought by reintroducing the hand under the neck flexure. When grasped, the introducer with attached snare is withdrawn, untied from the snare and the free end of the latter passed through the other 'eye' of Kühn's crutch. As the snare is pulled through, the instrument is passed into the uterus up to the lateral aspect of the neck. With the snare held moderately tight, the crutch is moved gradually forwards along the side of the neck by rotary to-and-fro movements of the handle outside the vulva. In this way the crutch is advanced towards the head, and when one of its branches is felt to abut against the solid head, the snare is pulled tightly and made fast to the crutch handle. The operator than repels the fetus by manual pressure on the pectoral muscles while the assistant pulls on the crutch handle. In this way the foal's head may be brought within reach of the operator's grasp and, with or without the aid of a mandibular snare, the muzzle is brought into the birth canal. With gentle pulling on the forelimbs and head delivery is then possible.

Blanchard's long-handled hook (which is not easy to sterilize) is designed to engage in the foal's orbit, commissure of the mouth, nostril or ear-canal. In an interval between bouts of straining the instrument is carefully inserted and, while guarded as far as possible by the other hand of the obstetrician, it is passed along very closely to the lateral surface of the neck. When the hook is felt to impinge on the fetal head an attempt is made, while still keeping the instrument against the fetus by pressure from the hand still in the uterus, to engage one of the aforementioned recesses of the foal's head. When a firm hold is obtained on the fetal head, gentle sustained traction on the hook, with retropulsion of the fetal trunk, should bring the head within the operator's grasp. Several readjustments of the hook may be required as progress is made.

In the case of a laterally displaced head of a dead foal, and possibly also permissible in a difficult dystocia with a living fetus, a pair of Krey–Schottler hooks may be used to bring the deviated head within reach. The method is to make as many applications of the hooks as are necessary to bring the head within reach by applying them consecutively forwards to the dorsal skin and muscles of the

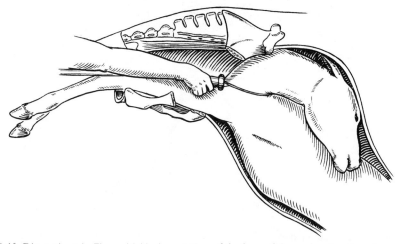

Fig. 14.12 Diangosis: as in Figure 14.11. Amputation of the base of the neck using the wire-saw fetotome.

neck. A grip with the first hook is taken on the nearest part of the neck, and while retropulsion is effected the snare of the hook is pulled on and the traction sustained while the second hook is applied as far as possible in front of the first one, and again retropulsion and traction are combined. In this way the head is finally brought within reach and delivery completed.

In cases of 'wryneck' where it is quite impossible to extend the neck, the head and neck must be amputated by means of the wire-saw fetotome (Figure 14.12). Finally, there are records of mares being foaled without correction of the displaced head, but this would seem to be a potentially dangerous procedure.

Downward deviation of the head

Downward deviation of the head is not so rare in horses as in cattle; nape posture is the most likely to be encountered. The methods of correction are the same as for the cow. Extension of the head requires the application of a mandibular snare, and while firm pressure is placed upon the fetal brow with one hand, the snare is pulled upwards and backwards by an assistant. If the operator can apply rotational as well as repellent force to the fetal head, lateral movement of the head — which is a necessary preliminary to its forward extension — is promoted. If this simple method does not soon succeed the veterinary surgeon should narcotize the mare, apply hobbles and place her in dorsal recumbency. Raising the hindquarters of the recumbent mare gives additional advantage. Retropulsion of the fetus and correction of the head posture are now greatly facilitated.

In view of the fact that spontaneous delivery of a foal in nape posture has been observed, it has been suggested that, where the head has projected so far into the vagina that the ears are visible at the vulva, traction without reposition is permissible. To aid traction, Krey's hooks should be attached to the nape and limb-snares are put on as usual.

In obstinate cases of nape posture with impaction at the pelvic brim, fetotomy is indicated. However, the introduction and correct placing of a wire- or chain-saw between the markedly flexed head and the neck would appear to be very difficult.

If the head is completely displaced between the forelimbs, so that it comes to lie under the chest or abdomen of the foal, reposition should be attempted by means of retropulsion and the application of Krey's hooks to the neck; traction is then applied with a view to raising the head to within reach of the hand. If this fails, a foreleg will have to be removed, preferably by the subcutaneous method, in order to give space for raising the head.

POSTURAL DEFECTS OF ANTERIOR PRESENTATION IN SHEEP

Postural defects are common causes of ovine dystocia. When affected sheep are promptly treated correction is relatively simple, and in many cases is successfully carried out by the shepherd. Manipulation is more difficult in the case of large single lambs, but delay in rendering obstetrical aid is the most frequent cause of difficulty. Repeated ineffectual maternal expulsive efforts cause dissipation of the fetal fluids, impaction of the fetus and close envelopment of the fetus by the uterus. Secondary uterine inertia supervenes, and in protracted cases the lamb dies and undergoes emphysematous decomposition. Thus even a simple postural defect in an unresponsive, inelastic, swollen fetus may be very difficult to correct. The veterinary surgeon is likely to see the more serious instances of postural abnormality in which there has been considerable delay and in which unskilful attempts at correction by a layman may have caused damage to the ewe.

Wherever possible, ewes which cannot lamb should be brought to the surgery, where they may be treated with due regard to cleanliness and asepsis. Gentleness of manipulation within the ovine genital tract is most essential; otherwise serious contusion or laceration of the gential organs may result and is especially liable to be followed by fatal shock or infection by organisms of the *Clostridium* group. The wool should be clipped from around the perineum and tail-base, and this area should be thoroughly washed. The ewe should then be placed on the operating table with the hindquarters overhanging one end. With the help of two assistants the patient may be placed in dorsal or lateral recumbency, as required. Alternatively the ewe may be held by an assistant so that its head and neck rest on the floor while the hindquarters are raised by grasping the hindlegs above the hocks. The assistant straddles the ewe and maintains her in the supine position with the hindquarters at a convenient height for the operator. In the case of heavy ewes the weight may be taken by cords which pass from the ewe's hocks to hooks in the ceiling, the assistant again straddling the ewe and controlling the hindlegs. Fetal fluid supplements, particularly the cellulose-based obstetrical lubricants as substitutes for amniotic fluid, should be infused. With the advantages provided by raising the ewe's hindquarters and instilling fluid, the majority of postural defects will be readily overcome. The principles of reposition adopted for the several varieties of postural aberration are the same as those used for the cow. Many cases can be rectified by the hand alone, but snares are frequently useful and should be of stout cotton parcel-string. Instruments are seldom required although forceps are occasionally employed in very small ewes. Epidural anaesthesia is not often required.

Carpal flexion posture

With the ewe held as previously described and with the instillation of fluid in delayed cases, retropulsion is easily achieved. The retained foot may then be grasped and gently brought into the pelvic entrance whence it is extended into the vagina. The ewe is then lowered on to her side and gentle traction applied each time she strains. After delivery of the fetus the uterus is searched for another lamb. Owing to uterine inertia a second (or third) lamb may fail to be advanced to the pelvic brim. The obstetrician should therefore bring the fore or hind extremity into the pelvis; expulsive efforts will recommence and gentle traction is then applied to help delivery.

Where there has been gross delay and it is found impossible to extend the leg of an emphysematous fetus, the carpus should be sawn through with the wire- or chain-saw. Copious lubrication is indicated and further fetotomy may be required as described for fetal oversize. As an alternative, unrelieved carpal flexion may be dealt with by the caesarean operation.

Incomplete extension of the elbow

Retropulsion of the fetus, followed by gentle extension of each limb in turn, is easily achieved. Gentle traction is then applied to the head and

forelimbs. An emphysematous case may require partial or complete dismemberment.

Shoulder flexion posture (Figure 14.13)

With adequate retropulsion, and fetal fluid supplement in delayed cases, it is usually possible to reach the forearm and to convert the defect to carpal flexion posture and then to proceed as previously described. In the case of a grossly oversized fetus where it is found impossible to advance the leg, caesarean section may be necessary; where the fetus is emphysematous the retained limb may be amputated by means of the wire-saw fetotome. Following the removal of one limb it is usually possible to deliver the fetus. In view of the fact that spontaneous delivery has been seen to occur despite complete retention of a forelimb it would seem proper where the ewe's pelvis is large and the lamb of small or moderate size to attempt delivery without rectification of posture. In such a case, however, it is likely that correction will be simple! In any case, inordinate force should not be used.

Lateral deviation of the head (Figure 14.14)

This is a very common cause of ovine dystocia. The methods used for correcting it are those described for cattle. With the hindquarters raised

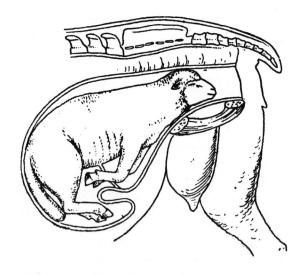

Fig. 14.13 Diagnosis: anterior presentation, dorsal position, bilateral shoulder flexion posture. (From a paper by H. Leeney in *Transactions of the Highland Agricultural Society*, c. 1890.)

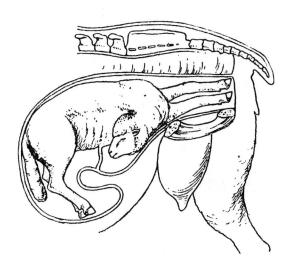

Fig. 14.14 Diagnosis: anterior presentation, dorsal position, lateral deviation of the head. (From a paper by H. Leeney in *Transactions of the Highland Agricultural Society, c.* 1890.)

and with the instillation of lubricant fluid, retropulsion and manual reposition are possible in most instances. Where there has been delay a mandibular snare may be used to good effect. Where there is insufficient room to correct the deviation the displaced head of an emphysematous lamb may be amputated with a wire fetotome protected by Glättli's spiral tubes, but a caesarean operation may be preferred.

POSTURAL DEFECTS OF POSTERIOR PRESENTATION

Faulty posture of the posterior limbs is more difficult to correct than abnormalities of the anterior limbs, particularly in horses. The defects now to be considered concern lack of extension of the hock and hip joints, which may affect one or both limbs. Also occasionally in calves it is found that the umbilical cord runs between the hindlimbs and over the posterior aspect of one or other. In this case it is necessary to create a hock flexion in order to replace the cord in its correct position. Failure to do this will result in the calf being born dead. Owing to the difficulty of extending the retained member, due to lack of space in front of the pelvis, three essentials figure prominently in the treatment, namely epidural anaesthesia, fetal fluid supplementation and retropulsion. All manipulations

should be conducted very carefully and gently for the danger of accidental perforation of the uterus is a real one. The variable factor exerting the greatest influence on the relative difficulty of the corrective procedure — as well as on the outcome of the operation — is the duration of dystocia prior to treatment. Cases attended in early second-stage labour, especially in cattle, may be delivered quite easily, but where there has been considerable delay, with consequent loss of fetal fluid, uterine contraction and death of the fetus, a most difficult and protracted fetotomy or a caesarean section may be necessary. There is a large proportion of stillbirths among fetuses presented posteriorly.

Hock flexion posture

Cattle

The condition is usually bilateral (Figure 14.15). The points of the hock may be felt in front of the pelvic brim or may be firmly engaged in the maternal birth canal. An estimate will be made of the likely degree of difficulty in correction and a decision made on whether epidural anaesthesia and/or fetal fluid replacements will be needed. The aim of the manipulative procedure is to extend the hock joint(s); the difficulty is in procuring sufficient space for this to be done. In recent cases, with or without epidural anaesthesia, the posture may be corrected by hand. The fetus is first repelled by pressing forward in its perineum, and the hand then grasps the fetal foot. As the foot is drawn back through an arc, the hock is firmly flexed and retropulsion maintained as far as possible; eventually, with the points of the digits in the cupped hand, the foot is lifted over the pelvic brim and the limb extended in the vagina. In cases in which it is found to be impossible to extend the hock owing to the lack of space, an assistant is directed to pass in an arm and to press forwards and upwards on the point of the hock while the operator again tries, as before, to bring the foot into the pelvic canal. An alternative method is to supplement manual extension by traction on a snare fixed to the retained foot in the following way. One end of an obstetric snare — to which may be attached Schriever's introducer — is passed into the birth canal, around the hock flexure, brought out and passed through the loop at the other end; the running noose thus formed is applied to the metatarsus. The noose is then

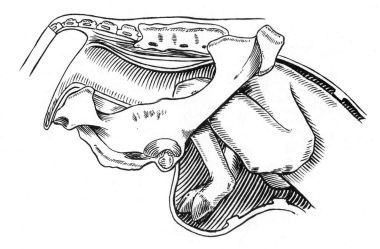

Fig. 14.15 Diagnosis: posterior presentation, dorsal position, bilateral hock flexion posture.

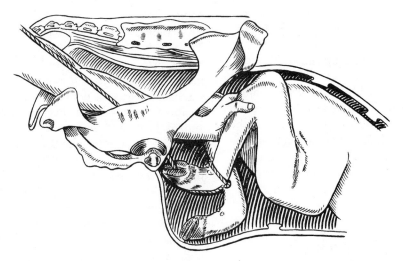

Fig. 14.16 Diagnosis: as in Figure 14.15. Correction using the hand and a digital snare.

manipulated down the limb until it lies in the pastern, the shank of the noose being placed from before backwards between the digits, so that when traction is applied to it the fetlock and pastern joints are flexed (Figure 14.16). After again repelling the fetus the obstetrician grasps the foot, and as the assistant pulls on the snare the extremity is lifted over the pelvic brim.

In the occasional case where it is impossible to extend the hock the calf will usually be dead and simple fetotomy may be performed. Either the Achilles tendon may be severed so as to make possible maximum flexion of the hock and thus allow the limb to be brought into the maternal pelvis; or the limb may be amputated below the

point of the hock by means of the wire-saw fetotome (Figure 14.17). A snare may then be applied above the hock and the limb extended.

Horses

The methods used are those described for cattle, but owing to the longer limbs of the foal the procedure is much more difficult and more frequent recourse to fetotomy will be required. If the foal should survive an unsuccessful manipulative attempt at correction it is worthwhile casting the mare and again trying to extend the limb with the mare in dorsal recumbency, preferably with the hind end raised by means of planks and bedding placed under the hindquarters.

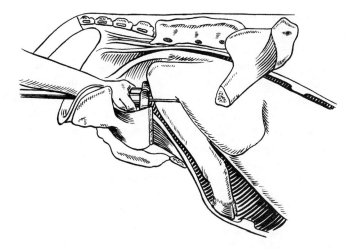

Fig. 14.17 Diagnosis: as in Figure 14.15. Fetotomy through the tarsus. Note that the fetotomy wire is below the os calcis.

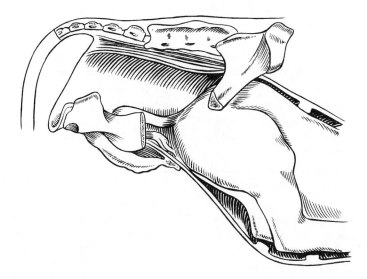

Fig. 14.18 Diagnosis: posterior presentation, dorsal position, bilateral hip flexion posture (breech presentation).

Hip flexion posture

Cattle

When both hindlegs are retained in the uterus — a commoner condition than unilateral retention — the case is described as 'breech presentation'; where much delay has occurred before aid is given, this constitutes one of the most difficult types of dystocia dealt with by veterinary obstetricians. Usually on vaginal examination, the calf's tail is recognized (Figure 14.18). The degree of engagement of the fetus in the maternal pelvis varies, and in some cases the hand cannot be passed to the hocks of the calf. The aim of the treatment is to convert the condition into one of hock flexion posture and then proceed accordingly. Again, the need for epidural anaesthesia and fetal fluid supplement will be primary considerations. In recent cases neither will be needed but in a protracted case both will be invaluable. The manipulative procedure is to repel the calf's perineum forwards and upwards with a view to bringing the retained limbs within reach, when the leg may be grasped as near to the hock as possible. Traction on the limb converts the posture into hock flexion, from which point the previously described procedure is carried out.

Occasionally, it is impossible to bring the hock within reach. In such cases the calf is almost invariably dead, and then fetotomy may be performed. The best method for removing the retained hindlimb is to use the wire-saw fetotome. One tube of the instrument is threaded, and the free end of the wire, attached to an introducer, is passed from above to below around the proximal part of the more accessible limb. The introducer is sought from below and brought out and the other tube of the fetotome is threaded. The fetotome is now passed along the vagina, and the head of the instrument placed against the fetal perineum. At this stage, a most important step in the procedure is to include the fetal tail in the loop of wire and to hold the head of the instrument firmly to the perineum while sawing takes place (Figure 14.19). In this way the femur is sectioned through its articular head. The detached limb is removed. The other hindlimb is similarly removed. An alternative procedure, after the amputation of one limb, is to apply traction — through the medium of an anal hook which is passed into the fetal anus and over the fetal pelvic brim — and to attempt to deliver the calf without extending the other hindlimb. Occasionally, after amputation of one hindlimb, it may be possible to extend the other limb and deliver the fetus by traction on the extended limb.

Although it is a somewhat cumbersome procedure and in most cases is not necessary when epidural anaesthesia is employed, there is little doubt that where difficulty is experienced in extending the legs of a breech presentation, the partial suspension of the cow by attaching its hindlegs to an overhead beam can be of tremendous help.

In the case of an impacted breech presentation of a dead fetus, an alternative procedure to percutaneous fetotomy, suggested by Graham (1979), is to cause fracture and collapse of the fetal pelvis by introducing a long-handled hook through an incision in the fetal perineum. The 75 cm blunt hook engages the pelvic brim and the fetal pelvis is fractured by abrupt backward traction. The procedure is repeated once or twice so as to ensure sufficient pelvic collapse. Traction on the unextended, lubricated breech, with the aid of Krey's hooks, may then succeed.

Horses

Occasionally a mare will foal unaided despite complete retention of the hindlimbs, and in many cases it is possible to deliver a breech presentation by traction without correcting the posture. But in recent cases, especially if the fetus is alive, an attempt should be made to extend the limbs, as described for cattle. Much greater difficulty will be experienced because of the longer limbs of the foal, and there is a very real danger of rupture of the uterus by the fetal foot. Serious consideration should be given to casting the mare and placing her in dorsal recumbency, as well as to inducing epidural or general anaesthesia (Figure 14.20).

If, after a proper effort, attempts to extend the hindlimbs are unsuccessful and the foal is still alive, no time should be lost before resorting to a caesarean operation. If, as is more likely, the foal is then

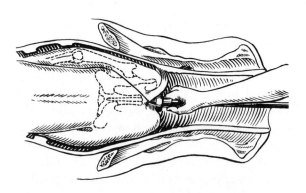

Fig. 14.19 Diagnosis: as in Figure 14.18. Percutaneous amputation of the hindlimb. Note that the fetal tail is within the wire loop.

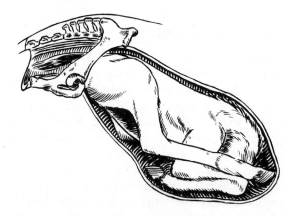

Fig. 14.20 Diagnosis: bilateral hip flexion posture in the mare (breech presentation).

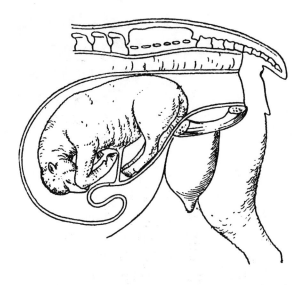

Fig. 14.21 Diagnosis: posterior presentation, dorsal position, bilateral hip flexion posture (breech presentation). (From a paper by H. Leeney in *Transactions of the Highland Agricultural Society c.* 1890.)

dead, deep narcosis or general anaesthesia should be induced. After the amputation of one hindlimb by means of the wire-saw tubular fetotome, as described for cattle, it should be possible to deliver the foal by traction through the medium of an anal hook or the Krey–Schottler double hook attached to the root of the tail.

Hock flexion posture and hip flexion posture in the ewe

A considerable proportion of twin lambs are presented posteriorly, and because of lack of uterine space, especially where both lambs occupy one uterine horn, one or both hindlegs may fail to extend into the vagina (Figure 14.21). Thus in flocks with a high proportion of twins, hock flexion and hip flexion postures will be common causes of dystocia.

These malpostures may be corrected in the manner described for cattle, but because twin lambs are smaller than singles and since it is a simple matter to raise the ewe's hindquarters, the requisite manoeuvres are much more easily performed than in cattle. In all delayed cases, fetal fluid supplement is indicated. The manipulation of the fetus, including its retropulsion, should be very gently performed.

In cases of irreducible malposture, section of the hock or hip can be conveniently carried out by means of the wire-saw protected by Glättli's spiral tubes.

Where breech presentation is accompanied by fetal oversize the caesarean operation is preferable to fetotomy.

REFERENCES

Graham, J. A. (1979) *J. Amer. Vet. Med. Assn,* **174**, 169.

15

Dystocia Due to Defects of Position or Presentation: Treatment

POSITION

Abnormal position of the fetus is encountered more frequently in horses than in cattle. This is considered to be due to the fact that in late gestation or first-stage labour in horses (but not in cattle) a physiological rotation of the fetus from the ventral to the dorsal position occurs and that occasionally this mechanism breaks down. The fetus then presents longitudinally — usually anteriorly, but sometimes posteriorly — either with its vertebral column applied to one side of the uterus (right or left lateral position) or facing the floor of the birth canal (ventral position). The process whereby the bovine or ovine fetus sometimes comes to lie in ventral position is not understood. It is hardly likely to be a gestational position; more probably it arises during the first stage of labour when the uterine peristaltic force generates a vigorous reflex response in the fetus that rotates it about its long axis. The mechanism would seem to be similar, or identical, to that which causes torsion of the uterus. Presumably the fetus moves with the amnion, the fetus and amnion revolving within the allantochorion. The greater freedom of the amnion within the allantois of the mare, as compared with the cow, would facilitate this change of position.

In order to make birth possible, fetuses in lateral or ventral position must be rotated into the normal (dorsal) upright position. This can be achieved by first repelling the fetus and then rotating it by appropriate force applied to the presenting extremity. Such rotation is easier to perform with the patient standing. In obstinate cases epidural anaesthesia is extremely useful.

Anterior presentation, lateral position (mare or cow)

In the case of a live calf, or foal, the obstetrician passes his or her hand to the fetal head and, by means of the thumb and middle finger, presses on the fetal eyeballs, the latter being protected by the eyelids. Firm pressure causes a convulsive reflex response in the fetus and, by applying a rotational force in the appropriate direction, it is easy to turn the fetus into the dorsal position. The fetal nose and forelimbs are then advanced into the maternal pelvis and the maternal expulsive efforts assisted by gently pulling on these appendages. Should the fetus be unresponsive, rotation is performed mechanically by means of Cämmerer's torsion fork. Epidural anaesthesia should be induced and snares applied to the forefeet and head. A canvas cuff is then passed over and along each foot-snare and pushed up the limb until finally it encircles the upper forearm. The fork is carefully passed into the vagina so that each of its prongs engages one of the cuffs. The operator then repels the fetus by pushing on the fork and, at the same time, turns it vigorously to the appropriate side. Provided there is sufficient uterine space (and if not fetal fluid supplement is indicated) the method is successful. Kühn's crutch can be used instead of Cämmerer's fork.

Anterior presentation, ventral position (mare or cow)

The same two methods, namely forceps grip and eyeball pressure with manual rotation or mechanical rotation by means of a torsion fork, are used. If the dam is down and will not get up, it should be placed in dorsal recumbency; raising the hindquarters will then be beneficial.

If the calf or foal should rest on its back with

the head and limbs flexed on to its neck and thorax, the fetus must first be repelled so that the head and forelimbs can be extended. Rotation is then carried out.

Posterior presentation, lateral position (mare or cow)

The operator introduces a hand and grasps the stifle region of the upper limb. Simultaneous retropulsion and downward pressure are applied to rotate the fetus through 90°. If this proves impracticable, Cämmerer's torsion fork should be applied to the hindlimbs.

Posterior presentation, ventral position (mare or cow)

The operator introduces a hand between the fetal hindlimbs and up to the inguinal region, where one of the thighs is grasped; then, pushing forwards, the operator rotates the fetus through a half circle. Failing this, the torsion fork should be used. An alternative procedure is to place a traction bar between the projecting hindfeet and to bind it to them by means of a snare; rotational force is then applied to the traction bar.

There is a grave risk that the hindfeet of a foal in posterior presentation, ventral position, will penetrate the vagina and rectum (Figure 15.1). In such a case the caesarean operation should be performed and the rectovaginal fistula repaired later.

Dystocia due to defects of position in sheep

The methods of treatment are those described for the mare and cow. By raising the ewe into the inclined supine position and infusing fetal fluid supplement, rotation is much easier in this species; instruments are seldom required.

PRESENTATION

Instead of the long axis of the fetus being in line with the birth canal it may be disposed vertically or transversely to the pelvic inlet. Owing to limitation of space in the sagittal plane, absolute vertical presentation is not possible but oblique vertical presentation occurs rarely, in mares rather than cows. According to whether the fetal vertebral column or abdomen is presented at the pelvic inlet, such dystocias are described as dorsovertical

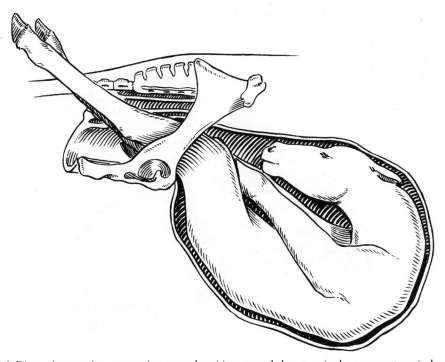

Fig. 15.1 Diagnosis: posterior presentation, ventral position, extended posture in the mare; rectovaginal rupture.

or ventrovertical presentations. Transverse presentations are also uncommon and are more likely to be encountered in the mare; they may be ventrotransverse or dorsotransverse and, again, oblique variants are more often seen.

All dystocias that arise from defects of presentation are serious, the special form of bicornual transverse presentation of the mare being notorious. The aim in all cases is to achieve version of the fetus so that a vertical or transverse presentation is converted into a longitudinal one. Obviously the nearer extremity should be moved towards the pelvic inlet, but where both extremities are equally distant it is usually simpler to convert to posterior presentation (two appendages being manipulated rather than three).

Oblique dorsovertical presentation (mare or cow)

According to whether the head or breech is nearer the pelvic inlet the presentation is converted into anterior or posterior longitudinal. An attempt is made to bring the fetal extremity (head and/or limbs) to the pelvic inlet and firstly to convert the defect into a ventral longitudinal presentation. The fetus can then be rotated to the dorsal position as described earlier. Retropulsion and the presence of copious fluid (natural or artificial) in the uterus are both essential. A grip is taken on the fetus by means of Krey's hook as near as possible to the more proximal fetal extremity. Then, while retropulsion is applied, the hook is pulled on with a view to bringing the fore or hind end of the fetus to the pelvic inlet. After adjustments of

position and posture the fetus is then delivered by gentle traction.

Should version not be practicable the caesarean operation should be performed.

Oblique ventrovertical presentation (mare or cow) ('dog-sitting position')

Whereas this abnormality (Figure 15.2) is more frequent than the preceding, it is still rare and is only likely to be encountered in the mare. However, when present it should cause no difficulty in diagnosis; if the veterinary surgeon is called to a foaling mare from which the fetal head and forelimbs protrude and to which lay traction has been applied without success, it is very probably a case of 'dog-sitting position', oversize being very unlikely in mares. 'Dog-sitting position' aptly describes the dystocia, the foal being disposed with its fore end advanced to a variable degree in the vagina and its hindparts in the uterus. It differs from normal anterior presentation in that the hindfeet also pass into the birth canal and rest on the pelvic brim. Thus the more the fetus is pulled the greater is the impaction. Most cases are severely impacted but after the induction of epidural anaesthesia and the infusion of lubricant fluid into the uterus an attempt should always be made to repel the fetus sufficiently to allow the hindfeet to be pushed off the pelvic brim into the uterus and thus to convert the dystocia into a simple anterior presentation. Traction is then applied. Should this attempt fail version should be tried, the aim now being to repel the front of the fetus and to convert

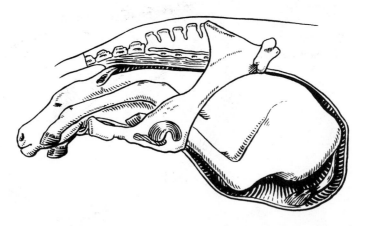

Fig. 15.2 Diagnosis: 'dog-sitting' position in the mare.

to posterior presentation, ventral position. To this end canvas cuffs are passed right up the forelimbs and engaged by Kühn's crutch or Cämmerer's torsion fork. Vigorous retropulsion is now applied and, as soon as practicable, snares are attached to the hindfeet; these snares are held taut while further retropulsion is effected. In this way, in a favourable case the fetus can be 'tipped over backwards' into the uterus so that it comes to rest in posterior presentation, ventral position. The fetus is then rotated from ventral to dorsal position and traction applied to the hindlegs.

In a case of dog-sitting position where the head, neck and forelimbs protrude from the vulva, retropulsion will not succeed. The mare should be narcotized, or preferably under general anaesthesia, and placed in dorsal recumbency and fetotomy begun immediately. The loop of the wire-saw should be placed as far back as possible around the fetal thorax, and the trunk bisected by sawing. Evisceration is then carried out. Next, snares are attached to the hindfeet, and while these are advanced the fetal vertebral column stump is repelled so that the remainder of the trunk is pushed into the uterus. Rotation is now performed, and the posterior half of the fetus delivered by traction on the hindfeet.

Where swelling of the vaginal mucosa prevents vaginal manipulation and fetotomy, a caesarean operation should be used.

Dorsotransverse presentation (mare or cow)

This is a rare cause of dystocia (Figures 15.3 and 15.4), but oblique variants of it occur in both the mare and cow. The obstetrician should ascertain the polarity of the fetus and decide which extremity is nearer the pelvic inlet. The technique of correction required involves repulsion of the fetus and the advancement of its nearer extremity to the birth canal. Unless one extremity is within easy reach, uterine version is likely to be an extremely difficult, or impossible, task in both the cow and mare. If there appears to be a chance of success, the cow should be given an epidural anaesthetic, and in the mare deep narcosis, or preferably general anaesthesia, should be induced so that she can be placed on her back. Fetal fluid supplement is then instilled and an attempt made by manipulation of the proximal fetal extremity to turn the fetus into

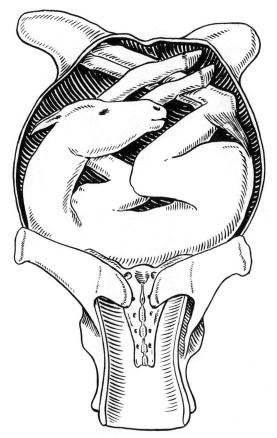

Fig. 15.3 Diagnosis: dorsotransverse presentation in the mare; uterine body gestation.

ventral position, anterior or posterior presentation. The next step is to rotate the fetus into dorsal position. Finally it is delivered by traction. If after a short determined effort it is obvious that version cannot be achieved, a caesarean operation should be performed immediately. Fetotomy is very difficult to carry out in this type of dystocia and consequently is not recommended.

Ventrotransverse presentation (mare or cow)

This presentation (Figure 15.5) is more likely to be seen in the mare than in the cow, and oblique variants of it are more usual. A variable number of fetal appendages may enter the maternal pelvis. It is possible that the head as well as the forelimbs are in the vagina, but it is usual for two or more legs only to be presented. The condition must be distinguished from twins and double monsters and from schistosoma reflexus. The aim of

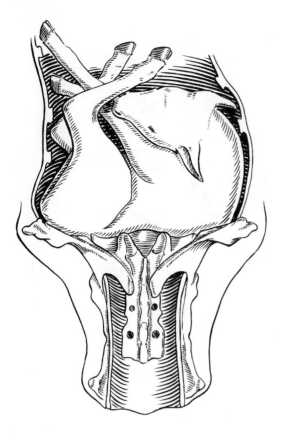

Fig. 15.4 Diagnosis: dorsotransverse presentation in the cow.

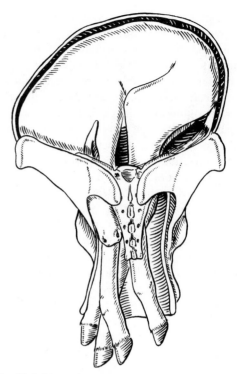

Fig. 15.5 Diagnosis: ventrotransverse presentation in the mare; uterine body gestation.

vaginal interference is firstly to convert the abnormality into longitudinal — usually posterior — presentation, ventral position; this means tht the posterior extremity must be advanced while the anterior extremity is repelled. Accordingly traction is applied to snares attached to the posterior digits while retropulsion of the fore part is effected through the medium of Cämmerer's (or Kühn's) crutch and cuffs, the latter being placed around the forearms. The presence of copious uterine fluid is essential; epidural anaesthesia will also be required for the cow. Deep narcosis, or preferably general anaesthesia, and dorsal recumbency is used for the mare. Unless progress with version is soon apparent the caesarean operation is recommended for both mare and cow. Fetotomy is likely to be arduous for the operator, dangerous for the dam and uncertain of success. Following successful version, the fetus is rotated from ventral to dorsal position and then delivered by traction on the hindlimbs.

In the *bicornual type of transverse presentation*

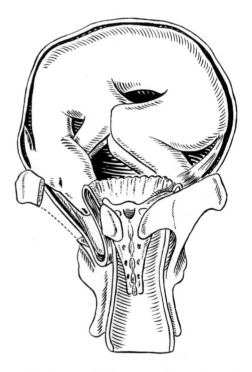

Fig. 15.6 Diagnosis: ventrotransverse presentation with ventral displacement of the uterus in the mare; bicornual gestation.

peculiar to mares the fetal extremities are disposed in the two horns and its trunk lies across the anterior portion of the uterine body (Figure 15.6). Ventral displacement of the uterus may have occurred, and, if so, it may be impossible to palpate the fetus. As soon as the presentation is recognized a caesarean operation should be performed.

Dystocia due to defects of presentation in sheep

The methods of treatment are those described for the mare and cow. By raising the ewe into the inclined, supine position and by infusing fetal fluid supplement, version is much easier in this species, but in protracted dystocia, caesarean section may provide an easier solution.

16

Dystocia Due to Twins
or Monstrosities

DYSTOCIA DUE TO TWINS

Twin gestation in cattle often culminates in dystocia but in mares abortion is a more likely sequel. It is arguable whether twin gestation predisposes to sheep dystocia because the increased likelihood of maldisposition and the added risk of simultaneous presentation dystocia are balanced by a reduction in fetopelvic disproportion. Twin dystocia is of three types:

1. Both fetuses present simultaneously and become impacted in the maternal pelvis (Figure 16.1).

2. One fetus only is presented but cannot be born because of defective posture, position or presentation; posture is often most at fault, the lack of extension of limbs or head being due to insufficient uterine space.

3. Uterine inertia; defective uterine contractions are caused, either by overstretching of the uterus by the excessive fetal load, or by premature birth. When inertia is present, birth of the first or second fetus does not proceed although presentation is normal.

The smaller size of twin fetuses facilitates manipulative correction and delivery; for the same reason natural or obstetric delivery may be possible despite defective posture.

In the treatment of twin dystocia the first essential is diagnosis. It is a *sine qua non* of obstetric practice that in all cases of difficult birth the presenting fetal appendages shall be identified. If this is made a rule the obstetrician will not blunder into applying traction simultaneously to two fetuses — as is commonly done by laymen — nor should twins be mistaken for a schistosomus, double monster or ventrotransverse presentation of a single fetus.

Where a twin is presented with an abnormality of posture it is treated as if it were a single fetus; in such cases the presence of twins is not known — but may be suspected on account of small fetal size and the history of the dam — until the uterus is searched after delivery and another fetus found. Again, the association of uterine inertia with

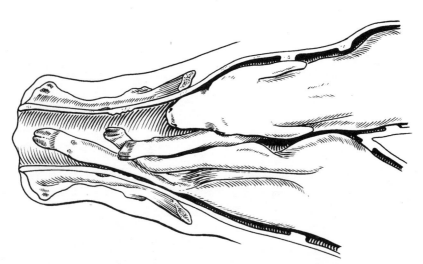

Fig. 16.1 Diagnosis: simultaneous engagement of twins. One twin is in anterior presentation, dorsal position, shoulder flexion posture; the other is in posterior presentation, dorsal position, extended posture.

twins may be known only after delivery of the first fetus.

Little attention has been given by veterinary surgeons to the relationship between the type of dystocia and the disposition of the twins within the uterus. Simultaneous presentation would seem probable when a twin from each cornu approached the pelvic inlet; abnormality of posture and inertia would be more likely when both fetuses occupied the same horn. However, Anderson et al. (1978) saw no dystocia in 16 cases of experimentally produced twinning in which a 5 day embryo was placed in each uterine horn. Their observations and the clinical experience of the authors indicate that dystocia is more likely with unicornual twinning.

When twins are known to be present and retropulsion is required — either of the presenting fetus to correct its posture or of the less advanced fetus to allow delivery of the first twin — it should be performed very carefully. There is a much greater likelihood of causing uterine rupture when twins are present, in both cattle and sheep. Spontaneous rupture has been seen when both fetuses were in the same horn.

There are many stillbirths among cattle twins; the second calf to be born is more likely to survive. Breech presentations are common.

Simultaneous presentation of twins (Figure 16.2) is treated in logical sequence. The polarity of the fetuses is determined, the more advanced fetus recognized and its presenting extremity appropriately snared. Any defect of presentation, position or posture must be diagnosed and treated; correction may be greatly facilitated by means of epidural anaesthesia. Then, with continuing retropulsion on the less advanced fetus, the nearer one is brought into the pelvis and delivered by simple traction. The other fetus, which may be presented in the opposite direction, is then appropriately manipulated. The delivery of ovine twins is more easily achieved if an assistant holds the ewe by its hindlegs in an inclined supine position. When the ewe is delivered of twins the uterus should always be examined for a third fetus.

In occasional cases of gross delay, corrective manipulation is impossible and fetotomy of the presenting fetus may be required. Severe pelvic impaction of dead fetuses may be more readily relieved by caesarean section.

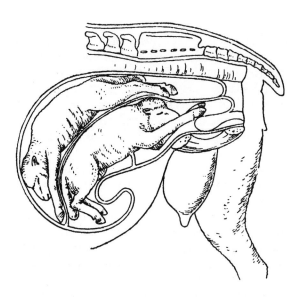

Fig. 16.2 Diagnosis: simultaneous engagement of twin lambs. One twin is in anterior presentation, dorsal position, extended posture; the other is in posterior presentation, dorsal position, extended posture. (From a paper by H. Leeney in *Transactions of the Highland Agricultural Society, c.* 1890.)

The afterbirth of bovine twins is likely to be retained.

Vandeplassche has recorded useful data on 44 cases of equine twin gestation. All pairs were of dizygotic origin (i.e. non-identical). In 33 of 34 twin pregnancies it was found that one fetus occupied each horn; in the remaining case the twins were in the same horn. Of 44 live foals born, 37 were reared. The study showed that there was a much smaller likelihood of viable twin foals being born to Thoroughbred mares than to Belgian draught mares and this difference might be related to a better uterine capacity in the draught mare (Vandeplassche et al., 1970).

Most cases of equine twin conception are followed by early death of one or both of the conceptuses. About 2% of equine gestations start as normal twin fetal development but mummification or abortion frequently occur so that less than 1% reach term.

DYSTOCIA DUE TO MONSTROSITIES

Monstrosities most often cause dystocia in dairy cattle, the commonest example being schistosoma reflexus; next in order of frequency are ankylosed calves including perosomus elumbis, double monsters, dropsical fetuses, including anasarcous and hydrocephalic calves, and anchondroplastic monsters (see Chapter 4). The same varieties occur, but to a lesser extent, in sheep. With the notable exception of wryneck, monstrosities are uncommon in mares. Instances of hydrocephalus, double monsters and perosomus elumbis are not rare in pigs.

With the exception of anasarcous fetuses, gross malformation is often associated with ankylosis of joints and muscular atrophy; consequently many monsters weigh less than normal calves. This, coupled with the fact that they are sometimes associated with abortion or premature birth, means that a monster may be sufficiently small to be passed spontaneously. However, the grossly irregular development, including bending or twisting of the vertebral column and ankylosis or duplication of limbs, means that a wider than normal fetal diameter presents at the pelvic inlet and that severe dystocia results.

Remarks on the delivery of monstrosities

Recognition of the exact disposition of the fetal extremities and an estimate of fetal size may be very difficult. The obstetrician must then consider whether careful traction — with due regard to lubrication and protection of the birth canal from irregularly disposed appendages — is likely to succeed. Prior to the attempt at vaginal delivery the diameter of anasarcous, ascitic and hydrocephalic fetuses may be reduced by appropriate multiple or single incisions with a fetotomy knife. If moderate traction does not soon succeed, fetotomy or caesarean section must be employed. In view of the worthless nature of monstrosities, fetotomy should be first considered, and in all cases where sufficient reduction of the fetal diameter may be achieved by simple section(s), fetotomy should be practised. Thus, for ankylosed fetuses, including wryneck and perosomus elumbis, for cases of anterior duplication and for schistosomes presented viscerally, fetotomy is indicated. The most suitable instrument will be the wire-saw fetotome. The hydrocephalic whose head is too rigid to be reduced by cranial puncture must have the dome sawn off by means of wire or chain.

Where it is obvious because of excessive fetal size — as in anasarca and extensive duplication — or because of very irregular presentation that several fetotomy sections will be required, the veterinary surgeon should resort to the caesarean operation. This will be less arduous for the operator and, in general, better for the immediate health and the future breeding potential of the cow.

Occasionally, monstrosities present baffling problems to the obstetrician. This happens when the presenting part of the fetus is normal and the distal extremity is grossly malformed; birth proceeds normally until the malformed portion engages the pelvic inlet. The cause is not apparent and may be impossible to ascertain. Examples are provided by perosomus elumbis where the front half of the calf negotiates the birth canal but the ankylosed and distorted hindlimbs become impacted; a hydrocephalic fetus in posterior presentation; and cases of anterior duplication presented posteriorly. In these instances heavy but unsuccessful traction has usually been applied before the arrival of the veterinary surgeon. This history, together with the normal appearance of the presenting portion, should make the veterinary surgeon suspicious that an abnormality is present in the distal portion. A caesarean operation provides the easiest solution.

Obstetric management of *schistosoma reflexus*

This most familiar bovine monstrosity requires special consideration. The features of the malformation were described in Chapter 4. The weight of the monster calf is usually around 22 kg. It may occur in ruminants and swine and may be presented viscerally or by its extremities. It is not uncommon for a fetus in visceral presentation to be naturally born.

With this type of dystocia, fetal viscera may be seen protruding from the vulva; if not they are soon located by vaginal exploration. The viscera may be mistaken for those of the mother and uterine rupture may be suspected, but it should not be difficult by careful examination to dispose of this suspicion, the absence of a uterine tear and the continuity of the viscera with the fetus being soon established. The viscera must be torn away from the fetus whose rigid vertebral angulation may then be felt at the pelvic brim. The fetal diameter is now compared with that of the birth

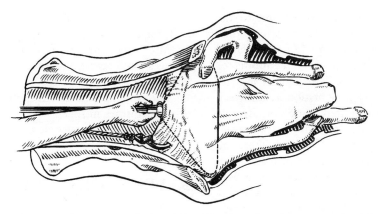

Fig. 16.3 Diagnosis: *schistosoma reflexus* in visceral presentation. The viscera have been removed and the calf is being divided by means of the wire-saw fetotome.

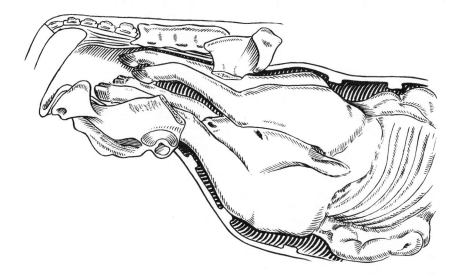

Fig. 16.4 Diagnosis: *schistosoma reflexus* presenting by the extremities. This dystocia is best relieved by caesarean section.

canal; where it seems favourable to birth, Krey's hooks are fastened to the presenting fetus. Reasonable traction, with adequate lubrication, is now applied, the veterinary surgeon paying particular regard to the possibility of damage by bony fetal prominences to the birth canal. In this way the expulsive efforts of the cow are gently aided, and smooth delivery may be achieved. Where, after a short period of such traction, it is obvious that safe vaginal delivery is not possible, the fetus should be bisected by means of the wire-saw fetotome. One arm of the instrument is loaded and the protruding wire is carried in on an introducer and passed around the spinal flexure of the fetus (Figure 16.3). Passing the introducer around the fetus

may be a tedious task; when accomplished, the other arm of the fetotome is loaded and the head of the instrument is passed into the vagina until it abuts on the fetus. The fetal vertebral column is then sawn through, and the smaller fetal moiety withdrawn by means of Krey's hooks. Should difficulty arise over withdrawal of the remaining portion it too may need to be divided perpendicularly to the first section, again using the wire-saw.

When a schistosome presents by its extremities — three or four legs, with or without the head — the excessive fetal diameter, together with the ankylosis of joints, is likely to prevent natural or obstetric delivery per vaginam (Figure 16.4), and unless the fetus is very small in relation to the maternal pelvis — as might occur in a schistosome twin to a normal calf — time should not be wasted on an attempt at vaginal delivery. Fetotomy or hysterotomy will be required. In general it is far easier to deal with such a presentation by caesarean section, the fetotomy required being considerable in amount and tedious of execution. Exceptions may be met in the case of small fetuses where the removal of a head or single limb will make birth possible. When performing the caesarean operation for the removal of a schistosome the veterinary surgeon should always consider the advantage of fetotomy from the laparotomy site; in this way the requisite length of the uterine incision may be kept within reasonable bounds and the risk of uterine rupture during extraction minimized (see Chapter 20 on the caesarean operation).

After successful removal of a schistosome the uterus should always be searched for injury and to ensure the absence of a second fetus.

The same considerations apply to the treatment of monstrosities in sheep.

REFERENCES

Anderson, G. B., Cupps, P. T., Drost, M., Horton, M. B. and Wright, R. W. (1978) *J. Anim. Sci.,* **46**, 449.

Vandeplassche, M., Podliachouk, L. and Beaud, R. (1970) *Can. J. Comp. Med.,* **34**, 281.

Dystocia is often accompanied by uterine inertia and followed by delay in uterine involution. Because of this interference with normal uterine function, retention of the afterbirth and puerperal metritis are especially likely to occur. Obstetric trauma to the genital tract also predisposes to infection, and where severe contusion has occurred there is a marked risk of infection by anaerobic organisms. Prolapse of the uterus is a serious complication of the third stage of labour but it is more likely to happen after normal birth than after dystocia. These three important conditions that follow delivery of the fetus, namely prolapse of the uterus, retention of the afterbirth and puerperal infection, are given special consideration in Chapters 19, 18 and 23. In addition, there are numerous accidents and diseases that accompany or follow parturition. Traumatic lesions of the soft tissues of the genital tract or bony pelvis may lead to fatal haemorrhage or infection, or to disability due to fractures, dislocations or paralysis. Other complications of parturition comprise displacement, hernia and rupture of the pelvic or abdominal organs. Parturition and the puerperium may also be complicated by metabolic diseases, particularly hypocalcaemia and ketonaemia, and by displacement of the abomasum. A difficult foaling may be followed by laminitis or tetanus, and in all species puerperal animals may incur embolic pneumonia, toxaemia, septicaemia and pyaemia as sequels to uterine infection. Endocarditis, unthriftiness and sterility are possible later sequelae.

While spontaneous trauma, rupture or displacement may occur in unassisted deliveries, the most frequent basic cause of parturient and postparturient disease is delay in giving obstetric aid to dystocia cases. Unskilled lay interference is another important cause of genital trauma. If skilled attention were given at the correct time in dystocia there would be relatively few difficult cases, and the amount of postparturient disease would be markedly reduced. Unfortunately, the time at which the veterinary surgeon is called is outside professional control; all the professional can do is to arrive as soon as possible in response to a request and carry out the required obstetric interference in a skilful manner. In the course of time the surgeon may educate his or her clients in the value of timely obstetric aid.

POSTPARTUM HAEMORRHAGE

Bleeding from the maternal side of the placenta in natural separation of the afterbirth is only likely in carnivora where breakdown of the marginal haematoma is accompanied by a green or brown discharge of altered blood. If, however, premature dehiscence occurs when the afterbirth is removed during premeditated caesarean section, severe and even fatal haemorrhage may follow. Because of the histological form of the epitheliochorial and synepithelial chorial placentae of horses, swine and ruminants, significant haemorrhage from the capillary plexuses around the crypts can occur only when there is considerable trauma of the endometrium as, for example, when marked force is used in early removal of a cotyledonary afterbirth. In veterinary obstetrics the usual cause of serious metrorrhagia is laceration of a uterine blood vessel by a fetal appendage, obstetric instrument or hand of the obstetrician. After removal of the fetus much blood may accumulate in the uterus before it begins to escape via the vagina; alternatively blood may drain through a rent in the uterine wall into the abdomen.

When, after delivery of the offspring, there is a profuse haemorrhage from the vulva, the most likely source is the broken ends of the vessels of the umbilical cord which have receded into the vagina. This is likely to occur in uterine inertia where, owing to poor uterine contractions, much of the blood from the fetal side of the placenta (allanto-chorion) is not expelled into the fetus during second-stage labour. Similar bleeding from mares is seen after the stud-groom has hastened a normal delivery by traction on the fetus and has immediately ligated the umbilical cord (near to the fetal abdomen) and then severed it. Such haemorrhage from the allantochorion does not affect the dam, but the young animal is thereby deprived of a natural blood transfusion which could be the cause of cerebral anoxia in newborn foals.

If, when the postparturient uterine examination is being conducted, profuse haemorrhage is occurring from a uterine laceration, prompt contraction of the uterus should be promoted by means of an injection of oxytocin. Next day the masses of clotted blood should be manually removed. Haemorrhage associated with uterine rupture is attended to when the uterine rent is repaired. When severe haemorrhage is occurring from a ruptured vaginal vessel an attempt must be made to close the vessel. Ligation is usually not practicable but artery forceps may be applied and left on for 24 hours. Where the vessel cannot be secured, an intravaginal pressure pack can be improvised from a freshly laundered bed-sheet. General symptoms of severe haemorrhage and shock should be counteracted by copious transfusion of blood (4–5 litres) from a neighbouring animal.

Fatal haemorrhage from vessels in the broad ligament has been seen in the mare and cow. Rooney (1964) recorded 10 cases of fatal haemorrhage from the ovarian, uterine or external iliac arteries in foaling (eight) or pregnant (two) mares. All were aged mares and nine of them were Thoroughbreds. The ruptures were associated with aneurysms or degenerative changes in the arteries and it was presumed that these lesions were predisposed to by age and that the actual ruptures were caused by stretching during pregnancy or pressure during parturition. Where such haemorrhage is suspected the only hope of saving the animal would be prompt laparotomy and ligation of the torn vessel.

CONTUSIONS AND LACERATIONS OF THE BIRTH CANAL AND NEIGHBOURING STRUCTURES

Any part of the birth canal may suffer contusion during forcible extraction of an oversized fetus, but the cervix and vulva are more likely to be lacerated than the dilatable vagina. The considerable fat content of the vagina of heifers of the beef breeds makes such animals particularly prone to vaginal contusion when the fetus is oversized. Infection by *Fusiformis necrophorus* is then probable, and a most severe necrotic vaginitis ensues. The condition is very painful and causes continuous, exhausting straining and marked toxaemia. Pyogenic infection is also possible. All vaginal contusions and lacerations should be treated with mild emollient and antibiotic preparations; parenteral antibiotics should also be given. Epidural anaesthesia gives temporary relief from straining.

Rupture of the vagina should be repaired, if possible, by suturing. Infection following rupture may give rise to peritonitis, to severe pelvic cellulitis with marked toxaemia and straining or to abscess formation with subsequent vaginal constriction. All vaginal injuries should be treated with due regard to the possible sequelae. Lacerations of the cervix may be sutured by applying vulsellum forceps to the organ and withdrawing it to the vulva. Wounds of the vulva and perineum are easily sutured. Mattress sutures of nylon should be used, devitalized tissue, including any loosely attached portions of adipose tissue, being first removed. If lacerations of the vulva and perineum are left unsutured, scar tissue formation and distortion impede the sphincter action of the vulva, with consequent aspiration of air, vaginitis and metritis; a special, and much more difficult, operation is then required.

When Caslick's operation to prevent vaginal aspiration has been performed in the mare, and the vulva has been incised at parturition to allow birth of the foal, the incised tissue should be resutured immediately after delivery. Repair of the vulva, perineum and cervix may be conveniently carried out under epidural anaesthesia.

In cows, previously unsuspected organizing haematomata of the vagina may suddenly prolapse from the vulva 4–6 weeks after parturition. These lesions resemble fibromata but are not neoplastic and are easily excised.

Haematoma of the vulva

This is a sequel to contusion of the submucous tissue during delivery. One lip of the vulva is usually affected and an obvious round swelling occupies the vulval orifice. The condition may arise spontaneously in the mare, but in both cows and mares it is likely to follow assisted delivery in which considerable manipulation, or forced traction, was required. Haematoma of the vulva may be confused with prolapse, tumour or cyst of the vagina. If left untreated, natural resolution usually occurs within a few weeks with resorption of fluid and regression of swelling; occasionally, pyogenic infection ensues and may be accompanied by fibrosis and distortion of the vulva, with vaginal aspiration. If left for 3 or 4 days after labour the haematoma may be safely incised and the clot removed without recurrence of haemorrhage. An abscess should be opened and drained.

Perineal injuries at parturition

Serious perineal injuries occur during the second stage of labour in both the cow and the mare, mostly in primiparous animals. These injuries may be classified as first-, second- and third-degree tears and rectovaginal fistulae.

Many heifers sustain slight tearing of the upper commissure because of vulval stretching during normal labour but such lesions heal satisfactorily by first intention without suturing. Tears which extend more deeply into the perineum do not close spontaneously, although epithelial repair is rapid. Such lesions destroy the sphincteric effect of the vulva and lead to aspiration of air into the vagina, even though the integrity of the anus is not impaired. With greater stretching and tearing during the second stage of labour, the wound may extend into and destroy the anal sphincter, thus

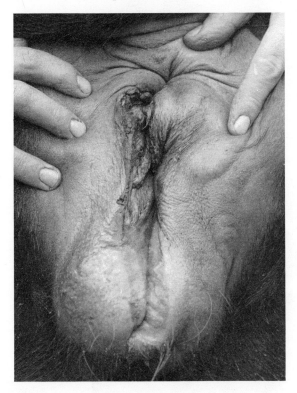

Fig. 17.1 Third-degree perineal laceration in a cow. Note swelling of the vulva and the tear extending from the dorsal commissure towards the anus.

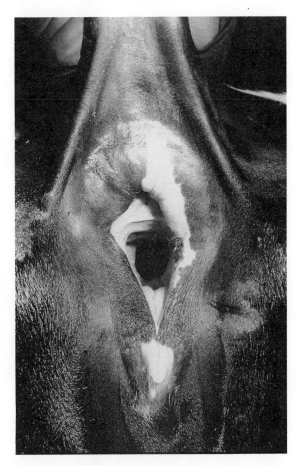

Fig. 17.2 Third-degree perineal laceration in a cow under caudal epidural anaesthesia to cause relaxation of the vulva and perineum. The shelf between the rectum and vagina is just visible.

creating a cloaca through which faeces fall into the terminal vagina (Figures 17.1 and 17.2). Despite rapid epithelialization, the abnormal communication between the terminal rectum and vagina persists, although its extent may be considerably reduced by wound granulation. Experience suggested that simple rectovaginal fistulae (Figure 17.3) without damage to the anal sphincter are uncommon spontaneous injuries to cattle, although they occur as developmental anomalies in cases of anal atresia. They may also result from

unsuccessful attempted closure of a third-degree perineal tear, as in the mare.

In the mare, the mechanism of perineal tearing is different. In this species, the initial injury is usually perforation of the vaginal roof by a fetal forelimb which may be deflected dorsally during the second stage of labour by a hymeneal rim. As a result of vigorous sustained straining, the limb is then likely to perforate the rectum and be forced, possibly with the fetal head, through the anal orifice, which in turn may be ruptured (Figure

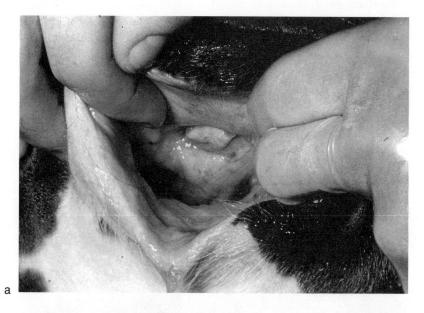

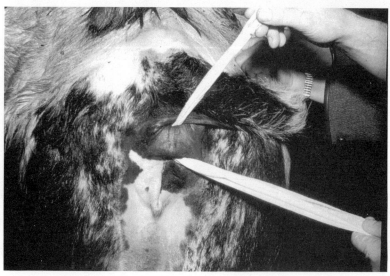

Fig. 17.3 Acquired rectovaginal fistula in a cow. (a) Vulva dilated to vaginal opening to fistula. (b) With a bandage passed through the fistula.

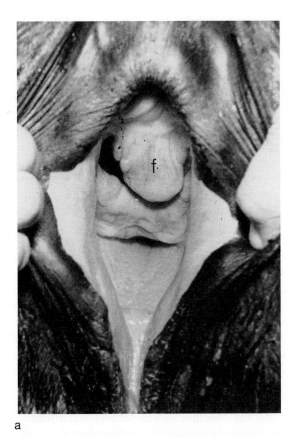

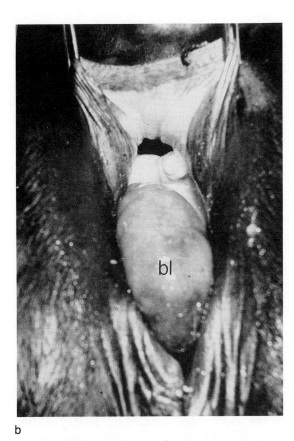

a

b

Fig. 17.4 Third-degree perineal defect in the mare. (a) Showing a flap of mucosa (f) attached to the roof of the vagina at the caudal border of the residual shelf. (b) Eversion of the bladder (bl).

17.4(a)). Early recognition of the injury may allow repositioning of the fetal extremities and normal vaginal delivery, but deliberate incision of the perineum and anal sphincter is usually expedient if the rectum is perforated because a third-degree defect is easier to repair surgically than a rectovaginal fistula which would otherwise result. Mares in which a Caslick closure of the upper vulval commissure is not reopened before foaling may sustain a similar injury in a slightly different way, the tear extending dorsally from the vulva, as in cows. Records of cases presented for repair indicate that third-degree tears are the most common perineal injury in the mare but rectovaginal fistula formation is still more frequent in the mare than the cow. By contrast, second-degree defects are rare in the mare but not uncommon in cows, simply because of the different mechanisms of tearing in the two species.

Perineal defects granulate and are epithelialized rapidly, but they are lacerated wounds with con-

siderable tissue damage and a degree of superficial sloughing is usual before granulation begins. The extent of inevitable tissue necrosis prejudices the likelihood of first-intention healing after immediate suturing. It is nevertheless advisable to stitch deep perineal wounds that have not perforated the anal sphincter as soon as possible. Third-degree tears with destruction of the sphincter and rectovaginal fistulae should be left to heal by granulation and surgical reconstruction can be undertaken later if necessary. The extent of such defects is considerably reduced by cicatrization and occasionally small, oblique fistulae in the mare close completely but in most cases a significant defect remains.

The clinical effects of a third-degree defect are two-fold: continuous aspiration of air into the vagina and contamination of the vaginal lumen with faecal fluids or, worse still, accumulation of faecal boluses in its terminal segment. Pneumovagina in turn, by distorting the lumen, may lead to pooling of urine cranial to the external urethral meatus. Inevitably in both the cow and the mare, these factors result in gross bacterial contamination and ascending infection in the genital tract. In both species, therefore, sizeable cloacal lesions result in infertility and affected mares are also aesthetically unsuited for other uses because of perineal incompetence.

In cases of rectovaginal fistula, the degree of faecal contamination of the vagina depends on the extent of the fistula. The occasional animals which are able to maintain a normal pregnancy are generally found to have a caudally sited lesion of very limited diameter.

Surgical intervention should be delayed until all tissue surfaces are covered by epithelium and this usually takes 6 weeks or so. In the mare, the urinary bladder is sometimes everted soon after the injury occurs (Figure 17.4(b)), but it is easily replaced and retained if necessary with sutures. There is no need for other treatment during the intervening period except perhaps for tetanus prophylaxis in the mare.

Second-degree defects are easily obliterated by stripping the vaginal mucosa from the normal level of the upper vulval commissure dorsally on both sides and suturing the submucosal tissues as in a Caslick operation.

For many years, surgical reconstruction of the perineum was based on the technique described by Götze in 1938, in which, after appropriate stripping of the mucosal surfaces, the residual shelf between rectum and vagina was mobilized and fixed as caudally as possible to separate the two cavities. The results were generally good but the operation resulted in considerable postoperative pain and sometimes faecal impaction because of reluctance to defaecate. The method has largely been superseded by the technique described by Aanes (1964), in which the rectum and vagina are separated by the construction of a new shelf from tissues *in situ* without undue tension on suture lines. Aanes advocated a two-stage operation, but the method to be described for repair of a third-degree defect is a one-stage procedure with other minor modifications of his suturing technique.

In cattle, the operation is ideally performed under epidural analgesia. The same technique can be used in the mare, but the operation can equally well be performed in this species with the animal

in dorsal recumbency and the hindquarters raised, under general anaesthesia. Cows require no dietary preparation. In the mare, a laxative diet without roughage is advisable for 3 days beforehand, followed by overnight starvation. After proper cleansing of the site, the rectum is gently packed with towelling; if the mare is anaesthetized, a vesical catheter may be inserted to divert urine from the operation site. In cows, the defect is usually no more than 6 cm deep from the perineum, but in the mare it is considerably longer and sometimes extends almost to the cervix. In both species, tissue forceps are placed on the cutaneous borders of the cloaca down to the normal level of the upper vulval commissure and on the caudal edge of the residual shelf. Bridges of skin across the defect are removed and it is then possible to see a sharp demarcation between the vaginal and rectal mucosae (Figures 17.5(a) and Plate 3(b) and (c)). The first stage of the procedure is to separate the vaginal mucous membrane from the tissues which will subsequently be apposed to create a shelf. The dissection begins at the level of the normal upper commissure and is extended dorsally on the mucocutaneous border and then cranially on both sides along the junction of vaginal and rectal mucous membranes until the incisions meet on the caudal edge of the residual shelf. The final stage of dissection is the separation of vaginal mucosa for 4 cm cranial to the edge of the shelf (Figure 17.5(b) and (c)). It is essential that all the vaginal mucous membrane is removed from the tissues which are to be sutured. There is minimal haemorrhage during the procedure and no need for haemostasis. In some cases, cicitrization results in considerable asymmetry of the cloaca which should be corrected before suturing is begun. The curtain of separated vaginal mucosa is then included in the purse-string-type sutures of polyglycolic acid which are placed and tied serially from the depth of the wound outwards. The method of suturing is illustrated in Figure 17.6, and a stage-by-state repair in a cow illustrated in Plate 3.

It is most important that the stitches tighten properly because dead space predisposes to wound breakdown. The operation is completed with mattress sutures in the perineal skin (Figure 17.7). Further minor closure of the upper commissure may be necessary under local anaesthetic infiltration when the integrity of the repair has been

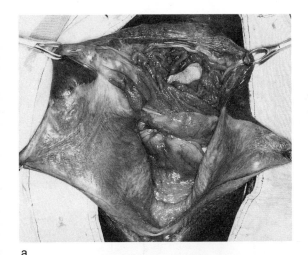

a

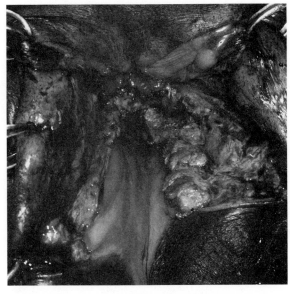

c

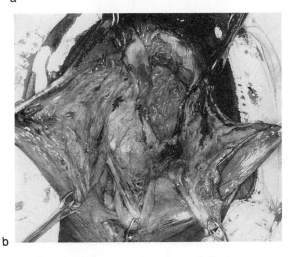

b

Fig. 17.5 (a) third-degree laceration in a mare exposed to demonstrate the clear demarcation between rectal and vaginal mucous membranes. Completed dissection of vaginal mucosa and the ventral surface of the shelf in (b) a cow and (c) a mare.

properly tested a month or so later. It should be emphasized that, although this operation restores breeding ability, it does not prevent air movement through the incompetent anal sphincter, a consideration which may be important in mares that are to be used for other purposes. In such animals a second operation to strengthen the sphincter can be attempted later by stripping mucocutaneous tissues in the defective segment and suturing what muscle remnants can be identified. The horse's anus is normally somewhat lax, and minor incompetence is no great detriment. If attempted reconstruction is unsuccessful, the operation can be repeated, but the prognosis is then less good because of local fibrosis and reduced vascularity.

Unless the vulval length is inadvertently shortened during reconstruction, subsequent parturition in both the cow and the mare usually occurs normally without the risk of vulval tearing or the need for episiotomy.

Paradoxically, a simple rectovaginal fistula is more difficult to repair than a third-degree defect. Aanes (1964) recommends that such lesions should first be converted into a cloaca and repaired as such after granulation stops. The deliberate destruction of perineum and anal sphincter can be avoided by adopting a different surgical approach to such lesions. Unless the fistula is deeply sited, it can be exposed satisfactorily by a dorsal commissure episiotomy which is extended cranially under the anal sphincter and rectal floor beyond the fistula (Figure 17.8). The rectal mucous membrane lining the lesion can then be securely inverted with sutures placed in a transverse direction in the submucosal tissues before the episiotomy is repaired in the conventional way.

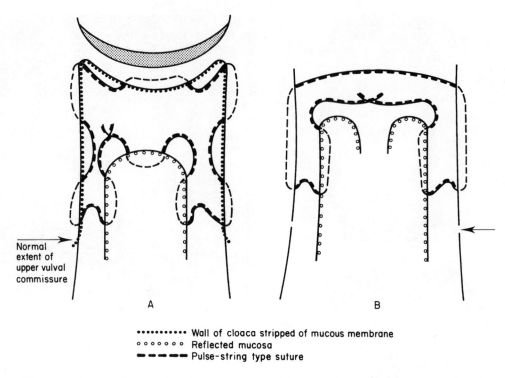

Normal
extent of
upper vulval
commissure

A

B

•••••••••••• Wall of cloaca stripped of mucous membrane
°°°°°°°° Reflected mucosa
━ ━ ━ ━━ Pulse-string type suture

Fig. 17.6 Diagram to show suturing technique for reconstruction of the perineum. (a) Below the shelf. (b) Caudal to the shelf.

Perineal defects are usually obvious in mares but are nevertheless sometimes not noticed by unwary purchasers. They are less obvious in cattle, particularly if the anal orifice remains intact.

Damage to the lumbosacral plexus

When a large fetus is forcibly drawn into the maternal pelvis the lumbar nerves which pass over the lumbosacral joint to form the anterior part of the lumbosacral plexus may be damaged; paralysis of the gluteal or obturator nerves is a possible result. This is particularly likely when an oversized fetus becomes impacted in a state of 'hip-lock', the nerves being trapped between the lumbosacral promontory of the mother and the iliac bones of the calf. In addition, the obturator nerve, as it passes down the inner surface of the iliac shaft, may be damaged by an oversized fetus.

Gluteal paralysis

Gluteal paralysis is seen in the mare and cow; in the mare it has followed spontaneous birth. It is recognized when the dam is found to have difficulty in rising and when she walks with 'weakness of the hindlimbs'. Later, atrophy of the gluteal muscles is apparent. Prognosis is favourable, the disability

usually disappearing in a few weeks, although occasionally complete recovery may take months. In warm weather the affected animal should be placed in a paddock which is free from ditches and obstacles; here a firmer foothold for getting up is more likely than in a barn or loose-box. The animal may be helped to rise by lifting on its tail and then steadying its hindquarters. In order that the mare may suckle the foal and also rest on its feet, slings may be usefully employed. If the mare or cow cannot get up within a few days of parturition the prognosis is grave.

Obturator paralysis

Obturator paralysis is more frequent in cows than mares. The obturator nerve supplies the adductor muscles of the thigh; thus when both nerves are damaged the legs will be splayed and the cow is unable to rise. If the cow is helped to its feet, the legs slide out laterally. When paralysis is one-sided the cow also requires assistance to get up but can stand readily, if the affected leg is prevented from sliding outwards. If the cow falls there is a risk of limb fracture or dislocation of the hip joint. Where there is complete and bilateral paralysis prognosis should be guarded; where it is unilateral and the

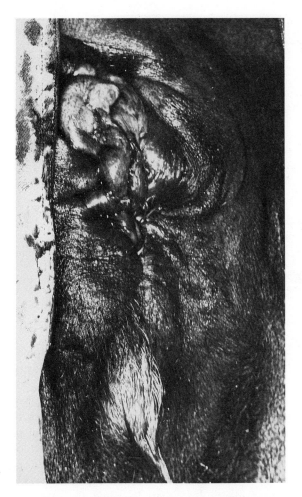

Fig. 17.7 Completed one-stage reconstruction of the perineum in a Friesian cow.

animal can walk with assistance the outlook is favourable. Hobbling together of the hindlegs with a strap applied above each fetlock prevents excessive abduction and secondary tearing of the adductor muscles or fracture of the femoral neck during attempts to stand. Most cases show rapid improvement within a few days and progress to a complete recovery. Unless there is marked improvement within a fortnight, recovery is unlikely. Treatment comprises good nursing. The cow should be well bedded with short litter on an earthen floor or on a concrete floor on which sand or grit has first been sprinkled. She must be assisted and maintained on her feet for milking or suckling and as often as possible at other times. The patient should be stimulated to walk but should be prevented from falling awkwardly. Slings are occasionally employed for cattle. Bedsores must be

prevented, the animal being turned from side to side, the hindquarters massaged, the bedding frequently changed and the cow's rear and udder kept clean and dry.

Rupture of the uterus or vagina

Rupture of the uterus may occur spontaneously, but faulty obstetric technique is a more frequent cause. Spontaneous rupture is most likely to arise in association with uterine torsion or with cervical non-dilatation but is also possibly due to the gross uterine distension that occurs with twins in one horn, with hydrallantois or with excessive fetal size. The most likely time of spontaneous rupture is in late gestation or during labour. Hopkins and Amor (1964) have remarked on the association of spontaneous uterine rupture and breech presentation: they encountered three cases and cited four other cases from the literature. In their cases (and in another spontaneous rupture with breech presentation seen by the present author) the dorsal aspect of the left uterine horn was torn and the split extended backwards to involve also the uterine body and cervix. They believe that breech presentation predisposes to rupture because the breech of the calf fully occupies the maternal pelvic inlet and allows no egress for the fetal fluid when the uterine and abdominal contractions build up the hydrostatic pressure within the uterus. In a review of 26 cases of uterine rupture, 18 of which were heifers, Pearson and Denny (1975) considered uterine torsion and fetopelvic disproportion to be the major predisposing factors. In this series, 14 of the 26 fetuses were mainly or entirely within the peritoneal cavity; four were still alive at the time of laparotomy. According to the size of the rupture — which may heal without incident or allow escape of the conceptus in the abdomen — and to whether or not infection occurs, there is great variation in the syndrome from cases in which no symptoms are shown to others in which shock and fatal toxaemia soon supervene. Thus in some instances the owner is unaware of the accident and the only evidence of it is the subsequent finding of a uterine adhesion or of a mummified fetus among the abdominal viscera — so-called extrauterine pregnancy. When rupture occurs during labour and the fetus passes into the abdomen, labour pains and straining cease and uterine inertia may be suspected until a uterine exploration proves

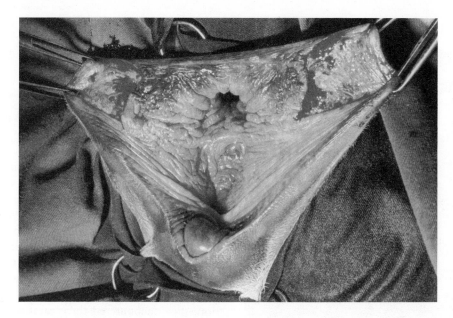

Fig. 17.8 A congenital rectovaginal fistula in a donkey exposed by episiotomy.

otherwise. Alternatively, the dam's intestines may prolapse into the uterus and even protrude from the vulva; the condition may then be confused with dystocia due to schistosoma reflexus in visceral presentation. Accidental rupture of the uterus is likely to occur in the most difficult dystocia cases: those in which the initial disposition of the fetus is markedly irregular and difficult to rectify and those in which there has been much delay in treatment with the development of unfavourable complications. Insufficient uterine space for the extension of a limb or head, inordinate traction on a wrongly disposed or oversized fetus and excessively vigorous retropulsion are the immediate causes of uterine rupture. When the cervix is incompletely dilated, traction on the fetus may cause rupture of that organ. Careless use of the obstetric forceps in the bitch is a cause of uterine rupture. Lastly, rupture of the uterus may be due to external violence as, for example, when the parturient dam falls heavily or receives a severe kick or horn-gore on its abdomen.

When making the initial examination of a dystocia case the veterinary surgeon must always explore the genital tract for traumatic lesions that may have been caused by unskilled lay interference or which, rarely, may have arisen spontaneously. If uterine rupture is found then, or occurs during subsequent manipulations, the obstetrician must decide — largely on considerations of size and

site of the lesion and the amount of manipulation, or traction, still required to effect delivery — whether to proceed with the delivery per vaginam or whether to perform laparotomy, extract the fetus and repair the uterine rupture from the laparotomy site. Except where a small dorsal rupture is discovered and the amount of obstetric interference still required is small, laparotomy is indicated. The procedure then adopted is almost identical to that described for caesarean section, the only complication being the possibly unfavourable site of uterine rupture in relation to the abdominal incision. The accidental rupture may be extended and the fetus extracted or, if the rent is unfavourably placed, another surgical incision must be made for delivery and then both it and the rupture must be repaired. The tear in the uterus is much more accessible for suturing after the fetus has been removed.

Since the 1960s more attention has been given to ovine obstetrics. White (1961) described a condition not previously noted in which, during late gestation, spontaneous rupture of the vagina occurs. Small intestine passes into the vagina and protrudes from the vulva. Ewes that are heavily pregnant with twins are most likely to suffer. The causes of the condition are probably the same as those which initiate vaginal prolapse. Preparturient straining is the immediate cause of the vaginal rupture, but the escape of abdominal viscera through the tear reduces abdominal pressure and prolapse of the vagina does not progress to its usual conclusion. Affected ewes soon die from shock. In one case, which was considered to have a similar aetiology, Fox (1962) noted complete prolapse of the intact pregnant uterus through a rent in the vaginal roof. O'Neill (1961) observed several parturient ewes that were unable to lamb in which rupture of the uterus was present. Prompt adoption of the caesarean operation and repair of the uterine tear gave good results.

Prolapse of the bladder

Prolapse of the bladder may follow a rupture in the floor of the vagina or eversion through the dilated urethra (Brunsdon, 1961) and may occur during or after parturition. The rounded organ protrudes from the vulva. The kink that forms in the urethra prevents micturition; thus the organ progressively distends with urine. The condition must be distinguished from prolapse of the vagina, cyst or tumour of the vagina, haematoma of the vulva and prolapse of perivaginal fat. The surface of the bladder is cleaned and the organ is punctured with a hypodermic needle to allow drainage of urine. It is then dressed with an antibiotic powder and gently pushed back into place through the vaginal rupture. The latter is then repaired. Epidural anaesthesia will greatly facilitate return of the prolapsed organ.

Eversion of the bladder

Eversion of the bladder is most likely in the mare. In this species the urethral opening is wide and parturient straining very forceful. The organ becomes everted during labour and may be injured during fetal expulsion. It should not be difficult to identify the everted bladder. It is pear shaped and attached to the vaginal floor; urine drips from the two openings of the ureters and the congested mucosa is apparent. Epidural anaesthesia should be induced. The bladder is first cleaned, and any lacerations are repaired by suture. The organ is then compressed between both hands and gradually forced back into the urethra. Further manipulation is then applied to the vaginal floor until the bladder is properly replaced. Antibiotic therapy, lasting several days should be prescribed. Tetanus antitoxin should be given. Eversion of the bladder is rare in cattle.

Brundson (1961) described a case which occurred during second-stage labour and which he successfully replaced.

Prolapse of perivaginal fat

Prolapse of perivaginal fat is most likely in fat heifers of beef breeds and is a sequel to a rupture of the vagina, often a small one. The fat should be snipped off with scissors, and, if possible, after the application of an antibiotic preparation, the vaginal tear should be sutured.

Prolapse of the rectum

Slight eversion of the rectum is a common accompaniment of powerful expulsive efforts. It recedes after delivery. Severe prolapse is likely only in the mare; if it is already present in a dystocia case when the veterinary surgeon arrives, an attempt should be made to reduce the prolapse and an assistant should be instructed to maintain the organ in position by pressing a towel against the mare's anus. Epidural anaesthesia may be needed to replace the rectum. When the prolapse has been present for some hours before veterinary assistance is available and the organ has become markedly oedematous and contused or torn, it may be difficult or impossible to replace it and maintain it in position. Submucous resection under epidural anaesthesia, or under a general anaesthetic, must then be carried out. In the mare, parturient prolapse of the rectum, no matter how transient, may prove fatal because stretching or tearing of the colic mesentery can result in infarction of the terminal colon (Figure 17.9). The affected segment of bowel becomes atonic, defaecation stops and the mare's condition deteriorates insidiously during the next few days.

PUERPERAL LAMINITIS

Puerperal laminitis is a troublesome complication of puerperal metritis. It is essentially an equine condition, but the other farm animals are occasionally affected. In the mare the condition is a likely sequel to retention of the placenta. Two to four days after foaling the typical stance of laminitis is seen, the hindlegs being placed well forward to ease the weight on the more severely affected forefeet. It is a most painful affection and causes

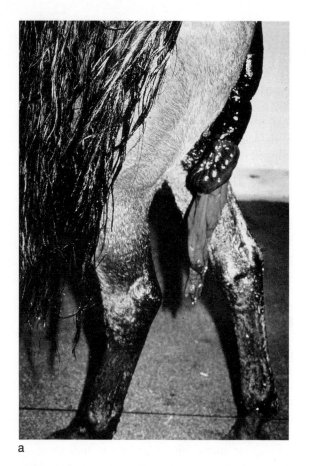

a

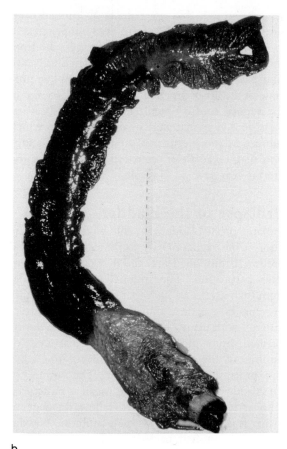

b

Fig. 17.9 Complications of second-stage rectal prolapse in a mare. (a) Infarction of prolapsed colon. (b) Infarction after reduction of the prolapse.

rapid loss of weight. Owing to the prolonged periods of recumbency and diminution in milk secretion the foal may require artificial feeding.

Avoidance of puerperal laminitis lies in preventing metritis by treating cases of dystocia and retention of the afterbirth with appropriate antimicrobial agents and by the timely removal of the retained fetal membranes (see p. 299).

In the treatment of puerperal laminitis attention to the uterus comprises removal of the retained afterbirth, if any, siphonage of the fetid exudate and the intrauterine infusion and systemic administration of appropriate antimicrobial agents; oxytocin is also indicated. When prompt treatment is applied, prognosis is favourable.

PARTURIENT RECUMBENCY

Recumbency, as a complication of parturition, is occasionally seen in all species but is essentially a bovine condition. Under this heading, cows which become recumbent in late gestation should first be considered; the cause here is nutritional, and two separate entities are seen. In one type, recumbency is associated with starvation. Cases occur towards the end of the winter when fodder is scarce or poorly saved. Cattle on hill farms are chiefly affected. Premature induction of calving with corticosteroids (see p. 149), or an elective caesarean section, can be used provided the animal is not too severely affected. Otherwise, in the interest of the animal's welfare, euthanasia should be performed and measures taken to ensure that similar cases do not re-occur. Prompt caesarean section and dietary supplementation are indicated. The other entity is a syndrome that appears to be identical to pregnancy toxaemia of ewes. Affected animals are in good bodily condition and are usually pregnant with twins. The general behaviour becomes sluggish, appetite is poor and ketosis, sometimes accompanied by icterus, is present. Premature induction of calving or termination of the pregnancy (see p. 149) is normally followed by rapid recovery. Cases which have been unsuccessfully treated therapeutically have shown marked fatty infiltration of the liver. The cause may be due to an excess of concentrated food in early pregnancy and to a deficient diet in late gestation.

Milk fever or parturient hypocalcaemia

Hypocalcaemia is the chief cause of recumbency in parturient and puerperal cows. Channel Island cattle, in which there is a high incidence of hypocalcaemia, may become recumbent before or during labour, but the majority of cattle show hypocalcaemia within 24 hours after labour. Recumbency of hypocalcaemia is associated with general paresis which usually progresses to coma or narcosis, the animal then being in lateral recumbency with a marked tendency to rumenal tympany. The condition is much more likely to follow normal birth than dystocia, and the history of rapid progression from normality through hyperaesthesia, paddling of hindlimbs and locomotor instability to final recumbency and coma is typical and makes diagnosis easy.

The coma or narcosis of milk fever may be confused with the final stage of severe puerperal toxaemia resulting from uterine infection. A proper consideration of the history and due regard to the symptoms should differentiate the conditions. Puerperal metritis usually follows dystocia and is often accompanied by retention of the afterbirth: there is a fetid vulval discharge and diarrhoea; straining is frequent and there is an expiratory grunt; the pulse is frequent but the temperature, although at first raised, may be falling in a case of advanced toxaemia and is therefore unreliable. A vaginal and uterine examination should verify the suspicion of metritis as a cause of recumbency. Other severe toxaemias that may cause parturient recumbency are septic mastitis, particularly that due to staphylococci, traumatic

pericarditis and peritonitis associated with uterine rupture.

True hypocalcaemia occurs occasionally in sows, but the most likely cause of postparturient recumbency is toxaemia due to metritis or mastitis. Incomplete parturition with retention of a fetus or a portion of the afterbirth should always be suspected. Failure of milk secretion is one of the symptoms of toxaemia and hypocalcaemia; it sometimes results from lack of the 'let down stimulus'. So-called agalactia of sows is thus not a specific syndrome but merely a symptom common to several quite different affections.

Physical inability to rise

Physical inability to rise may be due to muscular weakness or to lesions of the locomotor system. Inanition due to a variety of diseases may coincide with parturition. Locomotor lesions that may occur during labour and cause recumbency include dislocations of the hip and of the sacroiliac joints, fracture of the pelvis, femur or vertebral column, rupture of the gastrocnemius muscle and paralysis of the obturator or gluteal nerves. A diagnosis of disease of the locomotor system depends on a methodical clinical examination with a view to eliminating the several possibilities. The degree and form of the disability and the manner of the unsuccessful attempt to rise often give a strong indication of the cause. The examination includes the humane manipulation of the hindlimbs with the help of an assistant to determine the presence of excessive mobility or crepitus; it is combined with a rectal examination of the pelvic bones. Regional absence of peripheral sensation may verify nerve paralysis, including paraplegia associated with vertebral fracture. In cases of recumbency due to physical inability, or pain associated with attempts to rise, the affected animal is usually bright, its appetite is good and, when undisturbed, its temperature and pulse are unaffected. Each case must be treated on its merits, and the reader is referred to other texts for further information. It is not unusual in cattle practice to fail to discover the cause of recumbency despite a meticulous and complete examination; apart from recumbency such cases appear normal in every way. In these instances a brief application of the electric goad causes a determined attempt to rise. This is sometimes successful and in any case the extent of the disability may be then more clearly seen. The repeated application of the electric goad must be thoroughly deprecated.

Where no cause of recumbency can be found in an animal that appears normal in other respects, tissue swelling, oedema or haemorrhage in the vicinity of nerves is possible. If such were the case the normal recovery processes would diminish pressure on the nerves, and this would be reflected in progressively better attempts to rise. Experience in cattle practice shows that if a cow is still unable to rise after being recumbent for a week, the prognosis is grave. Slings, hoists, and other devices are sometimes used to encourage the patient to stand, but in general they are of little use. The best contribution that can be made to a recovery is the provision of first-class nursing. This comprises placing the recumbent animal on ample, soft, clean bedding which overlies a dry floor and which is frequently changed. The patient is turned from side to side as often as possible, with concurrent massage of the limb muscles. Meanwhile close veterinary attention is paid to the health of the cow's uterus and udder.

PUERPERAL TETANUS

Puerperal tetanus is a possible sequel to uterine manipulation for dystocia, retention of the afterbirth or prolapse of the uterus. It is most likely to be seen in mares 1–4 weeks after foaling.

All equine obstetric interference should be accompanied by prophylactic injections of tetanus antitoxin.

REFERENCES

Aanes, W. A. (1964) *J. Amer. Vet. Med. Assn,* **144**, 485.
Brunsdon, J. E. (1961) *Vet. Rec.,* **73**, 437.
Fox, M. W. (1962) Personal communication.
Götze, R. (1938) *Dt. Tierärztl. Wschr.,* **49**, 163.
Hopkins, A. R. and Amor, O. F. (1964) *Vet. Rec.,* **76**, 904.
O'Neill, A. R. (1961) *Vet. Rec.,* **73**, 1041.
Pearson, H. and Denny, H. R. (1975) *Vet. Rec.,* **97**, 240.
Rooney, E. F. (1964) *Cornell Vet.,* **54**, 11.
White, J. B. (1961) *Vet. Rec.,* **73**, 281, 330.

18 Retention of the Fetal Membranes

AETIOLOGY

The changes responsible for normal placental separation and expulsion have been described in Chapter 3.

Retention of the fetal membranes comprises a lack of dehiscence and a failure of expulsion of the afterbirth within the duration of physiological third-stage labour. It implies either an insufficiency of uterine contraction after the second stage of labour or a placental lesion which affects the normal physical union between the fetal villi and the maternal crypts. As regards the relative causative importance of these two possibilities opinion has veered from the view of Harms, and later Benesch, that retention was due to imperfect contraction of the uterus to the contention of Götze and others that a proliferative placentitis (particularly due to *Brucella abortus*) was the commonest cause. Because there is a higher incidence of retention in brucella-infected herds it has been assumed, without due reflection, that the brucella-induced placentitis was the cause of it. It is true that abortions in late gestation caused by *B. abortus* are likely to be followed by retention; however, in the majority of cattle abortions investigated no infection can be found and yet they seem equally likely to be associated with retention of the afterbirth. It is noteworthy that the birth of cattle twins — which are usually slightly premature — is often followed by failure of the third stage of labour. Morrison and Erb (1957) stated that 43% of cattle twin births were followed by retention, while Erb et al. (1958) reported that 37.4% of 760 cases of retention studied by them were accounted for by twin births and abortions. It seems, from the outcome of experimentally induced twinning by embryo transfer (Anderson et al., 1978) and from clinical experience, that unicornual and bicornual twinning, being associated with shortened gestation, are both conducive to retention. Also, if a calf is removed prematurely by elective caesarean operation there is delay in expulsion of the afterbirth. Heat stress can reduce gestation length and increase the incidence of retention of the afterbirth in dairy cattle. Thus Dubois and Williams (1980) found that cows which calved during the warm season in Georgia, USA, where the mean daily temperature was 26°C, had a reduction of 2.82 days in gestation length and an incidence of 24.05% retention, compared with 12.24% for the remainder of the year. The gestation lengths for retaining cows were, on average, 5.25 days shorter than those of non-retaining cows. One concludes from these observations that premature birth, irrespective of its cause, is a common factor in many cases of retention.

Premature parturition can be induced in cows by removal of the corpus luteum after about the seventh month of pregnancy; there is no infection but the afterbirth is usually retained (McDonald et al., 1953). If after removal of the corpus luteum adequate progesterone supplementation is provided the cows carry to term and expel their afterbirths. Similarly, if ovariectomy is performed between 200 and 230 days (Eastergren, 1967; Chew et al., 1979) or if the synthetic corticosteroids dexamethasone and flumethasone are administered to pregnant cattle in the last 40 days of gestation, premature parturition occurs and is extremely likely to be followed by retention of the fetal membranes, e.g. in 54% of 294 cows induced by Wagner et al. (1974).

Premature birth, whether induced by natural causes (known and unknown), experimental surgery or pharmacologically, implies either a failure of, or interference with, the endocrine control of parturition. It will be recalled from the discussion on parturition in Chapter 6 that the initiation and continuation of the myometrial contractions of birth are the outcome of an integrated sequence of endocrine events. If, therefore, the endocrine processes fail to control the time of parturition, as in premature births, myometrial dysfunction is to be expected and, as a consequence, there will be failure to expel the afterbirth.

With less severe impairment of endocrine control it can be visualized that the length of gestation will be normally governed and that parturition will begin but not proceed normally. This commonly occurs in the polytocous sow and bitch where several fetuses may be expelled and then, for no apparent reason, parturition does not progress; the failure is ascribed to uterine inertia. In the monotocous cow a comparable situation would be a failure of parturition to progress beyond the second stage.

Although there is veterinary consensus of an aetiological relationship between premature birth in cattle and retention of the afterbirth, a causative relationship between lack of uterine contractibility and failure to expel the fetal membranes is not universally accepted. Thus Zerobin and Sporri (1972) suggested that uterine atony was not a cause of retention, while the study by Martin et al. (1981) of retention in cows induced to calve prematurely (by means of dexamethasone and oestradiol benzoate) failed to establish a relationship between early postpartum uterine motility and retention. It is impossible to reconcile the conflicting findings of Benesch (1930), Jordan (1952) and Venable and MacDonald (1958) of a positive effect of uterine contractions on expulsion of the afterbirth with the negative results of Martin et al. (1981). However, Taverne (1984) stated that intrauterine pressure recordings made under clinical conditions should be interpreted with caution and he emphasized the need to record continuously over a 24 hour period from chronically implanted and multiple pressure and electrical sensors dispersed through the uterus. Martin et al. (1981) recorded at only three postpartum times, 1, 6 and 48 hours after fetal expulsion and for 20 minutes at each time.

An alternative explanation of retention and its association with premature birth is advanced by some workers. It is that the loosening process which normally occurs between the fetal villi and the maternal crypts depends on histological changes in the apposing surfaces, due to prevailing concentrations of certain hormones and enzymes. When birth is premature the hormonal changes may be asynchronous and therefore not favour-able to the occurrence of the requisite tissue changes (Bjorkman and Sollen, 1960; Grunert, 1984).

The role of the acellular layer between fetal and maternal epithelium at the level of the microvilli, the so-called 'glue line', may be important. This layer of adhesive protein probably undergoes some chemical change prior to normal separation. Maintenance of adhesion because of failure to undergo the prepartum changes has been shown using various staining techniques (Bjorkman and Sollen, 1960).

Confirmation of a probable endocrine explanation for retention associated with premature birth and for some of the cases that occur after a normal gestation length (followed by clinically normal first and second stages of labour) has come from investigations of hormone levels in both those groups of cattle (Agthe and Kolm, 1975; Chew et al., 1977; O'Brien and Stott, 1977; Stott and Rheinhard, 1978). Ovariectomy between days 200 and 230 usually does not cause abortion but leads to premature parturition, with a high incidence of dystocia and retention of the afterbirth. Similarly, premature parturition at 268 days, induced by injection of dexamethasone with oestradiol, predisposed to dystocia and retention. Concomitant hormone assays in both ovariectomized and induced cows indicated that dystocia and retention were likely if oestradiol-17β in maternal blood remained low until at least 4 days prepartum, particularly if plasma progesterone was chronically low for several weeks prepartum. Moreover, intact (control) cows which naturally retained the afterbirth showed higher than normal levels of oestradiol-17α and progesterone, together with abnormally low oestradiol-17β levels before parturition. Different types of abnormal change in progsterone levels, namely abrupt decreases or very slow decreases, were accompanied by 100% retention.

In other experiments in beef heifers, where prostaglandin $F_{2\alpha}$ ($PGF_{2\alpha}$) alone or with oestradiol was used at day 267 to induce premature parturition (Hendricks et al., 1977), the respective retention rates were 83 and 71%. Hormone assays were not done but it was known that $PGF_{2\alpha}$ caused a precipitous drop in progesterone levels.

The conclusion from these hormone studies of natural and induced retention of fetal membranes is that endocrine cases of retention depend on quantitative disorders of the normal preparturient hormonal ratios, particularly between oestrogens and progesterone, or on an asynchrony of endocrine events, or on temporal faults in the sequence of endocrine changes that precede parturition.

It should not be forgotten that factors other than hormone imbalance can cause uterine inertia: lack of blood calcium, particularly in dairy cattle; overstretching of the myometrium as with hydrops allantois or grossly oversized fetus; and degeneration of the myometrial fibres as a result of bacterial toxins. In addition to all these kinds of primary uterine inertia is the large category of secondary uterine inertia which results from exhaustion of the myometrium in obstructive dystocia; in these cases also, retention of the afterbirth is very common.

There is, as with primary uterine inertia, some evidence of an hereditary predisposition to retention of the fetal membranes. Cows of the beef breeds are much less often affected than those of dairy breeds and in the latter the incidence is higher in Ayrshires than Friesians. Old cows are more affected than young ones. Spring-time calving exerts a predisposing influence; it might be connected with a vitamin A deficiency which has been shown to produce retention under experimental conditions. Vinattieri et al. (1945) have shown that the incidence of retention in buffaloes is strikingly higher when the calves are removed at birth than when they are allowed to suckle. There is evidence of a high incidence of retained fetal membranes in areas deficient in selenium (Trinder et al., 1973; Julien et al., 1976a,b) and of a reduction of incidence after selenium supplementation of the diet. However, Gwazdauskas et al. (1979), in a careful study of 351 cattle over a 3 year period in an area not deficient, found no reduction in placental retention after 28 days of prepartum supplementation with selenium. It is concluded therefore that selenium deficiency may be a cause of endemics of retained afterbirth in certain deficient areas but that the generality of retention cases are not associated with selenium deficiency.

From an extensive clinical experience of parturition in American herds, which were known to be free at the time of observation from common gynaecological infections such as brucellosis, vibriosis, leptospirosis, IBR–IPV (infectious bovine rhinotracheitis–infectious pustular vulvovaginitis) and moulds, Roberts (1971) believes firmly that genital infection derived at or near the time of parturition is a potent cause of failure to cleanse. Retention occurred particularly when a number of cows calved in quick succession in the same calving quarters, and Roberts believed it was due to a build-up of virulence in the organisms which are usually present in bovine habitations such as group C *Streptococcus*, *Escherichia coli*, *Staphylococcus*, *Pseudomonas* and *Actinomyces* (*Corynebacterium*) *pyogenes*. These enzootics of retention were sometimes associated with metritis and calf scour. When there were intervals of months between consecutive calvings, or when cows in the same herds calved at pasture there was a dramatic drop in the incidence of the affection. The mechanism whereby the infections caused the retention is not clear: inflammatory swelling may affect the physical union between the maternal caruncle and fetal cotyledon; the involvement of the endometrium may interfere with the endocrine changes of the third stage of labour; or bacterial toxins may affect the myometrium. Clearly, the hygiene of calving pens must be strictly observed in the very large milking herds of the present day in order to prevent a build-up of parturient infection.

There is clinical evidence of an association between retention and parturient hypocalcaemia in Scandinavian herds, i.e. retention in one year is likely to be followed by milk fever the following year (Roine and Saloniemi, 1978). In Utah, USA, Lamb et al. (1979) found that Holstein heifers which were kept in confinement but which had been driven 1.5 km daily for 4–6 weeks before parturition had easier calvings and showed earlier expulsion of the fetal membranes and quicker involution of the uterus. Older cows showed no benefit from the exercise. Recently, Joosten and Hensen (1992) have shown a link between retained fetal membranes and MHC class 1 compatibility of the calf and dam, perhaps pointing to a failure of alloreactivity to the fetal membranes by the dam. In addition, retention may also be related to failure of the release of inflammatory mediators (Slama et al., 1993).

Before concluding the consideration of the causes of failure to expel the fetal membranes it is noteworthy that ruminants, particularly cows, which fail to deliver the placenta within 36 hours or so, are likely to retain it for 7–10 days. This is because substantial myometrial contractions do not proceed beyond 36 hours of the birth of the calf,

Table 18.1 Published incidences of retention of afterbirth

Study	Country	No. of calvings	Incidence (%)
Palmer (1932)	USA	375[a]	11.7
Kennedy (1947)	Scotland	431	8.3
Cohen (1956)	Israel	145 000	8.9
Erb et al. (1958)	USA	7 387	10.7
Leech et al. (1960)	Britain		3.8
Vandeplassche and Martens (1961)	Belgium	738[b]	8.0
Ben-David (1962)	Israel	24 000	8.4
Banerjee (1963)	Holland	2 276	11.2
Moller et al. (1967)	New Zealand	36 000	1.96
Vandeplassche and Martens (1961)	Belgium	64[c]	55.0
Geyer (1964)	Germany	1 200[c]	25.0

[a] Herds free from tuberculosis and brucellosis.
[b] Herds free from brucellosis, vibriosis and trichomoniasis.
[c] Dystocia cases.

and if the membranes have not been expelled by this time their subsequent dehiscence can occur only as a result of natural sloughing of the maternal caruncles or by putrefactive liquefaction of the fetal cotyledons, and their expulsion will thenceforward depend on uterine involution. When expulsion finally occurs, the membranes do not undergo inversion during the process as happens with physiological third-stage labour.

INCIDENCE

Dairy cattle are most prone to retention; sheep are occasionally affected. The condition occurs with the primary inertia complex of bitches and sows in which fetuses as well as membranes are retained; retention of separate afterbirths is rare. Failure to expel the membranes is an uncommon occurrence in mares but the heavy draught mares of former times were more prone to it. Tijskens (1972), in a study of 1322 warm-blooded mares, recorded a retention incidence of 4%. There are no figures for the frequency of the affection in other animals apart from dairy cows for which incidences as variable as 1.96 and 55% have been recorded, according to the sample of cows investigated (Table 18.1).

Commenting on the figures in Table 18.1, it is noteworthy that the lowest incidence was in New Zealand cows which were at pasture the whole year. Apart from this and the British figure of 3.8%, the average incidence for all calvings would seem to be about 11%; for normal calvings it is

about 8% and for dystocias 25–55%. Additional data relating to incidence are that retention tends to increase with parity, that there is an individual tendency to recurrent retention and that the incidence is very high with twins and with late abortions but not with early abortions (in which the whole conceptus is easily expelled). Also, genetically high-yielding dairy cows and cows on high nutritive planes at parturition are more prone to retention (Whitmore et al., 1974).

CLINICAL FEATURES

Since delayed involution of the uterus and a variable degree of metritis commonly accompany retention. Because of this association it is difficult to assess the pathogenic importance of retention *per se*.

Within 24 hours of its separation from the fetal blood supply the necrotic mass of fetal membranes begins to undergo bacterial putrefaction, and this process gradually frees the fetal villi from the maternal crypts. Irrespective of the presence of a concomitant metritis, therefore, there will be an accumulation of the toxic products of putrefaction within the uterus. The reaction to these toxins varies with the species: cattle, sheep and goats are least affected, mares and bitches show severe febrile reactions, while sows occupy an intermediate position. As the putrefactive process proceeds, a most disagreeable, fetid odour is produced which pervades the atmosphere and taints the milk. The milk from affected cows must not be sold for human consumption, and it is for this economic reason and for aesthetic considerations as much as for cow ill-health that farmers are concerned about retention.

When retention is accompanied by metritis there will be variable symptoms according to the severity of the uterine disease. In general, there will be increased pulse and respiratory rates, raised temperature, anorexia, diarrhoea, depression, reduced milk secretion, straining and fetid sanguinopurulent vaginal discharge; laminitis is an occasional complication. In mares, particularly the heavier draught type, laminitis commonly develops and tetanus has been known to follow.

The duration of retention seems to depend on several factors such as the extent of the areas of attachment of the fetal membranes, the rate of uterine involution, the amount of uterine exudate and the proportion of the afterbirth which had already passed through the cervix when retention began. In addition, experienced clinicians can detect differences in texture of the retained fetal cotyledons in cattle which are of prognostic significance; where they are fleshy and substantial they detach more readily than when they are thin and stringy, in which case they appear to be adherent to the maternal caruncles.

With respect to the amount of morbidity and mortality resulting from retention in cattle, there is little departure from health in cows which have calved spontaneously after a normal length of gestation. If the membranes are not passed within 36 hours they tend to be retained for 6–10 days, when they drop away as a putrescent mass. On the other hand, when retention follows extensive obstetric interference for dystocia, retention may be associated in 2–3 days with a severe metritis and toxaemia which, if untreated, can be fatal. However, similar cases may be equally ill if the placenta was removed at the time of delivery, so it seems that retention of itself is not necessarily the cause of the severe ill-health. Mortality is commonly put at 1–4% and morbidity, as denoted by some temporary impairment of appetite and reduction of milk yield, at 55–65% of cases. Palmer (1932) carried out careful observations on the pathogenicity of retention in 44 cattle: no treatment was given except to four cows which became quite ill and in which proflavine and saline were infused into the uterus. During the fortnight after calving appetite was good in 31.8%, fair in 54.5% and

poor in 13.6%; body weight was unaffected in 88.6%. When the 44 cases of retention were mated and compared with 44 cows in the herd which had cleansed normally there was no significant difference in the subsequent breeding records of the two groups. With respect to the latter aspect, although cases of retention commonly develop endometritis with a subsequent mucopurulent discharge (described by farmers as 'the whites') there is now a consensus of veterinary opinion which supports Palmer's findings that uncomplicated retention does not significantly affect the fertility of cows which are mated beyond 60 days of the last calving. Sandals et al. (1979) have provided clarification of this aspect by means of a retrospective analysis of computer-based records of 652 parturitions of 293 dairy cows in Canada. Their study revealed that the overall incidence of retained afterbirth was 11.2%. It was 4.6 times more likely after twin birth than after single birth and more common after autumn calvings. Metritis complex was diagnosed in 54.8% of retention cases. Furthermore, and most importantly, it was found that retained placenta alone did not impair subsequent reproductive performance but metritis complex alone, or with retained placenta, caused significant increases in 'days open', services per conception, calving to first heat interval and days from calving to first service. The conclusion was that the influence of retained placentae on fertility depends on the proportion of cows with retention that have the metritis complex.

Jordan (1948) found that the bacterial flora of the uterus in retention cases was the same as in cases of delayed involution without retention, streptococci (particularly *Streptococcus dysgalactiae*) appearing first and being followed next by staphylococci (often coagulase-negative) and finally by diphtheroids (*A. (C.) pyogenes* predominating). Coliform and anaerobic bacteria were also present. In all uncomplicated cases after the third day, Jordan found the characteristic blood leucocyte picture of pyogenic infection, with neutrophilia and 'shift to the left', but in toxaemic cases there was severe leucopenia, neutropenia and eosinopenia. It must be accepted that in the majority of cases of retention and of delayed involution without retention the uterus becomes and remains an infected focus for a month or even longer and that there is consequently a theoretical loss of breeding time. But in most of these animals natural resolution occurs and the breeding potential is normal 2–3 months later.

Any discussion of the pathology of placental retention would not be complete without reference to the possible harmful effects of treatment by manual removal. Ill-effects which have been ascribed to retention itself may have arisen from, or been aggravated by, injury resulting from such interference. Few veterinarians are not familiar with the cow whose well-being was distinctly reduced after manual removal of the membranes.

As regards the effects of retention of the allantochorion in the mare, orthodox teaching has been that in this species retention was likely to be followed after 12 hours by a rapidly developing metritis, severe toxaemia and laminitis. However, by carefully observing a small number of mares which held their afterbirths beyond 12 hours, Wright (1943) found that a majority of them cleansed in the succeeding 12 hours and up to that time there was no departure from health. It is possible that the riding mares and ponies which predominate in the horse population of today are less affected by retention than the heavy draught horses of former times. Because of the practice of early removal of the retained placenta of the mare there is little modern information on the natural outcome of retention in this species. However, in mares which had been subjected to elective caesarean operation the authors have seen no real ill-health in mares which have held the membranes for as long as 3 days.

The outcome of untreated cases of failure to cleanse in sheep is similar to that seen in cattle. Progressive putrefaction occurs, and the mass ultimately falls away in 5–10 days. It is unlikely that severe ill-health or death will ensue.

In the sow, retention is fortunately rare, but when it does occur it may give rise to a severe metritis. The fetal membranes comprise a variable number of component masses, and it is difficult in a given case to ascertain whether expulsion is complete. Retention is most likely after protracted labour. By the time a retention case has become noticeably ill with anorexia, fever and sanguinopurulent vaginal discharge, the cervix has become too small to admit the obstetrician's hand. In all assisted porcine deliveries the membranes should be examined and the number of umbilical cords compared with the number of fetuses. There may be a retention of a single after-birth or of an aggregated mass of several components. When there is retention the sow will not settle for long in lateral recumbency, there is consequent interference with suckling and a chorus of dissatisfied vocalizations from the piglets. The retained afterbirth is likely to be at the apex of a uterine horn which cannot be palpable by gynaecological examination.

In the bitch also, retention of the membranes is rare. Nevertheless, on occasion one or both of the placentae occupying the apices of the cornua are retained. The affection most often occurs in the 'toy' breeds, particularly when the litter has been large and labour long. Unless the condition is relieved early, either naturally or by assistance, it can prove fatal. One of the authors has performed several autopsies on Pekingese bitches which have died 4 or 5 days after whelping to find peritonitis resulting from necrotic perforation of the uterine wall at the site of an attached placenta.

The nature of the canine vulval discharge in the immediate postparturient period affords evidence of retention. The dark-green, mucoid discharge which is a feature of the second stage of labour in the bitch quickly ceases after the membranes have been expelled, and in the course of the next 12 hours changes to a blood-tinged, mucoid discharge. If it is noticed that the green discharge persists 12 hours or more after delivery of the last fetus, retention of a placenta should be suspected.

TREATMENT

General

The most rational treatment in all species would be to stimulate adequate myometrial contractions so that a 'natural' dehiscence and expulsion could occur. In cattle practice the veterinarian is not usually consulted until beyond 24 hours of retention because until then the farmer has hoped for a spontaneous expulsion. Because of the unpredictable and generally poor response to ecbolics, it is not surprising that veterinary surgeons have had recourse to manual detachment and traction, per vaginam. In any given case, it is very important not to adopt a rigid attitude of approach: one may *attempt* to remove the afterbirth if favourable circumstances are present: one should not *resolve* to remove the afterbirth at a particular time on every occasion. A good maxim is to remove the fetal membranes as soon as they will come readily; in this way no undue force will be used and the endometrium will not be damaged. It cannot be too strongly urged that all intrauterine manipulations must be effected with due regard to the principles of asepsis. Accordingly, the perineum of the affected animal must be thoroughly washed from one bucket of warm detergent and the obstetrician 'scrubs up' from another bucket of warm antiseptic solution, before putting on a plastic gauntlet which is then anointed with obstetric lubricant. Should the animal defaecate, the perineum must be washed again.

When an unusually high incidence of retention is occurring a whole-herd investigation is called for with a view to detecting a common cause. All retention cases, irrespective of the method of treatment, or no treatment, should be examined gynaecologically at about 30 days after calving and any showing evidence of endometritis should be treated (see Chapter 23).

Cattle

The arguments for and against manual removal have been reviewed by Boyd (1992).

No treatment

The authors are convinced that on the grounds of health of the retention case during the puerperium and with respect to its future fertility, uncomplicated cases require no treatment. (The other aesthetic aspect, which relates to the malodorous stench generated by a case of retention in a building where food for human consumption is being produced, cannot be ignored.) However, it requires courage to prescribe no treatment, and it would be imprudent to adopt a rigid attitude of non-interference. When called to treat a cow with retention the veterinarian must enquire about the animal's general health, and if there is any doubt from the attendant's answers a visit should be made and a clinical examination carried out. If the cow is ill with metritis, antibiotic treatment and uterine drainage are indicated. On the other hand, when the attendant's replies imply that the animal is normal, no visit need be made unless the patient's health deteriorates.

Manual removal

An ideal practice would be to carry out a careful aseptic exploration of the uterus of the affected cow within 1 day of parturition and to remove the membranes if the fetal cotyledons can be completely detached without injury to the maternal caruncles. If it is found impracticable to remove them on the first occasion, the examination may be repeated at daily intervals until the membranes could be removed. However, it is frequently found that attempts at removal during the first 48 hours are unsuccessful for the placenta is then too firmly attached and vigorous manipulation to free the afterbirth is likely to cause haemorrhage and even detachment of the maternal caruncles. Moreover, the apical parts of the gravid horn are at this time usually beyond the reach of the obstetrician's hand. For these reasons it has become a common practice to delay interference until day 3 or 4. By this time the progress of putrefactive liquefaction in the fetal components of the cotyledons makes their separation much easier to accomplish while the degree of uterine involution which has occurred brings the apex of the cornu — where the attachments are most firm — within reach. Even at this time after parturition, however, there will be failures, and, rather than resort to the use of undue force, the veterinarian should make a second attempt a few days later.

It will be recalled that there are about 120 functioning cotyledons in cattle gestations but in cases of retention a variable number of the more posterior members will have separated spontaneously and a variable bulk of the afterbirth will protrude through the cervix and hang from the vulva. The veterinarian twists the postcervical portion into a bulky 'rope' which is held in one hand at the vulva. With the other hand the 'rope' is gently followed through the cervix to the cotyledonary attachments in the uterus. The technique of detachment is to pick up the cotyledon and gently squeeze the base of the maternal caruncle so as to open the crypts on its convexity (as in the manner of opening a fan and thus simulating the separating effect of a natural myometrial contraction); while this gentle pressure is maintained the thumb is lightly passed over the periphery of the caruncle in order to complete the separation of the released villi. Succeeding cotyledons are approached in a circumferential order and similarly dealt with. Continuous steady traction and rotational force are applied with the other hand so that as succeeding portions of the membranes are detached they become incorporated in the continuous cord-like mass. The procedure tends to become progressively difficult as the more anteriorly situated cotyledons are approached, particularly when involution of the uterus has partially restored the coiled configuration of the organ. After the membranes have been freed from the pregnant horn there may be remaining attachments to be dealt with in the non-pregnant horn.

Cases vary immensely in the relative ease of their treatment from those in which the whole mass of afterbirth is found free in the uterus to others in which not even the most caudal cotyledons can be separated and for which further visits will be required. During the process of being cleansed the cow strains forcibly; consequently faeces and fetid uterine exudate are expelled on to the operator's arms which thus require to be frequently flushed by the attendant.

In all cases as much as possible of the uterine exudate should be removed by siphonage, as follows.

A sterile tube of rubber or plastic and somewhat wider than an equine stomach tube is passed well forward and held in the dependent part of the uterus. To the other end a funnel is attached and into this is poured clean hot water or saline (at about 49°C). The fluid is allowed to gravitate into the uterus. Just before the funnel empties it is quickly lowered to the ground in order to start the siphonage. The hand over the uterine end of the tube prevents placental debris from passing into and obstructing it. The tube is repeatedly filled and lowered until the fluid which returns from the uterus is clear; siphonage is complete when no more fluid can be drained away. Pessaries containing antibiotic may be placed in the uterus and a parenteral injection of a long-acting antibiotic given. If the cow is ill with toxaemia, further daily visits are indicated in order to repeat the removal of exudate which will have accumulated since the previous drainage.

Therapeutic treatment without manual removal
Oxytocin can be used within 24 hours of the birth of the calf, and it may be beneficial in some cases of retention which are due to primary uterine inertia.

It will exert little if any effect in cases due to secondary uterine inertia which follow dystocia.

In herds which experienced an unusually high incidence of retention of the afterbirth the administration of 10 ml (100 IU) of oxytocin to all cows immediately after calving was found by Shaw (1938) to reduce the rate of retention from 10 to 1%. However, using the same dose of oxytocin, but at 3–6 hours after calving, and injecting every other cow in a 200 cow herd, Miller and Lodge (1984) found no significant difference in rates of retention between treated and control cows.

Oestrogenic substances increase the sensitivity of the myometrium to oxytocin and enhance the natural uterine defence mechanisms. For these reasons the synthetic oestrogens stilboestrol dipropionate and oestradiol monobenzoate have been widely applied to cows with retained afterbirths in the form of parenteral injection, or uterine infusion and pessary, and their use has sometimes been followed by injections of oxytocin. Most of these clinical trials were uncontrolled and, accordingly, the results are impossible to appraise. Moller et al. (1967), in a well-documented record of the use of stilboestrol by parenteral injection on cows with retention in New Zealand, found that this treatment was of no value.

Uterine inertia is sometimes due to hypocalcaemia, and Fincher (1941) obtained benefit in some cases of retention by the administration of calcium gluconate.

A great variety of antiseptics and antimicrobial agents have in the past been introduced into the uterus in retention cases to check bacterial multiplication. Since a wide range of bacterial species, both aerobic and anaerobic, are present in the uterus of cows with placental retention (Noakes et al., 1991), broad-spectrum agents that are effective in an anaerobic environment should be used. Oxytetracyclines administered at therapeutic dose rates are frequently used. While they may exert a beneficial effect on the associated metritis, these compounds also reduce putrefaction and by retarding lysis may prolong retention. Many veterinarians now prefer not to attempt manual removal of the afterbirth but to apply treatment with tetracyclines until the membranes drop away. Effective control of uterine infection may require several visits and can thus be quite expensive. Moller et al. (1967), after treating in various ways 508 cows with retention, found that those which had received intrauterine tetracycline medication showed worse conception rates than others which had not been treated; whether the placenta was removed or allowed to drop spontaneously had no effect. Bannergee (1965) also studied intrauterine oxytetracycline treatment; his results led him to advocate the institution of oxytetracycline treatment within 72 hours of calving and non-removal of the placenta.

Other animals

Mare

Retention of the equine afterbirth is properly regarded by veterinary surgeons as a potentially more serious affection than the same condition in cattle. This attitude appears to have originated in former times when draught horses predominated; in them retention was likely soon to be followed by acute metritis and laminitis, and early manual removal was the rule. The riding horses and ponies of today are less frequently affected and seem to tolerate retention for at least 24 hours without noticeable departure from health. This knowledge, coupled with an appreciation of the risk of introducing extraneous organisms into the uterus by manual interference, has caused many veterinary surgeons to adopt a more conservative attitude to equine retention, which the authors fully support. If, therefore, within 24 hours of foaling the mare continues to eat and has a normal pulse rate and normal temperature, no gynaecological examination is made. Injections of 40–100 units of oxytocin may be given every 2–3 hours, beginning at the 12th hour, although, as Vandeplassche et al. (1972) have shown, the administration of 30–50 IU units by slow intravenous drip over a period of 1 hour is a more physiological and more successful method. Symptoms of colic often follow injections of oxytocin and commonly precede natural expulsion so that sedation may be required. Whether or not treatment has been given, it is not unusual for the membranes to be expelled between 12 and 24 hours, and no additional treatment is then needed.

If, after a lapse of 24 hours from foaling, the membranes are still retained an attempt should be made to remove them manually. This interference should be carried out with scrupulous regard to asepsis, and no undue force should be applied, for even moderate traction on the afterbirth may cause the uterus to become inverted and prolapsed (see prolapse of the equine uterus, p. 306). In most cases of retention some separation of the allanto-chorion has occurred and consequently a variable amount of the afterbirth hangs down from the vulva. The mare is effectively restrained and measures taken to protect the operator from being kicked. The tail is bandaged and held to one side by the attendant while the obstetrician thoroughly washes the perineum and rear of the mare. With the hand and arm protected by a clean plastic sleeve, the extruded mass, or failing that the freed part lying within the vagina, is grasped and twisted into a rope. The gloved hand, anointed with lubricant is gently introduced along the 'rope' to the area of circumferential attachment in the uterus. As the 'rope' is gently pulled and twisted, the tips of the fingers are pressed between the endometrium and the chorion. The villi are easily detached, and as the allantochorion is gradually freed it is taken up by further twisting of the detached mass. The process of separation usually proceeds quite smoothly, and the complete sac of allantochorion can be gradually detached from the pregnant horn. There is a tendency for attachment to be firmer in the non-pregnant horn, and occasionally retention is confined to this horn. If it is found impossible to detach the apical portions of the allantochorionic sac without tearing the membranes it is better to desist and to try again in 4–6 hours, by which time a successful outcome will be likely.

In all cases treated manually the afterbirth should be spread out on a table to check that the allantochorion has been completely removed. Any fluid exudate remaining in the uterus should be siphoned out and the mare treated with antibiotics (the dominant infective organism being *Streptococcus zooepidemicus*). Tetanus antitoxin should be given; injections of antihistamines may reduce the tendency to laminitis in the heavier type of mare.

In equine dystocias treated at the Ghent Veterinary School, Vandeplassche et al. (1972) found an incidence of 28% of retained placenta after fetotomy and 50% after caesarean operation; in the latter, the likelihood of retention was doubled if the foal was alive at the beginning of the operation compared with when it was dead. These authors emphasize the branching nature of the numerous chorionic microvilli which interdigitate strongly with the corresponding labyrinth of endometrial crypts. The microvilli are better developed in the uterine horns than in the body and are considerably more branched, as well as bigger, in the non-pregnant than in the pregnant horn. This latter property of the villi, coupled with the more marked folding of the allantochorion and endometrium as well as the slower involution of the non-pregnant horn, all combine to provide an explanation of the higher incidence of retention in the non-pregnant horn.

Vandeplassche and his colleagues refer particularly to the residue of microvilli which is present in the endometrium even after a normal expulsion of the afterbirth and which is vastly increased when manual removal is effected in a case of retention. During a difficult manual removal only the central branches of the chorionic villi are removed while practically all the microvilli are broken off and retained; rupture of endometrial and subendometrial capillaries may also occur. The consequences of difficult removal are: increased puerperal exudate, containing much tissue debris; endometritis and laminitis; uterine spasm and delayed involution of the uterus. It is for these reasons that Vandeplassche and his colleagues prefer to treat severe equine retention by means of intravenous drip administration of oxytocin rather than by persistence with manual removal. Moreover, they deprecate the use of any antiseptic solution to rinse the uterus after the expulsion of the afterbirth, because this depresses phagocytosis. To control the uterine bacterial flora they prefer a combination of penicillin and polymyxin.

Ewe

Veterinarians are seldom called to deal with retention of the afterbirth in the ewe. It is customary for the shepherd to apply traction from day to day to the exposed parts. If there is any sign of general ill-health, antibiotic pessaries or parenteral injections are indicated. The retained afterbirth is usually passed in from 2 to 10 days.

Sow

In all assisted deliveries where a count of the umbilical stalks on the voided membranes shows a deficiency as compared with the number of piglets born, a very careful and clean exploration of the uterus should be made. It will not be possible to reach the apex of the horn(s) where the retained membranes are likely to be attached.

In these cases it is usual to give an injection of 20–30 units of oxytocin in the hope that after the lapse of several hours it will be possible to reach the afterbirth and withdraw it manually. A course of antibiotics is prescribed.

In other instances of retention, by the time the sow has become noticeably ill with anorexia, raised temperature and a sanguinopurulent discharge, the cervix will have contracted too much to admit the obstetrician's hand. By this time also there will be little response to oxytocin and it is extremely difficult to give useful professional assistance. A course of antibiotic may save the sow's life.

Bitch

The persistence of a green genital discharge beyond 12 hours after the birth of the last puppy gives suspicion of a retained afterbirth. In such a case vaginal exploration with a finger may detect an umbilical cord, and by 'fiddling' it may be possible to bring its end out of the vulva. Gentle traction may result in the withdrawal of a placenta; if it does, it is likely that separation had already occurred and that its spontaneous expulsion was imminent. More often, however, gentle traction fails and if vigorous effort is applied the cord is torn away.

In any case the uterus should be palpated through the abdominal wall. In a comparatively small bitch it is usually possible to detect the retained placenta in the uterus for it forms an egg-like distension in the otherwise contracting organ. With the foreparts of the bitch raised, firm pressure should be applied to the distended part of the uterus. It is likely that by so doing separation will be effected and the placenta immediately expelled. At the same time gentle traction to any parts of the cord present at the vulva is helpful. If such treatment fails on the first occasion, it should be repeated after a few hours.

In the bitch also, if there is any doubt regarding the expulsion of the terminal placentae half an hour or so after the last fetuses have been delivered, oxytocin should be given. In the case of valuable toy bitches the veterinarian may well insist that the bitch shall be attended throughout the whole of her labour and that she shall be prevented from eating the placentae so they can be collected for subsequent inspection.

Radiography or ultrasonography of the abdomen may reveal the retained afterbirth.

If no response can be obtained from the administration of oxytocin, or from abdominal manipulation, a laparotomy is indicated in order to 'milk' the fetal membranes along the uterus towards the cervix where they may be grasped and withdrawn with forceps; if this fails, a hysterotomy can be performed to remove them.

REFERENCES

Agthe, D. and Kolm, H. P. (1975) *J. Reprod. Fertil.*, **43**, 163.

Anderson, G. B., Cupps, P. T., Drost, M., Horton, M. B. and Wright, R. W. (1978) *J. Anim. Sci.*, **46**, 449.

Banerjee, A. K. (1963) Thesis, University of Utrecht.

Banerjee, A. K. (1965) *Tijdschr. Diergeneesk.*, **90**, 531.

Ben-David, B. (1962) *Refuah. Vet.*, **19**, 16.

Bjorkman, N. and Sollen, P. (1960) *Acta Vet. Scand.*, **2**, 157.

Boyd, H. (1992) In: *Bovine Medicine: Diseases and Husbandry*, ed. A. H. Andrews, R. W. Blowey, H. Boyd and R. G. Eddy, p. 429. Oxford: Blackwells Scientific Publications Ltd.

Chew, B. P., Keller, H. F., Erb, R. E. and Malvern, P. V. (1977) *J. Anim. Sci.*, **44**, 1055.

Chew, B. P., Erb, R. E., Fessler, J. F., Callahan, C. J. and Malvern, P. V. (1979) *J. Dairy Sci.*, **62**, 557.

Cohen, P. (1956) Thesis, University of Utrecht.

Dubois, P. R. and Williams, D. J. (1980) *Proc. XIth Int. Congr. Dis. Cattle, Tel Aviv*, pp. 988–993.

Eastergren, V. L., Frost, O. L., Gomes, W. R., Erb, R. E. and Bullard, J. F. (1967) *J. Dairy Sci.*, **50**, 1293.

Erb, R. E., Hinze, P. M., Gildow, E. M. and Morrison, R. A. (1958) *J. Amer. Vet. Med. Assn*, **133**, 489.

Fincher, M. G. (1941) *J. Amer. Vet. Med. Assn*, **99**, 776.

Geyer, K. (1964) *Dtsch. tierärztl. Wschr.*, **71**, 5.

Grunert, E. (1984) *10th Int. Congr. Anim. Reprod. AI*, **IV**, xi–i.

Gwazdauskas, F. C., Bibb, T. L., McGilliard, M. L. and Lineweaver, J. A. (1979) *J. Dairy Sci.*, **72**, 978.

Henricks, D. M., Rawlings, N. C., Elliott, A. R., Dickey, J. F. and Hill, J. R. (1977) *J. Anim. Sci.*, **44**, 438.

Joosten, I. and Hensen, E. J. (1992) *Anim. Reprod. Sci.*, **28**, 451.

Jordan, W. J. (1948) Personal communication.

Jordan, W. J. (1952) *J. Comp. Path.*, **62**, 54.

Julien, W. E., Conrad, H. R., Jones, J. E. and Moxon, A. (1976a) *J. Dairy Sci.*, **59**, 1954.

Julien, W. E., Conrad, H. R., Jones, J. E. and Moxon, A. (1976b) *J. Dairy Sci.*, **59**, 1960.

Kennedy, A. J. (1947) *Vet. Rec.*, **59**, 519.

Lamb, R. C., Barker, B. O., Anderson, M. J. and Wallers, J. L. (1979) *J. Dairy Sci.*, **62**, 1791.

Leech, F. B., Davis, M. E., Macren, W. D. and Withers, F. W. (1960) *Disease Wastage and Husbandry in the British Dairy Herd*. London: HMSO.

McDonald, L. E., McNutt, S. H. and Nichols, L. E. (1953) *Amer. J. Vet. Res.*, **14**, 539.

Martin, L. R., Williams, W. F., Russell, E. and Gross, T. E. (1981) *Theriogenology*, **15**, 513.

Miller, B. J. and Lodge, J. R. (1984) *Theriogenology*, **22**, 325.

Moller, K., Newling, P. E., Robson, H. J., Jansen, G. J., Meursinge, J. A. and Cooper, M. G. (1967) *N. J. Vet. J.*, **15**, 111.

Morrison, R. A. and Erb, R. E. (1957) *Washington Agric. Exp. Stn. Bull.*, 25.

Noakes, D. E., Wallace, L. M. and Smith, G. R. (1991) *Vet. Rec.*, **128**, 440.

O'Brien, T. and Stott, G. H. (1977) *J. Dairy Sci.*, **60**, 249.

Palmer, C. C. (1932) *J. Amer. Vet. Med. Assn*, **80**, 59.

Roberts, S. J. (1971) *Veterinary Obstetrics and Genital Diseases*. Woodstock, VT.: Roberts.

Roine, K. and Saloniemi, H. (1978) *Acta Vet. Scand.*, **19**, 341.

Sandals, W. C. D., Curtis, R. A., Cote, J. F. and Martin, S. W. (1979) *Can. Vet. J.*, **20**, 131.

Shaw, R. N. (1938) *Lederle Int. Vet. Bull.*, **7**, 9.

Slama, H., Vaillancort, D. and Goff, A. K. (1993) *Can. J. Vet. Res.*, **57**, 293.

Stott, G. H. and Rheinhard, E. J. (1978) *J. Dairy Sci.*, **61**, 1457.

Taverne, M. A. M. (1984) *Proc. 10th Int. Congr. Anim. Reprod. AI*, **IV**, xi–i.

Tijskens, R. Personal communication.

Trinder, N. R., Hall, R. J. and Renton, C. P. (1973) *Vet. Rec.*, **93**, 641.

Vandeplassche, M. and Martens, C. (1961) *Proc. IVth Int. Congr. Anim. Reprod.*

Vandeplassche, M., Spincemaille, J., Bouters, R. and Bonte, P. (1972) *Equine Vet. J.*, **4**, 105.

Venable, J. and McDonald, L. E. (1958) *Amer. J. Vet. Res.*, **19**, 308.

Vinattieri, E., Hayward, A. H. S. and Artioli, D. (1945) *Vet. Rec.*, **57**, 509.

Wagner, W. C., Wilhelm, R. L. and Evans, L. E. (1974) *J. Anim. Sci.*, **38**, 485.

Whitmore, H. L., Tyler, W. J. and Casida, L. E. (1974) *J. Anim. Sci.*, **38**, 339.

Wright, J. G. (1943) *J. Comp. Path.*, **53**, 212.

Zerobin, K. and Sporri, I. (1972) *Adv. Vet. Sci. Comp. Med.*, **16**, 303.

Postparturient Prolapse of the Uterus

Prolapse of the uterus is a common complication of the third stage of labour in the cow and the ewe. It occurs less frequently in the sow and is rare in the mare and bitch. In the ruminant species the prolapse is generally a complete inversion of the gravid cornu, while in the sow and the bitch inversion is generally partial and comprises one cornu only. Cases are on record in which the bitch has everted one cornu before she has completely delivered the fetuses from the other. In the mare the rare cases of prolapse are generally partial only.

THE COW

The incidence varies from 2 per 1000 calvings in range beef cattle in America (Patterson et al., 1979) to 3 per 1000 cows per year in Scandinavian dairy cattle (Rasbech et al., 1967; Ellerby et al., 1969; Odegaard, 1977; Roine and Soloniemi, 1978).

The occurrence seems to be affected by seasonal as well as regional factors, the condition being commoner in some years and in some localities.

Multigravida (of the dairy breeds) are more often involved than are heifers. In the majority of instances the prolapse occurs within a few hours of an otherwise normal second-stage labour, although in some it may be delayed several days. In the latter group the condition is generally associated with a grossly protracted and assisted labour. Rarely, where delivery is achieved by heavy traction, the uterus prolapses immediately after the calf is withdrawn.

Aetiology

The cause of prolapse of the uterus is not clear, but there is no doubt that it occurs during the third stage of labour, within a few hours of the expulsion of the calf, and at a time when some of the fetal cotyledons have separated from the maternal caruncles. The only conceivable force that could lift the heavy uterus out of the abdomen into the pelvis and thence propel it to the exterior is abdominal straining. Gravity, through the medium of a sloping stand, bank or hillside, and traction by a variable weight of freed dependent afterbirth — containing variable loculi of retained uterine fluid and urine — are probable additional forces. Straining occurs normally during the third stage and is synchronous with the continuing peristaltic contractions of the uterus which occur every $3\frac{1}{2}$–4 minutes (Benesch and Steinmetzer, 1931, 1932). One can imagine the uterus being more affected by abdominal straining when it is relatively flaccid, and it is a particularly apt clinical observation that many cases of uterine prolapse show a simultaneous hypocalcaemia (milk fever) which is known to be conducive to uterine inertia. The authors believe, therefore, that uterine inversion and prolapse are associated with the onset of uterine inertia during the third stage when a portion of detached afterbirth occupies the birth canal and protrudes from the vulva. This concept of an association with inertia corresponds with the greater frequency of prolapse in cows than heifers, in dairy rather than beef cows and in closely confined and highly fed cows rather than those at range. One of the authors has confirmed the previous contention of Vandeplassche and Spincemaille (1963) that the pregnant horn does not undergo a progressive inversion from its anterior extremity; only the posterior two-thirds inverts. The actual ejection of this portion has been seen to occur very quickly in one bout of straining.

Some cattle with extreme laxity of ligaments and tissues around the vulva may prolapse immediately after every calving. In Australia, uterine prolapse is a feature of the disease seen in sheep grazed on clover pastures containing oestrogenic substances.

The signs of this condition are obvious. As a rule the affected cow is recumbent, and if in lateral recumbency rumenal tympany will be prominent,

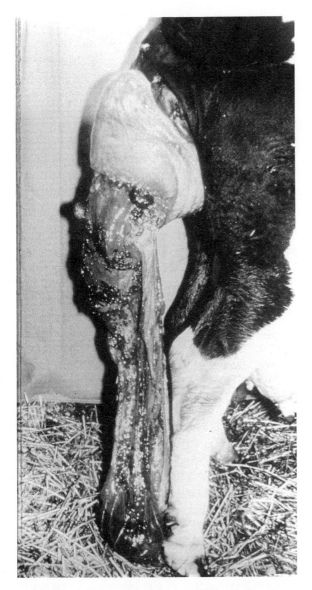

Fig. 19.1 Uterine prolapse in a cow. Note that in the placenta, which is still attached, fetal fluids have accumulated.

but occasionally the cow is standing with the everted organ hanging down almost to its hocks (Figure 19.1).

Prognosis

The prognosis will depend firstly on the type of case, secondly on the duration of the condition before treatment is forthcoming, and thirdly on whether the organ has sustained severe injury. Nevertheless, as the condition is generally encountered, that is, as a sequel to a normal parturition, and professional assistance is forthcoming within an hour or two of its occurrence, the prognosis is good. Replacement of the organ does not offer insurmountable difficulties and recurrence after replacement is uncommon. Moreover, such animals generally conceive again. Patterson et al. (1979) reported that 40% of cows became pregnant after uterine prolapse. Not infrequently, an animal which has everted her uterus at one parturition calves subsequently without trouble; in fact, repetition of the condition is the exception rather than the rule.

Occasionally prolapse of the uterus is followed in a matter of a hour or so by the animal's death. On post-mortem examination in such cases it is found that death was due to internal haemorrhage consequent on the weight of the everted organ having torn the mesovarium and the ovarian artery. Even in those cases in which there has been delay and in which the endometrium is grossly contaminated and deeply congested, the prognosis is not hopeless, for the recuperative powers of the organ are quite astonishing, and thus when dealing with dairy cattle amputation of the everted organ should be considered only when injury is gross and when resolution is clearly impossible.

Treatment

Replacement of the everted organ

On notification of the case, the farmer should be instructed to wrap the prolapsed viscus in a large towel or other suitable material to prevent further contamination, if, as is likely, the cow is recumbent; if she is standing, the organ should be supported by a large towel or sheet held by people on either side, until professional assistance is forthcoming. It is good practice to give a preliminary injection of calcium borogluconate (as for milk fever) and to relieve rumenal tympany, if present, by passing a stomach tube. In the past, the chief difficulties in replacement of the organ have been associated with the almost continuous straining which manipulation of the uterus provokes and to the fact that pressure had to be applied in an uphill direction. Numerous methods of overcoming these difficulties have been introduced: the tension of a rope around the posterior abdomen, raising the animal's hindparts on boards or on a truss of straw, or even casting her and raising her hindparts by means of a block and tackle hooked to a figure-of-eight rope around the hocks. Plender-leith (1980) described a method which is now in common usage amongst practitioners. The cow is placed in sternal recumbency with both hindlegs pulled out behind her (weight therefore being taken on her stifles). The assistant sits astride the cow, facing the rear, and holds the cow's tail up vertically. This manoeuvre causes the slope of the vulva to be upwards. The veterinary surgeon kneels between the cow's hocks and supports the weight of the prolapsed organ on his or her thighs, prior to replacement.

Whether the cow is standing or recumbent, an epidural anaesthetic should be given. This will prevent straining, and also has the advantage that defaecation is in abeyance during the operation. The everted organ should be thoroughly washed with warm normal saline solution. If the fetal membranes are already partially detached and their complete removal can be carried out easily and without injury to the caruncles, this should be done. But when attachment is complete or when attempts at detachment are associated with haemorrhage, it is better that the organ be replaced with the membranes still adherent. The subsequent management of the retained fetal membranes should be on the principles outlined in Chapter 18.

The prolapsed organ should be palpated in order to detect the possible presence within it of a distended urinary bladder; if such is the case, it should be relieved by the use of a catheter. The uterus should be supported by assistants holding the corners of a towel beneath the mass or upon a piece of board about 1 m long covered by a clean cloth or towel.

Smythe (1948) describes the operation of replacement as follows. Having well soaked the hands, the operator commences to replace the uterus little by little, starting with those portions nearest the vulval lips. By gentle pressure, the nearest cotyledons are pushed into the vagina, taking care that the lips of the vulva remain well apart and do not become turned inwards. It is generally best to replace portions of the upper and lower surfaces alternately. When the last portions only remain to be replaced, an assistant should press against these, using the palms of both hands, while the operator endeavours to draw the lips of the vulva over the prolapse. As the mass disappears through the lips of the vulva the operator, using a clenched fist, should then continue to press it forward to the full length of the arm. It is important that the uterus should be pressed forwards beyond the cervical ring; to ensure this the operator locates the margins of the dilated cervix, draws them towards him- or herself and, if possible, at the same time pushes the uterus in a forward direction with the other hand. In some cases it may be found helpful to grasp the cervical ring at several points in succession and with a piston-like movement of the hand and arm insinuate the uterine mass through it. When this has been accomplished the cervix should lie unoccupied at the level of the pelvic brim, and if the whole uterus has passed the cervix it will promptly regain its normal position. To ensure complete replacement of the uterus, 9–14 litres of clean warm water are delivered into the uterus by gravity feed and immediately removed by siphonage, the weight of water effacing any remaining inversion of the cornu. To help restore uterine tone, and thus to prevent recurrence of the prolapse, a postoperative injection of oxytocin should be given. Preoperative administration of oxytocin, by inducing firm contraction of the everted organ, markedly impedes replacement of the viscus. Calcium therapy should be given as necessary, and parenteral antibiotics should be administered.

A final advantage of epidural anaesthesia is that for an hour or so after replacement of the organ any tendency to strain will be removed. It has been customary in the past to insert a large pessary in the vagina after replacement and also to insert vulva sutures. It is unlikely that these practices serve much useful purpose. Many practitioners recommend the application of a tightly placed rope truss for 2 or 3 days. In uncomplicated cases it is generally found that within 24 hours of replacement the degree of cervical contraction present is such that recurrence is very unlikely.

Amputation of the everted organ

This operation is adopted as a last resort in those cases in which the uterus has undergone such severe changes that replacement of the organ must inevitably result in death and in occasional long-standing cases where it is found physically impossible to replace it because of the unfavourable texture of the organ. The prognosis is grave, its gravity being due not only to the magnitude of the operation but also the severity of the cases which prompts its adoption. Nevertheless, there are many records of recovery, and it has been possible to fatten the animal for the butcher. The operation, which is performed under sedation and epidural anaesthesia, comprises the application of a stout transfixing and encircling ligature immediately behind the region of the cervix and the subsequent excision of the prolapsed mass about 8 cm posterior to the ligature. For ligaturing, stout whipcord or elastic is generally used, encircling the mass three or four times and tying off after each encirclement. The ligature should be applied as tightly as possible, for it is necessary that it shall occlude not only the blood vessels in the uterine wall but also those present in the broad ligament which lies in the lumen of the everted organ. Amputation may be carried out with a knife or with the actual cautery. Clearly it is essential that none of the abdominal viscera shall occupy the interior of the prolapse, but accurate determination of this may be extremely difficult, for the size and density of the organ prevents any exact assessment by manipulation of what lies within it and thus most operations are carried out in the dark in relation to this factor. Fortunately, it is only rarely in the cow that this complication arises. To avoid this contingency, as well as to reduce subsequent peritoneal haemorrhage, Roberts (1949) suggests preliminary longitudinal incision of the dorsal wall of the uterus whereby the content of the prolapse can be seen and the vessels of the broad ligament ligated before the transfixing ligatures are placed around the anterior vagina. Having removed the organ, the vagina is replaced through the vulval lips into the pelvic canal. The operation may be followed by severe and continuous straining. If this is serious it is well to maintain epidural anaesthesia for as long as necessary.

OTHER SPECIES

Ewe (Figure 19.2)

The operation of replacement is similar to that described for the cow except that it is easier to perform because of the facility with which the hindquarters of the ewe can be kept raised by an attendant; epidural anaesthesia is not required but it does prevent straining after the organ is replaced. However, because of their different physical rela-

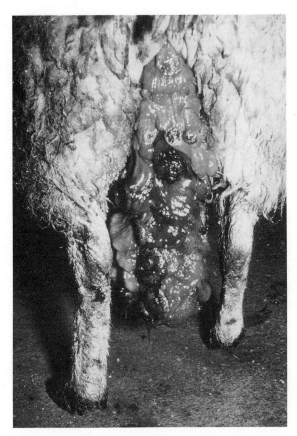

Figure 19.2 Uterine prolapse in a ewe.

tionship to the caruncles, the fetal cotyledons cannot readily be detached and rather than damage the uterus by persistent attempts to separate them, it is preferable to leave them attached and return them with the uterus; failure to detach them at this stage will not significantly affect the prognosis. When the uterus is grossly damaged, amputation can be performed after making sure there are no intestines in the 'lumen' of the prolapsed viscus. Anaerobic infection should be anticipated and a course of antibiotic prescribed.

Mare

There are few records of the condition in this species, but significant observations relating to its aetiology have been made at the Royal Veterinary College in mares which were subjected to elective caesarean operation at about 320 days of gestation. In three such cases, uterine eversion and prolapse occurred during expulsion of the afterbirth, and gynaecological examination of them revealed that the afterbirth had completely separated from the endometrium, except at the site of the hysterectomy wound, where it had become accidently attached to the uterus, or at the tip of the non-pregnant horn. It seemed that the weight of the separated and dependent portion had caused sufficient traction on the uterus to evert part of it and then, presumably, the mare strained and forced out a large volume of uterus. These observations are in line with notes made by one of the authors on three clinical cases of retention of the equine afterbirth in which uterine prolapse occurred while the membranes were being removed and was undoubtedly due to the traction applied to the allantochorion by the obstetrician; the eversion of the uterus thus caused at the point of attachment of the afterbirth was quickly converted into a prolapse when the mare strained. It is suggested therefore that in natural cases of uterine prolapse an important causative factor is the weight of that portion of free afterbirth which is dependent from the vulva and the traction which it exerts on the uterus during the passage of a peristaltic wave along that organ. (In view of these observations the authors would strongly advise against the use of undue traction on the detached portion of allantochorion while the more anterior retained portion is being freed.)

With regard to the treatment of equine prolapse, Heathcote (1933) recorded a case in a 3-year-old Shire mare which had foaled without assistance. After the fetal membranes had been detached, the mare was made to stand on a 30° slope, and replacement of the uterus was comparatively easy. She recovered completely and reared her foal. Firth (1947) reported a similar case in which complete prolapse occurred 24 hours after normal parturition in a multiparous cart mare in which replacement was comparatively easy with the patient placed on a bank and under chloral hydrate sedation. Roberts (1964) recorded easy replacement, without anaesthetic, of prolapsed vagina, cervix and both uterine horns which occurred 10 hours after the birth of a dead foal. Supportive therapy with oxytocin and antibiotic led to an uneventful recovery. If there is difficulty over restraint a general anaesthetic can be administered and the animal placed on its back with its hindquarters raised.

Sow

The consensus of veterinary opinion is that pigs are unable to tolerate uterine prolapse followed by manipulative reposition. The voluminous organ can be replaced if the sow is suspended by her hindlegs but there is a grave likelihood of her dying soon afterwards, apparently from shock. For this reason the prevailing practice is to recommend a prompt attempt to salvage the carcass. However, amputation of the prolapsed organ has been suggested, and Beswick (1964) has successfully performed this operation, using the technique described by Roberts for the cow (see p. 305). An alternative procedure which merits a trial is to 'float' the uterus back into the abdomen with the aid of water pressure. The sow is placed on her side, head downwards, on a slope and the end of a soft tube of rubber or plastic, of 2 cm diameter and 1.5 m long, is gently passed into the stoma of the prolapsed viscus and eased along as far as possible. Clean warm water, or saline, from a bucket is then very gently pumped into the uterus. The weight of the introduced water gradually draws the prolapsed organ back into the abdomen; the tube is introduced further and more fluid infused. By this means the whole uterus is not only returned but completely replaced without manipulation.

Penny and Arthur (1954) have described post-oestrual prolapse of the uterus in a gilt which was irreducible, despite abdominal taxis by means of a laparotomy.

Bitch and cat

A laparotomy can be performed, and with simultaneous external manipulation and abdominal taxis replacement can be attempted. It is more usual, however, to carry out 'external' hysterectomy on the prolapsed organ. The prognosis is favourable after amputation.

REFERENCES

Benesch, F. and Steinmetzer, K. (1931) *Wien. Tierärztl. Monatsschr.*, **18**, 1.

Benesch, F. and Steinmetzer, K. (1932) *Wien. Tierärztl. Monatsschr.*, **19**, 71.

Beswick, W. (1964) *Vet. Rec.*, **76**, 930.

Ellerby, F., Jochumsen, P. and Veiruplt, S. (1969) *Kgl. Vet.*, **77**, 154.

Firth, T. B. (1947) Personal communication.

Postparturient Prolapse of the Uterus

Heathcote, F. C. (1933) *Vet. Rec.*, **13**, 16.

Odegaard, S. A. (1977) *Acta Vet. Scand. Suppl.* **63**.

Patterson, D. J., Bellows, R. A., Burfening, P. J., Short, R. E. and Hitter (1979) *J. Anim. Sci.*, **49**(Suppl. 1), 325.

Penny, R. H. C. and Arthur, G. H. (1954) *Vet. Rec.*, **66**, 162.

Plenderleith, R. W. (1980) *Proc. Brit. Cattle Vet. Assoc. (1980–81)*, 55.

Rasbech, N. O., Jochumsen, P. and Christiansen, I. J. (1967) *Kgl. Vet.*, 265.

Roberts, C. F. (1964) *Vet. Rec.*, **76** 565.

Roberts, S. J. (1949) *Cornell Vet.*, **39**, 428.

Roine, K. and Soloniemi, H. (1979) *Acta Vet. Scand.*, **19**, 341.

Smythe, R. H. (1948) Personal communication.

Vandeplassche, M. and Spincemaille, J. (1963) *Berl. Mün. Tierarztle. Wochenschr.*, **76**, 324.

307

4

Part Four

Operative Interventions

20

THE COW

Caesarean section is now a routine obstetric procedure in cattle practice and is increasingly preferred to total fetotomy per vaginam in animals in which either technique may be adopted. Parkinson (1974) summarizes the advantages of laparohysterotomy as fetal survival, speedier, safer and less exhausting relief of dystocia and practicability in cases in which fetotomy is impossible.

Indications

The reasons for surgery include most causes of dystocia but analysis of published cases shows that the following five major indications account cumulatively for 90% of all caesarean sections:

1. Fetal oversize.
2. Incomplete dilatation of the cervix.
3. Irreducible uterine torsion.
4. Fetal deformity.
5. Errors of fetal presentation, position or posture.

In individual series, their relative frequency varies considerably depending primarily on the breed of cattle predominantly at risk and to a lesser extent on whether fetotomy is routinely practised. If the birth canal is fully dilated, fetal causes of dystocia may be amenable to relief by fetotomy but cervical failure and irreducible torsion are absolute indications for surgery. Non-surgical delivery may seem advisable if the fetus is grossly infected but, in fact, laparohysterotomy is often obligatory in such cases because of uterine involution or overdistension, or constriction of the birth canal.

Fetal oversize

Fetopelvic disproportion is consistently the most frequent overall indication for caesarean section in cattle. Even in dairy cattle practice, it accounts for approximately 25% of cases, but in beef breeding enterprises more than 90% of operations may be performed for this reason (Souques, 1968). Four particular forms may be encountered.

Physical Immaturity of the Dam. In herds in which bull and heifer calves are kept together or where a bull runs with suckling cows, calves may conceive at an unexpectedly early age. It is not uncommon for heifers to be parturient at term at only 14 months of age and, in exceptional cases, at only 1 year of age. Even at 18 months of age the maternal pelvis is still immature and usually too small for vaginal delivery.

Fetal Oversize. The vast majority of cases of disproportion are animals which may be regarded as mature and which are parturient at normal term with a normally developed fetus. Among British dairy breeds, the Friesian in particular has long been recognized to be more susceptible to this form of dystocia during the first pregnancy than, for example, the Ayrshire or Jersey; for this reason Friesian heifers are often bred to bulls of smaller breeds such as the Aberdeen Angus. Certain beef breeds are also frequently affected with fetopelvic disproportion and not only during the first pregnancy, largely on account of pronounced muscular development of the fetus. Double muscling or muscular hypertrophy is well recognized in certain breeds in Europe, where it is regarded as a desirable beef characteristic, and in the South Devon breed in Britain (MacKellar, 1960). Parkinson (1974), however, points out that not all cases of disproportion in breeds susceptible to muscular hypertrophy are attributable to the disorder. In his series of 105 caesarean sections, 80 operations were performed because of fetal oversize, mostly in South Devons. The importation of European breeds of cattle into Britain was widely expected to result in a greatly increased incidence of dystocia caused by fetal oversize. That this has not happened is due largely to the vigilance of cattle breeding organizations in recording incidences of dystocia associated with individual breeds and individual bulls. Data accumulated by the Milk Marketing Board and reviewed by Stables (1980) show clearly the influence of the sire on gestation length, calf birth weight and incidence of dystocia. On the basis of such information likely levels of dystocia can be predicted, and stud bulls are now given an 'ease of calving' rating.

The management of dystocia caused by feto-pelvic disproportion depends largely on experienced clinical assessment of how much traction can safely be exerted without risk of serious birth canal trauma or, worse still, impaction of the fetus after only partial delivery. This is the most worrying of all obstetric problems to be encountered in cattle practice, with ample scope for errors of judgement which may lead to death of the fetus and the dam. In many cases of oversize the fetal head cannot be drawn into the maternal pelvic cavity. In others, traction is more effective and, as a general rule, if the head can be brought through the vulva the rest of the fetus will follow provided that traction is synchronized with maternal straining. The difficulty lies in knowing when to abandon traction in favour of surgery. Excessive traction in such animals may merely exacerbate the degree of dystocia and compromise the success of an eventual caesarean operation. In an attempt to avoid this dilemma, techniques for pelvimetry have been described by Rice and Wiltbank (1972) and by Hindson (1978) (see p. 198). Hindson measured the force exerted on the fetus by various forms of manual and mechanical traction and also devised a 'traction ratio' which may be used to predict whether traction is likely to be safely successful or whether surgery should be undertaken at the start. The method is based on the fact that the digital diameter of the fetus and the interischial tuberosity diameter of the dam are reliable indices of fetal body weight and vertical and horizontal pelvic diameter, respectively. The ratio of these measurements, modified by correction factors to take account of parity, presentation and possible muscular hypertrophy of the fetus, indicates whether traction should be attempted.

In heifers particularly, precipitate traction early in second-stage labour is to be avoided unless dystocia has obviously developed, because the caudal vagina and vulva will not have been naturally dilated, and perineal damage is thus more likely. The frequent finding in hospital referrals of fractured limb bones in oversized calves suggests either an unreasonable degree of traction or traction in a wrong direction. Severe cases of this difficult form of dystocia are increasingly treated by surgery; such an attitude is entirely justified on clinical and humane grounds because the effects of injudicious traction cannot always be rectified. The deliberate adoption of breeding policies which require caesarean delivery is less justifiable in ethical terms.

A particularly serious form of sire-induced oversize is its occurrence in a group of heifers, all of which are pregnant to the same bull. Not uncommonly, several heifers in a batch may require more than normal assistance or have to be delivered by caesarean section. If the time interval permits, the induction of labour in the later calving animals within 10 days of anticipated term may be of considerable benefit (see p. 149).

Increasingly, caesarean section is carried out electively on transplant recipients. Ideally, it should be performed during the first stage of labour.

Fetal Deformity and Infection. The most extreme form of disproportion is sometimes encountered in fetal anasarca and achondroplasia in which the accumulation of fluid in the subcutaneous tissue spaces or serous cavities greatly increases the cross-sectional diameter of the fetus (see Chapter 4). Siamese twin defects are also usually too large for vaginal delivery. Commoner than all of these, however, is secondary putrefactive enlargement of the fetus which frequently develops in protracted dystocia.

Postmaturity. A moderate prolongation of pregnancy up to 290 days or thereabouts is a normal feature of certain breeds, but in occasional animals of any breed, gestation may last for considerably longer, even beyond 400 days. Postmaturity results in continued fetal growth in utero, particularly of the skeleton. In such cases dystocia at term is due not simply to fetal oversize, but also to inadequate parturient relaxation of the birth canal.

Incomplete cervical dilatation

Incomplete dilatation of the cervix is a common cause of dystocia in cattle, but it should be diagnosed only after careful assessment of the findings on vaginal exploration. Cervical dilatation during the first stage of labour is a gradual process and the presence of a cervical rim is not in itself an indication of dystocia, provided that the fetal membranes are still intact. Care should be taken in such cases not to perforate the membranes unless the cervix remains undilatated 2 hours or so later. Slow or arrested dilatation in multiparous cows may be associated with uterine inertia caused by hypocalcaemia; in these animals, the response to calcium therapy is rapid.

If, on initial or subsequent examination, the cervix is incompletely dilated and the membranes are already ruptured, with a fetal extremity presented against or through the cervix, or if the fetus is already dead, then further cervical dilatation is unlikely and a diagnosis of cervical dystocia is justified. If the cervical rim is shallow and membranous, or if it stretches sufficiently for the head to be drawn into the vagina, normal safe delivery may be possible, but in these cases, irrespective of the degree of dilatation, the cervix is usually too thickened and indurated for vaginal delivery to be safely attempted, and further delay results only in fetal death and a greater risk of intrauterine infection. There is little evidence to suggest that unequivocal cases of incomplete cervical dilatation in cattle respond to the administration of spasmolytic or hormonal agents, but convincing proof that delay and repeated vaginal examination in these animals lead to early intrauterine infection. In most caesarean operations performed for this indication, the fetus is dead, often because ineffective medical therapy has been attempted beforehand or uncertainty in the initial diagnosis has led to repeated vaginal examinations during the next few hours and fetal death in the meantime.

The presence of an incompletely dilated cervix after the birth of one twin with the other fetus still in utero, often in a breech presentation, clearly indicates that the cervix is able to constrict fairly soon after being fully dilated. The frequent finding of fetal malposture or malpresentation in cases of apparent failure to dilate may indicate that, in these cases at least, the cervix in fact is constricting and the dystocia is fetal rather than maternal in nature. Failure of the cervix to dilate or remain dilated is not uncommon in premature calvings and can result in the fetal head becoming trapped in the anterior vagina.

Incomplete dilatation of the cervix is an important complication of uterine torsion. After manipulative correction of the torsion, the cervix is often only partially dilated and seldom dilates further (Pearson, 1971). In such cases the cervical rim may be deep, but it is usually thin and stretches in response to traction on the fetus. Section of the cervical rim in the midline dorsally during traction may allow safe vaginal delivery but it should be remembered that the fetus (in cases of uterine torsion) is usually larger than normal and that a cervical incision may tear.

Irreducible uterine torsion

Torsion of the uterus in cattle constitutes a major indication for caesarean section, either because the torsion is irreducible or because the cervix remains inadequately dilated for vaginal delivery after reduction. In most cases of postcervical torsion, the degree of cervical dilatation and vaginal twisting permits the introduction of a hand into the uterus for manipulation of the fetus, but if the torsion affects the cervical canal or uterine body, the fetus is totally inaccessible. Such torsions are an absolute indication for caesarean section. Uterine torsion differs from all other causes of dystocia in cattle in that one or both of the fetal membranes usually remain intact even if the placenta separates, unless they are deliberately perforated. The presence of fetal fluids thus protects the fetus and the uterus from infection; in this respect the condition carries a favourable prognosis. Torsion, however, may still have seriously detrimental effects on the uterus. Rotation through 360° is common, and two or three complete revolutions of the uterus sometimes occur. The greater the degree of uterine rotation, the greater the interference with venous circulation within the uterus and its mesometrial and mesovarian attachments. The combination of uterine displacement and oedematous swelling of its wall may well result in perforation of the uterine body, especially by the fetal head. In exceptionally protracted cases, a fetal extremity may impinge, through a uterine tear, on the urethra or segments of large intestine and cause rupture of the urinary bladder or gut.

In most cases of uterine torsion, the prognosis is excellent, but paradoxically the operation may be technically difficult, firstly because small intestine is usually displaced and impedes access to the uterus and secondly because the presence of fetal fluids may make the uterus difficult to handle and impossible to exteriorize for suturing.

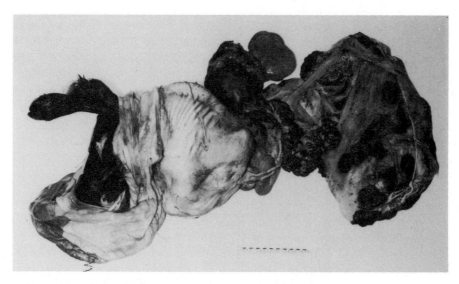

Fig. 20.1 *Schistosoma reflexus*. Incised skin pouch enveloping the trunk, head and limbs.

Fetal deformities

Cattle more than most species are susceptible to gross structural abnormalities of development. The incidence of some disorders such as achondroplasia and anasarca has decreased markedly during the last few decades, largely as the result of rigorous selection and culling of stud bulls, but other types of deformity still constitute a major indication for caesarean section or fetotomy if this method of delivery is preferred.

Schistosoma reflexus is by far the commonest gross structural defect in cattle. Occasional cases are born normally without assistance and others may be extracted with moderate traction. Most affected fetuses, however, cause dystocia because the characteristic angulation of the spine greatly increases the cross-sectional diameter, although the body weight may be less than normal for the breed. The fetus is presented in one of two ways: its exposed viscera may protrude from the vulva or the limbs and head may lie in the vagina and can be felt to be attached to the misshapen trunk. The latter presentation may be confusing in cases in which the appendages are enclosed in an inverted pouch of the skin which is all that can be palpated (Figure 20.1).

Cases of *schistosoma reflexus* occur sporadically in several breeds, sometimes as twin to a normal fetus (Figure 20.2), and are often still alive at delivery. It is noticeable that they are seldom associated with protracted parturition, presumably because they cause obvious manifestations of dystocia. The dystocia can be relieved by either fetotomy or caesarean section. If hysterotomy is performed, longer than normal abdominal and uterine incisions may be necessary and care is essential in manipulating the fetus from the uterus in order to avoid uterine tearing, which easily follows excessive traction. This manoeuvre is usually facilitated by the lubricant effect of residual amniotic fluid. The prognosis after caesarean section is

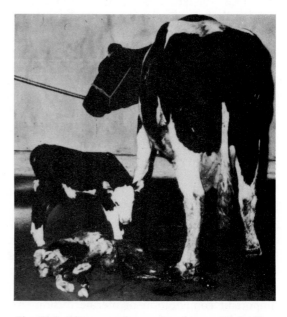

Fig. 20.2 *Schistosoma reflexus* twinned to a normal calf.

excellent, but the dam should not be rebred to the same sire.

Achondroplasia or bulldog calf deformity and anasarca or fetal dropsy, associated primarily with the Friesian and Ayrshire breeds, respectively, have decreased dramatically in incidence. Both disorders cause dystocia largely on account of the extensive subcutaneous accumulation of tissue fluids which greatly increases the cross-sectional diameter of the fetus and causes gross disproportion irrespective of the fetal body weight which may also be considerably increased. Both defects may also be associated with severe fetal ascites, placental oedema and hydroallantois.

Lesions of the fetal central nervous system may cause muscle contracture of the limbs which prevents normal extension in preparation for birth. Arthrogryposis, sometimes associated with torticollis and kyphosis, has been shown to result from viral infection of the dam during pregnancy and is also recognized as a genetic abnormality in the Charolais breed (Figure 20.3). Because the muscle contracture fixes limb joints in either flexion or extension, depending on the joint, the condition is sometimes called ankylosis, but the bones are not fused. Spina bifida is less common in cattle but causes similar contractures, usually of the hindlimbs only because the lesion is thoracolumbar in position. Fetal anencephaly and the deformity described as *perosomus elumbis* may also cause limb abnormalities. In most cases of muscle contracture, the musculature of affected limbs is palpably underdeveloped. The degree of contracture may be too severe for attempted delivery, but if the forelimbs in an anterior presentation can be brought into the vagina, traction may cause the flexed hindlegs to perforate the uterus below the pubic brim. Conjoined fetuses occur occasionally with varying degrees of fusion and generally require caesarean delivery unless only the head is duplicated.

Faulty fetal disposition

Provided that the cervix is fully dilated and remains so, most early cases of fetal malpresentation and malposture can be corrected manually or relieved by relatively simple fetotomy. However, the loss of fetal fluids followed by uterine contraction often makes these manipulations difficult and time-consuming and more likely to result in rupture of the uterus. In protracted cases, constriction of the

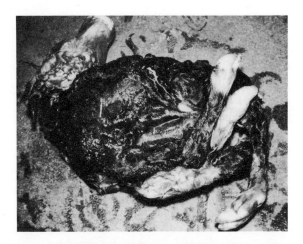

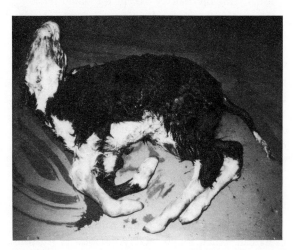

Fig. 20.3 Fetuses with varying severity of torticollis and muscle contracture of the limbs.

cervix may prevent vaginal correction of the dystocia and the fetus is then likely to become emphysematous.

Fetal emphysema

Fetal emphysema is a frequent complication of protracted parturition in cattle and, irrespective of the primary cause of dystocia, it is often the immediate indication for caesarean section. Such cases should be assessed realistically before the operation is undertaken because fetal putrefaction has a seriously adverse influence on maternal survival. Bacterial culture of such fetuses usually yields heavy growths of coliform, or coliform and clostridial organisms. The latter infection is associated with a high maternal mortality rate in the immediate postoperative period, probably because of endotoxaemic shock. On cursory examination, the clinical status of these cows may seem reasonable despite gross uterine distension; the pulse rate, however, is usually significantly raised and the animal noticeably quiet on handling. Such premonitory signs are likely to be followed, as soon as the uterus is incised, by the onset of rapidly deteriorating shock which is sometimes fatal within 24 hours, despite intensive supportive therapy. Experience suggests that coliform infection alone is less serious than clostridial putrefaction but preoperative differentiation is not possible. Despite the significant mortality rate in this group of cases, surgery is nevertheless worthwhile because there is usually no alternative, except for slaughter.

Miscellaneous indications

Occasional animals are encountered with full cervical dilatation and a normal-sized fetus, in which the caudal part of the birth canal is too constricted for delivery even after episiotomy. The condition is associated particularly with Friesian heifers which are sometimes older than is usual at the time of first calving. The natural termination of pathologically prolonged pregnancy may also be associated with absence of normal parturient changes in the vagina and vulva and a consequent need for caesarean section.

Abortion in late pregnancy sometimes requires caesarean relief for several contributory reasons such as incomplete birth canal dilatation, cervical constriction and fetal deformity, malpresentation, malposture or emphysema. Such cases are uncommon but they are nevertheless important because they may be associated with specific zoonotic infections such as salmonellosis (and, until recently, brucellosis) which can easily be contracted by the surgeon unless rigorous self-protective precautions are taken.

Fetal mummification and *hydrops uteri* may now be treated initially by inducing parturition, but caesarean section may still be necessary if induction fails or the birth canal is insufficiently dilated for vaginal delivery.

Laparotomy is essential in cases of uterine rupture. If this disorder occurs as a preparturient complication, the fetus usually lies totally within the peritoneal cavity and may survive, if the cord is not twisted, until the placenta separates at term. More frequently, rupture occurs as a complication of dystocia, particularly of uterine torsion, or as a result of manipulation of a fetus which is oversized or has faulty disposition. Uterine rupture during parturition may result in considerable uterine haemorrhage and hypovolaemic shock.

Repeated dislocation of the sacrococcygeal articulation during assisted delivery in successive parturitions can result in massive bony obstruction at the site and constitutes an uncommon indication for surgery.

Restraint and anaesthesia

The caesarean operation in cattle can be performed through a ventral, ventrolateral or sublumbar incision depending to a degree on the circumstances of the case but much more on the personal preference of the operator. Laparotomy in cattle is generally most easily performed on the standing animal because recumbency greatly increases intra-abdominal pressure. Caesarean section is not usually premeditated, and patients have not been starved beforehand. Animals anaesthetized for surgery are restrained in recumbency and may therefore develop considerable ruminal tympany and regurgitate ruminal fluid during the operation. These complications are avoided if the operation is performed under local analgesia with the animal standing. The left flank technique recommended by Formston in 1945 is highly satisfactory for cows which are accustomed to handling and restraint, and is now widely adopted as a routine approach to the caesarean operation. It should be remembered, however, if this method is used, that many heifers, and any animal which strains vigorously or develops shock, may become recumbent during the course of the operation. In such cases, the potentially serious risk of recumbency on the wrong side is readily overcome by traction on a rope applied above the right hind fetlock joint. For this reason too, the head should be tied or yoked in such a way that it can be released quickly. Beef cattle are sometimes not used to handling and can be difficult to restrain safely in the standing position; such cases are often cast, either conscious, sedated or anaesthetized. Occasional animals of a normally placid temperament become highly excitable and dangerously aggressive during transportation to a veterinary hospital for caesarean surgery. Hyperexcitability of this sort can be controlled by sedation, but proper restraint in recumbency may still be advisable for the safety of both personnel and patient. Fractious animals should always be adequately sedated to avoid potentially fatal visceral damage which may result from maniacal behaviour after the peritoneal cavity has been opened.

General anaesthesia, or heavy sedation with agents such as xylazine, may be indicated for exceptional cases but most caesarean operations are satisfactorily performed under local analgesia. Paravertebral nerve block of the last thoracic and first three lumbar spinal nerves provides excellent analgesia and relaxation for sublumbar incisions, with the only reservation that it induces marked hyperaemia in the muscle layers and a greater degree of haemorrhage which requires careful haemostasis. The technique is usually immediately effective but in occasional animals it is less successful even after repeated administration. Pain reflexes should therefore be tested properly before the operation is begun because the muscles and peritoneum may remain sensitive despite skin desensitization. Complete flaccidity of the abdominal wall and skin hyperthermia are more reliable signs of adequate analgesia than lack of response to pricking or even incision of the skin. Because paravertebral nerve block is not always entirely effective, local infiltration or field block may be preferred. Posterior epidural analgesia may also be indicated in animals which continue to strain vigorously, not only to control the straining and thus prevent prolapse of the rumen, but also to facilitate intrauterine manipulation of the presented parts of the fetus during surgery. It may, however, result in loss of hindlimb control and induced recumbency.

The preoperative administration of clenbuterol hydrochloride will relax the myometrium and facilitate handling and repair of the uterus.

Operative technique

After proper surgical preparation of the site, a vertical 30 cm incision is made in the sublumbar fossa (Figure 20.4) with careful haemostasis to prevent the formation of a postoperative haematoma in the wound. If the animal is straining vigorously, the peritoneum should not be incised until ligation is complete because the rumen is easily forced through the wound and can be difficult to replace. In multiparous cows which have continued to eat during the first stage of labour, the distended rumen may well bulge behind the

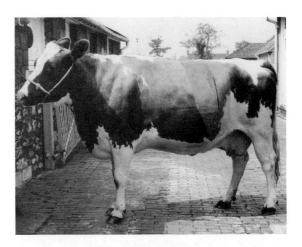

Fig. 20.4 Position of skin incision in the left sublumbar fossa.

costal arch and impede access to the uterus, but this difficulty does not justify rumenotomy to empty its contents. If the uterus is likely to be seriously infected, the incision may, alternatively, be sited more ventrally in the flank in order to minimize peritoneal contamination at hysterotomy.

After incision of the peritoneum (Figure 20.5), an excessive quantity of peritoneal fluid, sometimes blood tinged, may be immediately apparent in cases of uterine torsion or rupture. A preliminary examination of the uterus is made to determine which horn is gravid and how the fetus lies in relation to the greater curvature of this horn. Manipulation of the uterus towards the flank incision may seem advisable to reduce the risk of peritoneal contamination with uterine fluids (Figure 20.6). Except with gross intrauterine infection, these fluids are not irritant to the peritoneum and, in practice, this precaution is not necessary in fresh cases of dystocia and often not possible in protracted cases because the uterus involutes tightly on to the fetus after the fluids have escaped. In cases of fetal infection in which peritoneal contamination should theoretically be avoided at all costs, the uterus is often immovable and highly vulnerable to accidental perforation on handling. In any case, manipulation of the uterus causes stretching of the mesometrium and can quickly induce a marked pain response manifested by grunting and other signs of discomfort. Uterine torsion presents particular features at laparotomy in that there is usually excessive peritoneal fluid and almost always displacement of loops of small intestine to an abnormal position immediately

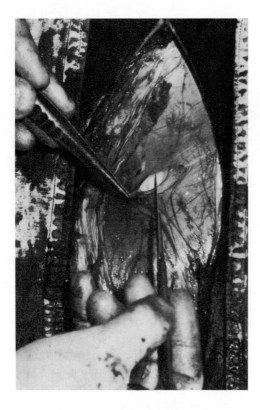

Fig. 20.5 Incision of the peritoneum.

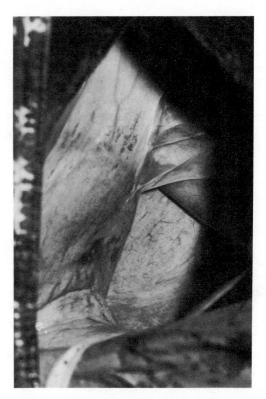

Fig. 20.6 The gravid uterus exposed by cranial displacement of the rumen.

caudal to the rumen, to such an extent that loops may spill through the wound. In these cases, it is desirable to reduce the torsion before hysterotomy simply to facilitate exteriorization of the uterus for repair after removal of the fetus but this is not always possible. Torsion is an exceptional form of dystocia because the membranes may still be intact and the presence of fetal fluid, combined with an oedematous, friable uterine wall, increases the risk of uterine perforation on handling. In attempting reduction of the torsion before hysterotomy, it may be easier to move the fetus 'nose after tail' in a horizontal plane rather than to rotate it through a vertical plane. It is often impossible to correct the twist before removal of the fetus, but as the fluids are not generally infected in these cases, peritoneal contamination is of little consequence.

The uterine incision should be made on the greater curvature of the gravid horn, extending caudally from the ovarian pole as far as possible on to the presented extremity of the fetus. An incision of inadequate length usually tears during extraction of the fetus and the tear may extend awkwardly into the vagina in such a way that it

cannot be sutured. If the membranes have not ruptured it is usually possible to bring a fetal limb to the lips of the abdominal wound and incise the overlying uterus virtually isolated from other viscera. In most caesarean cases, the fluids have escaped and the uterus is partially contracted. The hysterotomy is then performed blind with a scalpel blade or fetotomy knife as a single sweeping incision, beginning at the ovarian pole and with the knife guarded between finger and thumb which displace other viscera as the cut is extended caudally. A tentative incision may leave the endometrium intact, but care is essential with more forceful cutting not to incise a live fetus; such an injury is easily inflicted, usually along its dorsum, if the uterus is tightly contracted. Caruncles are seldom damaged by the uterine incision, which must sometimes be made boldly and quickly between bouts of abdominal straining. In extracting the fetus it is generally easier to grasp its presented parts, but this manoeuvre may provoke vigorous straining and thus predispose to tearing of the incision caudally. If the non-presented limbs are accessible, they should be extracted first (Figure

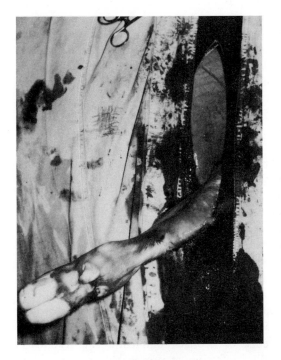

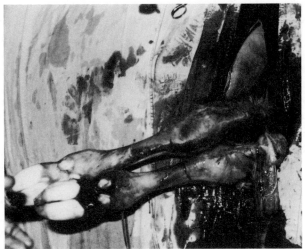

Fig. 20.7 Exteriorization of the hindlimbs.

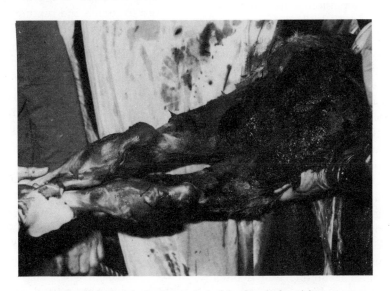

Fig. 20.8 Anticlockwise rotation of the fetus before delivery.

20.7). As in vaginal delivery, manipulation of the fetus *in utero* and in the peritoneal cavity should make maximum use of joint movements to minimize the risk of uterine damage (Figure 20.8). It is seldom necessary to snare the head in the uterus, but a finger and thumb grip in each orbit is often helpful in bringing the head into the peritoneal cavity. Particular hazards should be remembered in drawing the fetus from the uterus. Schistosoma calves often have a markedly increased diameter and may require additional traction on limb-snares. Such traction should be carefully controlled and synchronized with appropriate rotation of the trunk to ease the fetus not only through the uterine incision but through the abdominal wound, which may have to be extended. Again, as in vaginal delivery, fetal limbs affected with muscle contracture should be carefully eased through the hysterotomy with particular care that the hind digits do not damage the uterus if the fetus is extracted head first.

If fetal movements are perceptible during anterior delivery, the calf's head should be drawn quickly through the abdominal wound in case it begins to breathe. Irrespective of the position of the fetus in utero, it is most easily drawn through the abdominal wound if its vertebral column lies in the upper commissure of the incision, and appropriate rotation may therefore be necessary. With large fetuses, additional traction on sterile limb-snares is helpful provided that the direction of traction is carefully controlled, initially upwards and then forwards or backwards, depending on which fetal extremity has first been withdrawn from the uterus. Excessively vigorous pulling may result in serious uterine tearing.

On occasions, the fetus lies so far within the vagina that vaginal retropulsion is necessary. An extreme example is forelimb flexion with the head of a live fetus, often markedly swollen, with the tongue protruded, outside the vulva. A similar difficulty arises if presented extremities are far advanced in the vagina and the non-presented limbs cannot be easily withdrawn through the uterine incision because of myometrial contraction. In such cases the presented parts, after careful washing and lubrication, may have to be repelled by an assistant.

The emphysematous fetus presents unavoidable risks of peritoneal contamination, not least because its hair and hooves may already have been shed. In such cases, incision of the uterus is followed immediately by the escape of gas in the peritoneal cavity. All parts of the fetus may be grossly swollen and crepitate on handling. The uterine wall is often tightly stretched, and intrauterine manipulation can be difficult. Flank and uterine incisions of adequate length are therefore essential. Such fetuses often require considerable traction, not only on limb-snares but also with callipers applied in the orbits and at appropriate points on the trunk or upper limbs to secure additional purchase. It may be necessary to incise deeply at several sites on the thorax and abdomen to release gas and sometimes partially to eviscerate before extraction

is possible. In rare cases the fetus simply cannot be extracted from the uterus because a uterine incision of adequate length is not possible and, in such animals, fetotomy in utero may also be impracticable because the uterine wall is tightly stretched leaving no room for the introduction of fetotomy wires or blades. After the removal of a severely emphysematous fetus, the uterus is often noticeably ischaemic, of cardboard-like consistency and totally atonic. Incision of the fetal abdomen may also be necessary in occasional cases of anasarca complicated by ascites. Intrauterine fetotomy is otherwise seldom indicated during caesarean operation. The fact that many cows urinate immediately after extraction of a presented fetus suggests that urine has been retained because of urethral compression.

Caesarean delivery of a live calf provides the opportunity of ligating the umbilical cord before it is ruptured. Experience suggests that this procedure is associated with a disproportionately high incidence of neonatal omphalitis and secondary ascending infection; it is probably wiser to allow the cord to stretch and rupture spontaneously and to control any haemorrhage from the umbilical vessels by finger pressure or the temporary application of haemostatic clamps.

Before the uterus is sutured, it should always be examined for the presence of a second fetus. Repair of the hysterotomy is greatly facilitated by exteriorization of both cornua through the abdominal incision, but after removal of the fetus the healthy uterus contracts rapidly and may become markedly turgid. It is therefore advisable to bring the horns through the laparotomy before contraction begins. Torsions which cannot be reduced before hysterotomy should be untwisted at this stage, but these uteri may still be impossible to expose properly because of the volume and weight of fetal fluids. Exteriorization is accomplished by inserting a hand through the hysterotomy and drawing the gravid horn outside the abdomen. The smaller, non-gravid horn can then be lifted through the laparotomy (Figure 20.9). This manipulation stretches the uterine body and greatly aids in suture repair of the caudal part of the hysterotomy incision and tears extending from it. Exteriorization of the recently gravid uterus for repair places considerable tension on the broad ligaments, and the organ should always be care-

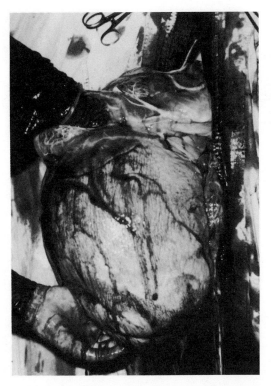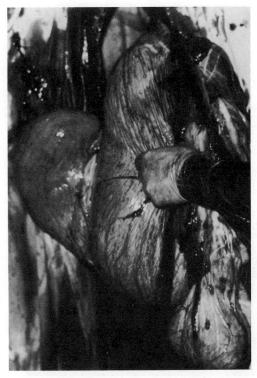

Fig. 20.9 Exteriorization of both uterine cornua for repair of the hysterotomy. Pockets of fetal fluid were drained but the placenta was left in utero and was expelled normally within 8 hours.

fully supported by an assistant unless the animal has become recumbent.

Before the uterus is stitched, consideration must be given to management of the placenta. If it has completely separated, it usually remains attached to the fetus and is removed with it. In a minority of cases it remains attached to only a few caruncles and can be separated quickly and with little haemorrhage. In all other cases it should be left in situ with no attempt at removal by traction or caruncular detachment. This approach is justified on two grounds. Firstly, it should be assumed that placentae which can physically be separated will be expelled naturally and more completely by uterine contraction within a few hours. If the calf is alive, or only recently dead, the placenta is almost always expelled within 24 hours, as a result of normal uterine contraction boosted by oxytocin therapy and endogenous oxytocin release if suckling occurs. Secondly, it is likely that deliberate detachment of placentae which would not be expelled normally always results in incomplete removal either of microvilli or of larger masses of placental tissue. Histological examination and bac-

terial culture of excised caruncles in such cases often confirm the presence of active endometritis and deep infection which prevent any form of physiological tissue separation. It is common practice to place antibiotic and other pessaries in the uterine lumen before repair of the hysterotomy, but the value of this procedure is questionable. If the placenta is subsequently expelled naturally, so too are the pessaries. If it continues to be retained, the drugs can have no more than a local action in the lumen and are probably ineffective in controlling deep infection. If intrauterine preparations are indicated at all in caesarean section, it is after the placenta has been expelled or manually removed, usually several days later.

Uterine repair (Figure 20.10) has conventionally been effected with sutures of plain or chromic catgut but, in recent years, polyglycolic acid and polyglactin have been used increasingly as alternative absorbable materials. In a comparison of the effects of suture materials on post-operative fertility rates in cattle subjected to caesarean operations, Boucoumont et al. (1978) found a significantly higher fertility after the use of polyglycolic acid

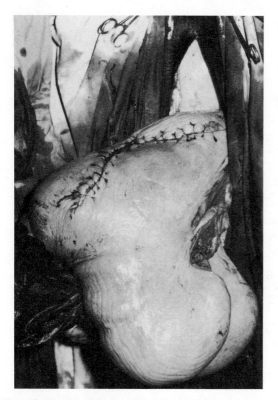

Fig. 20.10 The hysterotomy repaired with a continuous inversion suture of polyglycolic acid.

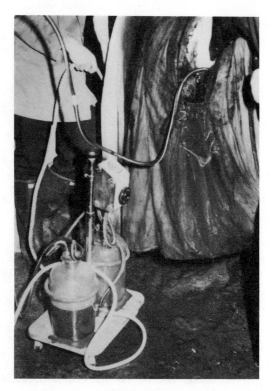

Fig. 20.11 Aspiration of fluid and blood clots from the peritoneal cavity.

and consider that catgut is more likely to cause inflammatory periuterine adhesions.

The suture pattern for hysterotomy repair is probably not important because normal uterine contraction necessarily results in a rapid overall reduction in size of the organ and consequent loosening of the stitches which serve only as a temporary scaffold for natural healing. Uterine incisions heal remarkably well and only rarely separate even with insecure sutures. A continuous inversion stitch results in good serosal apposition, but if the organ contracts rapidly and becomes turgid, inversion may be impossible, and the stitch then readily cuts through the tissues on tightening. A simple apposing suture is satisfactory in such cases. Although the uterus heals well it is not always easy to suture completely. The most common problem is repair of tears which extend deeply into the pelvic cavity. Unsutured vaginal defects, usually on the roof, are of little consequence, particularly if the placenta is expelled; very rarely does intestinal evisceration occur. Tears of the ovarian pole of the uterus are less common but may extend into the mesovarium

and cause considerable but rarely fatal haemorrhage. Other minor problems include serious oedema of the uterine wall in cases of protracted torsion and fibrosis of preoperative uterine ruptures.

During flank caesarean sections, fetal fluids inevitably enter the peritoneal cavity. If the fetus is alive or only recently dead such contamination is of no concern and the fluids need not be removed. Infected fluids, however, are harmful, and they can seldom be completely removed either by swabbing or by aspiration (Figure 20.11). This is perhaps the most serious disadvantage of a high flank approach. Soluble antibiotic preparations may be placed in the peritoneal cavity after copious saline lavage, and the abdominal wound is repaired by whatever method is preferred (Figures 20.12 and 20.13). At the end of all caesarean operations, oxytocin (40–50 IU) should routinely be administered parenterally to induce uterine contraction.

Postoperative management

Parenteral antibiotic therapy is generally recommended for 4 or 5 days, but if the fetus is alive

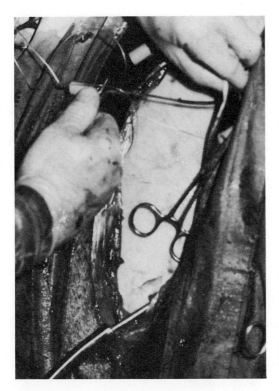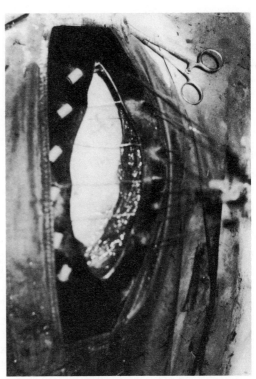

Fig. 20.12 Repair of the laparotomy with 'through-and-through' sutures of heavy gauge monofilament nylon.

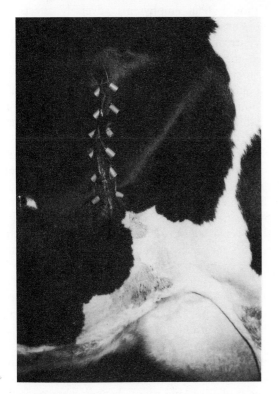

Fig. 20.13 The healing laparotomy 2 days later. The rubbers prevent pressure necrosis of the skin.

or only recently dead it should not be necessary. Cows which are recumbent before surgery and unable to stand afterwards may have obturator paralysis. Strapping together the hindlegs of these animals above the fetlock joints limits abduction during efforts to rise and prevents secondary complications such as fracture of the femoral neck and tearing of the adductor muscles.

Many cows show signs of surgical shock manifested by a respiratory grunt, drooping of the ears and even recumbency during the operation, but these are usually only transient. The recognition of worsening shock is not always easy but hypothermia with palpable coldness of the buccal mucous membranes and teats, tachycardia, respiratory grunting and unwillingness to rise are ominous signs which justify fluid supportive therapy before shock becomes irreversible. The need for such treatment should be anticipated preoperatively in cases of gross fetal putrefaction. Fluid therapy is crucially important in determining whether such cases live or die and entails the infusion of much larger volumes (20–30 litres per day) than are commonly administered. The control of pain with analgesics is also important on humane grounds, but spasmolytic agents prevent uterine contraction and, on occasions, their use has seemed to be responsible for fatal uterine haemorrhage. In cases of severe fetal impaction or birth canal trauma, persistent, forceful abdominal straining may be troublesome for 1 or 2 days after surgery and may threaten to interfere with healing of the abdominal wound. Sedation may be justified in these animals as an alternative to repeated epidural analgesic injections.

Expulsion of the placenta within 12 hours or so of the operation is a reassuring sign of uterine contraction, but in many cases it is retained for considerably longer. Provided that part of the placenta lies within the vagina and thus prevents complete cervical closure, such retention is less harmful than repeated premature attempts to remove it. Until caruncular necrosis has occurred, manual separation merely exposes highly vascular caruncular villi to invasion by pathogenic organisms which proliferate in uterine debris. Animals treated in this way often develop a sudden illness immediately afterwards, with severe pyrexia and anorexia, probably due to septicaemia. A better approach is to delay attempted removal until at least the fourth or fifth day, and every second or third day thereafter, and to leave the placenta until it can be removed completely simply by traction from the anterior vagina. Accumulated uterine fluids are then quickly discharged, and at this stage intrauterine antibiotic preparations may have a beneficial effect. Retention of the placenta, even for 2 weeks or more, is not a major contributory cause of death after caesarean section unless the uterus is grossly infected beforehand. In cases in which retention is associated with placentitis, the maternal caruncles may be shed with the placenta; such animals may still be capable of maintaining a normal pregnancy, probably by developing diffuse adventitious placentation.

After most caesarean sections the abdominal wound heals by first intention, but minor suppuration may follow inadequate haemostasis or operative contamination and cause surprisingly persistent pyrexia until drainage is established. Of much more concern is the occasional case of almost total failure of wound healing due probably to systemic rather than local causes. This complication is usually observed in animals with advanced fetal putrefaction which were critically ill before surgery. The peritoneum heals securely, but other tissues remain noticeably indolent with minimal suppuration and no granulation until the wound is stimulated by debridement.

It is remarkable how uncommonly clinical hypocalcaemia is observed after caesarean section, but the clinician should bear in mind that naturally resolving subclinical falls in plasma calcium may be present for 1 or 2 days after surgery.

Maternal recovery rate and causes of death

The maternal recovery rate after caesarean section in cattle is good. In a series of 1134 operations performed at the University of Bristol Veterinary School, 88% of the dams recovered despite the fact that in 37% the fetus was dead at the time of surgery (Pearson, unpublished data). This series included cases of protracted dystocia, many of which could not reasonably have been expected to survive because of the degree of fetal putrefaction and maternal toxaemia. The judicious selection of cases suitable for surgery would lead to an even higher recovery rate but would also condemn those animals which survive against expectation. Although fetal emphysema adversely affects the prognosis, Vandeplassche (1963) reported a recovery rate of 80% even in this group of animals. As a rule, the shorter the interval between the onset of dystocia and its surgical relief, the better is the prognosis. Recovery rates, of course, give no indication of subsequent productivity and take no account of animals which survive but remain unthrifty and infertile, generally because of chronic peritonitis and perimetritis. Such cases lose weight quickly and never regain bodily condition; there is often a chronic purulent uterine discharge and bouts of pyrexia despite prolonged but ineffective antibiotic treatment. Nevertheless, the overall recovery rate is high enough to justify routine caesarean section without selection of animals whenever vaginal delivery is impossible or likely to result in a serious degree of trauma to the birth canal. In many cases which carry a poor prognosis, the only alternative to surgery is casualty slaughter without hope of carcass salvage.

The majority of deaths occur within 36 hours of the operation and are attributable to endotoxaemic shock exacerbated by the effects of surgery. The finding at autopsy of changes characteristic of tissue hypoxia, in the liver particularly, suggests that in some cases death is inevitable, but others undoubtedly benefit from intensive fluid and antibiotic therapy. A less common cause of immediate postoperative death is intrauterine haemorrhage manifested by a slow but continuous trickle of unclotted blood, possibly followed by the expulsion of blood clots. Persistent blood loss from the vulva should not be ignored no matter how trivial it may seem, because it represents only an overflow from what might be a very large intrauterine accumulation of blood if the uterus fails to contract. In assessing the significance of such bleeding, the experienced clinician will be guided more by clinical signs of internal haemorrhage than by haematocrit values, which may remain normal until the time of death. Affected animals should receive oxytocin immediately and intravenous fluid or blood replacement therapy if their clinical status deteriorates. Packing of the vagina may be helpful provided that it does not stimulate abdominal straining.

The only other important cause of death after caesarean section is fibrinous peritonitis usually caused by *Actinomyces* (*Corynebacterium*) *pyogenes* infection with clinical manifestations from the third or fourth day onwards. Case records suggest that this complication is much less common nowadays, possibly because more effective antibiotics are now available, but occasional animals still fail to respond to treatment and die of an infection probably caused by inadequate asepsis rather than contamination with uterine contents.

Postoperative fertility

Postoperative productivity implies not only the maintenance of bodily condition and an acceptable level of lactation, but also the ability to conceive again and sustain a developing fetus to term. Numerous data are published on fertility rates after caesarean section but their significance is qualified by the fact that many animals are culled without being inseminated or served again. In 10 such series, the postoperative fertility rate ranged from 48 to 80%, with a mean value of 72% for 2368 animals, compared with a fairly uniform control figure of 89% after normal calvings (data cited by Boucoumont et al., 1978). Bouters and Vandeplassche (1986) report that in their series of caesarean sections only 75% of cows bred again after 'technically perfect' surgery and 9.7% of these

pregnancies ended in abortion. Vandeplassche (1985) has also compared various indices of fertility after spontaneous calvings and caesarean section. After surgery, the percentages of cows pregnant after the first, second and fifth insemination was markedly lower, the interval between calvings was longer, the abortion rate was higher, and the incidence of complications such as hydroallantois and cervical failure at subsequent parturitions was considerably increased.

It is not uncommon to have to perform a second caesarean section on the same animal, but rarely for the same indication. Endometrial herniation may then be apparent along the uterine scar with noticeable thinning of the uterine wall in this region, but spontaneous rupture of the uterus is unlikely. One exceptional cow in Germany survived six caesarean operations (Frerking and Santiago, 1976), while in Belgium, cows of the Belgian blue breed are subjected to repeated elective surgery.

In cases of dystocia which might be relieved by either fetotomy or caesarean section, the former technique has often been preferred on the assumption that it is significantly less likely to impair subsequent breeding ability. Debackere et al. (1959) reported a 7% greater conception rate after fetotomy, but this difference may be more apparent than real because their series included four times as many hysterotomies as fetotomies. It is also self-evident that caesarean section is often performed for the relief of severe dystocia that could not be tackled by fetotomy.

THE MARE

Because it is not often necessary, caesarean section in the mare is still widely regarded as a serious and, by inference, a dangerous operation. In fact, the mare tolerates this surgical interference as well as most other species and the generally good recovery rate after caesarean section has largely disproved the myth that the horse's peritoneal cavity is exceptionally vulnerable to infection or the development of dangerous postoperative adhesions. There is, however, little doubt that increasing familiarity with modern techniques for inducing and maintaining general anaesthesia has greatly improved the chances of maternal recovery.

Even in specialist equine hospitals in areas of high stud density, caesarean section is not a common procedure. In recording the results of a series of 71 operations performed at Ghent, Vandeplassche et al. (1977) also comment that they carry out 15 fetotomies for every caesarean section. Nevertheless, there are now a substantial number of reports of successful operations, many performed in the field under less than optimum conditions.

If the foal is alive, the operation should be performed with minimum delay. Arthur (1975) has observed that if the equine fetus lies in the maternal pelvic canal, it suffers fatal anoxia because of dehiscence of the allantochorion within 1 or 2 hours of the beginning of second-stage labour. This observation is corroborated by the fact that 70% of foals born by hysterotomy at Ghent were stillborn or died soon after birth (Vandeplassche, 1980). Intrepid surgery in the field may therefore be more expedient than referral to a specialist hospital.

Indications

The range of indications is more limited than in cattle. Cervical dystocia is not recognized in the mare, and disproportion and fetal deformities are less common than in other species. The major indication in the Ghent series, accounting for 39 of 71 cases, was bicornual pregnancy or transverse presentation, followed by other faulty dispositions complicated by injury, contraction or infection (13 cases) and uterine torsion (10 cases). In a much smaller series of 34 cases at the University of Bristol veterinary school, uterine torsion was the most frequent indication.

With considerable experience of equine dystocia, Vandeplassche et al. (1977) regard the following indications as absolute:

1. Cases which cannot be relieved by other means.
2. Cases which would otherwise require difficult, total fetotomy with severe risks to the dam.
3. Vulvovaginal trauma.
4. Advanced contraction and chronic metritis.
5. The saving of a live foal in irreducible malposture (with the reservation that the foal might be deformed).

In these forms of dystocia, caesarean section is considered to be the primary method of delivery rather than a last resort.

Significantly, these authors also specify forms of dystocia which they regard as contraindications for surgery; these include lateral deviation of the neck, hydrocephalus, breech presentation of a dead fetus, twin dystocia and prolapse of the maternal bladder.

Anaesthesia

Reposition of preparturient uterine torsions can be carried out by laparotomy in the standing animal under local analgesia or nerve block (Vandeplassche, 1980). The availability of potent inhalational anaesthetic agents and the means of administering them in a controlled manner enables the use of a balanced anaesthetic technique in horses as in other animals. The choice of anaesthetic drugs should have regard for the maintenance of maximum oxygenation of dam and fetus and the avoidance of central depression in both. Long-acting agents which are known to have a prolonged effect in neonates, or techniques which result in hypoxaemia such as usually follows neuroleptanalgesia, are to be avoided.

Premedication is rarely necessary in parturient mares suffering from dystocia and should be avoided if the foal is alive. Anaesthesia is best induced by the rapid intravenous administration of an ultra-short-acting barbiturate such as methohexitone sodium (5 mg/kg body weight) or thiopentone sodium (10 mg/kg body weight). Methohexitone sodium is preferred because of its more rapid redistribution and metabolism and consequent shorter action and lesser depressant effect on the fetus. After tracheal intubation, anaesthesia is maintained by the administration of halothane vaporized in oxygen or a mixture of oxygen and nitrous oxide delivered by an appropriate large animal anaesthetic apparatus. Vandeplassche et al. (1977) recommend the use of glycerol guiacolate for immobilization of the mare, followed by local infiltration analgesia. Although this drug is widely used alone in Europe for casting horses, it is not an anaesthetic agent.

Attention should be paid to the position of the mare after the induction of anaesthesia. Anaesthetized horses are susceptible to severe deleterious cardiopulmonary changes which occur in lateral recumbency but are more severe if the animal is placed on its back. These positions predispose to impaired oxygenation and alveolar hypoventila-tion, which are reflected in a widening alveolar arterial oxygen tension gradient (Hall, 1979). Failure to administer high concentrations of oxygen during anaesthesia can lead to severe arter-ial hypoxaemia not only of the dam but also of the fetus, with obvious adverse consequences. Dorsal recumbency may also induce 'supine hypotension' if the gravid uterus compresses the posterior vena cava and thus impedes venous return and reduces cardiac output. The mare should therefore be placed in lateral or dorsolateral recumbency what-ever laparotomy approach is adopted.

Operative technique

The operation can be performed through a mid-line, paramedian or ventral flank laparotomy. The midline approach is now widely adopted for gastrointestinal surgery and is even more satisfac-tory for caesarean section because this operation considerably reduces intra-abdominal pressure, and the wound can therefore be repaired easily without excessive tension on the sutures. All other approaches necessitate muscle division, which results in greater operative haemorrhage and post-operative oedema. Provided that the midline inci-sion is properly repaired, the risk of incisional hernia is negligible.

The mare's uterus is seldom so tightly con-tracted that a fetal limb cannot be grasped through the uterine wall and brought through the abdominal wound. For this reason a uterine incision of adequate length is easily made on the greater curvature of the gravid horn with little risk of tearing during manipulation of the fetus. In many cases, hysterotomy is followed immediately by profuse haemorrhage from the submucosal plexus of arteries and veins which are too numer-ous to be ligated individually. As a means of con-trolling such haemorrhage, Vandeplassche (1973) recommends the insertion of a continuous suture through all layers of uterine wall along the edges of the incision, after the placenta has first been detached from this area. The fetus is then extracted making maximum use of joint flexibility and gently supported outside the abdomen with its umbilical cord intact. The equine fetus is less sensitive than the fetal calf to 'pinching' stimuli *in utero* and, unless the placenta is separated, fetal viability should be assumed until cord or heart

palpation proves otherwise. If the foal is alive, the cord is left intact for several minutes until breathing begins. The cord is then ligated or preferably divided by stretching. If the foal is dead, the placenta may already have separated and is then easily removed through the hysterotomy. If the placenta remains attached to the endometrium, it is better not to attempt manual separation because this procedure results not only in diffuse endome-trial bleeding, but also in retention of microvilli which predisposes to subsequent endometritis. The uterine incision is repaired with polyglycolic acid inversion sutures in one or two rows, depending on whether the first row of stitches tears through the uterine wall, which is sometimes noticeably fragile. After the removal of clotted blood and other debris, a soluble antibiotic preparation may be sprinkled on the uterine incision.

After laparohysterotomy, the abdominal inci-sion is easy to suture because of flaccidity of the stretched abdominal musculature. It is important to insert closely spaced sutures of appropriate material in a continuous or interrupted pattern. The peri-toneum and subperitoneal fat need not be stitched. The laparotomy repair is completed with a continuous subcutaneous suture and appropriate stitches in the skin.

Postoperative management

After all cases of caesarean section, oxytocin should be administered to induce uterine contraction even when the placenta has been removed at surgery. Vandeplassche et al. (1971) recommend immediate oxytocin therapy followed by a supplementary slow intravenous infusion of 50 IU in saline if the placenta is not expelled within 4 hours. The latter method of administration probably has a more physiological effect. Experience suggests that oxytocin therapy in the mare is sometimes followed by excessively vigorous uterine contrac-tion and eversion of the cornua into the vagina and threatened eversion through the vulva even after the placenta has been expelled. Arthur (1975) has also encountered this complication after elective hysterotomy in pony mares. After oxytocin ther-apy, the placenta is usually expelled within 12 hours, but in occasional cases it may separate but remain within the uterus and anterior vagina and is then easily removed per vaginam. Retention for longer than 24 hours is no longer regarded as an indication for immediate manual separation provided that antibiotic therapy is maintained, but removal may still be justified in draught-type mares which are particularly susceptible to systemic reactions. After removal of the placenta, intrauterine antibiotic preparations may have a beneficial effect, but more important by far is siphonage of any uterine fluids which accumulate, especially in mares which show signs of anaphylactic response or which are not recovering satisfactorily. Vandeplassche et al. (1977) have commented on the 2–3 day delay in contraction after caesarean section and recommend division of perimetrial adhesions per rectum at the end of this period.

Antibiotic therapy is generally considered advisable after equine caesarean section, but on occasions it may be more harmful than beneficial. A potentially serious complication of this or any other stressful operation in the horse is the onset of severe diarrhoea, sometimes due to salmonellosis, during the immediate postoperative period. Owen (1975, 1980) has suggested that tetracycline therapy of stressed horses that happen to be salmonella carriers may induce clinical salmonellosis with enteric signs by removing the normal bacterial antagonists of the salmonellae. Salmonella infection in horses is not uncommon; the use of antibiotics which are excreted in bile may potentiate serious and sometimes fatal illness in unsuspected carrier animals. In such cases, stress associated with transportation or surgery may be aggravated by the induced diarrhoea. If the foal is alive, antibiotic therapy should not be necessary unless clinical signs of infection develop. If uterine infection and peritoneal contamination are likely, prophylactic treatment is indicated, but the antibiotic should be chosen with care.

Abdominal incisions in the horse are usually followed by local oedema of varying severity. After midline laparohysterotomy, diffuse subcutaneous oedema may extend along the ventral abdomen to the presternal region, but the swelling slowly subsides over a period of 7–10 days. The administration of diuretic agents appears to disperse the oedema more quickly, but the necessity for such treatment is questionable. Wound infection is treated by removal of appropriate skin sutures to provide drainage.

Maternal recovery rate and causes of death

If the dystocia is of short duration, the prognosis for maternal recovery is good. In the Ghent series of 77 operations, 62 mares (81%) recovered (Vandeplassche et al., 1977). The Ghent data suggest that most deaths occur during or very soon after surgery and are attributable to shock caused by uterine haemorrhage or gross uterine infection. Haemorrhage can be largely prevented by haemostatic suturing of the uterine incision and the effects of fetal emphysema and other forms of shock can be countered by intensive fluid therapy during and after the operation.

Because most deaths occur during the immediate postoperative period, the clinician is more likely to be worried by two particular complications which may develop within the next few days. The onset of diarrhoea should be viewed with the greatest concern because body fluid loss is rapid and severe and fluid reserves are soon depleted even if the mare continues to drink. The role of antibiotics in the pathogenesis of this disorder and their value in its treatment are unclear, but there is no argument about the necessity for immediate fluid replacement therapy to maintain hydration and normal electrolyte status. The other complication is laminitis, which has long been recognized as a sequel of placental retention in animals of the heavy draught breeds. The earliest sign of this supposedly anaphylactic reaction may be severe pulmonary oedema with dyspnoea and nasal regurgitation of fluids. Pedal pain is then manifested by reluctance to move or even to stand and, without careful clinical examination, the resultant recumbency during the early postoperative period may easily be mistaken for terminal illness justifying euthanasia. In such cases, accumulated uterine fluids should be removed immediately by siphonage. Diuretics are indicated for severe oedema, and the laminitis is treated by dietary restriction and the control of pain. The use of corticosteroids in such cases carries obvious risks.

Postoperative fertility

In the Ghent series of equine caesarean sections, only 14 mares conceived out of 27 which were covered again after surgery, and six of these aborted before term (Vandeplassche et al., 1977). The operation therefore has a markedly adverse effect not only on fertility but also on the ability to maintain a normal pregnancy because of uterine adhesions and fibrosis. The report by Arthur (1975), however, of two mares which each conceived after two elective operations suggests that the hysterotomy *per se* is less important in this respect than the state of the fetus and the uterus at the time of surgery.

THE SOW

The sow, like the bitch, is a difficult obstetrical patient because although the need for surgery may be clear, it is not always possible to identify a particular cause of dystocia even after the operation has been performed.

Indications

In a series of 57 operations reported by Renard et al. (1980) the major indications were irreducible vaginal prolapse (32%), fetopelvic disproportion including fetal emphysema (32%), secondary uterine inertia (23%) and, surprisingly, non–dilatation of the cervix (10%). Preparturient vaginal prolapse may be complicated by rectal prolapse and retroversion of the urinary bladder and even of the gravid uterus, and often undergoes considerable trauma and marked oedematous swelling. Fresh prolapses at term need not interfere with parturition but, if manual delivery is necessary, oedema rapidly develops, and the tissues then tear readily. Inertia of a primary or secondary nature is an important indication for surgery and, because of delay, the fetuses in such cases are often emphysematous. In secondary inertia, particularly, it is not always easy to be certain that fetuses remain in the uterus. If they cannot be palpated or ballotted through the uterine or abdominal wall, and if fetal heart sounds cannot be detected, radiography is advisable before surgery is undertaken. Less frequent clinical indications for caesarean section are maternal immaturity and pelvic deformity, uterine torsion of one or both cornua and fetal deformities such as hydrocephalus or conjoined piglets.

During the last few years, preparturient elective hysterotomy has been increasingly performed as an alternative to gravid hysterectomy to obtain disease-free piglets which are then fostered or reared artificially.

Anaesthesia

Because of difficulties in restraint, the operation is usually performed under deep sedation and local analgesia, or general anaesthesia. Herman and Vandeplassche (1968) reported the successful use of intravenous thiopentone sodium (150–200 mg/kg body weight) followed by local infiltration. If inhalational anaesthetic apparatus is available, this agent or methohexitone sodium may be administered intravenously to induce general anaesthesia, which is then maintained with halothane vaporized in oxygen or oxygen and nitrous oxide via a mask or endotracheal tube, but this method is potentially dangerous for certain present-day 'breeds' of pig. Stress-susceptible breeds such as the Piétrain and some Landrace often react adversely to halothane (and suxamethonium) by developing the syndrome of malignant hyperpyrexia, which is almost always fatal (Lucke and Hall, 1977). Increasing numbers of hybrid sows are now also vulnerable to this risk.

Techniques which may be more practicable in the field, for any sow, are a combination of intramuscular azaperone (2 mg/kg) and intravenous metomidate (2 mg/kg) with local infiltration analgesia or, alternatively, ketamine hydrochloride (15–20 mg/kg) alone or with azaperone or diazepam. Unfortunately, all these agents have a protracted depressant effect on the fetus. Renard et al. (1980) recommend the use of anterior epidural analgesia but also reported a very high incidence of postoperative hindlimb paresis which they attributed to lateral recumbency on a hard surface. Provided that the animal is adequately restrained under sedation, local analgesia or paravertebral nerve block may also be successfully employed.

Operative technique

The operation is performed through a vertical sublumbar or ventral flank incision on either side (Figure 20.14). The gravid horn(s) should be exteriorized for incision outside the peritoneal cavity in order to minimize peritoneal contamination. If the fetuses are not emphysematous, it is usually possible to evacuate both horns through a single incision as close to the uterine body as possible. The piglets in the ovarian poles of the cornua are squeezed down the horn and grasped through the incision. If the fetuses are

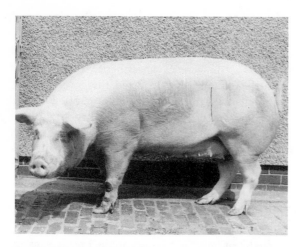

Fig. 20.14 Position of skin incision in the left sublumbar fossa.

emphysematous multiple incisions sited directly over or between them may be necessary. The piglet's umbilical cord is long and, even without placental separation, forceps clamping or ligation is possible before division. Placentae which have not separated should be left *in situ* and not forcibly removed by traction. Because the cornua are long, it is important to palpate the genital tract in its entirety to ensure that all piglets have been removed. The uterine incision(s) is repaired with inversion sutures of polyglycolic acid. The sow's uterus, like the mare's, is apt to tear if the suture is pulled too tight but this is of no consequence if rapid contraction is induced by postoperative oxytocin therapy.

Maternal recovery rate and causes of death

Unless the fetus and uterus are grossly infected, the maternal recovery rate after caesarean section in the sow is excellent. In a series of 78 unselected cases, Renard et al. (1980) reported a maternal recovery rate of 72%. Deaths are usually due to the combined effects of toxaemia and surgical shock and occur during the immediate postoperative period. Animals which are likely to die can often be identified before surgery because of a characteristic blotchy cyanosis of the limbs, ears and udder. The adverse effects of peritoneal contamination are more easily avoided in the sow than in larger animals because the uterus can be totally exteriorized during the operation. Other frequent complications recorded by Renard et al. (1980)

include constipation, locomotory problems exacerbated by the sow's tendency to remain recumbent, and the mastitis–metritis–agalactia syndrome. Severe preoperative vaginal prolapse may recur after surgery and require the insertion of a temporary retaining perivaginal suture.

THE EWE

The main indications for caesarean section in the ewe are failure of the cervix to dilate, irreducible or severely traumatized vaginal prolapse, fetopelvic disproportion, particularly in primiparous animals with a single fetus, and fetal emphysema after protracted dystocia. Less frequent indications are uterine torsion, vulvovestibular stricture and faulty fetal disposition which cannot be corrected because of maternal immaturity or uterine contraction. Vaginal prolapse should initially be treated conservatively by reposition and the insertion of vulval retention sutures, in the hope that pregnancy will continue to term, but many cases undergo early labour and incomplete dilatation of the cervix. Unfortunately, lambs from such animals frequently die of prematurity after showing characteristic convulsive limb movements and respiratory embarrassment.

Hysterotomy is usually performed through a left flank incision under paravertebral nerve block or local infiltration analgesia with the animal in right lateral recumbency (Figure 20.15). Care is essential in inducing local analgesia in sheep because accidental intravenous administration or the injection of an excessive quantity of anaesthetic agent may rapidly result in convulsions. It is also important in a high sublumbar incision to recognize the highly vascular mesometrial attachment to parietal peritoneum. The operation otherwise is performed as in the cow, but with even greater care to examine the uterus for multiple fetuses, which can always be removed through a single uterine incision. The sheep, more than any other species, is highly susceptible to the toxaemic effects of intrauterine clostridial infection, and most deaths are due to this complication.

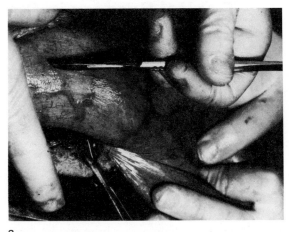

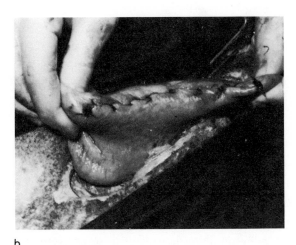

a   b

Fig. 20.15 Caesarean section in the ewe for the relief of incomplete cervical dilatation. (a) Incision of the exteriorized uterus over a fetal hind limb. (b) Hysterotomy repair with inversion sutures.

REFERENCES

Arthur, G. H. (1975) *Veterinary Reproduction and Obstetrics*, 4th edn. London: Baillière Tindall.

Boucoumont, D., Lecuyer, B., Rosenthiehl, D., Tisserand, R., Troccon, B. and Oullier, R. (1978) *Point Vét.*, **8**, 15.

Bouters, R. and Vandeplassche, M. (1986) Tierärztl. Prax., **14**, 205.

Debackere, M., Vandeplassche, M. and Paredis, F. (1959) *Vlaams Diergeneesk. Tijdschr.*, **28**, 1.

Formston, C. (1945) *Vet. Rec.*, **57**, 328.

Frerking, H. and Santiago, C. (1976) *Prakt. Tierarzt.*, **57**, 731.

Hall, L. W. (1979) *Equine Vet. J.*, **11**, 71.

Herman, J. and Vandeplassche, M. (1968) *Wien. Tierärztl. Monatsschr.*, **55**, 526.

Hindson, J. C. (1978) *Vet. Rec.*, **102**, 327.

Lucke, J. N. and Hall, G. M. (1977) *Proc. Ass. Vet. Anaesth. G. B. I.*, **7**, 114.

MacKellar, J. C. (1960) *Vet. Rec.*, **72**, 507.

Owen, R. ap R. (1975) *Vet. Rec.*, **96**, 267.

Owen, R. ap R. (1980) *Vet. Rec.*, **107**, 95.

Parkinson, J. D. (1974) *Vet. Rec.*, **95**, 508.

Pearson, H. (1971) *Vet. Rec.*, **89**, 597.

Renard, A., St-Pierre, H., Lamothe, P. and Couture, Y. (1980) *Méd. Vét. Québec*, **10**, 6.

Rice, L. E. and Wiltbank, J. N. (1972) *J. Amer. Vet. Med. Assn*, **161**, 1348.

Souques, J. C. (1968) Contribution a l'étude de l'opération caesarienne. Thesis, Alfort.

Stables, J. W. (1980) *Bovine Practnr*, **15**, 26.

Vandeplassche, M. (1963) *Schweiz. Arch. Tierheilkd*, **105**, 21.

Vandeplassche, M. (1973) *The Veterinary Annual*, p. 73. Bristol: John Wright.

Vandeplassche, M. (1980) *Equine Vet. J.*, **12**, 45.

Vandeplassche, M. (1985) *Pro Veterinario*, **2**, 5.

Vandeplassche, M., Spincemaille, J. and Bouters, R. (1971) *Equine Vet. J.*, **3**, 144.

Vandeplassche, M., Bouters, R., Spincemaille, J. and Bonte, P. (1977) *Proc. 23rd Ann. Conv. Am. Ass. Equine Practnrs*, p. 75.

21

Genital Surgery in the Bitch and Queen

THE CAESAREAN OPERATION

The bitch

Compared with larger animals, the bitch and cat are awkward obstetric patients in several respects. In the bitch, for instance, there is a much wider normal variation in the duration of pregnancy than is generally realized. In a survey of 4773 normal pregnancies Krzyzanowski et al. (1975) recorded a mean pregnancy length of 62.3 days, but the range extended from 54 to 72 days. In this series, 11.6% of animals whelped before the 60th day of pregnancy and 9.2% after the 65th day (see p. 98). These figures are of direct relevance to the timing of premeditated caesarean sections. In the bitch, there is also a wide variation in the durations of the first and second stages of labour and a dearth of data on which to base even arbitrary criteria of normality. In many bitches the first and second stages together last no longer than 3 or 4 hours, whereas in others the first stage alone may exceed 20 hours in length and still be followed by normal unassisted delivery of live fetuses. The occasional bitch which gives birth to one live puppy daily on three consecutive days is clearly exceptional, but intervals of this length could justifiably be taken to signify the onset of inertia.

The most serious obstacle to rational assessment of apparent dystocia is the physical impossibility of carrying out a proper internal examination of more than the terminal segment of the birth canal. Except in the smallest breeds, even the cervix is beyond reach on vaginal exploration. The clinician must therefore rely greatly on behavioural signs and the nature of the vaginal discharges, and interpret these observations on the basis of experience of normal whelping. In this respect the following generalizations may be helpful.

Failure of cervical dilatation is not recognized in the bitch or cat. In normal whelpings, the onset of voluntary abdominal straining signifies cervical relaxation and stimulation of the pelvic reflex by some part of the conceptus in the anterior vagina. As the second stage of labour progresses, the nature of abdominal contractions changes perceptibly. Initially, bouts of straining are brief and perfunctory, but as the fetus passes into the vagina the duration and intensity of straining increase. As the fetus distends the perineum, straining becomes forcefully sustained. The pattern of straining in cases of apparent dystocia may therefore indicate the likely position of the fetus in the birth canal.

Inertia of a primary or secondary nature is a common cause of dystocia in the bitch. Abdominal and uterine contractions are roughly synchronous but are not necessarily of equal intensity. The continuation of forceful involuntary straining cannot therefore be taken as evidence of continuing uterine contractions. This consideration is important because uterine contraction is by far the more effective of these expulsive forces and is essential for delivery, irrespective of the degree of abdominal straining. Uterine contraction is involuntary, but straining can be inhibited consciously, usually in anticipation of pain immediately before the birth of the first fetus of a litter. It is important, too, to realize that during normal whelpings there are periods of rest, indeed of sleep, when abdominal and presumably uterine contractions stop. Such behaviour does not necessarily indicate the onset of inertia. In this respect, it is interesting to consider the intervals between births in normal parturition. In a series of 11 whelpings involving 70 pups, the shortest interval was 10 minutes and the longest 135 minutes (Pearson, unpublished data). In polytocous species, it is unrealistic to expect all the fetuses to be born alive. In fact, in this series four of the five stillborn fetuses were the last in their respective litters. In many normal bitches, the period of straining before the birth of the first puppy may be considerably longer than the intervals between births, and 2 hours may safely elapse between rupture of the allantochorion and birth of the presented fetus. In general, the incidence of dystocia is lowest in young, primiparous animals. Many bitches which are affected with primary inertia later in life have a normal first parturition.

Indications

In larger animals the cause of dystocia can usually be identified, but this is often not possible in the bitch even after a caesarean operation has been performed. In practical terms, the decision to operate is therefore based largely on a subjective assessment of the circumstances of the case — the duration and progess of the whelping, the number and viability of fetuses born and still unborn, the nature of vaginal discharges, changes in the pattern of straining and the often uninformative findings on vaginal examination — rather than on a precise diagnosis of the cause of the dystocia. In fact, it is sometimes difficult to be sure that dystocia has supervened; the correct management of these cases, without resorting always to caesarean section, requires experience and sound clinical judgement. It is therefore more realistic to indicate when surgical interference may justifiably be considered than to catalogue the various maternal and fetal causes of dystocia, all of which may, on occasion, constitute a valid reason for caesarean section.

In explaining how canine dystocia may be recognized, Freak (1975) discusses three forms of delay.

1. Delay in the initiation of parturition.
2. Delay in propulsion.
3. Delay in delivery despite vigorous straining.

Most whelping problems present in exactly these ways.

Delay in the initiation of parturition may be due to several causes. There may, for example, be psychological inhibition in bitches suddenly transferred to a strange environment not conducive to the normal progress of labour. There may, in individual animals, simply be a long but normal first stage of labour. In such cases, it is helpful to know if allantoic fluid has been lost, but it is more important to appreciate the significance of the dark greenish-black discharge which arises from marginal areas of placentation. This fluid is not released until at least one placenta has separated, and its appearance before straining or the birth of a puppy signifies primary uterine inertia. In many such cases it is the only sign of cervical dilatation, and justifies immediate surgery if more than one or two fetuses are present. After the birth of one puppy, dead or alive, this discharge has less significance unless the bitch shows other signs of inertia.

In bitches which have undergone a normal first stage of labour, vigorous unproductive straining for more than 3 hours or so may indicate dystocia; such cases should be carefully assessed by abdominal auscultation and diagnostic ultrasonographs to confirm fetal viability and by vaginal examination to detect obstructive dystocia. Cases of this stage may be difficult to assess and offer ample scope for errors of judgement; a live fetus may well be born during preparation for surgery. Without positive signs of dystocia, such animals should be left a little longer unless straining abates or a placental discharge appears.

An excessively long interval since the birth of the last fetus may also be difficult to interpret. In bitches pregnant with only one or two fetuses, a delay at this stage may be normal, but if it exceeds 3 hours and is associated with vigorous straining, there is probably obstructive dystocia, the cause of which may be obvious on vaginal examination, abdominal palpation or even radiography and ultrasonography. An alternative explanation for continued straining without birth is the onset of inertia of a primary or secondary nature. The management of delay during the second stage of labour is plagued by difficulty in recognizing the signs of inertia, largely because abdominal straining may continue after inertia develops. A tentative diagnosis of inertia is more convincing if abdominal straining stops or is reduced in frequency and intensity, but this does not always occur. The assessment of these cases should be based on the assumption that, in primary inertia, the longer the delay, the more likely are the fetuses to die. The clinician learns by experience that it is better to perform an occasional hysterotomy unnecessarily than to delay until all the fetuses are dead. Primary inertia is occasionally due to hypocalcaemia or hypoglycaemia and responds spectacularly to appropriate therapy (Freak, 1975). Apparent inertia towards the end of the second stage of labour is likely to be secondary in nature and may respond quickly to the intramuscular administration of oxytocin.

The non-surgical relief of dystocia is admirably reviewed by Freak (1975). Certain forms of fetal dystocia may be corrected easily by finger, forceps or vectis manipulation per vaginam. Vaginal forceps delivery, under general anaesthesia if necessary, is particularly indicated in bitches in which the last one or two fetuses, usually dead, cannot be expelled naturally. In fact, in such cases, it is sometimes possible to milk the fetus into the birth canal by manipulation through the abdominal wall.

In some brachycephalic breeds, pregnancy is routinely terminated by caesarean section, largely on account of the exhaustive length of parturition and the high incidence of dystocia and stillbirths. Premeditated hysterotomy may also be indicated for other reasons such as pelvic deformity or gravid inguinal metrocele. Whatever the reason, surgery should normally be delayed until the onset of first-stage labour in order to avoid the risk of fetal prematurity. Prolongation of pregnancy beyond its expected termination is not an indication for immediate hysterotomy. Provided fetal movements and heart sounds are detectable, and the bitch remains healthy with no abnormal vaginal discharges, the case should be observed carefully but left until other signs develop.

Prolongation of pregnancy, sometimes up to 70 days or even more, in bitches carrying only one or two fetuses is a particular cause for concern. In the 'single-pup syndrome' fetal endocrine secretion may be inadequate to initiate the process of parturition, and the fetus may be larger than normal and therefore less likely to pass easily through the birth canal when labour begins. Many such pregnancies are terminated surgically, perhaps wisely, to avoid the risk of fetal death from primary uterine inertia.

Anaesthesia

The choice of anaesthetic technique is important in caesarean operations, either to ensure fetal viability or because of the condition of the bitch after a protracted or complicated whelping. Fetal viability can often be confirmed preoperatively by detecting fetal movements using ultrasonography or heart sounds through the abdominal wall, but the absence of such positive signs does not necessarily mean that all the fetuses are dead. The choice of anaesthetic agents should therefore be based on the assumption that live fetuses are present.

The delivery of live fetuses depends to a large extent on correcting or preventing fetal depression and hypoxia which may be due to:

1. Placental separation.
2. Maternal hypotension, usually caused by excessive doses of anaesthetic drugs.
3. Inadequate pulmonary ventilation of the bitch during anaesthesia due to the 'splinting' effect of the gravid uterus on the diaphragm or to the effects of anaesthetic drugs.

With the exception of depolarizing muscle relaxants, all anaesthetic agents cross the placental barrier.

After a protracted whelping, the bitch may already be dehydrated and even in hypovolaemic shock. Exacerbation of preoperative hypotension by the circulatory effects of exteriorization and evacuation of the uterus should be anticipated by intravenous fluid therapy from the outset, particularly if caesarean hysterectomy may be necessary. Blood loss during caesarean section is not usually severe, but uterine rupture or forcible removal of unseparated placentae, especially in small dogs, may cause life-threatening haemorrhage.

At the outset of parturition, bitches usually stop eating and often vomit. The stomach should remain empty thereafter except perhaps for ingested placentae, but after compulsive hyperventilation during labour some animals drink copiously. The possibility of vomiting should therefore be borne in mind, particularly if inhalation induction is to be carried out. In fact, vomiting at this stage is unusual and much more likely during recovery from anaesthesia at the end of the operation.

Small animals should be protected throughout the operation from the development of accidental hypothermia (Waterman, 1975).

Operative technique

The operation is performed through either a flank or a midline laparotomy. The *linea alba* offers an ideal approach to the gravid uterus. Veins between the rows of mammary glands immediately below the skin have to be ligated but there is no haemorrhage in the deeper tissues. The incision may be extended cranially as far as is necessary, and there is equal access to both uterine horns. A certain prejudice against this approach is probably based on the occasional occurrence of incisional hernia. This complication can be avoided by the use of non-absorbable suture material of adequate strength for the repair of the muscle layers of the incision. The proximity of the skin wound to the teats does not interfere with normal suckling.

The uterus can usually be exteriorized, but care is essential in this manipulation. The wall of the gravid uterus at term is thin and stretched and tears easily in a circumferential manner around the horn or body. It must therefore be exteriorized gently, as much by pressure through the abdominal wall as by direct traction. It is at this stage that respiratory and circulatory changes may be noticed. After exteriorization of the uterus, the peritoneal cavity is packed with swabs to prevent subsequent contamination with uterine fluids. (If small swabs are used for this purpose they should be counted before and after use.) If the uterus can be exteriorized, all the fetuses should be removed through a single, longitudinal incision on the dorsal surface of the uterine body. Those in the upper segments of the cornua are milked through the uterine wall until their membranes rupture and the fetal extremities, either the head or the loins, can be grasped with fingers through the hysterotomy incision. If the placenta slips out with the fetus, it is likely that the puppy is dead, but immediate palpation is still indicated for evidence of heart beat. Fetuses bathed in dark-green fluid are usually dead. On delivery of the fetus through the incision the membranes should be perforated with scissors and the fetal head exposed. The cord is then divided between two haemostatic clamps placed 3–4 cm from the umbilicus. The cord may alternatively be ligated, but ligatures pulled carelessly or tied too tightly cut through the tissues and predispose to bleeding. In breeds which are prone to cleft palate, this is the optimum time to inspect the mouth before the puppy, its cord clamp still attached, is transferred to an attendant for resuscitation.

When all the fetuses have been removed, the management of unseparated placentae should be considered. It is always possible, by traction and twisting of the cords and squeezing on the uterine wall, forcibly to detach the afterbirth, but the procedure leads to haemorrhage from the area of placental attachment. Such haemorrhage may be of little consequence in larger bitches, but in toy breeds the bleeding from even one or two such areas may be fatal. Attached placentae should be left *in situ*, and will be expelled by uterine involution, boosted by the parenteral administration of oxytocin, very soon after the operation is completed.

The uterine incision is closed with two rows of interrupted or continuous inversion sutures of polyglycolic acid or polyglactin.

In certain circumstances, this technique is modified depending on the disposition of the fetus(es) within the uterus. Impaction of a fetus in the uterine body and vagina may prevent exteriorization of the organ without serious risk of rupture. If the fetus cannot be eased out of the vagina into the uterus, an incision must be made *in situ* on the ventral presented surface. Collapse of that part of the tract leads to immediate escape of uterine fluids and considerable risk of peritoneal contamination, but this is of little consequence unless the fetus is infected. Remaining fetuses are removed through the same incision, which is then repaired. In cases of primary inertia with only one or two fetuses, they may lie in the upper segment of one or both uterine horns. Fetuses retained after the birth of most of the litter may lie in a similar position. A cornual incision may be expedient in such cases but care should be taken to avoid placental areas, not only to prevent excessive haemorrhage but also to avoid the risk of structural abnormalities in fetuses that develop at this site in subsequent pregnancies.

Laparohysterotomy will occasionally reveal unexpected findings such as uterine torsion (which is more common in the cat than in the dog) or rupture. The latter condition may cause serious haemorrhage and hypovolaemic shock, but if the uterus involutes the bleeding usually stops spontaneously. Uterine rupture probably accounts for most recorded cases of so-called extrauterine pregnancy in the bitch; it is remarkable how effectively such fetuses are encapsulated by the omentum and peritoneum and subsequently become heavily calcified, without apparent detriment to the dam.

After protracted, neglected dystocia, particularly with fetal putrefaction, the uterus may be irreversibly infarcted or infected with gas-producing coliform or clostridial organisms. Localized areas of ischaemia can be inverted by oversewing, but evidence of more extensive infarction or deep infection indicates the need for caesarean hysterectomy. The prognosis in such cases is serious, and intensive antibiotic and fluid therapy is essential. The widely adopted and valid view that a single retained fetus, no matter how decomposed, is best removed with forceps per vaginam might seem to disregard the fact that the uterus is an ideal medium for the proliferation of anaerobic organisms. The high recovery rate after such deliveries probably suggests that fetal putrefactive change in this species is due more often to coliform than clostridial infection.

Elective hysterectomy is often requested for bitches which require a caesarean operation. Whether the additional risk is warranted is entirely a matter for clinical judgement. Experience suggests that with proper supportive therapy the risk is not great. In cases of caesarean hysterectomy a preliminary hysterotomy incision should be avoided wherever possible, but it is sometimes necessary to remove an impacted fetus before the vagina can be ligated.

After completion of the uterine surgery, all packing swabs are removed and, if contamination has occured, an appropriate antibiotic preparation should be applied topically. The peritoneal and muscle layers of the laparotomy wound are repaired with interrupted stitches and the subcutaneous dead space is obliterated with a row of absorbable sutures, avoiding, if possible, islets of mammary tissue which, in lean bitches, may extend towards the midline. The skin sutures should be loosely but securely tied. The immediate administration intramuscularly of oxytocin (2–10 units) induces uterine involution and expulsion of remaining placentae and uterine debris.

Most caesarean sections result in uterine adhesions, not always confined to the area of incision. Such adhesions may seriously interfere with exposure and exteriorization of the uterus if a subsequent hysterotomy is necessary.

Postoperative management

Bitches which are allowed to eat their placentae usually have some degree of diarrhoea for a day or two afterwards. After caesarean section, most bitches accept their puppies and lick and suckle them normally, particularly if one or two were born naturally before surgery. Occasional bitches delivered entirely by caesarean operation may be less receptive and behave aggressively by threatening and even snapping at the pups. Such bitches should initially be gently restrained to allow the pups to suck, and most settle quickly. If the aggression persists, it may be necessary to protect the pups in a cage in the whelping box and place them on the bitch every few hours or so for feeding until she shows signs of normal maternal acceptance. The puppies' prime requirement immediately after birth is not food, but warmth and the maintenance of an ambient temperature of 30–32°C. Delay in feeding for up to 6 hours or so after birth is of no consequence.

Two particular problems may require veterinary attention during the initial postoperative period. It is normal after caesarean section for a considerable volume of blood and other uterine fluids to be voided as a result of uterine involution, but a continuing vaginal discharge of blood may indicate serious haemorrhage from areas of placental attachment if placentae have been forcibly detached. This is a life-threatening complication, especially in small animals, and indicates the need for further oxytocin therapy immediately. The animal's circulatory status should be carefully assessed by monitoring pulse and respiratory rates, and particular attention should be paid to pallor of mucous membranes and palpable uterine distension. Packed cell volumes have little meaning in rapid blood loss of this sort, and parenteral haemostatic agents are ineffective in arresting the haemorrhage. The correct and only beneficial treatment of these cases is immediate blood transfusion, or fluid repalcement therapy if whole blood is not available. If the blood loss continues, such therapy may have only a holding effect, and the need for hysterectomy may have to be considered once the animal's circulatory status has been stabilized. This is an avoidable but not uncommon cause of death after caesarean section in the bitch.

The second cause for concern may be the persistence of compulsive panting or hyperventilation, to the extent that it interferes with the bitch's natural inclination to suckle the puppies or even to sleep. It is occasionally caused by the unnecessary provision of extra heat from an overhead lamp or other appliance, but most often it develops naturally in bitches, especially of the brachycephalic types, which have behaved in a similar way during the first and second stages of labour. Apart from protecting the puppies, nothing can be done to allay this exhausting symptom except to sedate the bitch, but sedative drugs may be excreted in the milk and thus affect the young. It generally subsides over a period of 2 or 3 days.

Like all other species the bitch is susceptible to

infective peritonitis after laparohysterotomy, but the risk of this complication is minimized by good surgical technique and routine antibiotic therapy.

Intermittent uterine bleeding generally attributed to subinvolution may follow natural parturition or caesarean section and persist for several weeks afterwards. It has little effect on the bitch's packed cell volume and is best left to resolve spontaneously because drug therapy is ineffective, the uterus by this stage being no longer sensitive to oxytocin. Occasional animals with a haemorrhagic vulval discharge during the suckling period will be found, on closer examination, to have lesions of transmissible venereal tumour contracted at coitus.

Maternal recovery rate, causes of death and postoperative fertility

Mitchell (1966) reported a 13.3% maternal mortality in 120 bitches subjected to hysterotomy or caesarean hysterectomy. In this series, five of the 16 bitches which died failed to recover from the anaesthetic and the remainder died during the next 5 days. Only three of the animals which died had living fetuses *in utero*. Of equal interest in this report is the survival rate of 96.4% of puppies delivered from bitches anaesthetized without barbiturates compared with the 63.8% survival of pups from bitches which did receive barbiturates. The avoidance or minimal usage of barbiturate drugs therefore favours both maternal and fetal survival.

Deaths during or immediately after caesarean surgery are due principally to the combined effects of toxaemia and surgical shock or to uterine haemorrhage. The choice of a safe anaesthetic technique followed by routine fluid infusion and proper management of the placenta will reduce maternal deaths to a minimum.

There are no data on postoperative fertility in the bitch but it is certainly high, probably because the ovary and oviduct are completely protected by the bursa and are unlikely to be affected by adhesions.

The queen

The indications for caesarean section in the queen are not well documented, and it is likely that gravid ovariohysterectomy is performed more frequently than hysterotomy except in pedigree

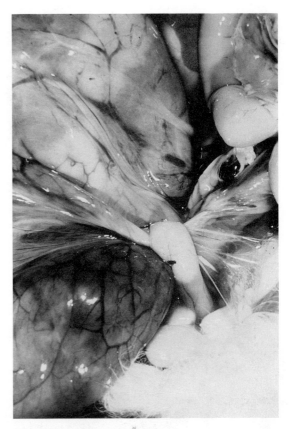

Fig. 21.1 Unicornual torsion in a queen.

animals. Joshua (1979) comments that inertia and oversize are less common in this species than faulty disposition or fetal deformities such as hydrocephalus and anasarca. Maternal causes of dystocia include pelvic distortion after fractures and uterine torsion affecting either the entire uterus or only one horn (Figure 21.1).

The operation is performed under general anaesthesia. The surgical approaches and technique described for the bitch are equally suitable for the queen. Except in animals intended for further breeding, gravid hysterectomy may be considered preferable to hysterotomy and is generally well tolerated in this species. Antibiotic and supportive fluid therapy is advisable after protracted dystocia or if the uterus is grossly infected. The presence of fetuses in the peritoneal cavity as a result of uterine rupture is usually of little consequence, and affected animals may survive indefinitely without surgery, the fetal remnants becoming encapsulated by the omentum or mesentery.

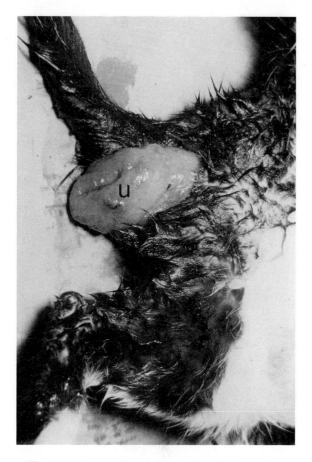

Fig. 21.2 Postparturient uterine eversion (u) in a queen.

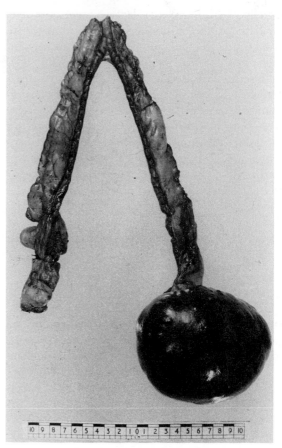

Fig. 21.3 Unilateral granulosa cell tumour in a bitch, responsible for a haemorrhagic vaginal discharge, vulval discharge and sexual attractiveness.

In the queen, the spaying operation performed electively or because of pyometritis or dystocia is rarely associated with postoperative complications such as sometimes develop in the bitch.

An unusual indication for ovariohysterectomy in the cat is postparturient eversion of the uterus (Figure 21.2), which can be removed *in situ* by exposure and ligation of blood vessels through a vaginal incision. Unless the tissues are grossly oedematous or traumatized the operation is better performed at laparotomy after the eversion has been reduced by gentle traction.

OVARIOHYSTERECTOMY IN THE BITCH

This operation is most frequently performed electively as a means of preventing unwanted pregnancies and the nuisances associated with heat periods in pet animals. An important clinical justification for spaying is its protective effects against the subsequent development of mammary tumours, but for this purpose it must be carried out during the first 30 months or so of life; thereafter its effectiveness declines rapidly (Schneider et al., 1969). It has no effect on mammary tumours which have already developed; the operation may also have a sparing effect on the development of vaginal leiomyomata later in life (Kidd and Burnie, 1986). The most important clinical indication for ovariohysterectomy is pyometritis. Surgery is still the treatment of choice for this disorder although there are reports of successful treatment with other methods (see Chapter 28). Non-surgical treatment by catheter drainage of the uterus per vaginam has also been described (Funkquist et al., 1983; Lagersted et al., 1987). Ovarian neoplasms are not common in the bitch but granulosa cell

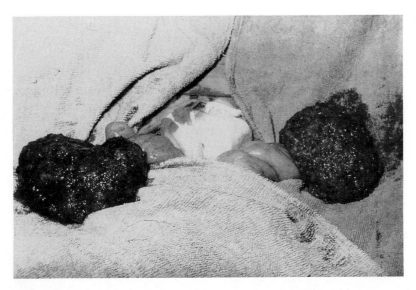

Fig. 21.4 Bilateral cystadenomata associated with haemoperitoneum in a bitch.

tumours and ovarian cystadenoma (Figures 21.3 and 21.4) are successfully treated by ovariectomy provided, with the latter tumour, that metastases are not evident, either locally on the serosa or in the lymphatics on the dome of the diaphragm. Spaying is also believed to be beneficial for cases of diabetes mellitus which can be difficult to stabilize at the time of oestrus and may be advisable in bitches with exaggerated or persistent manifestations of pseudo-pregnancy. Gravid hysterectomy is usually taken to imply removal of the uterus during caesarean surgery either electively or as an emergency procedure because of uterine infection or infarction, but it applies equally to spaying during pregnancy. It is a fact, paradoxically, that mid to late pregnancy is the safest time for elective spaying because the ovarian attachments are then stretched and haemostasis is easily achieved.

Elective ovariohysterectomy in the bitch should not be performed during oestrus because of the increased vascularity and turgidity of the genital tract at this time. It is also often considered to be premature before the first heat period on the dubious assumption that early spaying leads to the development of infantile vulva and consequent urine scalding.

It is customary in Britain to assume that hysterectomy is an indispensable part of the spaying operation, but for elective neutering there is no need to remove more than the ovaries because the only common spontaneously occurring uterine disorder, pyometritis, is dependent on cyclical ovarian activity. The technique of ovariectomy only prevents operative haemorrhage due to inadequate ligation of uterine vessels and the delayed but occasionally fatal bleeding associated with infection of the vaginal stump ligature. It also obviates the risk of accidental inclusion of ureters in the ligature and delayed uterine stump adhesions and can be performed more quickly and through a shorter incision than ovariohysterectomy. Both procedures are approached through the flank or linea alba depending on personal preference.

Spaying is a routine operation in small animal practice and it is often regarded as a simple procedure which can be performed quickly, without assistance, through as short a laparotomy as possible. The inexperienced surgeon soon learns that inadequate ligation of the ovarian and uterine vessels can result in fatal haemorrhage. It is therefore essential to have good relaxation of the abdominal musculature and an incision of adequate length. In cases of pyometritis and gravid hysterectomy, the distended uterus should be withdrawn carefully with simultaneous pressure through the abdominal wall in order to prevent tearing of the organ or the broad ligament (Figure 21.5). Careless handling may also induce the rapid formation of haematomata in the mesometrium. If the uterus is distended with pus or fetuses, the ovaries can generally be exposed without difficulty

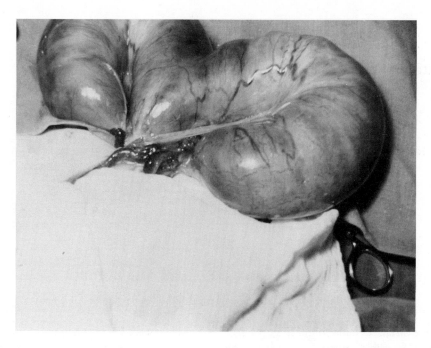

Fig. 21.5 Exteriorized uterus of bitch with pyometra. Note the grossly distended uterine horns causing increased fragility of the uterine wall.

for ligation, but in fat bitches undergoing elective spaying they may be impossible to expose without traction. In such cases, section of the ovarian ligament, which is easily recognized if the mesovarium is tensed, facilitates ligation, but the tissues are then more likely to tear on traction.

The choice of suture material for internal ligation is important because the use of non-absorbable multifilament ligatures may result in retroperitonitis with the formation of 'granulomata' especially on the ovarian stumps and sinuses discharging externally in the sublumbar region (Pearson, 1973). The material must also be of adequate calibre for proper tightening. During the process of ligation, crushing forceps may be of value if surgical assistance is not available but they should be used primarily as a means of elevating tissues for ligation rather than for crushing before the ligature is applied. A common technical fault is to ligate immediately adjacent to forceps placed below the ovary: tissues fixed in a clamp cannot be adequately compressed by ligation until the clamp is released. It is therefore essential to ligate well below the clamp or, alternatively, to place the instrument on the uterine side of the ovary and use it as a means of lifting the gonads and also of preventing

back bleeding until the uterine vessels have also been ligated. The broad ligament is relatively avascular but should be ligated in cases of pyometritis and in advanced pregnancy. The uterus is removed caudally below the cervix after the application of a tight encircling ligature on the anterior vagina. Transfixing ligatures are potentially dangerous because they may become contaminated in the vaginal lumen and subsequently act as a focus of infection and predispose to secondary haemorrhage. In cases of pyometritis and gravid hysterectomy, it is a wise precaution to ligate each pair of uterine vessels separately close to the main vaginal ligature. In caesarean hysterectomy, the vaginal stump is usually sealed with inversion sutures, but after pyometritis this procedure too may lead to lingering infection and haemorrhage at the site. The resultant vaginal blood loss is potentially fatal and may require further resection of the vaginal stump.

At laparotomy for pyometritis, the peritoneal cavity is sometimes bathed in pus which, in the absence of uterine perforation, can only be assumed to have passed up the uterine tubes because of increased intrauterine pressure. This complication is not usually serious but it may indicate the need for the insertion of a temporary in-dwelling peritoneal tube for drainage and irrigation.

The complications of ovariohysterectomy are well documented (Pearson, 1973; Dorn and Swist, 1977). After surgery for pyometritis and dystocia, the animal may require intravenous fluid therapy, the value of which in correcting or preventing dehydration cannot be overemphasized if vomiting persists or the blood urea level is markedly raised. Haemorrhage is an entirely avoidable complication but not a rare cause of death. Ovarian stump bleeding during surgery can be arrested by extending the abdominal incision, packing off the intestines and exposing the vessel for further ligation. Vaginal stump bleeding is less easy to deal with because the vessels retract into the pelvic cavity and sometimes cannot be located even when the vaginal stump is exposed. Such bleeding can usually be controlled by firm swab pressure over a period of several minutes. Clinical signs of internal haemorrhage after the operation is completed fully justify reopening of the laparotomy after appropriate fluid therapy or blood transfusion. Vaginal bleeding after hysterectomy is usually due to infection around the ligature of the vaginal stump and may become so severe that resection of the stump is necessary as a life-saving procedure. An embarrassing complication of elective spaying is continued evidence of ovarian activity manifested by signs of recurrent oestrus. The explanation in the bitch is usually a functional ovarian remnant, most often on the right side, and the correct treatment is extirpation of the tissue. Persistent lactation occurs when the bitch is spayed in metoestrus. It is important to delay surgery until the bitch is known to be anoestrus (see p. 31).

Possibly the most serious long-term complication of spaying is urinary incontinence. In a survey, Ruckstuhl (1978) recorded an overall incidence of 12% in 79 animals within 1 year of surgery and a frequency in larger breeds of almost 18%. In agreeing to spay animals of the larger types, especially perhaps the St Bernard and Old English sheepdog, the clinician should bear in mind that the likelihood of this condition is unpredictable and that the results of treatment may be disappointing.

The causal relationship between spaying and urinary incontinence is somewhat contentious but Thrusfield (1985), analysing a first opinion clinic population, found a positive association between all forms of acquired urinary incontinence and spaying in bitches aged 6 months or more. In a review of sphincter mechanism incontinence in the bitch, Holt (1985) found that 35 of 39 adult incontinent bitches in his series had been spayed. The onset of urinary incontinence within a few days of spaying in both the bitch and the cat may well be due to vaginoureteral fistula formation caused by inadvertent inclusion of a ureter in the vaginal ligature.

The description by Le Roux and Van der Walt (1977) of a technique for transplantation of ovarian tissue into an area of splanchnic venous drainage has received less clinical attention than it deserves as a possible means of maintaining a normal endocrine status for at least some time after ovariectomy. Transplantation of segments of one ovary into the wall of the stomach caused their secretions to be metabolized in the liver in such a way that cyclical signs of oestrus waned after a curtailed pro-oestrus phase.

Hysterectomy for pyometritis is occasionally complicated by incarceration of a segment of one horn in an inguinal metrocele. Simultaneous herniorraphy and laparotomy may be necessary, but preoperative aspiration of pus should first be attempted to relieve the incarceration and allow the uterus to be excised in the normal way. Conversely it may be possible to remove the entire uterus at herniorraphy, but this approach is not to be recommended.

REFERENCES

Dorn, A. S. and Swist, R. A. (1977) *J. Amer. Anim. Hosp. Assn*, **13**, 720.

Freak, M. (1975) *Vet. Rec.*, **96**, 303.

Funkquist, B., Lagerstedt, A.-S., Linde, C. and Obel, N. (1983) *Zentbl. Vet. Med. A.*, **30**, 72.

Holt, P. E. (1985) *J. Small Anim. Pract.*, **26**, 181.

Joshua, J. P. (1979) *Cat Owner's Encyclopaedia of Veterinary Medicine*. London: T. F. M. Publications.

Krzyzanowski, J., Malinowski, E. and Wojciech, S. (1975) *Med. Weter.*, **31**, 373.

Kydd, D. M. and Burnie, A. G. (1986) *J. Small Anim. Pract.*, **27**, 255.

Lagersted, A.-S., Obel, N. and Stravenborn, M. (1987) *J. Small Anim. Pract.*, **28**, 215.

Le Roux, P. H. and Van der Walt, L. A. (1977) *J. S. Afr. Vet. Med. Assn*, **48**, 117.

Mitchell, B. (1966) *Vet. Rec.*, **79**, 252.

Pearson, H. (1973) *J. Small Anim. Pract.*, **14**, 257.

Ruckstuhl, B. (1978) *Schweiz. Arch. Tierheilkd*, **120**, 143.

Schneider, R., Dorn, C. R. and Taylor, D. O. N. (1969) *J. Natl. Cancer Inst.*, **43**, 1249.

Thrusfield, M. V. (1985) *Vet. Rec.*, **116**, 695.

Waterman, A. E. (1975) *Vet. Rec.*, **96**, 308.

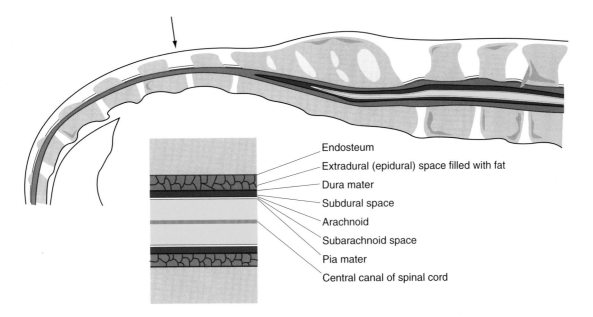

Endosteum
Extradural (epidural) space filled with fat
Dura mater
Subdural space
Arachnoid
Subarachnoid space
Pia mater
Central canal of spinal cord

Plate 1   The spinal meninges and the distribution of the spaces in the vertebral canal of the cow (region of the os sacrum).

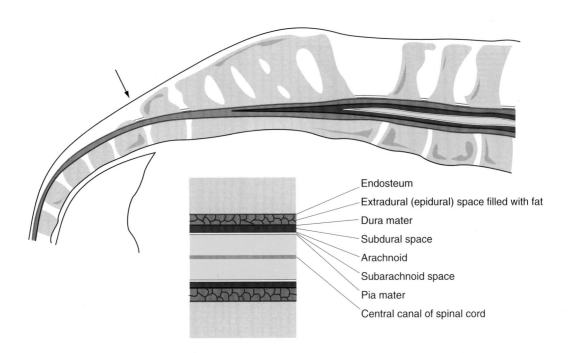

Endosteum
Extradural (epidural) space filled with fat
Dura mater
Subdural space
Arachnoid
Subarachnoid space
Pia mater
Central canal of spinal cord

Plate 2   The spinal meninges and the distribution of the spaces in the vertebral canal of the mare (region of the os sacrum).

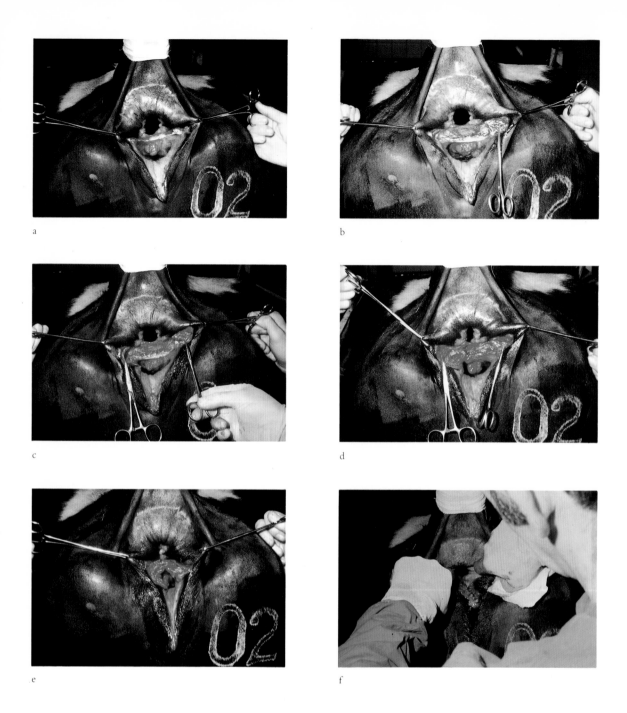

Plate 3 Repair of a third degree perineal laceration in a Friesian cow. (a) The perineal laceration exposed with cow under caudal epidural anaesthesia. (b) Commencement of dissection of vaginal mucosa. (c) Completion of dissection of vaginal mucosa; note exposed tissue ready for suturing. (d) Commencement of closure. (e) Closure almost completed. (f) Restoration of a complete shelf of tissue between rectum and vagina, the dorsal commissure of the vulva is subsequently repaired (see Figure 17.8).

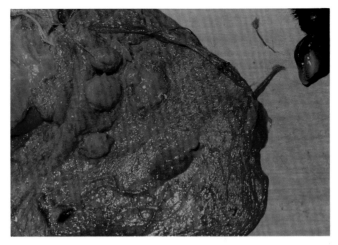

Plate 4   Placenta of lamb that had aborted due to infection with *C. psittaci (ovis)*. Note cotyledons covered with a light-brown deposit and similar material on the surface of the intercotyledonary chorionic surface. (Courtesy of A. J. Wilsmore.)

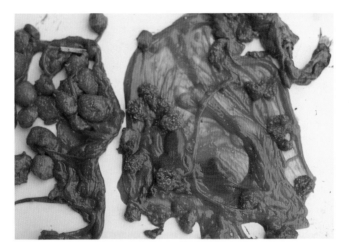

Plate 5   Placenta of lamb that had aborted due to infection with *T. gondii*. (Courtesy of A. J. Wilsmore.)

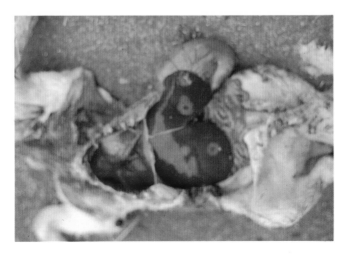

Plate 6   Aborted fetus showing characteristic lesion on the liver of *C. fetus* infection.

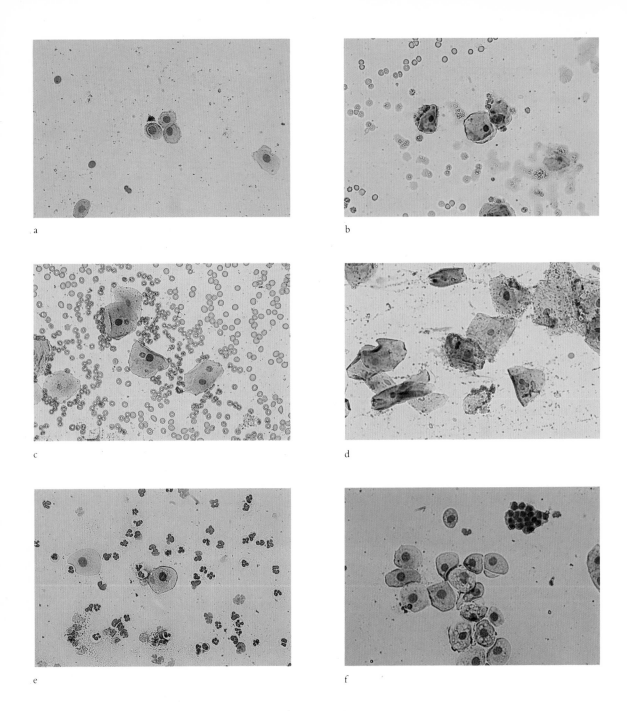

Plate 7 Photomicrographs of exfoliative vagina cells during various stages of the reproductive cycle. The smears have been stained with a modified Wright–Giemsa stain. (a) Anoestrus: parabasal epithelial cells and small intermediate epithelial cells. (b) Pro-oestrus: small intermediate epithelial cells, large intermediate epithelial cells and erythrocytes. Polymorphonuclear leucocytes are also found in low numbers during this stage of the cycle but are not demonstrated here. (c) Early oestrus: large intermediate epithelial cells, anuclear epithelial cells and erythrocytes. Polymorphonuclear leucocytes are generally absent during this stage of the cycle. (d) Oestrus: anuclear epithelial cells, large intermediate epithelial cells and erythrocytes. The percentage of anuclear cells is high. (e) Metoestrus (higher magnification than (a) − (d)): small intermediate epithelial cells and large numbers of polymorphonuclear leucocytes. During early metoestrus large intermediate epithelial cells may be present, and later numbers of parabasal epithelial cells increase. There is often a large amount of background debris. (f) Late metoestrus (higher magnification than (a) − (d)): parabasal epithelial cells and small vacuolated intermediate epithelial cells. Vacuolated cells are typical of this stage of the cycle but may also be found during anoestrus and more rarely during pro-oestrus.

5

Part Five

Infertility

22

The term 'fertility' as applied to the cow denotes the desire and ability to mate, the capacity to conceive and to nourish the embryo and finally the power to expel a normal calf and fetal membrane. Healthy cattle give expression to normal fertility by producing one viable calf per year. 'Sterility' means an absolute inability to reproduce, whereas 'infertility' is sometimes considered to be synonymous with sterility, or it implies a failure, or a delay, in producing the annual live calf. The term 'subfertility' is probably a more appropriate term for the latter. In the dairy cow not only does this interfere with the move from one generation to the other but it has an effect on efficient production of milk, since pregnancy and parturition are necessary for the initiation and maintenance of lactation in the species.

PREVALENCE AND COST OF INFERTILITY

Asdell (1952) estimated that at any time 10% of cows were experiencing some form of breeding trouble. In a survey carried out in the state of Kansas, 22% of cows were culled for breeding problems (Bozworth et al., 1972), and ranked second only to low production as a reason for disposal. In the UK, Grunsell and Paver (1955) estimated that 4% of cows per year were treated for infertility and other pathological conditions of the genital organs; Leech et al. (1960) found that 3.7% of cows were culled for infertility whilst for Northern Ireland, Gracey (1960) quoted a figure of 5.2%. Johannsson (1962) analysed the cow disposal figures for European and American dairy herds and concluded that about a third of all cows are culled because of reproductive disturbances, that 4–5%

of heifers are sterile and about 5% of calves are stillborn or die at birth. In two studies on the reasons for the disposal of dairy cows in England and Wales for the years 1972–1973 and 1976–1977 the percentages that were culled for reproductive conditions were as follows (Beynon, 1978):

	1972–1973	1976–1977
Friesians	44%	32.8%
All cows	43.2%	33%

In these two surveys there was evidence, when the 2 years were compared, of some reduction in the numbers which were suffering from breeding disorders; however, no specific explanation could be found for the apparent improvement since, when the figures are further examined, the individual subgroups are similar (Table 22.1).

It is generally assumed that infertility is less of a problem in beef cattle, although reliable data are unavailable.

The effect in Holsteins in the USA of extending the interval between successive calvings from 12 to 14 months on average resulted in a reduction of 8.8% in the annual financial return over feeding costs (Speicher and Meadows, 1967). The same extension of the calving interval resulted in an average loss of 144 kg milk per cow and 0.15 calves per cow (Lauderdale, 1964). In a study of

Table 22.1 Breeding problems in two groups of cows

Cause	1972–1973	1976–1977
Failure to breed (including long delays between calving and conception)	80%	78%
Brucella reactor/abortion	10%	11%
Other abortions	3.5%	3.4%
Bad calvings	6.5%	7.6%

32 dairy herds in South Ontario, Canada, comprising 2876 lactations, the records for 1979–1981 showed that the lactational incidence rate for reproductive disorders totalled 43.2% compared with 16.8 and 5.0% for mastitis and locomotor disease, respectively (Dohoo et al., 1983). In a series of studies undertaken in three areas of the USA the importance of reproductive disease and disorders was confirmed. In Michigan State, the mean incidence densities per 100 cow-years were 49.86, 33.06 and 13.81, for breeding problems, mastitis and birth problems, respectively. The total cost per cow per year was $24.46 for breeding problems, compared with $35.54 for mastitis (Kaneene and Hurd, 1990). In a study involving 43 herds in California a mean of 24.8% of the cows were culled each year, with reproductive failure the most common cause (Gardner et al., 1990). While in Ohio State the mean number of cases per 100 cow-years were: mastitis, 37 (21%); metritis, 32 (18%); infertility, 25 (14%); pneumonia, 19 (11%); cystic ovaries, 8 (5%); and retained placenta, 8 (5%) (Miller and Dorn, 1990). In the UK (Esslemont, 1992) has calculated that for dairy herds, at 1992 prices of milk, feed, calves, replacement heifers, culled cows, etc., the cost to the farmer for each day's extension of the calving-interval beyond 365 days can be as much as £3.35. If this is extrapolated to the UK National Herd, where the average calving-interval is 395 days, the annual loss is over £300 million.

Bozworth et al. (1972) state that 'infertility is one of the important economic losses in high producing herds and that modern feeding and management practices in large herds may accentuate the problem'. This comment is equally true today.

CAUSES OF INFERTILITY

Over the last 40–50 years there has been a noticeable change in the causes of infertility in cattle in many parts of the world. The recognition of *Tritrichomonas fetus* infection (Stableforth et al., 1937) and *Campylobacter fetus* infection (Sjollema et al., 1949) as causes of widespread infertility constituted major advances. Control measures, in particular the widespread use of artificial insemination, have largely eliminated these diseases from the UK

although world-wide they are both important causes of infertility. Similarly, the eradication programmes for bovine tuberculosis and brucellosis have reduced the importance of both of these diseases as causes of reproductive loss. Although non-specific infections due to opportunist pathogens are still important, by far the greatest cause of infertility is poor management of herds. In the dairy industry this has been largely due to the increase in herd size, the increases in the mechanization of farming and the concomitant reduction in the number of persons attending the herds. At the same time, the demands put upon the dairy cow to produce more milk and the genetic selection for high yield have inevitably resulted in functional aberrations of the reproductive and endocrine systems. Changes in fertility associated with such factors as those just described are illustrated by a study which evaluated the fertility of dairy herds in New York State which were under the Dairy Herd Improvement Testing Scheme (Butler and Smith, 1989). In 1951, the mean overall pregnancy (conception) rate was 66% for both cows and heifers, in 1973 the figure had fallen to 50% for cows, during which time the average annual milk production per cow had risen by 1500 kg (33%). In a more recent survey the same authors have shown that whereas milk production has increased by approximately 1500 kg from 1973 to 1985, mean overall conception rates in 1985 were 51%. Pregnancy rates for heifers are virtually the same as they were in 1951.

In this chapter it is now proposed to examine the various causes of cattle infertility under three main headings: anatomical factors, functional abnormalities and management problems. Infectious causes of infertility in cows are discussed in Chapter 23.

ANATOMICAL FACTORS AFFECTING FERTILITY

Both congenital and acquired abnormalities of the genital system can influence fertility. The latter type are more frequently encountered, as demonstrated in a survey by Kessy (1978) who found that in 2000 genital tracts that were examined from abattoirs only six specimens (0.3%) had evidence of congenital abnormalities compared with 194

(9.65%) with acquired lesions. Since most of the latter were identified in the tracts from parous specimens the importance of conditions that might occur during pregnancy, and especially at parturition and during the puerperium, is demonstrated. Anatomical abnormalities usually affect individual cows or heifers and are therefore unlikely to have a major influence on fertility in a herd.

Congenital anomalies

Ovarian agenesis
In rare instances one or both ovaries may be absent and in these cases the genital tract is infantile and cyclical behaviour is absent. An apparently hereditary condition of 'virtual absence of ovaries' was seen by Fincher (1946) in three maternal half-sister heifers.

Ovarian hypoplasia
In this condition one or both ovaries are small, narrow and functionless. Gonadal hypoplasia has been shown to affect both males and females of the Swedish Highland breed, and among 8145 cows Lagerlöf (1939) found an incidence of 13.1%. Of the affected cows, 87.1% had hypoplasia of the left, 4.3% of the right and 8.6% of both ovaries. Where both ovaries were hypoplastic the genital tract was infantile and oestrus cycles did not occur. Eriksson (1938) has stated that this affection is inherited as an autosomal recessive. There was a marked association of gonadal hypoplasia with white coat colour. Arthur (1959) reported a small number of cases in white Ayrshire heifers; they were acyclical. By the adoption of a vigorous control programme in which veterinary examination of breeding cattle led to the recognition and culling of cases of unilateral hypoplasia, the incidence of gonadal hypoplasia in Swedish Highland cattle was reduced from 17.5% in 1936 to 7.2% in 1952 (Lagerlöf and Boyd, 1953).

Although testicular hypoplasia affecting bulls of many breeds (see Chater 30) has been recognized in several countries no clear-cut entity of gonadal hypoplasia affecting males and females has been recorded as in the Swedish Highland breed.

Ovarian hypoplasia should be distinguished from functional anoestrus in heifers. In the latter the ovaries are not as small, their surfaces are smooth rather than furrowed and the shape is rounded rather than spindle-like; also the tubular tract is better developed. This is associated with poor body condition and is reversible when this improves. An extreme form of ovarian hypoplasia may be seen in the bovine freemartin.

Abnormalities of the uterine (fallopian) tubes
In Kessy's survey (1978) the uterine tube was the most frequent site identified as having congenital defects. Unilateral aplasia was identified in 0.1% of the specimens, duplication of the tube in 0.05% and segmental aplasia in 0.05%. Several other abnormalities were also identified which could not definitely be assumed to be congenital; 0.3% of the genital tracts from multiparous individuals had unilaterally or bilaterally occluded uterine tubes whilst one specimen showed evidence of hydrosalpinx (see below).

Intersexuality and freemartinism (see p. 117)
Freemartinism is a distinct form of intersexuality which arises as a result of a vascular anastomosis of the adjacent chorioallantoic sacs of heterozygous fetuses in multiple pregnancies (Lillie, 1916). As a result, although the external genitalia of freemartin heifers appear normal the internal genitalia frequently show masculinization. In extreme cases the gonads resemble testes, though spermatogenesis is not apparent, and there are well developed epididymides, vasa deferentia and vesicular glands (Short et al., 1969). However, in the least affected cases the female genital tract may be small, with a persistent hymen and hypoplastic ovaries (Wijeratne et al., 1977), whilst there are also reports of one freemartin heifer which showed signs of oestrus and the presence of a corpus luteum on one ovary (Wilkes et al., 1981), although the author doubts if this was a true freemartin but rather a congenitally malformed tubular genital tract. It is generally assumed that 92% of heifers which are born as co-twins to bulls are sterile (Biggers and McFeely, 1966).

The economic importance of early diagnosis of freemartinism has been shown by the survey of David et al. (1976) who found that a large number of heifers which were sold in markets for breeding were freemartins. This could also become important if induction of twinning by superovulation or embryo transfer becomes popular. The newborn freemartin can sometimes be recognized by its prominent clitoris with an obvious tuft of hair at the inferior commissure of the vulva, although these are not always reliable. Freemartins can be identified on the basis of the length of the vagina and the absence of the cervix. In the adult, the vagina is normally 30 cm in length compared with 8–10 cm in the freemartin. Rectal palpation will fail to identify the cervix. In calves of 1–4 weeks of age the vagina is normally 13–15 cm in length compared with 5–6 cm in a freemartin. Diagnosis at this age can be made using a blunt probe which should be inserted initially at an angle of 45° below the horizontal for 5 cm and then angled downwards to avoid impinging on the hymen (Long, 1990). It is easier when comparisons can be made between a number of animals.

The most accurate method of diagnosis, although not absolute, is the determination of sex chromosome chimerism by leucocyte tissue culture. Heifer calves which are born co-twins to males and which show morphological changes in their reproductive tracts invariably show sex chromosome chimerism in blood and blood-forming tissues. Unfortunately the distribution of male cell percentages in freemartins appears to be random, hence those with low male percentages in the blood will be as common as those with high male percentages (Wilkes et al., 1981).

Vascular anastomosis occurs as early as 30 days of gestation; thus if there is death of the male twin of a heterozygous pair after this time with the other being carried to term, it is possible for a single-born freemartin to occur. This has been demonstrated as a cause of infertility in heifers with apparently normal external genitalia but with sex chromosome chimerism (Wijeratne et al., 1977).

It is also possible to identify the presence of two populations of erythrocytes by haemolytic tests using a series of specific blood group reagents (Long, 1990).

Segmental aplasia of the müllerian ducts and 'white heifer disease'

Developmental defects of the Müllerian ducts lead to various anomalies of the vagina, cervix and uterus. The ovaries develop normally and, consequently, affected animals show normal cyclic behaviour with the usual secretory activity of the tubular genital tract. Hence, wherever a developmental obstruction of the tubular tract occurs in a

mature heifer the lumen in front of the obstruction becomes distended by cyclical secretions (Figures 22.1 and 22.2). The most common developmental aberration of the female tubular organs involves a variable degree of persistence of the hymen. This may appear as a vaginal constriction in front of the urethral opening, as a partition with a central aperture or as a complete partition between the vulva and vagina. The first type is likely to be discovered at parturition when it causes dystocia. The second and third types are likely to be found when investigating heifers which either strain forcibly after service or cannot be inseminated artificially. Where hymenal obstruction is complete there is an accumulation of cyclic secretions in front of the obstruction; this causes a fluctuating swelling of variable size which may be palpated per rectum. Following service, this retained secretion may become infected by pyogenic organisms. The less severe forms of hymenal obstruction may be

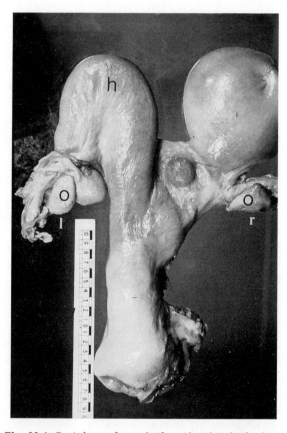

Fig. 22.1 Genital tract from a heifer with 'white heifer disease'. Note both ovaries (o) are normal with a corpus luteum present in the right and horns (h) distended with accumulated fluid.

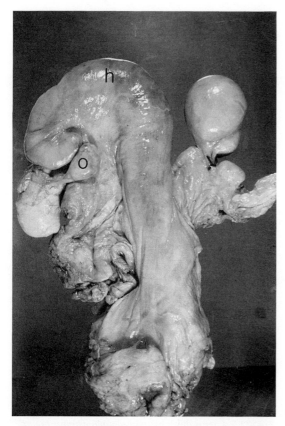

Fig. 22.2 Genital tract from a heifer with 'white heifer disease'. Note normal left ovary (o) and clearly distended left horn (h) with accumulated fluid.

rendered suitable for breeding by making cruciform incisions into the partition. Heifers with complete obstruction, which are ill because of retained pus, can be relieved by trocar and cannula and then fattened for slaughter. (In view of the probable hereditary origin of these developmental defects surgical intervention in order to make breeding possible is not advisable.)

The genital organs of most heifers with hymenal constriction are otherwise normal, but occasionally other defects of the tubular organs are present. Conversely, these other defects may occur independently of hymenal abnormality. The whole of the vagina, cervix and uterine horns may lack patency. In these cases, the genital tract is difficult to locate per rectum — as in the freemartin — but unlike the latter, the ovaries are normal. Instead of complete aplasia, there is more commonly partial, or segmental, aplasia of the Müllerian ducts; for example, in uterus unicornis only one uterine horn has a lumen, the other

appearing as a narrow, flat band. (Figure 22.3). Provided the remainder of the genital apparatus is normal these heifers may conceive to ovulations from the sound side. A more serious type of aplasia shows a small length of one cornua only with a lumen. Uterine secretion accumulates and causes a sac-like dilatation which may be confused with early pregnancy. Animals with this deformity are sterile.

In cases of *uterus didelphys* each uterine horn connects with the vagina by a separate cervical canal (Figure 22.4). These cases should conceive normally but may show dystocia due to fetal limbs entering each cervical canal. A similar complication may arise in heifers with a single cervix opening into a double *os uteri externum* (Figure 22.5) and in cattle showing a dorsoventral postcervical band. The expulsion of the afterbirth may also be

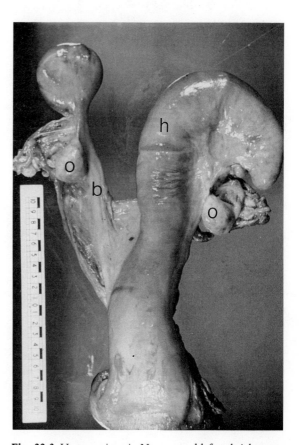

Fig. 22.3 Uterus unicornis. Note normal left and right ovaries (o) and complete right horn (h). The left horn comprises a flat band of tissue with no lumen (b) and a blind residual segment.

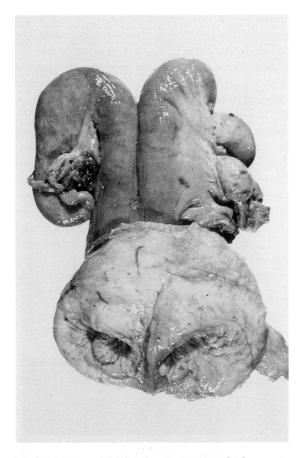

Fig. 22.4 Uterus didelphys showing two completely separate cervical canals.

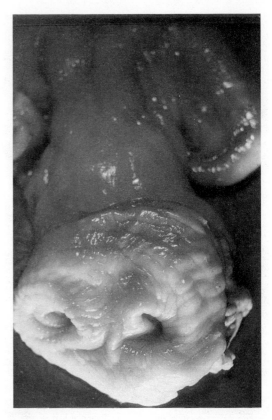

Fig. 22.5 Uterus didelphys with double external *os uteri*.

impeded by these structural aberrations. Vertical vaginal bands can be easily divided with an fetotomy knife.

The foregoing developmental anomalies may arise in all breeds but the hymenal defects occur particularly in white shorthorn heifers; thus the syndrome of straining and illness after service has become known as 'white heifer disease'. This condition is considered to be due to a sex-linked recessive gene with linkage to the gene for white coat colour. The other developmental defects of the Müllerian ducts are probably also due to sex-linked recessive genes; consequently they are likely to appear when in-breeding is practised and Fincher and Williams (1926) saw 56% of affected heifers in the progeny that results from the mating of a Friesian sire with his daughters.

Parovarian cysts
Commonly about 1 cm in diameter, these cysts are often present in the mesosalpinx of cattle. Unless

they impinge on the uterine tube and reduce its lumen (which they rarely do) they are unimportant.

Atresia of the vulva
An abnormally small vulva has been described as a cause of dystocia in Friesian and Jersey heifers. In such cases episiotomy or caesarean operation may be required to allow delivery. The defect has been seen to affect many of the progeny of a particular Jersey bull (Hull et al., 1940), thus indicating that it is of hereditary origin.

Cysts of Gaertner's canals
Cysts in linear series, which may be 6–8 cm in diameter, often occur on the floor of the vagina. They can be easily punctured and are not a cause of infertility.

Acquired abnormalities
Lesions of the uterine tube and adnexa
Since the early survey in 1921 by Carpenter et al. which showed that 15.3% of cows which were

examined at routine clinical work had lesions of the uterine tubes and adnexa, many similar studies have confirmed their high frequency of occurrence. The percentage incidence ranged from 0.95% in an abattoir study in Australia (Summers, 1974) to 100% in a similar study in Egypt (Afiefy et al., 1973).

The most frequently observed lesions are between the ovary and the ovarian bursa (Figure 22.6). The incidence of ovarobursal adhesions in the surveys described above ranged from 0.43% (Summers, 1974) to 46% (Afiefy et al., 1973). The extent of the adhesions varies; in some abattoir specimens they consist of fine web-like strands in the depth of the bursa, which do not involve the uterine tube; in others there is complete envelopment of the ovary in a closely applied fibrous bursa. Intermediate cases show fibrous strands of varying thickness which connect the fimbriae, or bursae, to the ovary; the site of ovarian attachment is frequently at the scar left from a regressed corpus luteum. Edwards (1961) found the web-like adhesions in 62% of slaughterhouse cattle; it is unlikely that such lesions would interfere with fertility and they will not be discussed further. Of the remaining more severe types, between 25 and 50% are bilateral and likely to interfere with ovulation or to impede sperm or egg transport through the uterine tube. Of the unilateral cases, the right side is more frequently involved. Conception is unlikely to occur to ovulations from the affected side. Where the bursa is diffusely applied to the ovary, ovulation is prevented and luteinization of the follicle occurs, the orange rim of the follicle being several millimetres thick. In some cases ovarian cysts can develop (see below); regressed luteinized follicles of past cycles are often present in the same ovary. Where the uterine tube is involved in the fibrous lesion, its lumen may become obstructed; Kessy (1978) found four specimens out of 2000 where it was impossible to insufflate the tube on the side adjacent to the adhesions. Perhaps a clue to the aetiology of this condition in these four cases is given by the fact that in two cases there was an associated pyometra and in the other two a macerated fetus. Another consequence of occlusion is the accumulation of secretions which causes distension and thinning of the wall, described as hydrosalpinx (Figure 22.7). Quite often they become secondarily infected by *Actinomyces (Corynebacterium) pyogenes* to produce a pyosalpinx; intraovarian and periovarian abscesses have also been seen (Arthur, 1962).

Knowledge of the cause of ovarobursal adhesions is incomplete. The condition is uncommon in heifers but its incidence increases with the age of the cow. The diffuse type of lesion, often with involvement of the uterine tube, was a relatively common accompaniment of tuberculous

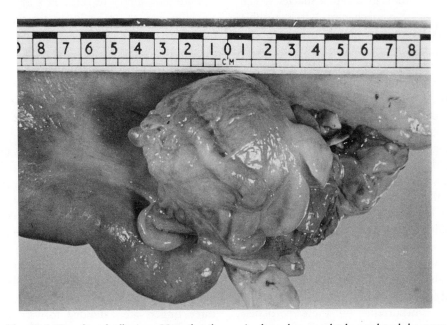

Fig. 22.6 Ovarobursal adhesions. Note that the ovarian bursa has completely enveloped the ovary.

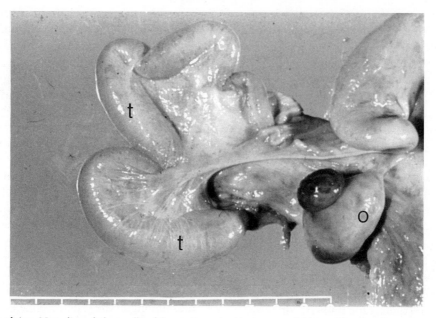

Fig. 22.7 Hydrosalpinx. Note distended ampulla of the uterine tube (t); the ovary (o) is unaffected and contains a corpus luteum.

peritonitis; similarly adhesions may occur as part of the more widespread peritonitis resulting from traumatic reticular penetration or from puerperal metritis. The strand-like adhesions arising from scars of old corpora lutea, which more commonly affect the right ovary, may be regarded as physiological hazards in that they may originate as slight haemorrhages from the site of ovulation. (They are not, however, common in sheep, a species which has a similar ovulating mechanism.) It is possible that a proportion of ovarobursal adhesions can occur as a result of rough palpation of the ovaries, particularly where manual enucleation of the corpus luteum or rupture of an ovarian cyst is attempted. In the former, massive haemorrhage and death of the cow can occur whilst in others, large haematomata attached to the surface of the ovary or filling the ovarian bursa have been identified. Since the availability of prostaglandins as luteolytic substances and with a more rational approach to the treatment of ovarian cysts, this cause should largely disappear. It is likely that there are additional, as yet unknown, causes of ovarobursal adhesions. Hoare (1967) has recovered mycoplasmas from a high proportion of ovarobursal and tubal lesions; although these organisms are commonly present in healthy cattle, the constancy of their occurrence in these particular lesions suggests an aetiological significance. It is

believed that mycoplasmas become pathogenic when the resistance of the host is lowered, for example as a result of a postparturient metritis or *Brucella* abortion. Hirst et al. (1966) have produced evidence of a causative relationship between mycoplasma-infected semen and infertility due to ovarobursal disease. In passing, it may be noted that ovarobursal adhesions are a feature of the viral epididymovaginitis of cattle in East Africa.

However, the most likely cause of ovarobursal adhesions in the pluriparous cow is a puerperal infection which arises from ascending infection or, in severe cases, perimetritis. The condition can also be induced by the intrauterine infusion of irritant substances such as Lugol's iodine in large volumes, particularly under pressure as might be achieved using an enema pump.

Diagnosis of ovarobursal adhesions in life is difficult and may be impossible; probably only one-third to one-half of the lesions that cause infertility are diagnosed by rectal palpation. Nielson (1949) has described a technique of rectal palpation which is designed to explore the patency of the ovarian bursa and to detect the uterine tube. Using the left hand, the method involves rotation of the right ovary so as to free it from the bursa; then while this is held lightly between thumb and forefinger, the other three fingers are extended forward medially and downwards to engage the anterior free edge of the ovarian bursa on the dorsal surface of one or more of these fingers. The fingers are then extended into the bursa and spread fan-wise to detect the presence of adhesions between the ovary and bursa. By turning the palm of the hand upwards the uterine tube may then be rolled between the fingers inside the bursa and the thumb outside the bursa. The left bursa may be examined by holding the left ovary between the last two fingers and thumb; by extending the forefinger and second finger forwards, downwards and medially it is possible to engage the edge of the bursa and then to explore the bursa and uterine tube as described for the right side. Using Nielson's method on 288 cows, Edwards (1961) was able to examine both bursae of 242 (84%).

In the more gross cases of ovarobursal adhesions the periphery of the ovary loses its clear definition. The ovarian outline is more bulky and irregular and the ovarian mass lacks mobility. In occasional difficult cases, laparotomy with direct vision or endoscopic examination of the ovaries may be used.

Two fairly simple tests are also available. The first one is based on a technique first described for use in women (Speck, 1948). He demonstrated that if phenolsulfonphthalene (PSP) was placed in the uterine lumen it was not absorbed and, if the uterine tubes were patent, it passed along them into the peritoneal cavity. From this site it was readily absorbed into the circulation and excreted by the kidneys into the urine where it produced a red or pink colour if alkaline. If the uterine tubes were occluded there was no passage of dye and hence no discoloration of the urine. The test has been used in the cow (Bertchtold and Brummer, 1968; Kothari, 1978); the latter author was able to demonstrate, using laparoscopy, the escape of the dye from the ostium. The test involves the infusion of 20 ml of a 0.1% sterile solution of PSP into the uterine lumen using a Nielson's catheter. This should be done carefully so as to avoid any trauma to the endometrium and thus enable absorption to occur. The bladder should then be catheterized and a small sample of urine kept for a control. A urine sample is then collected 30–60 minutes later, and to 10 ml a 0.2 ml volume of 10% trisodium orthophosphate buffer is added to make the urine alkaline. In the presence of PSP, the liquid becomes red or pink; in its absence the urine remains the same colour as the control. The test should be performed during the luteal phase of the cycle, preferably about day 10, since false negatives

can be obtained during the follicular phase (Kessy and Noakes, 1979a). False positives can arise if there is endometrial erosion due to infection and inflammation; it is not very effective in differentiating between bilateral and unilateral patency (Kessy and Noakes, 1979a).

A more accurate method of evaluating the patency of each uterine tube separately has been described by Coulthard (personal communication); it uses a Foley-type embryo flushing catheter (see Chapter 34). The catheter is introduced into one horn, the cuff inflated and a small volume of dye infused into the tip of the horn. If the tube is patent the dye will pass via that uterine tube to the peritoneal cavity and hence to the urine (the cuff prevents reflux of the dye to the other side). The procedure is repeated on the other side several days later.

The second test involves the use of starch particles to simulate the transport of the oocyte or zygote as first described in the cow by McDonald (1954) and subsequently described by Kessy and Noakes (1979a).

There is no doubt that ovarobursal disease is one of the major causes of individual cow infertility characterized by regular return to oestrus. There is no satisfactory treatment for the condition. Some cases may be prevented if rough manipulation of ovaries and irrigation of uteri with large quantities of irritant antiseptics are avoided. Prompt attention to cases of dystocia with a view to preventing puerperal metritis would also reduce the incidence of ovarobursal disease.

Several other acquired abnormalities of the uterine tubes can also cause infertility. A condition described as pachysalpinx has been identified in three genital tracts from parous animals (Kessy, 1978). The gross appearance of the tube resembles hydrosalpinx or pyosalpinx but no fluid is contained within the lumen; instead there is a mass of connective tissue. Enlargement and distension of the uterine tube can also occur as a result of the presence of multilocular mucosal cysts containing periodic acid–Schiff (PAS)-staining gelatinous material.

Kessy (1978), using air or carbon dioxide insufflation of the uterine tubes of abattoir specimens, found that 1.1% had occluded tubes in the absence of gross lesions; 17 were unilateral and five were bilateral. In the majority of cases the point of occlusion was about 25 mm from the uterotubal junction. Clinically these could be demonstrated only by using the PSP or starch grain test. Occlusion of the uterine tubes because of the bilateral adhesion of the fimbriae was demonstrated by laparotomy in a cyclic non-breeder (repeat breeder) cow which had shown evidence of tubal occlusion following the use of the PSP and starch grain test (Kessy and Noakes, 1979b). This cow subsequently conceived after the fimbriae were separated at laparotomy.

Adhesions of the uterus

A troublesome sequel to the caesarean operation is adhesion of the uterus to the omentum, intestines or abdominal wall. A similar lesion may follow uterine rupture. Such lesions may accompany ovarobursal disease and may follow tardy involution of the uterus and metritis. They are frequently associated with sterility.

Parturient trauma of the tubular genital tract

Dystocia due to fetal oversize is common in cattle, particularly in the Friesian breed. Delivery of large calves by heavy traction frequently damages the birth canal to such an extent that the animal is rendered sterile.

Rupture of the perineum

A third-degree perineal rupture may occur at calving, usually as a result of dystocia; the whole thickness of the vagina and rectal wall ruptures so that the rectum and vagina are confluent. The cow thus has a cloaca. This lesion does not heal; thus air and faeces are aspirated into the vagina causing vaginitis and metritis (see p. 279). Affected cows have a chronic mucopurulent vulval discharge but the general health is not impaired; normal cyclic behaviour resumes but conception does not occur because of the metritis (see below). The condition can be cured only by surgical reconstruction of the perineum using Götze's technique or that described by Aanes (see Chapter 17).

Rupture of the perineum may be prevented by sound obstetric technique, including episiotomy.

Parturient laceration or bruising of the vulva

This may be followed by cicatrization and distortion with imperfect closure of the vulval sphincter and aspiration of air. The sequelae are similar to but less severe than those of rupture of the perineum. Some of these cows are infertile to natural service but conceive to intrauterine insemination. At subsequent parturition, dystocia owing to fibrosis of the vulva may arise.

Cirrhosis of the cervix

Rarely, parturient laceration of the cervix is followed by fibrosis and obstruction of the cervical canal, with infertility. Occasionally, cirrhosis of the

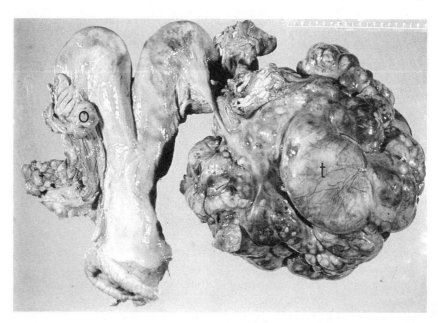

Fig. 22.8 A granulosa cell tumour (t) involving the right ovary. The left ovary (o) is normal.

cervix may prevent proper dilatation of the organ at parturition, but most cases of failure of cervical dilatation are of functional origin.

Prolapse of one or more of the cervical folds is commonly seen in the plurigravid cow. It is a physiological hazard of parturition and is not a cause of infertility.

Gross fibrosis of the vagina

This may follow laceration and pyogenic infection. It will cause a narrowing of the birth canal and dystocia. Caesarean section may then be required.

Tumours of the female genital organs

Granulosa cell tumours are the commonest neoplasms of the bovine ovary (Figure 22.8) but carcinomas, fibromas, thecomas and sarcomas have also been described. Most of the large and cystic neoplasms of the bovine ovary are granulosa cell tumours. They have been seen in pregnant as well as non-pregnant cattle. In the early stages of the tumour it presumably secretes oestrogen, for the affected animal is often nymphomaniacal. Later most of the tumour tissue undergoes luteinization and then anoestrus is usually present. In long-standing cases virilism may occur. The non-affected ovary is usually of the anoestrous type. The author saw a Friesian cow with a granulosa cell tumour which weighed 24 kg; the cow showed successive phases of nymphomania, anoestrus and virilism.

Tumours of the uterus are rare in cattle, although in the USA lymphosarcoma of the uterus is not uncommon. In all countries leiomyomata and fibromyomata are sometimes seen; pregnancy may occur in the neoplastic uterus. The larger uterine tumour may be confused on rectal palpation with a mummified fetus (Figures 22.9 and 22.10). A 2 year abattoir survey in Denver by Anderson and Davis (1958) revealed 24% of the cattle tumours (excluding 'cancer eye') to be in the genitalia; the latter were classified as follows: adenocarcinoma of the uterus, 26 cases; lymphosarcoma of the uterus, six; leiomyoma of the uterus, four; granulosa cell tumours of the ovary, six; cystadenoma of the ovary, one; and squamous

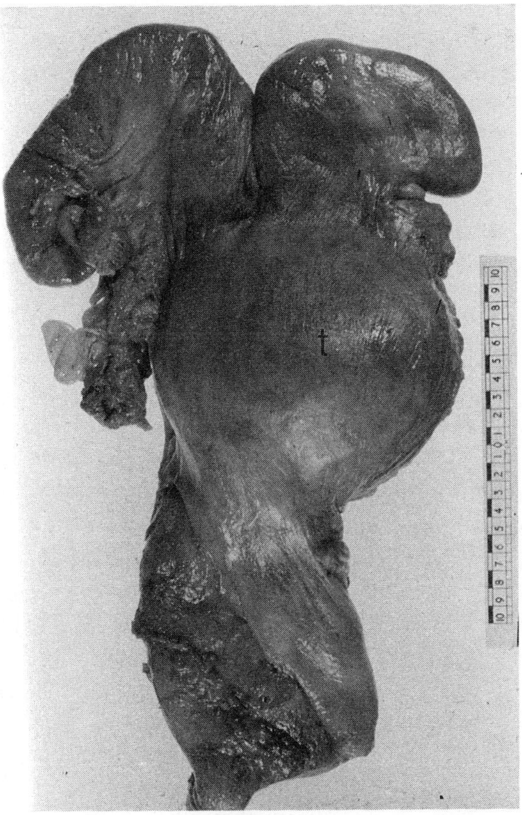

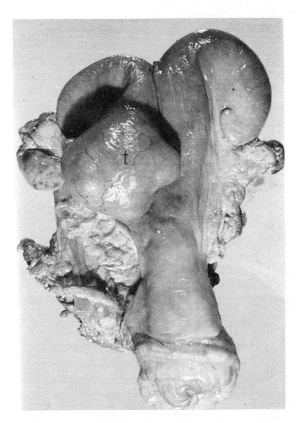

Fig. 22.9 Fibroma (t) involving the base of the uterine horns and body.

Fig. 22.10 Fibroma (t) involving the left uterine horn.

epithelioma of the vulva, one. The relative frequency of the uterine adenocarcinoma in this series and its rarity in Britain are noteworthy.

Tumours of the cervix are rare in cattle and the few recorded have been benign. Fibropapillomata of the vagina and vulva of cattle are not uncommon. They do not cause infertility but may interfere with birth. They are usually pedunculated and may be removed surgically. There is a possibility that one form of vaginal fibropapilloma is of viral origin and that it is transmitted venereally. It occurs in young cattle and undergoes spontaneous resolution.

FUNCTIONAL FORMS OF INFERTILITY

As a rule the functional forms of infertility tend to affect individual animals within a herd but in the aggregate they constitute an important cause of infertility; furthermore when they affect a large number of a particular subgroup in a herd they frequently reflect some other problem, especially nutrition.

Most functional aberrations occur because of some endocrinological abnormality which is frequently difficult to specify even with current methods of hormone assay, particularly when single, spot samples of blood or milk are examined. The abnormalities occur as a result of inherited factors; nutritional deficiencies or excesses; social influences which may arise from modern husbandry methods, for instance the grouping of large numbers of cows thus interfering with the establishment of a stable social hierarchy; and the stress of production.

No observed oestrus

After the onset of puberty, cyclic ovarian activity should be maintained continuously throughout the cow's life except during pregnancy and for a short period in the puerperium (see Chapter 7). The only way that the herdsman knows that this is occurring is the signs of oestrus at approximately 21-day intervals. It is possible that there are signs but that they are not being observed; in this case it is a management problem which is discussed elsewhere in this chapter. However, there are a number of other possible causes:

1. The ovaries may be quiescent and inactive; this is referred to as a true anoestrus.

2. There may be normal cyclic ovarian activity but the cow is not showing the normal behavioural signs; this is described as suboestrus or silent heat.

3. There may be a progesterone-producing structure in the ovary which is exerting an inhibitory effect upon the hypothalamus and anterior pituitary; this may be a persistent corpus luteum or a cyst.

True anoestrus

When this occurs the ovaries are quiescent with an absence of cyclic activity. The reasons for the failure of normal activity may be insufficient release or production of gonadotrophins to cause folliculogenesis, or it may reflect the failure of the ovaries to respond, but the latter is unlikely.

The clinical history will be of a cow or heifer which has not been seen in oestrus; rectal palpation will reveal small ovaries which are usually flat and smooth, especially in heifers, but since follicles up to prematuration size of 1.5 cm may be present the ovaries are sometimes rounded. The main feature will be the absence of a corpus luteum, either developing, mature or regressing. Old cows frequently have roughened irregular ovaries because of the presence of old regressed corpora lutea and corpora albicantia. Sometimes it may be difficult to identify a small developing or regressing corpus luteum and in ovaries these can be confused with anoestrus ovaries; however, the uterus in the former case will show some evidence of tone. Confirmation can be obtained by re-examination of the cow per rectum after 10 days, in which case the cow in true anoestrus will have virtually unchanged ovaries whilst a cow in late dioestrus or early dioestrus (metoestrus) will have a distinctly palpable corpus luteum. Milk or blood progesterone determinations are helpful in confirming a diagnosis; two samples can be taken at 10-day intervals or a single sample 10 days before a rectal palpation is made (Boyd and Munro, 1979). The more frequent use of milk progesterone assays from 25 days postpartum until the first service have been shown to be cost effective (McLeod, 1990).

Some cows resume cyclic ovarian activity within a few weeks of calving and then become anoestrus. In a study involving 535 dairy cows in four commercial herds, Bulman and Lamming (1978) found that 5.1% of the cows showed this pattern of activity, with the period of anoestrus exceeding 14 days. This compared with 4.9% which had not returned to oestrus 50 days or longer after calving. In a survey of 11 papers in a review by Stevenson and Call (1988), the mean percentage incidence was 5.5% (range 2.3–22.5%).

True anoestrus is most frequently diagnosed in high-yielding dairy cows, first-calf heifers which are still growing and beef suckler cows. There are a number of factors which predispose to the condition. The effect of the season of the year and environment is shown by its increased frequency in autumn calving herds which are housed indoors and fed on preserved fodder (Marion and Gier, 1968; Oxenreider and Wagner, 1971). The genetic influence is demonstrated by the longer period for the return of ovarian function postpartum in beef breeds (36–70 days) compared with dairy breeds (10–45 days). Suckling has a profound effect (Lamming, 1980). In an experiment with cross-bred beef cows, non-suckling cows exhibited their first oestrus 10-33 days postpartum, whilst identically bred and fed cows that suckled their calves did not return to oestrus for at least 98 days postpartum (Radford et al., 1978).

The anterior pituitary appears to be refractory to stimulation with gonadotrophin-releasing hormone (GnRH) in the immediate postpartum period; this lasts for 20 days in suckled beef cows compared with 9 days in milked Friesian cows (Lamming, 1978). The refractory period is probably due to the duration of progesterone-induced negative feedback during pregnancy (Lamming et al., 1979). The act of suckling stimulates bursts of prolactin secretion (Karg and Schams, 1974) which may be responsible for the extension of the period of anoestrus. Although no causal relationship has been established in the cow, there appears to be a reciprocal relationship between the hypothalamic control of luteinizing hormone (LH) and prolactin release: opioid antagonist treatments (see below) increase LH and decrease prolactin secretion whilst agonists have the opposite effect (Peters and Lamming, 1990). Radford et al. (1978) demonstrated that in suckled cows at 40 days postpartum the LH release in response to stimulation with an injection of oestradiol benzoate was reduced in comparison with that in non-suckled cows.

The effect of high milk yield on ovarian rebound is debatable. Some have demonstrated an effect (Oxenreider and Wagner, 1971) whilst others suggest that it is not a direct effect but a result of a concomitant loss of body weight and nutritional deficiency. An energy deficit is particularly important, exerting its effect by suppressing release of GnRH and LH (see p. 375), especially if there is excessive weight loss; this can be a problem especially in first calf heifers that are still growing. Deficiencies of phosphorus, copper, cobalt and manganese and the ingestion of phyto-oestrogens can cause anoestrus, whilst diseases which cause severe weight loss and debility or metabolic disturbances, such as ketosis, can have a similar effect.

It is generally accepted that suckling prolongs the period of acyclicity postpartum. Although this has been attributed to the negative energy balance and related weight loss that frequently occurs with multiple suckling, there is increasing evidence that endogenous opioid peptide release may be involved. These substances can suppress LH secretion by exerting an effect on GnRH release in the hypothalamus. Much of this work has involved the use of pharmacological dose rates of opioid antagonists which have increased LH secretion; whether the opioids are primary controllers of the secretion of this gonadotrophin is still open to question (Peters and Lamming, 1990).

In late autumn or winter calving cows that have been in anoestrus there is frequently a return to normal ovarian cyclic activity when the cows are turned out to grass in the spring. It is not known if this is due to increased energy intake, to a specific 'substance' in grass or to the effect of exercise and a new environment.

Treatment. Improved feeding, particularly increasing the energy intake, is important although it would be preferable to prevent the condition occurring by adequate feeding to maintain body weight. Temporary weaning and restricted suckling together with the use of progestagens (see below) during the time of calf removal has resulted in reducing the time to the first ovulation postpartum.

Equine chorionic gonadotrophin (eCG) can be used to stimulate ovarian activity; it can induce follicular growth and oestrus; a dose rate of 3000–4500 IU will frequently cause superovulation and therefore it is not advisable to serve or inseminate at the induced oestrus. If the cow is not inseminated there is a possibility that she will relapse into anoestrus.

The treatment of dairy cows with GnRH

causes the release of LH (Kittock et al., 1973). This has been used successfully to treat anoestrus dairy cows (Bulman and Lamming, 1978) with a single dose of 0.5 mg. Initiation of normal cyclical activity occurred if the injection of GnRH was followed by a rise in plasma progesterone. In suckled beef cows a second injection of GnRH, 10 days later, is necessary after the transient rise in progesterone to initiate normal cyclic activity (Webb et al., 1977). It has been suggested that the initial progesterone rise has a modulating effect upon endogenous gonadotrophin secretion (Lamming, 1978) and that the repeated dose may mimic the surges of LH that occur in normal cyclic activity (Kittock et al., 1973). The newer synthetic GnRH analogues such as buserelin at dose rates of 0.02 mg will stimulate oestrus in 1–3 weeks after treatment.

Progestogen treatment, often associated with oestrogens, has been used to induce ovarian activity postpartum (Foote and Hunter, 1964; Britt et al., 1974; Wisehart and Young, 1974). These are effective because they either simulate the short luteal phase that usually precedes the first normal oestrus cycle (Lamming, 1980) or else cause an accumulation of gonadotrophin by exerting a negative-feedback effect on the anterior pituitary. Whichever mechanism is responsible rapid and easy withdrawal is desirable, which is difficult with injections or implants. The progesterone-releasing intravaginal device (PRID) or controlled internal drug release (CIDR) (see Chapter 1) is easily inserted and readily removed. When these devices are placed in anoestrus cows for 10–14 days, most show oestrus within a few days of their removal; although conception rates are sometimes poor at the first oestrus (Bulman et al., 1978) there is a reduction in the calving conception interval, compared with untreated controls (Lamming, 1980). Several authors have found that the injection of low doses, viz. 750 IU of eCG, at the time of PRID or CIDR withdrawal improves the response (Mulvehill and Sreenan, 1977; MacMillan and Pickering, 1988). However, larger dose rates will probably have an undesirable superovulatory effect.

Oestrogens, both natural and synthetic, have been used to treat anoestrus. They will readily induce behavioural oestrus without inducing ovarian activity and ovulation; however, it is possible that in some cases they might disturb the gonadal–pituitary–hypothalamic axis so that cyclic activity is initiated.

Suboestrus or silent heat

A number of authors (Casida and Wisnicky, 1950; Morrow et al., 1966; King et al., 1976) have shown that the first and second ovulations postpartum are frequently not preceded by behavioural signs of oestrus and are thus truly 'silent heats'. After the second oestrus it is unlikely that many true 'silent heats' occur. When ovulation occurs in the absence of observed oestrus it is more likely to be the result of a failure of observation than to poor detection (see Management causes). Hall et al. (1959) reported an incidence of 10.6% of silent heats even when cows were examined four times in 24 hours, with no improvement in the detection rate when the frequency of observation was increased to every 2 hours. Labhsetwar et al. (1963) reported a figure of 23.7% in 3076 ovulations, and a similar figure of 27.3% was quoted by Kidder et al. (1952) when the herd was inspected every 12 hours; it was especially high (44%) during the first 60 days after calving but even during the subsequent 60 days it was 11%. Lamming and Bulman (1976) quoted a figure of 7% for silent or unobserved oestrus.

A genetic predisposition to silent heat has been identified (Labhsetwar et al., 1963), with certain sire lines showing a statistically significant effect. The same authors found that it was more common in the hotter months of the year, although in temperate climates it has been shown to be more common in the winter than in the summer months (Hammond, 1927). A number of nutritional deficiencies are also said to cause suboestrus: β-carotene, phosphorus, copper, cobalt. Overweight may also have an effect. Attempts have been made to identify an endocrinological reason for a cow failing to show behavioural signs but to date none has been identified.

Diagnosis of the condition is made on the clinical history and rectal palpation of the genital system. No differentiation can be made from non-observed oestrus, since the clinician will be checking for evidence of cyclic ovarian activity as demonstrated by a palpable corpus luteum or, if the cow is in late dioestrus, early dioestrus (metoestrus) or oestrus, by the presence of good uterine tone. The corpus luteum must be differentiated from a cyst; it may be persistent or the cow may be pregnant. If there is any doubt then a re-examination should be made in 10 days. Since the accuracy of identifying a corpus luteum by rectal palpation has been reported as 89% (Dawson, 1975) and 77% (Boyd and Munro, 1979) the determination of progesterone in milk or blood is a useful aid.

In respect of treatment, if a mature corpus luteum is present and the cow is not pregnant, prostaglandin $F_{2\alpha}$ ($PGF_{2\alpha}$) or an analogue followed by fixed-time insemination is indicated (see Chapter 1). If the corpus luteum is at a refractory stage (see Chapter 1) a double injection prostaglandin regimen at an 11 day interval could be used. Alternatively a PRID or other progestogen implant could be used followed by fixed-time insemination.

Non-detected oestrus

This is described elsewhere in this chapter under management faults.

Persistent corpus luteum

The mechanisms involved in the control of the lifespan of the corpus luteum are described in Chapter 1. Anything which interferes with the production or release of endogenous luteolysin will result in a persistent corpus luteum. Pregnancy is the condition which most frequently results in persistence of the corpus luteum, but in the presence of uterine infection and inflammation of the tissues there is interference with the production or the release of luteolysin (Ginther, 1968; Seguin et al., 1974). This condition can be self-perpetuating since progesterone domination of the uterus reduces its resistance to infection and prevents recurrent periods of oestrus when the uterus is more resistant (Rowson et al., 1953). One consequence of this is pyometra which, if untreated, can persist for several months.

There is little firm evidence that persistence of the corpus luteum can occur in the absence of uterine lesions. Although Lamming and Bulman (1976) identified 2% of the cows with elevated milk progesterone levels for more than 30 days, there was no critical examination of the uterus either clinically or by means of endometrial biopsy. However, all four cows which showed this feature in the study conceived at the first oestrus after treatment. It is the author's opinion that most cases of 'persistent corpus luteum', in the absence of uterine lesions, are incorrectly diag-

nosed and are due to silent heat or non-detected oestrus. The only sure way of reaching a true diagnosis would be sequential rectal palpation or the use of repeat milk or blood progesterone determinations. Gross uterine inflammation and pyometra can be identified on rectal palpation (see Chapter 23).

The condition, once diagnosed, is readily treated with $PGF_{2\alpha}$ or a synthetic analogue, provided that the clinician is confident that the cow is not pregnant; oestrus will occur in 3–5 days.

Ovarian cysts

These will be discussed in detail below under ovulatory defects.

Ovulatory defects

Ovulation in the cow is atypical since it occurs 10–12 hours after the end of behavioural oestrus and 18–26 hours after the ovulatory LH peak (see Chapter 1). During oestrus and after the end of oestrus, several follicles undergo development but usually only one, or occasionally two, ovulate; the other follicles regress and become atretic. A number of defects associated with ovulation can occur (Figure 22.11); these are outlined below. The consequences for fertility of an ovulatory defect are two-fold: either the oocyte is not liberated and hence cannot be fertilized or else it is liberated too late so that the spermatozoa are now incapable of fertilization or else the oocyte has aged and is not capable of normal development.

Ovulatory defects are due to: endocrine deficiency or imbalance, failure of the development of hormone receptors at the target tissue, mechanical

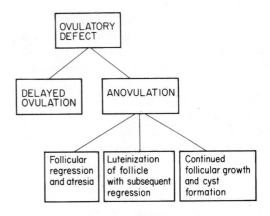

Fig. 22.11 Ovulatory defects in the cow.

factors. The endocrine control of ovulation is described in Chapter 1; it is a complex interaction between ovarian hormones, the anterior pituitary and the hypothalamus. Thus if the quantity of pituitary hormone released is insufficient or its timing is incorrect (this is particularly true of LH), then ovulation is delayed or fails to occur. In a minority of cases, because of extensive lesions involving adhesion of the ovarian bursa to the surface of the ovary, the physical process of ovulation is prevented.

Delayed ovulation

There is little information on the incidence of delayed ovulation as a cause of infertility. Hancock (1948) found that only 36% of cows that had ovulated by the second day after oestrus conceived to service during oestrus, compared with 65% conception in the majority (69%) which had ovulated by the first day after oestrus. An incidence of 18% delayed ovulation has been reported in South Africa (Van Rensburg and de Vos, 1962); the delay was less than 48 hours in 85% of the cases and more than 48 hours in 15%. These authors recommended that if ovulation had not occurred by 24 hours after service the cow should be reinseminated; and of 51 cases so treated 32 conceived, compared with no conceptions in 18 cows in which the follicle had failed to rupture within 24 hours of a single service. A much lower incidence of less than 2% in 'repeat breeder' cows has been reported by Zemjanis (1980). In a group of Holstein cows, Erb et al. (1976) (who assumed that ovulation normally occurred within 2 days of the LH peak) found that, of the seven cows that ovulated later than 2 days after this surge, none conceived.

Several authors have noted that certain cows have an apparent prolonged follicular phase of the oestrous cycle as determined by the presence of low progesterone concentrations in blood and milk (Erb et al., 1976; Bulman and Lamming, 1978; Jackson et al., 1979). However, there is no evidence that this is because of delayed ovulation; rather it is related to a delay in the corpus luteum assuming normal steroidogenesis.

Diagnosis of the condition is difficult since it requires either sequential rectal palpation of the ovaries or sequential transrectal ultrasound imaging, both of which might interfere with the process of ovulation and may cause premature rupture. It has been recommended that a diagnosis can be made if the same follicle can be detected in the same ovary on two successive examinations, one at peak oestrous and another 24–36 hours later (Zemjanis, 1980). Errors can easily be made, and the same author questions the value of a single examination.

Delayed ovulation is generally assumed to be one of the causes of failure of conception in cyclic non-breeders (American 'repeat breeders'). Treatment has consisted of using those hormones that might hasten the timing of ovulation. Results have frequently been equivocal as measured by improved pregnancy rates and reduced services per pregnancy. Results for human chorionic gonadotrophin (hCG) have often been disappointing (Hansel et al., 1976; Leidl et al., 1979). Those for GnRH have been rather more encouraging (Schels and Mostafawi, 1978; Lee et al., 1981; Nakao et al., 1983) especially by improving pregnancy rates for services other than the first (Maurice et al., 1982; Stevenson et al., 1984). GnRH administration causes a rapid rise in FSH and LH concentrations which peak within 30 to 60 minutes and return to pre-injection values within 4 hours. The pattern of release of LH resembles the pre-ovulatory one observed during late oestrous in normal cyclical animals (Leslie, 1983).

An alternative approach to treatment is to use two artificial inseminations — one at the normal time (see Chapter 24) and one 24 hours later.

Anovulation

Associated with those conditions which can predispose to true anoestrus (see below) it is sometimes observed that before this occurs it is preceded by an anovulatory oestrous, with the follicle regressing and becoming atretic. Similarly, during the puerperium, before the onset of normal cyclic ovarian activity, a similar situation may arise, which is comparable with that observed in seasonal polyoestrous species at the start of the breeding season. If cows are examined per rectum during the first few weeks after calving, a number of enlarged anovulatory follicles can often be detected; they are incorrectly described as being cysts (see later) but they are transient and do not persist even if no treatment is given.

Sometimes, however, a follicle does not regress but, having reached its maximum size of 2–2.5 cm in diameter, the wall becomes luteinized. This

Table 22.2 Fluid-containing structures in bovine ovaries

Follicles	Vacuolated corpora lutea	Luteinized follicles	Folicular cysts	Luteinized cysts
Transient, dynamic, soft, fluctuant structures	Occurs after up to 25% of normal ovulations	Follow anovulation of mature follicle	Follow anovulation of mature follicle	Follow anovulation of mature follicle
Usually identifiable clinically ≤1.5 cm diameter at all stages of oestrous cycle	Same size as non-vacuolated corpus luteum but may feel slightly softer on palpation	No evidence of ovulation point	Soft, thin-walled, fluid-filled structure ≥2.5 cm diameter which persists	Thick-walled, fluid-filled structure ≥2.5 cm diameter which persists
1.5–2.0 cm in diameter just before, during and for 12 hours after oestrus	Evidence of ovulation point	< 2.5 cm diameter	Frequently multiple in one or both ovaries	Usually single
	Central vacuole disappears during pregnancy	Larger cavity than vacuolated corpus luteum	Thickness of cyst wall < 3 mm	Thickness of cyst wall > 3 mm
	Associated with normal oestrous cycle	More likely to occur in immediate post partum period	Associated with low peripheral blood progesterone levels	Associated with high peripheral blood progesterone levels
		Associated with normal or shorter length of oestrous cycle	Affected cows will be either anoestrus or nymphomaniacal	Affected cows wil be anoestrous

structure functions in the same way as a corpus luteum either regressing after 17–18 days or, frequently, much earlier so that the cow returns to oestrus at a shorter than normal interval. After the demise of the luteinized follicle, the subsequent oestrus will probably be followed by a normal ovulation. Such a structure will be < 2.5 cm in diameter, fluid filled, with a rim of luteal tissue lining the follicle and with no evidence of a point of ovulation.

Evidence of this occurring in a living animal comes from a report by Watson and Harwood (1984). They found that in a Friesian cow ovulation failed to occur after the second oestrus 68 days after calving, as determined by twice weekly rectal palpation. Frequent sequential blood samples demonstrated a normal LH peak, lasting about 10 hours and reaching a maximum concentration of 24 ng/ml, which was preceded by a normal preovulatory oestradiol-17β peak the day before oestrus. Thus there was apparently no extra-ovarian endocrine abnormality and the cow ovu-

lated and conceived at the subsequent oestrus 22 days after the previous anovulatory one. Obviously it could have been confused with a luteal cyst (see later), but it was not larger than a mature follicle and did not persist. Others may also confuse it with a 'cystic' corpus luteum (see Chapter 1) which is a normal corpus luteum containing a central fluid lacuna and hence has an ovulation papilla. 'Cystic' corpora lutea are not abnormal; they accounted for 25% of the corpora lutea examined in ovaries obtained from the abattoir. They contain the same amount of progesterone as non-cystic corpora lutea (Donaldson and Hansel, 1968). Perhaps, to avoid confusion, the term 'vacuolated' corpus luteum would be preferable. These can often be identified using transrectal ultrasound imaging.

Diagnosis of anovulation can only be made retrospectively by noting on rectal palpation that a follicle persists longer than one would have suspected. In the case of the luteinized follicle it will remain for 17–18 days before regressing; the ovary containing it will be rounded, smooth and fluctuating rather than irregular and solid as it is with a corpus luteum. There is no information on the incidence of these conditions.

Treatment is directed towards ensuring that ovulation occurs at the next oestrous; hence hCG or GnRH administered as described for delayed ovulation are indicated. If ovarobursal adhesions are present there is no treatment.

Cystic ovaries

Ovaries are said to be cystic when they contain one or more persistent, i.e. longer than 10 days, fluid-filled structures larger than a mature follicle, i.e. > 2.5 cm diameter, in one or both ovaries resulting in aberrant reproductive function (details of fluid-containing structures in bovine ovaries are listed in Table 22.2). Sometimes the definition specifically excludes the presence of a corpus luteum; however, this is not always correct (Al-Dahash and David, 1977a; Carroll et al., 1990). Cysts arise as a result of anovulation of a Graafian follicle but, instead of regression and atresia, or luteinization followed by regression, the follicle increases in size, there is degeneration of the granulosa cell layer and it persists, usually for at least 10 days. The consequence of this is to alter the normal cyclical activity of the cow so that it becomes either acyclic or nymphomaniacal.

Cows frequently develop large, fluid-filled structures in the ovaries in the immediate postpartum period (see Chapter 7). It has been reported that up to 60% of cows develop cysts before the first postpartum ovulation (Morrow et al., 1966; Kesler et al., 1979). These will normally go undetected, unless the cow is examined by rectal palpation, and if they regress spontaneously without any extension in the interval to first oestrous or evidence of nymphomania, they should not be considered as true ovarian cysts. The point of distinction is that they do not cause aberrant reproductive function.

Incidence. It is universally accepted that cystic ovarian disease is an important cause of infertility. Many of the early studies, particularly abattoir surveys, may not have given a true impression of the incidence because the authors would not have known if the criteria of persistence and aberrant function had been satisfied. Studies in the USA have reported an incidence of 5.6–47.4% (Kesler and Garverick, 1982; Peralta and Ax, 1982). Day (1991) quotes four North American references giving figures ranging from 6 to 19% per lacta-

tion. Whilst in a study involving 34 dairy herds in Ontario there was a lactational incidence of 5% with a median time to first diagnosis postpartum of 90.5 days. Anecdotal evidence has frequently suggested that cystic ovarian disease is increasing in incidence: a 20 year retrospective study of a single dairy herd involving 923 cows and 2246 calvings showed a steady increase from 1963. In 1966 only 10% of cows were affected whereas in 1983 the comparable figure was 57%. Cystic ovarian disease depresses fertility in a number of ways: it extends the calving interval, decreases lifetime milk yields and increases the involuntary culling rate. The cost has been calculated to be $137 per lactation per cow (Bartlett et al., 1986).

Predisposing Factors. As the condition has become more common in recent years, it must reflect the effects of genetic selection for high yield, social problems related to large groups of cows and diet. That the condition is probably hereditary is shown by a significantly higher incidence in some families within a breed (Garm, 1949; Casida and Chapman, 1951), whilst the influence of the sire on the incidence of cystic ovaries has been shown by Palsson (1961); moreover beef breeds are seldom affected. In a study involving 390 000 cows of the Swedish Red and White (SRB) and Swedish Friesians (SLB), the SRB cows were twice as likely to have cystic ovarian disease than those of the SLB breed (Emmanuelson and Bendixen, 1991). In the SRB breed the probability of cystic ovaries increased with parity but not for SLB cows. Despite evidence for a genetic predisposition estimates of the heritability are low (Day, 1991). The relationship between incidence and yield has been demonstrated by Hendricksson (1956) and Marion and Gier (1968) who observed that the disease was more prevalent in high-yielding cows and that it occurs at the stage in the lactation curve when yield is at its peak. Recently, a relationship between milk volume and fat output has been shown (Ashmawy et al., 1992). The same authors also demonstrated that in the two groups of cows that they studied the repeatability of cyst development was 20% in Guernseys and 6% in Holsteins. The feeding of high-protein diets appears to be a contributory factor. Whilst the season of the year also appears to have some effect, since the disease is more prevalent in winter than at other times of the year (Bierschwal, 1966; Roine, 1973), this may reflect the fact that the majority of cows are calving in the autumn and thus will have reached peak yield at this time.

There was some evidence that β-carotene, the plant precursor of vitamin A, may be important in reducing the incidence of ovarian cysts (Lotthammer, 1979). However, this has not been supported by the work of others (Folman et al., 1979; Marcek et al., 1985) who found that supplementation of cows' diets with β-carotene had no beneficial effect in reducing the incidence of cysts. There is also a suggestion that postpartum uterine infection might predispose to the disease (Bosu and Peters, 1987).

Aetiology. As with all conditions associated with ovulatory failure there are two basic causes: mechanical interference with ovulation and endocrine abnormalities. The former is of least importance, although in a study by Al-Dahash and David (1977a) ovarobursal adhesions were present in 7.67% of the genital tracts with cystic ovaries, compared with 1.8% of the non-cystic population.

Many attempts have been made to determine the precise endocrine abnormalities that are responsible for cystic ovaries but there are many unanswered questions. Before discussing these it might be appropriate to review the neuroendocrine control of folliculogenesis and ovulation as succinctly summarized by Eyestone and Ax (1984).

Follicular development from antrum formation to ovulation is a hormone-dependent process. Small antral follicles contain FSH receptors, but few or no LH receptors. As the follicles grow, granulosa cells acquire the ability to aromatize androgens to oestrogens (primarily oestradiol-17β, E_2); however, individual follicles of similar size may vary considerably in this respect. LH receptors appear in the theca interna cells of most follicles, and in the granulosa cells of follicles containing high levels of aromatase activity. E_2, synthesized by the granulosa cells, is secreted into the follicular fluid and vasculature. Oestrogenic follicles with LH receptors in the granulosa are competent to develop to ovulation under the appropriate gonadotropic stimulus; the remainder are destined for atresia.

Oestrogenic follicles are the principal source of circulating E_2 prior to ovulation. As the follicles develop towards ovulation, peripheral E_2 increases to a point at which it exerts a positive feedback effect on LH release, resulting in the preovulatory LH surge. The effect of E_2 on LH release occurs at the hypothalamic and pituitary level. The increase in pulse frequency of LH release, due to E_2 stimulation, presumably reflects increased frequency of GnRH pulse release from the hypothalamus. E_2 also increases pituitary sensitivity to GnRH. The combined effects of high preovulatory E_2 levels on the hypothalamic–pituitary axis form the basis for the positive feedback of E_2 on LH release. LH then binds to its receptors in the preovulatory follicle, causing an increase in intracellular cAMP, decline of androgen and oestrogen synthesis, an increase in $PGF_{2\alpha}$ synthesis, an increase in follicular plasminogen activator, and down-regulation of its own receptors. Proteolytic enzymes break down the apical follicle wall and ovulation occurs.

Any defect or asynchrony in this complex process could lead to anovulation and cyst formation; as yet the primary defect has not been identified with certainty.

Ovarian cysts have been induced by the administration of LH antiserum (Nadaraja and Hansel, 1976). This suggests deficient LH release, either due to a failure of pituitary synthesis of LH or failure of pituitary response to GnRH. By administering progesterone either just before, or at the onset, of oestrus the preovulatory surge was suppressed and there was persistence of an anovulatory follicle (Lee et al., 1988). Some support for this hypothesis has come from the observation that in cows that develop cysts, LH concentrations during pro-oestrus and oestrus are lower than in ovulating cows (Kesler et al., 1979). The converse was found in a study involving chronic cystic ovarian diseased cows (Brown et al., 1986) and in a study in which cysts were induced experimentally with oestradiol-17β and progesterone treatments (Cook et al., 1991); in both, pituitary LH contents were the same as normal cyclical cows. In the latter study, not only were basal concentrations of LH higher in the peripheral blood during cyst development, but also pulse frequency and amplitude. The pituitaries of cows with follicular cysts respond to exogenous GnRH by secreting LH (Kittock et al., 1973), and when pituitary LH receptors were investigated no differences could be found in the numbers in cows with or without cysts.

Another explanation for LH release failure might be the absence of, or reduced, response to the positive feedback of the preovulatory oestrogen peak. However, by administering exogenous oestradiol benzoate, no difference in the magnitude of response in cows with or without cysts was demonstrated (Zaied et al., 1981). It was noted that there was a temporal delay between the oestrogen peak and the LH peak in cows with follicular cysts. Thus the development of cysts may be due to asynchrony of the hormonal events rather than the absence of any particular hormone.

The problem of ovulatory failure and cyst formation may be due to defects within the ovary. The ability of follicles to respond to the preovulatory LH surge is dependent upon the timely induction of LH receptors during follicular maturation; if too few receptors are available then ovulatory failure may occur. Studies in women have shown that in cells from cystic follicles the number of LH receptors was only 51% of that found in normal preovulatory follicles (Rajaniemi et al., 1980). Again it is important to stress that follicular cysts will respond to hCG and GnRH therapy by either ovulating or luteinization (Berchtold et al., 1980; Kesler et al., 1981); thus confirming the presence of adequate LH receptors in such stuctures.

Ovulation inhibition, followed by cyst formation, has been produced experimentally with injections of adrenocorticotrophic hormone (ACTH) (Liptrap and McNally, 1976). The authors were unable to produce a similar response with hydrocortisone treatment, suggesting a direct effect of ACTH upon the ovulatory mechanism. Since ACTH and adrenal hyperactivity has been described in the rat and sow (Liptrap, 1970; Baldwin and Sawyer, 1974), and since stress is associated with elevated ACTH (Christian et al., 1965) it might explain the influence of intensive husbandry and high production.

The administration of bromocriptine (a prolactin inhibitor) blocks cyst formation in hypothyroid rats (Copman and Adams, 1981). Hafez (1975) has suggested that ovulatory failure and cyst formation are related to high prolactin secretion, associated with high yeild. McNeilly (1980) has shown that prolactin may not be involved in FSH and LH release at ovulation, although Bartosik et al. (1967) suggest that prolactin may reduce the sensitivity of the ovary to normal concentrations of LH.

Since hypothyroidism has been associated with cystic follicles in a number of species (Eyestone and Ax, 1984), an association with cystic ovaries in cattle has been postulated by the same authors. Thyroxine concentrations are negatively corre-

lated with milk production, so that high yielding cows have lower concentrations than low yielding animals. Whilst it is tempting to speculate on the influence of thyroid function, the precise mechanism involved has not been described.

Since endogenous opioid peptides have been shown to modify GnRH release, and hence LH secretion, the role of these ubiquitous substances cannot be ignored in the aetiology of cystic ovaries.

Distribution, Classification, Diagnosis and Clinical Signs. More cysts are identified in the right ovary than in the left, thus reflecting the relative activities of the two ovaries, whilst in a number of cases cysts are present in both ovaries. Garm (1949) found that multiple cysts were more frequent than single cysts; however, Elmore et al. (1975) found that 75% were solitary cysts. In a large survey of over 8000 genital tracts of which 307 had cystic ovaries, 53.5% had a single cyst and 46.2% had multiple cysts (Al-Dahash and David, 1977b). The latter authors found that the majority of cysts were 2.5–3.0 cm in diameter, with very few larger than 5–6 cm. Most of the studies have been done on abattoir-derived material from cows after slaughter, which tends to suggest that ovarian cysts are static structures. However, there is good evidence that the ovaries of cows with cysts are dynamic, with cysts regressing spontaneously after a period of time, only to be replaced by others (Kesler and Garverick 1982; Carroll et al., 1990; Cook et al., 1990). There are also changes in the type of cyst, as determined by the degree of luteinization (see below). Cysts have been identified in association with a corpus luteum (Al-Dahash and David, 1977b; Roy et al., 1985; Carroll et al., 1990) (see Figure 22.12).

Traditionally, ovarian cysts have been classified, following rectal palpation, as either follicular cysts (Figures 22.12, 22.13 and 22.15(a)), which are thin-walled, frequently multiple and with little or no luteal tissue in the cyst wall, or luteal or luteinized cysts, which are thick walled, more usually single and with a large quantity of luteal tissue present in the cyst wall (Figures 22.14, 15(b) and 22.16). However, the accurate classification of cysts is difficult. It has generally been accepted that the definitive diagnostic test is the measurement of progesterone concentrations in blood plasma/serum or milk. In this method a discriminatory value of 2 ng/ml for milk (Booth, 1988) or

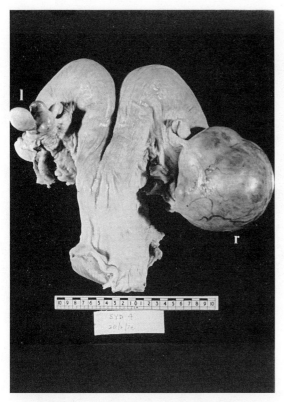

Fig. 22.12 Genital tract with large 10 cm thin-walled cyst in right (r) ovary and left (l) ovary with corpus luteum.

0.5–1.0 ng/ml for plasma/serum (Carroll et al., 1990; Farin et al., 1992) is used to determine the type of cyst. Thus, if it is equal to or above the discriminatory value it is a luteinized cyst, and if it is below it is a follicular cyst. Comparisons can be made with classifications based on rectal palpation and/or transrectal ultrasound imaging. Currently, follicular cysts are between two and three times more common than luteal cysts (Kesler and Garverick, 1982; Leslie and Bosu, 1983; Booth, 1988). However, the accuracy of progesterone assays as a method of diagnosing the type of ovarian cyst has been questioned by the study of Carroll et al. (1990), who showed, using transrectal ultrasound imaging, the dynamic state of ovarian structures, the fluctuations in plasma progesterone concentrations with time and the occurrence of ovulation with corpus luteum formation in the presence of cysts. Thus, a cow with a follicular cyst with a thin wall (Figure 28.15(a)) containing very little luteal tissue but with a corpus luteum on the same or other ovary would have a plasma or milk progesterone concentration above the discriminatory value, indicative of a luteal cyst. The accuracy of diagnosis can be improved by the use of transrectal ultrasound imaging. Luteal cysts will have a thicker wall comprising luteal tissue; a thickness of >3 mm is generally considered to be diagnostic (Figure 22.15(b)).

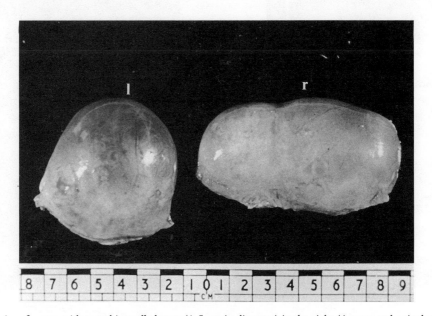

Fig. 22.13 Ovaries of a cow with two thin-walled cysts (4–5 cm in diameter) in the right (r) ovary and a single thin-walled cyst (5 cm in diameter) in the left (l) ovary.

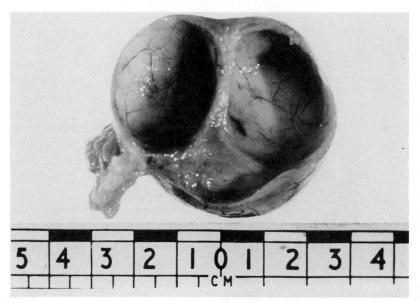

Fig. 22.14 Cross-section of an ovary of a cow showing three cysts with some degree of luteinization.

(a)   (b)

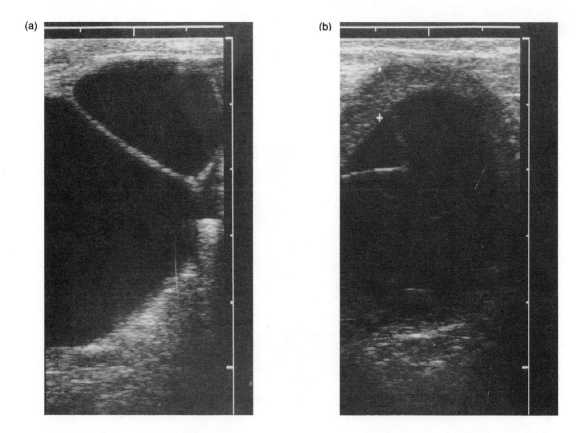

Fig. 22.15 (a) Ultrasound image of the ovary of a cow with a thin-walled cyst. (b) Ultrasound image of the ovary of a cow with a luteal cyst. Note thick wall of luteal tissue which is > 3 mm in thickness. (By courtesy of W. R. Ward.)

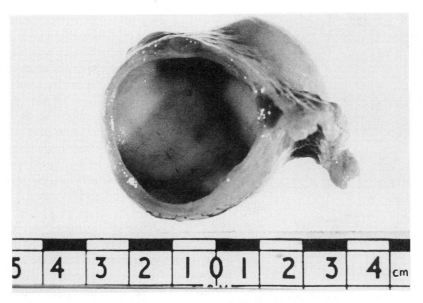

Fig. 22.16 Cross-section of an ovary of a cow showing a typical single, thick-walled, luteal cyst. Note that the wall comprises at least 3 mm of luteal tissue.

Even the oldest veterinary textbooks refer to nymphomania in cows. Roberts (1955), in a survey of 352 cows with cystic ovaries, found that 73.6% were nymphomaniac and 26.4% acyclical. In recent years there has been a change in behavioural patterns. Bierschwall (1966) reported 60% as acyclical, Dobson et al. (1977) found 73% acyclical and 27% nymphomaniacal; more recently, Booth (1988) in a survey of 200 cows with cystic ovarian disease reported that 38% of the 141 cows with follicular cysts (72.5% of the total) showed signs of nymphomania, whilst Carroll et al. (1990) identified nymphomania in 12.5% of 16 cows that developed ovarian cysts.

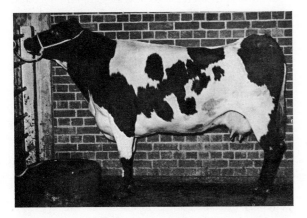

Fig. 22.17 An Ayrshire cow with the typical nymphomaniac configuration.

Cows with the follicular type of cyst are usually nymphomaniacal with excessive, prolonged signs of oestrous and a shortened interval between successive heats. There is oedematous swelling of the vulva, frequent and copious discharge of clear mucus, sinking of the sacrosciatic ligaments and upward displacement of the coccyx (Figure 22.17); affected cows have a nervous disposition with depressed milk yield and loss of bodily condition. They will attempt to ride other cows and, as with cows in oestrous, will stand to be mounted by other cows. Because of their excessive sexual activity they have a general disruptive effect upon the rest of the herd, making accurate oestrous detection difficult. Furthermore, owing to the relaxation of the pelvic ligaments, they are prone to pelvic and hip fractures. Cows with this type of cystic ovary do not have elevated blood oestrogen concentrations (Kittock et al., 1973; Dobson et al., 1977); hence the changes are likely to be due to an increased period of oestrogen domination rather than to excessive amounts of oestrogen (Dobson et al., 1977).

The luteal or luteinized cyst usually results in a cessation of cyclical activity; the structure functions as a persistent corpus luteum. It is difficult to understand why it does not regress under the influence of endogenous luteolysin, since it will regress under the influence of exogenous prostaglandin (see later). If cows with luteinized cysts

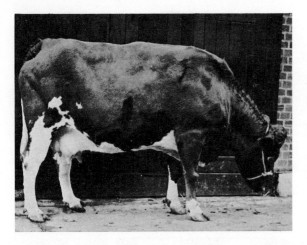

Fig. 22.18 Cow with masculine configuration and behaviour (virilism) associated with a long-standing luteal cyst.

are left untreated then a proportion of them will become virilized (Arthur, 1959). These individuals will develop a masculine conformation and will attempt to mount other cows, but unlike the nymphomaniacal cow they will not stand to be mounted by other cows (Figure 22.18).

An interesting effect of the presence of a cyst and an associated corpus luteum is that there is a greater tendency for the granulosa layer of the cysts to be absent (Al-Dahash and David, 1977c), which may have been due to the effect of progesterone from the corpus luteum or the age of the cyst. In the same survey 22.8% of the cysts which were examined showed evidence of luteinization, varying from small isolated patches to a continuous thick layer below the theca; usually it was seen as a thick crescentic layer at the base of the cyst. Luteinization was most frequently seen in the single thick-walled cyst, where 58% showed evidence.

Testosterone concentrations have been measured in cows with follicular cysts and nymphomania. These values were not different from those for normal cows and could not be correlated with the intensity of nymphomaniacal behaviour (Eyestone and Ax, 1984).

Treatment. The treatment of cystic ovarian disease in cattle has been reviewed in detail by Nanda et al. (1989). Spontaneous recovery can occur quite frequently; it has been reported to be as high as 50% in cows that develop cysts within 45 days of calving (Morrow et al., 1966), whilst others have reported recovery in the absence of treatment

in 13–29% of cases (Beck and Ellis, 1960; Whitmore et al., 1974; Bierschwal et al., 1975).

The earliest method of treating cysts was by manual rupture at rectal palpation. Although rupture sometimes occurs inadvertently it should not be done intentionally as it can cause trauma or haemorrhage which might result in ovarobursal adhesions (see p. 352). Surgical removal of one chronically affected ovary might be worth considering in a limited number of cases where other treatments have failed, or paracentesis using a long hypodermic needle through the sacrosciatic ligament.

The choice of treatment and its success will depend to some extent upon the diagnosis of the type of cyst. Failure of cows with supposed luteal cysts (see below) to respond to PGF$_{2\alpha}$ therapy is invariably due to misdiagnosis. Follicular cysts have been treated successfully using unfractionated sheep pituitary extracts (Casida et al., 1944). hCG has been used successfully since it was first described by Roberts (1955). The dose rate of hCG varies; in the UK doses of 3000–4500 IU are frequently used, whilst in the USA the usual dose rate is 10000 IU; it should be given intravenously. Sometimes hCG is used in conjunction with progesterone (see below).

GnRH has become available during the last few years, initially as a synthetic decapeptide of identical molecular structure to the naturally occurring hormone but also as a nonapeptide analogue with a longer biological half-life.

Both GnRH and hCG cause luteinization of the cyst, the latter by stimulating a rise in endogenous LH; as a consequence, plasma progesterone concentrations increase to at least 2 ng/ml 10 days after treatment. This has a negative feedback on the pituitary, thus causing a decline in endogenous LH and oestradiol-17β concentrations and is probably the most important factor in restoring normal cyclical activity (Kesler and Garverick, 1982). At the normal dose rates of GnRH, 100–250 μg, luteinization of the cyst occurs (Kesler et al., 1981); however, using larger dose rates of 0.5– 1.0 mg, ovulation of follicles appears to occur (Berchtold et al., 1980). If a synthetic nonapeptide such as buserelin is used, the dose rate is 10 μg. Results with GnRH and hCG treatment have generally been good. Dobson et al. (1977) reported a 90% response to GnRH and a 76% response to hCG, while 50% and 27% conceived at 1.4 and 2.25 services, respectively. Over 80% of cows treated with GnRH had resumed normal cyclical activity within 18–23 days of treatment (Kesler et al., 1978). In a large and detailed survey involving 225 cows with ovarian cysts and irregular oestrous cycles (Whitmore et al., 1979), 76% responded to a single injection of 100 μg of GnRH and only four failed to respond to up to three injections; 83% of the treated cows became pregnant with a 49% pregnancy rate to first service. In the study by Kesler et al. (1979) those cows that failed to respond to GnRH treatment had mean pretreatment peripheral progesterone concentrations of $0.4 \pm SE\ 0.2$ ng/ml; perhaps the degeneration of the cyst wall prevented the thecal cells from responding to LH stimulation. The use of hCG in combination with progesterone in various forms has been used, but the equivocal results obtained and the additional expense cannot justify its use.

In the author's opinion, one of the most successful methods of therapy is the use of a PRID (see p. 40). In a study in which it was used in 25 cows (18 of which had been treated unsuccessfully with other hormones), 68% recovered within 13–18 days after the insertion of the PRID and 88% of these conceived within three inseminations (Nanda et al., 1988). Signs of nymphomania abate within 24 hours, the cysts gradually regress and following removal after 10–12 days there is oestrous with ovulation and corpus luteum formation. Presumably progesterone absorbed from the PRID suppresses the gonadotrophin support that is required for the maintenance of the cyst, resulting in its demise. Following its withdrawal, there is a surge of gonadotrophin with ovulation and corpus luteum formation. In a study involving 116 cases of follicular cysts which were treated with either 500 μg of gonadorelin or 20 μg of buserelin intramuscularly, 52.6% recovered 3–15 days after treatment and 93.4% conceived within 1.55 inseminations. Only 7.8% had recurrent cysts. Some were treated with a second dose of GnRH (Nanda et al., 1988).

Luteal cysts have been treated with progesterone, hCG, GnRH and $PGF_{2\alpha}$ or an analogue. Results with progesterone have been variable; thus, Trainin (1964) reported that only 10% of cows showed regression of the cyst with only one cow conceiving, but Dobson et al. (1977) had a good response with eight of nine cows showing regression of the cyst, of which five conceived with a mean of 1.5 services per conception. They used a treatment regimen of 100 mg of progesterone in oil by intramuscular injection on three successive occasions at intervals of 48 hours. A PRID is an effective method of administering progesterone. hCG treatment was fairly successful, according to Bierschwal (1966), with 50% of acyclic cows conceiving to the first oestrus after treatment and the average interval to first oestrus being 24.5 days. Presumably hCG stimulates further luteinization and the heavily luteinized cyst then perhaps becomes susceptible to the action of endogenous luteolysin. Alternatively, since secondary ovulations with corpus luteum formation frequently occur, the subsequent release of luteolysin which causes regression of the corpus luteum might have a similar effect on the cyst. This is also probably the response after the injection of GnRH, since good results have also been reported following its use; 65% of cysts regressed and 50% of the cows thus treated conceived at a mean interval of 37 days after treatment (Dobson et al., 1977). The most logical way to treat a luteal cyst is the use of $PGF_{2\alpha}$, although there is still no explanation for the failure of cows to respond to their endogenous luteolysin. A predictable response was obtained by Dobson et al. (1977): 26 of 27 cows showed regression of the cyst, the majority coming into oestrus in 3–5 days, and 56% of the cows conceived at a mean treatment-to-conception interval of 27 days. Jackson (1981), in a survey involving several countries, reported over 80% response with disappearance of the cyst and oestrus within 3–5 days, with at least 60% and in most cases over 90% of these cows conceiving.

In discussing ovarian cysts, emphasis has been placed on the differentiation of the type of cyst, based on clinical history, rectal palpation, progesterone assay or ultrasound imaging. Perhaps such differentiation is not necessary, since in a survey of 84 cows with cystic ovaries, Elmore et al. (1975) treated the cows with GnRH or hCG irrespective of the type and excellent results were obtained. The majority of cows had luteal cysts, with first service conception rates of 55 and 46%, overall conception rate of 97 and 100% and at mean treatment-to-conception intervals of 37 and 48 days following GnRH and hCG, respectively. A further suggestion for routine treatment is to inject GnRH when the cyst is first diagnosed, followed by PGF$_{2\alpha}$ 9 days later (Kesler et al., 1978); this can then reduce the interval to first service and conception. However, in a study in which comparisons of subsequent fertility were made with GnRH therapy alone, the results were worse; in addition, such a treatment regimen is more expensive (Archibald et al., 1991). Similar disappointing results were reported by Nanda et al. (1988).

Uterine Changes. In discussing cystic ovarian disease most attention has quite properly been directed to the ovaries. However, one consequence of the disease is the development of mucometra in which there is distension of the uterus with mucoid fluid and thinning of the uterine wall. In a survey conducted by Al-Dahash and David (1977a) these uterine features were all associated with ovaries which contained thin-walled, follicular cysts and no corpora lutea. In the same survey several specimens showed marked dilatation of the uterine glands and this was associated with thick-walled luteal cysts with or without a corpus luteum.

Prevention. By careful genetic selection improvements have been made by eliminating bulls that have sired daughters which have subsequently suffered from cystic ovarian disease (see p. 362). Ideally, cows should not be treated for cystic ovaries and certainly the progeny should not be used for breeding. Unfortunately, this places the herdsman and the veterinarian in a dilemma since frequently those cows that are affected are the best producers.

Prophylactic use of GnRH has shown some success in reducing the prevalence of cysts in herds. It has been recommended that all cows should be treated with 100–200 μg of GnRH 12–14 days postpartum (Kesler and Garverick, 1982). Whether it is cost-effective has not been calculated.

Luteal deficiency

Progesterone is necessary for the maintenance of pregnancy. Until 150–200 days of pregnancy, and perhaps in some cases to term, the main source of the hormone is the corpus luteum so that if this is not completely formed or it is not functioning adequately then insufficient progesterone is produced and the pregnancy fails. Luteal deficiency has been suspected of causing infertility for many years and, although proof is difficult, cyclic non-breeders (repeat breeders) are frequently treated on this assumption.

It is impossible on rectal palpation to differentiate between a normal and abnormal corpus luteum; there is a natural variation in luteal size and the position of the corpus luteum within the ovary is variable and thus makes estimation of its size very difficult. By determining progesterone concentrations in blood or milk it has been possible to make some assessment of luteal function. Erb et al. (1976) found that in 50% of cows that ovulated, yet failed to conceive, the plasma progesterone values 6 days or more after ovulation were lower than in the group that conceived. Extended low progesterone concentrations during the early luteal phase have been reported in 2% of cows (Bulman and Lamming, 1978) and 18% of cows (Jackson, 1981) although some of the individuals which had this pattern conceived. In a study involving 91 cows postpartum (Edgerton and Hafs, 1973) the plasma progesterone values during the first dioestrus after calving were 34% lower in 10% of the cows than during the second cycle. In the same study, the progesterone levels were similar in both pregnant and non-pregnant cows up to 11 days of the cycle; however, in the former group they increased thereafter but in the group that had failed the levels reached a plateau before decreasing. Diagnosis of luteal deficiency, using single blood or milk samples, is unreliable since there are wide fluctuations in the same animal.

LH is luteotrophic in the cow (Simmons and Hansel, 1964; Donaldson et al., 1965). Thus if hCG or GnRH are injected after ovulation they may stimulate the development and function of the corpus luteum or, more likely, induce accessory corpus luteum formation. This is one of the 'holding injections' used in infertile cows; however, there is no statistically significant effect in improving pregnancy rates (Greve and Lehn-Jensen, 1982; Sreenan and Diskin, 1983).

Alternatively, hCG or GnRH might be given 11–13 days after service or AI since, in the absence of pregnancy it would be several days before the corpus luteum would be starting to regress (see Chapter 3), and if the stimulus for the maternal recognition of pregnancy is weak, it might prevent the corpus luteum regressing and provide sufficient time for pregnancy to become established. Studies with GnRH have produced equivocal results.

MacMillan et al. (1986) improved first- and second-service pregnancy (conception) rates by 11.5 and 15.6%, respectively, when cows were treated 11–13 days after insemination. Sheldon and Dobson (1993) improved pregnancy rates from 50.6% in untreated controls to 60.0% in cows treated with GnRH on day 11. Conversely, Jubb et al. (1990) were unable to show any significant improvement when used on day 12. If an improvement is obtained then it must occur either as a result of the formation of accessory corpora lutea, or by disrupting normal folliculogenesis. In the latter, this would delay the timing of the preovulatory rise in oestradiol until a new wave of follicles have developed, thus affecting the formation of oxytocin receptors and delaying luteolysis (see Chapter 1).

Progesterone implants have been used at a dose rate of 800 mg for an adult cow. They are expensive and, in the author's experience, of little value because of the low level of absorption.

Hormonal imbalance

There is much conflicting evidence concerning the relationships between hormonal imbalance and infertility, probably influenced to some extent by the errors inherent in measuring hormone concentrations in a limited number of peripheral blood samples.

It is known that the rate of transport of the oocyte and zygote along the uterine tube is under the influence of oestrogens and progesterone (Whitney and Burdick, 1936, 1938). Thus, if there is an incorrect balance of these hormones there may be accelerated or retarded passage of the zygote, so that it reaches the uterus at a time when the environment is hostile to its survival. It has also been known for some time that in order to have good embryo survival after embryo transfer the recipient's and donor's oestrous cycles must be synchronized within one day of each other (Rowson et al., 1969; Newcombe and Rowson, 1975).

Elevated plasma progesterone concentrations have been recorded in beef heifers that failed to conceive (Corah et al., 1974), in cows that were infused with ACTH (Gwazdauskas et al., 1972) and in Guernsey cows subjected to high environmental temperatures (Abilay et al., 1975). Abnormal plasma oestrogen concentration on days 3 and 4 of the oestrous cycle have been observed in cows

with abnormal embryos (Ayalon, 1973). Erb et al. (1976) found higher plasma oestrogen concentrations 8 and 12 hours after oestrous in fertile cows compared with others.

Even if an imbalance could be demonstrated it is doubtful if it could be sensibly and accurately corrected. The association with embryonic death is discussed further on p. 426.

A positive relationship between luteal phase progesterone concentrations in the peripheral blood or milk and embryo survival has been found by some workers, whilst others have found no such relationship.

Fatty liver syndrome

A number of reports (Morrow, 1976; McCormack, 1978; Reid, 1980) have described the frequent occurrence of fatty liver in high-yielding dairy cows. This condition is probably due to mobilization of body fat reserves, especially subcutaneous, to meet the energy deficit which occurs in milk production, particularly in relation to the supply of endogenous and exogenous protein (Roberts et al., 1981). The consequences of high fat mobilization have been reported as being ketosis, postpartum metritis and retained placenta (Sommer, 1975; Morrow et al., 1979). However, the latter authors described a high incidence of metabolic and infectious diseases in one herd of 600 cows.

In this syndrome there is also evidence of depressed fertility (Reid et al., 1979). In a study of two groups of cows, one with severe fatty liver (> 30% fat in liver parenchyma) and one with mild fatty liver (< 20% fat in the liver parenchyma), the mean calving intervals and services per conception were 395.5 days and 2.39 services and 359 days and 1.73 services, respectively. Five of 10 cows with severe fatty liver had calving intervals greater than 400 days, averaged over all the previous lactations, whilst more of the cows in the mild fatty groups had an average calving interval greater than 400 days. Similar effects upon fertility have been demonstrated in a 100-cow Friesian herd over a 2-year period with the calving indices for the two years being 402 and 397 days. The first service pregnancy rates were not too bad, being 58 and 55%, respectively, but the main factor responsible for the extended calving indices was the prolonged calving to first service interval which was 99 and 81 days for each of the 2 years (Higgins and Anderson, 1983). This may have been due to a delay in the time to first postpartum ovulation which, in cows with moderate and severe fatty liver, was shown to be delayed (Reid et al., 1983). Other evidence of impaired reproductive function in cows with mild and moderate fatty liver is a shorter interval, i.e. average of 16 days between the first and second ovulation, in the latter group compared with the former group, which was 21 days (Watson, 1985).

The presence of fatty liver can be shown by biopsy but this is a difficult and sometimes dangerous procedure. Evidence of impaired liver function and poor fertility has been obtained by measuring blood cholesterol and the enzyme aspartate aminotransferase in cows 8 weeks before calving; the former is lowered, the latter is elevated (Lotthammer, 1975; Sommer, 1975). Although serum albumin values normally decline in cows after calving, eventually returning to precalving values at 7–9 weeks (Rowlands et al., 1980), depressed values are associated with fatty liver (Reid et al., 1979). In the two groups of cows described above, mean serum albumen and plasma glucose values, respectively, between 1 and 8 weeks after calving, were 30.2 g/l and 2.33 mmol/l in the mild fatty liver group and 26.79 g/l and 2.14 mmol/l in the severe fatty liver group. These differences were significant ($P < 0.05$). Since albumen is synthesized in the liver, impaired liver functions will influence its production, whilst if fat has replaced glycogen in the liver parenchyma total glycogen reserves will be reduced. The evidence of an inverse correlation between serum albumen levels and fertility is conflicting; early work (Rowlands et al., 1977) demonstrated one, but subsequently this has not been substantiated (Rowlands et al., 1980), although it is likely that cows that are able to regulate their serum albumen levels should have better fertility.

Treatment is not possible; usually there will be eventual recovery. Some attempts to prevent the condition from occurring can be made by ensuring that cows are not excessively fat at calving and receive adequate energy thereafter to exclude the need for excess fat mobilization. Morrow et al. (1979) stress the importance of preventing excess energy intake during the end of the previous lactation and the dry period.

Lameness

Although some studies have failed to show any influence of foot disorders on fertility (Cobo-Abreu et al., 1979; Dohoo and Martin, 1984), a recent survey involving 770 cows over 1491 lactations has shown reduced fertility as measured by calving to first service interval, calving to conception interval and overall conception rates (Lucey et al., 1986). The greatest effect occurred in cows that had solar or white line lesions during the 36–70 days after calving, the time when cows would be served first; the calving to first service interval was extended by 17 days and the calving–conception interval by 30 days. Overall conception rates during the 63 days before the lameness was diagnosed were 31% compared with 40% at other times. Heel lesions had a particularly serious effect on conception rates. Treatment of lameness was followed by improved fertility (Lucey et al., 1986).

MANAGEMENT FACTORS

Nutrition

Studies into the effect of nutrition upon reproduction in cattle have increased in recent years because, with the elimination of specific infectious agents causing infertility, the move towards higher production and the use of new feedstuffs, its role has been considered to be more important. The main problem in determining the influence of nutrition is the time interval between the implementation of dietary change and its apparent effect. The response of the animal can also be complicated because of the interaction of a number of factors: the current and previous nutrition, the existing bodily condition and previous changes and the present and previous level of production.

At present, little is known about how nutritional deficiencies and excesses cause infertility. They may act via the hypothalamus and anterior pituitary, thus influencing the production of gonadotrophins, or directly on the ovaries, thus influencing oogenesis and endocrine function. Perhaps nutrition influences sperm transport, fertilization, early cell division and the development of the embryo and fetus.

It is not proposed to describe the nutrient requirements and feeding regimens of cattle; this information is described by experts elsewhere.

However, it is the aim of the author to highlight the important relationships between nutrition and reproductive function.

Effect on the time of puberty

Puberty, as determined by the appearance of the first oestrous, occurs between 5 and 20 months of age; body size rather than age is the main stimulus (Joubert, 1954; Asdell, 1955; Reid et al., 1964). At puberty, beef heifers are 50% and dairy heifers 35–45% of their mature weight; thus, pubertal weights for Friesians are 240–260 kg, Herefords 270–300 kg and Aberdeen Angus 230–250 kg.

The effect of dietary intake on the time of onset of puberty was clearly demonstrated by Asdell (1955), who found that when he fed Friesian heifers on high, medium and low planes of nutrition puberty occurred at 9, 11 and 15 months of age, respectively. As the feeding level increases, the age at puberty decreases; even the feeding level before weaning in beef heifers has a significant effect (Wiltbank et al., 1966). In Friesian heifers the age at puberty decreased 0.77 days for each additional 0.45 kg body weight at 6 months and 0.36 days for each additional 0.45 kg body weight between 6 and 12 months of age. These results demonstrate the importance of adequate feeding during calfhood to ensure the early onset of puberty.

Effect on the heifer from puberty to first calving

Although heifers can conceive at the onset of puberty it is not advisable for them to become pregnant because, since they are not fully grown, dystocia will be common at their first calving because of fetomaternal disproportion (see Chapter 11). The weights of Friesian heifers at their first service usually range between 325 and 440 kg. The precise weight will depend upon the breed of the sire and overall farm policy; inevitably it will be a compromise, since breeding at an early age can improve the lifetime productivity of an individual animal. Pinney et al. (1962) found that beef-breed heifers which calved at 2 years of age, rather than 3 years, produced 0.8 more calf per cow at 10% less cost over their entire production life.

Once cyclical activity has commenced at puberty it should continue uninterrupted, apart from pregnancy, throughout the life of the animal. There is no evidence that growth restrictions in early life will influence reproductive performance once the feeding of a normal diet has been implemented (Alden, 1970). However, dietary insufficiency or, in some circumstances, dietary excess can have profound effects upon reproductive function. During the immediate postpubertal period the heifer is under considerable stress, since she is continuing growing to physical maturity whilst conceiving and maintaining a pregnancy to term. The most severe effect of inadequate nutrition is the cessation of cyclical activity, although other less severe manifestations are silent oestrous, ovulatory defects, conception failure and fetal and embryonic death.

Some of the earliest studies on the effect of feeding levels on heifer fertility were reported by Asdell (1955), who demonstrated that Holstein heifers which were bred at 15 months of age and had been fed during the period before service on low, medium and high planes of nutrition required 1.89, 1.64 and 1.33 services per conception, respectively.

Although protein, vitamins and mineral deficiencies are capable of producing poor fertility, the main effect is that of deficient energy intake. This has been demonstrated in a study by Leaver (1977), involving Friesian heifers fed from 6 weeks before to 6 weeks after artificial insemination on three different levels of nutrition. These were referred to as high, medium and low, and gave mean growth rates of 0.68, 0.50 and 0.34 kg/day, respectively. The pregnancy rates to first service for the three groups were 65, 69 and 67%. When heifers were given a body score at the time of insemination and the pregnancy rates were corrected for the level of nutrition the results were 42, 72, 70 and 63% for poor, moderate, good and very good bodily condition, respectively, although it must be stressed that these results were not statistically significant. Heifers that are in poor or moderate condition achieve improved conception rates when dietary intake is increased but those in good condition show no response. This study also shows that if heifers are overfed and are fat there is a depression in fertility; the mechanism responsible is not known.

In a study involving 100 Friesian dairy heifers, Ducker et al. (1985) studied the effects of different levels of energy intake during the last 10 weeks of pregnancy and during early lactation on reproduction. They used 'high' (H) levels of feeding (83.6 MJ/day) and 'low' (L) levels (64.6 MJ/day)

Table 22.3 The relationship between loss of body condition during the first five weeks postpartum and reproductive performance

	Body condition score[a]		
	A	B	C
Number of cows	17	64	12
Mean days to first ovulation	27 ± 2	31 ± 2	42 ± 5
Mean days to first observed oestrus	48 ± 6	41 ± 3	62 ± 7
Mean days to first service	68 ± 4	67 ± 2	79 ± 5
Mean first service pregnancy (conception) rate	65	53	17
Mean services per conception	1.8 ± 0.4	2.3 ± 0.2	2.3 ± 0.4

After Butler and Smith (1989).
[a] Body condition scores: A = < 0.5 body condition score lost, B = 0.5–1.0 body condition score lost, C = > 1.0 body condition score lost.

during pregnancy, and 'high' (H) (146.8 MJ/day) and 'low' (L) (119.8 MJ/day) in weeks 6–18 of lactation. High levels of feeding during pregnancy reduced significantly the interval to first ovulation. However, the calving to first artificial insemination interval was not affected. Heifers that were on a HH regime suffered a greater level of embryonic death, the best fertility as measured by the first service pregnancy rate and calving to conception interval were those on a HL regime. None of the heifers suffered severe weight loss which probably would have depressed fertility if it had occurred.

Additional feeding after insemination improved conception rates only in those heifers growing at less than 750 g/day before insemination (Rochet, 1973). Drew (1978) found no effect of liveweight or condition score at the time of service on pregnancy rate. However, if she increased the energy intake by supplementary feeding with rolled barley, equivalent to 20 MJ/head/day for 6 weeks before the service date, so that liveweight gain increased from 0.23 kg/day to 0.43 kg/day, the conception rates increased from 50 to 60%. It is recommended that dairy heifers should be growing at a rate of 0.7 kg/day to achieve optimum fertility.

Long-term feeding at high levels has been shown to reduce pregnancy rates and increase the proportion of barren animals (Wickersham and Schultz, 1963; Reid et al., 1964). It also increases the prevalence of dystocia but, surprisingly, this risk can be reduced by restricting food intake in late gestation in beef heifers, so reducing the birth weight of the calf (Young, 1970); such an approach is fraught with danger. Provided that they are well fed postpartum there is generally no adverse effect

on subsequent fertility (Young, 1970), although the same author (Young, 1965, 1967, 1968) demonstrated that range heifers are particularly sensitive to the effects of malnutrition during the later stages of their first pregnancy if they have not reached physical maturity. This is demonstrated by delays in returning to oestrous after calving and poor conception rates at first service.

Energy requirements and body weight changes in pregnancy and lactation

In many dairy cows during early lactation the rate of increase in milk production exceeds feed intake. As a consequence, there is a negative energy balance which results in the cow mobilizing her energy reserves with a resultant loss of weight. The negative energy balance is at its maximum 1–2 weeks after calving and it can persist beyond the 5–6 week period when peak yields occur, and if it is not corrected it can extend well beyond the time when it would be appropriate to start serving cows, the earliest service date (see p. 431). In high-yielding cows, appetite, even when using energy density diets, may not be able to satisfy energy requirements until yields have started to decline.

It has been shown that there is a direct correlation between milk yield and negative energy balance and also a direct correlation between negative energy balance and the time interval after calving to the first ovulation; the latter becoming significant within the first 2 weeks of lactation (Butler and Smith, 1989).

How does inadequate energy intake affect fertility? It will reduce the time interval to the first ovulation, which normally occurs 17–42 days postpartum (see Chapter 7), thereby delaying the time interval to the first insemination if it extends beyond the earliest service date (Table 22.3) (Butler and Smith, 1989). However, in most dairy herds the main effect of inadequate energy intake and negative energy balance will be on conception rates. It is suggested that reduced conception rates also arise because of delays to first ovulation postpartum (Butler and Smith, 1989). While this might be true of high-yielding cows in severe negative energy balance, the author cannot accept that this is the reason in most cows.

McClure (1961) showed that cows which lost the least weight after calving and were gaining weight at the time of service had a higher chance of conceiving to first service than those cows which exhibited a lower recovery of body weight during early lactation. In a group of Ayrshire cows, those which gained weight over the service period had a 77.6% conception rate to first service compared with 16% for those which lost weight (King, 1968). The same author suggested that there is a change of 1% in conception rate to first service for every 1% change in liveweight. McClure (1970) reported that a 10% fall in liveweight postpartum was associated with low fertility. A more positive approach to the effect of energy-deficient diets in dairy cows is recommended by Morris (1976). He states that if the weight loss between calving and 60 days postpartum is 5% there should be concern; if it exceeds 10% then there is likely to be poor fertility. Action needs to be taken before the problem occurs, which means regular weighing, accurate body scoring or the use of a girth band measure regularly after calving. Some confirmation can be obtained by noting the response of the cows to the introduction of an energy supplement diet, such as barley, or of feeding above yield (Morris, 1976). Ward (1968) and Lamond (1968) agreed that there was a body weight below which fertility was lowered; the highest rates of infertility were found in the cows which were in the poorest condition. Warnick et al. (1967) found that beef cows were infertile when losing weight, whilst a 2% increase in liveweight in the 3 weeks before service improved conception rates (Moller and Shannon, 1972). Increasing the energy intake in Friesian cows during a 9 week period around the time of insemination did not improve pregnancy rates when compared with controls (Ducker et al., 1984). However, these same authors identified an

effect of milk yield, since those cows that were giving high yields at 21 days of lactation had poorer fertility when compared with those with more modest values. Conversely, those with high cumulative yields by day 21 of lactation became pregnant more readily.

Attempts have been made to assess the energy balance of lactating cows by estimating blood metabolites. A relationship between reduced blood glucose levels, excessive weight loss at the time of mating and depressed pregnancy rates was demonstrated by McClure (1968). He found that blood glucose values less than 30 mg/dl were associated with reduced fertility. Morris (1976) also recommends this as a method of identifying an energy deficit, using either this value or one less than twice the standard deviation below the mean for dry cows in the herd. However, the measurement of non-esterified fatty acids is a more accurate method of assessing energy status but the collection and processing is more difficult (Morris, 1976).

The mechanisms which are involved in mediating the effects of energy deficit on reproductive function are many and varied. Inadequate energy has been shown to reduce the pulse frequency of LH in the postpartum cow. This facet of gonadotrophin secretion has been shown to play an important role in the return of cyclical ovarian activity (see Chapter 7). There is some evidence that hypoglycaemia and hypoinsulinaemia occur with an energy deficit, both of which may directly or indirectly influence gonadotrophin release. In the rat, for example, it has been shown that an insulin receptor located in the hypothalamus may modulate GnRH output. In addition, insulin has been shown to exert an effect upon the ovary that is similar to that of gonadotrophins (Poretsky and Kalin, 1987). It has been postulated that low insulin concentrations may limit the responsiveness of the ovary to endogenous gonadotrophin secretion, thus affecting ovulation and corpus luteum formation (Butler and Smith, 1989). Finally, the role of neural opioid peptides must also be considered since an energy deficit will cause increased secretion of these substances which have been shown to reduce pulsatile GnRH, and hence LH secretion. Signs of energy deficiency are usually first shown in first calf heifers, followed by second calf heifers, with mature cows least affected.

Perhaps a further method of relating energy

intake and fertility may arise from changes in milk protein concentrations (Hagermeister, 1978); these are affected primarily by the energy intake not the protein intake of the cows. He demonstrated a significant inverse relationship between the calving–conception interval and milk protein concentration; thus mean values of 2.6% were related to a 105-day calving–conception interval compared with 3.4% for an interval of 94 days.

Protein. Evaluation of the protein requirements of cattle in relation to reproductive function are subject to the same limitations previously described for nutrition studies in general. Many early experiments failed to ensure that diets containing different levels of digestible crude protein were isocaloric (Tassel, 1967a). In addition, due to ruminal metabolism, crude protein dry matter (CPDM) intake alone does not adequately describe protein requirements of a dairy cow. The assessment of the supply of rumen degradable and undegradable protein probably is a more meaningful measurement with regard to fertility (Ferguson and Chalupa, 1989). Using logistic regression analysis, the same authors were able to show that the age of the cow, as well as dietary energy intake, modified the impact of protein intake on reproduction. For example, fertility was reduced in mature cows (4+ lactations) fed diets containing 19% compared with 16% CPDM and rumen digestible crude protein levels of 72 versus 62%. The fertility of cows in their second or third lactations was not affected greatly. First-lactation cows had better conception rates (65 versus 36%) when fed diets of 16% CPDM that contained more rumen degradable protein.

It is generally recommended that for a dairy cow producing more than 30 kg of milk per day, 16% crude protein per dry matter is the optimum. In a study involving high-yielding Friesian cows (Treacher et al., 1976), it was found that if cows were fed 75% of the recommended crude protein intake the mean calving to first oestrus interval was extended to 46 days compared with 35 days for the control group on a normal intake; however, the calving interval was shorter in the low protein group. In a more recent study involving high-yielding cows producing more than 30 kg of milk per day at peak lactation, a definite influence of different protein intake was demonstrated (Jordan and Swanson, 1979). For a period from 4 to 95 days postpartum, groups of cows were fed isocaloric diets containing three different levels of crude protein: 12.7%, 16.3% and 19.3%. Cows on the highest level had the shortest interval to first oestrus, but in all other aspects (services per conception, calving interval) the best results were obtained with the lowest level of protein intake. Similar results have been reported by Hagermeister (1980) who showed that if they fed two levels of crude protein (16 and 19%) conception rates were 56 and 44% and services per conception 1.79 and 2.25, respectively. However, in an experiment in which isocaloric diets containing 80 and 100% of the US National Research Council recommended levels of crude protein were fed during the last 60 days of gestation, there was no difference in the incidence of reproductive problems or performance, although pregnancy rates in both groups were poor (Chew et al., 1984). No evidence of impaired reproductive performance was detected in a small number of cows fed for three successive lactations on crude protein levels of 13, 15 and 17% (Edwards et al., 1980).

High levels of protein in the diet have been shown to adversely affect fertility (Gould, 1969). The feeding of excess degradable protein results in increased ammonia and urea production in the rumen. These substances are toxic to spermatozoa, oocytes and embryos, so that elevated blood concentrations might influence the uterine environment. In addition, they may also have an effect upon the hypothalamic–pituitary–ovarian axis. Others have reported that 20% dietary CPDM increased the incidence of retained placenta, dystocia and postpartum metritis compared with a 13% level. It had been suggested that there was also impaired intrauterine leucocyte function in cows fed the higher level (Anderson and Barton, 1987). In many cases it is exacerbated by feeding inadequate dietary energy so that the rumen flora are unable to utilize the available protein.

The mechanisms involved in the effects of dietary protein on reproductive function have not been studied in detail. It is likely that it does so via the hypothalamic–pituitary–ovarian axis. Jordan and Swanson (1979) reported that cows fed diets of 19% CPDM had increased basal blood LH concentrations and an exaggerated LH response to GnRH stimulation. Some effect on basal LH concentrations was also found in non-lactating ovariectomized cows (Blauwiekel et al., 1986). The influence of levels of dietary protein on blood progesterone concentrations have been shown to be variable; however, Ferguson and Chalupa (1989), using logistic regression analysis, found that serum progesterone concentrations decreased as CPDM was increased from 13 to 15% but changed little when it was increased from 15 to 20%. The source of dietary protein can also affect peripheral progesterone concentrations (Garverick et al., 1971).

Results from attempts to correlate serum urea nitrogen concentrations and fertility have generally been equivocal, so that interpretation of such values can be difficult.

Minerals and Vitamins. While it is generally agreed that micronutrients (minerals and vitamins) have an effect upon fertility of cattle there are conflicting opinions about the significance of apparent deficiencies. This is because of the inherent difficulties of accurately determining nutrient requirements; our lack of knowledge of the interaction of micronutrients in the alimentary tract; and because many of the studies that determined nutrient requirements were done 40 or more years ago when yields were much lower.

Phosphorus. It has been estimated that the normal requirements for phosphorus in the cow for the maintenance of pregnancy are about 13 g/day, with about 7 g extra for each 4.5 litres (1 gallon) of milk (Deas et al., 1979). Normal diets that are fed to cows are adequate and should ensure normal fertility; however, because of the interaction with calcium, deficiencies may occur. The evidence for the importance of hypophosphataemia as a cause of infertility is conflicting.

The provision of supplementary phosphorus has been shown to improve the breeding performance of grazing cattle (Sheehy, 1946; Hart and Mitchell, 1965; Tassel, 1967b). A number of authors have described infertility as shown by anoestrus, suboestrus, irregular cycles and low conception rates (Hignett and Hignett, 1951; Morris, 1976) in the absence of other clinical signs of phosphorus deficiency. Morris (1976) suggests that a blood phosphorus level of less than 4 mg/dl in affected or susceptible animals, i.e. those at peak production, confirms the diagnosis. He found that deficiency normally occurs when the phosphorus content of the feed is less than 0.20% or even 0.26%. High-yielding cows need phosphorus in excess of that available in pasture but since cereal grains contain large amounts, deficiencies are unlikely to occur.

In a controlled experiment with Ayrshire and Friesian heifers, Littlejohn and Lewis (1960) found no evidence of reduced fertility associated with an imbalance of calcium and phosphorus.

If hypophosphataemia is suspected, a rapid response can follow the feeding of dicalcium phosphate (150–200 g/day) or bone meal. It is important to ensure that the ratio of calcium to phosphorus is 1:1.

Copper. Copper deficiency, either direct or indirect (the latter being due to excessive molybdenum or iron intake and also possibly excess dietary sulfur, calcium and zinc) has been said to cause delayed puberty, anoestrus, suboestrus or poor pregnancy rates. When this occurs in association with other signs of hypocuprosis, such as anaemia, poor growth, bleached coat colour and diarrhoea, a diagnosis is likely. However, opinions differ as to the relationship between copper status and reproduction. A number of studies have demonstrated poor fertility associated with low blood copper concentrations followed by improvements after copper supplementation (Bennets et al., 1948; Munro, 1957; Pickering, 1975). However, there are an equal number of studies suggesting that fertility is not related to blood copper concentrations (Littlejohn and Lewis, 1960; Larson et al., 1980) and that copper supplementation has no positive effect (Whitaker, 1980). Frequently, the plasma or serum value used to diagnose hypocupraemia is incorrect. Suttle (1993) emphasizes the need to use a threshold value of 9.4 μmol/l (0.6 mg/l) and states that values below 4 μmol/l are probably required before health or fertility is compromised.

Hypocuprosis induced by high molybdenum intake in the diet has been recognized for many years in the so-called 'teart' pastures in south-west England. However, it is only where pastures contain levels > 500 μmol or 5 mg/kg is there likely to be a copper-responsive infertility problem (Suttle, 1993). This has been confirmed in Canadian studies of dairy herds fed on silage where a positive correlation between fertility and the copper:molybdenum ratio in the diet was found. Liming of pastures to maintain the correct pH for the growth of grass and other forage crops can affect the uptake of molybdenum by plants, so that even at normal rates of application it is possible to change the pH sufficiently to increase the uptake of molybdenum (Phillipo, 1983).

Whilst the effect of high molybdenum has always been assumed to be due to hypocuprosis, a study by Phillipo et al. (1982a,b) has provided evidence that molybdenum may have a direct effect upon reproduction. In their study, prepubertal heifer calves subjected to diets with molybdenum and iron supplementation, both of which produced comparable levels of hypocuprosis, were compared with a normal control group without supplementation, and a reduced food intake group. Neither growth rate nor time interval to first oestrus nor pregnancy rates at the fourth oestrus were affected in the iron-induced hypocuprosis group. However, in the molybdenum supplemented group (+5 mg Mo/kg dry matter) the interval to first oestrus was extended, and the pregnancy rates at the fourth oestrus were reduced. Furthermore, there was evidence of a direct effect of molybdenum on the hypothalamus–pituitary, since plasma LH pulse frequencies were reduced. Molybdates have also been shown to interact with steroid hormone receptors (Dahmer et al., 1984).

Perhaps in the light of recent studies we need to reconsider the role of copper deficiency *per se* in causing infertility. In a study involving 17 beef-suckler herds in which average herd plasma copper concentrations ranged from 0.16 to 0.92 mg/l within one month of mating, average pregnancy rates for the herds ranged from 37 to 65%, and showed no correlation. In fact the herd with the lowest plasma copper value had a pregnancy rate of 63% (Phillipo et al., 1982). Furthermore, in four farms with low copper status, supplementation with 100 mg of copper before mating did not improve the pregnancy rates compared with untreated controls. Thus, copper *per se* does not appear to be a major factor in influencing the fertility of beef suckler herds (Phillipo et al., 1982).

Cobalt. Deficiency of this element can occur in association with copper deficiency. Usually poor fertility will be present at the same time as other obvious signs of deficiency such as anaemia and poor bodily condition; the only accurate diagnostic procedure is the estimation of liver vitamin B_{12} (Morris, 1976). As with many supposedly occurring trace element deficiencies it exerts its effect upon fertility in a number of different ways, viz. increased number of 'silent' oestruses, poor conception rates, and irregular interoestrus intervals. Sometimes poor fertility in apparently normal cows can be corrected following cobalt supplementation.

Manganese. Manganese has a ubiquitous role in reproductive function being involved in steroid synthesis. Both the pituitary gland and ovaries are relatively rich in this trace element. A variety of reproductive disorders which depress fertility in cows have been blamed on manganese deficiency; these include: anoestrus, poor follicular development, delayed ovulation, silent oestrus, and reduced conception rates. Under normal circumstances it is likely that normal pasture will provide the necessary requirement of 80 ppm in the food (Alderman and Stranks, 1967); however some foods (maize silage) are low in manganese. In addition, there is an interaction with the calcium: phosphorus ratio in the diet, with some evidence that high liming of pasture can cause manganese deficiency.

Iodine and goitrogens. Reproductive failure resulting from iodine deficiency is invariably related to impaired thyroid function in the dam, embryo or fetus, and in the last two it can cause embryonic death, abortion, stillbirth, or weak goitrous calves. A high level of stillbirth, sometimes associated with a delayed second stage of parturition, has been observed in herds fed high-quality succulent grass heavily treated with nitrogen. There is good evidence that treatment with iodized oil injection can improve the deficient status (Logan et al., 1991; Mee, 1991). Simple iodine deficiency can occur because of an intake below 0.8 ppm (Alderman, 1970).

Disturbance of thyroid function can also be due to goitrogenic substance present in kale, lentils, soya bean, linseed and certain strains of white clover (Tassell, 1976b). High level of goitrogenic substance can produce anoestrus in heifers (David, 1965).

Zinc. Zinc deficiency has been shown to have an adverse effect upon reproductive function in the male of many species. Its influence on reproductive function in the cow and heifer is not clear.

Phyto-oestrogens. When cows ingest large quantities of these substances they become anoestrus, with large ovarian cysts, vulval and cervical enlargement and poor conception rates (Morris, 1976). Such substances are found in subterranean clover, certain strains of red and white clover and lucerne.

Selenium and vitamin E. It is difficult to separate the effects of selenium and/or vitamin E deficiency since both have a ubiquitous antioxidant function which protects a wide range of biological systems from oxidative degradation. In addition, they can exert a sparing effect upon each other. Probably because it is now possible to measure the selenium status of cows, by estimating the enzyme glutathione peroxidase in heparinized blood, the influence of selenium on reproductive function has been investigated.

In early studies (Trinder et al., 1969) it was shown that selenium and vitamin E injections reduced the incidence of placental retention, and as a consequence would improve the fertility of herds. However, since this initial study, the results published have been decidedly equivocal. Some studies have confirmed the beneficial effect of supplementation (Julien et al., 1976; Harrison et al., 1984), whilst others have failed to identify a positive response (Gwazdauskas et al., 1979; Schingoeth et al., 1981; Segerson et al., 1981; Hidiroglou et al., 1987). Selenium and vitamin E supplementation has also been shown to reduce the incidence of metritis and cystic ovaries when administered prepartum (Harrison et al., 1984). However, in this latter study it is worth stressing that even after the supplementation with vitamin E and selenium the incidence of postpartum metritis was 57% and that of cystic ovarian disease 19%, both values being very high. To demonstrate the contradictions in many of the studies comparisons were made of blood selenium concentrations and cystic ovarian disease (Mohammed et al., 1991). In cows with cystic ovaries the mean blood selenium concentration was 141 ng/ml compared with 136 ng/ml in normal cows. When a logistic regression analysis was performed, cows with selenium concentrations in blood that were greater than 169 ng/ml had twice the risk of developing cystic ovaries than cows with selenium values less than 108 ng/ml.

More recent studies involving selenium-deficient Friesian–Holstein heifers have shown improved pregnancy rates after treatment (Mac-Pherson et al., 1987).

Vitamin A. It is difficult to separate the effects of vitamin A and β-carotene since β-carotene is the plant precursor of vitamin A.

Vitamin A deficiency has been known to delay the onset of puberty in heifer calves and to cause cows to give birth to weak and abnormal calves (Byers et al., 1956). Madsen and Davis (1949) fed cows at different levels of carotene ranging from 30 to 240 mg/kg body weight per day over a number of years. They found that at the lowest level of 30 mg/kg no pregnancies occurred; at the 45 mg/kg level pregnancies occurred but the calves were born with clinical signs of vitamin A deficiency. A response with improved fertility was apparent when cows were fed at a level of 90 mg/kg. Evidence of a direct effect of vitamin A deficiency on reproduction is given by the study of Kuhlman and Gallup (1942), who reported 1.99 services per pregnancy in 21 cows receiving 86 μg of β-carotene per kilogram of body weight during the 90 days before service. The fertility was improved when β-carotene intakes were increased.

β-Carotene. In recent years there has been much interest in the direct influence of β-carotene (not as a precursor of vitamin A) on reproduction in cattle. This has arisen because of the feeding of maize silage, which is known to have a low β-carotene content of 2–4 mg/kg dry matter (Lotthammer, 1979), in association with poor-quality hay and straw. Diets deficient in β-carotene but adequate in vitamin A have been shown to increase the prevalence of extended follicular phases, and cause delayed ovulation, silent oestrus and anovulation with follicular cysts (Lotthammer et al., 1978). Cooke (1978) compared two groups of cows, one fed on maize silage which contained 2.22 μg/ml of β-carotene and the other on grass silage which contained 7.3 μg/ml. The fertility for the two groups showed that the first service pregnancy rates were 45 and 62%, and the number of services per pregnancy were 2.12 and 1.64, respectively. Reduced pregnancy rates were identified by Lotthammer et al. (1978). Bovine luteal tissue has one of the highest β-carotene content of any tissue (Friesecke, 1978) and it has been suggested that β-carotene may be involved in ovarian steroid production or corpus luteum formation (Jackson, 1981).

As with many studies involving the influence of specific nutrients on reproduction, conflicting results have been obtained. In Israel, Folman et al. (1979) reported that rations deficient in β-carotene had no adverse influence on reproductive performance in dairy heifers. In a similar study, involving 160 Friesian heifers (Ducker et al., 1984) fed on a diet based primarily on maize silage, although plasma β-carotene concentrations were low in the control group and high in the β-carotene-supplemented group, reproductive performance and growth rates were similar. β-Carotene supplementation of maize silage-fed cows did not alter the concentrations or variations in plasma LH or progesterone (Bindas et al., 1983). The reproductive performance for the supplemented and control groups were similar, i.e., the average intervals from calving to first oestrus were 74 and 64 days, the average calving to conceptions intervals were 95 and 102 days and the average numbers of services per pregnancy were 1.7 and 1.9, respectively. β-Carotene deficiency was reported to have no effect on the incidence of ovarian cysts or their responsiveness to treatment (Marcek et al., 1985).

The reasons for the different responses are difficult to explain. Perhaps in those studies where reduced reproductive performances occurred there was a concurrent vitamin A deficiency. Alternatively, perhaps β-carotene deficiency occurs at levels well below those normally found in practice, or perhaps the association between β-carotene deficiency and fertility is a reflection of some other unspecified deficiency (Ducker et al., 1984).

Investigation of nutritional factors as a cause of infertility

Frequently, it is not possible to determine accurately the specific cause of infertility because the clinical signs appear some time after the deficiency has occurred. Even when there is an improvement in response to a change in diet it is not possible to assume success, since changes in the season of the year and management can also have an effect, as seen when cows are turned out to grass in the spring.

In most cases the most important factor responsible for poor fertility is unknowingly underfeeding. This is due to:

1. Over-evaluation of the feeding value of forages: for this reason it is important to obtain accurate analysis of the major food components from truly representative samples.

2. Overestimation of feed intake under self-feed conditions: this is especially true of silage.

3. Failure to appreciate the reduction of forage intake caused by high concentrate intake (Alderman, 1970).

4. Underfeeding of concentrates due to the automatic dispensers giving short measure. Parker and Blowey (1976) found errors greater than 50% in some cases.

It is necessary to calculate the requirements of the cows for maintenance and production and then obtain accurate information about the precise quantities fed. Contributions from mineral licks and other free access sources are difficult to quantify. Weighing, the use of a girth band measure or condition scoring of a representative number of animals are also useful.

Metabolic profiles

Since the introduction of metabolic profile lists in 1970 (Payne et al., 1970) they have frequently been used to help in the evaluation of the nutritional status of a herd, particularly in relation to fertility. Although some are enthusiastic about them (Morris, 1976), others (Parker and Blowey, 1976) point to the importance of using them in conjunction with other more direct methods, particularly since there are dangers of using single blood concentrations to assess the metabolic status of an animal. The author has found them useful in persuading a reluctant farmer to improve feeding. Details of the tests and their evaluation are available elsewhere (Payne et al., 1970; Parker and Blowey, 1976; Morris, 1976).

Poor oestrus detection

In the absence of a bull, although the cow shows signs of being in oestrus, she may not be seen by the herdsman. It is generally accepted that oestrus detection rates are rarely better than 60%; in many cases they are less than 50%. Williamson et al. (1972) found that in one herd in Australia the herdsman correctly selected only 56% of cows that were known to be in oestrus as determined by continuous veterinary observation. King et al. (1976) found that the rate of oestrus detection preceding the third postpartum ovulation was 100% by continuous observation, but it was reduced to 64% when casual observations were made by the herdsman. The importance of trained staff to identify oestrus correctly was shown by Esslemont (1974); he found that in four units where such personnel were used the detection rate was 82–97%, yet with untrained staff it was 67%. How is the oestrus detection rate calculated? It has to be an estimate since it refers to the percentage of oestrous periods observed in relation to the number of oestrous periods that can be assumed to have occurred in that time (see p. 433)

Reasons for poor detection

There is frequently confusion between undetected oestrus and silent oestrus or suboestrus, the former referring to the situation where a cow shows behavioural signs but is not seen in oestrus whereas the latter refers to the cow not showing behavioural signs. King et al. (1976), using continuous observation of dairy herds, found that at the time of the third postpartum ovulation and for subsequent ovulations 100% of cows showed signs of oestrus. At the first postpartum ovulation only 50% showed signs and at the second 94% were detected. Similar figures have been reported by Morrow et al. (1966). When the same herds were subjected to casual observations, 64% of cows were seen in oestrus preceding the third ovulation, 44% for the second and 20% for the first ovulation (King et al., 1976). It is therefore unusual for normally fed, healthy cows to fail to show signs of behavioural oestrus once normal cyclical activity has been re-established postpartum.

What are the reasons for poor detection rates? These are outlined below:

1. *Ignorance of the 'true signs' of oestrus.* The true signs are described in Chapter 1; however, it is worthwhile stressing that the most reliable sign of oestrus, with the exception of a few cows which show head mounting, is standing to be mounted. Mounting of other cows is frequently a sign of approaching oestrus.

2. *The problems of herd size.* Most observers agree that closely associated with increased herd size there is a reduction in the accuracy and efficiency of oestrus detection (Fallon, 1962; Esslemont, 1974; Wood, 1976). In large herds cows lose their individual identity, they are not so accurately identified and hence the slight changes in behaviour which in a small herd might warn the herdsman of approaching oestrus are not seen. In large herds with increased mechanization there is a reduction in the man:cow ratio.

3. *The relatively short duration of oestrus.* Esslemont (1974) found that although the mean duration is 15 hours, 20% of cows are in oestrus for less

than 6 hours. Furthermore, because of the reduction in general farm activity, there is greater mounting activity during the hours of darkness (Williamson et al., 1972; Hurnick et al., 1975; Esslemont and Bryant, 1976).

4. *The nature of the housing.* Crowded collection areas, confined spaces and muddy floors sometimes prevent cows that are not in oestrus escaping from the attentions of other mounting cows and may not permit the ready grouping of sexually active individuals. A suitable 'loafing' area should be provided to enable cows to show oestrous behaviour.

Methods of improving oestrus detection

It is important to ensure that the cows in the herd are in fact undergoing cyclic reproductive activity; this can be done by careful rectal palpation as described earlier in this chapter.

A variety of methods can be used to improve the detection rate:

1. *Improved identification of the cows.* Good freeze-branding on the rumps, together with numbered collars or large ear tags, should preferably be used so that it is possible readily to identify the individual from all aspects. The herdsman must then be able to record the animal number immediately and permanently.

2. *The provision of adequate lighting.* This is most important at night but also during the day when cows are housed in dark yards; it enables cows to be seen showing behavioural signs and allows their accurate identification.

3. *Increased and regular observation of cows.* Esslemont (1973) recommends a rigid regimen involving three or four periods of observation for 15 or 30 minutes. In his study, the poorest detection rate of 69.6% was achieved by making three observations of 15 minutes at 8.00, 14.00 and 21.00 hours. Increasing the duration to 30 minutes improved the rate to 81.2%, whilst the best result of 84.1% was obtained by making four observations of 30 minutes at 8.00, 14.00, 21.00 and 24.00 hours. The absolute times are not critical and can be varied to suit the timetable of the farm, but they should not be made at milking, in the collecting yards, when concentrates are being fed or whilst mucking out is occurring.

4. *Use of oestrus-detection aids.* A 'heat mount' detector such as the KaMaR can be used. This

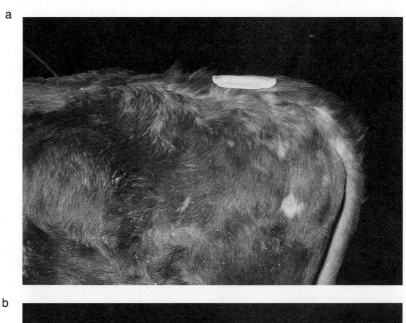

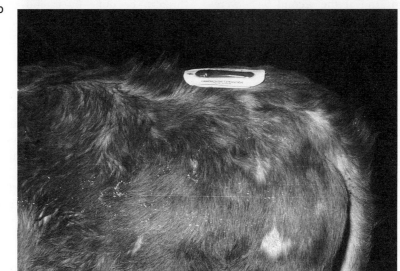

Fig. 22.19 KaMaR heat mount detector attached to the sacrum of a cow (a) before, (b) after activation.

consists of a soft, translucent plastic dome attached to a rectangle of canvas in which there is placed a soft plastic vial of red dye which is fixed with adhesive just cranial to the base of the tail (Figure 22.19). When a cow is mounted and the vial subjected to sufficient pressure, i.e. at standing oestrus, it is compressed, the dye escapes and the dome becomes red.

False positives can occur when the detector is activated by a cow rubbing the underside of a rail or in crowded collecting yards when a cow that is not in oestrous cannot escape the attentions of mounting cows. They can also become detached

when placed on wet coats or when the winter coat is being shed.

In 1977, Macmillan and Curnow in New Zealand reported on the use of the technique of tail-painting using brittle high-gloss, enamel paint to improve the detection of oestrus in cows after $PGF_{2\alpha}$ therapy. The paint was placed as a thick layer in the mid-line over the sacrum and base of tail. When a cow is in standing oestrus the mounting by other cows will result in the abrading and removal of the paint. In their study, an additional 6% of cows that were not observed in standing oestrus by the herdsman were correctly identified

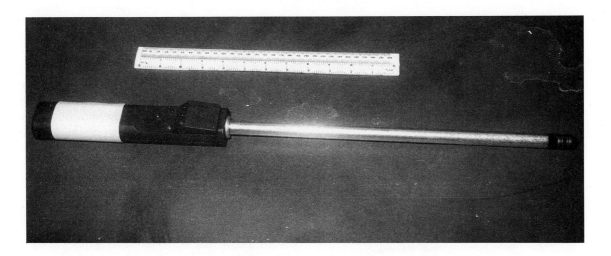

Fig. 22.20 Vaginal probe for measuring changes in electrical impedance in order to detect oestrus.

as being in oestrous using tail paint; incorrect diagnosis was made in 4.8% of cows and was assumed to be due to shedding of the coat. Improvements in detection have been found to be 11.2% (Ball et al., 1983). Although some false-positive detections of oestrous were made in cows and heifers when between 25 and 75% of paint remained (Kerr and McCaughey, 1984), pregnancy rates of 60% were obtained following artificial insemination on the observation of the condition of the tail paint.

Water-based paints or pastes have been used in the UK. It is important that these should be applied using a brush against the line of the hair to ensure good adhesion before smoothing in the direction of the hairline. There should be regular inspection of the paint so that repainting can be done if necessary.

5. *Use of teaser bulls, androgenized steers or cows.* Vasectomized or other sterile entires or androgenized steers can be used, either equipped with some form of marking device or in association with 'heat mount' detectors. They have not been very popular in the UK, largely because teaser bulls with good libido present a major safety hazard when allowed to run loose with the herd. Furthermore, where venereal diseases are present they represent a major health hazard because of their ability to transmit such diseases.

Androgenized cows can also be effective 'teasers' (Britt, 1980). By administering testosterone propionate in oil, by intramuscular injection every week for 3 weeks, a suitable teaser is prepared which can be used about 2 weeks after the last injection. Maintenance of sexual activity requires repeat treatment at intervals, but these androgenized cows have distinct advantages since they are safer and do not transmit venereal disease.

6. *Use of pedometers.* During oestrus the cow shows greater movement and activity (see p. 18). One method that has been used to identify this is the attachment of pedometers to the individual animals (Kiddy, 1977). Since then a number of devices have been made to record the frequency of movement; as yet their reliability is not good and they are expensive. With the rapid developments that are occurring in electronics, it is likely that some simple, inexpensive and reliable instrument will be developed.

7. *Use of closed-circuit television.* Television cameras, recorders and monitors are now much cheaper and more reliable than before. During the night, provided that there is adequate lighting and good animal identification, a continuous video recording can be made of the 'loafing' areas of the yard where cows are housed. The herdsman can then rapidly scan the recording in the morning and identify cows that are in oestrus.

8. *Use of dogs.* Dogs can be trained to detect odours associated with oestrous in cows. The sources of the odours are widespread throughout the genital tract and also appear in milk and urine (Kiddy et al., 1984).

9. *Vaginal probes to measure electrical resistance.* Since the early 1970s there has been considerable interest in measuring the changes that occur in the

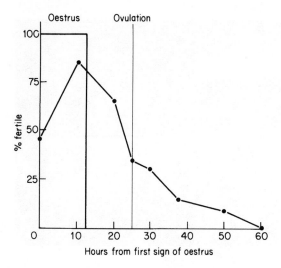

Fig. 22.21 Conception rates in the cow; the effect of the time of insemination in relation to oestrus and ovulation. (After Trimberger (1948).)

electrical resistance of vaginal mucus during the oestrous cycle. At oestrus it falls, and is associated with the rise in oestrogen. Generally, results have been disappointing (Foote et al., 1979; Cavestany and Foot, 1985). The reason for the variability in the measurements may well be related to the fact that the tip of the probe with its associated electrode is not in contact with vaginal mucus. In addition, the author has obtained aberrant results when the cow has recently urinated before the probe was inserted. An example of one such commercially available instrument is shown in Figure 22.20.

10. *Use of milk progesterone assays.* The return to oestrus in non-pregnant cows can be anticipated by the measurement of progesterone concentrations in sequential milk samples (see p. 449).

11. *Use of prostaglandins and progestogens.* Immediate improvements can be achieved by using either of these hormones. Since it is possible to anticipate approximately when oestrus will occur following their use (see Chapter 1) the herdsman can be extra vigilant at these times and can inseminate cows that are observed in oestrus. Failing this, no attempt need be made to detect oestrus and cows can be inseminated either once or twice at fixed times as outlined in Chapter 1.

Incorrect timing of artificial insemination

Oestrus is short in the cow, with ovulation occurring 10–12 hours after the end of oestrus. During the next six hours the oocyte travels about a third of the way down the uterine tube during which time fertilization occurs, about 30 hours after the onset of oestrus (Robinson, 1979). The best conception rates occur if insemination is made in the middle to the end of standing oestrus, i.e. 13–18 hours before ovulation. Cows may conceive if they are inseminated at the beginning of oestrus or even 36 hours after the end of oestrus but conception rates are reduced (Figure 22.21) (Trimberger, 1948).

When natural service is used there are no problems, since a cow will only stand for the bull when she is in oestrus, and under free-range conditions a cow may be served several times at each oestrus. The correct timing of artificial insemination is thus dependent upon true, accurate and early identification of oestrus, the accurate identification of the individual animal and informing the artificial insemination organization at the correct time. A cow that is first seen in oestrus in the morning is usually inseminated in the afternoon of the same day, whilst a cow that is first seen in oestrus in the afternoon is inseminated early the next day.

A number of observers (Hoffmann et al., 1974; Appleyard and Cook, 1976), using the determination of milk progesterone concentrations, have shown that between 10 and 15%, or perhaps even 22%, of cows are inseminated during the luteal phase of the oestrus cycle. It is not surprising that these animals fail to conceive. However, these figures do not include those animals which are inseminated during the follicular phase of the cycle at times that are not optimum for good conception rates. The main reasons for these errors are incorrect identification of animals that are in oestrus and failure to appreciate the true signs of oestrus. Frequently, where large numbers of cows are inseminated at the incorrect time, the oestrus detection rate is poor, thus generally reflecting a poor standard of herd management. The methods that should be used to obtain an improvement are those outlined above to improve the oestrus detection rate of the herd.

REFERENCES

Abilay, T. R., Johnson, H. D. and Nadan, M. (1975) *J. Dairy Sci.*, **58**, 1836.

Afiefy, M. M., Abu-Fadle, W. and Zaki, W. (1973) *Zentbl. Vet.*, **20A**, 256.

Al-Dahash, S. Y. A. and David, J. S. E. (1977a) *Vet. Rec.*, **101**, 296.

Al-Dahash, S. Y. A. and David, J. S. E. (1977b) *Vet. Rec.*, **101**, 323.

Al-Dahash, S. Y. A. and David, J. S. E. (1977c) *Vet. Rec.*, **101**, 342.

Alden, G. W. (1970) *Nutr. Abstr. Revs.*, **40**, 1167.

Alderman, G. (1970) *Vet. Rec.*, **70**, 35.

Alderman, G. and Stranks, M. H. (1967) *J. Sci. Food Agr.*, **18**, 151.

Anderson, G. W. and Barton, B. (1987) New England Feed Dealers Conference cited by Ferguson and Chalupa (1989).

Anderson, W. A. and Davis, C. L. (1958) In: *Reproduction and Infertility, 3rd Symposium*, ed. F. X. Gassner, New York: Pergamon Press.

Appleyard, W. T. and Cook, B. (1976) *Vet. Rec.*, **99**, 253.

Archibald, L. F., Norman, S. N., Tran, C., Lyle, S. and Thomas, P. G. A. (1991) *Vet. Med. US*, 1037.

Arthur, G. H. (1959) *Vet. Rec.*, **71**, 598.

Arthur, G. H. (1962) Unpublished data.

Asdell, S. A. (1952) *Vet. Rec.*, **64**, 831.

Asdell, S. A. (1955) *Cattle Fertility and Sterility*. Boston, Mass.: Little, Brown.

Ashmawy, A. A., Vogt, D. W., Garverick, H. A. and Young-quist, R. S. (1992) *J. Anim. Breed. Genet.*, **109**, 129.

Ayalon, N. (1973) *Annual Report Research No. 2*. Beit Dagan, Israel: Kimron Veterinary Institute.

Baillie, J. (1980) Ph.D. Thesis, University of Reading.

Baldwin, D. M. and Sawyer, C. H. (1974) *Endocrinology*, **94**, 1397.

Ball, P. J. H., Cowpe, J. E. D. and Harker, D. B. (1983) *Vet. Rec.*, **112**, 147.

Bartlett, P. C., Ngategize, P. K., Kaneene, J. B., Kirk, J. H., Anderson, S. M. and Mather, E. C. (1986) *Prev. Vet. Med.*, **4**, 33.

Bartosik, D., Romanoft, E. B., Watson, D. J. and Scricco, E. (1967) *Endocrinology*, **81**, 186.

Beck, C. C. and Ellis, D. J. (1960) *Vet. Med.*, **55**, 79.

Bennets, H. W., Beck, A. B. and Hartley, R. (1948) *Aust. Vet. J.*, **24**, 237.

Bertchtold, M. P. and Brummer, H. (1968) *Berl. Mun. Tierarztl. Wochenschr.*, **81**, 238.

Berchtold, M, P., Rusch, P., Thun, R. and King, S. (1980) *Zuchthg.*, **15**, 126.

Beynon, V. H. (1978) *The Disposal of Dairy Cows in England and Wales 1976–1977*. Exeter: University of Exeter Agricultural Economics Unit.

Bierschwal, C. J. (1966) *J. Amer. Vet. Med. Assn*, **149**, 1951.

Bierschwal, C. J., Garverick, H. A., Martin, C. E. and Youngquist, R. S. (1975) *J. Anim. Sci.*, **41**, 1660.

Biggers, J. D. and McFeely, R. A. (1966) *Adv. Reprod. Physiol.*, **1**, 29.

Bindas, E. M., Gwazdauskas, F. C., Aiello, R. J., Herbein, J. H., McGilliard, M. L. and Polan, C. E. (1983) *J. Dairy Sci.*, **67**, 1249.

Blauwiekel, R., Kincaid, R. L. and Reeves, J. J. (1986) *J. Dairy Sci.*, **69**, 439.

Booth, J. M. (1988) *Vet. Rec.*, **123**, 437.

Bosu, W. T. K. and Peter, A. T. (1987) *Theriogenology*, **28**, 725.

Boyd, H. and Munro, C. D. (1979) *Vet. Rec.*, **104**, 34.

Bozworth, R. W., Ward, G., Call, E. P. and Bonewitz, E. R. (1972) *J. Dairy Sci.*, **55**, 334.

Britt, J. H. (1980) In: *Current Therapy in Theriogenology*, ed. D. A. Morrow. Philadelphia: Saunders.

Britt, J. H., Morrow, D. A., Kittock, R. J. and Sequin, B. E. (1974) *J. Dairy Sci.*, **57**, 89.

Brown, J. L., Schoenemann, H. M. and Reeves, J. J. (1986) *Theriogenology*, **17**, 689.

Bulman, D. C. and Lamming, G. E. (1978) *J. Reprod. Fertil.*, **54**, 447.

Bulman, D. C., McKibbin, P. E., Appleyard, W. T. and Lamming, G. E. (1978) *J. Reprod. Fertil.*, **53**, 289.

Butler, W. R. and Smith, R. D. (1989) *J. Dairy Sci.*, **72**, 767.

Byers, J. H., Jones, J. R. and Bone, J. F. (1956) *J. Dairy Sci.*, **39**, 1556.

Carpenter, C. M., Williams, W. W. and Gilman, H. L. (1921) *J. Amer. Vet. Med. Assn*, **59**, 173.

Carroll, D. J., Pierson, R. A., Hauser, E. R., Grummer, R. R. and Combs, D. K. (1990) *Theriogenology*, **34**, 349.

Casida, L. E. and Chapman, A. B. (1951) *J. Dairy Sci.*, **34**, 1200.

Casida, L. E. and Wisnicky, W. (1950) *J. Anim. Sci.*, **9**, 238.

Casida, L. E., McShane, W. H. and Meyer, R. K. (1944) *J. Anim. Sci.*, **3**, 273.

Cavestany, D. and Foote, R. H. (1985) *Cornell Vet.*, **75**, 441.

Chew, B. P., Murdock, F. R., Riley, R. E. and Hillen, J. K. (1984) *J. Dairy Sci.*, **67**, 270.

Christian, J. J., Lloyd, J. A. and Davis, D. E. (1965) *Recent Prog. Hormone Res.*, **21**, 501.

Cobo-Abreu, R., Martin, S. W., Willoughby, R. A. and Stone, J. B. (1979) *Can. Vet. J.*, **20**, 191.

Cook, D. L., Parfet, J. R., Smith, C. A., Moss, G. E., Youngquist, R. S. and Garverick, H. A. (1991) *J. Reprod. Fertil.*, **91**, 19.

Cooke, B. C. (1978) *Anim. Prod. Abstr.*, 356.

Copmann, T. L. and Adams, W. C. (1981) *J. Amer. Vet. Med. Assn*, **101**, 1095.

Corah, L. R., Quealey, A. P., Dunn, T. G. and Kaltenbach, C. C. (1974) *J. Anim. Sci.*, **39**, 380.

Dahmer, M. K., Housley, P. R. and Pratt, W. B. (1984) *Ann. Rev. Physiol.*, **46**, 67.

David, J. S. E. (1965) Ph.D. Thesis, University of Bristol.

David, J. S. E., Long, S. M. and Eddy, R. G. (1976) *Vet. Rec.*, **98**, 417.

Dawson, F. L. M. (1975) *Vet. Rec.*, **96**, 218.

Day, N. (1991) *Vet. Med.*, 753.

Deas, D. W., Melrose, D. R., Reed, H. C. B., Vandeplassche, M. and Pidduck, H. (1979) In: *Fertility and Infertility in Domestic Animals*, ed. J. A. Laing, p. 137. London: Baillière Tindall.

Dobson, H., Rankin, J. E. F. and Ward, W. R. (1977) *Vet. Rec.*, **101**, 459.

Dohoo, I. R. and Martin, S. W. (1984) *Prev. Vet. Med.*, **2**, 755.

Dohoo, I. R., Martin, S. W., Meek, A. H. and Sandals, W. C. D. (1983) *Prev. Vet. Med.*, **1**, 321.

Donaldson, L. E. and Hansel, W. (1968) *Aust. Vet. J.*, **50**, 403.

Donaldson, L. E., Hansel, W. and Van Vleck, L. D. (1965) *J. Dairy Sci.*, **48**, 331.

Drew, B. (1978) In: *Control of Reproduction*, ed. J. M. Steenan, p. 475. The Hague: Martinus Nijhoff.

Ducker, M. J., Yarrow, N. H., Bloomfield, G. A. and Edwards-Webb, J. D. (1984) *Anim. Prod.*, **39**, 9.

Ducker, M. J., Haggett, R. A., Fisher, W. J. and Morant, S. V. (1985) *Anim. Prod.*, **41**, 1.

Edgerton, L. A. and Hafs, H. D. (1973) *J. Dairy Sci.*, **56**, 451.

Edwards, J. S., Bartley, E. E. and Dayton, A. D. (1980) *J. Dairy Sci.*, **63**, 243.

Edwards, M. J. (1961) Thesis, University of Liverpool.

Elmore, R. G., Bierschwal, C. J., Youngquist, R. S., Cantley, T. C., Kesler, D. J. and Garverick, H. A. (1975) *Vet. Med. Small Anim. Clin.*, **70**, 1346.

Emmanuelson, U. and Bendixen, P. H. (1991) *Prev. Vet. Med.*, **10**, 261.

Erb, R. E., Gaverick, H. A., Randel, R. D., Brown, B. L. and Callahan, C. J. (1976) *Theriogenology*, **5**, 227.

Eriksson, K. (1938) *Scand. Vet.*, **28**, 409.

Esselmont, R. J. (1973) Ph.D. Thesis, University of Reading.

Esselmont, R. J. (1974) *ADAS Q. Rev.*, **12**, 175.

Esselmont, R. J. (1992) *Daisy Dairy Information System. Report No. 1.* Reading: University of Reading.

Esselmont, R. J. and Bryant (1976) *Vet. Rec.*, **99**, 472.

Eyestone, W. H. and Ax, R. L. (1984) *Theriogenology*, **22**, 109.

Fallon, G. R. (1962) *Brit. Vet. J.*, **118**, 327.

Farin, P. W., Youngquist, R. S., Parfet, J. R. and Gaverick, H. A. (1992) *J. Amer. Vet. Med. Assn*, **200**, 1085.

Ferguson, J. D. and Chalupa, W. (1989) *J. Dairy Sci.*, **72**, 746.

Fincher, M. G. (1946) *Trans. Amer. Soc. Study Sterility*, **1**, 17.

Fincher, M. G. and Williams, W. L. (1926) *Cornell Vet.*, **16**, 1.

Folman, Y., Ascarelli, I., Herz, Z., Rosenberg, M., Davidson, M. and Halevi, A. (1979) *Brit. J. Nutr.*, **41**, 353.

Foote, W. D. and Hunter, J. E. (1964) *J. Anim. Sci.*, **23**, 517.

Foote, R. H., Oltenacu, E. A. B., Mellinger, N. R., Scott, N. R. and Marshall, R. A. (1979) *J. Dairy Sci.*, **62**, 69.

Friesecke, H. (1978) Cited by Jackson (1981).

Gardner, I. A., Hird, D. W., Utterback, W. W., Danye-Elmi, C., Heron, B. R., Christiansen, K. H. and Sischo, W. M. (1990) *Prev. Vet. Med.*, **8**, 157.

Garm, O. (1949) *Acta Endocrinol.*, **11**(Suppl. 3), 1.

Garverick, H. A., Erb, R. E., Randel, R. D. and Cunningham, M. D. (1971) *J. Dairy Sci.*, **54**, 1669.

Ginther, P. J. (1968) *J. Amer. Vet. Med. Assn*, **153**, 1656.

Gould, C. M. (1969) *Vet. Rec.*, **85**, 662.

Gracey, J. F. (1960 *Survey of Livestock Diseases.* Belfast: HMSO.

Greve, T. and Lehn-Jensen, H. (1982) *Theriogenology*, **17**, 91.

Grunsell, C. S. and Paver, H. (1955) *Vet. Rec.*, **60**, 974.

Gwazdauskas, F. C., Thatcher, W. W. and Wilcox, C. J. (1972) *J. Dairy Sci.*, **55**, 1165.

Gwazdauskas, F. C., Bibb, T. L., McGilliard, M. L. and Lineweaver, J. A. (1979) *J. Dairy Sci.*, **62**, 678.

Hafez, E. S. E. (1975) In: *Reproduction in Farm Animals*, 3rd edn, ed. E. S. E. Hafez, p. 24. Philadelphia: Lea and Febiger.

Hagermeister, M. (1978) *Muhle Mischfutterechnik*, **115**, 324.

Hagermeister, M. (1980) In: *Recent Advances in Animal Nutrition*, ed. W. Haresign, p. 81. London: Butterworth.

Hall, J. B., Branton, C. and Stone, E. J. (1959) *J. Dairy Sci.*, **42**, 1.

Hammond, J. (1927) *The Physiology of Reproduction in the Cow.* London: Cambridge University Press.

Hancock, J. L. (1948) *Vet. Rec.*, **60**, 513.

Hansel, W., Spalding, R. W., Larson, L. L., Laster, D. B., Wagner, W. and Braun, R. K. (1976) *J. Dairy Sci.*, **59**, 751.

Harrison, J. H., Hancock, D. D. and Conrad, H. R. (1984) *J. Dairy Sci.*, **67**, 123.

Hart, B. and Mitchell, G. L. (1965) *Aust. Vet. J.*, **41**, 305.

Hendricksson, B. (1956) *Acta Agric. Scand.*, **7**, 1.

Hidiroglou, M., McAllister, A. J. and Williams, C. J. (1987) *J. Dairy Sci.*, **70**, 1281.

Higgins, R. J. and Anderson, W. S. (1983) *Vet. Rec.*, **113**, 461.

Hignett, S. L. and Hignett, P. G. (1951) *Vet. Rec.*, **63**, 603.

Hirst, R. S., Nielson, S. W. and Plastridge, W. N. (1966) *Path. Vet.*, **3**, 616.

Hoare, M. (1967) *Vet. Rec.*, **85**, 351.

Hoffmann, B., Hamburger, R., Gunzler, O., Korndorfer, L. and Lohoff, H. (1974) *Theriogenology*, **2**, 21.

Hull, F. E., Dimock, W. W., Ely, F. and Morrison, H. R. (1940) *Buyll. Ky Agric. Exp. Stn.*, 462.

Hurnic, J. F., King, G. J. and Robertson, H. A. (1975) *Appl. Anim. Ethol.*, **2**, 55.

Jackson, P. S. (1981) Thesis, University of London.

Jackson, P.S., Johnson, C. T., Bulman, D. C. and Holdsworth, R. J. (1979) *Brit. Vet. J.*, **135**, 578.

Johannsson, I. (1962) *Genetic Aspects of Cattle Breeding.* Edinburgh: Oliver and Boyd.

Jordan, E. R. and Swanson, L. V. (1979) *J. Dairy Sci.*, **62**, 58.

Joubert, D. M. (1954) *J. Agric. Sci., Camb.*, **44**, 5.

Jubb, T. F., Abhayaratne, D., Malmo, J. and Anderson, G. A. (1990) *Aust. Vet. J.*, **67**, 359.

Julien, W. E., Conrad, H. R., Jones, J. E. and Moxon, A. K. (1976) *J. Dairy Sci.*, **59**, 1954.

Kaneene, J. B. and Hurd, H. S. (1990) *Prev. Vet. Med.*, **8**, 103.

Karg, H. and Schams, D. (1974) *J. Reprod. Fertil.*, **39**, 463.

Kastli, F. and Hall, J. G. (1978) *Vet. Rec.*, **102**, 80.

Kerr, O. M. and McCaughey, W. J. (1984) *Vet. Rec.*, **114**, 605.

Kesler, D. J. and Garverick, H. A. (1982) *J. Anim. Sci.*, **55**, 1147.

Kesler, D. J., Garverick, H. A., Caudle, A. B., Bierschwal, C. J., Elmore, R. G. and Youngquist, R. S. (1978) *J. Anim. Sci.*, **46**, 719.

Kesler, D. J., Garverick, H. A., Bierschwal, C. J., Elmore, R. G. and Youngquist, R. S. (1979) *J. Dairy Sci.*, **62**, 1290.

Kesler, D. J., Elmore, R. G., Brown, E. M. and Garverick, H. A. (1981) *Theriogenology*, **16**, 207.

Kessy, B. M. (1978) Ph.D. Thesis, University of London.

Kessy, B. M. and Noakes, D. E. (1979a) *Vet. Rec.*, **105**, 414.

Kessy, B. M. and Noakes, D. E. (1979b) *Vet. Rec.*, **105**, 489.

Kidder, H. E., Barrett, G. R. and Casida, L. E. (1952) *J. Dairy Sci.*, **35**, 436.

Kiddy, C. A. (1977) *J. Dairy Sci.*, **60**, 235.

Kiddy, C. A., Mitchell, D. S. and Hawk, H. W. (1984) *J. Dairy Sci.*, **67**, 388.

King, G. J., Hurnick, J. F. and Robertson, H. A. (1976) *J. Anim. Sci.*, **42**, 688.

King, J. O. L. (1968) *Vet. Rec.*, **83**, 492.

Kittock, R. H., Britt, J. H. and Convey, E. M. (1973) *J. Anim. Sci.*, **37**, 985.

Kothari, B. U. (1978) Thesis, University of Glasgow.

Kuhlman, A. H. and Gallup, W. D. (1942) *J. Dairy Sci.*, **25**, 688.

Labhestwar, A. P., Tyler, W. J. and Casida, L. E. (1963) *J. Dairy Sci.*, **46**, 843.

Lagerlöf, N. (1939) *Proc. 5th Int. Vet. Congr., Copenhagen*, p. 609.

Lagerlöf, N. and Boyd, H. (1953) *Cornell Vet.*, **43**, 52.

Lamming, G. E. (1978) In: *Control of Ovulation*, ed. D. B. Crighton, N. B. Haynes, G. R. Foxcroft and G. E. Lamming, p. 335. London: Butterworth.

Lamming, G. E. (1980) *Proc. IX Int. Congr. Anim. Reprod. Artif. Insem., Madrid.*

Lamming, G. E. and Bulman, D. C. (1976) *Brit. Vet. J.*, **132**, 507.

Lamming, G. E., Foster, J. P. and Bulman, D. C. (1979) *Vet. Rec.*, **104**, 156.

Lamond, D. R. (1968) *Aust. Vet. J.*, **57**, 348.

Larson, L. L., Marbruck, H. S. and Lowry, S. R. (1980) *J. Dairy Sci.*, **63**, 283.

Lauderdale, J. W. (1964) *J. Dairy Sci.*, **57**, 348.

Leaver, J. D. (1977) *Anim. Prod.*, **25**, 219.

Lee, C. N., Ax, R. L., Pennington, J. A., Hoffman, W. F. and Brown, M. D. (1981) *J. Dairy Sci.*, **64**(Suppl. 1), Abstr. 163.

Lee, C. N., Cook, D. L., Parfet, J. R., Smith, C. A., Youngquist, R. S. and Garverick, H. A. (1988) *J. Dairy Sci.*, **71**, 3505.

Leech, F. B., Davies, M. E., Macral, W. D. and Withers, F. W. (1960) *Disease, Wastage and Husbandry in British Dairy Herds.* London: HMSO.

Leidl, W., Bostedt, H., Lamprecht, W., Prinzen, R. and Wendt, V. (1979) *Tierarztl. Umsch.*, **34**, 546.

Leslie, K. E. (1983) *Can. Vet. J.*, **24**, 116.

Leslie, K. E. and Bosu, W. T. K. (1983) *Can. Vet. J.*, **24**, 352.

Lillie, F. R. (1916) *Science, N. Y.*, **43**, 611.

Liptrap, R. M. (1970) *J. Endocrinol.*, **47**, 197.

Liptrap, R. M. and McNally, P. J. (1976) *Amer. J. Vet. Res.*, **37**, 369.

Littlejohn, A. and Lewis, G. (1960) *Vet. Rec.*, **72**, 1137.

Logan, E. F., Smyth, J. A., Kennedy, D. G., Rice, D. A. and Ellis, W. A. (1991) *Vet. Rec.*, **129**, 99.

Long, S. E. (1990) *In Practice*, **12**, 208.

Lotthammer, K. H. (1975) *Prakt. Tierarzt.*, **56**(Suppl), 24.

Lotthammer, K. H. (1979) *Feedstuffs*, **51**, 16.

Lotthammer, K. H., Schams, D. and Scholz, H. (1978) *Zuchthygiene*, **13**, 76.

Lucey, S., Rowlands, G. J. and Russell, A. M. (1986) *Vet. Rec.*, **118**, 628.

McClure, T. J. (1961) *N.Z. Vet. J.*, **9**, 107.

McClure, T. J. (1968) *Brit. Vet. J.*, **124**, 126.

McClure, T. J. (1970) *Res. Vet. Sci.*, **11**, 247.

McCormack, J. (1978) *Vet. Med. Small Anim. Clin.*, **73**, 1057.

McDonald, L. E. (1954) *Proc. 91st Ann. Congr. Amer. Vet. Med. Assn, Seattle, Washington.*

Macmillan, K. L. and Curnow, R. J. (1977) *N.Z. J. Expt. Agr.*, **5**, 357.

MacMillan, K. L. and Pickering, J. G. E. (1988) *Proc. XI Int. Congr. Animal Reproduction AI*, Abstr. 442.

MacMillan, K. L., Taufa, V. K. and Day, A. M. (1986) *Anim. Reprod. Sci.*, **11**, 1.

McLeod, B. (1990) *Farmers Weekly*, Feb., 51.

McNeilly, A. S. (1980) *J. Reprod. Fertil.*, **581**, 537.

MacPherson, A., Kelly, E. F., Chalmers, J. S. and Roberts, D. J. (1987) In: *Trace Substances in Environmental Health — XXI*, ed. D. D. Hemphill, University of Missouri.

Madsen, L. L. and Davis, R. E. (1949) *J. Anim. Sci.*, **8**, 625.

Marcek, J. M., Apell, L. H., Hoffman, C. L., Moredick, P. T. and Swanson, L. V. (1985) *J. Dairy Sci.*, **68**, 71.

Marion, G. B. and Gier, H. T. (1968) *J. Anim. Sci.*, **27**, 1621.

Maurice, E., Ax, R. L. and Brown, M. D. (1982) *J. Dairy Sci.*, **65**(Suppl. 1), Abstr. 179.

Mee, J. F. (1991) *Vet. Rec.*, **129**, 201.

Miller, G. Y. and Dorn, C. R. (1990) *Prev. Vet. Med.*, **8**, 171.

Mohammed, H. O., White, M. E., Guard, C. L., Smith, H. C., Mechor, G. D. and Booker, C. W. (1991) *J. Dairy Sci.*, **74**, 218.

Moller, K. and Shannon, P. (1972) *N.Z. Vet. J.*, **20**, 47.

Morris, R. S. (1976) *Diagnosis of Infertility in Larger Dairy Herds.* Proc. No. 28. Refresher Course for Veterinarians, Sydney.

Morrow, D. A. (1976) *J. Dairy Sci.*, **59**, 1625.

Morrow, D. A., Roberts, S. J., McEntee, K. and Gray, H. F. (1966) *Cornell Vet.*, **59**, 173.

Morrow, D. A., Hillman, D., Dade, A. W. and Kitchen, H. (1979) *J. Amer. Vet. Med. Assn*, **174**, 161.

Mulvehill, P. and Sreenan, J. M. (1977) *J. Reprod. Fertil.*, **50**, 323.

Munro, I. B. (1957) *Vet. Rec.*, **69**, 125.

Nadaraja, R. and Hansel, W. (1976) *J. Reprod. Fertil.*, **47**, 203.

Nakao, T., Narita, S., Tanaka, K., Hara, H., Shirakawa, J., Nashiro, H., Saga, N., Tsunoda, N. and Kawata, K. (1983) *Theriogenology*, **20**, 11.

Nanda, A. S., Ward, W. R., Williams, P. C. W. and Dobson, H. (1988) *Vet. Rec.*, **122**, 155.

Nanda, A. S., Ward, W. R. and Dobson, H. (1989) *Vet. Bull.*, **7**, 537.

Newcombe, R. and Rowson, L. E. A. (1975) *J. Reprod. Fertil.*, **43**, 539.

Nielson, F. (1949) *Proc. 14th Int. Vet. Congr. London*, Sect. 4(c), p. 105.

Oxenreider, S. L. and Wagner, W. C. (1971) *J. Anim. Sci.*, **33**, 1026.

Palsson, E. (1961) *Proc. IV Int. Congr. Anim. Reprod. Artif. Insem., The Hague.*

Parker, B. N. J. and Blowey, R. W. (1976) *Vet. Rec.*, **98**, 394.

Payne, J. M., Dew, S. M., Manston, R. and Faulks, M. (1970) *Vet. Rec.*, **87**, 150.

Peralta, R. U. and Ax, R. L. (1982) *J. Dairy Sci.*, **65**(Suppl. 1), Abstr. 182.

Peters, A. R. and Lamming, G. E. (1990) In: *Oxford Reviews of Reproductive Biology*, ed. S. R. Milligan, Vol. 12. Oxford: Oxford University Press.

Phillipo, M. (1983) In: *Trace Elements in Animal Production and Veterinary Practice*, ed. N. F. Suttle, p. 51. British Society for Animal Production.

Phillipo, M., Humphries, W. R., Lawrence, C. B. and Price, J. (1982a) *J. Agr. Sci., Camb.*, **99**, 359.

Pickering, J. P. (1975) *Vet. Rec.*, **97**, 295.

Pinney, D. O., Pope, L. S., Van Cotthem, C. and Urban, K. (1962) Cited by Young, J. S. (1974) *Proc. Aust. Soc. Anim. Prod.*, **10**, 45.

Poretsky, L. and Kalin, M. F. (1987) *Endocrine Rev.*, **8**, 132.

Radford, H. N., Nancarrow, C. D. and Mattner, P. E. (1978) *J. Reprod. Fertil.*, **54**, 49.

Rajaniemi, H. J., Ronnbell, L., Kauppila, A., Ylostalo, R. and Viako, R. (1980) *J. Clin. Endocrinol. Metab.*, **51**, 1054.

Reid, I. M. (1980) *Vet. Rec.*, **107**, 281.

Reid, I. M., Roberts, C. J. and Manston, R. (1979) *Vet. Rec.*, **104**, 75.

Reid, I. M., Dew, S. M., Collins, R. A., Ducker, M. J.,

Bloomfield, G. A. and Morant, S. V. (1983) *J. Agr. Sci., Camb.*, **101**, 499.

Reid, J. T., Loosli, J. K., Trimberger, G. W., Turk, K. L., Asdell, S. A. and Smith, S. E. (1964) *Cornell Univ. Agric. Exp. Stn. Bull.*, 987.

Roberts, C. J., Reid, I. M., Rowlands, G. J. and Patterson, A. (1981) *Vet. Rec.*, **108**, 78.

Roberts, S. J. (1955) *Cornell Vet.*, **45**, 497.

Robinson, T. J. (1979) In: *Reproduction in Domestic Animals*, 3rd edn, ed. H. H. Cole and P. T. Cupps, p. 433. New York: Academic Press.

Rochet, M. (1973) *Ann. Zootech.*, **22**, 227.

Roine, K. (1973) *Nord. Vet.*, **25**, 242.

Rowlands, C. J., Little, W. and Kitchenham, B. A. (1977) *J. Dairy Sci.*, **44**, 1.

Rowlands, G. J., Manston, R., Stark, A. J., Russell, A. M., Collis, K. A. and Collis, S. C. (1980) *J. Agr. Sci., Camb.*, **94**, 517.

Rowson, L. E. A., Lamming, G. E. and Fry, R. M. (1953) *Vet. Rec.*, **65**, 335.

Rowson, L. E. A., Moor, R. M. and Lawson, R. A. S. (1969) *J. Reprod. Fertil.*, **18**, 517.

Roy, J. H. B., Perfitt, M. W., Glencross, R. G. and Turvey, A. (1985) *Vet. Rec.*, **116**, 370.

Sheldon, I. M. and Dobson, H. (1993) *Vet. Rec.*, **133**, 160.

Schels, H. F. and Mostafawi, D. (1978) *Vet. Rec.*, **103**, 31.

Schingoeth, D. J., Kirkbride, C. A., Olson, O. E., Owens, M. J., Ludens, F. C. and Tucker, W. L. (1981) *J. Dairy Sci.*, **64**(Suppl. 1), Abstr. 120.

Seguin, B. E., Morrow, D. A. and Louis, T. H. (1974) *Amer. J. Vet. Res.*, **35**, 57.

Sheehy, G. J. (1946) *Nature, Lond.*, **157**, 442.

Short, R. V., Smith, J., Mann, T., Evans, E. P., Hallet, J., Fryer, A. and Hamerton, J. L. (1969) *Cytogenetics*, **8**, 369.

Simmons, K. E. and Hansel, W. (1964) *J. Anim. Sci.*, **23**, 136.

Sjollema, P., Stegenga, T. and Terpstra, J. (1949) *Rep. 14th Int. Vet. Congr. London*, Sect. 4(c).

Sommer, H. (1975) *Vet. Med. Revs.*, **1**, 42.

Speck, G. (1948) *Amer. J. Obstet. Gynecol.*, **55**, 1048.

Speicher, J. A. and Meadows, C. E. (1967) *Proc. 62nd Ann. Meet. Amer. Dairy Sci. Ass., Cornell Univ., N. Y.*

Stableforth, A. W., Scorgie, N. J. and Fould, G. N. (1937) *Vet. Rec.*, **49**, 248.

Stevenson, J. S., Schmidt, M. K. and Callow, E. P. (1984) *J. Dairy Sci.*, **67**, 140.

Stevenson, J. S. and Call, E. P. (1988) *J. Dairy Sci.*, **71**, 2572.

Summers, P. M. (1974) *Aust. Vet. J.*, **50**, 403.

Suttle, N. (1993) *Vet. Rec.*, **133**, 123.

Tassell, R. (1967a) *Brit. Vet. J.*, **123**, 12.

Tassell, R. (1967b) *Brit. Vet. J.*, **123**, 459.

Trainin, D. (1964) *Proc. Vth Int. Congr. Anim. Reprod. Artif. Insem.*

Treacher, R. J., Little, W., Collis, K. A. and Stark, A. J. (1976) *J. Dairy Res.*, **43**, 357.

Trimberger, G. W. (1948) *Nebr. Univ. Agric. Exp. Stn. Res. Bull.*, 129.

Trinder, N., Woodhouse, C. D. and Rentan, C. P. (1969) *Vet. Rec.*, **85**, 550.

Van Rensburg, S. W. J. and de Vos, W. H. (1962) *Onderstepoort. J. Vet. Res.*, **29**, 55.

Ward, H. K. (1968) *Rhod. J. Agr. Res.*, **6**, 93.

Warnick, A. C., Kirst, R. C., Burns, W. C. And Kroger, M. (1967) *J. Anim. Sci.*, **26**, 231.

Watson, E. D. (1985) *Brit. Vet. J.*, **141**, 576.

Watson, E. D. and Harwood, D. J. (1984) *Vet. Rec.*, **114**, 424.

Webb, R., Lamming, G. E., Havnes, N. B., Hofs, H. D. and Manns, J. G. (1977) *J. Reprod. Fertil.*, **50**, 203.

Whitaker, D. (1980) *Brit. Vet. J.*, **136**, 214.

Whitmore, H. L., Tyler, W. J. and Casida, L. E. (1974) *J. Amer. Vet. Med. Assn*, **165**, 693.

Whitmore, H. L., Hurtgen, J. P., Mather, E. C. and Seguin, B. E. (1979) *J. Amer. Vet. Med. Assn*, **174**, 979.

Whitney, R. and Burdick, H. O. (1936) *Endocrinology*, **20**, 643.

Whitney, R. and Burdick, H. O. (1938) *Endocrinology*, **22**, 63.

Wickersham, E. W. and Schultz, L. H. (1963) *J. Dairy Sci.*, **46**, 544.

Wijeratne, W. V. S., Munro, I. B. and Wilkes, P. R. (1977) *Vet. Rec.*, **100**, 333.

Wilkes, P. R., Wijeratne, W. V. S. and Munro, I. B. (1981) *Vet. Rec.*, **108**, 349.

Williamson, N. B., Morris, R. S., Blood, D. C. and Cannon, C. M. (1972) *Vet. Rec.*, **91**, 50.

Wiltbank, J. N., Gregory, K. E., Swiger, L. A., Ingalls, J. A., Rothlisberger, J. A. and Koch, R. M. (1966) *J. Anim. Sci.*, **25**, 744.

Wisehart, D. F. and Young, I. M. (1974) *Vet. Rec.*, **95**, 503.

Wood, P. D. P. (1976) *Anim. Prod.*, **22**, 275.

Young, J. S. (1965) *N.Z. Vet. J.*, **13**, 1.

Young, J. S. (1967) *N.Z. Vet. J.*, **15**, 167.

Young, J. S. (1968) *Aust. Vet. J.*, **44**, 350.

Young, J. S. (1970) *Vet. Rev.*, **9**, 22.

Zaied, A. A., Garverick, H. A., Kesler, D. J., Bierschwal, C. J., Elmore, R. G. and Youngquist, R. S. (1981) *Theriogenology*, **16**, 349.

Zemjanis, R. (1980) *Current Therapy in Theriogenology*, ed. W. Morrow. Philadelphia: Saunders.

23

Infections of the bovine genital tract affect fertility by altering its environment so that there may be impaired sperm transport, sperm death or, since there is a hostile environment to the subsequent development of the conceptus, embryonic and fetal death, stillbirth or weakly calves. Both specific and non-specific infections occur naturally. Specific infections develop without predisposing causes, and such diseases are usually of an enzootic type. Non-specific infections, on the other hand, require a predisposing cause and tend to affect individual cows. The organisms involved are opportunist pathogens which normally inhabit the environment of the cow and are present on its integument and in the faeces, such as group C streptococci, staphylococci, *Actinomyces* (*Corynebacterium*) *pyogenes* and *Escherichia coli*.

NON-SPECIFIC INFECTION

The mechanisms which prevent opportunist pathogens from colonizing the genital tract are, firstly, the physical barriers of the vulval sphincter and cervix and, secondly, the natural defence mechanism of the tissues which is influenced significantly by the endocrine system.

There are only two occasions when the physical barriers are breached; these are at coitus, or insemination, and at the time of parturition, especially immediately postpartum. The endocrine system has an important influence on the resistance of the genital tract to infection, and it is not surprising that on the two occasions when the physical barriers are breached the genital tract is in its most resistant state. In general, it can be assumed that under oestrogen dominance the genital tract is more resistant to infection, whilst under progesterone dominance it is more susceptible.

At oestrus and parturition massive contamination with opportunist pathogens usually occurs, yet there is rarely impairment of health and this contamination is soon eliminated (see Chapter 7). At both these stages oestrogens are the dominant hormones since oestrus is part of the follicular phase of the oestrous cycle (see Chapter 1) and before parturition there is a significant rise in oestrogens and conversely a decline in progesterone. At oestrus and at parturition, there is a numerical change in the peripheral blood picture with a relative neutrophilia and 'shift to the left'. At oestrus the blood supply to the uterus is increased under the influence of increased oestrogen concentrations, whilst at parturition there is a massive blood supply to the gravid uterus. This, coupled with the migration of white cells from the circulation to the uterine lumen, enables vigorous and active phagocytosis of bacteria to occur. The increase in the quantity and nature of vaginal mucus also plays an important role by providing a protective physical barrier and flushing and diluting the bacterial contaminants; the presence of secretory immunoglobulins is also important.

Since the genital tract is generally able to overcome the potential challenge of massive non-specific bacterial contamination it is important to consider the reasons for failure. Firstly, if there is damage to the vulva, impairing the 'sphincter-like' barrier, there will be aspiration of air, ballooning of the vagina, dehydration of the mucosa and the development of vaginitis. At oestrus when the cervix relaxes, or if the cervix is damaged, it may allow heavy contamination of the uterine lumen and the creation of an endometritis. Both these conditions usually result from poor obstetric practice, and are largely preventable (see Chapter 6). Vulval injury and perineal lacerations can be repaired, as described in Chapter 17, and thus the physical barrier is restored, enabling the cow to overcome the infection. Surgical repairs to the cervix are virtually impossible.

Failure of the natural defence mechanisms at and after calving is due to a number of factors:

these include dystocia, placental retention, metabolic diseases and fatty liver disease. Injured and devitalized tissue is less resistant and is readily infected; as a result, a severe and sometimes fatal puerperal metritis can occur. Other factors which delay uterine involution have been described in Chapter 7.

Since progesterone domination of the genital system increases its susceptibility to infection, any condition which results in prolongation of the luteal phase can enable non-specific contaminants to become pathogenic. A persistent corpus luteum either of dioestrus or of a degenerate pregnancy, and luteal cysts, can sometimes result in pyometra. The pathogenesis of the latter will be discussed later in greater detail.

Puerperal metritis

Puerperal metritis occurs within a few days of parturition. It usually follows an abnormal first or second stage of labour; it is associated with uterine inertia and is frequently accompanied by retention of the fetal membranes. The infecting organisms are *A. (C.) pyogenes*, group C streptococci, haemolytic staphylococci, coliforms, and Gram-negative anaerobes, particularly *Bacteroides* spp.; exceptionally, clostridia are present and soon produce serious, and often fatal, disease. The bacterial invaders colonize the non-involuted uterus whence their toxins are absorbed and cause severe symptoms. Not uncommonly, septicaemia and pyaemia occur. Affected animals show both local and general symptoms. There is a fetid, reddish serous, vaginal discharge, accompanied by frequent expulsive straining efforts. The uterus contains a large volume of this toxic exudate; the cotyledons are swollen and the fetal membranes usually remain firmly attached.

The cervix remains partly open with the posterior portion of the membranes passing through it to the vagina and exterior of the body, but it is difficult for the obstetrician to pass a hand into the uterus after the third postparturient day. The vulva and vagina are swollen and deeply congested. Vaginal and uterine exploration of an affected case causes acute discomfort and is accompanied and followed by the most severe and persistent expulsive efforts. Symptoms of toxaemia are anorexia, elevation of body temperature to 40–41°C and a frequent pulse rate in the region of 100/

minute. The respirations are frequent and often suggest a respiratory disease. Diarrhoea is common. Not infrequently the disease extends from the uterus to the peritoneum; the cow then shows an arched back, walks with a stiff gait and grunts with each expiration. Peritonitis may be followed by uterine and ovarian adhesions. Complications of metritis include pneumonia, polyathritis and endocarditis. In pyaemic cases, abscesses may develop in the lungs, liver, kidney or brain. Puerperal metritis must be differentiated from (primary) pneumonia, traumatic reticulitis and pericarditis, and from milk fever and acute mastitis.

The treatment of puerperal metritis calls for a humane and conservative approach. The animal should first be made comfortable by transferring it to a well bedded and warm loose-box. A very gentle attempt should be made to remove the fetal membranes by gentle external traction, but no attempt should be made to explore the vagina and uterus with the hand. It should be appreciated that the uterus is particularly friable and that it contains a voluminous mass of septic material. Rough attempts at removal of the fetal membranes or even careful exploration of the vagina and uterus can cause severe damage and predispose to the absorption of toxins and entry of bacteria. If the cow is continually straining, posterior epidural anaesthesia should be used; this will give only transient relief for 1–2 hours, but sometimes it will 'break the cycle' and stop the straining, which is often self-perpetuating and debilitating. If the case is seen within 3 days of parturition 50 IU of oxytocin by intravenous injection may cause contraction of the uterus and expulsion of fluid and debris. Otherwise the condition is best treated by the systemic administration of broad-spectrum antibiotics and other supportive therapy, in particular fluids. The author is of the opinion that intrauterine antibiotics are of little value. The use of oestrogens is debatable, since although it has previously been shown that they increase the resistance of the genital system, it must also be remembered that they increase the blood flow to the uterus and therefore hasten the absorption of bacterial toxins. Oestrogens should not be used in cases of acute puerperal metritis.

Once the temperature has subsided, and the cow shows some signs of improvement, some benefit can be obtained by uterine lavage and drainage. This can be done with a soft rubber tube of 5 cm diameter, at one end of which a large number of holes are made (a horse's stomach tube is ideal), to which is attached a large funnel. The perforated end is carefully inserted through the cervix into the uterine lumen and several litres of warm (49°C) sterile saline are poured down the tube through the funnel. The funnel end is quickly lowered before the tube empties, thus establishing the siphon. The interior end inevitably becomes blocked but the obstructing material is flushed out with more saline and the siphonage repeated over and over again, until the uterus is as empty as possible. The warm saline solution is believed to exert both a soothing and a stimulating effect on the uterus, and this, together with the evacuation of exudate, promotes involution. Antibiotic pessaries may then be inserted and a course of parenteral antibiotics continued. Ideally, the patient should be given daily treatment as outlined above. A favourable turn is shown by resumption of appetite, more formed motions and less fetid, but thicker, vaginal discharge.

Recovered cases inevitably show a mucopurulent discharge or leucorrhoea due to chronic endometritis; this will be discussed in detail below. Unfortunately the prognosis for subsequent fertility should always be guarded, since cows that have suffered a severe puerperal metritis inevitably develop lesions such as ovarobursal adhesions, uterine adhesions and occluded uterine tubes as described in Chapter 22.

Endometritis

Endometritis implies inflammation of the endometrium; it is a common condition in the cow, and although it has a profound effect upon the fertility of the animal it does not affect its general health. The causal organisms usually reach the uterus from the vagina at coitus, insemination, parturition or postpartum, although it is possible in some circumstances for infection to arrive by the circulation. Specific pathogens such as *Campylobacter fetus* and *Tritrichomonas fetus* affect fertility because, having entered the genital tract at coitus, they cause endometritis. These will be discussed in greater detail later in this chapter and, although important, they do not have a major role in causing endometritis. In the UK and northern Europe the non-specific, opportunist pathogens are the

most important cause of endometritis and have a significant effect upon fertility.

Endometritis influences fertility in two ways, firstly, in the short term, it reduces fertility by extending the calving to conception interval and increasing the number of services per pregnancy (see Chapter 24) and, secondly, in the long term, it can result in sterility due to irreversible changes of the genital tracts (see pp. 350–354). With regard to the short-term influence, Studer and Morrow (1978) found a significant correlation between the state of the uterus, as determined by rectal palpation, and the calving–conception interval, especially in relation to the amount of pus in the discharge. Extension of the calving to conception interval has been shown to be an average of 12 days (Tennant and Peddicord, 1968), 20 days (Erb et al., 1981), 10 Days (Bretzlaff et al., 1982) and 31 days (Borsberry and Dobson, 1989), whilst the services per conception have been increased from 1.67 and 2.16 to 2.0 and 2.42, respectively (Tennant and Peddicord, 1968; Bretzlaff et al., 1982).

The long-term effect is clearly shown by the increased culling rate, which, in the survey of Bretzlaff et al. (1982), changed from an average of 5% for the herd in general to 20.6% for those which suffered from metritis. Comparable figures of 6.2 and 13.6%, respectively, were obtained by Tennant and Peddicord (1968). Other workers have demonstrated pathological evidence of endometritis in cows culled for infertility, particularly the repeat-breeder cow (Brus, 1954; Fujimoto, 1956; Dawson, 1963).

World-wide figures for the prevalence of endometritis are varied, ranging from 43 to 35% in France (Andriamanga et al., 1984; Martinez and Thibier, 1984); 37% in Israel (Markusfeld, 1984) to 10% in Belgium (Bouters and Vanderplassche, 1977) and 6.25 and 10.3% for Jersey and Holstein cows, respectively, in the USA (Fonseca et al., 1983). In the UK an incidence rate of 10.1% was recorded (Borsberry and Dobson, 1989), whilst in a study involving 20 000 cows in 63 herds during the calving season 1989–1990, a mean incidence rate of 15% was reported for cows with a vulval discharge. The lowest and highest quartile values were 3.7 and 26.9%, respectively (Esslemont and Spincer, 1992).

Although the differences in incidence rates may be genuine and related to predisposition factors (see below), they may be due to differences in clinical opinion about what constitutes endometritis. In most cases a diagnosis is based upon the presence of an abnormal vulval discharge; however, this may be due to a vaginitis. In addition, some cows produce a more copious than normal volume of postpartum lochial discharge (see Chapter 7).

Endometritis reduces the profitability of a dairy enterprise; the cost can be calculated by relating it to the increase in the calving–conception interval (se p. 431). In the study by Esslemont and Spincer (1992) an average of 1.42 cases per cow at a total cost of £160.80 was calculated: the latter was mainly due to an extended calving–conception interval, increased culling rates, reduced milk yield and the cost of treatment.

How does endometritis develop? In Chapter 7 it was shown that the great majority of cows suffer from bacterial contamination after calving; the flora is frequently changing because of elimination and recontamination. In cows that develop endometritis the bacterial flora colonize the uterus and cause the endometrium to respond. A number of factors have been shown to predispose to endometritis (Andriamanga et al., 1984; Markusfeld, 1984, 1985):

1. *Dystocia*. Endometritis, frequently following an acute puerperal metritis, is more prevalent in cows and heifers that have had severe dystocia.

2. *Retained placenta*. This is probably the major cause of endometritis.

3. *Season of year*. Cows calving during the winter or spring are more prone to endometritis than those calving at other times.

4. *Twins and induction of calving*. Since retained placenta is a problem in both these situations, it is not surprising that metritis is more prevalent.

5. *Return of cyclical ovarian activity*. It has been known for some time that the uterus of the cow is more resistant to infection at oestrus than during the luteal phase of the cycle (Rowson et al., 1953). Since cellular defence mechanisms are potentiated during oestrus (Frank et al., 1983) it has been generally assumed that a delay in return to cyclical activity would predispose cows to endometritis. This has been shown by Andriamanga et al. (1984) who found that 34% of the cows that were cyclical by 37 days postpartum had endometritis compared with 49% that were acyclical by the same stage. However, Olson et al. (1984) found

that in the cows that developed pyometra (see below) the average interval from calving to first ovulation was 15.5 days compared with 21.8 days for the normal, non-infected animals. In these cows that ovulated early, the bacterial contamination was such that it was probably not eliminated at the oestrus, so that when there followed a luteal phase the bacteria were able to proliferate and colonize the uterus.

6. *Bacterial loading*. The environment which the parturient and postparturient cow occupies can also have an effect. A number of observations have shown that a dirty, unhygienic calving environment can predispose to endometritis. This is probably the explanation for the effect of season of year, since cows calving in the winter or indoors in the spring are likely to be in a more heavily contaminated environment. Although in a study in which uterine swabs from cows from two hygienically contrasting farms were cultured aerobically and anaerobically, and where the incidence rates of endometritis were between 2–3 and 15%, there was no qualitative or quantitative difference in the bacterial flora (Noakes et al., 1991).

The nature of the flora is also important. In the studies of Hartigan et al. (1974a) it was found that endometritis is almost invariably a sequel to invasion with *A. (C.) pyogenes*; histopathological lesions of endometritis were observed in 97.4% of the uteri infected with this organism. Furthermore, the consequences of uterine contamination with *A. (C.) pyogenes* depended upon the duration of the infection. More recently, the role of obligate anaerobes in the pathogenesis of endometritis has been demonstrated (Ruder et al., 1981; Olson et al., 1984). There is good evidence that there is synergism between *A. (C.) pyogenes* and *Fusobacterium necrophorum*, the latter organism apparently producing a leucocidal endotoxin which would interfere with the host's ability to eliminate *A. (C.) pyogenes*. *Bacteroides* spp. also produce substances that interfere with phagocytic ingestion and bacterial kill.

7. *Milk yield*. Markusfeld (1984) found that postpartum metritis was more prevalent in first calvers that yielded less in the last 5 months before calving than those that yielded average or above. This was probably because they were overfed and became fat.

8. *Metabolic diseases*. Ketosis, hypocalcaemia and overfeeding during the dry period can predispose

the endometritis. This is probably associated with the fatty liver syndrome (Reid et al., 1979).

Clinical signs of endometritis are the presence, in the postpartum cow, of a white or whitish yellow mucopurulent vaginal discharge, leucorrhoea or 'whites'. The volume of the discharge is variable but frequently increases at the time of oestrus when the cervix dilates and there is copious vaginal mucus. The cow rarely shows any signs of systemic illness, although in a few cases milk yield and appetite may be slightly depressed. Rectal palpation frequently shows a poorly involuted uterus which has a 'doughy' feel. Studer and Morrow (1978) found a close correlation between size and texture of uterus and cervix, the nature of the purulent exudate and the degree of endometritis determined by biopsy and the nature of the bacterial isolation.

Opinions vary on the significance of subclinical endometritis. It is possible to obtain biopsies, and an instrument modified from that described by Hartigan et al. (1974b) and used by Ayliffe (1979) is quite satisfactory for this procedure (Figure 23.1). In a study by Hartigan et al. (1972), 12.5% of the genital tracts obtained from an abattoir showed gross lesions at post-mortem examination yet 50% showed evidence of endometritis histologically, and 77% of infertile cows had clinically diagnosed endometritis, when biopsies were obtained; 80% showed evidence of lesions, and bacterial infection was found in 64% of cows with clinical endometritis (Sagartz and Hardenbrook, 1971). A group of 49 infertile cows which had been clinically diagnosed to be infertile from causes other than endometritis were found, upon biopsy examination, to have lesions of endometritis in 92% of cases (Schmidt-Adamopolou, 1978). Interpretation of biopsy material requires considerable experience of the normal cyclical changes that occur in the endometrium.

There are many studies describing the bacterial flora associated with endometritis. There is little value in performing routine swabbing and bacterial sensitivity tests before treatment. This is because of the variable nature of the flora and the problems associated with the collection of uncontaminated uterine swabs; material for anaerobic culture requires considerable care.

A wide range of antimicrobial agents, including sulfonamides and antibiotics in various combina-

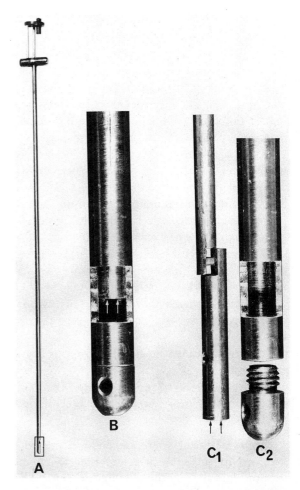

Fig. 23.1 Biopsy instrument. A, whole instrument showing window with cutting edge; B, 'close-up' with edge partially withdrawn (arrowed); 'close-up' views C_1 and C_2 showing the cutting edge (arrowed) and interchangeable tip C_1.

tions and hormones, such as oestradiol benzoate and prostaglandin $F_{2\alpha}$ (PGF$_{2\alpha}$) or analogues have been used as treatment. In addition, antiseptic agents such as 'Lotagen', chlorhexidine and Lugol's iodine solution have been popular at times; however, the last can cause severe endometrial damage and requires critical evaluation of its efficacy.

The following criteria should be considered before using a particular antimicrobial agent:

1. Its efficacy against the wide range of aerobic and anaerobic, and Gram-positive and Gram-negative bacteria that will be present.

2. Its efficacy within the generally anaerobic environment of the uterus. Such antibiotics as the aminoglycosides are rendered ineffective; in

addition, the penicillinases produced by some bacteria will destroy penicillins.

3. An effective bacteriostatic or bactericidal concentration at the site of infection can probably be best achieved by the intrauterine route of administration. The substance must be evenly and rapidly distributed throughout the uterine lumen with good penetration into the endometrium.

4. It must not inhibit natural uterine defence mechanisms, particularly the cellular component.

5. It must not traumatize the endometrium. Several of the vehicles used in the formulation of pharmaceutical preparations, namely propylene glycol, can cause a necrotizing endometritis.

6. Details of its absorption from the uterus and excretion in the milk must be known so that appropriate withdrawal times can be followed.

7. Treatment must not reduce fertility by producing irreversible changes in the reproductive system.

8. Treatment must be cost-effective by enhancing fertility.

9. If substances by mistake enter the food chain, then they must not adversely affect human health.

In the treatment of chronic endometritis with antimicrobial substances it is preferable to administer the substance by the intrauterine route. This will result in effective minimum inhibitory concentrations (MICs) reaching the endometrium and being established in the intraluminal secretions, provided an adequate dose rate is used. The latter is important in the effective treatment of the disease since frequently subtherapeutic dose rates are used. A broad-spectrum antibiotic, such as oxytetracyline, used at a dose rate of up to 22 mg/kg, will provide effective MICs in the lumen and uterine tissues. Considerable concentrations of antibiotic reach the endometrium following intravenous or intramuscular injection (Ayliffe and Noakes, 1978; Masera et al., 1980).

Several intrauterine therapeutic preparations also contain oestrogens, whilst others recommend the use of oestrogens administered by intramuscular injection at the same time as intrauterine infusion of antibiotics. Such hormones increase uterine blood flow and stimulate the changes that occur during the follicular phase of the oestrous cycle. There would appear to be a rationale for such use

but there is no reliable information on their true efficacy.

The best method of treating clinical endometritis, when there is a palpable mature corpus luteum on the ovary, is the use of $PGF_{2\alpha}$ or its synthetic analogues. The theory behind their use is that when administered during the luteal phase of the oestrous cycle they hasten the return of oestrus and at the same time reduce the period during which the genital system is under the influence of progesterone. Frequently, clinical signs of endometritis, as characterized by leucorrhoea, are seen by the herdsman at oestrus; in such a case no responsive corpus luteum will be present and the cow will require re-examination in 6–8 days when prostaglandin therapy can be used. The cow will return to oestrus 3–5 days after treatment, and unless the purulent discharge is severe it is advisable to serve or inseminate at the induced oestrus. Good results, as determined by conception at the induced oestrus, have been reported by Gustafsson et al. (1976), Coulson (1978) and Jackson (1981). Alternatively, if no corpus luteum can be palpated, the cow is probably best treated with 3–5 mg of oestradiol benzoate intramuscularly. High dose rates of natural and synthetic oestrogens can result in irreversible changes such as ovarian cysts. Although endometritis is frequently self-limiting, with spontaneous recovery after a spontaneous oestrus, there is a danger that it will lead to pyometra.

Pyometra

Pyometra is characterized by a progressive accumulation of pus in the uterus and by the persistence of functional luteal tissue in the ovary, which is usually a corpus luteum or rarely a luteal cyst. The condition arises in two ways. In most cases it occurs as a sequel to chronic endometritis, as noted above; as a result of the inflammation the uterus ceases to produce or release the endogenous luteolysin (see Chapter 1). The corpus luteum of dioestrus persists, and since the genital tract is now under the continuous influence of progesterone, without the intervening oestrus, the infective process progresses. Because the cervix remains fairly tightly closed the purulent exudate accumulates within the uterine lumen; but occasionally there is a slight purulent discharge. In a small number of cases pyometra results from embryonic or fetal death in which the corpus luteum of pregnancy persisted, with subsequent invasion by *A. (C.) pyogenes* and the production of a purulent exudate; in some instances it is possible to identify the remains of the embryo.

Cows which suffer from pyometra show little or no signs of ill health; the main reason for them being examined is the absence of cyclical activity and perhaps the presence of an intermittent vaginal discharge. The uterine horns are enlarged and distended (Figure 23.2), quite often to an unequal degree, owing to incomplete involution of the previously gravid horn or to recent conceptual death. Differentiation of pyometra from a normal pregnancy can sometimes be difficult, but there are a number of distinguishing points:

1. The uterine wall is thicker than at pregnancy.
2. The uterus has a more 'doughy' and less vibrant feel.
3. It is not possible to 'slip' the allantochorion.
4. No uterine caruncles can be palpated.

Pyometra associated with *T. fetus* infection presents features which are different from those previously described. Uterine pus is, as a rule, much more copious and may attain a volume of many litres. It is generally more fluid, with the consistency of pea-soup, and is greyish-white or white. The uterus undergoes much greater distension. The mucus occupying the cervix is moist and slippery, rather than sticky and tenacious, and in it motile trichomonads can generally be demonstrated.

If there is any doubt about the diagnosis of pyometra the cow should be left untreated and re-examined 2 weeks later for evidence of change.

The best treatment is the use of PGF$_{2\alpha}$ or its analogues. They result in regression of the corpus luteum, dilatation of the cervix, expulsion of the purulent fluid and oestrus 3–5 days later. Provided that the condition is not too long-standing and therapy is instituted quickly there is a reasonable possibility that the cow will eventually conceive again.

Salpingitis

A chronic salpingitis, invariably resulting from an ascending infection from the uterus, can result in infertility if unilateral, and sterility if bilateral. The

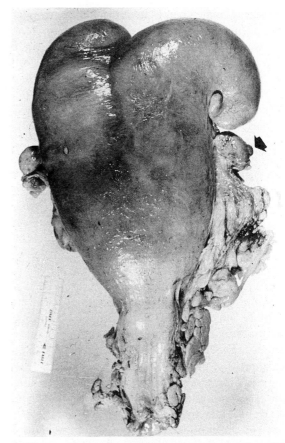

Fig. 23.2 Cow's uterus with pyometra. Note the distended horns and a corpus luteum present in the right ovary, indicated by the arrow, and fibrin tags over the dorsal surface of the uterine horns and body.

resulting lesions have been described in Chapter 22.

Cervicitis and vaginitis

Inflammation of the vagina and cervix is likely to follow obstetric trauma incurred during the relief of difficult dystocia, and in these circumstances, as well as with delayed involution of the uterus and retention of the afterbirth, it usually accompanies puerperal metritis. The organisms present in these infections are those normally found in the posterior vagina and include *E. coli*, streptococci, staphylococci and *A. (C.) pyogenes*, the latter organism being most prominent in established infections. Obstetric contusion of the vagina, especially in fat heifers of the beef breeds, is particularly likely to be followed by necrotic vaginitis associated with *F. necrophorum* infection, while in other instances involving the removal of dead, emphysematous calves in unhygienic circumstances, parturient trauma may be followed by severe toxaemia due to invasion by other anaerobic bacteria. Treatment will involve parenteral broad-spectrum antibiotics parenterally and possibly, if severe, supportive fluid therapy. Local emollient creams are also helpful. Since vaginitis will cause persistent straining, particularly if severe, caudal epidural anaesthesia will provide temporary relief.

Third-degree perineal lacerations due to severe calving trauma will invariably result in vaginitis and cervicitis due to faecal contamination, whilst second-degree perineal lacerations may give rise to a pneumovagina if the conformation of the vulva is compromised. Surgical correction of the former by Aanes's method, and of the latter by Caslick's operation, are described in Chapter 17.

An increasng number of cows are now diagnosed as having vaginal urine pooling or urovagina. In such animals urine accumulates in the anterior vagina impinging upon the cervix, and causes inflammation of both these organs. The inflammation then extends into the uterus, causing endometritis. There seems to be a greater prevalence in certain breeds, particularly the Charolais and Holsteins. The cause of the condition is not known, although stretching of the suspensory apparatus of the genital tract as a result of several pregnancies may be a factor. Surgical treatment has been described (Hudson, 1972) but the author has found it impossible to perform.

SPECIFIC INFECTIONS

In the UK over the last 40–50 years there has been a distinct change in the importance of the different specific pathogenic organisms that influence reproductive function in cattle. With the increased use of artificial insemination and close monitoring of bulls at artificial insemination studs many of the venereally transmitted diseases such as vibriosis and trichomoniasis have assumed less importance. Similarly, specific eradication programmes with vaccination, blood testing and slaughter schemes have been instrumental in reducing the prevalence of diseases such as brucellosis. Conversely, other diseases such as IBR–IPV (infectious bovine rhinotracheitis–infectious pustular vulvovaginitis), bovine viral diarrhoea (BVD) and leptospirosis

have assumed much greater importance, either because of a genuine increase in prevalence or better diagnosis, whilst the prevalence of some abortifacient organisms remains fairly static. The results from the Veterinary Investigation Service of the Ministry of Agriculture, published in the Veterinary Investigation Diagnosis Analysis (VIDA II) for the year 1977 and the years 1984–1992 (inclusive) are summarized in Table 23.1 to illustrate several of these points. One problem, which is clearly shown in this report, is the small percentage (4.3–7.4%) of fetopathies from which a specific infectious agent is identified. Rather better results have been reported elsewhere, with firm diagnosis being made in 23–37% of cases (Kirkbride et al., 1973; Jerrett and McOrist, 1985). The relatively low diagnostic rate can be attributed to a number of factors: inadequate samples sent to the laboratory; delay between infection and abortion occurring; destruction of the causal organism after fetal death, abortion and recovery of material; no infectious organism involved.

Even though there has been a change in the importance of different specific infectious agents in causing infertility, the author firmly believes that adequate attention must be paid to all infectious agents. Those that have been eliminated can cause catastrophic effects if they gain entry to a herd with a low immune status to that disease.

BACTERIAL AND PROTOZOAL AGENTS

Genital vibriosis

Infection due to *Campylobacter fetus* (formerly *Vibrio fetus*) has long been recognized as a cause of abortion in sheep and cattle (McFadyean and Stockman, 1913). Although its importance has declined with the use of artificial insemination, because of bull screening at artificial insemination studs and antibiotic in semen extenders, it must always be considered as a cause of infertility where natural service is used since it is most frequently transmitted venereally from carrier bulls to susceptible cows and heifers. In many countries it is still a major cause of reproductive disease. In a 15 year study in Argentina involving over 11 300 bulls, 22% were found to be immunofluorescent-positive (Villar and Spina, 1982); whilst

Table 23.1 Percentage frequency of isolation of pathogens from bovine fetopathies examined by Ministry of Agriculture Veterinary Investigation Centes (source VIDA II)

	1977	1984	1985	1986	1987	1988	1989	1990	1991	1992
BVD	NR	7.6	7.8	10.3	10.8	8.0	8.3	14.5	8.0	8.7
Brucella abortus	52.3	2.0	2.9	1.7	0.3	0.2	0.5	0.1	0.1	NR
Campylobacter spp.	0.4	1.1	1.3	0.6	0.4	0.8	1.1	0.7	1.3	1.3
A. (C.) pyogenes	20.2	25.5	17.0	8.1	5.3	3.7	2.9	3.5	4.0	3.8
Leptospira	NR	10.9	22.7	32.1	33.5	46.4	50.1	45.6	42.1	43.2
Listeria monocytogenes	0.6	1.2	1.5	2.1	1.2	1.7	1.2	1.3	1.2	1.4
Salmonella dublin	9.3	10.5	13.3	9.5	15.4	14.4	9.7	9.4	11.8	11.8
Salmonella typhimurium	0.5	1.3	1.7	1.5	0.9	0.4	0.5	0.6	0.7	0.5
Other *Salmonella* serotypes	0.8	1.4	1.8	0.6	1.0	0.8	1.1	1.2	1.7	1.5
Bacillus licheniformis	NR	NR	NR	NR	NR	NR	NR	NR	8.2	8.2
Coxiella burnetii	0	0.6	0.2	0.3	0.5	0.1	0.2	0.3	0.4	0.5
Fungi	8.2	15.3	7.9	14.5	9.7	6.1	7.5	6.9	6.1	6.0
IBR–IPV	NR	4.5	4.5	4.9	5.4	6.1	4.1	4.9	4.3	5.2
Other pathogens	7.6	18.0	17.4	13.8	15.7	11.3	12.8	11.0	10.0	7.9
Total identified	1 675	1 402	1 792	1 743	1 524	2 297	2 019	2 205	1 617	1 604
Total submitted	38 967	29 511	30 657	32 390	28 740	31 401	31 930	29 749	27 889	27 802
Percentage diagnosed	4.3	4.8	5.8	5.4	5.3	7.3	6.3	7.4	5.8	5.8

NR, not recorded

in 400 cows in three dairy herds in California 47% were seropositive for *C. fetus* (Ahktar et al., 1993). About 90% of infertility due to *C. fetus* is due to the subspecies *venerealis*; however, the subspecies *fetus*, of which there are two serotypes, can cause sporadic abortion but is not normally associated with infertility and is not spread venereally. Saprophytic organisms such as *Campylobacter bulbus* and *C. faecalis* may be present in the alimentary tract of cattle and in the prepuce of the bull. In the latter site, they may complicate diagnosis by direct bacteriological examination and fluorescent antibody tests.

Clinical signs and course of disease

Lawson and MacKinnon (1952) have studied bovine genital vibriosis under experimental conditions and have provided an excellent account of the symptoms, course and diagnosis of the disease. Boyd (1955) has produced data from Sweden on the natural history of *C. fetus* infection. In the bull, the organism is confined to the glans penis, prepuce and distal urethra. In the cow the site of infection is the vagina, cervix, uterus and uterine tubes. Unless treated, a bull is likely to carry the infection for life without any interference with its reproductive behaviour or seminal qualities. The bull acts simply as a carrier and transmits the infection at service to the vagina of the female; there are no lesions.

As might be expected, the organisms do not interfere with the fertilization process, but following their colonization of the uterus, a tissue reaction occurs which is inimical to nidation of the embryo, or to its continuing nourishment in the uterus. In a majority of susceptible females served by an infected bull, therefore, fertilization occurs but is followed by early embryonic death. In a much smaller proportion of infected cows, later abortion occurs at from 4 to 7 months.

C. fetus infection also causes inflammation of the cervix with increased secretion of mucus which may become mixed with uterine exudate to form a mucoflocculent vulval discharge after service. This, however, is not nearly so conspicuous a symptom as in trichomoniasis (see below). The endometritis is of a mild nature and cannot be appreciated by rectal palpation of the uterus.

If death of the embryo occurs before the maternal recognition of pregnancy (Chapter 3) the cow will return to service at 3 weeks; later death of the embryo will be followed by irregular return to heat, often at around 30 days. Hence the first signs of genital vibriosis to be seen by the stockman will be a number of females returning, some regularly, and some irregularly, to service by a newly introduced bull. A small proportion of susceptible cows and heifers conceive to first service by an infected bull and carry their calves to full term. With continued service by the infected bull, reinfection occurs, but the cows gradually develop an immunity as a result of which the uterine reaction is reduced and early abortion does not occur. In some of these cases, however, quite extensive disease of the fetal membranes is present; it is very similar to that caused by *Brucella abortus* and comprises necrosis with yellowish-brown discoloration of the fetal cotyledons and leather-like thickening, or oedema, of the inter-cotyledonary allantochorion. Such lesions are likely to lead to abortion at from 4 to 7 months of gestation.

As the disease progresses in the herd and immunity is gradually built up, the length of interval between infected service and return to service tends to increase. Eventually, after an average of five services, the majority of cows become safely pregnant and carry their calves to term. It is always possible, however, that the occasional cow will abort and, at parturition, a few cows may retain the fetal membranes as a result of the disease. Most cows which have had normal gestations to an infected bull will be free of infection at the time they are next required to be served. In this way a closed herd, after experiencing serious infertility for about 6 months, will gradually become immune and thereafter undergo normal gestation at the end of which there will be freedom of infection. It is likely that reinfection of some cows will occur if bred again after normal parturition to the same bull and a similar, but very much smaller, infertility problem recurs. Within 2 or 3 years, however, normal fertility is probable. But in ordinary circumstances, few milking herds remain closed for long, it being usual to introduce a number of heifers to the milking herd each year. In this way, non-immune animals are added, and the disease may remain troublesome for years either in the maiden heifers, or in the first-calf heifers, if the latter had been served for the first pregnancy by a separate clean bull. In the same way, in a 'flying' herd the symptoms of vibriosis may be perpetuated by the non-immune bought-in females.

Diagnosis

Genital vibriosis will be strongly suspected when a majority of cows or heifers are returning regularly or irregularly to service, especially if the infertility coincides with the introduction of a new bull. The possibility that the breeding trouble is due to defective semen of the newly introduced bull should first be eliminated and then specific enquiry for the presence of C. fetus should be made.

A variety of diagnostic tests can be used to diagnose C. fetus infection. These are: (1) the identification of the organism following direct smear or culture, (2) serological tests, (3) vaginal mucus agglutination and (4) fluorescent antibody tests.

In bulls suspected of infection, preputial washings and subsequent aspiration of the fluid or scraping of the penile or preputial mucosa can be used for subsequent bacteriological examination (Bartlett, 1948; Dufty and McEntee, 1969; Tedesco, 1977). Ideally, a selective enriched transport medium should be used; this contains polymyxin B, which inhibits the growth of contaminants, obviates the need for refrigeration, and at temperatures over 38°C — and even after a delay of 2–5 days — can result in good recovery of the organism (Eaglesome and Garcia, 1992). Tissues from an aborted fetus (lung, spleen, liver) and abomasal fluid should be removed aseptically and maintained at 4°C until they reach the laboratory. Direct smears of abomasal contents should be examined using phase contrast or dark field microscopy. If the selective enriched transport medium is used this is normally incubated for 4 days at 37°C before transfer to blood agar plates. In the case of fresh samples, these are streaked on to the plates.

Serological tests are of little or no value, since genital campylobacteriosis does not engender measurable serum antibody levels.

A vaginal mucus agglutination test was first described by Kendrick (1967) and has been used extensively since. Mucus can be collected by a variety of different methods; however, it is important not to use the copious mucus of oestrus in which the agglutinins will be diluted, but mucus from a cow in dioestrus, which can be difficult to

collect in sufficient quantities. A variety of methods have been used; these include a glass or plastic pipette to which is attached a mouth piece, and a small portable vacuum pump. Probably the simplest and most effective method in cows, as opposed to heifers, is to insert a clean, gloved hand into the vagina and to scoop mucus into the palm of the hand from the ventral fornix. This can be transferred to a wide-mouth collecting bottle. The vaginal mucus agglutination test should be used for herd diagnosis rather than for individual cows. False positives can be obtained if the mucus is contaminated with blood. It is important to ensure that sufficient time has elapsed since animals would have been exposed to infection; thus in investigating a herd it is important to ensure that all non-pregnant cows that were first exposed to service more than 60 days previously should be sampled. One positive reaction is sufficient to establish a herd infection; for this reason, confirmation of an infected bull can be made by allowing test mating of two virgin heifers and performing a mucus agglutination test 60–80 days later. Recently, a method has been developed in which a piece of Whatman filter paper is placed on the lateral wall of the vagina cranial to the urethral opening until it is saturated; secretory immunoglobulin (IgA) is then detected using enzyme-linked immunosorbent assay (ELISA) (Hum et al., 1991).

Preputial samples from suspect bulls can be examined using fluorescent antibody techniques. At present it is not possible to differentiate between the two subspecies venerealis and fetus although it can distinguish them from other species of Campylobacter. Dufty (1967) advised that a bull can be declared non-infected after four consecutive negative fluorescent antibody tests.

Treatment and control

Control is based on three epidemiological facts: first that transmission is venereal, secondly that bulls remain permanently infected and thirdly that infected cows overcome the infection, or become immune, in a period of 3–6 months from service. Thus if infected service is replaced by artificial insemination, 'self-cure' of the cows will occur. Non-infected semen may be obtained from the local artificial insemination centre or from a newly purchased clean bull; the latter may be a virgin bull or one that has been proved to be free of infection; alternatively the herd bull himself may be cured of infection and subsequently used artificially. Such an artificial insemination scheme proves highly successful and poses no problem in the case of the non-exposed females — including the annual intake of clean heifers, these being effectively shielded from infection. The drawback is that in some herds artificial insemination is not easily applicable to the type of husbandry followed; also some pedigree herds require a special blood-line that is not available in bulls at the artificial insemination centre. A question the attending veterinary surgeon will soon be required to answer is 'how long is it necessary to persist with artificial insemination?' It seems certain that in a majority of cows *C. fetus* will not survive a normal gestation, but Frank and Bryner (1953) recovered *Campylobacter* spp. from a few cows as long as 196 days beyond the end of a pregnancy initiated by infected semen. It would seem wise therefore to continue insemination until every exposed cow has completed two normal pregnancies. Natural breeding can then be resumed. In the above scheme it is, of course, safe to use a clean bull on the virgin heifers and to protect him from infection by using him artificially for the infected part of the herd. After the heifers have calved they may again be mated naturally to the clean bull. Such a departure from a total insemination programme requires a very strict supervision to ensure that accurate service records are kept and thus to avoid accidental contamination of the clean bull by a cow from the infected group.

A less satisfactory method is to breed the heifers and any non-exposed cows artificially or to a clean bull — as outlined above — and to continue service by the herd bull on the infected group. In addition to the risk of accidental contamination of the clean bull there is always the possibility that reinfection of recovered cows may thus occur and that a minor degree of infertility may persist; the much more serious aspect is that such a herd will never be free of infection so long as the infected bull continues to be used.

C. fetus is sensitive to streptomycin (Binns, 1953), and this antibiotic has been used to treat the disease in bulls. Dihydrostreptomycin at a dose rate of 22 mg/kg subcutaneously, together with the local application of the same antibiotic to the penis and prepuce (50% solution) is effective,

although it must be remembered that the bulls will be susceptible to reinfection. The use of the same antibiotic in the cow has no beneficial effect, whether administered locally or parenterally.

Vaccination has been used to cure infected bulls. Bouters (1973) reported that by giving two doses of vaccine at a month's interval, 51 known infected bulls were cured, and this, together with annual vaccination programmes, greatly reduced the incidence of genital vibriosis in areas of Belgium where ambulant stud bulls were used. Some have expressed concern that it may only modify the carrier status (Hoerlein, 1980).

Vaccination programmes have been successful in controlling the disease in situations where artificial insemination cannot be practised. Using oil adjuvant bacterins with high cell counts of immunogenic strains of *C. fetus* subsp. *venerealis* good results have been obtained. Preferably vaccination should be carried out 30–90 days before breeding commences and, since the immunity wanes annually, revaccination is recommended for optimum protection as close to the time of service as possible (Hoerlein, 1980).

Brucellosis (contagious abortion)

Brucellosis in cattle is most commonly caused by *Brucella abortus*. *Brucella melitensis*, which occurs in sheep and goats, can also be transmitted to cattle.

B. abortus occurs in most countries of the world where cattle are kept in any significant numbers except for those that have implemented eradication schemes. Thimm and Wundt (1976) showed that the disease occurs in 95 out of 153 countries where information was available.

Clinical signs

Where the disease occurs it causes serious economic loss due primarily to abortion in the second half of gestation, although earlier abortions occur at the beginning of an outbreak. In addition, some calves will be born alive but they will be weak and unthrifty. Infected cows usually abort once and seldom more than twice, although in subsequent pregnancies the uterus may be reinfected from the udder but the cow then carries the fetus to term. Infected cows that abort in later gestation and those that carry to term often retain their fetal membranes; this is partly due to uterine inertia and partly to placentitis. Such animals show delayed involution of the uterus and are prone to secondary bacterial invasion with resultant puerperal metritis. Whereas the *Brucella* organisms are usually expelled from the uterus within 2 weeks of parturition or abortion, i.e. well before the next mating, it is possible that they are still present at this time and a chronic endometritis which will cause infertility until it resolves after a few oestrous cycles. Inasmuch as it initiates many cases of puerperal metritis, *B. abortus* may predispose to the formation of ovarobursal adhesions.

Leaving aside abortion and puerperal infection (which is usually due to secondary bacterial invasion), is *B. abortus* a cause of bovine infertility? This seems unlikely, for the organism does not naturally colonize the non-pregnant uterus. A bull with a *Brucella* lesion in its testicle, epididymis or seminal vesicle can transmit organisms to the vagina and cervix, but it seems unlikely that the uterus becomes infected thereby. If, however, intrauterine insemination with infected semen is applied, a uterine infection may become established and cause infertility; in view of the measures taken to ensure that artificial insemination bulls are free from brucellosis, this eventuality is very improbable under present-day conditions.

Epidemiology

Cattle become infected by ingesting *B. abortus* on contaminated pasture, or in food and water, or by licking an aborted fetus, infected afterbirth or genital exudate from a recently aborted or recently calved cow. Infection may also occur via the teat from infected milk of another cow and via the vagina from infected semen. In experimental studies of brucellosis, conjunctival inoculation is usually employed. Although infected cows often shed the organism in the milk (thereby endangering the public health) and thus infect calves, the main danger of spread to other cattle is at the time of abortion or parturition. For a day or two before, during and for about a fortnight after delivery, the genital discharge of the infected female is highly dangerous. When the fetal membranes are retained the uterus may not free itself until about a month after delivery. After the completion of uterine involution the organisms colonize the udder and supramammary lymph nodes, whence, in the next gestation, infection of the placenta again occurs.

Calves that derive milk-borne infection throw off infection from the lymph glands of the gastro-intestinal tract in 50–80 days. The infantile uterus does not become infected.

The uterus of pregnant cattle becomes infected from the bloodstream, and the organisms parasitize the allantochorion whence fetal and amniotic infections occur. The changes caused in the placenta and fetus lead to abortion. Occasionally, fetal death occurs and is not followed by abortion, the retained fetus undergoing mummification or maceration. Fetuses from late abortions are often born alive but are frequently weakly and may consequently contract white scour.

Outside the animal body *B. abortus* may live for months in aborted fetuses or fetal membranes, but when exposed to drying and sunshine it is soon killed.

Diagnosis

The organism can be identified in stained smears prepared from suspected contaminated material. Special staining techniques using a modified Koster and Ziehl–Neelson method is quite successful (Brinley Morgan and MacKinnon, 1979). A more specific method of direct identification is a fluorescent antibody technique, and enables differentiation from other infectious disease such as Q fever (Brinley Morgan and MacKinnon, 1979). *B. abortus* can be cultured from the fetal stomach of an abort or from fresh afterbirth or uterine exudate. Because culture of the organism is time-consuming and expensive, new methods of identification have been devised. A colony blot ELISA using monoclonal antibodies provides a rapid, inexpensive and reliable method of identifying *B. abortus* (Eaglesome and Garcia, 1992). Where contamination is probable, the suspected material is inoculated into guinea-pigs, in which characteristic lesions occur and from which the organisms can be cultured. (The organisms can also be recovered by guinea-pig inoculation from milk and from semen.)

Numerous serological tests have been used to diagnose brucellosis using a wide range of biological materials such as milk, whey, serum, vaginal mucus and semen. These have then been subjected to agglutination test, the complement fixation test, the antiglobulin test, the fluorescent antibody test and immunodiffusion or electroimmunodiffusion tests (Brinley Morgan and MacKinnon, 1979).

The rose bengal plate test was introduced into the UK in 1970 as the main initial screening test of serum samples in the brucellosis eradication scheme (Brinley Morgan and Richards, 1974). It is recognized that it is oversensitive and may identify non-infected animals as being positive. For this reason the positive samples are re-examined using the serum agglutination test (SAT) or complement fixation test (CFT); rose bengal-negative samples are not normally retested.

An SAT is very widely used, provided that the antigen is standardized against the international standard *anti-Brucella abortus serum*. It has some deficiencies: (1) it detects non-specific antibodies as well as specific antibodies from *Brucella* infection and vaccination; (2) during incubation it is the last of all the possible tests to indicate the presence of infection, however after abortion it may be the last to detect diagnostically significant levels; (3) in the chronic stage of the disease the agglutinins wane, thus giving a negative result when other tests would give a positive result (Brinley Morgan and MacKinnon, 1979).

The CFT is a more definitive test than the SAT, especially in differentiating titres arising from infection from vaccination. The CFT identifies infected adults before the SAT, and, as the disease becomes chronic, the titres detected by the SAT tend to fall below diagnostic levels whereas titres detected by the CFT persist at diagnostically significant levels. In calves vaccinated with strain 19 (see below), titres detected by the CFT become negative in most cases by 6 months after vaccination, whereas an 18 month period is required for the SAT. The milk ring test, which detects *Brucella* antibodies in milk, is very useful in screening the presence of brucellosis in herds by collecting bulk milk samples or in individual animals. Positive results can then be followed up by using other diagnostic tests on individual animals.

The vaginal mucus agglutination test can be used on samples from individual cows; it is not very reliable.

It must be conceded that during an active infection of a herd the blood agglutination test is an unsatisfactory means of recognizing individual infection; during the period of incubation negative reactions will occur and, furthermore, it is quite common for a negative reaction to be given at the time of, and for a few days after, an abortion due to *Brucella*. Infected bulls sometimes fail to react to the blood test, and it is considered that if the agglutination test is performed on semen plasma, rather than blood, a better indication of infection

will be obtained. In recent years, because of the purification of specific *B. abortus* antigens and the production of corresponding monoclonal antibodies, enzyme immunoassays have been developed. Using some competitive ELISAs, it is possible to discriminate between vaccinated and non-vaccinated infected animals (Nielsen et al., 1989). Such methods play an important role in the control of the disease (see below).

Control

There is confusion over the veterinary and public health aspects of control. From the animal husbandry viewpoint an immunized herd in which abortions are eliminated is a fairly satisfactory position which may be readily achieved by calfhood vaccination, using *B. abortus* S19 live antigen. But from the public health standpoint such a state of affairs is unsatisfactory in that vaccination does not eliminate herd infection and, as a consequence, there is a perpetual risk of undulant fever in those who consume the raw milk.

To meet both requirements enlightened governments have followed a two-stage policy in respect of brucellosis control. In the first place widespread vaccination is encouraged in order to reduce losses due to abortion and its sequelae and, secondly, a programme of national eradication of the disease is initiated. In some countries, states, areas or even herds where rigorous measures of hygiene can be enforced, eradication has been achieved without recourse to vaccination. Norway, in 1952, was the first country to eradicate the disease, and Sweden and Denmark are now free; in Britain, USA and New Zealand immunization has been widely practised. Britain became free of *Brucella* in 1983.

The EU considers a bovine herd to be officially brucellosis-free if it contains no animals vaccinated against brucellosis (except females vaccinated at least 3 years previously), if all bovine animals have been free from clinical signs for at least 6 months and if all cattle over 12 months old have passed the SAG test at less than 30 IU. Animals in these herds are subject to twice yearly blood tests. In those herds where milk is collected into churns, the milk ring test may be used. Replacement cattle must be certified from a brucellosis-free herd and officially tested if over 12 months old. Testing replacement cattle need not be required if infected herds have not exceeded 0.2% for at least 2 years and certification need not be required if at least 99.8% of herds are officially free, and infected herds are under supervision.

Vaccination. In 1941, S19 vaccine was officially introduced into the USA, since when it has been employed in Great Britain and other countries. S19 is a smooth variant of a strain of *B. abortus* of reduced virulence but of high antigenic quality. It is intended for use on calves 4–8 months old before the onset of puberty in which it causes a febrile reaction and a low blood agglutination titre, the latter being usually lost before the heifer reaches breeding age. In self-contained herds calfhood vaccination is sufficient for life but where adult cattle are brought in, and in the presence of active infection, cows should be revaccinated after the first calf. When infection is introduced to an unvaccinated herd all adult female stock, except those with possible blood agglutination titres, as well as calves, and cows pregnant up to 4 months, should be vaccinated. S19 gives a better immunity when used on cows rather than calves, but in sexually mature cattle higher and more persistent agglutinating titres are produced; also, a greater general reaction occurs with serious interference with subsequent milk yield. Vaccinal titres occurring in adult cows may be confused with natural infection but they seldom rise above 1:200 and decline with passage of time. It is not usual to vaccinate bull calves, mainly because brucellosis of bulls is uncommon and also because a vaccinal titre might throw suspicion on the bull and would preclude its purchase for artificial insemination or for export. In addition, it has been reported that S19 may produce permanent infection in bulls which is similar to the natural disease, and thus should not be used (Nicoletti, 1986).

The widespread application of S19 vaccination has greatly reduced the losses from contagious abortion, and when its use is restricted to calves — as originally intended — the results are excellent. But although infection is reduced, vaccination will not eradicate the disease.

The titres produced by S19 in cattle vaccinated as adults constitute a serious disadvantage when an eradication programme is dependent on the interpretation of the SAT. For this reason, vaccines prepared from killed cultures of McEwan's *B. abortus* S45/20 with adjuvant, which cause only insignificant titres, have been recommended for use on cattle of all ages; pregnant cows may also be safely vaccinated. When the brucellosis eradication scheme was introduced in Britain (Brucellosis Accredited Herds Scheme) the use of S19 vaccines was restricted to calves between 90 and 180 days of age. Herds were not accepted into the scheme until at least a year after the last use of the vaccine.

Eradication. In order to tackle the problem of eradication, statutory powers are required to implement a compulsory programme. In Britain this was preceded by a voluntary scheme with incentives to encourage herd owners to become brucellosis-free at an earlier date.

The scheme which has proved successful in Britain is illustrated in Figure 23.3, which is modified from that of Brinley Morgan and MacKinnon (1979). Once the herd has become a Brucellosis Accredited Herd only accredited animals can be introduced into the herd, and it becomes subject to the requirements of the Brucellosis Orders of 1979 (Scotland) and 1981 (England and Wales). Under these regulations *all* births before 271 days constitute an abortion, and the following measures must be taken:

1. A veterinary inspector or officer (usually the Divisional Veterinary Officer) of the Ministry of Agriculture, Fisheries and Food (MAFF) must be notified.
2. The cow that is aborting or has aborted must be isolated, together with the fetus or calf and placenta.
3. The fetus or calf and placenta must be retained on the premises.

Where there are no statutory powers implementing such an eradication scheme then interim measures, similar to those used in Britain, can be used in an attempt to become brucellosis-free.

In positive herds with no recent history of abortion, repeated herd blood samples are taken and if these disclose inactive infection with a small proportion of reacting animals, it is advisable to sell the reactors. Further herd blood samplings are undertaken with a view to obtaining a certificate of freedom from the disease. Such herds become controlled as in the first category. If there are too many reactors for immediate disposal to be an economical proposition, the disease is controlled, as far as possible, on the farm; reactors are separated from non-reactors and are strictly isolated when they calve or if they abort. Rigorous cleaning, disinfection and disposal of infective material is

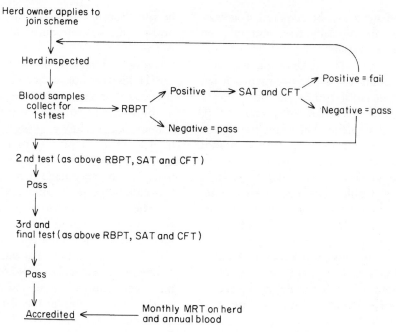

Fig. 23.3 Brucellosis eradication scheme used in Britain. RBPT, rose bengal plate test; MRT, milk ring test; other abbreviations defined in text. (After Brinley Morgan and MaKinnon).

practised. The complete isolation of the reactor from 4 days before calving or abortion to 14 days aterwards is the key to successful reduction in incidence of the disease on the farm. Calfhood vaccination should be performed in these infected herds. When the incidence of infection is sufficiently reduced, the reactors may be slaughtered.

Lastly, in heavily infected herds with current abortion, the spread of infection must be controlled in every possible way. It is best to isolate all parturient or aborting animals from 4 days before to 14 days after parturition. Disposal of infected material, thorough cleansing and disinfection after an abortion and segregation of reactors is practised. There will be a shortage of young stock on such a farm, and this can be made good by buying in calves from free herds; these calves and all other young stock are vaccinated. When the disease becomes quiescent — as shown by further blood tests — disposal of reactors may begin.

Cows in controlled herds should be served only by non-reacting bulls, or inseminated with semen from *Brucella*-free bulls.

By employing the above measures in Denmark between 1946 and 1954 the incidence of infected herds was reduced from 25 to 2.4% (Nielsen, 1955). In roughly the same period the number of

human cases of undulant fever fell from 325 to 35. In the USA, control measures for bovine brucellosis reduced the numbers of human cases from 2000 in 1947 to 248 in 1967. New Zealand began its national eradication scheme in 1971: in 1973, brucellosis accounted for 17% of all bovine abortions; by 1977 this figure had been reduced to 2.2%. The success of the scheme in Britain can be seen in the figures for abortions due to *B. abortus* and listed in Table 23.1.

Tuberculosis of the genitalia

In many countries throughout the world bovine tuberculosis has been eradicated. However, before eradication schemes were implemented it was an important cause of infertility and thus, where bovine tuberculosis still exists, it should always be considered as a possible cause. Infection may reach the tract either by spread from the peritoneum via the uterine tubes or by penetration of the serosa, or by bloodstream invasion, in which case the endometrium may be involved in the absence of serous or tubal lesions. Occasionally, primary uterine infections may arise from contaminated instruments or hands during gynaecological or obstetrical interferences.

Uterus

Williams (1939) classified uterine tuberculosis as being of three clinical types — peritoneal, glandular and epithelial.

Peritoneal. The outstanding feature is extensive adhesions of the cornua to themselves, the parietal peritoneum and adjacent organs. The adhesions often contain multiple abscesses up to the size of a hen's egg or even larger.

Glandular. This type involved chiefly the glandular layer of the mucous membrane and is characterized by marked hypertrophy of a diffuse or nodular nature. Caseous or caseopurulent foci of variable size are found throughout.

No clear line of demarcation exists between these types, but one generally predominates. The condition is generally bicornual and to a degree symmetrical. The presence of a vulval discharge varies, depending on the degree to which the mucous membrane is involved. In advanced cases there is a profuse mucopurulent discharge, pyogenic infection being added to the tuberculous one. In these cases the uterine tubes are almost invariably involved.

Epithelial. This type generally originates in the bloodstream and the lesions take the form of multiple pin-head-sized granulomata. Often there is no appreciable enlargement of the uterus, but a vulval discharge, from which acid-fast organisms can readily be isolated, is the rule. The discharge may be serosanguineous or frankly purulent.

Tuberculosis of the uterus is not an inevitable barrier to reproduction, for quite frequently a calf is born from a grossly infected uterus (the calf itself being affected by the congenital form of the disease), but it is probable in such cases that the uterine infection was acquired or, at least, rapidly developed during pregnancy. The epithelial form is especially liable to develop after parturition.

The uterine tubes are generally involved in types 1 and 2. They become progressively thickened, often attaining a diameter of 1 cm and may contain local abscesses. There are generally adhesions of the bursa to the ovary. An ovary itself may be the site of tuberculous abscesses. The cervix is rarely affected.

The diagnosis by rectal examination of early cases may be difficult, but particular attention should be paid to the uterine tubes, for the detection of thickened, tortuous tubes is diagnostic. (In this connection care must be taken that the ter-

minations of the cornua are not confused with the uterine tubes.) In advanced cases, diffuse or nodular enlargement of the uterus will be readily detected. In infected herds, an animal showing a chronic vulval discharge continuing beyond the puerperium should always be examined for acid-fast organisms and abortions or premature births should be regarded with suspicion.

Trichomoniasis

The recognition of *Tritrichomonas fetus* infection as a cause of infertility was an important advance in our understanding of the role of specific venereal pathogens in cattle (Riedmuller, 1928; Abelein, 1938; Stableforth et al., 1937). Since the 1950s, with the widespread use of artificial insemination, the disease has been reduced dramatically in many countries; it is probably non-existent in Britain at the present time. However, world-wide it is a major cause of reproductive failure. In California, recent surveys have shown that between 5 and 38.5% of beef bulls are infected and 8.7% of dairy cows (Skirrow and BonDurant, 1988; BonDurant et al., 1990). Similar high levels of infection have been reported elsewhere in the USA and South Africa (Eaglesome and Garcia, 1992). Whenever natural service is used it must always be considered as a cause of infertility.

Clinical signs

The causal organism is a flagellate protozoan (Figure 23.4). In the female, infection is characterized by low pregnancy rates, a profuse mucoflocculent vulval discharge, early abortion and pyometra. Irregularities of the oestrous cycle are common in infected herds.

Cows and heifers which have been exposed to infected service fall into the following clinical groups:

1. Conceive and carry to term without clinical signs of infection developing.

2. Return to multiple services, but show no obvious signs of infection. Oestrous periods may be regular or irregular.

3. Fail to conceive and develop an oedematous condition of the endometrium with a mucoflocculent discharge.

4. Conceive but abort at from 2–4 months of gestation.

5. Develop pyometra and become acyclic.

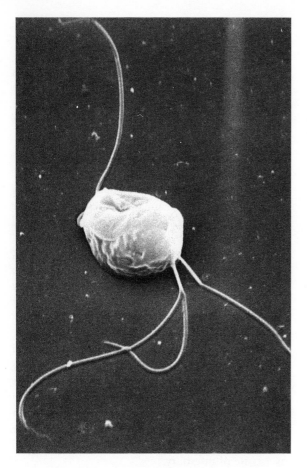

Fig. 23.4 Scanning electron micrograph of *T. fetus* (×16 500).

The clinical picture has been clearly described by Wright and Arthur (1945). The disease had been introduced into a herd by a bull 10 months prior to the commencement of the investigation, by which time 77 cows and heifers had been exposed to infection by one or more services. The results of exposure to infection were as follows: 21% conceived and carried to term and no evidence of infection was found; 49% failed to conceive but the parasite was not isolated from them; 30% showed the presence of the parasite. This last group comprised 23 animals; four of them aborted and four others developed pyometra.

The organism produces a catarrhal endometritis and vaginitis with oedema of vulva, perivaginal tissue and uterine wall. Affected animals show an intermittent vulval discharge and on rectal palpation the uterus is found to be enlarged and flaccid. Manipulation of the uterus often provokes a discharge from the vulva and motile trichomonads

can generally be demonstrated in it. Kerr and Robertson (1941, 1943) showed that both naturally and artificially infected cows develop specific agglutinins against the parasite in their blood serum, while Pierce (1946) found that similar agglutinins developed in the vaginal discharge of infected animals. There is evidence that animals which develop a clinical infection may subsequently conceive to infected service and carry to term, but it would appear that immunity is lost after a normal gestational period. In the female, the disease is essentially self-limiting and infection confers a relative degree of temporary resistance. The effect of *T. fetus* on conception varies according to the activity of the infection. Initial infections generally terminate pregnancy almost from the outset and they are followed by a variable degree of uterine involvement. Less active infections, influenced in measure by resistance acquired from previous infections, may not prevent pregnancy proceeding to a more advanced stage and the abortion of visible fetuses or the development of pyometra more often follows repeated than primary infection. Nevertheless, both initial and reinfection are occasionally followed by normal pregnancy.

Visible abortion generally occurs at 2–4 months, and it is significant that in those cases which expel the fetus at the later limit its size is smaller than that appropriate to the period of gestation; this is due to growth retardation. In such abortion cases the fetus, which is grey in colour, is generally expelled complete in its membranes. There are no signs of putrefaction and *T. fetus* can readily be demonstrated in the fetal fluids. After the act of abortion, however, parasites quickly disappear from the vaginal discharges, and it is unlikely they will be found later than 7 days after the act. The author has had an animal conceive normally to artificial insemination using non-infected semen 67 days after abortion. Pyometra, which can occur in up to 10% of cows in an outbreak, probably occurs following late embryonic or early fetal death with persistence of the corpus luteum. Administration of $PGF_{2\alpha}$ will cause regression of the corpus luteum, and the uterus will empty itself, and recovery may occur. The pus in these cases is teeming with trichomonads in association with pyogenic corynebacteria.

There appears to be great variation in the intensity and duration of infection in individual females. In some, no clinical signs of infection are seen after exposure, yet their subsequent conception to the use of carrier semen indicates they have a tolerance. In those in which an oedematous condition of the uterus develops, the parasite may be found for as long as 4 months after infected service, while in cases which ultimately abort or develop pyometra the parasite continues to flourish in the uterus as long as the uterus is occupied by conceptus or pus, but once it is evacuated the organism quickly disappears.

The author has never found persistence of infection throughout a normal pregnancy, and this is confirmed by the experience of Bartlett and his coworkers in the USA (Bartlett et al., 1947). It may thus be taken that any animal which has carried to term subsequent to infection is free from disease.

Diagnosis

Although clinical signs and history frequently strongly support a diagnosis of trichomoniasis, a positive diagnosis can be made following identification of the organism. The best source of material are the fetal membranes or the organs of an aborted fetus (especially the abomasum). Failing this, the organism can be identified in vaginal mucus or mucopurulent discharge; the former can be collected as previously described for *C. fetus*, although following abortion the organisms often disappear within 48 hours. In cases of pyometra the pus should be examined since, unlike other discharges, large numbers of trichomonads will be present. Material contaminated with faeces should be discarded because non-pathogenic trichomonads may be present. It is also possible to culture *T. fetus* on modified Diamond's medium; however, a period of up to 9 days is required (BonDurant, 1990). Agglutinating antibodies are developed locally in the vagina and uterus in response to infection, their identification can be used as a herd test in the same way as described previously for *C. fetus* (see p. 399). There is no suitable serological test available at present.

In the bull, the presence of infection can be demonstrated by the identification of the organism in preputial washing or preferably following vigorous scraping of the preputial mucosa to obtain as much smegma as possible (Eaglesome and Garcia, 1992). The bull should be allowed a period of 5–10 days of sexual rest before sampling so that the

number of trichomonads can increase. Alternatively, the presence of the infection in a bull can be demonstrated using a test mating with a virgin heifer (Ball et al., 1983). Cervical mucus should be collected 10–20 days later to demonstrate the presence of *T. fetus* by direct examination or culture.

Whatever the source of the material which might contain trichomonads, it should be examined as soon as possible after collection.

Treatment and control

Control is based on the assumption that recovery in the female is spontaneous, and that infection of healthy animals cannot occur if natural service is replaced by artificial insemination with semen from non-infected bulls.

When it is established that *T. fetus* infection exists in a herd, the females should be grouped as follows:

1. Those actually or potentially infected by service from a carrier bull.
2. Those which have not been exposed to infection. This group will comprise recently calved cows not served since the introduction of an infected bull, and maiden heifers.

When more than one bull is being used in the herd the general attitude should be that they are carriers despite the fact that examination of service records indicates that one or other of them has not been exposed to infection. Experience leads to a strong suspicion of the reliability of service records, and thus the general rule should be that no bull on the farm shall be used to serve non-infected cows and heifers. This attitude may be relaxed when, for example, a young bull is running with heifers on some remote part of the farm and has made no contact with the general herd. Again, the farmer must be made to understand that it is imperative that there shall be no errors in regard to group 2 and that animals about which there is any doubt must be included in 1.

A non-infected bull should be obtained, and it is imperative that there is no possibility that he is exposed to infection. The regimen must be continued until all the adult animals in the herd at the time the infection was demonstrated have conceived and 'carried' to insemination. Or it may be decided to allow him to serve naturally animals in group 2 and use his semen for the insemination of those in group 1. Needless to say, the time the infection has been in existence and hence the proportion of animals exposed will influence one in this matter.

Treatment. As a general principle, carrier bulls should be culled since, unlike the infection in the female, it persists indefinitely. However, in a valuable animal whose blood-line it is desirous to maintain, treatment may be considered.

Since the recognition of *T. fetus* as a cause of herd infertility a great variety of agents have been used for the treatment of the infected bull. The original method used by Abelein (1938) and Swangard (1939) involved the thorough manual application to the penis and prepuce — withdrawn under epidural anaesthesia — of an ointment which contained trypaflavine and a protozoacidal agent. The penis may also be extruded under bilateral internal pudendal nerve block or with the aid of a tranquillizing drug. Several other compounds have been used, these include acriflavine, diminazene aceturate and metronidazole. The technique is time-consuming and the results are unreliable.

Bartlett (1948) used sodium iodide in a dosage of 5 g/45 kg body weight in 500 ml water, by intravenous injection on five occasions at 2 day intervals.

In the USA, where trichomoniasis is still a problem in beef herds, bulls have been cured by oral dimetridazole at a dose rate of 50 mg/kg body weight for 5 days (McLaughlin, 1968) or intravenous metronidazole as a single injection at a dose rate of 75 mg/kg every 12 hours on three occasions. Ipronidazole, in a single intramuscular dose of 30 g has been demonstrated to be effective in a substantial percentage of bulls. Pretreatment with a broad-spectrum antibiotic improves the response. Unfortunately, these therapeutic substances are not licensed for use in cattle in the UK and USA.

A new antibiotic, trichostatin, has been found to be effective against *T. fetus in vitro* and *in vivo* (Otoguro et al., 1988). There is no evidence that the treatment of cows or heifers hastens the time to self-cure.

Whichever treatment is used for *T. fetus*-infected bulls, the only criterion of cure is the uninfected impregnation of several maiden heifers.

Leptospirosis

Leptospirosis is an important zoonotic disease of cattle caused by parasitic spirochaetes classified within the genus *Leptospira* (Eaglesome and Garcia, 1992). Its distribution is world-wide, and cattle can be infected with a number of serogroups and serovars, several of which have a specific effect upon the genital system causing fetal death with abortion, stillbirth and weakly live calves.

Several surveys have shown how common the disease is in cattle. For example, following a bacteriological examination of 60 cows and heifers seleted at random at an abattoir, *Leptospira interrogans* serovar *hardjo* was isolated from 65% of the animals. In these the spirochaete was isolated from the vagina in 21.7%, the ovary and tubular genital tract in 57% and the urinary system in 62% of the animals. When the results from the microscopic agglutination test (MAT) of sera collected from the same animals were studied, the prevalence of antibodies to the serovar *hardjo* was lower than that from the microbiological study. Overall, 48% (1 in 10) and 27% (1 in 100) had detectable titres to the serovar *hardjo* (Ellis et al., 1986). In 109 herds surveyed in New South Wales using the MAT on serum at a dilution of 1:100 only 28% were negative, with a prevalence of 27% positive to the serovar *pomona*, 16% positive to the serovar *hardjo*, and 31% positive to both (King, 1991). Infection due to the serovar *pomona* is greater in Australia, New Zealand and the USA, whilst in parts of Africa, Russia and Israel infection with the serogroup *grippotyphosa* is the most important incidental leptospiral infection of cattle (Ellis, 1986).

Clinical signs

There are a number of different manifestations of *Leptospira* infection:

1. An acute febrile disease with temperatures of 40°C or more, together with haemoglobinuria, icterus and anorexia. Although the mortality rate in adult cows is low, pregnant animals will abort. This is usually caused by serovars such as *pomona* and *canicola*, and serogroups such as *icterohaemorrhagiae* and *grippotyphosa*.

2. A less acute type of disease where there is no pyrexia is most frequently associated with the serovar *hardjo*, which was first isolated from cattle in 1960 (Roth and Galton, 1960) and has now been shown to be endemic in the cattle population of the

UK (Ellis et al., 1981) and many other countries (Ellis, 1984).

The resultant reproductive effect of infection with the serovar *hardjo* is abortion, stillbirth or the birth of weakly calves. Abortion can occur at all stages of gestation from the fourth month to term; it is most common after 6 months. It can occur in the absence of any clinical signs of disease (Thiermann, 1982).

In some herds, abortions have occurred after a 'leptospiral mastitis' or agalactia has been observed during the previous 3 months (Ellis and Michna, 1976). The clinical history is as follows. There is a precipitous fall in milk yield, especially in cows that are in early lactation. From all four quarters the milk that is obtained is thick and colostrum-like with clots, and is frequently blood tinged; the udder is soft and flaccid, not hard as is characteristic of mastitis. There is a bacteraemia with or without a concurrent pyrexia. The agalactia lasts about 2–10 days, after which milk production usually returns close to normal although, in cows near the end of their lactation, milk production may not recover. Agalactia may not be so obvious in suckler cows although careful inspection of the calves may show reduced growth rates.

The number of animals infected in any one herd will vary from over 50% of cows during the 2 month period of an epidemic in a highly susceptible herd, to sporadic problems amongst first and second calf cows in a resistant herd (Hathaway and Little, 1983).

Abortion occurs all year round but, after correcting for any seasonal variations in calving, it is most prevalent in September and October.

The importance of the serovar *hardjo* as a cause of reproductive failure is clearly shown in the study of Ellis (1984) in which he found that, following the examination of 472 aborted fetuses, 20 stillborn calves and 13 weakly calves, it was isolated from 56, 70 and 85% of the cases, respectively.

Diagnosis

There are no lesions that are specific for leptospirosis, thus diagnosis of leptospirosis as a cause of abortion is based almost entirely upon demonstrating specific antibodies in fetal sera or by demonstrating leptospires in fetal organs, particularly lungs, kidneys, and adrenal glands, by culture or immunofluorescence.

The MAT is used extensively in the diagnosis of leptospirosis using serum from animals that have aborted or are suspected of being infected. It is of limited value in individual animals, but it can be useful as a herd screening test for both serovars *pomona* and *hardjo*, particularly in herds where the infection is endemic without clinical signs of the disease, and where certain groups might be at risk, i.e. heifers, newly purchased animals and farm staff. The screening of all animals in a herd is expensive; however, it is possible to sample a minimum number in order to obtain reliable information on the disease status. The following is recommended (Anon., 1992):

Total herd size	Number to be sampled
20	16
40	21
60	23
90	25
120	26
160	27
300	28
450+	29

The various categories within the herd, i.e. heifers, dry cows, cows in milk, should be sampled proportionately. When a partial or herd test reveals *hardjo* seropositive animals, then if the titres are below 1:400 and are confined to older animals in the herd which have mixed freely in the herd, then the infection can probably be considered to be historical rather than active.

Where more than 20% of the herd are seropositive or if titres are over 1:1600, then an active infection is present and further spread of the disease is possible (Anon., 1992).

Single samples from individual cows are of little value and it is impossible to separate infected from vaccinated animals. However, a high titre in a cow (> 1:1000) at the time of abortion is generally proof of infection; unfortunately, low titres < 1:100 can occur in infected animals (Ellis et al., 1982). Paired samples from individual animals are of no value, since there is usually an interval of 6–12 weeks between infection of the dam and fetal expulsion, by which time the dam's antibody titre is either falling, static or not detectable (Ellis, 1984–1985).

Transmission and pathogenesis

Infection of susceptible cattle can occur through mucous membranes and abraded skin. In all leptospires, excretion in urine is a common source of transmisison of the disease; normally it occurs for several weeks but it has been reported to be as long as 542 days (Thiermann, 1982) and it could be for a lifetime (Ellis, 1984). It can be present in the puerperal discharge for up to 8 days (Ellis, 1984), and can persist in the pregnant and non-pregnant uterus for up to 142 and 97 days after infection, respectively. Most beef heifers become infected as calves because of contact with adult cattle, and for this reason leptospiral abortions are less common in these breeds. Dairy heifers usually become infected at 2–3 years of age, either from older cows or an infected bull; sometimes they become infected when they are introduced into the main herd after calving (Ellis 1984–1985). The role of the bull in the transmission of the disease has been questioned since, according to Ellis et al. (1986), outbreaks of *hardjo* infection have frequently been associated with the introduction of a bull into a herd. The same authors, using material collected from seven stock bulls slaughtered at an abattoir, were able to demonstrate leptospires subgroup *sejroe* in the genital tracts of three bulls, particularly the vesicular glands, as well as the urinary system. Venereal transmission is thus a possibility.

Treatment and control

General control measures related to good hygiene, thus minimizing the risk of infection with leptospires from other host species, should be implemented. These include the strict segregation of cattle from pigs, rodent control and the draining or fencing off of contaminated water sources. The role of sheep in the epidemiology of the serovar *hardjo* is still not clear; however, since they have been shown to excrete the organism in their urine, it seems prudent not to graze them together.

There are two methods of specific treatment and control: they are the use of a vaccine or parenteral streptomycin/dihydrostreptomycin, or a combination of both. The antibiotic should be used at a dose rate of 25 mg/kg by intramuscular injection with no greater a volume than 20 ml at any one site. Milk should be withdrawn for 7 days and meat for 28 days. Repeated doses may be necessary. In closed herds, vaccination of all members of the herd should be done annually. In open herds the frequency should be increased to 6 monthly intervals; this is particularly important for heifers between 6 months and 3 years of age (Ellis, 1984). In an acute outbreak, combined treatment should be used.

Salmonellosis

Salmonellosis-induced abortion has been reported from many countries. In Britain it has persisted as a continuing, although not a major, problem for some time (see Table 23.1). The main organism involved is *Salmonella dublin* which is responsible for 80% of salmonella abortions (Hinton, 1983).

It is more prevalent in certain areas of Britain, notably Dorset, Somerset and south-west Wales. The disease is contracted following the grazing of pasture possibly contaminated with slurry from animal units, human sewage or infected river water.

Clinical signs

The classical sign of salmonellosis in adult cattle is dysentery, which may be associated with abortion. More frequently, salmonella abortions occur in late pregnancy in the absence of any other clinical signs, although malaise, pyrexia and inappetance have been recorded (Hinton, 1983).

Salmonella abortions are more prevalent in the period June to December; Hinton (1983) recorded 81% of salmonella abortions occurring during this time of the year. In most outbreaks only one or two animals are affected on each farm although occasionally five or six cases may be reported at one particular time.

Placental retention is a common sequel although there is no adverse effect upon fertility (Hall and Jones, 1976).

Pathogenesis

Following experimental infection of pregnant heifers with *S. dublin*, the organism rapidly spreads to the liver, spleen, lungs and adjacent lymph nodes of the dam; this is associated with pyrexia. Six to eight days later it spreads to the placentomes causing a second bout of pyrexia. The placentome is damaged, probably by endotoxin, causing necrosis, placental failure, fetal death and abortion (Hall and Jones, 1977).

Diagnosis

A definite diagnosis depends upon the isolation of the organism from fetal tissues and membranes, uterine discharges or vaginal mucus. Serological tests can be used, especially the SAT, although agglutinins fall to low titres fairly soon after the event (Hinton, 1983).

Control

Cows that have aborted only excrete the organism for a very short perid of time, unlike the continuous or intermittent excretors that occur following enteric infection. Potential excretors need to be isolated until vaginal discharge ceases; fetuses and fetal membranes together with contaminated bedding should be disposed of safely. Adequate cleansing and disinfection of premises should be performed.

Since the problem is inevitably a sporadic one, expensive prophylactic measures, such as vaccination, are not necessary.

Bacillus abortion

It is only in the last decade that abortion due to *Bacillus* spp., in particular *B. licheniformis*, has been demonstrated. In some parts of the UK, notably northern Scotland and Cumbria, *B. licheniformis* is the most commonly diagnosed cause of abortion in cattle (Counter, 1984–1985).

Clinical signs

Sporadic cases occur in late gestation although there are reports of small outbreaks in two consecutive years (Counter, 1984–1985). Sometimes live calves can be born with some evidence of placental lesions.

The placentitis due to *B. licheniformis* is similar to that following mycotic infection. The allantochorion is dry, leathery and yellow or yellowish-brown in colour. Often, there is oedema of the allantochorion, especially around the cotyledons, which appears almost as if there are vesicles present. The cotyledons are haemorrhagic and necrotic.

The fetus may be infected and, if so, there will usually be evidence of a fibrinous pleurisy, pericarditis and peritonitis. There are no systemic signs of disease in the cow (Counter, 1984–1985).

Diagnosis

This depends upon the appearance of the placenta and the culture of *Bacillus* from the fetus, especially the abomasum, placenta and vaginal swab.

Transmission and pathogenesis

B. licheniformis is ubiquitous; however, a common source of infection is silage, especially when water, other foodstuffs and bedding are contaminated with silage effluent. Wet spoilt hay can be a source.

The method of infection is not known, but it is probably haematogenous following entry via the gastrointestinal tract.

Control

Infected silage or hay should not be fed.

Listeriosis

Listeria monocytogenes is primarily a parasite of the central nervous system in sheep and cattle, causing encephalitis; however Table 23.1 shows that it is consistently, if not frequently, isolated from bovine abortuses; it is also a cause of abortion in sheep and goats (Chapter 25).

Clinical signs

Usually abortion is sporadic, occurring towards the end of gestation; however, there are reports of minor outbreaks in some herds. In some individuals there may be pyrexia before, or at the time of, or after abortions have occurred. The aborted fetus frequently has characteristic multiple yellow or grey necrotic foci in the liver and cotyledons, which is similar to that described in sheep.

Diagnosis

This is dependent upon the identification of the organism in the abomasum and liver of the fetus and in the placenta and vaginal discharges by a direct smear or by immunofluorescence. Culture of the organism is not easy, although a series of subcultures following refrigeration has proved to be successful. Serological tests are not used in its diagnosis.

Transmission and pathogenesis

L. monocytogenes is ubiquitous in the environment, being present in the soil, sewage effluent, bedding and foodstuffs; it is particularly resistant to the effects of drying, sunlight and extreme temperature, thus it persists. There is good evidence that there is an association between listeriosis and the feeding of poor quality silage of higher than normal pH. Cross-infection between sheep and cattle is possible.

The organism gains entry by ingestion or penetration of mucous membranes of the respiratory system or conjunctiva, as well as the central nervous system. *L. monocytogenes* has a predilection for the placenta, causing a placentitis, and affects the fetus to cause abortion. A latent infection can occur with abortion occurring after a time lag and triggered by stress.

Treatment and control

The possibility of preventing further abortions occurring in a herd might be considered by using oxytetracycline or penicillin; however, this is rarely practicable. If silage is being fed this must be considered to be a potential source of infection and, if possible, withheld from pregnant cows. There is evidence that some individuals become asymptomless carriers, excreting the organism in faeces and milk.

Actinomyces (Corynebacterium) pyogenes

Table 23.1 shows that *A. (C.) pyogenes* is frequently isolated from bovine fetopathies, although it would appear to be less prevalent than in the 1970s and early 1980s. The significance of the presence of this organism is difficult to assess since *A. (C.) pyogenes* is a frequent secondary invader following the effect of the primary pathogen. Nevertheless, its presence in a fetopathy is usually significant.

A. (C.) pyogenes is believed to reach the uterus by a haematogenous route to produce a suppurative placentitis. Organisms found in the fetal bronchioles probably originate from aspiration of contaminated amniotic fluid. A fetal septicaemia can occur by transplacental passage (Smith, 1990).

Abortion may occur at any stage of gestation, although the organism is most frequently isolated from those that occur in the last trimester.

Diagnosis is usually made by the isolation of the organism from the placenta, abomasal contents or fetal tissues. There are no serological tests. Since the abortions are sporadic there are no suitable methods of treatment or control.

Escherichia coli

Sporadic abortions due to *E. coli* have been reported (Rowe and Smithies, 1978; Moorthy, 1985). It is suggested that, following stress, the organism reaches the fetus and placenta via haematogenous spread or ascending the genital tract.

Neospora caninum

Surveys of abortion in the USA, New Zealand, Japan and The Netherlands have reported an incidence rate of between 1.5 and 19.0% due to the protozoon *N. caninum*. It has not been recorded in the UK.

Abortion occurs in late gestation, although congenitally defective live calves can be born. Diagnosis is made on characteristic lesions, especially in the brain, and identification of the parasite in fetal tissue. The definitive host is likely to be a carnivore and hence oocyst-contaminated food is likely to be the source of infection. Access to cattle food by dogs should be prevented.

VIRAL, MYCOPLASMA AND FUNGAL AGENTS

Bovine viral diarrhoea (BVD)

Whilst BVD has been recognized as a disease of cattle for some time, its importance as a cause of infertility has been recognized only more recently. Since 1980, when it was first recorded as causing abortion in cattle, it has risen from 1.2% of isolations to a peak of 14.5% in 1990 (see Table 23.1).

The BVD virus is a member of the togavirus family and is fairly closely related to the virus of Border disease of sheep and less closely to the classical swinefever virus; there are two biotypes.

Clinical signs

These are described in detail elsewhere (Blood et al., 1989) but will be summarized briefly. BVD-affected animals may show a transient pyrexia with leucopenial viraemia for up to 15 days; in susceptible herds there will be diarrhoea with a high morbidity but low mortality rate, oculonasal discharge and mouth ulcers. In dairy cattle there is usually a drop in milk yield. The virus has a profound immunosuppressive effect which can increase the susceptibility of the host to other diseases. Frequently the disease is subclinical.

The mucosal type of disease occurs in herds that are chronically infected, where calves have a persistent infection. There is pyrexia, anorexia, watery diarrhoea, nasal discharge, buccal ulceration and lameness; the mortality rate is high.

The effect of the BVD virus on reproduction is varied, and is as follows.

Acute virus infection, with either biotype, can severely affect the embryo or fetus. Infection during the first month of gestation will result in embryonic death and resorption with no external signs of reproductive disease and with the cow or heifer returning to oestrus at a normal or extended interval. This will result in reduced pregnancy rates. In a study involving the insemination of BVD virus, seronegative cows before seroconversion due to exposure to a persistently infected cow, had first service pregnancy rates of 22.2% compared with 78.6% in those that were seropositive when inseminated (Virakula et al., 1993). Houe et al. (1993) found evidence of improved pregnancy rates in a study involving dairy herds with persistently infected animals, associated with increased immunity to the disease. From the second to the fourth month of gestation, infection will be followed by abortion, death with mummification, growth retardation, developmental abnormalities of the central nervous system and alopecia; some infected cows or heifers will carry calves to term, but these may well become persistently infected. It has generally been assumed that infection before 125 days of gestation is necessary for the carrier state to occur in calves (McClurkin et al., 1984), although Roeder et al. (1986) found an earlier time of 81 days or less.

From the fifth and sixth months of gestation there can be abortion, congenital abnormalities of the central nervous system and eyes. Infection after the sixth month of gestation may result in abortion. There is a time interval of several days to 2 months between infection with BVD virus and abortion (Bolin, 1990a).

Irrespective of the biotype, the fetus will develop measurable antibodies by 5–6 months of gestation (Bolin, 1990b). Fetal infection can also be followed by normal premature live, stillborn or weakly calves as well as those with congenital abnormalities.

Diagnosis

There may be a history of the overt disease. However, since in most cases there may only be slight pyrexia, inappetence and respiratory distress which may go undetected, the first signs are likely to be abortions and birth of congenitally deformed calves. The fetuses may be fresh, autolysed or mummified (Bolin, 1990a). Some histological lesions are characteristic of the infection.

The virus can be isolated from the fetus, particularly lymphoid tissue such as the spleen. Immunocytochemical identification of BVD viral proteins in fetal tissue, especially kidney, lung or lymphoid tissue, can sometimes be detected, even though the virus cannot be demonstrated. A substantial rise in neutralizing antibodies in herds experiencing abortions and in the serum of newborn calves or the thoracic fluids of abortuses is diagnostic of infection. In the case of live calves serum must be obtained *before* colostrum is ingested.

The recent introduction of a persistent infected cow or heifer into a susceptible herd should be viewed with concern (Duffell and Harkness, 1985).

Transmission and pathogenesis

Bulls have been shown to excrete the virus in their semen following spontaneous, persistent, chronic infection (Barlow et al., 1986; Revell et al., 1988) and also following experimental infection (Kirkland et al., 1991). In the latter study, the virus was shed after the viraemia had subsided; the vesicular glands and prostate were the main sites of virus replication.

Carriers or persistently infected animals are a source of infection and although numerically it probably occurs once for every 100–1000 calves born, they are important in maintaining the BVD virus in nature (Bolin, 1990a). Persistently infected cows transmit the disease vertically through transplacental infection to their calves, although the majority of infected calves are born to normal cows that were susceptible to infection during the first 4 months of gestation. Although the acute systemic form of the disease is the most prevalent, it is the mild clinical form that is likely to have the greatest effect upon reproductive function, since the mild pyrexia and modest mucosal lesions can go undetected.

Affected animals shed large amounts of virus continuously, which in the case of persistently infected animals will be over their entire lifetime. The virus will be excreted in oculonasal discharges, saliva, urine and faeces.

In countries where vaccination has been used,

contaminated modified-live-virus vaccines or poorly attenuated modified-live BVD virus vaccines have been responsible for the introduction of the infectious agent on to a farm (Baker, 1987). In addition, where virus-contaminated fetal calf serum has been used in embryo transfer techniques there is also a possibility of disease transmission.

Control

This can be expensive and may not be cost-effective if it requires extensive culling of persistently infected animals which are a continuous source of infection and their removal is essential. The basic principles are: (1) that farms do not breed from persistently infected cows; (2) only immune animals are introduced to the breeding herd — this can be achieved by deliberate exposure to persistently infected cattle before breeding; (3) any purchased animals introduced into the herd should be screened beforehand. Since there is some suggestion that cross-infection can occur between cattle and sheep and goats (Duffell and Harkness, 1985), the species should be separated.

The absence of antibody titres is generally assumed to indicate the absence of infection. With BVD this is not the case: a seropositive animal would be a safe purchase but a seronegative one requires to be free of virus to assure freedom from risk (Duffell and Harkness, 1985).

Vaccines are used in many countries as a control measure. Killed-virus vaccines can be used in pregnant cows, modified-live-virus vaccines cannot. Concern at the use of the latter has been expressed. Details of vaccination programmes have been described by Ames and Baker (1990).

Infectious bovine rhinotracheitis virus (IBR)

The bovine herpesvirus (BHV-1) is present worldwide and causes an acute respiratory disease of cattle with conjunctivitis. It also causes a disease of the genital organs of the bull and cow; this has been reported for many years, long before the respiratory form of the disease was recognized and the causal organism identified. The disease of the genital system has been variously called infectious pustular vulvovaginitis (IPV), vesicular venereal disease, coital vesicular exanthema and a disease peculiar to the continent of Africa — specific

bovine venereal epididymitis and vaginitis or 'epivag'. As the latter name implies, it causes epididymitis in the bull; more frequently the organism produces a vesicular balanoposthitis. 'Epivag' may be due to a different virus strain.

Although the virus has an obvious effect upon the mucosa of the vulva, vagina, penis and prepuce, it also affects reproduction by causing infertility in cows and heifers and also produces abortion. BHV-1 causes both the respiratory and genital forms of the disease; they usually occur independently, but abortion frequently occurs following the acute rhinotracheitis.

Clinical signs

The onset of vulvovaginitis is sudden and acute. If it is transmitted venereally it appears 24–48 hours after mating; heifers tend to be more severely affected than cows. The vulval labia become swollen and tender and, in light-skinned animals, deeply congested. This is quickly followed by the development of numerous red vesicles on the mucosa. These may rupture early or develop into pustules which give rise to haemorrhagic ulcers 3 mm or so in diameter.

The quantity of vulval discharge is variable, ranging from small quantities of exudate, which adheres to the vulval and tail hairs, to a copious mucopurulent discharge. A speculum is useful to examine the vaginal mucosa but, because of the pain and discomfort, posterior epidural anaesthesia is worthwhile. The lesions are obviously painful since affected animals are restless with swishing of the tail, frequent urination and straining. There may be transient pyrexia and reduced milk yield, but the systemic effects are variable depending upon the presence of respiratory problems.

When females show the presence of the lesions, the bull must be examined. Similar lesions to those described for the cow will be seen on the penile integument and preputial mucosa. The bull may be reluctant to serve, and there may be a preputial discharge with matting of the preputial hairs (see Chapter 30).

In both the male and female the acute phase of the disease will subside in about 10–14 days with a few animals showing a persistent vulval discharge for several weeks.

Infertility. Opinions have varied over the role of BHV-1 as a cause of infertility. Early studies by Parsonson (1964) and Hellig (1965) suggested that it had no effect, whereas Kendrick and McEntee (1967) found that, if semen infected with the virus was used for artificial insemination, there were reduced pregnancy rates, endometritis and short-ened interoestrus intervals. Experimentally, when infected semen is deposited in the uterus it causes a severe, necrotizing endometritis but lesions remain localized to the site of virus deposition; they were resolved in 1–2 weeks (Miller and Van Der Maaten, 1984). It is now accepted that, following natural service with an infected bull, the cow or heifer will develop lesions but fertility will be unaffected. However, if virus-infected semen is introduced into the uterus, as would occur at artificial insemination, infertility as shown by poor pregnancy rates occurs (Parsonson and Snowdon, 1975).

The virus also causes embryonic death by direct invasion of cells as early as 7 days (Bowen et al., 1985; Miller and Van Der Maaten, 1986) after passing through the endometrium. Furthermore, the virus can also cause a necrotizing oophoritis involving both ovaries. The corpus luteum appears to be particularly susceptible, especially during the first few days after ovulation. This damage to the devel-oping corpus luteum must affect its immediate func-tion, perhaps resulting in lower than normal progesterone production. The consequence is embryonic death (see p. 424) with the cow return-ing to oestrus at a normal interval after insemination.

Abortion. This is a common sequel to infec-tion with or without previous respiratory tract signs of disease, and also following vaccination with a modified live vaccine. The age of gestation at the time of infection appears to be critical, since cows that are $5\frac{1}{2}$ months pregnant, or less, do not abort, whilst those older than this have a 25% probability of aborting (Huck and Lamont, 1979). In beef herds, abortion 'storms' occur with between 5 and 60% of cows aborting. In dairy herds it is generally sporadic. Abortions occur from 4 months of gestation to term.

The time interval from infection to abortion varies from a few days to 100 days; in the latter case the fetus is extensively autolysed. Some calves are stillborn, and a few may be born alive, but succumb subsequently.

Diagnosis
The genital tract lesions are fairly characteristic of the disease, but it must be differentiated from granular vulvovaginitis due to *Ureaplasma* spp. and catarrhal vaginocervicitis.

Some investigators consider that a severely autolysed fetus strongly suggests BHV-1 infec-tion. There is frequently a liquefactive necrosis of the whole of the kidney cortex with perirenal haemorrhagic oedema. Histologically, there is always focal necrosis of the liver and in many cases there are necrotic lesions in the brain, lungs, spleen, adrenal cortex and lymph nodes. There are characteristic virus inclusion bodies at the periphery of these necrotic lesions in fresh experi-mental cases but, because of autolysis, they are not always demonstrable in field cases of abortion. The virus has been found in all fetal tissue and is concentrated in the cotyledons.

Nettleton (1986) has recommended that the following samples should be submitted for labora-tory examination: following abortion, paired serum samples from the dam are taken at the time of abortion and a second 2–4 weeks later. However, since cows may have been infected up to 4 months before abortion occurs, a significant rise in antibody titres is unlikely to be demon-strated. Serological examination of paired serum samples from at least 10 cows in the herd should reveal seroconversion or a four-fold increase in titres if IBR infection is active in the herd (Kirkbride, 1990a).

For subsequent fluorescent antibody tests, pieces of fetal tissue, particularly kidney and ad-renal gland, should be taken together with a piece of placenta. Such tests that demonstrate specific focal fluorescence are diagnostic of the disease. Virus isolation is not particularly reliable but should be used if only placental tissue is available (Kirkbride, 1990a).

Following the presence of genital lesions, va-ginal swabs, preputial washings and semen should be placed in virus transport medium. Paired serum samples should be taken from the affected cows.

Pathogenesis and transmission
The disease is readily transmitted venereally, but this is not the only route, since it can occur via contaminated bedding and the mutual licking and sniffing of the vulva and perineum of infected and non-infected animals. Also, it can be trans-mitted by virus contaminated semen. Once it has gained entry it is transported haematogenously in leucocytes.

Some animals can become lifelong latent carriers of the virus, despite the formation of specific antibodies. The infection enters a latent phase in the ganglion cells of the central nervous system. Under certain circumstances, such as stress, calving, transportation, vaccination or corticosteroid therapy, the latent infection can be reactivated so that the virus migrates along nerves to the periphery, where it multiplies and is excreted. These animals represent a reservoir of the virus.

Treatment

Spontaneous recovery of the genital lesions will occur and hence treatment is not really necessary; however, the administration of emollient creams to the vulva, vagina and penis may be useful. Vulval stenosis and penile/preputial adhesions and phimosis can occur (see Chapter 30).

Control

Infected animals should be isolated and natural service suspended. Vaccination is the most effective way of controlling the disease; a number of live, attenuated vaccines are available, often combined with a bovine parainfluenza virus vaccine. Heifers should be vaccinated after 6 months of age and before their first service, thereafter annual vaccination is preferable. Pregnant animals should only be vaccinated with a killed vaccine. Both the intranasal and intramuscular routes are used. Vaccination of bulls is questionable, since on blood testing they will be seropositive and may be rejected for sale as being infected. Routine examination of semen for the presence of the virus is preferable as a method of control.

Catarrhal vaginocavititis

This contagious, mainly venereally transmitted disease was first described in South Africa (Van Rensburg, 1953); since then it has been reported in many countries. It is caused by an enterovirus from the enteric cytopathic bovine orphan (ECBO) group.

Clinical signs

Affected animals have a profuse, postcoital, nonodorous, yellow, mucoid vulval discharge. The cervix and vagina are inflamed but there are no pustules, as occur in IPV infection, and no fever. The typical yellow gelatinous exudate frequently accumulates in the vagina, varying in quantity from a few to several hundred millilitres. The disease persists for a few days to a few weeks. Only a few animals show clinical signs of the disease at any one time and, as a consequence, pregnancy rates are reduced and there are prolonged, irregular returns to oestrus, presumably due to late embryonic death. In some herds, fetal mummification, abortion and stillbirth have been reported as being a problem.

Bulls may or may not become clinically infected but, in Belgium, Bouters et al. (1964) have provided definite proof of the association of two ECBO serotypes with seminal vesiculitis and infertility lasting up to 90 days. The penis and prepuce do not show the lesions that occur following BHV-1 infection.

Diagnosis

The most reliable method of diagnosis is serological examination of paired blood samples, collected at least 15 days apart, for evidence of rising antibody titres; the first sample should be collected as soon as possible after the disease is suspected.

The virus can be isolated from vaginal mucus, but the recovery rate is frequently low (Huck and Lamont, 1979).

Transmission and pathogenesis

Although the disease is transmitted venereally it can also be spread by faecal contamination of the vulva, or by animals licking the perineum of infected and non-infected individuals; hence the disease can occur in virgin heifers.

Treatment and control

There is no specific treatment or vaccine. Infected bulls should not be used for service for several months, even after clinical signs of disease have disappeared. Potentially infected animals should be isolated after purchase and, in closed herds, serological examination of potential additions to the herd might be contemplated.

Parainfluenza 3 (PI3) virus abortion

This widely distributed virus has been recovered from aborted fetuses in which it caused a septicaemic disease (Sattar et al., 1968). Experimentally it can cause fetal death and abortion after intrafetal inoculation but it has not done so after introduction into the respiratory system.

Vaccines to PI3 virus are available commercially, often combined with IBR vaccines. Vaccination can be done during calfhood, or in adult cattle to give lifelong protection.

Epizootic bovine abortion (EBA)

This disease was first identified in the mid-1950s in California. It is characterized by a high abortion rate of 30–40% during the last trimester of gestation in cows and heifers newly introduced to beef herds in particular areas of the state of California. The dam shows no clinical signs other than abortion.

Early studies suggested that the disease was due to *Chlamydia psittaci*; however, there is considerable debate about the authenticity of the isolation of the organism and its role in the pathogenesis. It has been recognized that the argasid tick *Ornithodoros coriaceus* is a vector, with abortion occurring 100 days or more after exposure. Lesions in aborted fetuses are characteristic and are used in its diagnosis.

Bovine chlamydial abortion

C. psittaci is a pathogen of both the bovine male and female genital tract. In the former it affects the testes, epididymides and other accessory glands, in particular the vesicular glands, where it is believed to be involved in the seminal vesculitis syndrome (see Chapter 30); the organism can be excreted in the semen of affected bulls, although it has also been isolated from bulls that were clinically normal (Eaglesome and Garcia, 1992).

Apart from the effect of chlamydial infection on bull fertility, it has an influence on fertility in the female. If contaminated semen is used, then after fertilization has occurred there will be embryonic death due to either a direct effect upon the embryo or, more likely, via its effect upon the endometrium. *C. psittaci* also causes abortion; this has been demonstrated in the USA and southern Europe. Characteristically, abortion occurs at 7–9 months of gestation without any other clinical signs, although experimental infection is followed by a short period of pyrexia and a leucopenia.

The lesions following abortion are fairly characteristic; the intercotyledonary areas of the placenta are more frequently affected, being thickened and leathery in appearance with a reddish-white opaque discoloration; oedema is quite common. In the aborted fetus the liver is enlarged with a coarsely nodular surface, firm consistency and a mottled reddish-yellow colour (Shewen, 1986). The organism can be cultured from aborted fetuses and discharges following the use of transport media. Giemsa-stained smears for the identification of elementary bodies or inclusions is also useful. Serological tests such as the CFT have been used but are generally too insensitive. It is likely that the ELISA tests, used to detect the infection in sheep, will be developed for use in cattle.

Tetracyclines could be used to treat pregnant cows that have been exposed to infection; it is not really practicable because it requires knowing that the secondary chlamydaemia has not occurred, and animals must be treated until normal calving. Pregnant animals should be segregated from potential sources of infection. Vaccines are available for use in sheep but none have yet to be developed for use in cattle. Following abortion there should be a natural immunity.

As mentioned above, there is still doubt about the role of *C. psittaci* in epizootic bovine abortion. Shewen (1986) considers that chlamydial abortion in cattle is probably underdiagnosed.

Transmissible genital fibropapillomas

Wart-like tumours commonly occur on the penis of young bulls (see Chapter 30) and occasionally similar growths occur on the vulva, perineum and vestibulovaginal epithelium of heifers. They are caused by a virus of the papovavirus group and are transmitted by contact with infected animals.

These fibropapillomata regress spontaneously in 2–6 months, the speed of regression may be expedited by the use of a wart vaccine (formalized tissue). Except in so far as the larger tumours (which may be removed surgically) might interfere mechanically with coitus, they do not cause infertility in female animals.

Blue tongue

Blue tongue is mainly a disease of sheep, but in cattle the virus is markedly fetopathic and is an occasional cause of seasonal abortion particularly in Africa, where the transmitting agent is *Culicoides varriipennis*.

Genital mycoplasmosis

There has been much controversy concerning the relationship between mycoplasmas and genital disease in cattle ever since *Mycoplasma bovigenitalium* was demonstrated in the genital tract of infertile cows and the semen of bulls (Edward et al., 1947; Blom and Erno, 1967). Evidence for pathogenicity has mainly been indirect, based frequently on their isolation from diseased rather than healthy tissue, and with limited experimental studies (Eaglesome and Garcia, 1992). The mycoplasmas that have been implicated are *M. bovigenitalium*, *M. bovis*, *Acholeplasma laidlawii* and *Ureaplasma diversum*. These cause two specific reproductive disorders, granular vulvovaginitis and abortion. Granular vulvovaginitis has been recognized for many years, and until recently was assumed to have no other adverse effect upon reproduction.

Granular vulvovaginitis

There is a sudden onset of a purulent vulval discharge 4–10 days after service or artificial insemination. The vaginal mucosa is inflamed with numerous raised granular lesions, especially on the ventral surface of the posterior vagina, vulva and around the clitoris (Wright, 1982–1983). The infected animals show discomfort, especially after urination, but there is no pyrexia or systemic influence. Few lesions occur cranial to the urethral opening. Pregnancy rates are reduced.

Other reproductive disorders

Mycoplasmas are frequently isolated from bulls' semen since they can colonize the accessory reproductive organs, particularly the vesicular glands where they cause seminal vesiculitis. *M. bovis* has been shown to cause salpingitis, which may explain its relationship with the repeat breeder syndrome (see p. 429). *U. diversum* can also cause salpingitis and endometritis.

Abortion. Mycoplasmas have been implicated as a cause of abortion and neonatal death in calves. The organisms have been isolated from spontaneously aborted fetuses, for example Langford (1975) cultured them from 8.7% of aborted fetuses but none from normal fetuses. In a study of 245 bovine abortions in Northern Ireland, Ball et al. (1978) recovered mycoplasmas from 23.7% of aborted placental material and none from normal controls, and from 4.4% of aborted fetuses and 1.3% from non-aborted controls. In this latter study, *A. laidlawii* was most frequently isolated; however, it is particularly ubiquitous, and this may reflect post-abortion contamination; they are generally considered saprophytic. *M. bovis* has been shown experimentally to consistently cause abortion when inoculated into pregnant cows. Since it is seldom found in the reproductive tract of normal cows, its isolation from the placenta or aborted fetus can be considered significant (Kirkbride, 1990b).

Diagnosis. Most bovine mycoplasmas are easily recovered in conventional mycoplasma media, although some may require special supplements or conditions for optimum growth (see Eaglesome and Garcia, 1992). The development of ELISA and other diagnostic tests are likely in the near future.

Transmission and pathogenesis

Surveys have shown that mycoplasmas are frequently isolated from bovine semen, and several of these have been shown to be capable of colonizing the male and female genital systems. In addition, certain species, such as *M. bovigenitalium*, *M. bovis* and *U. diversum*, have been associated with naturally occurring and experimentally induced infections. Since it is known that the absence of a cell wall enables them to adhere intimately with the host cells, they readily colonize the genital tract; the local concentration of toxic metabolic products may injure the host cells (Eaglesome and Garcia, 1992). Thus, these organisms, when deposited in the cow's or heifer's genital tract in semen or transferred mechanically by the bull's penis or artificial insemination pipette, can readily cause infection.

Treatment and control

Natural service, if used, should be suspended and semen should be collected and cultured for the presence of mycoplasmas.

If artificial insemination is used the standard Cassou pipette should be protected by a disposable polythene sheath to prevent vulval or vaginal contamination before it is introduced through the cervix.

The uterus can be infused with a solution

containing 1 g of tetracycline or spectinomycin 1 day after insemination; this has been shown to improve pregnancy rates.

Infected bulls should be rested for 3 months and treated systemically for 5 days with tetracyclines, together with sheath irrigation.

Stress, associated with intensive management systems, is said to predispose to the disease, thus transfer to pasture of affected animals should be considered. This may reduce spread by direct contagion.

A number of antibiotics have been incorporated in semen; a combination of lincomycin, spectinomycin, tylosin and gentamicin added to raw semen and non-glycerolated whole milk or egg yolk-based extenders has been shown to control *M. bovis*, *M. bovigenitalium* and *Ureaplasma* spp. (Shin et al., 1988).

Haemophilus somnus abortion and infertility

H. somnus is a fairly common inhabitant of the genital tracts of male and female cattle without evidence of macroscopic lesions. The organism can be routinely isolated from the mucosal surfaces of the urogenital tract of normal healthy cattle (Eaglesome and Garcia, 1992). Figures of 28% of normal cows (Slee and Stephens, 1985) and 90% of normal bulls (Jansen et al., 1981) have been published in the literature.

H. somnus has been reported to adversely affect reproduction in a number of different ways. It has been shown to cause abortion, endometritis, vaginitis and cervicitis; it may be one of the organisms responsible for granular vulvovaginitis (see above).

Diagnosis can be made following culture of the organism, which can be difficult because of overgrowth by contaminants. Serological tests are currently unreliable.

There are few reports on the treatment of infected cows. Penicillin and streptomycin have been reported to have been used successfully in treating cows where *H. somnus* was frequently isolated from cervicovaginal mucus and where fertility was depressed (Eaglesome and Garcia, 1992). Since the organism colonizes the genital tract of the bull and can be isolated from semen, this may well be an important source of infection of cows and heifers. Good hygiene and the use of

combinations of antibiotics should control infection following artificial insemination.

Mycotic abortion

Fungal invasion of the placenta and fetus is a frequent and consistent cause of abortion in cattle (see Table 23.1). Abortions are normally sporadic, although in some herds the incidence may be as high as 5–10%. Elsewhere, the frequency of diagnosis is high; in the north-eastern states of the USA mycotic abortions accounted for 22% of all infectious abortions and 5.1% of all abortions investigated (Hubbert et al., 1973). Similarly in South Dakota, USA, a survey over a 5 year period found that 14.6% of all infectious abortions were due to fungi; this was 4.8% of the total number of abortions (Kirkbride et al., 1973).

Mycotic abortion is much more prevalent during the months of December, January, February and March in the UK compared with the rest of the year.

The fungi that are most frequently isolated following abortion are *Absidia* spp., *Rhizopus* spp., *Mucor* spp. and *Aspergillus* spp., particularly *A. fumigatus* (Pepin, 1983). Other fungi such as *Mortiella wolfii* and *Petriellidium boydii* have also been implicated.

Clinical signs

Infection does not always cause abortion, since infected live calves can be born. When abortion occurs it is usually sporadic in nature between 4 and 9 months of gestation, although it is more prevalent between 7 and 8 months.

There are no other clinical signs of disease in the dam but the appearance of the lesions on the placenta and the calf are fairly characteristic of mycotic infection. The whole or part of the placenta usually appears discoloured when shed, it is either grey, yellow or reddish-brown; the intercotyledonary areas of the allantochorion are thickened, wrinkled or leathery. Those cotyledons that have attached portions of the corresponding caruncle, after the placenta has been shed, appear thickened and have a cup-like or coffee bean appearance (Pepin, 1983). Between 25 and 33% of the fetuses are infected (Austwick, 1968; Kendrick, 1975). In a proportion of these, characteristic fetal skin lesions are present which are circumscribed, greyish-white thickened patches similar in appearance to skin ringworm in calves and young cattle.

Diagnosis

The appearance of the placenta is fairly typical in fungal abortion although some bacteria can produce similar lesions. The fetal skin lesions are almost pathognonomic.

Laboratory confirmation requires submission of placental tissue, preferably the whole organ (Pepin, 1983). Culture from placental tissue is of no value since the placenta is usually contaminated after it has been expelled. Culture from fetal lungs and abomasum is more reliable but contamination can occur.

The reliable and traditional method of diagnosis is the identification of fungal cells in histological sections of the placenta. Since fungal infections are frequently localized, resulting in focal lesions, selection of suitable material is important. Another technique is the potassium hydroxide 'crush' mount of non-fixed tissue (Pepin, 1983).

According to Kirkbride (1990c), conclusive diagnosis of mycotic placentitis can be made if: (1) the characteristic lesions of placentitis are present in association with the presence of mycotic elements, (2) the characteristic lesions of fetal dermatomycosis are present in association with the presence of mycotic elements, and (3) there is a fetal bronchopneumonia associated with mycotic elements.

Serological tests are, at present, unreliable and cannot be used for routine diagnosis.

Transmission and pathogenesis

Many of the species of fungi are ubiquitous in the air and environment in which cattle live; however, there is good evidence that mouldy hay and straw and other food such as silage and sugar beet pulp are important sources of infection. It is most prevalent in the winter months when the cattle are housed. This was demonstrated in a survey in south-west Wales involving 531 herds over a 5 year period (Williams et al., 1977). When hay was fed to cows housed in sheds the percentage of mycotic abortions was 7.14%, compared with that for other systems of management, including the feeding of hay in loose housing, where it was between 1.32 and 0.19%.

There is still speculation about how the organism reaches the uterus and infects the placenta and fetus. It is generally agreed that there is haematogenous spread following entry into the vascular system from the respiratory or alimentary tracts. There is some evidence that fungal-contaminated semen can cause uterine lesions (Kendrick et al., 1975), although it is unlikely to be important.

The fetus and placenta are much more susceptible to mycotic invasion than maternal tissues; this may be due to growth enhancement of fungi by the products of conception. Once the fungus has colonized the uterus it probably spreads in two ways. (1) After initial infection of a few placentomes it spreads slowly throughout the placenta until sufficient is affected to cause abortion; at the same time the mycelium will invade the fetus. (2) After initial infection there is rapid invasion of the placenta with abortion occurring before the fetus is affected.

Control

The feeding of mouldy forage or the use of mouldy bedding should be avoided.

REFERENCES

Abelein, R. (1938) *Mun. Tierartzl. Wochenschr.*, **80**, 683.

Ahktar, S., Riemann, H. P., Thurmond, M. C. and Franti, C. E. (1993) *Vet. Res. Commun.*, **17**, 95.

Ames, T. R. and Baker, J. C. (1990) *Vet. Med-US.*, **85**, 1140.

Andriamanga, S., Steffan, J. and Thibier, M. (1984) *Ann. Rech. Vet.*, **15**, 503.

Anon. (1992) *Guideline for the Diagnosis and Control of* Leptospira hardjo *infection in cattle*, the British Cattle Veterinary Association. Frampton-on-Severn, Gloucestershire.

Austwick, P. K. C. (1968) *Vet. Rec.*, **82**, 236.

Ayliffe, T. R. (1979) Ph.D. Thesis, University of London.

Ayliffe, T. R. and Noakes, D. E. (1978) *Vet. Rec.*, **102**, 215.

Baker, J. C. (1987) *J. Amer. Vet. Med. Assn*, **190**, 1449.

Ball, H. J., Neill, S. D., Ellis, W. A., O'Brien, J. J. and Ferguson, H. W. (1978) *Brit. Vet. J.*, **134**, 584.

Ball, L., Ott, R. S., Mortimer, R. G. and Simons, J. C. (1983) *Theriogenology*, **12**, 57.

Barlow, R. H., Nettleton, P. F., Gardiner, A. C., Grieg, A., Campbell, J. R. and Bonn, J. H. (1986) *Vet. Rec.*, **118**, 321.

Bartlett, D. E. (1947) *Proc. US Live Stk. Sanit. Assn*, 170.

Bartlett, D. E. (1948) *Amer. J. Vet. Res.*, **9**, 33.

Bartlett, D. E., Hassan, E. V. and Teeter, K. G. (1947) *J. Amer. Vet. Med. Assn*, **110**, 114.

Berg, R. L. and Firehammer, M. S. (1980) *J. Amer. Vet. Med. Assn*, **173**, 467.

Binns, W. (1953) Thesis, Cornell University.

Blom, E. and Erno, H. (1967) *Acta Vet. Scand.*, **8**, 186.

Blood, D. C. and Radostits, O. M. (1989) In: *Veterinary Medicine*, 7th edn, pp. 847–851. London: Baillière Tindall.

Bolin, S. R. (1990a) *Vet. Med.*, **85**, 1124.

Bolin, S. R. (1990b) In: *Laboratory Diagnosis of Livestock Abortion*, 3rd edn., ed. C. A. Kirkbride, p. 121. Ames: Iowa State University Press.

BonDurant, R. H., Anderson, M. L., Blanchard, P. and Hird, D. (1990) In: *Laboratory Diagnosis of Livestock Abortion*, 3rd edn, ed. C. A. Kirkbride, pp. 161–164. Ames: Iowa State University Press.

Borsberry, S. and Dobson, H. (1989) *Vet. Rec.*, **125**, 103.

Bouters, R. (1973) Personal communication.

Bouters, R., Vandeplassche, M. and Florent, A. (1964) *Vlaams Diergeneesk. Tijdschr.*, **33**, 405.

Bowen, R. A., Elsden, R. P. and Seidel, G. E. (1985) *Amer. J. Vet. Res.*, **46**, 1095.

Boyd, H. (1955) Thesis, University of Uppsala.

Bretzlaff, K. N., Whitmore, H. L., Spahr, S. L. and Ott, R. S. (1982) *Theriogenology*, **17**, 527.

Brinley Morgan, W. J. and MacKinnon, D. J. (1979) In: *Fertility and Infertility in Domestic Animals*, ed. J. A. Laing, 3rd edn, pp. 171–198. London: Baillière Tindall.

Brinley Morgan, W. J. and Richards, R. A. (1974) *Vet. Rec.*, **94**, 510.

Brus, D. H. J. (1954) Ph.D. Thesis, University of Utrecht.

Coulson, A. (1978) *Vet. Rec.*, **103**, 359.

Counter, D. E. (1984–1985) *Proc. BCVA*, p. 269.

Dawson, F. L. M. (1963) *J. Reprod. Fertil.*, **5**, 397.

Duffell, S. J. and Harkness, J. W. (1985) *Vet. Rec.*, **117**, 240.

Dufty, J. H. (1967) *Aust. Vet. J.*, **43**, 433.

Dufty, J. H. and McEntee, K. (1969) *Aust. Vet. J.*, **45**, 140.

Eaglesome, M. D. and Garcia, M. M. (1992) *Vet. Bull.*, **62**, 743.

Edward, D. G. F., Hancock, J. L. and Hignett, S. L. (1947) *Vet. Rec.*, **59**, 329.

Ellis, W. A., O'Brien, J. J., Neill, S. D. and Hanna, J. (1982) *Vet. Rec.*, **110**, 178.

Ellis, W. A. (1984) *Prev. Vet. Med.*, **2**, 411.

Ellis, W. A. (1984–1985) *Proc. BCVA*, pp. 267–268.

Ellis, W. A. (1986) In: *Current Therapy in Theriogenology*, ed. D. A. Morrow, 2nd edn, p. 267. London: W. B. Saunders.

Ellis, W. A. and Michna, S. W. (1976) *Vet. Rec.*, **99**, 430.

Ellis, W. A., O'Brien, J. J. and Cassells, J. A. (1981) *Vet. Rec.*, **108**, 555.

Ellis, W. A., Songer, J. G., Montgomery, J. and Cassells, J. A. (1986) *Vet. Rec.*, **118**, 11.

Erb, H. N., Martin, S. W., Ison, N. and Swaminathan, S. (1981) *J. Dairy Sci.*, **64**, 272.

Esslemont, R. J. and Spencer, I. (1992) *The prevalence and costs of diseases in dairy herds*. Report No. 2, The Dairy Information System (DAISY), University of Reading.

Fonseca, F. A., Britt, J. H., McDaniel, B. T., Wilk, J. C. and Rakes, A. H. (1983) *J. Dairy Sci.*, **66**, 1128.

Frank, A. H. and Bryner, J. H. (1953) *Proc. US Live Stk. Sanit. Assn.*

Frank, T., Anderson, K. L., Smith, A. R., Whitmore, H. L. and Gustafsson, B. K. (1983) *Theriogenology*, **20**, 103.

Fujimoto, Y. (1956) *Jpn. J. Vet. Res.*, **4**, 129.

Gasparini, G. W., Vaghi, M. and Tardini, A. (1963) *Vet. Rec.*, **75**, 940.

Gustafsson, B., Backstrom, G. and Edquist, L. E. (1976) *Theriogenology*, **6**, 45.

Hall, G. A. and Jones, P. W. (1976) *Brit. Vet. J.*, **135**, 75.

Hall, G. A. and Jones, P. W. (1977) *J. Comp. Pathol.*, **87**, 53.

Hartigan, P. J., Murphy, J. A., Nunn, W. R. and Griffin, J. F. T. (1972) *Irish Vet. J.*, **26**, 225.

Hartigan, P. J., Griffin, J. H. T. and Nunn, W. R. (1974a) *Theriogenology*, **1**, 153.

Hartigan, R. J., Nunn, W. R. and Griffin, J. F. T. (1974b) *Brit. Vet. J.*, **130**, 160.

Hathaway, S. C. and Little, T. W. A. (1983) *Vet. Rec.*, **112**, 215.

Hellig, H. (1965) *J. S. Afr. Vet. Med. Assn*, **36**, 219.

Hinton, M. H. (1973) *Vet. Rec.*, **93**, 162.

Hoerlein, A. B. (1980) In: *Bovine Medicine and Surgery*, ed. W. J. Gibbons, E. J. Catcott and J. F. Smithcors, p. 231. Wheaton, Ill.: American Veterinary Publications.

Houe, H., Pedersen, K. M. and Meyling, A. (1993) *Prev. Vet. Med.*, **15**, 117.

Hubbert, W. T., Booth, G. D., Bolton, W. D., Dunne, H. W., McEntee, K., Smith, R. E. and Tourtellott, M. E. (1973) *Cornell Vet.*, **63**, 291.

Huck, R. A. and Lamont, P. H. (1979) In: *Fertility and Infertility in Domestic Animals*, p. 160. London: Baillière Tindall.

Hum, S., Stephens, S. and Quinn, C. (1991) *Aust. Vet. J.*, **68**, 272.

Jackson, P. S. (1981) D.Vet.Med. Thesis, University of London.

Jansen, E. D., Cates, W. F., Barth, A., Nechala, L., Pawlyshyn, V., Saunders, J. R. and Osborne, A. D. (1981) *Can. Vet. J.*, **22**, 361.

Jerrett, I. V. and McOrist, S. (1985) Proceedings No. 78, Dairy cattle production, Sydney, 169–189.

Kendrick, J. W. (1967) *J. Amer. Vet. Med. Assn*, **150**, 495.

Kendrick, J. W. (1975) *Proc. Amer. Assn Vet. Lab. Diagn.*, October, 331.

Kendrick, J. W. and McEntee, K. (1967) *Cornell Vet.*, **57**, 3.

Kendrick, J. W., Harlan, G. P., Bushnell, R. B. and Kronlund, N. (1975) *Theriogenology*, **4**, 125.

Kerr, W. R. and Robertson, M. (1941) *Vet. J.*, **97**, 351.

Kerr, W. R. and Robertson, M. (1943) *J. Comp. Pathol.*, **53**, 280.

King, S. (1991) *Aust. Vet. J.*, **68**, 307.

Kirkbride, C. A. (1990a) In: *Laboratory Diagnosis of Livestock Abortion*, 3rd edn., ed. C. A. Kirkbride, p. 91. Ames: Iowa State University Press.

Kirkbride, C. A. (1990b) In: *Laboratory Diagnosis of Livestock Abortion*, 3rd edn., ed. C. A. Kirkbride, p. 17. Ames: Iowa State University Press.

Kirkbride, C. A. (1990c) In: *Laboratory Diagnosis of Livestock Abortion*, 3rd edn., ed. C. A. Kirkbride, p. 136. Ames: Iowa State University Press.

Kirkbride, C. A., Bicknell, E. J., Reed, D. E., Robi, W. U., Knutltson, M. G. and Wohlgemuth, K. (1973) *J. Amer. Vet. Med. Assn*, **162**, 556.

Kirkland, P. D., Richards, S. G., Rothwell, J. T. and Stanley, D. F. (1991) *Vet. Rec.*, **128**, 587.

Langford, E. V. (1975) *Can. J. Comp. Med.*, **39**, 133.

Lawson, J. R. and McKinnon, D. J. (1952) *Vet. Rec.*, **64**, 763.

McClurkin, A. W., Littledike, E. T., Cudlip, R. C., Frank, G. H., Covia, M. F. and Bolin, S. R. (1984) *Can. J. Comp. Med. Vet. Sci.*, **48**, 156.

McFadyean, J. and Stockman, S. (1913) *Rep. Depl. Commun. Epizootic Abortion*.

McLaughlin, D. K. (1968) *J. Parasitol.*, **54**, 1038.

Mare, D. J. and Van Rensburg, S. J. (1961) *Onderstepoort J. Vet. Res.*, **26**, 479.

Markusfeld, O. (1984) *Vet. Rec.*, **114**, 539.

Markusfeld, O. (1985) *Vet. Rec.*, **116**, 489.

Martinez, J. and Thibier, M. (1984) *Theriogenology*, **21**, 583.

Masera, J., Gustafsson, B. K., Afiefy, M. M., Stowe, C. M. and Bergt, G. P. (1980) *J. Amer. Vet. Med. Assn*, **176**, 1099.

Miller, J. M. and Van Der Maaten, M. J. (1984) *Amer. J. Vet. Res.*, **45**, 790.

Miller, J. M. and Van Der Maaten, M. J. (1986) *Amer. J. Vet. Res.*, **47**, 223.

Moorthy, A. R. S. (1985) *Vet. Rec.*, **116**, 159.

Nettleton, P. F. (1986) *Vet. Ann.*, **26**, 90.

Nicoletti, P. (1986) In: *Current Therapy in Theriogenology*, ed. D. A. Morrow, Vol. 2, pp. 271–274. Philadelphia: W. B. Saunders.

Nielson, F. W. (1955) *Vet. Rec.*, **67**, 939.

Nielsen, K., Cherwonogrodzky, J. W., Duncan, J. R., Bundle, D. R. (1989) *Amer. J. Vet. Res.*, **50**, 5.

Noakes, D. E., Wallace, L. and Smith, G. R. (1991) *Vet. Rec.*, **128**, 440.

Olson, J. D., Ball, L., Mortimer, R. G., Farin, P. W., Adney, W. S. and Huffman, E. M. (1984) *Amer. J. Vet. Res.*, **45**, 2251.

Otoguro, K., Oiwa, R., Iwai, Y., Tamaka, H. and Omura, S. (1988) *J. Antibiotics*, **41**, 461.

Parsonson, I. M. (1964) *Aust. Vet. J.*, **40**, 257.

Parsonson, I. M. and Snowdon, W. A. (1975) *Aust. Vet. J.*, **51**, 365.

Pepin, G. A. (1983) *Vet. Ann.*, **23**, 79.

Pierce, A. E. (1946) *Vet. Rec.*, **58**, 16.

Reid, I. M., Roberts, C. J. and Manston, R. (1979) *Vet. Rec.*, **104**, 75.

Revell, S. G., Chasey, D., Drew, T. W. and Edwards, S. (1988) *Vet. Rec.*, **123**, 122.

Riedmuller, L. (1928) *Zentbl. Bakt. ParasitKde*, **108**, 103.

Roeder, P. L., Jeffrey, M. and Cranwell, M. P. (1986) *Vet. Rec.*, **118**, 24.

Roth, E. E. and Galton, M. M. (1960) *Amer. J. Vet. Res.*, **21**, 422.

Rowe, R. F. and Smithies, L. K. (1978) *Bovine Practitioner*, **10**, 102.

Rowson, L. E. A., Lamming, G. E. and Fry, R. M. (1953) *Vet. Rec.*, **65**, 335.

Ruder, C. A., Sasser, R. G., Williams, R. J., Ely, J. K., Bull, R. C. and Butler, J. E. (1981) *Theriogenology*, **15**, 573.

Sagartz, J. W. and Hardenbrook, H. G. (1971) *J. Amer. Vet. Med. Assn*, **158**, 619.

Sattar, S. A., Bohl, E. H., Trapp, A. L. and Hamdy, A. H. (1968) *Amer. J. Vet. Res.*, **122**, 45.

Schmidt-Adamopolou, B. (1978) *Dt. Tierartzl., Wochenschr.*, **83**, 553.

Shewen, P. G. (1986) In: *Current Therapy in Theriogenology*, ed. D. A. Morrow, 2nd edn, p. 279. Philadelphia: W. B. Saunders.

Shin, S. J., Lein, D. H., Patten, V. H. and Ruhnke, H. L. (1988) *Theriogenology*, **29**, 577.

Skirrow, S. Z. and Bondurant, R. H. (1988) *Vet. Bull.*, **58**, 591.

Slee, K. J. and Stephens, L. R. (1985) *Vet. Rec.*, **116**, 215.

Smith, R. E. (1990) In: *Laboratory Diagnosis of Livestock Abortion*, 3rd edn, ed. C. A. Kirkbride, pp. 66–69. Ames: Iowa State University.

Stableforth, A. W., Scorgie, N. J. and Gould, G. N. (1937) *Vet. Rec.*, **49**, 211.

Studer, E. and Morrow, D. A. (1978) *J. Amer. Vet. Med. Assn*, **172**, 489.

Swangard, W. M. (1939) *J. Amer. Vet. Med. Assn*, **95**, 146, 749.

Tedesco, L. F., Errico, F. and Baglivi, L. P. D. (1977) *Aust. Vet. J.*, **53**, 470.

Tennant, B. and Peddicord, R. G. (1968) *Cornell Vet.*, **58**, 185.

Thiermann, A. B. (1982) *Amer. J. Vet. Res.*, **43**, 780.

Thimm, B. and Wundt, W. (1976) Cited by Brinley Morgan, W. J. and Mackinnon, D. J. (1979) In: *Fertility and Infertility in Domestic Animals*, ed. J. A. Laing, 3rd edn, pp. 171–198. London: Baillière Tindall.

Van Rensburg, S. W. J. (1953) *Brit. Vet. J.*, **109**, 226.

Villar, J. A. and Spina, E. M. (1982) *Gaceta veterinaria*, **44**, 647.

Virakula, P., Fagbubgm, M. L., Joo, H. S. and Meyling, A. (1993) *Theriogenology*, **29**, 441.

Williams, B. M., Shreeve, B. J. and Herbert, C. N. (1977) *Vet. Rec.*, **100**, 382.

Williams, W. L. (1939) *The Diseases of the Genital Organs of Domestic Animals*, 2nd edn. Baltimore: Williams and Wilkins.

Witte, K. (1962) *Dt. Tierartzl. Wochenschr.*, **69**, 394.

Wright, C. L. (1982–1983) *Proc. BCVA*, p. 265.

Wright, J. G. and Arthur, G. H. (1945) *J. Comp. Pathol.*, **55**, 49.

In dealing with fertility and infertility of cattle the veterinarian has two tasks to perform: first, he or she may be asked to investigate and determine the cause of infertility in individual animals or in the herd; second, he or she may be required to assist in the maintenance of optimum fertility so that the livestock enterprise functions as efficiently and profitably as possible. In the dairy herd, the main source of income is from the sale of milk although, except for Channel Island breeds, the calf will also provide a substantial additional source. In beef suckler herds, the calf is the source of income. In both types of farming, enterprise income will also be generated from the sale of cull cows; however, this is likely to result in a net loss since the cost of a replacement, either purchased or reared on the farm, will be greater.

NORMAL EXPECTATIONS OF FERTILITY

It is well recognized that although a cow may have an apparently normal reproductive system and is inseminated or served at the correct time with fertile semen she may fail to conceive. The herdsman should identify this in the first instance that the cow has returned to oestrus. In the UK the mean non-return rate to artificial insemination at 30–60 days is just under 80%. However, the calving rate to a single insemination is probably no better than 55% (Diskin and Sreenan, 1986). The results following natural service are probably higher.

The reasons for the discrepancy between the non-return rate to artificial insemination or natural service and calving rate are as follows:

1. In the case of the artificial insemination non-return figures, it is likely that a proportion of cows that return to oestrus are not reported.

2. Some cows which return are culled and the data not recorded.

3. Oestrus may not be detected.

4. There may be a persistent corpus luteum associated with uterine infection.

5. Luteal cysts.

6. Some cows may abort.

However, there is another important explanation for the discrepancy which has been briefly discussed, namely embryonic or early fetal death (see Chapter 4).

EMBRYONIC LOSS

Since Corner's (1923) discovery of the phenomenon of conceptual death or loss in sows it is established that there is an incidence of 20–50% embryonic and fetal death in apparently normal healthy animals of all domestic species, including cattle. Extensive studies have shown that there are a number of factors which may cause embryonic death but the aetiology of a large part of the problem remains unexplained. The existence of this unexplained moiety in rather constant degree in all species led Hanly (1961) to suggest that it was due to a more universally active factor than any of those so far investigated. Bishop (1964) proposed that because embryonic loss appeared to be a general feature of mammalian reproduction it probably conferred some biological advantage which might allow the elimination of undesirable genetic material at a low biological cost. If this were so, then a considerable part of embryonic death should be regarded as a normal occurrence and thus unavoidable. This concept of inevitable conceptual loss implies a limit to the chance of a successful outcome to each mating or insemination which will not be significantly affected by previous success or failure.

This concept of the inevitability of embryonic

loss, thus limiting the successful outcome of each service or insemination, has been generally accepted. However, there is little evidence that inherent genetic abnormalities are the main cause since the work in humans, from which the theory has been extrapolated, has been done on aborted human fetuses, not embryos (Land et al., 1983). Furthermore, there is now good evidence that it is possible to select mice genetically for a high rate of embryo survival (Bradford, 1969) and that mammalian gametogenesis and syngamy do not necessarily lead to a high incidence of mortal damage (Land et al., 1983). Perhaps the genetic selection of domestic species for high embryonic survival rates might be a profitable way to increase the overall fertility rate.

There is increasing evidence that the major reason for embryonic loss is spontaneous asynchrony between dam and embryo which would appear to be largely mediated by endogenous ovarian steroids (Wilmut et al., 1985).

How can the incidence of embryonic loss be determined? If fertilization occurs the developing conceptus prevents the return to oestrus by inhibiting the production or release of endogenous luteolysin (see Chapter 3). If the embryo dies before 13 days of age then the cow will return to oestrus at the normal interoestrus interval. If, however, the embryo dies after this age then the interoestrus interval will be extended beyond the generally accepted figure of 18–24 days. It is therefore impossible to differentiate, by observing the occurrence of oestrus, between fertilization failure and embryonic death before 13 days of age. This is particularly important since it has been postulated that most embryos die before 15 days of age (Boyd et al., 1969; Ayalon, 1972). For many years the only method available for the study of embryonic death was slaughter at known time intervals after service or insemination, followed by flushing of uterine tubes and horns. In such studies, using first-service heifers, Bearden et al. (1956) reported a fertilization failure of only 3.4% and an embryonic loss up to 35 days of 10.5%; in 'repeat breeder' heifers, Tanabe and Almquist (1953) reported a fertilization failure of 40.8% and an embryonic loss of 28.7%. In normal fertile cows Ayalon (1978) and Boyd et al. (1969) found fertilization failure rates of 17 and 15% and embryonic loss rates up to 35 days of 14 and 15%, respectively. In 'repeat breeder' cows similar figures for these two categories were 39.7 and 39.2% (Tanabe and

Casida, 1949) and 29 and 36% (Ayalon, 1978), respectively. In a large survey of 4286 randomly selected cows the greatest incidence of embryonic loss (14.9%) occurred between 30 and 60 days; at 60–90 days it was 5.5% and at 90–120 days it was 2.8% (Barrett et al., 1948). In a study using milk progesterone determinations, it was found that the incidence of fertilization failure, together with conceptual loss up to 20 days after artificial insemination, was almost equal to fetal loss between 20 and 80 days (Pope and Hodgeson-Jones, 1975).

There is good evidence that the critical period for embryonic demise is on day 7 after fertilization when the morula develops into the blastocyst (Ayalon, 1973), and that embryonic loss at this time is greater in 'repeat breeder' cows (Ayalon, 1978). In a review using composite data for heifers from nine publications, Sreenan and Diskin (1986) calculated the mean fertilization rate to be 88%; for cows from four sources the mean fertilization rate was 90%. The same authors calculated the mean embryonic death rate using data from nine sources involving 468 heifers and cows; the percentage pregnant 2–5 days after artificial insemination was 85%, between 11 and 13 days it was 73%, and for 25–42 days, 67%.

The development of embryo transfer techniques for the non-surgical flushing of embryos (see Chapter 34) have enabled a large number of studies to be performed (Sreenan and Diskin, 1983; Roche et al., 1985). Using these methods it is possible to flush cows and heifers repeatedly at varying time intervals after insemination, to recover the embryos. These can be examined critically microscopically, thus allowing differentiation between unfertilized oocytes, normal embryos and abnormal and dead embryos. Furthermore, doubts about embryo viability can also be confirmed by in vitro culture. Karyotyping of cells can also be performed to determine chromosome abnormalities (Gustafsson et al., 1985) (see Chapter 4).

The factors responsible for embryonic death have been divided into two main groups, genetic and environmental factors (Boyd, 1965). These have been reviewed in detail by Ayalon (1978).

Genetic factors

Intrinsic genetic factors
Support for the role of genetic or intrinsic factors as the major cause of embryonic death in domestic

species has waned in recent years, largely because the techniques of embryo recovery, evaluation, culture and transfer have enabled studies to be performed on developing embryos. The role of intrinsic factors has been reviewed by King (1985). Among the intrinsic factors that are known to adversely affect the embryo are chromosome abnormalities and single gene mutations. More recently, mutagen-induced irreversible changes of DNA have been suggested as being responsible for embryo loss (King, 1985).

Chromosome abnormalities are known to be one of the major causes of fetal death in humans (Simpson, 1980). Their involvement in embryonic death in cattle was shown by McFeely and Rajakoski (1968), who found tetraploid cells in one of eight bovine blastocysts at 12–16 days of age. When they occur it is likely that there will be early loss of the embryo with return to service, in polytocous species there will be reduced litter size. Chromosome abnormalities are either inherited or arise *de novo* during gametogenesis, fertilization and early cleavage of the embryo (Hamerton, 1971) (see Chapter 4). During gametogenesis, abnormal meiosis can produce gametes with unbalanced chromosome composition such as duplication and deletion of segments of chromosome, whole chromosomes or the failure of the reduction division. Although abnormal, these gametes are capable of participation in fertilization so that the embryo has chromosome abnormalities. Chromosome abnormalities can occur because of polyspermic fertilization, failure to extrude one or both polar bodies, fertilization of the oocyte and the polar body, at the first cleavage division or because of failure at meiosis. Whilst it has been clearly demonstrated that superovulated oocytes quite frequently have cytogenetic abnormalities (up to one-third) due to polyspermic fertilization and/or mitotic activity of the polar body (King, 1985), those derived from a single ovulation do not. Recent work on virgin and repeat breeder heifers indentified two animals, out of a total of 42 from the latter group, which had 1/29 gene translocations, but the remainder had normal karyotypes (Gustafsson et al., 1985). Gayerie de Abrea et al. (1984) reported that 9% of cow embryos had abnormal karyotypes compared with 6% in heifers.

Single genes that affect embryological development have not been identified in domestic animals although they are known to cause fetal death and congenital abnormalities in humans.

Acquired genetic factors
Handling of embryos during embryo transfer has been shown to cause increased embryonic loss due to permanent alterations in DNA induced by exposure to substances described as mutagens. The known mutagenic factors have been listed by King (1985), and include superovulatory hormones, culture media and serum, ultraviolet light and DNA-binding dyes, radioactivity, ethylene oxide and viral genes. As yet, no endogenous mutagens have been identified in cattle or other domestic species, although they are likely to occur and are probably responsible for mediating the effects of some of the environmental factors described below.

Environmental factors

Nutrition
It is generally agreed that dietary deficiencies and excesses can influence the level of embryonic death, particularly at the time of cleavage and blastocyst elongation (Gustafsson et al., 1985). However, there is little work to distinguish this from fertilization failure as a cause of poor pregnancy rates.

In a study of beef heifers on a high- and low-energy dietary regimen there was a reduction in the pregnancy rate in the latter group which was shown to be due to early embryonic death and not fertilization failure (Spitzer et al., 1978). This loss did not appear to be mediated through abnormal progesterone or luteinizing hormone levels as determined in the peripheral blood. Conversely, reduced fertilization rates and lower circulating progesterone concentrations were identified in heifers subjected to undernutrition (Hill et al., 1970).

Age of dam
Opinions vary about the effect of the age of the dam on the embryonic death rate. Studies by Bearden et al. (1956) and Ayalon (1978) suggested that there was very little difference between old and young animals. However, Boyd and Reed (1961) found that interservice intervals of 25–35 days were more prevalent in older cows, which is suggestive of late embryonic death. More recently,

Ball (1978) identified a higher rate of embryo loss at 28–43 days in cows that have had four or more lactations (15.1%) compared with those inseminated during their first lactation (3.3%). By contrast, the pregnancy rate at 21 days after artificial insemination, as determined by milk progesterone, showed no age effect. At this stage of gestation, i.e. 28–43 days, placental attachment is occurring; perhaps the influence of previous pregnancies has some deleterious effect upon this process.

Temperature

There is evidence that high environmental temperatures can depress fertility, with a high incidence of embryonic death before 35 days (Stott and Williams, 1962). In dairy cows the first 4–6 days after service are the most critical (Wiersma and Stott, 1969).

Infection

This has been described earlier (Chapter 23).

Hormonal asynchrony and imbalance

There is much conflicting evidence on the importance of hormonal imbalance in causing embryonic death. However, experimental work in sheep using ovariectomized ewes as recipients for ovine embryos has clearly shown that a rigid sequence of hormonal treatment must be used: (1) progesterone to simulate the previous luteal phase; (2) oestradiol to simulate oestrus; (3) low progesterone concentrations to simulate early dioestrus; and (4) high levels of progesterone to simulate dioestrus, to ensure that the embryos survive (Wilmut et al., 1985). There are no comparable studies yet published in the cow, but it would be reasonable to extrapolate to this species that a similar situation would arise. It has been known for some time that in order to get normal embryo survival following embryo transfer the recipients and donor must have their oestrous cycles closely synchronized (Rowson et al., 1969; Newcombe and Rowson, 1975). Thus the embryo is highly susceptible to the direct influence of the hormonal status of the cow or, indirectly, to the uterine environment produced by the hormonal status.

Evidence for progesterone influencing embryo survival is conflicting. A positive relationship between luteal phase progesterone concentrations in peripheral blood or milk samples has been found (Hendricks et al., 1971; Erb et al., 1976; Holness et al., 1977; Bulman and Lamming, 1978; Lukaszewska and Hansel, 1980). Others have found no such relationship (Shemesh et al., 1968; Pope et al., 1969; Hasler et al., 1980; Sreenan and Diskin, 1983; Roche et al., 1985). Others have found that progesterone concentrations in the luteal phase before service were important (Folman et al., 1973).

Failure of pregnancy has also been ascribed to oestrogens. Erb et al. (1976) found that plasma concentrations were higher in fertile cows, particularly 12 and 8 hours after oestrus. Conversely, Ayalon (1973) found that embryos obtained from cows in which plasma oestrogen concentrations were high at oestrus and on days three and four of the oestrous cycle were abnormal. It must be stressed, however, that single blood samples are of little or no value because of the rapid fluctuations in the levels in the peripheral circulation.

Attempts have also been made to reduce embryonic death by the administration of exogenous hormones to correct apparent insufficiencies, particularly progesterone.

As an alternative to direct progesterone supplementation, human chorionic gonadotrophin (hCG) has been administered as a luteotrophic agent in mid- to late dioestrus. It has been shown to significantly increase peripheral blood progesterone concentrations either by stimulating secondary ovulations causing the formation of accessory corpora lutea (Christie et al., 1979; Holness et al., 1982) but also by increasing progesterone synthesis from the existing corpus luteum (Santos-Valadez et al., 1982). In a review of six papers describing the effect of hCG on conception rates in cows there was some improvement after use but it was not statistically significant (Diskin and Sreenan, 1986). More recently, gonadotrophin-releasing hormone (GnRH) analogues have also been used in an attempt to improve embryo survival and hence conception (pregnancy) rates when administered around the time of the maternal recognition of pregnancy. Equivocal results have been obtained. In a study involving 1720 dairy cows in New Zealand treated with 10 µg of buserelin between days 11 and 13 after insemination, a significant improvement in pregnancy rates was obtained (MacMillan et al., 1986). Conversely, in a study involving 2050 cows in Australia, the use of 10 µg of buserelin on day 12 after insemination had no significant effect on pregnancy rates compared with placebo-treated controls (Jubb et al., 1990). Peters (personal communication) has shown a positive effect of treatment.

It must be concluded that other, as yet unknown, causes are involved other than a simple endocrine deficiency.

Uterine environment
Embryo transfer experiments have shown the importance of the correct uterine environment for the successful survival and development of the embryo (Rowson et al., 1972). The nature of the uterine secretions is under the influence of the ovarian steroid hormones (Heap and Lamming, 1961). The possible role of mutagens has already been discussed above in relation to the development of acquired genetic defects. However an adverse uterine environment may cause embryonic death by other means, particularly at the critical 6–8 day stage. Differences in the composition of uterine washings and secretions have been identified in repeat breeder cows compared with normal fertile cows.

INVESTIGATION OF THE INDIVIDUAL INFERTILE COW

History
Before performing a detailed gynaecological examination it is important to obtain a detailed and accurate history, particularly a breeding history, of the cow. The following should be obtained:

1. Age.
2. Parity (there are certain conditions which can be excluded in nulliparous as opposed to parous individuals).
3. Date of last calving, together with information on the occurrence of dystocia, retained placenta or puerperal infection.
4. Dates of observed oestrus since calving, if recorded.
5. Presence of any abnormal discharge.
6. Numbers and dates of services or inseminations.
7. Dates of observed oestrus since service or artificial insemination.

8. Previous fertility records, particularly calving conception intervals and services per conception.
9. Details of feeding, management and milk yield; in suckler cows the number of calves suckled.
10. Details of health, i.e. signs of milk fever, mastitis or ketosis.
11. Details of fertility of other cows or heifers in the group or herd.

Clinical examination
A good general clinical examination should be undertaken with assessment of body condition and/or live weight. The genital system should then be examined in detail. Where it is available, transrectal ultrasonography should be used.

1. Inspect the vulva, perineum and vestibule for evidence of current or healed lesions and discharges.
2. Examine the base of the tail for signs of rub marks, and back and flanks for hoof marks, which might indicate that the individual has been ridden by other cows.
3. Explore the vagina by hand or speculum to examine the mucosa and to inspect the mucus.
4. Palpate the cervix per rectum to determine its size and position in relation to the pelvic brim, and of the uterine horns to determine if involution is complete (see Chapter 7). Assess the texture of the uterus, the degree of tone, the mobility of the horns and the absence of adhesions. *The absence of signs of pregnancy should be confirmed.*
5. Palpate the uterine tubes for evidence of induration or increased size.
6. Palpate the ovarian bursa for evidence of adhesions.
7. Palpate the ovaries to note their position, mobility and size and to identify the presence of any structures.

Diagnostic tests
Most diagnostic tests are of limited value, although single blood or milk progesterone assays are useful to identify the presence of luteal tissue if concentrations are high (4–6 ng/ml in plasma or 12–18 ng/ml in milk). Specific serological tests, for example the mucus agglutination or fluorescent antibody tests for *Campylobacter fetus* (see p. 399) are diagnostic for this disease. Bacterial swabbing

and culture and endometrial biopsy are of limited value. The PSP (phenolsulphonphthalein) test for tubal patency can also be used to demonstrate occluded uterine tubes.

Summary of the signs of infertility: the diagnosis, cause and treatment

The following summary describes a procedure for investigating an infertile animal on the basis of the clinical history, signs and examination, with an indication of a possible diagnosis of the cause and its treatment.

No observed oestrus

Rectal palpation or diagnostic ultrasonography should establish the presence or absence of pregnancy. If the individual is pregnant it should be recorded; however, if there is any doubt or if it might be an early pregnancy then a re-examination at a later date is required. If there is no pregnancy then palpation of the ovaries is the next step.

Absence of Ovaries. Uncommon: due to ovarian agenesis or freemartinism and hence will be seen only in a nulliparous animal. There is no treatment, and thus the animal should be culled.

Small Inactive Ovaries. If the ovaries are small, narrow and functionless, in a heifer, then this is due to delayed puberty, ovarian hypoplasia or, possibly, freemartinism. There is no treatment; if delayed puberty is suspected, normal cyclic activity should eventually occur.

If the ovaries are flattened, smooth, small and inactive then this is true anoestrus; if there is a need for confirmation then a milk progesterone determination 10 days later will help. The condition may be due to high yield, suckling, inadequate energy intake, intercurrent disease, severe postpartum weight loss or trace element deficiency.

Check feeding and assess bodily condition; improve deficiencies if present. Insert a PRID or a CIDR (p. 358) for 12 days; oestrus should occur several days after withdrawal. Alternatively, GnRH analogues can be used with oestrus occurring in 1–3 weeks. In beef cattle whose milk is not used for human consumption, a norgestamet (Crestar) implant and injection, together with 400–600 IU of equine chorionic gonadotrophin (eCG) at the time of implant removal can be used.

Presence of One or More Corpora Lutea. A number of situations are possible:

1. The animal may be pregnant: if in doubt re-examine later and check records.

2. Non-detected oestrus: if this is the case, improve detection with increased frequency of observation, heat mount detectors or tail paint or induce luteolysis with prostaglandin $F_{2\alpha}$ ($PGF_{2\alpha}$) or an analogue, followed by artificial insemination at observed oestrus or at a fixed time.

3. Suboestrus or 'silent heat': this is only likely if soon after calving. Treat with $PGF_{2\alpha}$ or an analogue as above.

4. Persistent corpus luteum: thoroughly palpate the uterus, using retraction forceps if necessary, to check for the absence of pregnancy. It may be due to pyometra, chronic endometritis, mummified fetus or, rarely, a non-specific cause. Treat with $PGF_{2\alpha}$ or an analogue.

Small Active Ovaries. The palpation of small follicles, and perhaps a regressing corpus luteum or evidence of recent ovulation associated with good uterine tone, indicates that the animal is coming into oestrus, is in oestrus or has been in oestrus. Careful inspection of the vulva at the time of palpation may reveal clear mucus. Re-examination in 10 days should reveal the presence of a corpus luteum.

Ovarian Cysts (Luteal). The presence of one or both enlarged ovaries, containing one or more fluid-filled, thick-walled structures more than 2.5 cm in diameter, particularly if confirmed using ultrasonography (see p. 366), should confirm the diagnosis. A repeat examination several days later will confirm their persistence, and a milk or blood progesterone determination will show the presence of luteal tissue. Treat with $PGF_{2\alpha}$ or an analogue.

Prolonged interoestrus interval

The ovaries and genital tract should be examined per rectum. If the ovaries are normal, infertility may be due to:

1. Non-detected oestrus: if the interval between successive heats is approximately twice the interoestrus interval, i.e. 36–48 days, then this indicates that one oestrus has not been observed or recorded. Irregular intervals that are not the product of the normal interval are likely to be due to incorrect identification of oestrus (see p. 384). If large numbers of animals are reported then this suggests that the oestrus detection rate is poor (see p. 381).

If a susceptible corpus luteum is present, $PGF_{2\alpha}$ can be used to cause luteolysis and oestrus in 3–5 days time. Methods of improving oestrus-detection should be implemented (see pp. 381–384).

2. Embryonic or fetal death: the interval between successive heats is unlikely to be an approximate multiple of 21 and thus will be some other interval such as 35 or 46 days. In an individual cow it is probably of no significance, but if a number of animals are involved, especially if natural service is used, specific pathogens should be eliminated and other causes sought.

Regular return to oestrus (repeat breeder or cyclic non-breeder)

The ovaries and genital tract should be examined per rectum to determine the presence of gross abnormalities such as severe adhesions or uterine infection. This condition can occur only if there is a failure of fertilization or embryonic death before day 12 of the oestrous cycle. There are a number of possible causes:

1. Infertile bull: if a number of cows and heifers are involved he should be examined as described in Chapter 30. If artificial insemination is used from an approved centre this can be excluded although it must be stressed that there is considerable variation in the fertility of bulls standing at artificial insemination studs, although they will be above a minimal level. A bull with a high fertility should be selected.

2. Incorrect timing of service or artificial insemination: this is unlikely to occur repeatedly unless the time of ovulation is asynchronous. If a number of animals are involved, advice on the correct time may be worthwhile or else fixed time artificial insemination after the administration of $PGF_{2\alpha}$ or progestogens.

3. Nutritional deficiency or excess: check diet.

4. Occluded uterine tubes: palpate carefully and use the PSP test to confirm.

5. Anatomical defects: palpate carefully, if the animal is nulliparous, look for segmental aplasia; if it is a parous animal, check for ovarobursal or uterine adhesions.

6. Endometritis: if there are clinical signs, diagnosis is simple but subclinical disease can be diagnosed only by biopsy. If suspected, treat with antibiotics after insemination or by $PGF_{2\alpha}$ to shorten the luteal phase preceding insemination.

7. Delayed ovulation: diagnosis is difficult. Treat with GnRH or hCG at the time of insemination or repeat insemination on the subsequent day.

8. Anovulation: diagnosis depends on ovarian palpation or transrectal ultrasonography 7–10 days after oestrus to demonstrate failure of ovulation by absence of a corpus luteum. Treat with GnRH or hCG at the time of insemination.

9. Luteal deficiency: there is no absolute proof that it occurs, but if other causes have been eliminated the use of a luteotrophic agent, such as hCG, might be worthwhile at 2–3 days after subsequent inseminations to improve corpus luteum formation, at mid-cycle to stimulate accessory corpus luteum formation. Alternatively, GnRH analogue can be administered at day 12 or 13 after insemination.

Short interoestrus interval

This condition is usually identified by other signs of nymphomania and palpation or imaging of ovaries. The cause may be:

1. Enlarged ovaries: if either one or, more likely, both contain one or more thin-walled, fluid-filled structures this should confirm the diagnosis of follicular cysts. Treat with GnRH, hCG or a PRID.

2. Artificial insemination at the wrong time due to incorrect oestrus detection. This is often preceded or followed by an extended interval so that the sum of the two intervals is 36–48 days. If large numbers of cows have the same history, oestrus detection should be improved (see p. 381–384).

Abortion

This is defined as the production of one or more calves between 152 and 270 days of gestation; they are either born dead or survive for less than 24 hours.

The cow should be isolated, the fetus and fetal membranes should be retained and the case treated as a suspected *Brucella* abortion under the brucellosis scheme. In the UK, this requires any abortion occurring less than 271 days after insemination to be reported to the Divisional Veterinary Officer of the Ministry of Agriculture, and clotted blood, milk and a vaginal swab submitted for laboratory examination. The physical appearance of the fetus and fetal membranes should be noted, the fetus aged approximately and this confirmed by the service or insemination date if available. Elimination of infection as a cause is made by being unable to demonstrate organisms in the fetus, fetal membranes, vaginal and uterine discharges and/or by the demonstration of specific antibodies in body fluids. Where possible the whole fetus should be submitted to the laboratory for cultural examination.

Possible infectious causes of abortion are:

1. *Brucella abortus*: occurs at 6–9 months of gestation.
2. *Leptospira* spp.: occurs at 6–9 months of gestation.
3. *Listeria monocytogenes*: sporadic outbreaks at 6–9 months of gestation.
4. *Campylobacter fetus* (*venerealis*): occurs at 5–7 months of gestation.
5. *Tritrichomonas fetus*: occurs before 5 months of gestation.
6. *Salmonella* spp.: especially *S. dublin*; usually sporadic with no specific time, although usually about 7 months of gestation.
7. *Actinomyces* (*Corynebacterium*) *pyogenes*: usually sporadic and occurs at any stage.
8. *Myobacterium tuberculosis*: occurs at any stage.
9. Mycotic agents, *Aspergillus* spp., *Absidia* spp., *Mucoralis* group: occurs from 4 months to term.
10. *Bacillus licheniformis*: sporadic late abortions.
11. *Neospora caninum*: late abortions.
12. Infectious bovine rhinotracheitis–infectious pustular vulvovaginitis (IBR–IPV) virus: occurs at 4–7 months of gestation.
13. Bovine viral diarrhoea (BVD) virus: occurs at any stage.

The approach to investigating the cause of abortion will depend upon the frequency. If sporadic, then a full laboratory investigation is probably unnecessary because many abortions are not associated with infection. However, if it exceeds 3–5% of the herd — and it is important to consider stillbirths and premature calvings (excluding twins) in this calculation — then a thorough investigation should be implemented. The approach recommended by Pritchard (1993) should be followed:

Sporadic abortions

1. Perform statutory brucellosis investigation.
2. Determine if all abortions have been reported and that it is a true sporadic case. If so,

proceed to (3), if not, or if there is any doubt, then follow the procedure for an outbreak investigation (see below).

3. Clinical examination of cow.
4. Examine placenta for evidence of obvious lesions, particularly fungi or *Bacillus licheniformis* (see Chapter 23).
5. Submit serum for *Leptospira* serovar *hardjo* serology unless it is a vaccinated herd.
6. Request culture of vaginal swab for *Salmonella dublin*.
7. Obtain detailed history of changes in husbandry, movement of livestock, purchase of animals, hiring of bulls, signs of ill-health, and age of aborting cows.

Abortion outbreak

1. Repeat (1), (2), (3), (4) and (7) above.
2. Ideally, submit one or more fresh whole fetuses and placentas — *or*
3. Several complete fresh cotyledons.
4. Fetal stomach contents (2 ml) aseptically collected using vacutainer or syringe and needle.
5. Fluid from thorax or abdomen (2 ml) using methods described in (4).
6. About 5 g of fresh lung, liver, thymus and salivary gland. All tissues and other samples should be refrigerated and packed with ice, but not frozen.
7. Air-dried, acetone-fixed impression smears from fresh cotyledons, lung, liver and kidney.
8. Formal-saline-fixed cotyledon, fetal liver, heart and lung.
9. Two 7 ml vacutainers of clotted blood from all cows that have recently aborted.
10. Repeat samples from the same cows as in (9) 2–3 weeks later for possible rising antibody titres in the serum.

If an infectious cause is not identified using routine diagnostic tests it may be necessary to extend the investigation in an attempt to confirm the presence of a less common infectious agent. However, abortions can be caused by many other factors: congenital defects due to genetic factors or teratogens; trauma; allergies; dietary excesses such as high protein pastures (Norton and Campbell, 1990), or deficiencies such as iodine; poisonous plants such as brassicas, hemlock and, in the USA, pine needles (*Pinus ponderosa*); chemicals such as nitrates and chlorinated naphthalene; and hormones such as prostaglandins. Diagnosis is generally based on circumstantial evidence, and in some cases the presence of pathognomonic lesions.

NB. The cause of many abortions is not ascertained despite meticulous investigation (see Table 23.1).

EVALUATION OF DAIRY HERD FERTILITY

Regular, accurate evaluation of the fertility status of the dairy herd is an essential part of a control programme and should be done at least twice a year. It is also an important prerequisite when investigating a suspected herd infertility problem (Eddy, 1980).

In order to evaluate fertility it is necessary first of all to quantify certain reproductive values, and in order to do this it is necessary to have access to records of reproductive events. This presents few problems if details are recorded as described later (pp. 436–440); however, on many farms the information is incomplete and is dispersed in many places such as on milk record sheets, artificial insemination receipts or the farm diary. Obviously, the accuracy and value of such calculations will depend upon the quantity and quality of the information provided, and it will be necessary to modify one's assessment accordingly, depending upon clinical judgement, the history of the herd and the primary complaints of the herdsman or owner.

The minimum information required is: (1) identity of cow; (2) last calving date; (3) first and subsequent service or insemination dates; (4) confirmation of pregnancy.

The following measurements of fertility can be made (the terms and definitions used are those stated in *Dairy Herd Fertility: Reproductive Terms and Definitions* (Ministry of Agriculture, Fisheries and Food, Booklet 2476)).

Non-return rate to first insemination
This is the percentage of cows or heifers, in a particular group over a specified period of time, which have not been presented for a repeat insemination within a specific period of time. The periods are usually 30–60 days or 49 days. This is used, particularly in artificial insemination centres, to monitor the fertility of bulls and the performance of inseminators. Figures of 79% are frequently obtained at 30–60 days, which is often more than 20% better than the calving rate to first insemination. The discrepancy is due to: (1) failure to identify, record and report if the cow returns to oestrus; (2) culling the cow after she has returned to oestrus; (3) subsequently using natural service; (4) prenatal death. It is therefore an imperfect measure of fertility but can be useful if no pregnancy diagnosis is performed.

Calving interval and calving index
The calving interval is the interval in days for an individual cow between successive calvings; the calving index is the mean calving interval of all the cows in a herd at a specific point in time, calculated retrospectively from their most recent calving date. These two measurements have been used traditionally as a measure of fertility, since they indicate how closely the individual cow or herd approximates to the accepted optimum of 365 days.

The disadvantages of these measurements are that they are historical in that they are calculated retrospectively; furthermore, the calving index can give an overoptimistic assessment of fertility when many of the cows that fail to become pregnant are culled.

More contemporary measurements are the *predicted calving interval or index*, where the estimated date of the next calving is calculated by counting 280 days (mean gestation length) from the assumed date of conception (last recorded service date). This assumes that pregnancy will be maintained; both values should be 365 days.

Calving to conception interval
The calving interval (or index, CI) is the sum of two components, the interval from the last calving date to the date of conception (*a*) and the length of gestation (*b*), thus:

$$CI = a + b$$

therefore

$$CI = 85 \text{ days} + 280 \text{ days} = 365 \text{ days}$$

The calving to conception interval (CCI) is calculated by counting the number of days from calving to the service which resulted in pregnancy (effective service); this is usually the last recorded service date. The CCI is a useful measurement of fertility but requires a positive diagnosis of pregnancy to be made. It is influenced by two factors: how soon after calving the cows are served or inseminated and how readily they become pregnant when they have been served. The CCI can be expressed thus:

$$\text{Mean CCI} = c + d$$

where c is the mean calving to first service interval and d is the mean first service to conception interval, therefore

$$\text{Mean CCI} = 65 \text{ days} + 20 \text{ days} = 85 \text{ days}.$$

The mean CCI is a useful measure of fertility, provided that the interval from calving to first service is stated, since this probably will have the greatest influence upon its length.

Days open

This is defined as the interval, in days, from calving to the subsequent effective service date of those cows that conceive, and from calving to culling or death for those cows that did not conceive. Numerically, it will always be greater than the mean CCI unless all cows that are served conceive, in which case it would be the same. Days open is a popular measurement of fertility in North America.

Calving to first service interval

In the case of a herd that calves all the year round a mean value of 65 days should result in a mean CCI of 85 days (see above). The factors that influence the calving to first service interval are:

1. Breeding policy of the farm. Although cows will return to oestrus after calving as early as 2–3 weeks, they should not be served before 45 days, and in the case of first calvers, high-yielding cows and those that have had dystocia and problems during the puerperium (see Chapter 7) slightly longer should elapse. Thus, in a seasonal calving herd, those that calve early in the season will have their first service delayed and, for those that calve late, it may be necessary to advance the date of first service, thereby tightening the calving pattern.

2. Delayed return of cyclical activity after calving, i.e. true anoestrus (see Chapter 22).

3. Failure to detect oestrus in those cows that have resumed normal cyclical activity.

Factors (2) and (3) can be improved by ensuring that cows have returned to cyclical activity post-

partum. This can be done by regular and routine examination of those cows, per rectum, that have failed to be seen in oestrus by 42 days postpartum and by the use of milk progesterone assays (see p. 448). Detection of oestrus depends upon the herdsman knowing the true signs of oestrus, having a regular routine, recording the events and using oestrus detection aids (see Chapter 22).

Overall pregnancy rate

This (originally called the overall conception rate) is the number of services given to a defined group of cows or heifers, over a specified period of time, which result in a diagnosed pregnancy not less than 42 days after service; the figure is expressed as a percentage of the total number of all services and should include culled cows. The method of pregnancy diagnosis should be specified. The *first service pregnancy rate* is usually calculated separately and obviously refers to first services only. Thus in a 12 month period, if 100 cows receive 180 services, of which 90 resulted in a confirmed pregnancy, the overall pregnancy rate would be 50%.

The pregnancy rate is influenced by:

1. The correct timing of artificial insemination (see Chapter 22) which will be dependent particularly on the accuracy of oestrus detection.

2. Correct artificial insemination technique, handling and storage of semen, especially if 'do-it-yourself' artificial insemination is used.

3. Good fertility of the bull if natural service is used, and the absence of venereal disease.

4. Adequate nutritional status of cows and heifers at the time of service and afterwards (see Chapter 22).

5. Complete uterine involution and absence of uterine infection (see Chapter 23). Especially relevant to first-service conception rates.

The pregnancy rate to first service and overall pregnancy rate are very useful measures of fertility; the latter is used to calculate the *reproductive efficiency* of the herd (see below). The rates for the first service are usually slightly higher than those for all services because the latter group will include those cows that may be sterile and receive many services before they are culled. Mean values of 60 and 58%, respectively, are obtainable, although nationally the figures are much lower.

In order to identify the influence of management changes, particularly nutrition, it is worthwhile calculating these two parameters on a monthly basis provided that there are a minimum of 10 services per month, or expressing them as Cu-Sums (see below).

Oestrus detection

Improving the detection of oestrus has a much greater influence upon reducing the calving to conception interval than improving the pregnancy rates; the latter can only be improved up to a certain level (Esslemont and Ellis, 1974; Esslemont and Eddy, 1977). It is generally assumed that in the UK it is rarely better than 60%, yet it is possible to achieve a figure of 80%. It is important that *all* observed heats are recorded even though they occur before the earliest date for service (before 45 days). This enables herdsmen to anticipate the time of a subsequent oestrus and thus improves the detection rate. It also enables the early detection of acyclic cows.

It is possible to estimate the oestrus detection rate but it is important to stress that it is an estimate and not an accurate measurement. A number of different methods are used and they all have some measure of inaccuracy (Esslemont et al., 1985). One method is to determine the number of supposed missed oestrous periods. Thus an interval of 36–48 days (2 × 18–24) suggests that one oestrus has been missed and an interval of 54–72 days (3 × 18–24) suggests that two have been missed, although this latter range is fairly wide and can lead to errors. The percentage oestrus detection rate (ODR) is calculated thus:

$$ODR = \frac{\text{No. of interservice intervals recorded}}{\text{No. of interservice intervals recorded + No. of missed oestrous periods}} \times 100$$

This overestimated the heat detection by about 5% (Esslemont et al., 1985).

Another method is to calculate the mean interservice interval for the herd, so that the ODR is calculated thus:

$$ODR = \frac{21}{\text{Mean interservice interval}} \times 100$$

A large number of short interservice intervals due to inaccurate oestrus detection (see below) can overestimate the oestrus detection rate.

One simple method of assessing the oestrus detection rate at routine sessions of pregnancy diagnosis will be the number of cows that are assumed by the herdsman to be pregnant, and thus submitted for examination, but are found to be non-pregnant. Non-pregnant cows should have returned to oestrus since service or artificial insemination, and hence should have been seen in oestrus.

In many apparently well-managed dairy herds where the calving to first service interval is on target, there is a failure to detect returns to oestrus in non-pregnant cows. This will result in a large number of interoestrus intervals that are two or three times the normal interval. Milk progesterone assays can be helpful (see p. 449).

Poor oestrus detection may be due to:

1. Poor accommodation inhibiting cows from exhibiting overt signs of oestrus.
2. Poor lighting or identification of animals.
3. Failure to record signs of approaching oestrus and signs of true oestrus.
4. Inadequate regimen for observing cows for signs of oestrus (see Chapter 22), perhaps due to the herdsman being overworked. Methods of improving and aiding the detection of oestrus are described in Chapter 22.

Distribution of interoestrus intervals

Analysis of the distribution of interoestrus and interservice intervals will provide useful information about a number of aspects of the reproductive status of the herd. These intervals are subdivided into the following groups: (a) 2–17 days, this excludes those intervals of 1 day associated with double fixed-time artificial insemination (see Chapter 3); (b) 18–24 days, the normal interoestrus interval; (c) 25–35 days; (d) 36–48 days, twice the normal interoestrus interval; and (e) more than 48 days. In a well-managed herd, with accurate detection of oestrus and presentation for service, at least 45% of intervals should be within the 18–24 day range, thus 12% for (a), 53% for (b), 15% for (c), 10% for (d) and 10% for > 48 days (Anon., 1984). If the percentage for the 36–48 day interval is high and the figures for the 18–24 day interval are low then this is indicative of poor oestrus detection.

A large number of intervals in groups (a) and (c) suggests inaccurate identification of oestrus, whilst a large number of intervals in groups (c), (d) and (e) could be associated with a late embryonic or early fetal death problem (see p. 423). As with all fertility measurements they should be evaluated together with other parameters.

Using the percentage distribution of the inter-oestrus and interservice intervals, a single figure referred to as the *oestrus detection efficiency* (ODE) is sometimes calculated as follows:

$$\text{ODE} = \frac{b + d}{a + b + c + 2(d + e)} \times 100$$

A good ODE would be 50% or more.

First service submission rate

Measurements of oestrus detection rates are not very accurate, and for this reason the first service submission rate is calculated; this is a measure of how quickly cows are served after they have become eligible for service. It is defined as: the number of cows or heifers served within a 21 or 24 day period expressed as a percentage of the number of cows or heifers that are at, or beyond, the earliest date at the start of the 21 or 24 day period.

Thus once a cow has reached the earliest time after calving that she is ready for service, i.e. above 45 days in all-the-year-round calving herds, then she should be served or inseminated within the next 21 or 24 days. However, pregnancy rates will probably not reach their optimum for at least 90 days postpartum (DeKruif, 1975; Williamson et al., 1980; Esslemont et al., 1985). Furthermore, cows that have suffered dystocia or an abnormal puerperium should not be served before 60 days postpartum and should be examined routinely before service. It has been shown that there is a good correlation between the physical state of the uterus, as determined by rectal palpation and the amount of mucopurulent discharge and the regeneration of the endometrium (Studer and Morrow, 1978).

Heifers, and cows yielding more than 40 litres per day, should not be served before 50 days postpartum.

The submission rate is influenced by: (1) the time interval to the resumption of normal cyclical activity after calving, and (2) the detection of oestrus in those cows that have resumed normal cyclical activity, and their presentation for service or artificial insemination. A good submission rate is

80%. In seasonally calving herds it will tend to be higher in those cows that calve earlier than in the later calvers. This is because, with the former, the presence of more non-pregnant cows will ensure greater interaction when they are in oestrus, which should improve its detection (Anon., 1984). The calculation of a rolling average submission rate can be difficult unless it is part of a computer programme. A relatively simple method of obtaining a fairly accurate measurement is to list all cows that are ready for service (at or beyond the earliest service date of 45 days since calving) at the start of each 21 or 24 day service period. At the end of this period identify all those that have been served. The percentage submission rate is calculated thus:

$$\frac{\text{No. of cows served that are listed}}{\text{No. of cows that are listed}} \times 100$$

Another method is to list all cows chronologically in order of the calving date. Add 21 days to the earliest date on or after which they are ready for service, i.e. 45 + 21 (24) = 66 (69) days. Thus every cow should be served before the target date of 66 or 69 days postpartum. The submission rate is calculated thus:

$$\frac{\text{No. of cows served on or before the target date}}{\text{No. of cows that should have been served on or before the target date}}$$

In a tight seasonally calved herd, the earliest service date will be selected in relation to when the cows are required to calve down the following year. Thus, cows that calve early in the season will have a longer time interval before they need to be served compared with those that calve late in the season. The choice of 21 days is based on the assumption that this is the mean interoestrus interval. However, 24 days can be used as it is the normal maximum interval. It is irrelevant which is selected as long as its use is consistent.

Reproductive efficiency

Attempts have been made to calculate a single index that provides an overall measurement of fertility and takes into account many different parameters. One such measurement is the reproductive efficiency (RE) of the herd (Anon., 1984); it is calculated thus:

$$\text{RE} = \frac{\text{Submission rate} \times \text{Overall pregnancy rate}}{100}$$

Thus if the submission rate is high, i.e. 80%, and the overall pregnancy rate is good, i.e. 55%, then the RE is 44. In a herd with a more modest submission rate of 70% and an overall pregnancy rate of 50%, the RE is 35.

The advantage of this measurement is that an artificially high submission rate, obtained by an overzealous herdsman presenting cows for artificial insemination when they are not in oestrus, will be compensated by a reduced pregnancy rate. Conversely, an overcautious herdsman may have a reduced submission rate but although the pregnancy rate may rise to 65%, producing a reasonable RE value, it is not possible to increase this further (see pp. 423–424).

Fertility factor

Another composite measurement can be obtained by calculating the fertility factor (FF) (Esslemont et al., 1985). This is obtained following the calculation of the overall pregnancy rate (OPR) and the estimation of the oestrus-detection rate (ODR). It is calculated thus:

$$FF = \frac{ODR \times OPR}{100}$$

Thus if the ODR is 60% and the OPR rate is 50%, then the FF is:

$$\frac{50 \times 60}{100} = 30$$

Another way of calculating this factor is to estimate how many cows in the herd become pregnant during a 21 day period after being detected in oestrus and inseminated; using the figures above it would be 30%. As Esslemont et al. (1985) comments: 'Most farmers estimates would be higher'.

Culling rate

One method of achieving a CI around 365 days is by culling those cows that are slow to get in calf. This is rarely cost-effective because it will be necessary to replace the culled cow with a heifer. The purchase price or the cost of rearing such a replacement is much greater than the price obtained for the cull. Overall culling figures for infertility should not exceed 5%; thus 95% of the cows that calve and are served should become pregnant again.

Fertility index

Another single index that can be calculated and takes into consideration the pregnancy rate to first service, services per conception, calving to conception interval and culling rate, is the fertility index (De Kruif, 1975; Esslemont and Eddy, 1977; Esslemont et al., 1985).

The cost of fertility in dairy herds

Poor fertility reduces the profitability of a dairy enterprise. Various figures have been quoted for the financial loss to the dairy farmer for every day that the calving interval for each cow is extended. In the USA, Bartlett et al. (1986) quoted $2.60, in the UK the quote was £3.00 per day (Anon., 1984). The most recent figure for the UK is £3.35 per day (Esslemont and Spincer, 1992). This latter figure is obtained by calculating the value of the net reduction in milk yield, the cost of keeping a dry cow which obviously is non-productive, the reduced number of calves per annum and the slip in the calving pattern.

More recently, an attempt has been made to incorporate other fertility parameters in the cost of reduced fertility by using the FERTEX (fertility index) score for a dairy herd (Esslemont, 1992). This takes into account the mean calving interval (calving index), the total percentage culling rate and the overall pregnancy rate. Each of the three indices is adjusted using a financial score which gives a penalty or bonus for the herd. This is best explained using the example illustrated by Esslemont (1992), given in Table 24.1.

Using data obtained from 63 dairy herds involving 20 000 cows in the calving season 1989–1990 in the UK that used DAISY — the Dairy Information System — Esslemont and Spincer (1992) have attempted to measure the cost of disease. This has been done by calculating both the direct and indirect costs. Direct costs, which are much easier to identify, include: veterinary time, herdsman's time, pharmaceutical agents and medicines, milk discarded for human consumption, reduced milk yield, and calf mortality. Indirect costs include: reduced fertility, increased culling rate of adult cows, increased likelihood of the same disease or other diseases occurring, and extra services per conception.

Using these data, the costs for some common

Table 24.1 The FERTEX score for a dairy herd (Esslemont, 1992)

(a) Standard indices and the penalty or bonus incurred for divergence

	Standard values	Divergence from standard values: penalty or bonus
Calving index (days)	360	£3.00/day
Percentage culling rate	22	£590/cull
Services/conception	2.0	£20/service

(b) Worked example for a herd. A figure of approximately £82 per cow is obtained

	Actual herd value	Financial score
Calving index (days)	380	(+20) × £3 × 100 = £6000
Percentage culling rate	25	(+3) × £590 = £1770
Services/conception	2.2	(+0.2) × £20 × 100 = £400
		Cost/100 cows = £8170

Table 24.2 Costs for some common diseases, based on DAISY

Reproductive disorder or disease	Percentage mean incidence	Direct costs (£)	Indirect costs (£)	Total per case or per cow (£)
Twins	3.89	−79.14	212.27	133.13
Calf mortality	7.29	137.53	176.36	313.89
Retained placenta	3.89	65.66	221.16	286.82

diseases involving the reproductive system are given in Table 24.2.

In the case of twins, the benefits from the value of an extra calf and the increased milk yield (Eddy et al., 1991) is offset by the greater indirect costs such as an extended calving interval, increased culling rate, increased calf mortality, increased incidence of retained placenta and vulval discharge, and increased number of oestruses-not-observed.

Recording systems

Irrespective of the recording system used there are certain basic requirements. Perhaps the most important is the ability to easily and accurately identify every cow from virtually any point whether she is standing or recumbent. This enables all persons working on the farm to identify cows in oestrus, thus assisting the herdsman. Each cow should have a permanent freeze brand on the rump which must be kept clean and clipped, together with a collar or large ear tag with number.

It will be necessary to record, at least, the following: calving date; dates of oestruses although not served; all service or artificial insemination dates; bull identity; results of pregnancy diagnosis; parturient and periparturient problems and diseases.

There are many varied recording systems ranging from simple manual ones involving the use of notebooks and diaries to sophisticated on-farm computers with a keyboard and VDU adjacent to the milking parlours and cattle housing. Most systems fall between these two extremes.

The investigation of infertility problems and the maintenance of good fertility requires the keeping of accurate records of the reproductive history of each and every cow in the herd. The absence of accurate and accessible records makes the task of the veterinarian difficult, if not impossible. Some information is often available in an apparently unpromising situation, for example, artificial insemination receipts and milk recording sheets, especially if the herd is involved in milk recording schemes.

CLIP WHEN CULLED

1 2 3 4 5 6 7 8 9 10 11 12

HERD _____   COW NAME _____

BREED _____   EAR NO. _____

DAM _____   SIRE _____

DATE OF BIRTH _____   DATE S.19 _____

DATE	REARING RECORD

LIFE SUMMARY

Lact. No.	Calved	Conceived	D.off	Days open	Length Lact.	No. dry days	C.I.	Milk (lb)	B.F.	

MASTITIS RECORD

Date	Quarter	Treatment	Date	Quarter	Treatment

NOTES

Fig. 24.1 An example of a simple individual cow record card suitable for permanent recording.

A	B	C	D	E	F	G	H	I	J	K	L	M	N	O	P	Q	R	S	T	U	V	W
Name	Lactation No.	Calving date	Bulling date (not served)	Bull mpd	Target date to serve	Interval to 1st A.I. or N.S.	1st service	Int	2nd service	Int	3rd service	Int	4th service	Int	5th service	Int	6th service	No. serves	Calving/conception days	Next calving date	Dry off date	Remarks
A 94	3	1/9	5/10	PJ	26/10	55	27/10	21	16/11										2	76	25/8		PREGNANT
A 105	2	3/9	14/10	H	28/10	61	3/11												1	61	11/8		PREGNANT
A 54	5	4/9		H	29/10	73	16/11	22	7/12	23	30/12								3	118	8/10		NON-OBSERVED OESTRUS PRD PREGNANT
X 514	8	5/9		-	-													0				CULL. CHRONIC LAMENESS
A 176	1	7/9		PJ	1/11	60	30/11												1	84	8/9		RFM. METRITIS PREGNANT
A 32	6	7/9	19/11	PJ	1/11	70	10/12	40	9/1	22	31/1								3	146	9/11		PREGNANT
X 499	9	10/9	19/11	PJ	4/11	55	4/11												1	55	12/8		PREGNANT
A 60	4	10/9	19/10	H	4/11	59	8/11												1	59	16/8		PREGNANT
A 81	3	11/9	23/10	PJ	5/11	63	14/11	21	5/12										2	84	13/9		MASTITIS . PREGNANT
A 98	2	12/9	17/10	ZT	6/11	56	7/11												1	56	15/8		PREGNANT
A 88	3	17/9		ZT	11/11	65	21/11	9	30/11	33	2/1								2	107	11/10		PREGNANT

Total / Mean

```
HERD :   2 -                                                                      DAISY    A7
                                                                                  DATE 30MAR95
                                                                                  PAGE     1


--------------------------------------------------------------------------------------------------
COWS FOR VET TO SEE : WORKLIST
--------------------------------------------------------------------------------------------------


Number of checks =  16

Date of last visit = 28MAR95
Date of next visit = 30MAR95
Calving-1st serve interval = 63 days
Service-P.D. interval =      42 days
Calving-1st heat interval =  42 days
PD negative,no action for    21 days


Sorted by Reason
       then Cow name


*=more than one reason

--------------------------------------------------------------------------------------------------
   COW    GRP  REASON TO BE SEEN              Days    ----CRUCIAL EVENT----    FURTHER DETAILS        Latest 2
                                             Calved  Type    Date  Days to                           Heats/Serves
                                             at visit             visit                              Days to visit
   -----+-----+-------------------------------+-----+------+---------+-----+-------------------------------------------
   74*    0  For revisit(PD? )               262    PD?    3MAR95   27                                :SE140
   74*    0  For vet P.D.                    262    SERV  10NOV94  140                                :SE140
   366    0  For vet P.D.                    274    SERV   9DEC94  111                                :SE111
   315    0  P.D. neg, no action for 21 days 169    PD-   23FEB95   35                                :SE107
   316    0  P.D. neg, no action for 21 days 172    PD-   23FEB95   35                                :SE117
   -----+-----+-------------------------------+-----+------+---------+-----+-------------------------------------------
   406    0  P.D. neg, no action for 21 days 266    PD-    3MAR95   27    T PRID                      :SE 91
    55    0  No serve 63 days since calving  185    ONO   15DEC94  105    F ACY    T PRID
    56    0  No serve 63 days since calving   79    VLD   28FEB95   30    F FC
    68    0  No serve 63 days since calving   73    ONO   28MAR95    2    F CLLO   T PG
   154    0  No serve 63 days since calving   70    VLD   28FEB95   30    T PG
   -----+-----+-------------------------------+-----+------+---------+-----+-------------------------------------------
   204    0  No serve 63 days since calving   77    CALV  12JAN95   77
   312    0  No serve 63 days since calving   80    ONO   28MAR95    2
   486    0  No serve 63 days since calving   90    ONO   10FEB95   48    F INV
   513    0  No serve 63 days since calving   92    CALV  28DEC94   92
 T 64    0  No serve 63 days since calving    87    VLD   28FEB95   30
   -----+-----+-------------------------------+-----+------+---------+-----+-------------------------------------------
 T 85    0  No serve 63 days since calving    87    CALV   2JAN95   87
--------------------------------------------------------------------------------------------------


END OF REPORT
```

Fig. 24.3 An example of a computerized work or action list identifying cows that require veterinary examination at the next routine fertility visit (DAISY).

2. Heifers should be served at 14–15 months of age so that ideally they calve about 1 month before the cows in a seasonally calving herd. This enables them to have a longer calving to conception interval and calve for the second time at the same time as the rest of the herd. They should be approximately 325 kg liveweight and growing at 0.7 kg/day. It is advisable to 'flush' them by increasing the feed intake from before the service period until diagnosed pregnant.

3. A bull with a low probability of causing dystocia due to fetomaternal disproportion should be used whether by artificial insemination or natural service.

4. Pregnancy diagnosis by rectal palpation at 5–6 weeks. Adequate feeding should be maintained.

HEAT DETECTION ANALYSIS - BY INTERVAL BETWEEN SERVES   COWS CALVING   1JUL85 - 24FEB86   ALL COWS

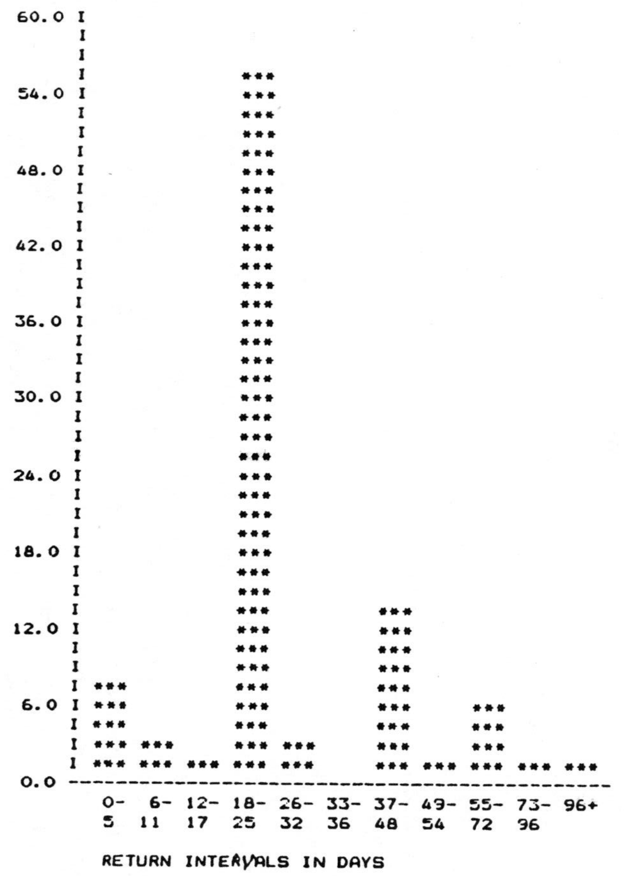

```
60.0 I
     I
54.0 I   ***
     I   ***
     I   ***
48.0 I   ***
     I   ***
     I   ***
42.0 I   ***
     I   ***
     I   ***
36.0 I   ***
     I   ***
     I   ***
30.0 I   ***
     I   ***
     I   ***
24.0 I   ***
     I   ***
     I   ***
18.0 I   ***
     I   ***
     I   ***
12.0 I   ***   ***
     I   ***   ***
     I   ***   ***   ***
 6.0 I***  ***  ***  ***
     I***  ***  ***  ***
     I***  ***  ***  ***  ***
 0.0 I***  ***  ***  ***  ***  ***  ***  ***
      0-   6-  12-  18-  26-  33-  37-  49-  55-  73-  96+
      5   11   17   25   32   36   48   54   72   96

            RETURN INTERVALS IN DAYS
```

X

END OF REPORT

Fig. 24.4 (a) An example of a computer produced histogram illustrating the distribution of interservice intervals. Note that in this program the daily intervals are quite short (DAISY).

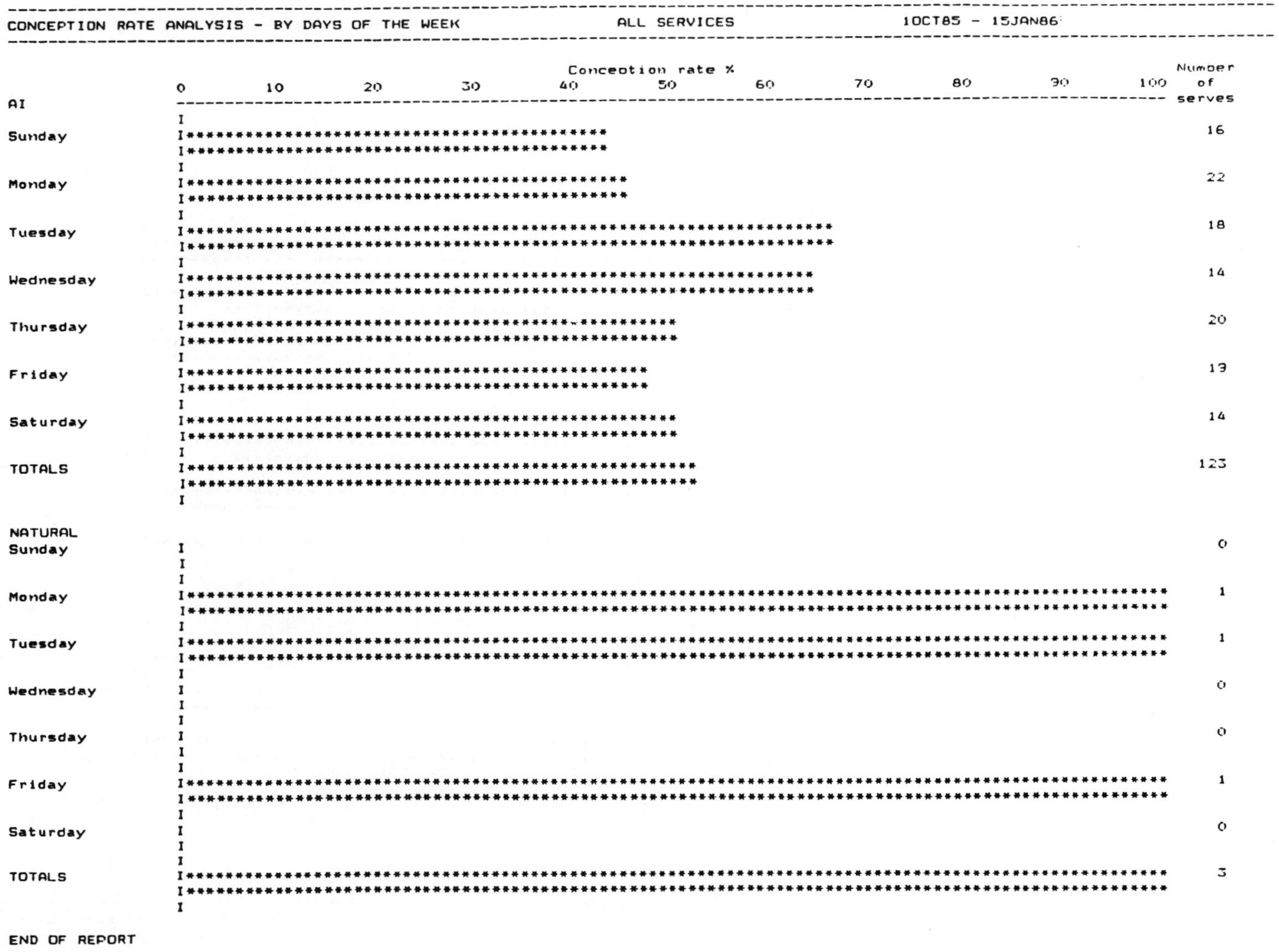

Fig. 24.4 (b) An example of a computer-produced histogram illustrating pregnancy (conception) rates by the days of the week when cows were inseminated (DAISY).

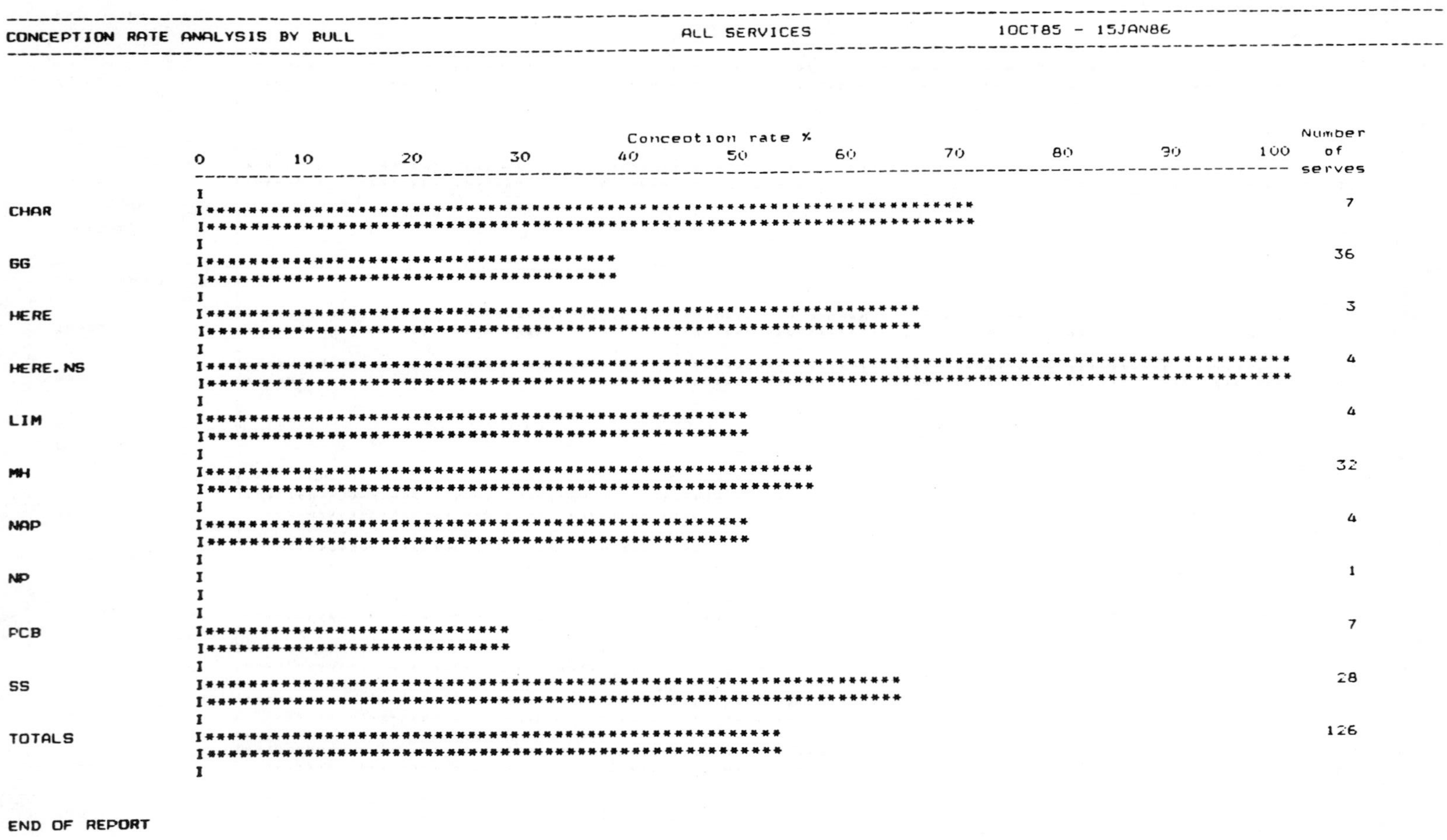

CONCEPTION RATE ANALYSIS BY BULL   ALL SERVICES   1OCT85 – 15JAN86

Conception rate %

| | 0 | 10 | 20 | 30 | 40 | 50 | 60 | 70 | 80 | 90 | 100 | Number of serves |

CHAR ... 7
GG ... 36
HERE ... 3
HERE.NS ... 4
LIM ... 4
MH ... 32
NAP ... 4
NP ... 1
PCB ... 7
SS ... 28
TOTALS ... 126

END OF REPORT

Fig. 24.4 (c) An example of a computer-produced histogram illustrating pregnancy (conception) rates to individual bulls whose identities are listed by abbreviations or initials (DAISY).

HERD :   2 -

CONCEPTION RATE ANALYSIS - Q-SUM   ALL SERVICES   1JAN91 - 31DEC91

Key : %=to be CUlled @=Not to be Served $=left herd w=P+ unknown serve x2=double insemination

Date	Cow	Lac	Srv	Bull	Res	Int	Ca-S	Type	Comments	Grp	Cow
								CR tending to be under 50%*CR tending to be over 50%			
3JAN	6	3	1	LOD	+V	0	36	.*		0	6
9JAN	37$	2	2	LOD	-O	49	93	*		1	37
13JAN	55	4	1	LOD	+V	0	79	.*		0	55
18JAN	97	5	1	LOD	-	0	49	*		0	97
24FEB	37$	2	3	LLY	-O	46	139	*.	SE FOR PROF NOAKES	1	37
27MAR	28	2	2	LLY	+V	98	139	*		0	28
27MAR	79	6	1	LLY	-	0	91	*.		0	79
29MAR	31	4	1	LLY	+V	0	58	*		0	31
30MAR	69	4	1	LLY	+V	0	70	.*		0	69
30MAR	102	1	1	LLY	+V	0	89	. *		0	102
30MAR	4$	3	1	LLY	-O	0	112	.*		1	4
30MAR	44	5	1	LLY	-	0	73	*		0	44
31MAR	68	8	1	LLY	+V	0	54	.*		0	68
7APR	96	5	1	LLY	+V	0	82	. *		0	96
7APR	104	1	1	LLY	+V	0	98	. *		0	104
7APR	39	3	2	LLY	+V	118	192	. *		0	39
7APR	97	5	2	LLY	-	79	128	. *		0	97
8APR	53	9	1	LLY	+V	0	96	. *		0	53
9APR	87$	4	1	LLY	-V	0	127	. *		0	87
11APR	24	5	1	LLY	+V	0	107	. *		0	24
11APR	47	3	1	LLY	+V	0	54	. *		0	47
14APR	89$	4	1	LLY	-V	0	95	. *		0	89
14APR	51$	2	2	LLY	-V	106	186	. *		0	51
14APR	98$	5	1	LLY	?	0	152	. *		0	98
15APR	79	6	2	UN	+V	19	110	. *		0	79
18APR	95	5	1	LOD	+V	0	66	. *		0	95
5MAY	51$	2	3	LLY	-V	21	207	. *		0	51
9MAY	89$	4	2	LOD	-V	25	120	. *		0	89
12MAY	44	5	2	LOD	+V	43	116	. *		0	44
12MAY	43$	4	1	LOD	?	0	131	. *		0	43
19MAY	80	6	1	LOD	+V	0	73	. *		0	80
20MAY	101	1	1	LOD	-	0	117	. *		0	101
21MAY	38$	4	1	LOD	-V	0	100	.*		0	38
21MAY	4$	3	2	LOD	-O	52	164	*		1	4
21MAY	37$	2	4	LOD	-O	86	225	*.		1	37
26MAY	97	5	3	LOD	-	49	177	* .		0	97
26MAY	51$	2	4	LOD	-V	21	228	* .		0	51
1JUN	89$	4	3	LOD	-V	23	143	* .		0	89
5JUN	103	1	1	LOD	-	0	135	* .		0	103

Fig. 24.5 An example of a computer-produced 'Cu-Sum' for pregnancy (conception) rates to all services (DAISY).

5. They should be at a condition score of $2\frac{1}{2}$–3 and about 480–500 kg liveweight at the time of calving.

Visual presentation of data

Simple methods involving the use of herd record sheets (see Figure 24.2) or rotary boards, especially if they have some form of colour symbols, are good methods of presenting data so that they can assist the herdsman in managing the herd.

Computerized systems often produce graphic print-outs, for example histograms of frequency of interoestrus/service intervals (Figure 24.4(a)) or pregnancy rates for different days of the week (Figure 24.4(b)), or for different bulls (Figure 24.4(c)).

One useful method of monitoring the contemporary fertility of a herd is to record the pregnancy rates to all services, or first services, as a Cumulative sum or Cu-Sum (Gould, 1974) recorded in chronological order. Although several computer programs will produce a print-out of Cu-Sums for overall pregnancy rate (Figure 24.5) it is quite straightforward to produce one manually; all that is required is a sheet of squared graph paper preferably marked in 0.1 inch squares.

Half-way down the vertical axis 'ink in' or cross the first small square; this represents the first service for the year or season. Move along one column and repeat the same procedure for the next small square; this represents the second service of the season or year. If this resulted in conception, as determined by pregnancy diagnosis, then the square in the line above is marked. If the cow does not conceive then the square in the line below is marked. This procedure is repeated for all the services with each vertical small column representing a cow (Eddy, 1980). If more than

one cow is served on the same day then several squares will be marked. The Cu-Sum graph can be completed only after the presence or absence of conception has been confirmed by pregnancy diagnosis. Such a graph is shown in Figure 24.6; a rising graph represents a period when conception rates are greater than 50%, a falling graph a period when conception rates are less than 50%. The dates of the services should be placed on the horizontal axis and any changes in feeding, environment, management or service procedure recorded as well. This will then give a good visual record of factors which might influence conception rates.

Cu-Sums can be used to represent other fertility parameters. Figure 24.7 is a computer print-out for the first service submission rate.

MANAGING FERTILITY AND ROUTINE VISITS IN BEEF SUCKLER HERDS

Veterinary involvement in assisting the herdsman in the management of fertility in beef suckler herds is minimal. However, since good fertility, together with correct nutrition, is a major influence on the profitability of suckled calf production, there is a

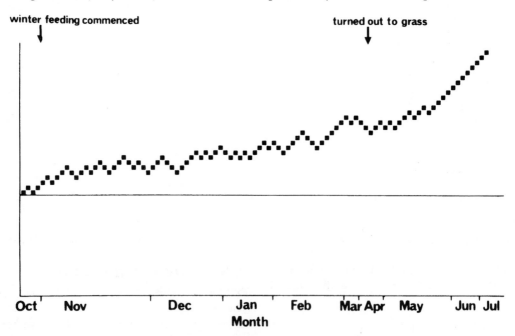

Fig. 24.6 An example of a manually produced 'Cu-Sum' of pregnancy (conception) rates to all services throughout a breeding year; the overall pregnancy rate was 65%.

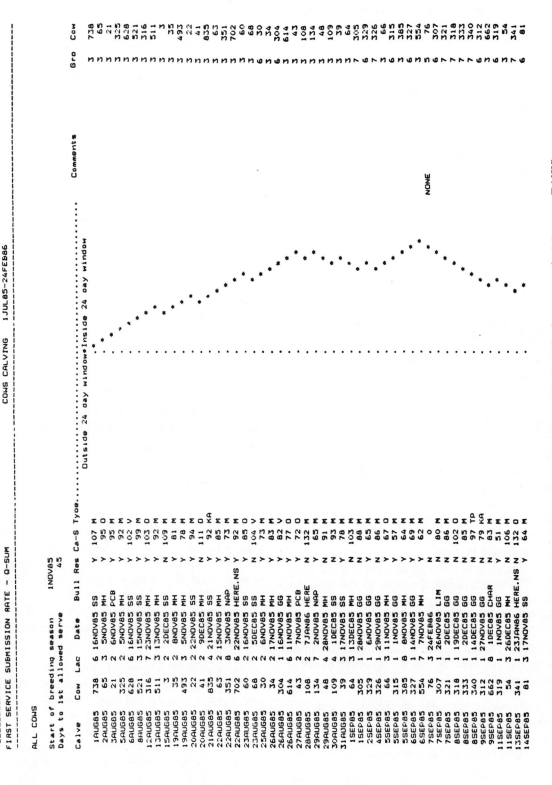

Fig. 24.7 An example of a computer-produced 'Cu-Sum' for first service submission rates (DAISY).

need for veterinary input with the implementation of fertility control schemes and routine visits, although it will not be at the level required for dairy herds.

Apart from the obvious differences, suckler cows have a greater longevity than dairy cows, 9 years compared with 6 years, and produce 6–7 calves in a lifetime. In addition, natural service rather than artificial insemination is generally used, which means that the male has a greater direct influence on fertility and could transmit venereal diseases.

The requirements for good reproductive performance in a suckler herd are as follows:

1. A calf per year, thus a 365 day calving index. The calving indices for some of the best herds in the UK exceed this figure (Meat and Livestock Commission Report, 1992).

2. A compact calving period of 2 months. This ensures that calves are of similar age and weight at weaning and improves their overall health and reduces calf mortality by ensuring that late-born calves do not acquire infection from older, earlier-born animals. In addition, cows are at a similar stage in their production cycle, thus their feeding and other aspects of management will be the same.

3. Cows should calve at the best time of year to utilize the available feed, thus in spring, summer and autumn but not winter.

4. Cows should calve at a condition score of $2\frac{1}{2}$–3.

5. It is important to use a fertile bull, running with a reasonable number of cows and heifers. Particularly in heifers, a sire which produces easy calvings should be used.

6. Ideally, heifers should be served so that they calve 2–3 weeks before the cows in the herd, to provide the opportunity for a longer calving to conception interval.

7. Primipara may lose excessive weight, hence they should be fed separately and additionally from the rest of the herd. It may be necessary to wean the calves slightly earlier.

A scheme for managing the fertility of a suckler herd to satisfy the requirements previously listed is as follows, and can be modified depending on the time of the proposed calving season:

1. The herd is calving during September and October. Details of dystocia, retained placenta,

uterine infection and other non-reproductive diseases should be recorded.

2. Early to mid-December: assess condition score of all cows — they should be at least $2\frac{1}{2}$ — and examine per rectum all cows that had reproductive disorders and disease. Ideally all cows should be examined for return of cyclical ovarian activity.

3. Early December: examine the bull or bulls for health, bodily condition and fertility. Ensure that there are adequate numbers and that they are free from venereal disease.

4. Mid-December: introduce bull or bulls for 8 weeks and remove in mid-February.

5. Examine per rectum all cows for pregnancy from the time that the bull was removed and for the next 6–8 weeks. Estimate gestational age and predict calving date for each animal.

6. Calves weaned in June: assess condition score of cows and modify feeding if necessary.

7. Calving during September to October at condition score 3.

THE USE OF MILK (OR PLASMA) PROGESTERONE ASSAYS IN COW FERTILITY MANAGEMENT

In Chapter 3 (see p. 83), the milk or plasma progesterone assay is described as a method of diagnosing pregnancy in cows 24 days after service. However, the same assay can in other ways assist both veterinarian and herdsman in managing the fertility of the herd. The assays are expensive, require some degree of laboratory skill and thus they should be used judiciously rather than as a non-selective procedure on all cows at all times. Possible applications have been described by Drew (1986) and are as follows:

1. *To identify, or confirm, postpartum anoestrus before the target service date.* At a single rectal palpation of a cow that has not been observed in oestrus since calving it may not be possible to make a definite diagnosis of anoestrus (acyclicity) (see p. 357). A high progesterone concentration in the milk 10 days before (or after) the palpation of ovaries without a corpus luteum is indicative of a non-observed oestrus. A low (or zero) milk

Table 24.4 Timing of insemination in relation to milk progesterone concentration

Day of previous insemination	17	18	19	20	21	22
Milk progesterone concentration	High	High	Low	Low	Low	Low ↑ AI

AI, artificial insemination.

progesterone concentration at the same time interval before (or after) palpation when no corpus luteum was identified is indicative of anoestrus. Furthermore, two consecutive low (or zero) milk progesterone concentrations in samples collected 7–10 days apart confirms that the cow is anoestrus.

2. *To ensure that a cow is close to, or is in oestrus, on the day of insemination.* Milk progesterone concentrations should be low on the day of insemination. Thus, this test enables the accuracy of oestrus detection to be checked. If it is done before the cow is due to be inseminated it can prevent the wastage of a dose of semen. It can be used to investigate a herd where poor overall pregnancy rates are obtained and prevent the insemination of cows that are already pregnant.

A single low progesterone sample does not necessarily show that the cow is at the optimum time for insemination but rather that the cow is not in dioestrus. A more accurate assessment of optimum timing (see p. 384) can be achieved if milk samples are collected and assayed every day from day 17 after the last recorded oestrus. Normally the samples on days 17 and 18 will have high progesterone values, day 19 intermediate and days 20, 21 and 22 will have low values. The timing of the high:low values will depend upon the normal cycle length (see p. 18). If oestrus has not been observed, then the cow should be inseminated on the third consecutive day of low progesterone concentrations (Table 24.4); using such a scheme acceptable pregnancy rates have been obtained.

3. *To anticipate the return to oestrus in the absence of pregnancy.* If the milk progesterone concentration is low on day 19 after service or insemination, then the cow can be assumed to be non-pregnant, and her return to oestrus can be anticipated. This can improve the oestrus detection rate after service.

Despite the expense of performing more frequent milk progesterone assays, it has been shown that it can be cost-effective (Eddy and Clarke, 1987). In a study involving four dairy herds, milk samples were collected at either 18, 20, 22 and 24 days or 19, 21 and 23 days after service. The calving to conception intervals in two herds were reduced from 115 to 84 days and from 85 to 74 days with a potential cost benefit of 7.4:1 and 3.4:1, respectively.

4. *To confirm ovarian structures identified at rectal palpation.* Confirmation of the presence of a corpus luteum or luteal cyst (see pp. 364–368) can be made by the presence of concurrently high milk progesterone concentrations.

5. *To assess the response of cows to therapy.* The assessment of the response to therapy is frequently entirely empirical. The assay of progesterone concentrations in milk at the time of treatment and at varying time intervals afterwards can be used to assess the luteolytic response after prostaglandin treatment or the luteotrophic response after GnRH or hCG therapy.

The regular collection of large numbers of milk samples and their assay is another task that, if imposed upon an already overworked herdsman by an overenthusiastic veterinarian, can result in loss of enthusiasm for this and other chores. For this reason selectivity of sampling should be a major aim so that the demands for large numbers of samples should be reduced.

SURGICAL PREPARATION OF TEASER BULLS AND RAMS

In intensively managed dairy herds, teaser bulls fitted with marking devices are sometimes used to enhance the efficiency of oestrus detection (see Chapter 22). Teaser rams are used for slightly different purposes, firstly to guarantee a short lambing period by ensuring that all ewes in the flock are undergoing oestrous cycles before the stud ram is introduced and secondly to induce, and, to some extent, synchronize, cyclical activity in anoestrous females.

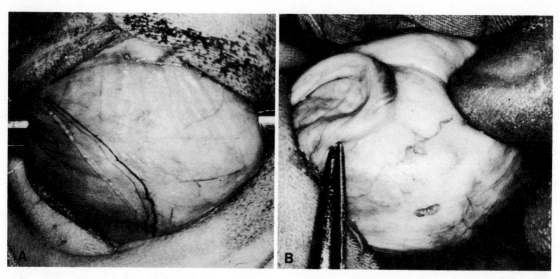

Fig. 24.8 Vasectomy in the bull. (A) The spermatic cord is elevated through the skin incision in the neck of the scrotum. (B) The vas deferens is exposed after incision of the tunica vaginalis reflexa.

Table 24.5 Effect of bilateral vasectomy (at day 0) on semen quality of daily ejaculates in a bull

Semen	Days before and after vasectomy						
	−2	−1	+1	+2	+4	+6	+8
Motility	5+	4+	−1	0	0	0	
Density ($\times 10^6$)	3605	2200	1465	70	10	5	0
Volume (ml)	3.5	1.5	1.5	3.0	1.0	1.5	1.0
Sperm count (%)							
Normal live	86	70	8	0	0	0	
Normal dead	14	20	84	78	92	80	All
Abnormal live				1	4		dead
Abnormal dead				20	4	20	

Teaser bulls are prepared by surgical manipulations of the penis or prepuce to prevent intromission or by vasectomy or by the occlusion of other genital ducts induced by the injection of chemical irritant agents. Surgical procedures include penectomy (Straub and Kendrick, 1965), fixation of the penis to the ventral abdominal wall (Belling, 1961) and partial occlusion of the preputial orifice (Bieberly and Bieberly, 1973), but these techniques prevent protrusion and ejaculation and are thought, for these reasons, to lead to frustration and rapid loss of libido. Moreover the Farm Animal Welfare Council in Britain has indicated that penectomy at least is an unacceptable mutilation. A more sophisticated technique for surgically deviating the prepuce from the ventral midline has been described by Rommel (1961) and Jöchle et al. (1973), but it has not been adopted in Britain.

In Great Britain, vasectomy is still the most widely practised invasive method of preparing teaser bulls. With the reservations that coitus may transmit venereal diseases and that vasectomized animals retain a normal masculine aggressiveness and can lose libido because of overwork, teasers prepared in this way perform satisfactorily for an indefinite period of time. The technique is reviewed by Pearson (1978), with particular emphasis on the possible legal implications of improper surgery. In ruminants, which have a pendulous scrotum, the spermatic cord is exposed through an incision in the scrotal neck and, after splitting of the tunica vaginalis reflexa, the vas deferens is identified as a distinctively dense tubular structure lying in its own separate fold of mesorchium (Figure 24.8). At least 3 cm of the vas is resected between non-absorbable ligatures, and the scrotal skin is sutured after the testis has first been pressed into the scrotum to draw the cord back within the tunica which need not be closed. The prudent clinician will submit the excised tissues for biopsy, perhaps examine ejaculates for sperm quality and certainly ask to be informed immediately if females running with the teaser fail to return to service. The effect of vasectomy on sperm quality is immediate (Table 24.5); in the bull, viable extragonadal sperm reserves can probably be completely exhausted by one or two natural or artificial services, but the ram may continue to ejaculate immotile sperm from ampullary reserves for a considerable period afterwards. Vasectomy is not often requested in the boar, but in this species the vas is approached by an inguinal or scrotal incision.

A non-invasive method of chemical sterilization without loss of libido was described by Pineda et al. (1977), who found that the injection of chlorhexidine in dimethyl sulfoxide into the epididymides of dogs induced long-lasting and probably irreversible azoospermia. The effect of this technique was tested by Pearson et al. (1980) in bulls and rams. Four bulls became aspermic within 2 weeks of the injection into each cauda epididymis of 5 ml of a preparation containing 3% chlorhexidine gluconate in 50% dimethyl sulfoxide in aqueous solution and remained aspermic throughout a trial period of at least 54 weeks. Experimental and clinical trials of the same technique in rams are equally encouraging.

REFERENCES

Anon. (1984) In: *Dairy Herd Fertility*, Reference Book 259, pp. 13, 15, 20. London: HMSO.

Ayalon, N. (1972) *Proc. VIIth Int. Congr. Reprod. Artific. Insem., Munich*, **1**, 741.

Ayalon, N. (1973) *Ann. Rep. Res.*, No. 2, Kimron Veterinary Institute Beit Dagan (Israel).

Ayalon, N. (1978) *J. Reprod. Fertil.*, **54**, 483.

Ball, P. J. H. (1978) *Res. Vet. Sci.*, **25**, 120.

Barrett, G. R., Casida, L. E. and Lloyd, C. A. (1948) *J. Dairy Sci.*, **31**, 682.

Bartlett, P. C., Ngategize, P. K., Kaneene, J. B., Kirk, J. H., Anderson, S. M. and Mather, E. C. (1986) *Prev. Vet. Med.*, **4**, 33.

Bearden, H. J., Hansel, W. and Bratton, R. W. (1956) *J. Dairy Sci.*, **39**, 312.

Belling, T. H. (1961) *J. Amer. Vet. Med. Assn*, **138**, 670.

Bieberly, F. and Bieberly, S. (1973) *Vet. Med. Small Anim. Clin.*, **68**, 1086.

Bishop, M. W. H. (1964) *J. Reprod. Fertil.*, **7**, 383.

Boyd, H. (1965) *Vet. Bull.*, **35**, 251.

Boyd, H. and Reed, H. C. B. (1961) *Brit. Vet. J.*, **117**, 18.

Boyd, H., Bacsich, P., Young, A. and McCracken, J. A. (1969) *Brit. Vet. J.*, **125**, 87.

Bradford, G. (1969) *Genetics*, **61**, 905.

Bulman, D. C. and Lamming, G. E. (1978) *J. Reprod. Fertil.*, **54**, 447.

Christie, W. B., Newcomb, R. and Rowson, L. E. A. (1979) *J. Reprod. Fertil.*, **56**, 701.

Corner, G. W. (1923) *Amer. J. Anat.*, **31**, 523.

De Kruif, A. (1975) *Tijdschr. Diergeneesk*, **100**, 1089.

Diskin, M. G. and Sreenan, J. M. (1986) In: *Embryonic Mortality in Farm Animals*, ed. J. M. Sreenan and M. G. Diskin, pp. 142–158. Dordrecht: Martinus Nijhoff.

Drew, B. (1986) *In Practice*, **8**, 17.

Eddy, R. G. (1980) *In Practice*, **2**, 25.

Eddy, R. G. and Clark, P. J. (1987) *Vet. Rec.*, **120**, 31.

Eddy, R. G., Davies, O. and David, C. (1991) *Vet. Rec.*, **129**, 526.

Erb, R. E., Gaverick, H. A., Randel, R. D., Brown, B. L. and Callahan, C. J. (1976) *Theriogenology*, **5**, 227.

Esslemont, R. J. (1992) *DAISY, The Dairy Information System*, Report No. 1. Reading: University of Reading.

Esslemont, R. J. and Eddy, R. G. (1977) *Brit. Vet. J.*, **133**, 346.

Esslemont, R. J. and Ellis, P. R. (1974) *Vet. Rec.*, **95**, 319.

Esslemont, R. J. and Spincer, I. (1992) *The Prevalence and Costs of Diseases in Dairy Herds.* Report No. 2, The Dairy Information System (DAISY), University of Reading.

Esslemont, R. J., Baillie, J. H. and Cooper, M. J. (1985) *Fertility Management of Dairy Cattle*, pp. 71, 85. London: Collins.

Folman, Y., Rosenberger, M., Herz, Z. and Davidson, M. (1973) *J. Reprod. Fertil.*, **34**, 367.

Gayerie de Abrea, F., Lamming, G. E. and Shaw, R. C. (1984) *Proc. 10th Int. Congr. Anim. Reprod. AI*, **II**, 82.

Gould, C. M. (1974) Cited by Eddy, R. G. (1980) *In Practice*, **2**, 25.

Gustafsson, H., Larsson, K. and Gustavsson, I. (1985) *Acta Vet. Scand.*, **26**, 1.

Hamerton, J. L. (1971) *Human Cytogenetics*, cited by King, W. A. (1985) *Theriogenology*, **23**, 161.

Hanly, S. (1961) *J. Reprod. Fertil.*, **2**, 182.

Hasler, J. F., Bowen, R. A., Nelson, L. D. and Seidel, G. E. (1980) *J. Reprod. Fertil.*, **58**, 71.

Heap, R. B. and Lamming, G. E. (1961) *Proc. IVth Int. Congr. Anim. Reprod. Artif. Insem.*, The Hague, **II**, 300.

Hendricks, D. M., Lamond, D. R., Hill, J. R. and Dickey, J. F. (1971) *J. Anim. Sci.*, **33**, 450.

Hill, J. R., Lamond, D. R., Henricks, D. M., Dickey, J. F. and Niswender, G. D. (1970) *Biol. Reprod.*, **2**, 78.

Holness, D. H., Ellison, J. A. and Wilkins, L. M. (1977) *Rhodesian J. Agr. Res.*, **15**, 3.

Holness, D. H., McCabe, C. T. and Sprowson, G. W. (1982) *Theriogenology*, **17**, 133.

Jöchle, W., Gimenezi, T., Esparza, H. and Hidalgo, M. A. (1973) *Vet. Med. Small Anim. Clin.*, **68**, 395.

Jubb, T. F., Abhayaratne, D., Malmo, J. and Anderson, G. A. (1990) *Aust. Vet. J.*, **67**, 359.

King, W. A. (1985) *Theriogenology*, **23**, 161.

Land, R. B., Atkins, K. D. and Roberts, R. C. (1983) In: *Sheep Production*, ed. W. Havesign, p. 515. London: Butterworth.

Lukaszewska, J. H. and Hansel, W. (1980) *J. Reprod. Fertil.*, **59**, 485.

McFeely, R. A. and Rajakoski, E. (1968) *Proc. Int. Congr. Anim. Reprod. Artif. Insem., Paris*, **II**, 905.

MacMillan, K. L., Taufa, V. K. and Day, A. M. (1986) *Anim. Reprod. Sci.*, **11**, 1.

Newcombe, R. and Rowson, L. E. A. (1975) *J. Reprod. Fertil.*, **43**, 539.

Norton, J. H. and Campbell, R. S. F. (1990) *Vet. Bull.*, **60**, 1137.

Pearson, H. (1978) *Vet. Ann.*, **18**, 80.

Pearson, H., Arthur, G. H., Rosevink, B. and Kakati, B. (1980) *Vet. Rec.*, **107**, 285.

Pineda, M. H., Reimers, J. J., Hopwood, M. L. and Seidel, G. E. (1977) *Amer. J. Vet. Res.*, **38**, 831.

Pope, G. S. and Hodgeson-Jones, L. S. (1975) *Vet. Rec.*, **96**, 154.

Pope, G. S., Gupta, S. K. and Munro, I. B. (1969) *J. Reprod. Fertil.*, **20**, 369.

Pritchard, G. (1993) *Cattle Pract.*, **1**, 115.

Roche, J. F., Ireland, J. J., Boland, M. P. and McGeady, T. M. (1985) *Vet. Rec.*, **116**, 153.

Rommel, W. (1961) *Mh. Vet. Med.*, **16**, 19.

Rowson, L. E. A., Moor, R. M. and Lawson, R. A. S. (1969) *J. Reprod. Fertil.*, **18**, 517.

Rowson, L. E. A., Lawson, R. A. S., Moor, R. H. and Baker, A. A. (1972) *J. Reprod. Fertil.*, **28**, 427.

Santos-Valadez, S. de, Seidel, G. E. and Elsden, R. P. (1982) *Theriogenology*, **17**, 85.

Shemesh, M., Ayalon, N. and Lindner, H. R. (1968) *J. Reprod. Fertil.*, **15**, 161.

Shemesh, M., Ayalon, N., Lavi, S., Mileguir, S., Shore, L. S. and Toby, D. A. (1983) *Brit. Vet. J.*, **139**, 41.

Simpson, J. L. (1980) *Fertil. Steril.*, **33**, 107.

Spitzer, J. C., Niswender, G. D., Seidel, G. E. and Wiltbank, J. N. (1978) *J. Anim. Sci.*, **46**, 1071.

Sreenan, J. M. and Diskin, M. G. (1983) *Vet. Rec.*, **112**, 517.

Sreenan, J. M. and Diskin, M. G. (1986) In: *Embryonic Mortality in Farm Animals*, ed. J. M. Sreenan and M. G. Diskin, pp. 1–11. Dordrecht: Martinus Nijhoff.

Stott, G. H. and Williams, R. J. (1962) *J. Dairy Sci.*, **45**, 1.

Straub, O. C. and Kendrick, J. W. (1965) *J. Amer. Vet. Med. Assn*, **147**, 373.

Studer, E. and Morrow, D. A. (1978) *J. Amer. Vet. Med. Assn*, **172**, 489.

Tanabe, T. Y. and Almquist, J. O. (1953) *J. Dairy Sci.*, **36**, 586.

Tanabe, T. Y. and Casida, L. E. (1949) *J. Dairy Sci.*, **32**, 237.

Wiersma, F. and Stott, G. H. (1969) *Trans. Amer. Soc. Agr. Eng.*, **12**, 130.

Williamson, N. B., Quinton, F. W. and Anderson, G. A. (1980) *Aust. Vet. J.*, **56**, 477.

Wilmut, I., Sales, D. I. and Ashworth, C. J. (1985) *Theriogenology*, **23**, 107.

SHEEP

The level of fertility in sheep is usually expressed as the reproductive performance of the flock. This can be defined as the number of lambs weaned per ewe per year. Three factors will influence the reproductive performance: (1) the fertility, which is whether the ewes are pregnant and lamb; the reciprocal of the number of barren ewes in the flock; (2) the fecundity, which is the number of lambs born per pregnancy; (3) the survival rate, which is the number of lambs that survive to weaning.

The information that is available on the reproductive performance of sheep generally comes from studies on lowland flocks. Figures published by the Meat and Livestock Commission (MLC), involving over 400 flocks over 5 years, quote 6% barren ewes. Other studies carried out in the 1960s and 1970s in the UK quote similar figures of 6–7%. Average figures for ewe productivity in lowland and upland flocks in 1994 have been published by the MLC. For 217 lowland flocks the percentages of lambs born, born live and weaned were 170, 160 and 152 respectively. For 128 upland flocks, the values were 153, 146 and 121%. In both lowland and upland flocks there were 5% barren ewes. In a detailed study of 5488 ewes in 34 flocks involving 10 pure breeds or crosses, Smith (1991) found that of the 348 ewes that suffered true reproductive losses 52.9% were barren and 37.6% aborted. Before the advent of accurate and inexpensive methods of pregnancy diagnosis, especially B-mode ultrasound (see Chapter 3), barren ewes were frequently not identified until they had failed to lamb when anticipated. Barren ewes are usually culled and as a consequence there is some genetic selection against poor fertility. Fecundity is influenced by genetic selection, age of the ewe, nutritional status and environment. It has been estimated that the number of lambs born per ewe per year can be increased by between 0.01 and 0.02 by genetic selection. The survival rate will be influenced mainly by management factors and the environment but also by genetic selection for such traits as good mothering behaviour.

The better level of fertility of sheep compared with cattle is a reflection of the more natural breeding environment that the former are subject to. Ewes are generally allowed to run with the ram during the breeding season and not segregated, thus oestrus detection problems are not encountered. Furthermore, most breeds of sheep have a longer period of acyclicity after parturition than the cow, thus allowing the reproductive system time to recover from the effects of pregnancy. The fertility of ewes, as measured by pregnancy (conception) rates to first service was 91.6% (Smith, 1991). In the same study, 99.4% had conceived by the third mating. Poorer results are generally obtained using artificial insemination, although the use of intrauterine insemination by laparoscopy has been much more successful with pregnancy rates of over 70%, using fresh extended semen (Gourley and Riese, 1990). The main factors responsible for infertility in sheep are specific infectious agents that usually result in abortion; not surprisingly, much veterinary research into sheep reproduction concentrates on these problems. Structural, functional and managemental factors are of limited importance.

Structural defects

Structural defects of the genital organs are uncommon in sheep. In an abattoir survey of 2081 sheep genitalia, Emady et al. (1975) found 0.72% with macroscopic abnormalities. In a more recent and extensive survey, involving 33 506 bovine genital tracts (9970 parous) examined at two abattoirs in the West Country (UK), Smith (1993) identified 6.57% of parous and 1.95% of nulliparous tracts with pathological lesions. Most involved the ovaries and its associated bursa with fibrin tags, and paraovarian cysts being most frequently identified. However, it is unlikely that these lesions alone would have caused infertility (and hence culling). There is no doubt that many of the other lesions identified in this survey would have caused infertility or sterility. Owing to the rarity of anastomosis of the adjacent allantoic vessels of twins, the freemartin condition is likely to be rare but incidences of 0.23–1.22% have been recorded (Dain, 1971; Long, 1980; Smith, 1993). Cases of intersexuality are seen, mainly at the time of lamb castration; they are male pseudohermaphrodites and are referred to by shepherds as 'wilgils'. The fact that several may be seen at once in a flock tends to point to a hereditary cause. Occlusion of the uterine tubes and hydrosalpinx is an occasional cause of ovine infertility. Other developmental defects of the genital organs of sheep are rare, although there is good evidence of an association between ovarian hypoplasia and breeds with high fecundity (Smith and Vaughan, personal communication).

Functional factors

Except in the case of unthrifty ewes (which are usually culled) anoestrus is uncommon in sheep; Smith (1991) identified the condition in 0.3% of 5488 lowland ewes. In fact, when the rams are turned out with the flock it is usual for most of the ewes to be mated within a month. The first heats of the breeding season of some ewes are not accompanied by ovulation and, according to Dutt (1954), ewes more frequently fail to become fertilized at early than at later matings. Apart from anovulation, the cause of this poor fertility is not known. Ovarian cysts, which are commonly encountered in cattle (see Chapter 22) are of limited importance in sheep. Smith (1993) identified follicular cysts in 2.9 and 10.02% of abnormal parous and nulliparous genital tracts, respectively. Luteal cysts were rare.

It is possible that a greater degree of embryonic death follows early matings. It is certain that embryonic death, or resorption, is a conspicuous feature of sheep infertility and by comparing the number of corpora lutea with the number of fetuses the incidence of the condition has been estimated to be between 8 and 13% (Hammond, 1921; Winters and Feuffel, 1936; Arthur, 1956).

Such pathological reproduction is more often associated with multiple than with single conception.

Early embryonic death has been associated with infectious diseases such as toxoplasmosis and Border disease (see below). In a survey by Johnston (1988), 35.2% of barren ewes had elevated antibody titres to *Toxoplasma* compared with 19.2% of fertile ewes.

Sporadic cases of obvious abortion and of fetal mummificaton are occasionally seen. A specific environmental cause of sheep infertility due to grazing on pastures of subterranean clover was described by Bennetts et al. (1946) in Australia. This clover contains large amounts of oestrogenic substance (genistein) the ingestion of which leads to cystic degeneration of the endometrium and permanent sterility. Although oestrogenic substances in small amounts have been identified in other plants, no comparable degree of infertility due to such substances has been seen outside Australia.

Asynchrony or imbalance of the hormonal changes that occur around the time of oestrus and during the early luteal phase probably results in embryonic death. In an experimental study involving ovariectomized ewes as recipients for sheep embryos, a rigid regimen of steroid hormone replacement is necessary to ensure embryo survival (Wilmut et al., 1985). The sequence is: (1) progesterone supplementation to simulate the previous luteal phase; (2) oestradiol to simulate oestrus; (3) low levels of progesterone supplementation to simulate early dioestrus, followed by (4) high levels of progesterone to simulate the normal luteal phase.

Management factors

Oestrus detection and artificial insemination

Artificial insemination in sheep has not assumed the popularity achieved in cattle. A number of factors has been responsible, notably the disappointing results using frozen/thawed semen deposited intracervically. Much better results (pregnancy rates of up to 65%) have been achieved following intrauterine insemination with frozen/thawed semen using a laparoscope and local anaesthesia (see pp. 645–647).

Oestrus is best detected with a raddled vasectomized ram or the examination of the appearance of the vaginal mucus. Artificial insemination is best used in midoestrus or 12–14 hours after onset.

Teasing

The introduction of vasectomized teasers into the flock, before fertile rams, had no effect on pregnancy (conception) rates (Smith, 1991). However, in his study, they had a profound effect upon the onset of cyclical activity and hence a compact lambing season. Of teased ewes, 84.8% exhibited oestrus in the first 16 days after exposure to the fertile ram. Two 16 day cycles were required for the unteased ewes to show comparable activity. The author of this study also demonstrated the necessity of adequately isolating ewes and rams before teasing.

Ram:ewe ratio

The number of rams per ewe will vary and will depend upon a number of factors: (1) the age of the ram; (2) the age of the ewes; (3) whether more than one ram is to be used with the group of ewes; (4) the terrain and size of the enclosure; (5) the weather. Ram:ewe ratios of 1:25 to 1:40 are suitable in non-synchronized flocks; however, where synchronization is attempted a ratio of at least 1:10 should be available.

Nutrition

It is important that ewes should be in good bodily condition at tupping time. Increasing the energy intake several weeks before tupping so that the ewes are gaining weight (flushing) will increase the fecundity in those ewes with the genetic potential and, provided the level of feeding is maintained for a month after mating, should ensure good pregnancy rates. Some reduction in food intake is reasonable during the second and third months of gestation but feeding should be increased in the last 6–8 weeks before lambing.

Increasing fecundity

Increased ovulation rates can be achieved by the administration of equine chorionic gonadotrophin (eCG) on the 12th or 13th day of the oestrous cycle. Good results have been obtained by immunization against androstenedione.

Infectious agents

Non-specific infections of the genital tract, especially the uterus, are of minimal importance in ewes, probably because in most breeds of sheep there is a long period of anoestrus following lambing. Bacteria that enter the uterus at the time of parturition are eliminated before the genital tract can be exposed to a period of progesterone influence, which will occur during dioestrus. However, there are a number of specific infectious agents that can have a profound effect upon fertility, particularly by causing abortion and perinatal mortality.

Table 25.1 Percentage frequency of isolation of pathogens from ovine fetopathies examined by Ministry of Agriculture Veterinary Investigation Centres (source: VIDA–II)

	1977	1984	1985	1986	1987	1988	1989	1990	1991	1992
Brucella abortus	0	0	0	0	0	0.02	0	0	0	NR
Actinomyces (Corynebacterium) pyogenes	0.5	1.6	1.3	1.9	1.5	1.0	0.8	0.8	1.2	1.1
Campylobacter spp.	13.2	14.3	9.0	8.8	7.2	7.3	6.9	9.1	8.6	6.7
Chlamydia	32.2	39.5	43.4	41.3	45.2	40.1	41.9	43.8	41.0	46.9
Listeria monocytogenes	0.7	2.1	1.9	3.0	2.6	2.6	3.2	2.9	2.6	3.0
Salmonella abortus ovis	0.5	0.1	0.1	0.1	0.1	0.07	0.05	0.1	0.3	NR
Salmonella dublin	1.7	0.3	0.3	0.4	0.6	0.6	0.6	0.3	0.1	0.4
Salmonella typhimurium	0	0.3	0.6	0.4	0.3	0.1	0.1	0.2	0.3	0.2
Other Salmonella serotypes	2.2	1.8	1.9	1.5	2.6	1.7	1.3	2.2	3.1	1.2
Toxoplasma spp.	36.2	31.3	34.7	34.6	32.0	40.3	38.4	35.3	37.4	35.4
Coxiella burnetii	NR	0.1	0.04	0	0.2	0.05	0.03	0.3	0.1	0.2
Fungi	0.7	0.1	0.08	0.1	0.1	0.3	0.4	0.05	0.2	0.2
Other pathogens	12.0	8.4	6.5	8.0	7.6	5.9	6.3	4.8	5.2	4.7
Total identified	583	2419	2667	2685	3214	4116	3774	3749	2940	2529
Total submitted	1349	4790	5288	4984	6081	7292	6712	6325	5006	4184
Percentage diagnosed	43.2	50.5	50.4	53.9	52.9	56.4	56.2	59.3	58.7	60.4

NR, not recorded.

Figures collected by the Ministry of Agriculture, Fisheries and Food Veterinary Investigation Service listing the infectious causes of fetopathy identified in material submitted to their laboratories for 1977 and from 1984 to 1992 are summarized in Table 25.1. In comparison with figures published for bovine fetopathies (see p. 397) it is noticeable the greater percentage of cases where an infectious agent is identified, namely over 22.0%.

Ovine vibriosis (Campylobacter fetus infection)

This disease caused by *C. fetus*, subsp. *intestinalis* and subsp. *jejuni*, is a common cause of abortion in Great Britain and throughout the sheep-raising areas of the world. Unlike bovine vibriosis the disease is not transmitted venereally.

Clinical Signs. The only clinical signs of the disease are abortion in late gestation, usually the last 6 weeks, or stillbirth or the birth of weakly lambs at term. Ewes rarely show any other clinical signs apart from some vulval swelling and the presence of a reddish-coloured vulval discharge in some animals. Metritis may develop after abortion so that some ewes may become ill and even die. The subspecies *jejuni* can cause diarrhoea in lambs.

Diagnosis. When there is abortion in late gestation campylobacter infection must be suspected. There are signs of placentitis with oedema and necrosis of the fetal cotyledons, although these are not pathognomonic; the aborted fetus looks fresh. In some fetuses there is subcutaneous oedema and blood-stained serum in the body cavities. The most characteristic fetal lesion is the presence of pale necrotic foci 0.5–2.0 cm in diameter (Plate 4) randomly distributed throughout the liver with a raised periphery and depressed centre (Dennis, 1991).

The organism can be identified in Gram- or modified Ziehl–Neelsen-stained smears of the placenta, fetal liver and fetal stomach contents, or by culture. Isolation of the organism from vaginal discharges of the ewe is not very helpful and serological tests are of little value.

It is important to stress that *C. fetus* can be isolated in association with abortions due to *Toxoplasma gondii* and *Chlamydia psittaci* (see below).

Transmission and Pathogenesis. The disease is transmitted following ingestion of the organism, particularly following the introduction of chronically infected carriers into the flock which excrete

C. fetus in their faeces. It is a particular problem of intensively housed flocks. It can also be transmitted by carrion birds such as magpies and crows that eat infected abortuses on one farm and then feed from food troughs on a clean farm. Once abortions occur, there is lateral spread within the flock to other susceptible pregnant ewes. The organism survives well in cold moist conditions but soon perishes in hot, dry weather.

Experimental infection of ewes that are less than 3 months pregnant does not cause abortion; the incubation period is 7–25 days.

Treatment and Control. As soon as vibriosis is suspected, precautionary sanitary measures should be implemented. Aborting ewes should be isolated from pregnant ewes and, where there is a possibility of extensive lateral spread of infection, pregnant ewes shuld be treated with intramuscular injections of 300 000 IU of penicillin and 1 g of dihydrostreptomycin on two consecutive days.

In a natural outbreak of the disease, an average of 15–20% of pregnant ewes will either abort, produce stillborn lambs or weakly lambs. There is no associated infertility due to fertilization failure or embryonic death. In the second year, there is a dramatic fall in the number of abortions to about 2–3%. Thus, most ewes from an infected flock acquire an immunity in the first year irrespective of whether or not they aborted. This acquired immunity lasts for about 3 years, which, in most circumstances, will be equal to the expected breeding life of the individual. For this reason it is sensible to retain all of the ewes within a flock although the infection will remain. Therefore, newly purchased ewes can be exposed to the infection and hence should be mixed with the infected animals before tupping and up to mid-gestation, but they should be separated in late pregnancy.

In the USA a formalin-killed adjuvant vaccine incorporating the most prevalent serotypes, I and V, has been used. Two injections, 15–30 days apart, are given either before the breeding season or during the first half of pregnancy. The immunity will last for about 3 years but each annual batch of replacement ewes must be vaccinated. There is some evidence that, in the early stages of an outbreak of vibriosis in a flock, vaccination of all remaining pregnant ewes might be worthwhile. Since there is a 10–14 day delay before immunity develops after vaccination, early diagnosis is imperative. No such vaccine is available at present in the UK.

Salmonellosis

Salmonella abortus ovis is a cause of enzootic abortion in sheep in Britain and Europe. Its relative importance has declined and in Britain it is largely restricted to Devon and Cornwall. Other salmonella species, such as *S. dublin*, *S. typhimurium* and *S. montevideo*, cause occasional abortion in sheep and are world-wide in their distribution. The latter organism is now a significant cause of reproductive failure in some parts of Britain.

Clinical Signs. These vary depending on the species of salmonella. In the case of *S. abortus ovis* and *S. montevideo* the predominant sign is abortion in the last 6 weeks of gestation with occasionally a mild transitory pyrexia and temporary inappetance which frequently goes unnoticed. Some ewes develop a severe postpartum metritis. Diarrhoea is not a feature in those lambs that are born alive. (Linklater, 1983). With *S. dublin* and *S. typhimurium* the ewes are typically very ill with pyrexia, inappetance, severe diarrhoea and sometimes death. Where lambs are born alive they also show signs of severe illness with diarrhoea and a high mortality rate up to about 1 month of age.

Diagnosis. Diagnosis is usually fairly straightforward with the identification of the organism following culture of fetal stomach contents, placental tissue or vaginal discharges. In addition, fluorescent antibody techniques are also used for the rapid diagnosis of the organisms in the same tissues. Serological tests can be used to diagnose infection with *S. abortus ovis*.

Transmission and Pathogenesis. *S. abortus ovis* is host-specific and is usually introduced into a flock by an infected sheep; however, the other species of salmonella are not host-specific and can be introduced into the flock through contaminated food or water, by wild birds such as seagulls, or by other infected livestock. Once the disease has become established it will be readily spread laterally within the flock by ingestion of contaminated food or water. There is always a danger with salmonella infections that symptomless carriers may remain in the flock, providing a persistent reservoir of infection. There is some suggestion that *S. abortus ovis* may be spread by infected rams at coitus although it is more likely that the infected ram will shed the organism in the faeces.

After experimental infection of ewes with *S. abortus ovis*, abortion occurs 6–25 days later and the organism may continue to be excreted from the vagina for at least 18 days after abortion. Infection causes a fetal bacteraemia, placentitis, followed by fetal death and abortion.

S. montevideo appears to have a predilection for sheep and could become established in the sheep population of the UK (Linklater, 1983). It has been isolated from mesenteric lymph nodes of sheep slaughtered at abattoirs all the year around, and thus the carry-over of infection from year to year occurs in the sheep themselves.

Treatment and Control. In an attempt to reduce lateral spread within a flock at the beginning of an abortion outbreak, good hygiene with isolation of potentially infected animals should be practised.

In natural outbreaks of abortion due to *S. abortus ovis* 15–25% of ewes may abort in the last 6 weeks of gestation. However, ewes that have aborted become immune so that in subsequent years the problem is largely confined to ewe lambs or new additions to the flock. For this reason the customary mixing of non-immune non-pregnant female with aborting ewes can result in their acquiring an active immunity. Vaccines have been developed and are used in some countries, whilst some protection has been achieved by using a vaccine against *S. cholera suis*. Chemotherapeutic substances such as chloramphenicol, furazolidone and trimethoprim have been used to control salmonellosis once it has been introduced into the flock.

A number of general principles have been suggested for the control of *S. montevideo* which are applicable to other salmonella species (Linklater, 1983):

1. Turn over troughs to prevent faecal contamination from birds.
2. Move the feeding areas frequently to prevent the build up of infection; this is particularly true in severe weather.
3. Do not feed off the ground.
4. Try to avoid having sheep drinking out of streams and open ditches by using piped fresh water.
5. If abortions occur, isolate ewes.
6. Reduce stresses on the flock such as frequent moving and disruption.

It is important to stress that *Salmonella* spp. other than *S. abortus ovis* are zoonoses and hence care should be exercised when dealing with affected material.

Chlamydial (enzootic) abortion

For many years, in Scotland and the English border counties shepherds and veterinarians have been familiar with an enzootic abortion in flocks, the causal organism being identified by Stamp et al. (1950). The disease is now known to be widespread in Britain, where it is the most frequently identified infectious cause of abortion in sheep (see Table 25.1), Europe and the western USA. The organism, now called *Chlamydia psittaci (ovis)*, has a highly specialized life-cycle which involves alternate intra- and extracellular phases which confer advantages for evasion of host immune responses and facilitates the maintenance of low-grade asymptomatic infection (Aitken, 1986). Although the organism has a predilection for the placenta during pregnancy, it can also cause pneumonia and polyarthritis.

Clinical Signs. The ewes show no signs of systemic illness, the first indication normally being abortion in the last 3 weeks of gestation; a few ewes may show evidence of a vaginal discharge for several days beforehand. A small number of ewes will abort in the first third of gestation but this usually passes unnoticed; some lambs are carried to term and are stillborn or weakly.

The placenta shows typical signs of a placentitis which gives a gross appearance that is similar to that following *Brucella abortus* infection in cattle (see p. 401). The intercotyledonary allantochorion is oedematous or thickened and leathery in appearance; there is degeneration and necrosis of the fetal cotyledons and a thick yellow deposit on the chorion. The essential lesion is a subacute chorionitis (Plate 5).

The aborted lambs are in most cases fresh, although occasionally some will undergo mummification and maceration. There are no characteristic lesions but the abdominal cavity is sometimes distended with blood-stained fluid. A small number of ewes may develop a post-abortion metritis (Aitken, 1986).

Diagnosis. The necrotic changes that occur in the cotyledons in ewes that are aborting close to term is fairly indicative of *C. psittaci* infection, although it must be differentiated from abortion due to *Toxoplasma gondii* (see below). It is also important to stress that abortion problems in some flocks may be due to more than one organism.

Confirmation of the diagnosis requires microscopical examination of Ziehl–Neelson-stained smears made from the affected parts of the placenta. If no placental tissue is available, stained smears obtained from vaginal discharges within 24 hours of abortion can be useful (Aitken, 1986). The stained organism *C. psittaci* can be confused with *Coxiella burnetii*, which causes Q fever and is occasionally a cause of abortion in sheep (see below). Isolation of the organism requires that a small piece of affected cotyledon or fresh vaginal swabs should be placed in a suitable transport medium and sent to the laboratory for culture (Aitken, 1986).

The disease can be confirmed, retrospectively if necessary, serologically using the complement fixation test, an enzyme-linked immunosorbent assay (ELISA) or indirect immunofluorescent antibody test. Paired samples should be taken at the time of abortion and 2–3 weeks later, which, in aborting ewes, should show a significant rise in antibody titres. Vaccinated ewes will have lower titres with no evidence of a rise.

Transmission and Pathogenesis. In a flock infected for the first time up to one-third of the ewes may be affected; however, when endemic, the numbers affected will be between 5 and 10%.

The disease is usually brought into an unaffected flock by infected, newly purchased ewes suffering from asymptomatic enteric infection. These ewes may abort and, as a consequence, cause lateral spread within the flock following ingestion of food and pasture contaminated with vaginal discharges and placental material. Ewe lambs can be infected at birth or at a later age and, when they become pregnant, they may abort and disseminate the infection in vaginal discharges and placenta. Since *C. psittaci* is a common parasite of a wide range of animals, interspecies transmission is a possibility.

C. psittaci has also been isolated from the epididymis, testis and Cowper's glands of two rams (Rodalakis and Barnard, 1977); it may be possible for the disease to be transmitted venereally.

Treatment and Control. As with all cases of abortion, good hygiene is important so that dangers of lateral spread of infection can be reduced; thus, ewes that are aborting or have aborted should be isolated from the rest of the flock for about 3 weeks until vaginal discharges have ceased. These ewes should not be used as foster mothers and should be separated from ewe lambs (note that this is a totally different recommendation compared with ovine vibriosis and toxoplasmosis). Although ewes that have aborted are ususaly immune, it must be remembered that they are likely to become asymptomatic carriers of the organism; thus in flocks where small numbers of ewes are infected it may be preferable to cull these animals.

Ewes purchased as replacements should be free from the disease; however the existing serological tests are not always sensitive enough to detect carrier animals. A delayed hypersensitivity skin test may become a feasible method of diagnosis (Aitken, 1986).

A formalin-inactivated vaccine, recently modified with current commonly isolated strains of *C. psittaci*, has been shown to prevent abortion without eliminating infection. It provides an immunity which lasts about 3 years. It should be used on all breeding ewes in the late summer just before tupping, and thereafter on new and replacement animals brought into the flock. It can be used during an outbreak of abortion where there are ewes that are at risk and are more than 8 weeks from term. This will provide sufficient time for them to develop an immunity and thus prevent abortion.

Another procedure that can be used in flocks with an extended lambing season, to reduce rather than eliminate abortions, is the use of antibiotics. Although infection may be acquired at any stage of pregnancy the placenta is particularly receptive to chlamydia at 80–110 days. Thus ewes exposed to infection when 3–4 months pregnant are particularly at risk and are liable to abort 5–6 weeks later. Long-acting oxytetracycline, at a dose of 20 mg/kg repeated every 10–14 days until lambing, has been used, although it is expensive (Aitken, 1986).

It is important to stress that *C. psittaci* is a zoonosis causing flu-like symptoms and abortion in pregnant women. For this reason, protective disposable gloves should be used and good hygiene employed. Pregnant women should avoid contact with lambing ewes.

Toxoplasmosis

Toxoplasmosis has a world-wide distribution in domestic animals and humans. Infection with

Toxoplasma gondii has been shown to cause abortion, stillbirths and weakly offspring in many domestic species including sheep. Table 25.1 shows that in the years listed it was isolated from about one third of the fetopathies investigated by the Ministry of Agriculture Veterinary Investigation Services. Toxoplasmosis in non-pregnant sheep is typically mild and inapparent (Blewett and Watson, 1983) but in pregnant ewes it is essentially a disease of the conceptus, and in sheep the seasonal breeding pattern results in large numbers of susceptible animals being present together at the same time.

The causal organism is a protozoon, *T. gondii*; it has a complex life cycle which involves an asexual cyle which can occur in any species of mammal or bird, and a sexual cycle which can only be completed in cats and wild Felidae. In the cat family, the parasite multiplies within the epithelial cells of the intestine and, as a consequence, oocysts will be excreted in the faeces. This can continue for about 8 days during which time tens of thousands of oocysts can be shed. These sporulate within a few days and are then ingested by sheep. (Frenkel, 1973).

Clinical Signs. The effect upon reproduction is dependent upon the stage of pregnancy when infection occurs. If it occurs early in gestation, i.e. before 60–70 days, there is usually fetal resorption with ewes returning to oestrus or remaining barren. Infection in mid-gestation will result in abortion or mummification; sometimes in the case of the latter, one member of a set of twins or triplets will be involved. Infection in late gestation, after 120 days, will usually result in stillbirth, weakly or normal lambs. The ewes show no signs of illness apart from rare neurological signs. The gross appearance of the placenta, particularly the cotyledons, is fairly typical of the disease. The cotyledons are bright to dark-red in colour with multiple small white nodules 1–3 mm in diameter. These nodules may be sparse or so numerous that they become confluent; sometimes normal cotyledons are present whilst the intercotyledonary areas of the allantochorion appear normal (Plate 6) (unlike infection with *C. psittaci*).

Diagnosis. The history and clinical signs, especially the appearance of the placenta, is suggestive of the disease. Confirmation can sometimes be made using Giemsa- or Leishmann-stained smears of the cotyledons containing the white nodules; alternatively histological sections of the cotyledons may be required to demonstrate the presence of the parasite. Examination of the brain, especially in those lambs that die soon after birth, may reveal foci of glial cells and leuco-encephalomalacia which are characteristic of the infection (Buxton et al., 1981a). Immunofluorescent staining of cotyledon sections can also be used.

The organism can best be isolated using mouse inoculation techniques; these are described in detail elsewhere (Buxton, 1983).

A number of satisfactory serological tests on the maternal serum have been used including the dye test of Sabin and Feldman, the indirect fluorescent antibody (IFA) test, radioimmunoassay and the ELISA test (Buxton, 1983); the last test has been modified to detect anti-toxoplasma immunoglobulin G (IgG) (Buxton et al., 1988) in body fluids (Buxton, 1983). The indirect haemagglutination test (IHA) has been developed so that kits are available for use by veterinarians in practice laboratories. A single serum sample with an elevated titre may well only indicate past infection; for this reason paired serum samples at 14 day intervals which show a rising titre are indicative of an active infection.

Serological diagnosis in newborn lambs is preferably done on precolostral serum or cerebrospinal fluid. If postcolostral samples only are available it is necessary to demonstrate IgM and IgG antibody (Buxton, 1983).

Transmission and Pathogenesis. Although toxoplasmas have been demonstrated in the semen of experimentally infected rams (Spence et al., 1978) and naturally infected rams, infection of the ewe at tupping would be unlikely to cause abortion. Similarly, lateral spread within a flock from aborting ewes is likely to be relatively unimportant. However, lambs that are born alive and survive from infected ewes can be congenitally infected.

Without doubt, the principal vector in the spread of toxoplasmosis is the cat and its related wild species which excrete oocysts in their faeces, and as a consequence, contaminate pasture, forage and other foodstuffs. Passive spread of oocysts by birds, flies and other insects can occur, whilst wild rodents, especially mice, remain the main source of infection for the cat.

Treatment and Control. It is possible to treat ewes during the acute phase of the disease with sulfonamides and potentiated sulfonamides such as trimethoprim, but it is expensive. A recent study has demonstrated the efficacy of a combination of sulfamethazine and pyrimethamine, which is used to treat the disease in humans (Buxton et al., 1993).

Although there is virtually no danger of lateral spread from aborting ewes, isolation in the early stages of an abortion outbreak should have been implemented before a firm diagnosis would have been made. Since there is a possibility that other infectious agents may be present there is no harm in maintaining an isolation policy.

The main thrust of any control measure is dependent upon the fact that ewes that have aborted will be immune and should be retained in the flock. New additions should be exposed to possible infection with oocysts from contaminated food as early as possible before the start of the breeding season.

Recently, an effective vaccine has been developed using living tachyzoites of the S48 strain of *T. gondii* (O'Connell et al., 1988; Buxton et al., 1991). Ewe lambs should be vaccinated from 5 months of age while ewes and shearlings should be vaccinated during the 4 month period prior to tupping; pregnant animals must not be vaccinated. Recent studies have shown that the degree of protection produced by the S48 tachyzoites was as good at 18 months as 6 months after vaccination.

It is advisable to control the numbers of feral cats that have access to farm buildings and to control vigorously the vermin (especially mice) that are the main source of infection for the cats. Where possible, foodstuffs should be protected from possible faecal contamination by cats, although this can be very difficult to ensure. *T. gondii* is a zoonosis and thus potentially contaminated material should be handled with care. There is evidence that sheep infected with *T. gondii* are less responsive to vaccination procedures due to an apparent immunosuppressive effect of the parasite (Buxton et al., 1981a).

Listeriosis

Listeriosis due to *Listeria monocytogenes* has a worldwide distribution in several domestic species, especially ruminants (see p. 411), and in humans. Infection in sheep causes encephalitis, abortion and septicaemia although, whilst there has been some increase in prevalence of the disease in recent years (see Table 25.1), it is rare for the nervous disease and abortions to occur together.

Clinical Signs. The neurological signs characteristic of listerial encephalitis are of circling with evidence of unilateral facial paralysis with tilting and turning of the head.

Abortions due to *L. monocytogenes* generally occur in late gestation, and there is frequently a heavy brown vaginal discharge (Low and Linklater, 1985). Death of the ewe may follow due to metritis and septicaemia.

The gross appearance of the aborted lambs and the placenta, although not pathognomonic of the infection, is nevertheless a useful indicator of possible infection with *L. monocytogenes*. The aborted lambs frequently show small grey or yellow areas of focal necrosis of the liver and oedema and congestion of the meninges. The placental villi are necrotic and the chorion is covered with a brownish-red exudate.

Diagnosis. This is based upon isolation in culture of *L. monocytogenes* from the fetal stomach, liver or the placenta; but this may require repeated subculture from refrigerated material (see p. 412). Smith et al. (1968) have used fluorescent antibody techniques, whilst inoculation of mice with necrotic liver, and keratitis in rabbits are additional tests.

Transmission and Pathogenesis. *L. monocytogenes* is a ubiquitous organism frequently found in soil but also isolated from feedstuffs and faeces of healthy animals. Whilst pasture contamination with human sewage is probably quite important in the spread of the disease, the most likely source of infection is soil, especially following the feeding of soil-contaminated silage where poor fermentation has occurred.

Sheep are probably frequently exposed to infection but presumably it requires some other factors to precipitate clinical listeriosis. Following ingestion in late pregnancy, the organism penetrates the gut mucosa and infects the fetus causing a septicaemia and placentitis, both of which kill the fetal lamb. As a consequence abortion occurs.

Treatment and Control. Aborting ewes should be isolated to reduce the possibility of the lateral spread of infection. If silage is being fed it should be withheld pending confirmation of the causal agent. A variety of antibiotics, chloramphenicol, tetracyclines and penicillin, are effective *in vitro*,

however there is little documented evidence of the value of such therapy to prevent abortions occurring.

No vaccines are available at present, so prevention is dependent upon a number of management procedures involving silage feeding to sheep (Low and Linklater, 1985). These are: (1) do not use soil-contaminated grass for silage; (2) use additives to reduce the pH of the silage; (3) do not feed obviously mouldy silage; (4) do not feed silage to sheep if the pH exceeds 5, or the ash content exceeds 70 mg/kg dry matter; (5) empty uneaten silage from the feed trough after 24 hours.

Brucellosis

Sheep can be infected with both *Brucella melitensis* and *B. ovis*. The former infection is endemic in many Mediterranean countries, Africa and Central America; it does not occur in Great Britain. The latter infection has been reported in parts of Europe, South Africa, western states of the USA, New Zealand and Australia.

B. melitensis, which affects many species, including humans, causes abortions in late pregnancy, stillbirths or weak lambs. The placental lesions are similar to those identified in cattle with *B. abortus* infection, notably a placentitis with oedematous and necrotic cotyledons with the intercotyledonary parts of the chorion being thickened and leathery in appearance. The disease is diagnosed by direct examination or culture of placental smears, fetal stomach contents or vaginal discharges; serological tests such as the complement fixation test are used. The disease can be controlled by using *B. melitensis* or *B. abortus* S19 vaccines.

B. ovis is host-specific. Its main effect on sheep breeding is its effect upon the ram, where it causes an epididymitis and subsequent infertility or sterility. The organism causes placentitis followed by abortion in ewes in late gestation; however, according to Hartley et al. (1954), the incidence of abortion is usually low, i.e. 7–10% of ewes. Whilst a ram can be infected after serving a ewe that has been previously served by an infected ram, ewes themselves are not infected venereally. The method of infection of ewes is not fully understood.

Border disease (Hypomyelinosis congenita)

This disease was first recognized in flocks along the English–Welsh border in the 1950s (Hughes et al., 1959) affecting newborn lambs which showed neurological symptoms such as tremor and a coarse fleece and which were generally weakly with a high mortality rate. Since then it has been recognized in many other places in the UK (Barlow and Dickinson, 1965; Acland et al., 1972; Sweasey et al., 1979). It has now been shown to cause reproductive failure.

The disease is due to infection with a pestivirus similar to that which causes bovine viral diarrhoea (BVD) in cattle (see p. 412) and European swine fever.

Clinical Signs. The clinical signs in lambs are well documented elsewhere (Barlow and Gardiner, 1983). In adult ewes infection results in a mild pyrexia which would probably go undiagnosed. However, if ewes are pregnant the virus will affect the fetus causing fetal death with mummification, abortion or, if early on in fetal life, death with resorption, and the birth of weakly affected lambs. Abortion can occur at any stage of gestation although it is most common around 90 days of gestation with the voiding of a brown, mummified, or swollen anasarcous fetus (Barlow and Gardiner, 1983). The conceptus is most susceptible to experimental infection between 16 and 80 days of gestation; hence, at an early stage, the only clinical sign will be barrenness.

Diagnosis. This can be made on clinical signs in lambs, supported by histopathological examination of the brain and spinal cord and of virus isolation from the lamb or fluorescent antibody staining technique. Serological tests on ewes which abort, or are barren, have to be examined in relation to antibody levels in other ewes in the flock.

Transmission. The most likely source of infection is from ewe lambs, which have recovered from border disease, being introduced into the flock. These individuals remain chronic excretors of the virus for a long period of time and yet appear healthy; although likely to have reduced fertility, they can give birth to infected progeny which themselves are a source of infection. Some ram lambs can excrete the virus in their semen although they may have poor fertility associated with small soft testes (Barlow and Gardiner, 1983).

Treatment and Control. There is no treatment and, as yet, there is no commercially available vaccine; although one may become available eventually. The disease is best controlled by ensuring that the flock remains closed and hence the disease does not gain entry. Once it is present in a flock it is important, in the early stages of the outbreak, to attempt to segregate pregnant ewes from those that have given birth to clinically affected lambs. At the same time, to ensure that non-pregnant ewes develop an immunity, they should be exposed to infection and thereafter any surviving lambs from the infected flock should not be retained for breeding and should be sent for slaughter, so that symptomless carriers do not remain.

Leptospirosis

Despite not being listed as an identifiable cause of abortion in sheep (Table 25.1) there is evidence from the UK and the rest of the world that leptospires, including *L. interrogans* serovar *hardjo*, which is a common pathogen of cattle (see p. 408), can have an adverse effect upon reproductive performance by causing late abortion and stillbirth.

There is still debate whether or not sheep are a maintenance host for the infection, or whether there is a requirement for cattle as an established maintenance host to be closely involved (Cousins et al., 1989). Nevertheless, it is generally recognized as good practice in the control of the disease to minimize contact between the two species.

Diagnosis is based on the methods previously described for cattle (see p. 409); this involves the demonstration of the organism in aborted fetuses or fetal membranes using fluorescent antibody techniques or the presence of rising antibody titres in paired blood samples.

Treatment in an acute outbreak involves the use of dihydrostreptomycin at a dose rate of 25 mg/kg for all pregnant ewes. Where an outbreak of the disease is anticipated, vaccination at tupping time with a quarter dose of the cattle vaccine with a boost 2–4 weeks later is recommended (Ellis, 1992).

Ureaplasmosis

Ureaplasma spp. have been isolated from normal ewes (Ball et al., 1984) and from ewes with granular vulvitis (Doig and Ruhnke, 1977); there is some suggestion that they are common inhabitants of the urogenital tract of sheep. Ureaplasmas have been identified as a cause of infertility and abortions in cattle (see p. 418) and in other non-domestic species. Although a possible role in infertility and abortion has been identified in sheep

(Livingstone et al., 1978), this is not, as yet, conclusive.

Tick-borne fever (TBF)

The disease is caused by a small, Gram-negative bacterium *Rickettsia phagocytophilia* or *Cytoecetes phagocytophilia*, and is known in Scotland, Scandinavia, The Netherlands and South Africa. The organism is transmitted by a parasitic tick, which in Europe is usually *Ixodes ricinus*.

In susceptible ewes, it causes an acute febrile disease which lasts for about 10 days; recovery in non-pregnant ewes is generally uneventful. The majority of pregnant ewes will abort generally 2–8 days after the start of the fever. A proportion of pregnant ewes may die.

Diagnosis can be confirmed by identifying the organism in the leucocytes of ewes that have aborted or during the septicaemic phase.

Infected ewes that survive develop an immunity, whilst the majority of all sheep from tick-infected areas will have acquired an immunity at an early age. Newly purchased non-acclimatized sheep should be introduced to the farm before tupping, preferably when the tick numbers are at their highest in April to June and September/October. The ticks are also controlled by the appropriate dipping routine.

Q fever

This is due to infection with a rickettsia, *Coxiella burnetii*, which can affect a wide range of mammals and causes abortion in cattle and goats. It can sometimes be transmitted by ticks.

FEMALE GOATS

Infertility in the goat is generally not a major problem with, in the absence of any major infectious cause of abortion (see below), only a small number of barren does remaining at the end of the breeding season.

Structural defects

Abnormal sexual differentiation during embryological and fetal development, resulting in intersexes, is relatively common in the goat, especially in breeds such as the Alpine, Saanen and Toggenburg. It is much more prevalent in polled individuals where polledness is a simple dominant character with full penetrance but it is associated with a recessive hermaphrodite effect with incomplete penetrance (Baxendell, 1985). Intersexes can also occur as a result of freemartinism where placental fusion occurs in twins of dissimilar sex (see Chapter 4).

Intersexes vary in the degree of external structural abnormality. Most of them are generally female-like in appearance at birth but, as they grow and mature, there will be evidence of an enlarged clitoris, perhaps testes in the inguinal region and the development of male secondary sex characteristics, including the typical male odour.

Functional factors

The goat is a seasonal breeder responding to the effects of declining day-length. It is possible to advance the onset of the breeding season with the use of progestogen sponges and eCG treatment (see p. 42).

Hydrometra or pseudopregnancy ('cloudburst')

Hydrometra is the accumulation of sterile uterine secretions in the uterine lumen associated with persistence of a corpus luteum. As a consequence, there is a cessation of cyclical activity, variable degrees of abdominal distension and thus a pseudopregnancy.

The incidence of the disease varies between herds and within the same herd from year to year. Studies involving 71 dairy herds in France found an overall incidence of 2–3% (Mialot et al., 1991), although on one farm in the study it was 20%. In Holland, Hesselink (1993a) found a mean incidence in three herds totalling 550 does of 9%. The disease occurs more frequently in older does and is uncommon in yearlings. In Hesselink's study (1993a) there appeared to be an association with the use of progestogen sponges and eCG treatment to advance the onset of cyclical activity before the start of the normal breeding season.

Differentiation from normal pregnancy can be made using B-mode ultrasound imaging because of the presence of a fluid-filled uterus in the absence of a fetus or placentomes. If untreated, pseudopregnant does will expel an appreciable volume of cloudy uterine fluid around the time that kidding would have occurred in a normal pregnancy; hence the term 'cloudburst'.

Treatment with $PGF_{2\alpha}$ or an analogue will be followed by expulsion of the fluid and oestrus in about 4 days. Hesselink (1993b) reported a recurrence in one doe. By using a second injection 12 days after the first, good levels of fertility can be achieved, with 85% conceiving compared with 95% of unaffected animals (Hesselink, 1993b).

Cystic ovarian disease

Cystic ovarian disease has been described in dairy breeds of goats, particularly where they graze oestrogenic clovers and legumes (Baxendell, 1985). The typical clinical signs are those of continuous oestrus and short interoestrus intervals with a failure to conceive. The best treatment is probably 1500–2500 IU of human chorionic gonadotrophin (hCG) or, alternatively, gonadotrophin-releasing hormone (GnRH).

Abortion in Angora goats

Since the turn of the century abortion has been a problem amongst the Angora goats in eastern Cape Province in South Africa. In recent years it has reached such proportions that it has threatened the viability of the mohair industry. Since the increased interest in mohair production in many other parts of the world this problem has remained with the Angora goat.

The cause of the condition was for some time believed to be due to premature regression of the corpora lutea of pregnancy because of the decline in trophic stimulation from the anterior pituitary (Van Heerden, 1963). However, recent studies have identified two types of abortion. The most common is a 'stress-induced' abortion which occurs in poorly grown and immature does. It has been suggested by Wenzel et al. (1976) that hypoglycaemia in pregnant does stimulates the immature fetal adrenal to produce oestrogen precursors which result in the placental synthesis of oestrogens and subsequent abortions.

The less common type of abortion is referred to as 'habitual' abortion which is probably a genetically-determined hyperactivity of the maternal adrenal cortex prematurely initiating the process of parturition (see Chapter 6). Habitual aborters should be culled, together with any live offspring that might survive.

Management factors

Timing of service or artificial insemination

Optimum pregnancy rates are obtained when does are mated towards the end of oestrus (which lasts 1–2 days) and just before ovulation. Baxendell (1985) suggests that some goat owners serve their does only in the first 12 hours of oestrus to supposedly increase the number of female kids but with a consequential reduction in pregnancy rates.

Nutrition

Vitamin A, certain minerals (manganese and iodine) and energy deficiencies will reduce fertility.

Stress

Stress-induced abortion has been described above in Angora goats; however, there is evidence that other breeds of goats will abort if subjected to stress. This can result from inadequate feeding, transportation and adverse weather, particularly during the fourth month of gestation (Shelton, 1986).

Infectious agents

Non-specific infections appear to play a minor role in causing infertility in does, probably for similar reasons discussed above for the ewe (see p. 455). However, specific infectious agents are important in causing abortion; unfortunately no information of their relative importance in Great Britain is available. Many of these specific infectious agents are also important in sheep. Details of the isolation of specific pathogens isolated from the small number of caprine fetopathies examined by the Veterinary Investigation Service of the Ministry of Agriculture, Fisheries and Food are listed in Table 25.2.

Brucellosis

The organism most frequently involved is *Brucella melitensis* which is endemic in many Mediterranean countries, Africa and Central America; it does not occur in Britain. *B. abortus* occasionally causes problems but *B. ovis* has not been isolated from goats.

B. melitensis causes abortion in late pregnancy, stillbirths or weakly kids. The disease can be diagnosed by culture of fetus, fetal membranes or vaginal discharges, and can be controlled by

Table 25.2 Percentage frequency of isolation of pathogens from caprine fetopathies examined by Ministry of Agriculture Veterinary Investigation Centres (source: VIDA-II)

	1984	1985	1986	1987	1988	1989	1990	1991	1992
Actinomyces (Campylobacter) pyogenes	7.1	7.7	3.6	5.4	3.5	0	0	0	NR
Chlamydia	28.6	38.5	10.7	40.5	19.3	19.1	17.1	3.8	NR
Campylobacter spp.	7.4	0	0	0	3.5	0	5.7	3.8	5.0
Listeria monocytogenes	0	15.4	10.7	2.7	8.8	7.4	5.7	15.4	35.0
Salmonella serotypes	0	0	0	2.7	0	0	0	0	NR
Toxoplasma spp.	42.9	23.1	57.1	37.8	43.9	45.6	57.1	38.5	30.0
Coxiella burnetii	0	0	0	0	3.5	0	0	0	NR
Fungi	0	0	0	0	1.8	0	0	3.8	NR
Other pathogens	14.3	15.4	17.9	10.8	15.8	27.9	14.3	34.6	30.0
Total identified	14	13	28	37	57	68	35	26	20
Total submitted	62	59	89	134	161	164	98	90	61
Percentage diagnosed	22.6	22.0	31.5	27.6	35.4	41.5	35.7	28.9	32.8

NR, not recorded.

routine vaccination. It is important to remember that *B. melitensis* is a zoonosis.

Vibrosis

This is caused by infection with *Campylobacter* spp. probably *C. jejuni* and possibly *C. fetus*; abortion occurs in late gestation or there are stillborn or weakly kids. The diagnosis, treatment and control is similar to that described for sheep. It is uncommon.

Chlamydial (enzootic) abortion

This is an important cause of infertility in goats in many countries. It is due to infection with *Chlamydia psittaci* which is similar to, or identical with, the strain responsible for enzootic abortion in sheep (see p. 457).

Abortions usually occur in the last 4 weeks of gestation but stillborn and weakly kids can occur. The diagnosis and treatment are similar to that described above for sheep (see p. 458). Does infected in late pregnancy usually abort during the subsequent pregnancy and can produce infected lambs which, after a latent phase, abort during their first pregnancy.

The disease is best controlled by good hygiene to prevent lateral spread to susceptible animals, exposure of young non-pregnant does to infection and the use of a vaccine, which has been made compulsory in some countries where the disease has been widespread (Polydorou, 1981).

C. psittaci is a zoonosis causing abortion in pregnant women and generalized influenza-like symptoms; care should be exercised in handling potentially infected material.

Leptospirosis

Although it is not a frequently diagnosed cause of abortion there are reports in the literature (Van der Hoeden, 1953; Baxendell, 1985), particularly associated with *Leptospira grippotyphosa*. There is usually systemic illness preceding the abortion associated with septicaemia.

Diagnosis is based upon the identification of the organism and serological tests. The disease can be treated in the acute phase with streptomycin but it is doubtful if this would prevent abortion occurring. Control measures involving the use of vaccines might be tried in an outbreak.

Listeriosis

Encephalitis due to infection with *Listeria monocytogenes* is quite common in goats. The same organism can cause abortion in late gestation or stillbirth.

As in sheep and cattle, poorly fermented, soil-contaminated silage is a source of infection. The pathogenesis, diagnosis, treatment and control are similar to those described for sheep.

Salmonellosis

There are no host-specific salmonella species in the goat. However, the ubiquitous salmonellae have been reported to cause abortion (Baxendell, 1985).

Toxoplasmosis

This is a widespread disease of goats due to infection with *Toxoplasma gondii*. It causes fetal death with resorption if infection occurs early in gestation, or abortion. However, unlike sheep, fetal death is preceded in some cases by a period of severe illness with pyrexia, anorexia, diarrhoea and muscle weakness (Daubney et al., 1980).

The placental lesions are very similar to those described in sheep. Diagnosis is dependent upon identification of the organism in placental tissue or serological tests. There is currently no vaccine available but aborting does develop an immunity and does that have aborted should be retained within the herd whilst young, non-pregnant does should be exposed to infection before they become pregnant.

Infection of domestic cats and wild Felidae is essential for the completion of the sexual cycle of *T. gondii* and hence they play a critical role in the spread of the disease.

Treatment and control measures are similar to those described for sheep (see above).

T. gondii is a zoonosis and thus care should be taken in handling possibly infected material.

Q fever

Q fever is caused by *Coxiella burnetii*. It causes abortion and stillbirth in goats, either without any previous clinical signs or following a few day's illness where there is dullness, depression and anorexia. The abortion rate can be as high as 93% in some infected herds, but normally it is 5–50% (Miller et al., 1986).

Diagnosis is made upon the identification of the organism in smears of the placenta or the organs of the abortus, and serological tests demonstrating a rising antibody titre. Frequently, the appearance of placental lesions will confirm a diagnosis; this is particularly true of the intercotyledonary areas where there is an abundant inspissated or fluid red or white exudate. The underlying placental tissue is thickened and may be diffusely red or brown with multiple foci or confluent areas that are chalky white in appearance (Miller et al., 1986).

There is no vaccine and does can remain chronic carriers of the organism.

C. burnetii is a zoonosis and is excreted in milk.

Mycoplasmosis

A number of *Mycoplasma* spp. have been identified as causing abortion.

REFERENCES

Acland, H. M., Gard, G. P. and Plant, J. W. (1972) *Aust. Vet. J.*, **48**, 70.

Aitken, I. (1986) *In Practice*, 236.

Arthur, G. H. (1956) *J. Comp. Pathol.*, **66**, 345.

Ball, H. J., McCaughey, W. J. and Irwin, D. (1984) *Brit. Vet. J.*, **140**, 347.

Barlow, B. A. and Dickinson, A. G. (1965) *Res. Vet. Sci.*, **6**, 230.

Barlow, R. M. and Gardiner, A. C. (1983) In: *Diseases of Sheep*, ed. W. B. Martin, pp. 129–133. Oxford: Blackwell Scientific.

Baxendell, S. A. (1985) *Proceedings of Refresher Course No. 73.* University of Sydney Postgraduate Committee in Veterinary Science, pp. 355–362.

Bennetts, H. W., Underwood, E. J. an Shier, F. L. (1946) *Aust. Vet. J.*, **22**, 2.

Blewett, D. A. and Watson, W. A. (1983) *Brit. Vet. J.*, **139**, 546.

Buxton, D. (1983) In: *Diseases of Sheep*, ed. W. B. Martin, pp. 124–128. Oxford: Blackwell Scientific.

Buxton, D. (1993) *Vet. Ann.*, **33**, 45–52.

Buxton, D., Gilmour, J. S., Angus, K. W., Blewett, D. A. and Miller, J. K. (1981a) *Res. Vet. Sci.*, **32**, 170.

Buxton, D., Reid, H. W., Finlayson, J., Pow, I. and Anderson, J. S. (1981b) *Vet. Rec.*, **109**, 559.

Buxton, D., Blewett, D. A., Trees, A. J., McColgan, C. and Finlayson, J. (1988) *J. Comp. Pathol.*, **98**, 225.

Buxton, D., Thomson, K. M., Maley, S., Wright, S. and Bos, H. J. (1991) *Vet. Rec.*, **129**, 89.

Buxton, D., Thomson, K. M., Maley, S., Wright, S. and Bos, H. J. (1993) *Vet. Rec.*, **133**, 310.

Cousins, D. V., Ellis, T. M., Parkinson, J. and McGlashan, C. H. (1989) *Vet. Rec.*, **124**, 123.

Dain, A. (1971) *J. Reprod. Fertil.*, **24**, 91.

Daubney, J. P., Sharma, S. P. and Lopes, C. W. G. (1980) *Amer. J. Vet. Res.*, **41**, 1072.

Dennis, S. M. (1991) In: *Laboratory Diagnosis of Livestock Abortion*, 3rd edn, ed. C. A. Kirkbride, pp. 82–85. Ames: Iowa State University Press.

Doig, P. A. and Ruhnke, H. L. (1977) *Vet. Rec.*, **100**, 179.

Dutt, R. H. (1954) *Anim. Sci.*, **13**, 464.

Ellis, W. A. (1992) In: *Diseases of Sheep*, 2nd edn, ed. W. B. Martin and I. D. Aitken, pp. 78–80. Oxford: Blackwell Scientific.

Emady, M., Noakes, D. E. and Arthur, G. H. (1975) *Vet. Rec.*, **96**, 261.

Frenkel, J. K. (1973) Cited by Buxton, D. (1983) In: *Diseases of Sheep*, ed. W. B. Martin, p. 125. Oxford: Blackwell Scientific.

Hammond, J. (1921) *J. Agr. Sci., Camb.*, **11**, 337.

Haretley, W. J., Jebson, J. L. and McFarlane, D. (1954) *N. Z. Vet. J.*, **2**, 80.

Hesselink (1993a) *Vet. Rec.*, **132**, 110.

Hesselink (1993b) *Vet. Rec.*, **133**, 186.

Hughes, L. E., Kershaw, G. F. and Shaw, I. G. (1959) *Vet. Rec.*, **71**, 313.

Johnston, W. S. (1988) *Vet. Rec.*, **122**, 283.

Johnston, W. S., McClachan, G. K. and Murray, I. S. (1980) *Vet. Rec.*, **106**, 238.

Linklater, K. (1983) *Proc. Sheep Vet. Soc.*, **7**, 16–18.

Livingstone, C. W., Gauer, B. B. and Shelton, M. (1978) *Amer. J. Vet. Res.*, **39**, 1699.

Long, S. E. (1980) *Vet. Rec.*, **106**, 175.

Low, C. and Linklater, K. (1985) *In Practice*, 96.

Mialot, J. P., Saboureau, L., Gueraud, J. M., Prengere, E., Parizot, D., Pirot, G., Duquesmel, R., Petat, M. and Chemineau, P. (1991) *Rec. Med. Vet.*, **167**, 383.

Miller, R. B., Palmer, N. C. and Kierstad, M. (1986) In: *Current Therapy in Theriogenology*, ed. D. A. Morrow, pp. 607–609. Philadelphia: W. B. Saunders.

O'Connell, E., Wilkins, W. F. and Te Punga, W. A. (1988) *N. Z. Vet. J.*, **36**, 1.

Polydorou, K. (1981) *Brit. Vet. J.*, **137**, 411.

Rodalakis, A. and Bernard, K. (1977) *Bull. Acad. Vet. Fr.*, **50**, 65.

Shelton, M. (1986) In: *Current Therapy in Theriogenology*, 2nd edn, ed. D. A. Morrow, pp. 610–612. Philadelphia: W. B. Saunders.

Smith, K. C. (1991) Diploma in Sheep Health and Production, Dissertation, Royal College of Veterinary Surgeons.

Smith, K. C. (1993) Personal communication.

Smith, R. E., Reynolds, I. M. and Harris, J. C. (1968) *Cornell Vet.*, **58**, 389.

Spence, J. B., Beattie, C. P. and Faulkner, J. (1978) *Vet. Rec.*, **102**, 38.

Stamp, J. T., Watt, J. A. and Nisbuet, D. I. (1950) *Vet. Rec.*, **62**, 251.

Sweasey, D., Patterson, D. S. P., Richardson, C., Harkness, J. W., Shaw, I. G. and Williams, W. W. (1979) *Vet. Rec.*, **104**, 447.

Van der Hoeden, J. (1953) *J. Comp. Pathol.*, **63**, 101.

Van Heerden, K. M. (1963) *Onderstepoort J. Vet. Res.*, **30**, 23.

Wenzel, D., Le Roux, M. M. and Botha, L. J. J. (1976) *Agro Anim.*, **8**, 59.

Wilmut, I., Sales, D. I. and Ashworth, C. J. (1985) *Theriogenology*, **23**, 107.

Winters, L. M. and Feuffel, G. (1936) *Univ. Minn. Agric. Exp. Stn. Bull.*, 118.

26

Infertility in the Mare

Since the early nineteenth century, when 1st January was declared the official birthdate for Thoroughbred foals, irrespective of their actual birth dates within that year, horsemen have been plagued with problems attempting to breed mares in the winter and early spring. The promotion of yearling sales in the autumn also contributes to the pressure for early breeding, since well-grown older yearlings tend to sell for higher prices.

'Infertility' is an absolute term, and in most cases 'subfertile' would be a more accurate description. Very few mares are permanently and completely infertile, but subfertility of varying degrees is a major problem. To understand subfertility, some understanding of normal expectations of fertility are useful.

For Thoroughbred mares in the UK the pregnancy rate has increased from a low of 61.2% in 1971 to a high of 72.4% in 1989 (date of pregnancy determination not specified). Similarly, the live foal rate has increased from a low of 53% in 1971 to a high of 66% in 1989 (Ricketts and Young, 1990). For the Hunter Improvement Scheme the current live foal rate is around 60%. Ponies tend to have better rates.

Pregnancy rates at the end of the season will depend on: (1) the fertility of the stallion; (2) the fertility of mares; (3) and the management of the pregnant mare.

This last factor is often related to the value of the horses involved, i.e. frequent veterinary attention in cases where it is justified by the potential value of the foal, results in better fertility. Very expensive stallions tend to attract more fertile mares, or the stud may accept only young, fertile mares. Well-managed studs tease mares regularly and individually; this is very time consuming. An experienced stud manager knows, for example, the reasons why some mares fail to exhibit oestrous behaviour. In turn, the length of time that a mare fails to show oestrus before being presented to the veterinary surgeon for examination depends on stud policy and the owner's wishes.

A clinical protocol for the investigation of an infertile or subfertile mare is outlined in Table 26.1.

CAUSES OF INFERTILITY AND SUBFERTILITY

Many factors, acting either alone or in combination with others, can cause infertility or subfertility. Broadly, they can be categorized into infectious or non-infectious factors, with the latter being further divided into structural abnormalities and functional aberrations. This format will be used to discuss the various causes in this chapter. The factors are outlined in Table 26.2.

Table 26.1 Outline of a step by step protocol for the clinical examination of an infertile mare

1. Obtain the mare's previous breeding history
2. Assess her physical condition, general health and perineal conformation
3. Culture swab samples collected from the vestibule, clitoral fossa and sinuses
4. Examination per vaginam using a speculum, and collection of endometrial swabs for bacterial culture and stained smear
5. Manual vaginal examination
6. Examine the reproductive tract by rectal palpation
7. Transrectal real-time ultrasound examination of the reproductive tract
8. Endometrial biopsy
9. Endoscopic examination of the endometrium
10. Peripheral venous blood sample for hormone/chromosome analysis

Table 26.2 Summary of the causes of mare infertility

Non-infectious

Structural
- Defective vulva
- Defective vestibulovaginal constriction
- Vesicovaginal reflux
- Vaginal bleeding
- Persistent hymen
- Abnormal cervix
- Uterine tumour
- Uterine haematoma
- Uterine abscess
- Uterine adhesions
- Uterine cysts
- Partial dilatation of the uterus
- Abnormal oviduct
- Ovarian tumour
- Ovarian haematoma
- Gonadal dysgenesis
- Developmental abnormalities

Functional
1. No oestrous behaviour
   a. Anoestrus caused by ovarian quiescence
      (i) Winter anoestrus
      (ii) Poor body condition
      (iii) Disease
      (iv) Chromosomal abnormality
      (v) Pituitary abnormality
      (vi) Ovarian tumours
      (vii) Lactation related
   b. Anoestrus caused by prolonged luteal function
      (i) Prolonged dioestrus
      (ii) Dioestrous ovulation
      (iii) Pyometra
      (iv) Pregnancy/pseudopregnancy
   c. Anoestrus caused by behaviour
      (i) Silent heat
      (ii) Erratic postpartum behaviour
2. Shortened luteal phase — endometritis
3. Irregular or prolonged oestrus
   a. Transitional ('spring') oestrus
   b. Ovarian neoplasia
   c. Chromosomal abnormalities
4. Ovulatory dysfunction
5. Multiple ovulation
6. Gestational failure
   a. Early embryonic death
   b. Fetal death/abortion
      (i) Infectious: viral/bacterial/fungal
      (ii) Non-infectious: twins, uterine body pregnancy
      (iii) Placental/developmental abnormalities

Infectious

Endometritis: bacterial/fungal
Metritis
Pyometra

STRUCTURAL ABNORMALITIES OF THE FEMALE REPRODUCTIVE TRACT

Vulva

In the normal mare the vulva provides an effective barrier to protect the uterus from ascending infection. If the vulval seal is incompetent, pneumovagina may occur and the reproductive tract can become infected. The initial vaginitis may lead to cervicitis and acute endometritis resulting in subfertility. Caslick (1937) first pointed out the importance of this condition in relation to genital infection. Interestingly, it is most commonly found in Thoroughbreds, and, in the author's experience, is almost unknown in Shires and native ponies. Defective vulval conformation can be (1) congenital, which is very rare or (2) acquired, which is due to (a) vulval stretching following repeated foalings, (b) injury to perineal tissue or (c) poor bodily condition.

Older, pluriparous mares are more commonly affected with pneumovagina. However, young mares that are in work and have little body fat and/or poor vulval conformation, can develop pneumovagina. In some mares, pneumovagina may only occur during oestrus when the perineal tissues are more relaxed. A 'Caslick index' has been described in an attempt to determine which mares require treatment (Pascoe, 1979), but its use is not widespread. Some mares make an obvious noise whilst walking, but in other mares the diagnosis may be more difficult. The presence of a frothy exudate in the anterior vagina on examination with a speculum is pathognomic. Rectal palpation of a ballooned vagina or uterus from which air can be expelled confirms the diagnosis. Real-time ultrasound examination of the uterus may reveal the presence of air as hyperechoic (white) foci. Cytological and histological examination of the endometrium may demonstrate significant numbers of neutrophils and eosinophils indicative of an endometritis.

Treatment should be directed at correcting the physical pnemovaginitis and concurrently treating the acute endometritis. The former can be done surgically by Caslick's operation. However, when the angle of the vulval surface relative to the vertical is the primary deformity, Caslick's operation is ineffective, and perineal resection should be used to achieve a satisfactory vulval conformation (Pouret, 1982). In the author's opinion many mares are subjected to Caslick's operation unnecessarily: the operation should be reserved for mares with a true vulval defect rather than just because the mare has failed to become pregnant.

Vagina

Vesicovaginal reflux, also known as urovagina and urine pooling, is the retention of incompletely voided urine in the vaginal fornix due to an exaggerated downward cranial slope of the vagina. Pneumovagina from a defective vulval conformation also predisposes to the condition. Transient urine pooling, which is sometimes found in postpartum mares, usually resolves after uterine involution has occurred. Uterine infection with an accumulation of exudate in the vaginal fornix can be confused with the condition. It can be treated surgically by vaginoplasty (perhaps more correctly termed caudal relocation of the transverse fold, as surgical intervention is in the vestibule) (Monin, 1972), urethral extension (McKinnon and Belden, 1988) or perineal resection (Pouret, 1982).

Vaginal bleeding from varicose veins in the remnants of the hymen at the dorsal vestibulovaginal junction is occasionally seen in older mares, particularly during oestrus. Treatment is not usually necessary as the varicose veins normally shrink spontaneously, although diathermy can be used.

Manual vaginal examination of maiden mares often reveals the presence of hymen tissue which generally breaks down with pressure. A complete persistent hymen can also occur which can result in the accumulation of fluid within the vagina and uterus due to impaired natural drainage. Sometimes the hymen may be so tough that it can only be ruptured using a guarded scalpel blade or scissors. The small incision can then be enlarged using the fingers and hand. Rarely, failure of proper fusion of the Müllerian ducts may result in the presence of dorsoventral bands of fibrous tissue in the anterior vagina and fornix. They do not interfere with fertility and are easily broken down manually.

Cervix

The cervix, whilst forming an important protective physical barrier to protect the uterus, must also relax during oestrus to allow intrauterine ejaculation of semen at coitus and drainage of uterine fluid. A cervicitis is usually associated with endometritis and/or vaginitis.

Fibrosis of the cervix often occurs in older mares, particularly maiden mares. Adhesions of the cervix arise from trauma at parturition or mating; they can be broken down manually, but this must be done daily to prevent recurrence. Artificial insemination has been used successfully in mares with an abnormally narrow cervix. Impaired cervical drainage of uterine fluid can predispose to chronic endometritis.

Cervical lacerations may need surgical repair if severe. Developmental abnormalities of the cervix have been described; these include aplasia and a double cervix.

Uterus

Uterine cysts

Uterine cysts are the most common type of uterine lesion identified in the mare. Two distinct morphological types are recognized: (1) endometrial cysts, which are usually 2 cm or less in diameter, and (2) lymphatic cysts, which are generally larger. They can be diagnosed at post-mortem examination; however, the use of ultrasonography has

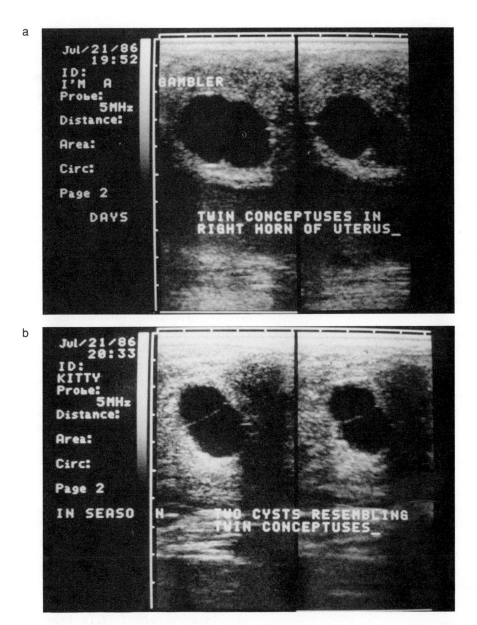

Fig. 26.1 Ultrasonographic images of (a) unilateral 16-day-old twin conceptuses and (b) two endometrial cysts. Specular reflections can be seen in (a), but note the remarkably similar appearance. Prior knowledge of the cysts due to routine ultrasound examination is vital.

shown that the incidence is much greater than was originally suspected.

The relationship between subfertility and uterine cysts is not clear. Some authors suggest that uterine cysts can reduce pregnancy rates (Adams et al., 1987). However, it is difficult to be sure of their primary role as they are a common sign of uterine disease in general, including senility and previous endometritis. The author's experience is that only mares that are severely affected have a reduced pregnancy rate.

Endometrial cysts can be confused with an early conceptus. Differentiation is based on previous cyst mapping, but also the early mobility of the conceptus, the presence of specular reflections, the conceptus's spherical appearance and growth rate (Figure 26.1).

Larger lymphatic cysts may impede the early

mobility of the conceptus, whilst later in pregnancy, contact between the cyst wall and yolk sac or allantois may prevent absorption of nutrients.

Partial dilatation of the uterus

The discrete collection of fluid in ventral dilatations of the uterus which can be palpated per rectum was first reported by Knudsen (1964). Ventral uterine enlargements have subsequently been discussed by Kenney and Ganjam (1975), who suggested that they originated by one of four mechanisms: mucosal atrophy, myometrial atony, lymphatic lacunae or endometrial cysts. Their precise relationship to subfertility is not clear, but mares which fail to eliminate the fluid and debris which accumulate in these sacculations after mating are susceptible to the establishment of chronic endometritis (see later).

Uterine adhesions

Uterine adhesions are occasionally diagnosed on endoscopic examinations of the uterus. It has been suggested that the incidence may be greater than was previously thought (Stone et al., 1991). Multiple adhesions adversely affect fertility by causing fluid accumulation or by affecting the mobility of the conceptus. Treatment is by manual breakdown, or the use of an endoscope and electrocautery laser.

Uterine neoplasia (Madwell and Theilen, 1987), abscesses (Van Camp, 1993) and haematomata (Shideler et al., 1990; Pycock, 1994a) are rarely reported in the mare. Uterine foreign bodies (e.g. fetal remnants), which may act as a nidus for the establishment of chronic endometritis, have been documented (Ginther and Pierson, 1984), but are uncommon.

Uterine tubes and periovarian structures

Uterine tube abnormalities are rare in the mare. Anomalies are usually due to remnants of embryological structures. Cysts lying within the ovulation fossa of the ovary are of paramesonephric origin and generally have no adverse effect upon fertility; however, they are termed ovarian cysts by some authors, which may account for the diagnosis of 'cystic ovaries' in the mare (see below). It is possible that sometimes, particularly if they are numerous as can occur in older mares, they could impede the release of the oocyte from the ovulation fossa. Paraovarian cysts (mesonephric in

origin) are fairly common, especially in Shires and Clydesdales, but they do not affect fertility. There has been a recent report of the presence of collagenous masses within the uterine tube which might occlude its lumen (Liu et al., 1990).

Ovarian neoplasia

Ovarian neoplasia is uncommon in the mare although many types of tumour have been described, with the granulosa theca cell tumours (CTCTs) (Figure 26.2) being by far the commonest (Meagher et al., 1977). Of the other types, teratomata and cystadenomata are the next most frequently identified (Bosu et al., 1982). Teratomata, which are composed of different tissue types, are difficult to differentiate clinically from GTCTs.

GTCTs arise from the sex cord stromal tissue within the ovary and are frequently hormonally active, producing variable amounts of steroids which cause behavioural changes and alteration to normal cyclical activity. Mares may exhibit nymphomania, anoestrus or aggresiveness with signs of virilism (clitoral enlargement, stallion-like conformation). There appears to be no breed predisposition for GTCTs, and there is a wide range of age distribution (Meagher et al., 1977). One grossly enlarged ovary (> 10 cm diameter) and with the opposite ovary small and inactive, together with behavioural changes and raised serum testosterone levels are usually sufficient evidence to confirm the diagnosis of a GTCT. However, there can be other reasons for a large ovary: (1) a normal ovary during the breeding season with large follicles; (2) other tumours; (3) haematomata, and abscesses, haemorrhagic and anovulatory follicles (these will be considered later).

In mares with GTCTs, behavioural changes alone can be misleading since not all affected mares show virilism, and tumours other than GTCTs can also result in elevated plasma testosterone values. It has been the author's experience that occasionally owners express the opinion that their mare is 'awkward' when in oestrus, and request veterinary treatment. Frequently such mares are required to perform to a high level, e.g. advanced dressage. Examination during the period of abnormal behaviour has shown them to be in dioestrus with two normal ovaries. Owner pressure to perform an ovariectomy on suspicion of a GTCT should be resisted, at least until the mare has

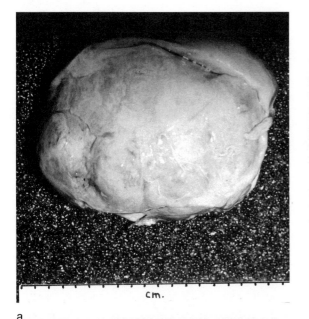

a

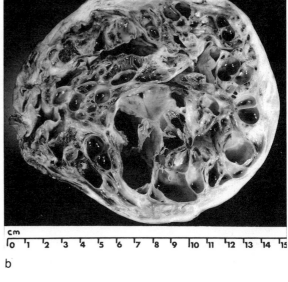

b

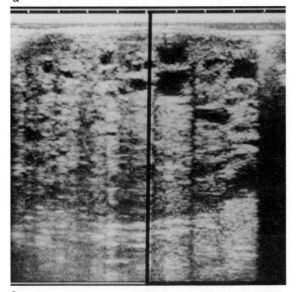

c

Fig. 26.2 Granulosa theca cell tumour. (a) Gross characteristics. Note the large size and smooth surface. (b) Cross-section of an affected ovary showing the 'honeycomb' or multilocular appearance. (c) Ultrasonographic image showing the 'honeycomb' appearance with multiple, small, non-echogenic areas separated by large areas of dense stroma.

been monitored throughout one complete cycle. Transrectal ultrasonography generally assists a diagnosis — often the GTCT appears as a large (7–40 cm) mass, spherical and with a multicystic or 'honeycomb' appearance (Figure 26.2(c)). However, Hinrichs and Hunt (1990) caution that there is no typical ultrasonographic appearance of GTCTs, since they can vary from being uniformly homogenous to having one or several large fluid-filled cysts. The echogenicity of the cyst wall differentiates it from persistent, large anovulatory follicles. Teratomata, melanomata and dysgerminomata are solid neoplastic lesions appearing uniformly echogenic. However, the ultrasonic appearance of some GTCTs seen by the author can be similar to that of luteinized, unruptured ('haemorrhagic') follicles (see below).

It is important to diagnose accurately the reason for the enlarged ovary. For example, in one report, 39% (11 out of 28) of surgically excised enlarged ovaries did not warrant removal (Bosu et al., 1982); these authors concluded that histopathological examination of ovarian tissue and plasma hormone concentrations are needed for a definitive diagnosis.

Recently, it has been suggested that the identification of the hormone inhibin (see p. 7) may be more reliable than testosterone in confirming the presence of a GTCT (Piquette et al., 1990). The secretion of high amounts of inhibin by the neoplastic granulosa cells inhibits follicle-stimulating hormone (FSH) secretion, and is thought to be the reason for atrophy of the contralateral ovary.

Unilateral ovariectomy is the only satisfactory treatment for GTCTs, since the prospect of breeding from the mare is extremely poor unless the neoplastic ovary is removed. Most mares return to normal cyclical ovarian activity during the next breeding season and are fertile.

Most GTCTs are benign and unilateral although a bilateral case has been reported. Metastasis of the tumour is rare, but does occur (Meagher et al., 1977).

Ovarian haematoma

The follicle in the mare normally fills with blood after ovulation (Allen et al., 1987). A form of apparent ovulatory failure (see ovulatory dysfunction later) has been described in the mare in which the preovulatory follicle grows to an unusually large size (7–10 cm), apparently fails to ovulate, but fills with blood and then gradually regresses. These haematomata persist for a variable period of time, often beyond the next ovulation and corpus luteum formation, and normal cyclic ovarian activity continues. They normally resolve spontaneously and no treatment is required.

Ultrasonographic imaging is useful, although the haematomata may have a similar appearance to that of a GTCT. Typically, ovarian haematomata have a uniformly echogenic appearance, but this homogeneity may only be present before clotting has occurred. After clotting, the non-echogenic areas are separated by trabeculae and are similar to those of a multicystic GTCT. The diagnosis of a haematoma may be made on the basis of clinical signs, namely maintenance of cyclicity, a normal contralateral ovary, the presence of an ovulation fossa and speed of enlargement and regression of the ovary with time.

Gonadal dysgenesis (see Chapter 4)

This is not common; however, in a maiden mare, once winter anoestrus has been eliminated as a cause of acyclicity, XY ovarian dysgenesis must be considered as a possible cause. Examination of the reproductive system will show the presence of very small ovaries (< 1 cm in diameter), and a poorly developed tubular genital tract which is similar to those with X0 chromosomes (Turner's syndrome). There is no treatment and the mare is sterile.

FUNCTIONAL INFERTILITY

Mares are seasonally polyoestrous, and environmental and other factors can exert a profound effect on reproductive function particularly during the transitional period between winter anoestrus and the onset of cyclical activity in the spring. Irregularities of follicular development, ovulation and behavioural patterns are also observed during the normal breeding season; in addition, endometritis can also cause cyclical irregularities.

Anoestrus due to ovarian acyclicity

Winter anoestrus

The onset of cyclic activity is stimulated by increased day length (see Chapter 1). During winter months mares are normally acyclical.

Diagnosis. On rectal palpation or transrectal ultrasound imaging both ovaries will be small (< $3 \times 2 \times 2$ cm), and in some mares there will be a number of small follicles. Plasma progesterone concentrations are less than 1 ng/ml.

Treatment. Although increasing day length is the primary controlling factor, ensuring freedom from disease and good body condition by stabling, adequate nutrition, anthelmintic therapy and attention to dental conditions can hasten the onset of cyclical ovarian activity. Thus, prolonged anoestrus can be prevented by good management. Progesterone/progestogen withdrawal therapy has been used successfully. Progesterone can be administered as an oil-based intramuscular injection, orally as the synthetic progestogen altrenogest (Equine Regumate) or by using a silastic progesterone-releasing intravaginal device (PRID). However, such therapy is effective only in anoestrous mares that are already well into the transitional phase to the resumption of cyclical ovarian activity. Repeated daily injections of equine pituitary gland extract to mares in winter anoestrus leads to follicular development, whilst Hyland et al. (1987) have reported success using a mini-pump which infused gonadotrophin-releasing hormone (GnRH) intravenously over a period of 28 days.

These last two treatments are impractical for routine use.

In aged mares, the delayed initiation of normal cyclical ovarian activity may reduce the number of oestrous cycles during the breeding season and, therefore, it is particularly important to prevent poor body condition from occurring in such animals.

Pituitary abnormalities

Rarely Cushing's syndrome caused by adenomatous hyperplasia of the intermediate pituitary has been associated with anoestrus in aged mares. This is presumably due to destruction of the cells secreting luteinizing hormone and follicle-stimulating hormone.

Lactation-related anoestrus

Lactation-related anoestrus is commonest in mares foaling early in the season. Affected mares may have a normal postpartum oestrus after 6–12 days, but fail to return to oestrus at the end of the first dioestrus. Alternatively they may not even have a normal 'foal heat'.

Diagnosis. The ovaries resemble those of a mare in deep winter anoestrus, i.e. small and inactive; the condition can last for several months. Originally it was thought to be due to prolactin suppressing pituitary gonadotrophin release, but this is now in doubt. In the author's experience, the condition is most likely to be seen in early foaling mares which normally live in the south of the UK (where it is generally warmer), but are sent to the north of the UK for service. Affected mares should be teased and examined weekly per rectum to assess their ovarian status.

Treatment. Treatments similar to those described above for winter anoestrus have been used, but with little success. In the last few years, twice daily injections of 0.04 mg (10 ml) of a synthetic GnRH analogue (buserelin; Receptal) have been found to induce the development of a follicle within 7–14 days of commencing therapy. The author has successfully treated seven out of 14 mares using this regimen, but it is expensive, the pregnancy rate at the induced oestrus is reduced and the mare may return to anoestrus following the induced ovulation.

Anoestrus caused by a prolonged luteal phase

Persistence of luteal activity

Persistence of luteal activity in the non-pregnant mare is a major cause of subfertility. Traditionally, the term 'prolonged dioestrus' has been used to describe a condition where the function of the corpus luteum continues beyond its normal cyclical lifespan of 15/16 days, resulting in the maintenance of elevated circulating progesterone concentrations for longer than expected. Recently, Ginther (1990), in reviewing the condition, has suggested that the term 'prolonged luteal activity' should be used, as 'persistent dioestrus' implies that the corpus luteum persists, whereas it is possible that others are formed sequentially from dioestrous ovulations. These occur in up to 20% of oestrous cycles in Thoroughbred mares (less frequently in ponies) and are not accompanied by oestrus; the cervix will remain pale in colour, dry and tightly closed. If dioestrous ovulations occur late in the luteal phase they will be refractory to the effect of endogenous luteolysins, resulting in a persistent luteal phase.

True persistence of the corpus luteum occurs in approximately 20% of ovulations. These mares present great difficulty to the stud manager as they can be assumed incorrectly to be pregnant.

Diagnosis. Plasma progesterone profiles are indistinguishable from those of pregnant animals. The uterus becomes firm and tubular (tonic) and the cervix is typical of that of pregnancy. Transrectal ultrasound imaging fails to detect a conceptus.

Treatment. Failure of synthesis and/or release of prostaglandin $F_{2\alpha}$ ($PGF_{2\alpha}$) at the end of dioestrus is the most likely cause of persistence of the corpus luteum. Recently, Ginther (1990) has suggested that it might also be due to failure of the corpus luteum to respond to $PGF_{2\alpha}$, or failure of $PGF_{2\alpha}$ to reach the corpus luteum. Treatment is by the injection of a luteolytic dose of $PGF_{2\alpha}$ or a synthetic analogue. The interval between treatment and ovulation varies considerably depending upon the size of follicles at the time of treatment. Therefore, it is advisable always to examine mares using ultrasonography before treatment in order to assess the status of folliculogenesis.

Pyometra

Pyometra (see also later) is the accumulation of substantial quantities of inflammatory exudate in

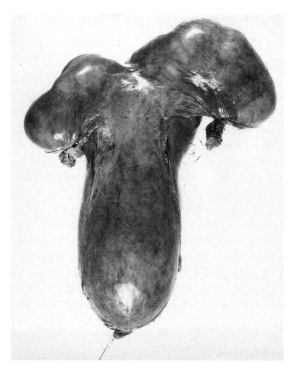

Fig. 26.3 Uterus of mare with pyometra treated by ovario-hysterectomy.

the uterus causing its distention (Hughes et al., 1979). When the endometrium is severely damaged, there is extensive loss of surface epithelium, severe endometrial fibrosis and glandular atrophy causing a prolonged luteal phase, presumably due to interference with the synthesis or release of $PGF_{2\alpha}$. This is in contrast to mild endometritis with collection of small amounts of intraluminal uterine fluid, which is more likely to cause premature release of $PGF_{2\alpha}$ and luteolysis (see p. 486). An example of the distended uterus of a mare with pyometra, treated by ovariohysterectomy is shown in Figure 26.3.

Pregnancy/pseudopregnancy

Pseudopregnancy is a term used to describe a syndrome in which non-pregnant mares that have been served do not return to oestrus. It occurs if there is early embryonic death after 15 days of gestation with persistence of the corpus luteum verum resulting in a prolonged luteal phase. The cervix remains tightly closed and the uterus is tense and tubular. It is differentiated from pregnancy by the absence of a conceptus on ultrasound examination. If early fetal death occurs after endometrial cup formation at 36 days (see p. 65–66), mares will either become anoestrus or come into oestrus. However, in the latter, follicular luteinization without ovulation is thought to occur and therefore the oestrus is not fertile; this will last until the endometrial cups regress spontaneously at 90–150 days. There is currently no practical way of destroying endometrial cups prematurely.

Behavioural anoestrus — silent oestrus

Some mares either do not show oestrus, or are slow to show detectable signs using standard teasing methods despite the fact that ovulation occurs; this is called silent oestrus. The degree of reduced expression of oestrus varies from partial (suboestrus) to complete (anoestrus). The incidence of silent oestrus has been reported to be 6% (Nelson et al., 1985); it is thought to have a higher incidence in maiden mares early in the breeding season and in mares with a young foal 'at foot'. Other factors which affect oestrous behaviour include being at grass with very dominant mares, and stallion preferences. Fillies that are in training and have been treated with anabolic steroids may be more likely to suffer from the condition due to 'androgenization'.

Diagnosis. Rectal and vaginal examinations confirm that the mare is in oestrus and has follicles of an ovulatory size. It is essential to distinguish the condition from a prolonged luteal phase in which there is also follicular development.

Treatment. In order to breed mares during a silent oestrus some form of restraint may be necessary. In Australia, where many fillies are bred whilst they are in training, they are treated with an intramuscular injection of oestradiol benzoate (10 mg); however, there is a reduction in the pregnancy rates, and it should be used only as a last resort. In many cases it is a failure of the detection system rather than a true reproductive disorder of individual mares. However, it has been associated with reduced oestradiol concentrations in the peripheral circulation and a shorter interval from luteolysis to ovulation (Nelson et al., 1985). There is no suggestion that aberrant morphological abnormalities in follicular development are involved.

Shortened luteal phase — endometritis

At coitus the mare's uterine lumen becomes contaminated with microorganisms and debris. In most mares there is a transient endometritis which usually resolves spontaneously within 72–96 hours. However, if the endometritis persists after day 4 or 5 of dioestrus, the premature release of $PGF_{2\alpha}$ results in luteolysis and a rapid decline of progesterone and an early return to oestrus. Endometritis will be considered fully later.

Irregular or prolonged oestrus

True persistent oestrus appears to be rare in mares other than during the transitional period from winter anoestrus or in association with steroid hormone-producing ovarian tumours. Some cases that are presented as having persistent oestrus may actually represent normal behaviour, or other types of behaviour may be misinterpreted as being persistent oestrus. Mares that are anoestrus due to disease, or old mares whose ovaries have ceased to function normally, may be receptive to a stallion. Frequent urination due to hindlimb or back pain, or a urogenital problem, may be mistaken for persistent oestrus.

Transitional 'spring' oestrus
Pressure to breed mares early in the year before the onset of their natural breeding season can cause difficulties for the veterinarian, particularly because of erratic and unpredictable reproductive function during the period when the mare is emerging from winter anoestrus. Shortly after the winter solstice, changes in the pineal/hypothalamic/pituitary axes result in some follicular growth; however, they remain small, do not ovulate, and regress. Eventually, after a variable transitional period of up to 2 months, larger follicles (> 35 mm) will develop and ovulate, usually heralding the onset of normal cyclical ovarian activity. During the transitional period the behaviour is variable, ranging from total rejection of the stallion, to interest but resistance to him mounting, to normal acceptance. These behavioural signs can be consistent or inconsistent.

Diagnosis. Ultrasonic examination and rectal palpation will reveal transitional follicles reaching a preovulatory size of > 30 mm. Visual identification of a corpus luteum confirms that the first ovulation has occurred and hence the onset of normal ovarian cyclical activity.

Treatment. Progesterone or progestogens, with or without the addition of oestradiol esters,

have been used, involving several parenteral routes of administration including intramuscular injection, in-feed medication and intravaginal coils. Treatment is based on progesterone exerting a negative feedback on gonadotrophin secretion which is followed by a surge release of FSH and luteinizing hormone (LH). When the source of progesterone is withdrawn or its effect wanes there is follicular growth, maturation and ovulation. Progesterone treatment is more effective in mares that are in late transitional anoestrus and is ineffective in mares with minimal follicular activity, particularly during deep anoestrus. Currently, the most effective treatment is the use of in-feed medication with the potent progestogen altrenogest (Equine Regumate). This liquid, which contains 2.2 mg/ml of the active substance, should be added to the food once per day at a dose rate of 0.044 mg/kg body weight for 10 consecutive days; oestrus should occur within 8 days and ovulation between 7 and 13 days after the last treatment. Because of the possibility of ovulation occurring during treatment, an injection of $PGF_{2\alpha}$ on the last day of in-feed medication may be necessary to cause luteolysis of any corpus luteum that may be present.

There has been much interest recently in using GnRH or its analogues to hasten ovulation in transitional or even anoestrus mares (Harrison et al., 1990). GnRH or an analogue can be administered by injection, infusion or subcutaneous implant. The author has successfully used 0.04 mg of buserelin (Receptal) given twice daily by intramuscular injection. It is expensive, as treatment is necessary for at least 1–2 weeks — a mean of 15.8 days is cited by Ginther and Bergfelt (1990). It is noteworthy that these authors found a high multiple ovulation rate associated with GnRH treatment.

Irrespective of the hormones used, mares that are being treated early in the season need 16 hours of adequate light and good housing and nutrition to ensure success.

Because of the considerable variation in the duration of oestrus during the transitional period, efficient breeding of the mare can be difficult. It is recommended that the interval between matings should not exceed 2 or 3 days, although there have been no critical studies on the survival time of sperm in the mares' genital tract. It is important not to begin mating too early or this will result in the mare being mated many times. The appearance of uterine oedema is an indication that the follicle should ovulate within a few days.

Cystic ovarian disease comparable to that described in cattle (see p. 362) does not occur in the mare. The persistent follicles which occur during the transitional and other periods are structurally normal; however, their presence may explain why the diagnosis of this condition has been made in the past.

Ovarian neoplasia
This has been considered earlier under structural infertility.

Chromosomal abnormalities
The normal chromosome complement for the domestic horse is $2n=64$. Various sex chromosome anomalies have been described in the horse, and these are described in detail in Chapter 4. The incidence of chromosomal abnormalities is difficult to assess, but must be suspected in mares with small, inactive ovaries and an immature tubular genital tract. However, some genetically normal young fillies in training can be acyclic, and thus they must be given more time to mature and karyotyping must be performed before making a final diagnosis.

Ovulatory dysfunction
Anovulatory haemorrhagic follicles
The most common form of ovulation failure in mares is when the preovulatory follicle fails to rupture, but fills with blood. The condition is known as 'haemorrhagic anovulatory follicle syndrome'. In one recent study, 12 cases occurred in eight mares during 213 ovulatory intervals monitored by ultrasound (Ginther and Pierson, 1989). Where this occurs, the preovulatory follicle fills with blood and is initially recognized, using transrectal ultrasound, by the presence of scattered free-floating echogenic spots within the follicular antrum. As the blood coagulates, the ultrasonic appearance varies from a speckled to a uniformly echogenic mass (Figure 26.4), These structures can be as large as 8–10 cm, occasionally much larger, and develop an outer wall of luteal tissue. Functionally, they gradually regress in the same way as a normal corpus luteum, but they remain visible ultrasonically over subsequent oestrous cycles.

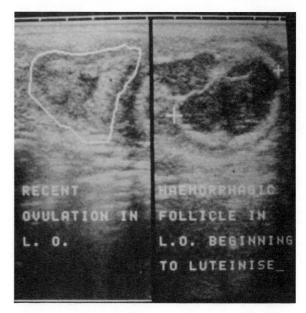

Fig. 26.4 Ultrasound image of a haemorrhagic follicle. A thick (4–7 mm) outer wall with an echotexture consistent with that of luteal tissue is visible.

The cause of these haemorrhagic follicles is not known. Similar structures are seen under continued equine chorionic gonadotrophin (eCG) stimulation during days 40–150 of pregnancy.

Anovulatory follicles in aged mares
Some aged mares, particularly over 20 years of age, fail to ovulate despite showing oestrous behaviour, and hence it may not be detected. On ultrasound examination their ovaries resemble those of seasonally anovulatory mares with a few small (< 10 mm) follicles. Endometrial biopsy shows evidence of gland atrophy. Currently there is no treatment, but identification of such mares is important to avoid unnecessary services.

Multiple ovulation
Double ovulations occur during 8–25% of oestrous cycles, the frequency depending upon the breed and type of the mare (Thoroughbreds, highest rate; ponies, lowest rate). Accurate detection of such ovulations is important as twinning is undesirable, firstly because it accounts for 10–30% of abortions and, secondly, even if both fetuses survive and are carried to term, many are dysmature, resulting in a high neonatal mortality rate. A further complication is that if embryonic/fetal death occurs after the formation of the endometrial cups (see

Chapter 3) these latter structures persist until they spontaneously regress as if pregnancy had been maintained, resulting in pseudopregnancy.

The reason for the low survival rate of twins is due to competition for placental space. Recent studies using transrectal ultrasound imaging has shown that the mare has an embryo reduction mechanism (see the review by Ginther, 1988) so that there is a wide disparity between the number of double ovulations and twin births. Most embryo reduction occurs after fixation at day 17 (see Chapter 3), and it is greatest when it occurs in the same horn and when the conceptuses are of unequal size. A deprivation hypothesis has been suggested (Ginther, 1989).

Management of twin ovulation

There are two approaches to dealing with twins:

1. If the initial examination of the mare is done before fixation (day 16/17) the twin embryos are reduced to a singleton by the manual destruction of one, either by pressure with the transducer or the use of the hand (Figure 26.5). The author prefers to gently separate the conceptual vesicles using the transducer to enable the procedure to be imaged. Where the conceptual vesicles are of dissimilar sizes, the smaller one should be ruptured. This is easier at days 14–16 when they are 14–20 mm in diameter than days 11–13 when they are 6–11 mm in diameter. Disadvantages of this method include expense, as all mares are scanned before the time of return to oestrus. In addition, if ovulations which occur more than 3 days apart have not been detected, a mistaken diagnosis of a single pregnancy may be made if the second vesicle is too small to detect. However, with experience, this technique is highly effective, and it is the method of choice of the author.

2. If initial examination is done after fixation, but before day 30, then if both conceptuses are in one horn they cannot be separated at this stage and the pregnancy can be terminated by use of $PGF_{2\alpha}$, the mare can be re-examined 5 days later in the event that reduction has occurred, or transvaginal ultrasound-guided allantocentesis can be attempted. Management of twin pregnancies after this period is complicated by the formation of endometrial cups at approximately day 37/38 of gestation. Endometrial cups remain functional until around days 90–130 of gestation in the pre-

sence or absence of a viable fetus. Therefore, if twin pregnancies are not successfully managed before the cups are formed or both embryos die after day 37, the mare usually will not return to a fertile oestrus for a prolonged period of time.

Methods of managing twins after day 37 of gestation are variable and unreliable. Dietary energy restriction, surgical removal of one vesicle, intracardiac injection of potassium chloride using transabdominal ultrasound and, most recently, transvaginal ultrasound-guided allantocentesis have all been attempted. The latter would appear to offer the best approach and has been successfully used by the author on several occasions.

Although accurate interpretation of the ultrasound image of early pregnancies in the mare and the technique of crushing a conceptus are skills which need experience, the advent of B-mode ultrasound imaging has provided a method of more readily managing twin pregnancy in the mare. Consequently, multiple ovulation in the mare should not be regarded as a reason for withholding mating. In fact, pregnancy rates are improved after twin ovulation.

Pregnancy failure

Pregnancy failure is a source of major economic loss to the horse industry. Embryonic death occurs before 40 days of gestation when organogenesis is complete, with early embryonic death (EED) occurring before the maternal recognition of pregnancy (see Chapter 3). Early fetal death occurs before 150 days of gestation; thus, late fetal death occurs afterwards. Abortion is defined as expulsion of the fetus and its membranes before 300 days, whereas a stillbirth is expulsion of the fetus and its membranes from day 300 onwards.

Embryonic death

In normal fertile mares the fertilization rate is over 90%, which is comparable with other domestic species, with estimates of the EED rate at between 5 and 24%. In subfertile mares, the rate is higher. The differences in the estimates are due to varying methods of pregnancy detection, and the animals studied. The period of greatest embryonic death in subfertile mares occurs in the interval before pregnancy can be detected with ultrasound (day 11), particularly at the time the embryo enters the uterus. Between days 14 and

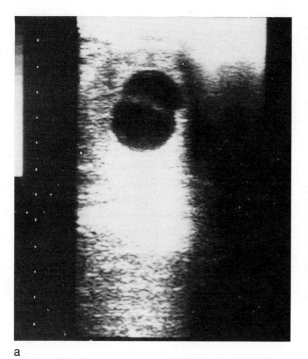

a

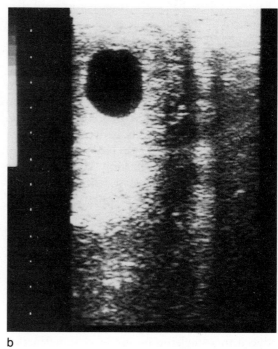

b

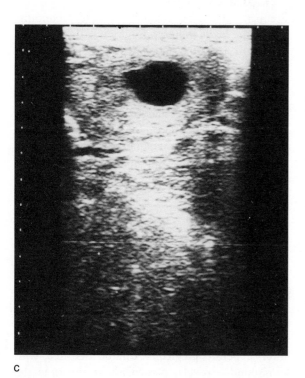

c

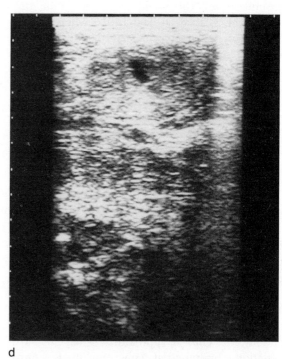

d

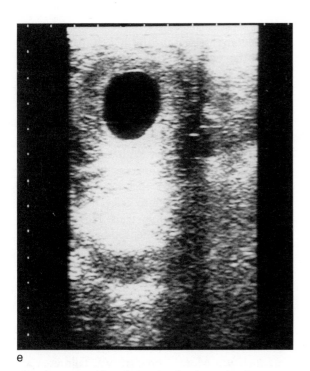

e

Fig. 26.5 Ultrasound images of a unilateral set of twin 16 day pregnancies. (a) Unilateral twin pregnancy. (b) By gentle pressure with the transducer, one of the conceptuses has been moved apart from the other. (c) Pressure is put on the selected conceptus using the transducer. The spherical shape is lost and then a distinct popping sensation is felt. (d) The small amount of fluid visible is rapidly resorbed. (e) The normal-looking remaining conceptus.

40, the rate of embryonic death varies between 10 and 17%. EED is multifactorial, in which external factors such as the environment and management as well as pathophysiological factors are involved. However, the evidence for many of these associations are anecdotal and frequently contradictory.

External Factors. These include stress, nutrition, season of the year, climate, sire effects and rectal palpation.

Maternal stress due to severe pain, malnutrition and transport has been implicated as a cause of EED. Frequently, mares at stud are transported at various stages of pregnancy; recent work failed to demonstrate any difference in pregnancy rates between transported and non-transported mares. Transporting pregnant mares home from stud a distance of 300 miles (500 km) in less than 9 hours of travelling time can be stressful, but should not result in embryonic death. If a longer journey is necessary, the journey should be broken after 8 hours. Waiting until the fifth week of pregnancy, or later, to transport broodmares may be advisable when critical events such as descent of the embryo into the uterus and transition from the yolk sac to the chorioallantoic placentation has occurred. The common practice of transporting mares to stud for mating and returning home the same day should not be detrimental to their fertility as long as the transport is safe and comfortable.

Far from being avoided, regular exercise is important during pregnancy, although during the latter half, forced exercise should be decreased. Rectal palpation and ultrasound examinations should be considered safe procedures when performed correctly, and recent evidence (Vogelsang et al., 1989) gives no indication that ultrasound examination damages the embryo.

Maternal Factors. A number of maternal factors including hormone deficiencies and imbalance, uterine environment, age and lactation have been implicated.

Hormonal deficiencies and imbalance. Progesterone is critical for the maintenance of pregnancy in mares. The only source of progesterone during the embryonic period is the primary corpus luteum. On the assumption that luteal insufficiency is important in EED, many mares are given exogenous progesterone or progestogens in an attempt to prevent it occurring. However, the rationale for this widespread practice is highly questionable, although primary luteal insufficiency as a cause of EED has been reported by Bergfelt et al. (1992). Progesterone supplementation has been recently reviewed by Allen (1993), who is sceptical of any benefit. Many dosage regimens used do not effectively elevate or maintain plasma progesterone levels. Withdrawal of supplementary progesterone therapy during midgestation may leave the clinician open to criticism if the mare subsequently aborts. In the author's opinion, progesterone therapy is most appropriate in mares which have uterine oedema and an indistinct corpus luteum at the time of first examination for pregnancy (15 days).

Uterine environment. An abnormal uterine environment is detrimental to embryonic survival. Endometritis may result in EED by inducing premature luteolysis or because of its direct effect on the embryo. Ideally, it would be preferable to avoid mating mares with acute endometritis; however, with the development of more effective treatments for postmating endometritis, in certain cases it may be preferable to mate mares even if there is evidence of the acute disease (see p. 486).

Severe periglandular fibrosis of the uterine glands may reduce the chances of embryo survival. Not only is this a response to persistent endometritis, but it also increases with age. This is one of the reasons for the reduced fertility of mares over 12 years of age, for despite similar fertilization rates, detected pregnancy rates are on average 33% lower. Paradoxically, increased embryonic death is occasionally seen in mares that are bred at a young age (11–16 months); the reasons for this are not known.

The mare normally resumes cyclical ovarian activity very shortly after parturition so that they are sometimes served as early as 7–10 days postpartum (at the foal heat). There is conflicting evidence about the level of embryonic death if fertilization occurs at this time, with some studies showing a higher rate and others no effect. A clear advantage of breeding at the first oestrus postpartum is that the foaling to conception interval is significantly shorter; 25 versus 44 days has been reported.

The reasons for the apparent decreased fertility in mares mated at the foal heat is the hostile uterine environment due to delayed uterine involution or persistent endometritis. However, pregnancy rates are clearly influenced by how strict the selection criteria are for mating at the foal heat. Traditionally, such factors as a normal foaling, placental expulsion, minimal vaginal bruising and absence of infection have been used. Endometrial cytology and ultrasonic scanning of the genital tract of each mare may be more reliable methods on which to base a decision.

Lactation. More pregnancy failures are detected in lactating than non-lactating (maiden or barren) mares; this also increases with the age of the mare.

Embryonic Factors. Embryonic abnormalities are also important to consider in relation to embryonic death. Embryos recovered from subfertile mares are smaller and have more morphological

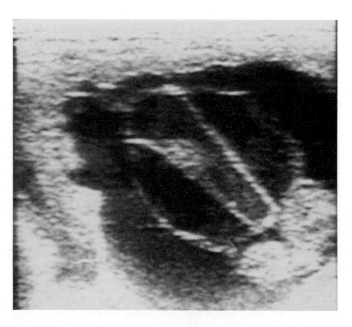

Fig. 26.6 Ultrasound image illustrating gestational failure in a 42 day pregnancy. Note the disruption of the fetal membranes (amnion and allantochorion).

defects than embryos from fertile mares; however, this may be due to an abnormal uterine environment.

Ultrasonic scanning has provided a valuable tool in studying embryonic death. Because pregnancy is often diagnosed at an early stage, it is important to inform owners that not all pregnancies detected with ultrasound will survive, even in apparently normal mares. There are certain morphological features detected with ultrasound that are typical of mares in which embryonic death is occurring. Some of the consistent features include: (1) presence of fluid within the uterine lumen; (2) prominent endometrial oedema; (3) decreased or prolonged conceptus mobility; (4) undersized or irregularly shaped conceptus; (5) cessation of embryonic heart beat; (6) reduced volume of placental fluids; (7) disorganization of placental membranes (Figure 26.6); (8) hyperechogenic areas in the embryo and membranes.

Fetal death/abortion

An overall abortion rate after 60 days of gestation of 10% is usually cited for the horse. In practice, it is important to distinguish infectious from non-infectious causes. Vaginal discharge, premature lactation and colic in pregnant mares may indicate an impending or recent abortion. Whatever the suspected cause, the general approach to the management of an aborting mare should always follow the UK Code of Practice as drawn up by the Horserace Betting Levy Board. All veterinary surgeons must have a copy of this code, which is updated annually.

When abortion occurs, the mare should be isolated, a history obtained and the fetus sent to an approved laboratory for autopsy. If a veterinary surgeon wishes to perform a post-mortem examination, small but representative samples of liver, lung, thymus, spleen and chorioallantois (two samples, one of which is from the cervical star, which is the irregular, star-shaped avillous area of the chorion that lies over the internal os of the cervix) (see p. 59) should be sent in formal saline for histological examination. In addition, frozen samples of fresh fetal liver and lung should be stored in a deep freeze at −20°C should viral isolation investigation be required at a later stage. Paired serum samples from the mare and close companions should also be taken for serological investigation. Swabs from fetal heart or liver and

the cervical pole of the chorion are used to screen for bacterial infection.

The fetus and fetal membranes (amnion, chorioallantois and umbilical cord) must be carefully examined for the presence of abnormalities and areas of discoloration.

The causes of equine abortion can be broadly divided into non-infectious (70%), infectious (15%) and unknown (15%).

Non-infectious Causes of Abortion and Stillbirth. *Twinning.* Historically, twins have been the single most important cause of abortion in Thoroughbreds (see p. 478). However, it is now much less common due to the widespread use of ultrasonography. The diagnosis of twin pregnancy can be made even if only one fetus is found, as examination of the placenta reveals an area devoid of villi where the two placentas were in contact. Twins should still be submitted to a diagnostic laboratory as twin pregnancies are not protected from equine herpes virus (EHV) infection.

Umbilical cord abnormalities. In mares, the umbilical cord is twisted, usually in a clockwise spiral. The normal length ranges from 36 to 83 cm (mean 55 cm). Increased cord length has been associated with excessive cord torsion, which can cause vascular obstruction of the urachus. This can result in abortion of an autolysed fetus. Decreased cord length can cause premature tearing of fetal membranes, leading to fetal asphyxia.

Premature placental separation. In mares, the interdigitating microvilli are connected by an unidentified electron-dense material. Placental separation involves dissolution of this substance. Causes of premature placental separation are largely unknown although maternal stress and endophyte-contaminated tall fescue have been implicated. When placental separation occurs shortly before parturition, the thickened placenta often does not rupture through the cervical star, and the allantochorion bulges out of the vulva ('redbag' delivery). The foal can become hypoxic, resulting in the neonatal maladjustment syndrome.

Body pregnancy. In this condition almost the entire chorionic surface of the placenta contained within the uterine body is without villi, while that contained within the horns is covered with an excessive number of villi. The proportion of the placenta corresponding to the two uterine horns is small, and the fetus is situated entirely within the uterine body. The fetus is frequently aborted completely contained within its placenta; its growth has been retarded. The abortion occurs when the nutritional demands of the fetus exceed the ability of the placenta to meet them.

Fetal abnormalities. Severe developmental anomalies involving the central nervous system or development of body cavities have been reported in aborted fetuses (see Chapter 4).

Maternal disease. Pyrexia, and malnutrition during pregnancy, have been implicated as causes of abortion.

INFECTIOUS CAUSES OF INFERTILITY

Viral abortion

Equine herpesvirus (EHV)

EHV is the single most important infectious cause of equine abortion. The disease is caused by EHV-1 and, rarely, EHV-4. EHV-1 is also capable of causing respiratory disease (most noticeable in foals and yearlings) and paralysis. EHV-4 normally causes respiratory disease, but occasionally has caused abortion. Clinical signs of herpesvirus infection of the respiratory tract are not distinguishable from those caused by other viruses (and secondary bacterial infection), namely nasal discharge, transient pyrexia and depression. The source of the virus is:

1. Clinically affected animals with nasal secretions.
2. Aborted fetuses and their membranes.
3. Infected foals born live at term.
4. Mares which have aborted, although they only shed virus from the genital tract for a short period.
5. Asymptomatic virus excreters.

Naturally acquired immunity after EHV-1 infection is short lived, so that even after only a few weeks or months reinfection is possible. Evidence has also been found of latent EHV-1 infection, with the virus remaining dormant in the reticuloendothelial cells of clinically normal animals for an unspecified length of time. Stress can activate the virus.

The majority of EHV-1 abortions occur in the last 4 months of gestation. The mares shows no signs of impending abortion or clinical disease. The fetus is usually fresh and still enclosed in its membranes, and typically has excess serosal fluids, minute spots on the liver, jaundice of the mucous and placental membranes, enlarged spleen, perirenal oedema and pulmonary haemorrhages. Rarely, some foals survive for up to 7 days, but they are weak, jaundiced and have a marked leucopenia. Histological lesions include foci of necrosis and eosinophilic intranuclear inclusion bodies seen in degenerating hepatocytes and/or bronchiolar epithelial cells. Virus isolation is possible from lung, liver and thymus samples which have been submitted in viral transport medium. Fluorescent antibody tests can be performed on frozen sections of liver and lung. Unfortunately, there is no test to detect latent carriers.

Control of EHV-1 infection is considered in detail in the Code of Conduct. Groups of mixed ages and reproductive status are most at risk from virus abortion, thus racehorses, hunters, weaned foals and yearlings should be kept away from pregnant mares. The pregnant mares should be kept in small groups, isolated from each other. All abortions and stillbirths should be investigated and the mare isolated pending the results. Newly arrived animals should never be mixed with pregnant mares on a farm.

A killed-virus vaccine and an attenuated live-virus vaccine are available commercially. However, only the killed-virus vaccine (Pneumabort-K, Willows Francis Ltd) is licensed for the prevention of abortion in mares in the UK, and the manufacturer advises that it is given during the fifth, seventh and ninth months of pregnancy. Results following vaccination are conflicting. It would seem most likely that, while vaccination does not prevent an individual animal aborting, if the stud has a vaccination policy, than the likelihood of an abortion storm is much reduced.

Equine viral arteritis (EVA)

Equine viral arteritis is a contagious viral disease of the horse that in recent years has become important for the Standardbred and Thoroughbred industries in the USA. An EVA outbreak was identified for the first time in the UK in 1993. The principal focus of the infection was an Anglo-Arab stallion imported from Poland.

The two important routes of EVA transmission are venereal, and aerosol via the respiratory secretions of an acutely infected horse. After an average incubation period of 7 days, EVA is excreted in all bodily secretions, including respiratory secretions and urine for up to 21 days (possibly longer in urine); close or direct contact is required for aerosol transmission to occur. Venereal transmission is believed to be the major cause of widespread dissemination of the virus. Stallions that become persistently infected with EVA shed the virus in the semen, which appears to be the sole route. In breeds that permit the use of artificial insemination, the virus can be transmitted through the use of fresh, chilled or frozen semen. Interestingly, marked changes in semen quality in stallions experimentally infected with EVA have recently been described (Neu et al., 1992). The recent outbreak in the UK was initially suspected after a semen sample from the affected stallion was routinely evaluated prior to its use to artificially inseminate a mare.

At present, there is no effective treatment for a chronically infected stallion. Such animals can remain persistently infected with the virus in the reproductive tract for variable periods of time, from several months to a period of years and, in some cases, the lifetime of a particular stallion. Up to now, there is no evidence that mares, geldings or foals that acquire the infection congenitally become carriers.

Clinical signs of EVA are very variable, and subclinical infections are the most common sequel. The classic clinical signs are of an influenza-like illness with pyrexia for 1–5 days, depression, a nasal discharge, conjunctivitis, anorexia, a focal dermatitis and oedema of the limbs, ventral abdomen, scrotum, prepuce and periorbital regions. Abortion may occur during, or shortly after, an acute illness or subclinical infection. Abortion occurs as a result of myometrial necrosis and oedema leading to placental detachment, and hence fetal death. Abortions tend to occur in the latter half of pregnancy.

A definitive diagnosis, based on clinical signs alone, is not possible due to their variable nature. Acute EVA can be confirmed by virus isolation from nasopharyngeal swabs, heparinized blood samples, and urine and semen samples. Serological evidence of EVA exposure can be found by taking an initial serum sample as soon as possible after clinical onset, followed by a convalescent sample 10–14 days later to detect a rise in the EVA antibody titre. Diagnosis of abortion due to EVA is largely dependent on virus isolation from the placenta or fetal tissues; there are no pathognomonic gross lesions. Mares infected with EVA will usually abort partially autolysed fetuses, in contrast to fresh fetuses aborted by mares infected with herpesvirus.

Since virtually all acutely infected horses recover uneventfully after EVA, any treatment is symptomatic. In the UK, the Code of Practice considers control measures for EVA and provides guidance in the event of an outbreak. A modified live-virus vaccine is available in North America, whereas a killed vaccine (Artervac, Willows Francis Ltd) is available in the UK. It must be remembered that certain countries will not accept the importation of seropositive animals. If an animal is to be vaccinated, a blood sample for serology should be taken prior to vaccination. A second blood sample should be taken 10 days after the second vaccination to ensure a serological response to vaccination. From the start of the 1994 breeding season many studs in the UK are requiring confirmation that mares are seronegative to EVA prior to arrival at stud. Vaccination of stallions is being widely adopted.

Bacterial abortion

A large number of bacterial species which gain access to the placenta can cause abortion in the mare. The ascending pathway via the cervix is the primary route of infection, and most infections occur in early pregnancy. Rarely, bacteria may be in the uterus at the time of conception or arrive haematogenously. Bacteria which spread rapidly through the allantochorion often infect the fetus, causing acute bacterial septicaemia. More chronic ascending infections are often localized around the cervical star and cause a focal or local placentitis. The placentitis often leads to placental insufficiency with abortion of a growth-retarded fetus, or the birth of a dysmature foal. The placenta is often thickened and covered with exudate and the fetus septicaemic. Bacteria that cause placentitis are similar to the organisms that cause endometritis (see below). They are often opportunist pathogens that can be isolated from the caudal genital tract of normal mares, i.e. *Streptococcus* spp. and *Escherichia coli*. Others are considered to be venereal pathogens, i.e. *Pseudomonas* spp. and *Klebsiella* spp.

Recently, leptospirosis has been diagnosed in association with abortion in Kentucky in the USA and Ireland. Leptospiral abortion is difficult to confirm because there are no clinical signs in the mares prior to abortion. Demonstrations of leptospires in fetal tissues and the placenta by immunofluorescence, and serology in mares, are needed for a diagnosis. Treatment of carriers with antibiotics is generally considered useful, but may not eliminate the shedding of the organism.

Fungal abortion

Aspergillus spp. are the most common cause of mycotic placentitis and mycotic abortion in the mare. Much less common is placentitis due to *Candida* spp. infection. Fungal disease has a similar pathogenesis to bacterial abortion with inflammation of the chorion beginning at the cervical pole.

Endometritis

Cause and Pathogenesis

Reduced fertility associated with endometritis, both acute and chronic, has been recognized for many years in broodmares. The term 'endometritis' refers to the acute or chronic inflammatory changes involving the endometrium. These changes frequently occur as a result of microbial infection, but they can also be due to non-infectious causes.

It is generally assumed that the uterine lumen of the normal fertile mare is bacteriologically sterile or may have a temporary, non-resident microflora, although bacteria have been seen in healthy uteri by scanning electron microscopy. Ricketts and Mackintosh (1987) suggested that the equine uterus may harbour obligate anaerobes as surface commensals.

The environment of the uterine lumen must be compatible with embryonic and fetal life. This presents a particular problem for the mare as a transient endometritis is an inevitable sequel to coitus. Ejaculation occurs through the dilated cervix, contaminating the uterine lumen with microorganisms and debris. Parturition and a defective perineal conformation can also result in contamination. In the normal healthy mare, the induced postcoital endometritis resolves within 24–72 hours. Microorganisms and inflammatory by-products disappear from the uterus to leave the endometrium in a satisfactory state to receive the fertilized ovum. Timing is critical, as the embryo descends from the uterine tube into the uterine lumen about $5\frac{1}{2}$ days after ovulation. In addition to being incompatible with embryonic survival,

endometritis persisting after day 4 of dioestrus also causes lysis of the corpus luteum due to premature endogenous prostaglandin release so that the mare has a shortened luteal phase.

In some mares the inflammation persists; these are referred to as susceptible individuals. The concept of susceptibility to endometritis was first suggested by Farrely and Mullaney (1964), who stated that infective endometritis is essentially the failure of as individual mare to limit the uterine and cervical microflora to a non-resident type. Hughes and Loy (1969) developed this concept and confirmed that resistant mares could eliminate induced infection without treatment; susceptible mares could not. In general, reduced resistance to endometritis is associated with advancing age and multiparity. Susceptibility to endometritis is not, however, an absolute state since failure of uterine defence mechanisms need only slow the process of eliminating infection.

Studies on immunoglobulins, opsonins and the functional ability of neutrophils in the uterus of susceptible mares have not confirmed the presence of an impaired immune response (see the review by Allen and Pycock, 1989). Evans et al. (1986) first suggested that reduced physical drainage may contribute to an increased susceptibility to uterine infection. The physical ability of the uterus to eliminate bacteria, inflammatory debris and fluid is now known to be a critical factor in uterine defence. Since the first description of the identification of the collection of small volumes of intrauterine fluid using ultrasound, which could not be palpated per rectum (Ginther and Pierson, 1984), general awareness of the frequency of this abnormality has increased. The detection of uterine fluid during both oestrus (Figure 26.7) and dioestrus has been reported (Allen and Pycock, 1988). Endometrial secretions and the formation of the small volume of free fluid may be associated with the same mechanism which causes normal oestral oedema. Small volumes of intrauterine fluid during oestrus do not affect pregnancy rates (Pycock and Newcombe, 1995a), but in mares that are susceptible to endometritis there is an accumulation of more fluid than in resistant mares. Intrauterine fluid during dioestrus is indicative of inflammation, and associated with subfertility, due to early embryonic death and a shortened luteal phase.

Initially, although a sterile transudate, fluid may

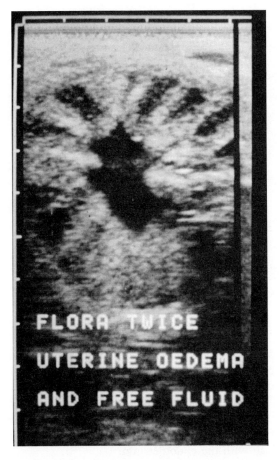

Fig. 26.7 Ultrasound image of fluid in the uterine body during oestrus. The depth is 20 mm, and the fluid is non-echogenic. The mottled appearance of the uterus suggests the mare is in oestrus.

act as a medium for bacteria which gain entry to the uterus at mating to multiply; it may also be spermicidal.

The bacterial species which cause bacterial endometritis are numerous, and can be classified as follows: (1) contaminants and commensals; (2) opportunist, causing an acute endometritis; and (3) venereally transmitted. Normally, the vestibular and clitoral area has a harmless and constantly fluctuating bacterial population. In association with benign saprophytic organisms, opportunistic organisms such as *Streptococcus zooepidemicus*, *E. coli* and *Staphyloccocus* spp. can be found. The stallion's penis is colonized by similar organisms. *S. zooepidemicus* is the most commonly isolated bacterial species from acute endometritis, particularly in the initial stages. *E. coli* is the next most common isolate.

In addition to these opportunist pathogens,

there are three bacteria which are venereally transmitted: *Taylorella equigenitalis* (contagious equine metritis organism, CEMO), *Klebsiella pneumoniae* (capsular types 1, 2 and 5) and *Pseudomonas aeruginosa* (some strains).

Symptomless carriers of both sexes allow persistence within the horse population. Carrier mares, which may or may not have shown signs of previous endometritis, harbour the organisms in the vestibular area, particularly the clitoral fossa and sinuses. Mating or gynaecological examination may result in their transfer into the uterus. Stallions may harbour the organisms over the entire surface of the penis and in the distal urethra. Control is by routine screening of swabs taken before mating by laboratories experienced in the isolation and identification of these specific organisms. Details of the control procedures for contagious equine metritis (CEM) and the other venereal pathogens are in the Horserace Betting Levy Board's Code of Practice.

Anaerobic bacteria have been isolated from the mare's uterus, with *Bacteroides fragilis* the most frequent. Further work is needed to assess the importance of anaerobes in endometritis.

Culture techniques and diagnosis of endometritis

Venereal Disease Screening. Before the breeding season, swabs should be taken from the clitoral fossa and clitoral sinuses (only the central sinus may be obvious), and the vestibule. The perineal area of the mare should not be cleaned except for the removal of gross contamination of the vulva with faeces using a dry paper towel. A protective disposable glove should be worn by the veterinary surgeon on the hand used to evert the ventral commisure of the vulva and expose the clitoris. The swabs should be placed in transport medium, clearly labelled with the mare's name and sent to an approved laboratory. It is important to penetrate the clitoral sinus, and therefore a large swab tip should not be used. Swabs are cultured aerobically on blood and MacConkey agar to screen for the presence of *K. pneumoniae* and *P. aeruginosa*. Microaerophilic culture on chocolate blood agar (with and without streptomycin) must also be done for the detection of CEMO. In addition, in stallions two sets of swabs must be taken from the pre-ejaculatory fluid (if possible), penile sheath, urethra and urethral fossa.

In the UK, this screening has been successful in

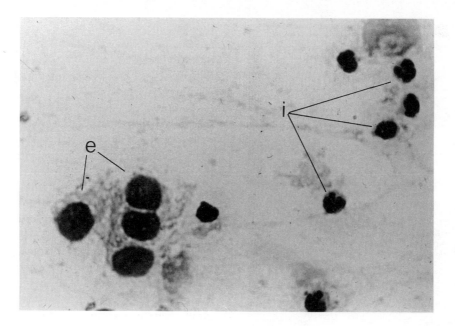

Fig. 26.8 Stained endometrial smear (Diff-Kwik, American Hospital Supplies) showing inflammatory (i) and endometrial (e) cells.

virtually eradicating CEM and vastly reducing the incidence of venereal disease.

Diagnosis of Endometritis. A diagnosis of endometritis can be made by collection of concurrent endometrial swab and smear samples during early oestrus for bacteriological culture and cytological examination, respectively. This allows time for resolution prior to mating, and maximizes the chances of pregnancy. The ideal technique should ensure that the swab enters the uterus and collects bacteria from only the uterine lumen. Two methods can be used:

1. A non-guarded endometrial swab on a sterile extension rod is carefully passed via a sterile speculum through the cervix into the uterine body and, after withdrawal, is placed in transport medium. A second swab is taken immediately afterwards for the endometrial smear.

2. A guarded swab is passed into the uterine lumen using a sterile speculum or enclosed in a disposable plastic arm-length glove. The swab tip is exposed only when it is in the uterine lumen. A second swab for cytological examination should again be taken. Swabs for culture should be plated on blood and MacConkey agar, and incubated at 37°C for 48 hours. Cultures should be examined at 24 and 48 hours. An air-dried smear is made by gently rolling the second swab either on a Test-simplet (Boehringer Corporation), which is a pre-stained slide or a clean dry microscope slide. The smear can be differentially stained with a rapid stain such as Diff-Kwik (American Hospital Supplies). The stained smear should then be examined for the presence of inflammatory and endometrial cells (Figure 26.8), the latter confirming contact of the swab with the endometrium.

Interpretation. A positive culture result, with no evidence of inflammatory cells in the smear (usually neutrophils), is likely to be due to contamination during collection. Diagnosis is based on the presence or absence of significant numbers of neutrophils in the smear. Very rarely, neutrophils can be detected, usually at the 'foal heat' or the first oestrus of the breeding season in maiden mares, although there is no endometritis.

Detection of Intraluminal Uterine Fluid Using Transrectal Ultrasound Imaging. Transrectal ultrasonography provides a non-invasive method of assessment of the uterus. In a study involving the ultrasonic examination and cytological and bacteriological sampling of the uterus in 380 broodmares premating, the author concluded that:

1. If no free fluid is detected during oestrus, then acute endometritis as detected in cytology is absent in 99% of cases.

2. Free fluid does not indicate inflammation.

3. Endometrial cytology and culture fails to detect sterile fluid accumulations.

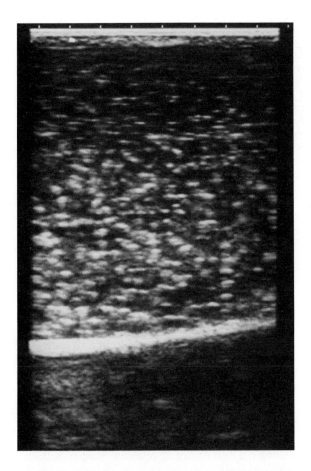

Fig. 26.9 Ultrasound image obtained with the transducer in a bucket of clean water. The hyperechoic foci are air bubbles which would wrongly be interpreted as cellular debris. Intrauterine fluid must not be assumed to be cellular because of hyperechoic foci.

It is suggested that intraluminal uterine fluid can be graded according to the degree of echogenicity, so that there is likely to be endometritis if the fluid is hyperechogenic rather than non-echogenic (McKinnon et al., 1987). In many cases, the author has found that interpretation of the cellular content of fluid on the basis of its ultrasonic appearance is difficult. Echogenicity may be proportional to the size and concentration of particulate matter within the fluid, rather than the viscocity of the fluid; for example, purulent exudates can appear non-echogenic. Air has hyperechoic foci, and the fluid with air bubbles appears cellular (Figure 26.9). Urine often appears echogenic.

Endometrial Biopsy. In some cases, endometrial biopsy may be a useful diagnostic aid. For detailed reviews of the clinical application and pathological findings in acute and chronic endometritis and endometrosis readers should consult Kenney (1978) and Ricketts (1978). The technique involves the insertion of a biopsy instrument through the cervix and into the uterus. With the biopsy instrument in the uterine lumen, a gloved hand is inserted into the rectum to allow manipulation of the instrument into the desired position. The sample is taken by closing the jaws of the instrument and tugging sharply. To avoid damage, the tissue is carefully transferred into a fixative solution by dislodging it from the jaws of the punch with a fine hypodermic needle. The instrument most commonly used today is the Yeoman (basket-jawed) biopsy forceps (Figure 26.10), ideally 60–70 cm in length, with which tissue specimens 2 × 1 cm (about 0.2% of the whole endometrial surface) are obtained. If the uterus appears normal on palpation, the sample should be taken from one of the areas of embryo fixation, i.e. the uterine horn–body junction on either side. Single samples are usually representative of the entire endometrium. If the uterus is abnormal on palpation per rectum, biopsy samples should be taken from both the affected area and a normal area. Biopsy specimens should be fixed in Bouin's fluid followed by sectioning and staining with haematoxylin and eosin. The endometrial biopsy sample should be sent to a laboratory that is experienced in evaluating samples.

Treatment of endometritis

Antibiotic Therapy. The traditional approach to treating endometritis has been the infusion of various antibiotics, dissolved or suspended in water or saline, into the uterine lumen during oestrus. The intrauterine route is preferable to systemic therapy as most acute endometritis cases are localized. Systemic treatment alone or in combination with local application is suitable in a few circumstances. Ideally, the choice of antibiotic for local treatment should be based on *in vitro* antibiotic sensitivity tests. However, in many cases this is not possible and a broad-spectrum combination is used. A particularly successful preparation has been a water-soluble mixture of neomycin (1 g), polymyxin B (40 000 IU), furaltadone (600 mg) (Utrin Wash; Univet) and crystalline benzylpenicillin (5 megaunits) dissolved in 30 ml of sterile water and then instilled into the uterus via a sterile irrigation catheter. This is inserted through the

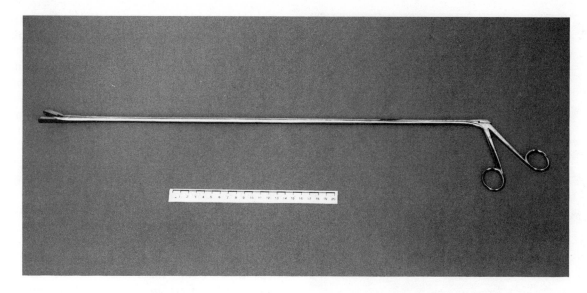

Fig. 26.10 Yeoman (basket-jawed) endometrial biopsy forceps.

cervix into the uterus along the index finger which has been introduced through the external os uteri. If the tip cannot be advanced once it has passed through the cervix, it may be helpful to direct the tip of the catheter downwards. The use of this extremely broad-spectrum preparation, has not resulted in superinfection with *Pseudomonas* spp., *Klebsiella* spp. or fungi. The number of infusions required depends on individual circumstances. The success of this treatment can be monitored using ultrasonography to identify the presence of intrauterine fluid. When antibiotics are combined with oxytocin (see later) a single daily treatment for three days has, in many cases, proved successful. Repeated endometrial swab/smear examinations may be used to monitor the response to therapy; however, every time the cervix is breached there is the risk of introducing more bacteria. An indwelling intrauterine device has been used which can retain a narrow–diameter infusion catheter within the cervix; however, there is a risk of ascending infection.

Since within 2 hours of service the spermatozoa necessary for fertilization are present within the uterine tube, and since the embryo does not descend into the uterus for about 5.5 days, mares may be treated safely from 12 hours after mating until 3 days from ovulation, providing non-irritant therapy is used. However, progesterone concentrations rise rapidly following ovulation in the mare and it is preferable to avoid treatment involving uterine interference beyond 2 days after ovulation. Both coitus and artificial insemination can be a source of uterine contamination; therefore, the successful management of susceptible mares should logically require some form of postmating therapy such as intrauterine antibiotic infusion and intravenous oxytocin.

Intrauterine Plasma and Colostrum Infusions. Plasma is a rich source of opsonin. Studies, following intrauterine infusion, have shown improvements in fertility, and it was suggested that the plasma had an enhancing effect on phagocytosis by uterine neutrophils. However, in a controlled experiment, it was not found to be efficacious in treating endometritis, and pregnancy rates were not improved (Adams and Ginther, 1989).

Colostrum is a rich source of immunoglobulins, and has been used by intrauterine infusion as a treatment. Since mares that are susceptible to endometritis do not possess a quantitative deficiency of immunoglobulins, it is questionable if such treatment should be used. In addition, transfer of infectious agents is also possible.

Curettage. Improved fertility after endometrial curettage of barren mares has been reported. This has involved the use of mechanical and chemical agents (namely povidone–iodine and kerosene).

Hormonal Therapy. Exogenous oestrogens have been used as a treatment of endometritis and have been shown to enhance natural uterine defence mechanisms. Repeated treatment with

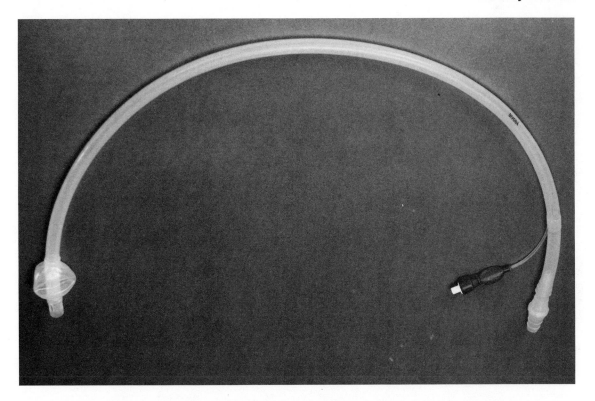

Fig. 26.11 Large-bore (30 French) embryo flushing catheter, 80 cm in length. Note inflated cuff.

PGF$_{2\alpha}$ increases the frequency of the follicular phases thus allowing intrauterine therapy to be used more readily. In addition, it also reduces the duration of the luteal phase where progesterone increases the susceptibility to infection.

Uterine Lavage. Recently, uterine lavage has become a popular treatment of endometritis. The technique involves the mechanical suction or siphonage of 1–2 litres of previously warmed saline infused into the uterus via a catheter that has been retained within the cervix by a cuff. The most convenient is a large-bore (30 French) (80 cm) equine embryo flushing catheter (EUF-80; Bivona) (Figure 26.11).

The rationale for such an approach are: (1) the removal of accumulated uterine fluid and inflammatory debris which may interfere with neutrophil function and the efficacy of antibiotics; (2) stimulation of uterine contractility; and (3) recruitment of fresh neutrophils through mechanical irritation of the endometrium.

The washings can also be inspected to provide immediate information concerning the nature of the uterine contents.

Oxytocin. The ideal method of treatment will involve the use of a non-invasive technique with early and complete elimination of any intrauterine fluid. Oxytocin stimulates uterine contractions in the cyclical and postpartum mare. Preliminary reports of its use to promote uterine drainage in mares susceptible to endometritis found that there was no adverse effect on fertility when used as an intravenous bolus of 10 IU (Allen, 1991). Subsequently, much success has been achieved with the use of 25 IU of oxytocin given as an intravenous bolus (Pycock, 1994b,c). No untoward effects have been noted apart from a very occasional mild and transient discomfort. Although the half-life of oxytocin has not been reported for the mare, it is likely to be between 2 and 10 minutes. In most mares the response is rapid, with fluid voided almost immediately. The process of drainage is illustrated (Figure 26.12).

The author has found the following regimen to be an effective treatment in the mare highly susceptible to endometritis, i.e. the mare that will pool much uterine fluid after mating: (1) a single mating must be arranged 2–3 days before the anticipated time of ovulation; (2) ultrasound examination of the uterus 3–12 hours after mating is used to assess the amount and echogenicity of any intrauterine fluid; (3) intravenous administration of

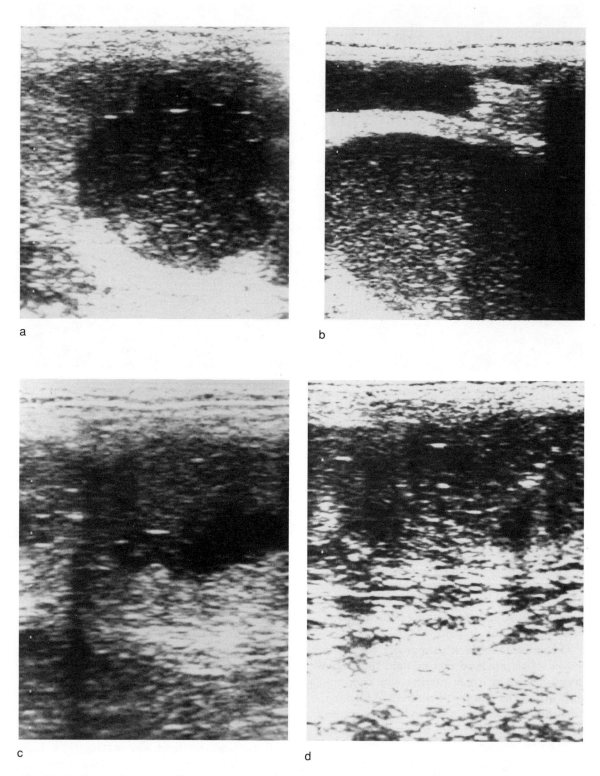

Fig. 26.12 Ultrasound images to illustrate intrauterine fluid removal with oxytocin. (a) Uterine body containing several centimetres of non-echoic fluid with hyperechoic foci. (b) Two minutes after oxytocin injection: fluid has been expelled via the cervix and can be imaged in the vagina; the cervix is to the right of the fluid. (c) Five minutes after oxytocin injection only a small depth of fluid remains in the uterus. (d) Thirty minutes after oxytocin injection the uterus is almost free of fluid. Air is seen as hyperechoic foci.

25 IU of oxytocin and manual dilation of the cervix in mares that exhibit intrauterine fluid; (4) infusion of a low volume of water-soluble broad-spectrum antibiotics into the uterus.

Asbury (1992) stated that there has been no corresponding improvement in the efficacy of the treatment of bacterial endometritis, despite the advances in the number and type of pharmacological agents available. Large field studies including proper controls are needed to critically evaluate therapy for endometritis. A recent clinical trial in over 1400 mares has shown that treatments with broad-spectrum antibiotic intrauterine infusions and intravenous oxytocin injection were effective in the treatment of endometritis and in the improvement of pregnancy rates (Pycock and Newcombe, 1995b).

Prevention
Good management also plays a vital role in the control and prevention of infectious infertility. Attention to hygiene at mating by using a tail bandage and washing the mare's vulva and perineal area with clean water (ideally from a spray nozzle which avoids the need for buckets) and limiting the number of matings are particularly important. Minimal contamination techniques in which semen extender containing antibiotics is infused into the uterus immediately before mating may be helpful.

Good hygiene at foaling is also essential and all mares should be thoroughly examined postpartum for the presence of trauma which might compromise the physical barriers to uterine contamination.

Gynaecological examinations, particularly of the vagina, should be performed as aseptically as possible. Since air in the vagina can cause irritation of the mucosa it should be expelled by applying downward pressure with the hand through the rectal wall.

Treatment of venereal infections
Any mare that is suspected of having a venereal infection must not be mated. In the case of clitoral or vestibular infections, topical treatment is used. This involves thorough cleaning with chlorhexidine surgical scrub followed by the application of 0.2% nitrofurazone ointment (*T. equigenitalis*), 0.3% gentamicin cream (*K. pneumoniae*) or silver nitrate and gentamicin cream (*P. aeruginosa*). These pathogens, particularly *P. aeruginosa*, are difficult to eliminate from the clitoris, hence clitoral sinusectomy or clitorectomy may have to be used in refractory cases. A broth culture containing a mixture of growing organisms prepared from the normal clitoral flora can suppress venereal pathogens in some cases. Evidence for the successful elimination of infection is based on three negative sets of clitoral and endometrial swabs, taken at weekly intervals.

Fungal infections
Mycotic endometritis is not as common as that of bacteriological origin, but recognition of a fungus as the causal agent is important since commonly used intrauterine antibiotic therapy is ineffective. In cases of fungal endometritis, mares may have a history of normal or abnormal oestrous cycles, they may be anoestrus or barren, and they may have had a recent abortion or a fetal membrane retention; in addition there may be a history of repeated intrauterine antibiotic therapy. Yeasts more frequently cause endometritis than moulds; *Candida albicans* is the most common isolate.

Diagnosis
This is based upon the presence of fungal elements and inflammatory cells in endometrial smears. In addition, yeasts can also be identified following staining with 'Diff-Kwik' (American Hospital Supplies) using a magnification of 400. Fungal elements are more readily identified in endometrial biopsies following staining with Gomori's methenamine silver or periodic acid–Schiff (PAS).

Successful culture of endometrial smears for fungi can be difficult because the organisms may be present in low numbers, and furthermore they require a long incubation period. For example, studies in Florida, USA, where *C. albicans* infection is very common, have shown that despite the identification of yeast buds in stained smears in the presence of neutrophils, the organism was frequently not detected following culture.

Treatment
These infections are very difficult to treat. Intrauterine lavage with 2–3 litres of warm saline, followed by antimycotic preparations such as povidone–iodine (1–2% solution daily for 5 days); nystatin (200 000–500 000 units daily for 5 days) or clotrimazole (400–600 mg every other day for 12 days) has been used with limited success. Selection of the correct treatment should be based on sensitivity results.

Prognosis

The prognosis for the subsequent fertility of mares with mycotic endometritis is poor. It is suggested that a normal healthy uterus can eliminate mycotic infection.

Viral infectious disease — equine coital exanthma

In addition to EHV-1, EHV-4 and equine viral arteritis infection which cause abortion (see above), EHV-3 causes a relatively benign venereal disease referred to as coital exanthema; it affects both sexes. There have been reports of its transfer during gynaecological examination.

The virus can remain dormant until conditions favour its proliferation with the development of the characteristic clinical signs. Normally, following coitus, they develop after an incubation period of 4–7 days. Multiple vesicles appear on the vulval mucosa and perineum, resulting in a short period of local irritation. These rupture, leaving small ulcers 3–10 mm in diameter which are painful to touch. In the absence of infection with opportunist pathogens, healing occurs in 10–14 days, when it ceases to be contagious. There is permanent loss of pigmentation at the site of the healed lesions. Pregnancy rates are not reduced. In the stallion, the vesicles develop on the shaft of the penis and the prepuce; if severe, he may be reluctant to serve.

Treatment consists of immediate sexual rest and the application of an antiseptic powder or spray to prevent secondary bacterial infection; this allows the ulcers to heal. The disease is controlled by withholding breeding of all affected stallions and mares and taking hygienic precautions when handling these animals.

Protozoal infections — dourine

Trypanosoma equiperdum causes a venereal disease called dourine, which is currently prevalent in Africa, the Middle East and Central and South America; it has been eradicated from Europe and North America. The incubation period is 1–4 weeks and the disease has an extremely protracted course which can extend over a period of weeks or months. It affects horses, mules and donkeys of either sex. The initial sign is a non-painful swelling of the external genitalia of both stallions and mares; mares show a vaginal discharge and stallions have a paraphimosis. Some weeks later, depigmented areas and urticaria-like raised plaques 2–10 cm in diameter appear over the body surface. The disease is characterized by a low morbidity, but a high mortality of 50–75%.

Diagnosis of dourine is made from the clinical signs, particularly the skin plaques, together with demonstration of the trypanasome in the discharges and in the skin lesions. A complement fixation test is also available. Treatment using quinapyramine sulfate has been attempted, but stallions that recover may become carriers. Therefore, strict screening using a complement fixation test, with slaughter of positive and affected animals, as well as the institution of quarantine programmes, should be used to control this disease.

Metritis

Metritis is the inflammation of the entire thickness of the uterine wall. It occurs when there is massive contamination of the uterus, frequently in association with trauma or retained placenta during foaling. It has a grave prognosis, particularly in heavy horses, since the absorption of toxins from the uterine lumen into the general circulation results in systemic signs including pyrexia, depression, loss of appetite and laminitis. Toxin production is associated with rapid bacterial growth, frequently involving Gram-negative organisms. Treatment involves repeated lavage of the uterus with warm sterile saline (2–3 litres) several times per day until it is free of inflammatory exudates and placental debris. Bacterial growth should be controlled, so as to limit toxin production, with a broad-spectrum antibiotic effective against *E. coli*, which is invariably present. Supportive therapy with parenteral antibiotics, antihistamines (in cases of retained placenta), oxytocin and intravenous fluid therapy is indicated in many cases.

Systemic signs such as pulse rate and mucous membrane colour are used to monitor the response to therapy in conjunction with examination of the uterine fluid.

Despite all efforts, some mares die due to toxaemia or irreversible changes in the foot following laminitis such as pedal-bone rotation.

Pyometra

Pyometra describes the accumulation of large volumes of inflammatory exudate in the distended uterus. It must be distinguished from the smaller, and intermittent, accumulations of fluid that can be detected by ultrasonography in acute endometritis. Pyometra occurs because of interference with natural drainage of fluid from the uterus which may be due to cervical adhesions or an abnormally constricted, tortuous or irregular cervix. In some cases, the fluid accumulates in the absence of cervical lesions presumably due to an impaired ability to eliminate the exudate. Other predisposing factors are chronic infection with *P. aeruginosa* or fungi.

Some clinicians restrict the term 'pyometra' to cases where, in addition to the accumulation of exudate within the uterine lumen, the corpus luteum persists beyond its normal lifespan. Some mares with pyometra have normal, regular cyclical ovarian activity. Persistence of the corpus luteum is probably due to the failure of the synthesis and/or release of prostaglandins from the uterus. Mares which have prolonged luteal activity have the greatest endometrial damage.

The mare with pyometra seldom shows overt signs of systemic disease even when there is up to 60 litres of exudate in the uterine lumen. Very occasionally there is weight loss, depression and anorexia. A vulval discharge is often observed, especially at oestrus, which may vary in consistency from watery to cream-like. Although the culture of endometrial swabs can sometimes result in the growth of mixed organisms or sometimes no bacterial growth at all, in most cases the organism isolated is *S. zooepidemicus*.

Diagnosis

The diagnosis of pyometra is based upon rectal palpation, ultrasonic examination of an enlarged fluid-filled uterus and analysis of the uterine fluid. Pregnancy must be eliminated together with rare conditions such as mucometra and pneumouterus.

Due to the lack of systemic illness, cases of pyometra have often become chronic before treatment is sought. In such cases the prognosis is poor because of severe endometrial damage which is unlikely to be able to sustain a normal pregnancy.

Treatment

In the absence of systemic illness or an unsightly vulval discharge, treatment of chronic pyometra may not be indicated; although some mares can show signs of discomfort during exercise. Hysterectomy can be performed following aspiration of the exudate from the uterus, although great care has to be taken to prevent contamination of the peritoneal cavity (see p. 476).

Many cases can be significantly improved without surgery by repeated large-volume lavage with warm saline. Initially, $PGF_{2\alpha}$ can be used to induce luteolysis of the corpus luteum if present, which should allow the cervix to relax sufficiently for digital exploration for the presence of any adhesions. Oestradiol or PGE_2 may also help relax the cervix. The broad-spectrum combination of antibiotics used to treat endometritis (see earlier) should be infused after repeated large-volume lavage and oxytocin to achieve drainage of exudate, and an endometrial biopsy is useful in assessing the degree of endometrial damage. The mare must be treated as a susceptible mare if she is to be mated (see p. 489).

REFERENCES

Adams, G. P. and Ginther, O. J. (1989) *J. Amer. Vet. Med. Assn,* **194**, 372.

Adams, G. P., Kastelic, J. P., Bergfelt, D. R. and Ginther, O. J. (1987) *J. Reprod. Fertil. Suppl.,* **35**, 445.

Allen, W. E. (1991) *Vet. Rec.,* **128**, 593.

Allen, W. E. and Pycock, J. F. (1988) *Vet. Rec.,* **122**, 489.

Allen, W. E. and Pycock, J. F. (1989) *Vet. Rec.,* **125**, 298.

Allen, W. E., Arbeid, P. E., Kooros, K. and Pycock, J. F. (1987) *Vet. Rec.,* **121**, 422.

Allen, W. R. (1993) *Equine Vet. J.,* **25**, 90.

Asbury, A. C. (1992) *Equine Vet. J.,* **24**, 416.

Bergfelt, D. R., Woods, J. A. and Ginther, O. J. (1992) *J. Reprod. Fertil.,* **95**, 339.

Bosu, W. T. K., Van Camp, S. C., Miller, R. B. and Owen, R. ap R. (1982) *Can. Vet. J.,* **23**, 6.

Caslick, E. A. (1937) *Cornell Vet.,* **27**, 178.

Evans, M. J., Hamer, J. M., Gason, L. M. and Irvine, C. H. G. (1986) *Theriogenology,* **26**, 37.

Farrely, B. Y. and Mullaney, P. E. (1964) *Ir. Vet. J.,* **18**, 201.

Ginther, O. J. (1988) *J. Equine Vet. Sci.,* **8**, 101.

Ginther, O. J. (1989) *Amer. J. Vet. Res.,* **50**, 45.

Ginther, O. J. (1990) *Equine Vet. J.,* **22**, 152.

Ginther, O. J. and Bergfelt, D. R. (1990) *J. Reprod. Fertil.,* **88**, 119.

Ginther, O. J. and Pierson, R. A. (1984) *Theriogenology,* **21**, 505.

Ginther, O. J. and Pierson, R. A. (1989) *J. Equine Vet. Sci.,* **9**, 4.

Harrison, L. A., Squires, E. L., Nett, T. M. and McKinnon, A. O. (1990) *J. Anim. Sci.,* **68**, 690.

Hinrichs, K. and Hunt, P. R. (1990) *Equine Vet. J.,* **22**, 99.

Hughes, J. P. and Loy, R. G. (1969) *Proc. 15th Ann. Conv. Amer. Assn Equine Pract.,* p. 289.

Hughes, J. P., Stabenfeldt, G. H., Kindahl, H., Kennedy, P. C.,

Edqvist, L. E., Neely, D. P. and Schalm, O. (1979) *J. Reprod. Fertil. Suppl.*, **27**, 321.

Hyland, J. H., Wright, P. J., Clarke, I. J., Carson, R. S., Langsford, D. A. and Jeffcot, L. B. (1987) *J. Reprod. Fertil. Suppl.*, **35**, 211.

Kenney, R. M. (1978) *J. Amer. Vet. Med. Assn*, **172**, 241.

Kenney, R. M. and Ganjam, V. K. (1975) *J. Reprod. Fertil. Suppl.*, **23**, 335.

Knudsen, O. (1964) *Cornell Vet.*, **54**, 423.

Liu, I. K. M., Lantz, K. C., Schlafke, S., Bowers, J. M. and Enders, A. C. (1990) *Proc. 36th Ann. Conv. Amer. Assn Equine Pract.*, p. 41.

McKinnon, A. O. and Belden, J. O. (1988) *J. Amer. Vet. Med. Assn*, **192**, 647.

McKinnon, A. O., Squires, E. L., Carnevale, E. M., Harrison, L. A., Frantz, D. D., McChesney, A. E. and Shideler, R. K. (1987) *Proc. 33rd Ann. Conv. Amer. Assn Equine Pract.*, p. 605.

Madwell, B. R. and Theilen, G. H. (1987) In: *Veterinary Cancer Medicine*, 2nd edn, ed. G. H. Theilen, pp. 583–600. Philadelphia: Lea and Febiger.

Meagher, D. M., Wheat, J. D., Hughes, J. P., Stabenfeldt, G. H. and Harris, B. A. (1977) *Proc. 23rd Ann. Conv. Amer. Assn Equine Pract.*, p. 133.

Monin, T. (1972) *Proc. 18th Ann. Conv. Amer. Assn Equine Pract.*, p. 99.

Nelson, E. M., Kiefer, B. L., Roser, J. F. and Evans, J. W. (1985) *Theriogenology*, **23**, 241.

Neu, S. M., Timoney, P. J. and Lowry, S. R. (1992) *Theriogenology*, **37**, 407.

Pascoe, R. R. (1979) *J. Reprod. Fertil. Suppl.*, **27**, 229.

Piquette, G. N., Kenney, R. M., Sertich, P. L., Yamoto, M. and Hsueh, A. (1990) *Biol. Reprod.*, **43**, 1050.

Pouret, E. J. (1982) *Equine Vet. J.*, **14**, 249.

Pycock, J. F. (1994a) *Equine Vet. Educ.*, **6**, 132.

Pycock, J. F. (1994b) *Equine Vet. Educ.*, **6**, 36.

Pycock, J. F. (1994c) *Proc. 40th Ann. Conv. Amer. Assn. Equine Pract.*, p. 19.

Pycock, J. F. and Newcombe, J. R. N. (1995a) *Equine Pract.* (in press).

Pycock, J. F. and Newcombe, J. R. N. (1995b) *Vet. Rec.* (submitted).

Ricketts, S. W. (1978) Fellowship Thesis, Royal College of Veterinary Surgeons.

Ricketts, S. W. and Mackintosh, M. E. (1987) *J. Reprod. Fertil. Suppl.*, **35**, 343.

Ricketts, S. W. and Young, A. (1990) *Vet. Rec.*, **126**, 68.

Shideler, R. K., Squires, E. L., Trotter, G. and Tarr, S. (1990) *Equine Vet. Sci.*, **10**, 187.

Stone, R., Bracher, V. and Mathias, S. (1991) *Equine Vet. Educ.*, **3**, 181.

Van Camp, S. D. (1993) In: *Equine Reproduction*, ed. A. O. McKinnon and J. L. Voss, pp. 392–396. Philadelphia: Lea and Febiger.

Vogelsang, M. M., Vogelsang, S. G., Lindsey, B. R. and Massey, J. M. (1989) *Theriogenology*, **32**, 95.

27

Infertility in the Sow and Gilt

Pig producers expect high levels of fertility, and any shortfalls represent a serious economic loss (Glossop and Foulkes, 1986). The efficiency of a pig operation may be described in terms that take into account a financial component, e.g. the number of pigs sold per sow place per year, or the number of kilograms of pigmeat sold per square metre of pig unit (Douglas and Mackinnon, 1992). Consideration of reproductive efficiency, however, requires an evaluation of fertility level, which may be expressed in various ways (definitions taken from PIC, 1990–1991):

1. *Farrowing rate* — the number of sows which farrow to a given number of services, normally expressed as a percentage, i.e.

$$\frac{\text{Number of farrowings}}{\text{Number of services}} \times 100$$

2. *Farrowing index* — the number of farrowings per sow per year, i.e.

$$\frac{\text{Total number of farrowings per year}}{\text{Average sow inventory}}$$

3. *Conception rate* (or non-return rate) — the number of sows that conceive to service expressed as a percentage of those served. The conception rate is usually estimated as the non-return rate to oestrus (28 days after service) or identified by pregnancy diagnosis at 30 days or more, after service. These terms are by no means as precise as the farrowing rate, but can provide an earlier warning of a problem.

4. *Empty days* — the number of days on which a sow is not pregnant per year. There are, of course, days during which it is not possible for a sow to be pregnant, for example in lactation, or during the weaning to oestrus interval, and these must be taken into account.

5. *Piglets born per sow per year* — this figure should be divided into two components: total numbers born, and numbers born live.

All fertility parameters interrelate, and Figure 27.1 illustrates the relationship between them (Douglas and Mackinnon, 1992). Each producer must establish targets for reproductive performance. In order to do this a realistic way it is first necessary to consider the physiological potential of the sow (Glossop, 1992). The reproductive cycle of the sow comprises:

Gestation	= 115 days
Lactation	= 21–28 days
Interval from weaning to oestrus	= 5 days
Total no. days per reproductive cycle	= 141–148 days

From these calculations the maximum realizable farrowing index is 2.5–2.6 (Glossop, 1992), although this assumes a farrowing rate of 100%, which is rather optimistic. The calculation does, however, highlight factors that will influence the farrowing index: these include gestation length (which is, of course, fixed), lactation length and weaning to oestrus interval along with conception rate and farrowing rate.

Analysis of reproductive data from any of the bureau recording schemes demonstrates the shortfall between the physiological potential and the reality. Table 27.1 details fertility data for herds in the UK recording with the Pigtales bureau (PIC, 1993). It is interesting to compare overall herd performance with that achieved by the top-performing herds. Clearly, some herds are getting close to the potential farrowing index of 2.5–2.6. The aim must surely be to raise *overall* herd performance in line with this.

Any discrepancy between the targets and the reality represents an economic loss resulting from suboptimal fertility. Targets set for a particular unit must take into account management factors which influence fertility. Realistic performance targets for most herds are set out in Table 27.2. The reproductive performance of a herd relies upon the

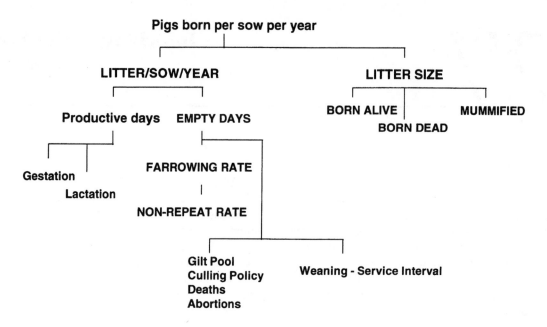

Fig. 27.1 Flow chart showing reproductive factors influencing fertility (Douglas and Mackinnon, 1992).

Table 27.1 UK Herd performance — 1992 (averages weighted by sow herd size)

	All farms	*Bottom 33%*	*Top 33%*	*Top 10%*
No. farms	110	36	37	12
No. sows	23 611	6192	8067	2370
Farrowing rate	80%	74%	85%	88%
Farrowing index	2.29	2.18	2.39	2.43
Live births per litter	10.74	10.43	11.04	11.22
Live births per sow per year	24.64	22.74	26.34	27.27

PIC (1993).

exercise of tight control over, and optimization of, such factors. The purpose of this chapter is to examine these factors and to gain an understanding of how they may be controlled.

FACTORS WHICH AFFECT FERTILITY

In Wrathall's (1977) classification of factors that affect fertility the importance of management and stockmanship are emphasized; it is vital to recognize this when attempting to solve a fertility problem. Any investigation of herd infertility should take into account management factors before making a detailed study of other issues.

The quality of stockmanship will be reflected in such basic procedures as oestrus detection, supervision of service, general hygiene and record-keeping. As units grow larger and as management systems change in response to consumer demands, stockmanship characteristics and requirements may have to be adjusted, but remain, nonetheless, of paramount importance. English (1991) discusses this subject in great detail, pointing out that good stockmanship involves a combination of sound basic knowledge, patience, empathy, sensitivity, organizational skills and an appreciation of priorities.

Management determines the nature of the sow's environment and monitors the operation through observation and record-keeping. The environment, in turn, affects the endocrine control of reproduction. In large intensive units, irregularities of reproduction are often more apparent

Table 27.2 Targets for reproductive efficiency

Litters/sow/year	> 2.3
Farrowing rate	> 85%
Non-repeat rate	> 90%
Litter size	
Born live	> 11.0
Born dead	< 0.5
Mummified	< 0.5

Douglas and Mackinnon (1992).

than in less intensive systems. The keeping of large numbers of breeding animals together favours the build-up and spread of microbial and viral diseases that may interfere with fertility.

An investigation of a fertility problem in the pig is rarely, if ever, considered on an individual sow basis. The parameters of reproductive performance demonstrate this with fertility being expressed in terms of percentages of the herd, and averages. Sows that deviate from the norm invariably are removed from the herd rather than being treated or being allowed to continue in a subfertile way. Herd fertility investigations are therefore exactly as they sound — investigations of overall reproductive performance. This being so, it must be remembered that a herd comprises a number of individuals: in order to understand and fully appreciate a fertility problem it is essential to consider individual sow records.

Any investigation of herd infertility must begin with an evaluation of the problem. This requires an initial understanding of the history of the problem (Douglas and Mackinnon, 1992), and examination of the records (Muirhead, 1976), which may be presented in a variety of ways. Ideally, the unit will record fertility data along with all other performance data on an in-house or bureau computer system, and Figure 27.2 shows examples of records maintained in this way. Where this is not the case, time must first be spent handling the raw data that may be in the form of pocket record books for the service house and the farrowing house. This is an extremely laborious process but the information is vital to any investigation.

Parameters of relevance to the investigation include:

- Herd size.
- Age profile.
- Return rate/conception rate.

- Distribution of return intervals.
- Weaning-to-oestrus interval.
- Farrowing rate.
- Total numbers born.
- Total numbers born live.
- Lactation length.
- Number of empty days.

It is of particular importance to evaluate the data with reference to:

- Reproductive performance of the herd before the problem.
- Reproductive performance of other herds (Meredith, 1983).
- Physiological potential reproductive performance (Glossop, 1992).

Examination of records should provide a definition of the nature and extent of the problem. This exercise is followed by a clinical appraisal of the stock, post-mortem examination and laboratory diagnosis as appropriate (Douglas and Mackinnon, 1992). At the outset it should be recognized that the route of a fertility problem is often multifactorial.

The problem will probably fall into one or more of the following categories:

- Anoestrus.
- Conception failure.
- Pregnancy failure.

ANOESTRUS

Anoestrus is defined as 'the absence of oestrous behaviour (standing to a boar or to a riding test) but excludes the normal interval (dioestrus) between two successive oestrous periods' (Meredith, 1984). By definition, delayed oestrus is included in this category (Douglas and Mackinnon, 1992). Anoestrus is inevitable at certain stages in a sow's life (e.g. before puberty, during pregnancy and lactation), and this should be taken into account in any investigation. It must be recognized, however, that even 'normal' periods of anoestrus represent non-productive days and should be kept to a minimum in the non-pregnant sow (Meredith, 1984).

Anoestrus is considered to be one of the commonest reproductive disorders of sows and gilts (Meredith, 1979). In an American survey of

C:\PIGS\REPORTS\27A02204.014

EFFICIENCY REPORT

Farm Number

Run on 28 Sep 1993

Dated 16-May-93 in Week No.19 - Second Quarter 92

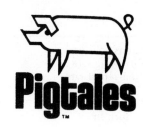

	PERIOD 1 From 15-Nov-92 To 16-May-93 (ACTUAL)	PERIOD 2 From 17-May-92 To 16-May-93 (ACTUAL)	 (TARGET)
SERVICES Total	302	581	554
Repeat %	8	8	10
Matings/Service	2.0	2.0	2.0
Matings/Boar/Week	2.1	1.9	1.6
FARROWINGS Total	240	469	471
Livebirths/Litter	2686/11.2	5299/11.3	5652/12.0
Mummified % Total	1.2	1.4	0.0
Stillbirths % Total	9.5	9.0	2.5
Index (Interval)	2.25(162)	2.25(162)	2.25(162)
Born/Sow/Year	25.2	25.4	27.0
Born/Female/Year	23.5	23.7	25.3
LOSSES Total	395	747	678
Losses % of Liveborn	14.7	14.1	12.0
WEANINGS Normal (& Late)	237(0)	470(0)	471
Pigs Weaned/Litter	2265/ 9.6	4561/ 9.7	4974/10.6
Late Foster % Weaned	0.0	0.0	0.0
Sub-Standard % Weaned	0.0	0.0	0.0
Weaned/Sow/Year	21.5	21.8	23.8
Weaned/Female/Year	20.1	20.4	22.4
STOCK Sows	214	209	210
Boars	11	12	13
Sow:Boar Ratio	19.5	17.4	16.0
Gilts	15	15	14
Sow:Gilt Ratio	14.3	13.9	15.0

(a)

C:\PIG5\REPORTS\23102203.014

FARROWING CONTROL CHART

Farm Number

Run on 28 Sep 1993

Dated 16-May-93 in Week No.19 - Second Quarter 93

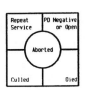

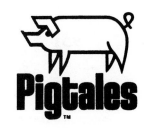

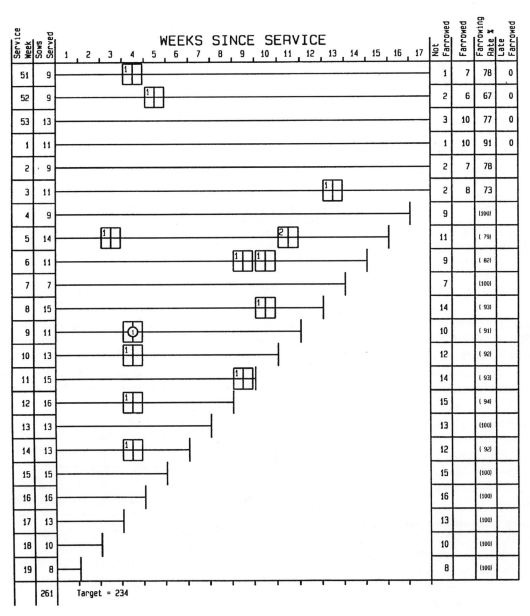

Farrowing Rate (from week 30 to week 2) = 85% -- Target = 85%

(b)

SOW **951**

Sire:
Dam:

LAST FARROWED 06-05-93   BORN/YR **32.5**
SOW'S AGE   2 Yrs 10 Mths   WEAN/YR **26.9**

LITTER NUMBER	1	2	3	4	5	AVGE		6
BOAR(S) USED	**1xMIX**	**1xMIX**	**1x**	**1x**	**1x**		**1x**	
FARROWING INTERVAL ·		146	143	147	140	144		
SERVICES/MATINGS	1/3	1/3	1/3	1/2	1/3	1.0		1/3
PROBLEMS								
STILLBIRTHS	1	0	0	0	0	0.2		
MUMMIFIED	0	0	1	1	0	0.4		
LIVEBIRTHS	7	12	15	15	15	12.8		
FOSTERED ON	1	0	0	1	0	0.4		
FOSTERED OFF	-1	0	-2	-3	0	-1.2		
PRE-WEANING DEATHS	-1	0	-2	-2	-3	-1.6		
WEANED	9	12	11	10	11	10.6		0
SUB-STANDARD	0	0	0	0	0	0.0		0
AV.BIRTH WEIGHT	1.1	1.3	1.1	1.5	0.0	1.3		
AV.WEANING WEIGHT	5.3	6.7	7.0	5.3	5.4	5.9		
AGE AT WEANING	23	24	28	21	28	24.9		

Boars Used (Breed)............ **LEN(   )**   **ZAK(   )**   **WILL(   )**
Service date.................. **15-06-93** (Wk 24)
3 Week date.................. **06-07-93** PD _____
Due to Farrow................ **08-10-93**
Date Farrowed................ _____
Date Weaned.................. _____

(c)   07-10-93

Fig. 27.2 Herd fertility records. (a) Efficiency report. (b) Farrowing control chart. (c) Sow record card.

more than 11 000 sows in eight herds, Hurtgen et al. (1980) confirmed that this condition was more common in sows that had been weaned from their first litter (i.e. second-litter gilts). The same authors also indicated that anoestrus is more prevalent in summer: in their study the percentage of sows showing oestrus within 7 days of weaning was 68.6% from July to September compared with 82% during the remaining 9 months.

The term 'sub-oestrus' refers to a condition in which cyclic animals show no obvious external signs of oestrus; in such cases it is necessary to ensure that the problem is not merely one of poor oestrus detection. Sub-oestrus is characterized by the presence of corpora lutea. Meredith (1977) demonstrated by rectal palpation that the cervix is relatively small and firm in anoestrus and softer in sub-oestrus under the influence of this luteal tissue.

It is important first to establish that the problem is truly one of anoestrus and not simply inadequate oestrus detection. Accurate oestrus detection involves time and effort, in conjunction with good record-keeping. Oestrus detection appears to be an even greater problem in gilts. Observations in Australian piggeries have indicated that there is considerable room for enhancement in reproductive efficiency by improving oestrus detection in this particular group of breeding females. Hemsworth (1988) suggests that the detection rate of oestrus in gilts can be as low as 50–60%.

The average weaning to oestrus interval is 4–6 days, and any delay in this results in loss of production due to an increase in empty days. A confounding factor is that fertility appears to be lower in sows with an extended weaning-to-oestrus interval (unpublished observation). The net result of anoestrus is economic loss, and every effort should be made to minimize the interval.

Investigation of anoestrus

Having established from the records and from observation on the actual unit that anoestrus really is a problem, it is necessary to investigate the situation further.

Ovarian function tests

The ovaries of sows which demonstrate no physical signs of oestrus may be truly inactive (anoestrus), active with oestrus inapparent (suboestrus) or even pregnant (Meredith, 1983). Tests for ovarian function will differentiate between these conditions. Ovarian activity has been identified in apparently anoestrus gilts by plasma progesterone assay (Einarsson et al., 1978; Christensen, 1981). It is, therefore, important to investigate ovarian activity before attempting to treat an anoestrus female. Progesterone may be measured in plasma or whole sow's blood by enzyme-linked immuno-assay (ELISA) as described by Glossop and Foulkes (1986). Weekly blood progesterone assay will differentiate between truly inactive, pregnant and normally cyclical ovaries (Glossop and Foulkes, 1990).

An incidence of sows which have normal cyclical ovaries but which are apparently suboestrus may result from inadequate oestrus detection, perhaps due to lack of emphasis on this important stage of the breeding cycle, or to suboptimal conditions for observing signs of oestrus. Ideally, the producer should be encouraged to observe for oestrus in the presence of the boar (Almond and Dial, 1987) at least once (and preferably twice)

each day from the day of weaning. Oestrus may be may be inhibited by stress, unsuitable environment, psychological inhibitions, exogenous hormones or lameness (Meredith, 1979). The presence of the boar appears to be a key issue in the identification of oestrus in both sows and gilts (Glossop, 1992).

Post-mortem examination

Ovarian function may be assessed by post-mortem examination of the reproductive tracts of cull sows from the herd under investigation. This type of study can reveal a whole range of abnormalities:

1. Acyclic ovaries: inactive, with some small follicles (< 5 mm diameter), absence of corpora lutea.

2. Cystic ovaries:

- Multiple large cysts (usually < 14 mm in diameter), generally containing some luteal tissue that produces progesterone. These may regress, but some persist and can inhibit oestrus (Figure 27.3).
- Multiple small cysts — these often produce oestrogen, which results in sows having markedly irregular cycle lengths and exhibiting intense signs of oestrus (nymphomania).
- Single cysts — these rarely affect sow fertility and tend to be incidental findings at post-mortem.

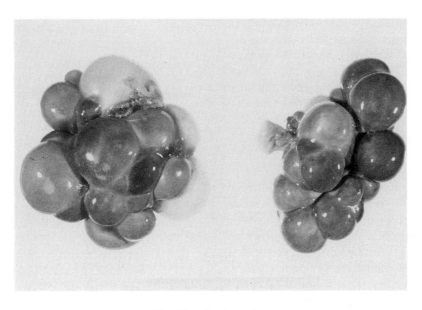

Fig. 27.3 Cystic ovaries.

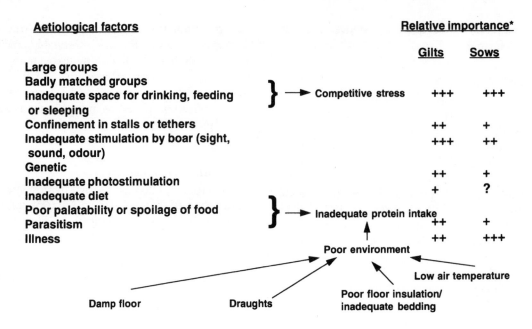

* Author's estimate for UK conditions of husbandry

Fig. 27.4 Factors that influence the appearance of oestrus in sows and gilts. (From Meredith, 1979.)

Real-time ultrasound

This is a relatively new technique which can be used to observe changes in the size and shape of the ovaries by a non-invasive method in the live animal (Weitze et al., 1990a). Such investigations are time-consuming and require expensive equipment and a considerable level of expertise. They do provide, however, a valuable tool for diagnosis of infertility and research into ovarian activity.

Factors that influence the appearance of oestrus in sows and gilts are summarized in Figure 27.4 (Meredith, 1979). Walton (1986) considers exposure to mature boars to be the single most important feature of the post-weaning environment to ensure rapid return to oestrus and ovulation.

Treatment of anoestrus

Anoestrus is of such economic significance that it must be treated promptly by identifying and remedying all contributing factors as a matter of urgency. In serious cases where ovaries are truly inactive it may be worth considering hormone therapy as a means of restoring cyclical activity as rapidly as possible. Various hormone preparations are available but a combination of equine chorionic gonadotrophin (eCG) and human chorionic gonadotrophin (hCG) is still probably the preparation of choice (Meredith, 1979). Injection of a

preparation containing 200 IU hCG and 400 IU of eCG (PG600, Intervet) into 363 anoestrus sows resulted in 87.6% showing signs of oestrus within 3–8 days (Schilling and Cerne, 1972).

CONCEPTION FAILURE

This problem is recognized by an increased number of regular returns to service (i.e. returns at 18–24 days after service). The conception rate (or non-return rate) in breeding herds should be at least 90% (see Table 27.2) and an incidence of returns higher than 10% may be regarded as abnormal and unacceptable. Conception failure suggests that viable ova did not come into contact with viable spermatozoa at the appropriate time. The result of this will be either total conception failure (i.e. regular return to service) or partial conception failure (i.e. reduction in litter size). Assuming that ovulation has taken place, conception failure must be due to one or more of the following factors.

Timing of service

The sow ovulates, on average, 36–44 hours after the onset of standing oestrus (Hunter, 1988a; Weitze et al., 1990b). Ova have a finite lifespan following ovulation and must come into contact with the spermatozoa at an early stage after ovulation, and in any event within 8 hours. Spermatozoa can survive for up to 40 hours inside the sow's reproductive tract (Hunter, 1988a). A service regimen must take all these factors into account and aim to ensure that the uterus contains viable spermatozoa in advance of, and during, the time when ovulation may occur (Glossop, 1991). Inappropriate timing of service may result in total conception failure (i.e. regular return to service) or partial conception failure (i.e. reduced numbers born).

For this reason, an optimal service management regimen should ensure that each sow is served on the day of onset of standing oestrus and at least once more, 18–24 hours later. Lynch and O'Grady (1984) said that 'A single mating at the appropriate stage of oestrus should be sufficient to get a high proportion of ova fertilized at the optimum time to ensure a high embryonic survival rate and large litter size at birth' — the problem comes in identifying this moment correctly. Existing service regimens seek to compensate for inaccuracies in timing. The single most important factor in achieving an acceptable conception rate is timing.

Quality of service

One cannot assume that service has been performed properly without careful supervision to ensure that the boar has actually achieved intromission (Douglas and Mackinnon, 1992). Service pen design, particularly with reference to the floor surface is of direct relevance to the quality of service.

Semen quality

This aspect of fertility is often overlooked although semen quality can be affected by a wide range of factors such as age, environmental temperature, frequency of use and disease (see Chapter 30 on male fertility for a more detailed discussion on this subject). Where semen quality is affected in terms of ejaculate volume, sperm count, sperm motility or morphology, it is possible that conception rates may be affected. Where boars are used for natural service, particularly in a cross-service regimen, it may be that subfertile or infertile individuals are missed. Consideration of boar fertility should also take into account physical breeding soundness,

paying particular attention to feet and leg conformation.

Having established an abnormally high incidence of regular returns to service, it is necessary to consider the pattern of the problem. For example, is the problem prevalent within a particular group of individuals differentiated by parity, lactation length, weaning-to-oestrus interval, day of service or service regimen? All of these factors can be related to conception rates and should be considered with care by categorizing each return and attempting to establish a pattern.

The next essential step in the investigation is to visit the unit on a busy service day to observe routine procedures. The following questions should be asked:

- Are service pens adequate in terms of size, shape, construction, floor surface?
- Are services properly supervised?
- Are boars being worked in rotation or are some boars being overworked?
- Is semen quality acceptable?
- Are the boars physically sound for breeding?
- What is the physical condition of the sows?
- Is sufficient time spent on oestrus detection?
- Are conditions adequate for oestrus detection? (For example, is there sufficient light in the service house?)
- When are sows served in relation to the onset of standing oestrus?
- What service regimen is used?
- Where artificial insemination is used, do staff understand all the procedures involved?
- Is there evidence of an infectious disease?
- Do the staff have any idea of the cause of the problem?

Despite the reference to infectious disease, regular returns to service, particularly in the absence of other reproductive signs, are more likely to be due to a management problem. It is important to remember that where oestrus detection is suboptimal, a proportion of first returns may be missed, becoming apparent at the second return. For this reason, emphasis should be placed on continued careful observation for signs of oestrus throughout pregnancy bearing in mind that a significant proportion of returns occurs outside the 'normal range' of 18–24 days after service (Glossop and Foulkes, 1988). Boar presence is of great

Table 27.3 Use of hormone assay to identify anoestrus, cycling or pregnant sows

	Day 21: progesterone	Day 28: progesterone	Day 28: oestrone sulfate
Anoestrus	Low	Low	Low
Cycling	Low	High	Low
Pregnant	High	High	High
Early embryonic death	High	High/low	Low

Glossop and Foulkes (1990).

importance in the accurate detection of returns (Almond and Dial, 1987).

PREGNANCY FAILURE

Pregnancy failure may be divided into two main sections:

- Failure to establish pregnancy.
- Failure of an established pregnancy.

The reaction of the conceptus to an adverse factor varies markedly with age, and it is helpful to categorize the various stages accordingly. Wrathall (1975) classifies the stages as pre-attachment (before days 13–14), embryonic (from days 14 to 35) and fetal (after day 35).

Failure to establish pregnancy

Unattached conceptuses within the uterus are susceptible to damage by many factors. Where pregnancy fails around the time of maternal recognition of pregnancy (see p. 63) (i.e. around days 12–13) sows tend to return to oestrus outside the normal range for 'regular returns'. In an experiment where blastocysts were flushed from the uterine horns of pigs on days 10–13 after service, those flushed on day 12 or 13 returned on days 26–30. Those flushed on day 10 or 11 returned at the 'normal' time (Meulen et al., 1987). A proportion of so-called 'late returns' have been recorded on herds with fertility levels within the normal range, and it has been suggested that failure of establishment of pregnancy is the cause of this (Glossop and Foulkes, 1988). In a study of 2472 return intervals, 25.6% of returns before day 31 occurred after the time when oestrus is commonly expected. The relatively high incidence of this phenomenon in apparently normal herds represents a financial loss that may be avoidable. The exact mechanism of action for this has not yet been clarified, but it is

likely to involve a problem with the maternal recognition of pregnancy that commences on about day 12 after conception; any form of stress should be avoided around this period of time. Moving sows, regrouping, exposure to extremes of temperature or changes of diet may all contribute to such problems. An infectious challenge at this time may also have a deleterious effect on the establishment of pregnancy. Failure of pregnancy at this stage may be total (resulting in an irregular return to service) or partial (resulting in resorption of some embryos, and consequent reduction in litter size) (Wrathall, 1975).

Investigation of early pregnancy failure is extremely difficult from clinical signs alone. It is necessary to establish the presence of a pregnancy that subsequently fails, and strategic use of hormone assays can be of value in this situation (Glossop and Foulkes, 1990). These authors describe a regimen for measuring progesterone on days 21 and 28, and oestrone sulfate on day 28 after service. By using such strategic hormone assays it is possible to differentiate between sows that have failed to conceive and those which have suffered early loss of pregnancy (Table 27.3). Identifying that conception has probably taken place (by progesterone assay) but that the pregnancy has terminated by day 28 (by a negative result for oestrone sulfate) provides useful information as to the possible cause of events.

Failure of an established pregnancy

Death of conceptuses during the embryonic stage tend to result in resorption if abortion does not occur. Dissolution of embryos in the absence of anaerobic bacteria appears to be an aseptic, autolytic process resulting in complete disappearance of the products, or a vaginal discharge (Wrathall, 1975). Partial failure of pregnancy may therefore result in a reduction in numbers born being the

Table 27.4 Percentage frequency of isolation of pathogens from porcine fetopathies examined by Ministry of Agriculture Veterinary Investigation Centres (source: VIDA–II)

	1984	1985	1986	1987	1988	1989	1990	1991	1992
Erysipelothrix rhusiopathiae	0.8	3.0	1.7	3.6	8.2	5.2	5.5	3.1	4.1
Leptospira spp.	NR	NR	NR	NR	NR	NR	NR	21.0	24.0
Listeria monocytogenes	0	0	0.2	0	0	0.7	0	0	0.6
Streptococcus spp.	5.4	3.6	4.3	3.0	6.2	3.9	5.5	8.0	8.2
Parvovirus	70.2	70.2	76.8	68.0	57.4	68.0	56.4	38.3	40.0
Other pathogens	23.6	23.2	17.0	25.4	28.2	22.2	32.5	29.6	23.4
Total identified	500	534	466	303	195	153	163	162	171
Total submitted	1410	1376	1101	869	661	482	445	529	527
Percentage diagnosed	35.5	38.8	42.3	34.9	29.5	31.7	36.6	30.6	32.4

NR, not recorded.

only presenting sign. Once pregnancy has been confirmed (e.g. by the Doppler ultrasound technique on days 28–35) fetal death is more likely to result from an infectious disease. Beyond 35 days, fetal death will result in mummified fetuses at farrowing. Mummification is the most common clinical manifestation for a viral infection, e.g. Aujeszky's disease, porcine parvovirus (PPV), porcine reproductive respiratory syndrome (PRRS) or swine fever. Under such viral attack it may be only a small number of fetuses that are affected. Environmental conditions may have an effect on the maintenance of pregnancy. Social interaction with boars has been shown to enhance the maintenance of pregnancy in a study in Australia during the period of seasonal infertility (Wilson and Love, 1986).

INFECTIOUS CAUSES OF INFERTILITY

An infectious form of infertility can be of great economic significance to a unit. It is vital, however, to ensure that management and stockmanship are adequate before searching for an infectious agent in any investigation into infertility. It should also be recognized that a whole range of management factors (e.g. environment, stress and nutrition) may lower the natural defence mechanisms, rendering an animal population more susceptible to disease (Fiennes, 1970). In other words, all factors must be taken into account even when it is likely that an infectious agent exists. UK Veterinary Investigation Centre records demonstrate the frequencies of pathogens isolated from fetuses pre-

sented for examination; such information is of value when assessing the relative importance of individual pathogens (Table 27.4).

Wrathall (1971) classified infectious causes of infertility into three groups:

- *Group 1* — Infections associated with ubiquitous microorganisms that are present in the majority of pig populations.

   Under normal circumstances such organisms are generally harmless but may act as opportunist pathogens when other predisposing factors allow them to gain access to a susceptible reproductive tract. An episode of this type would tend to be sporadic in nature. Examples of this type of organism include:

   — *Escherichia coli.*
   — *Erysipelothrix rhusiopathiae.*
   — *Listeria* spp.
   — *Mycoplasma* spp.
   — *Pasteurella* spp.
   — *Salmonella* spp.
   — *Klebsiella* spp.
   — *Corynebacterium* spp.
   — *Staphylococcus* spp
   — *Streptococcus* spp.
   — *Campylobacter* spp.

Clinical signs could include conception failure, abortion, stillbirths, perinatal death and endometritis. Diagnosis and control of group 1 infections can be difficult due to the ubiquitous nature of these organisms in normal healthy populations. Control measures must include removal of all predisposing factors, enhancement of resistance to susceptible animals and reduction of the weight of infection to exposed individuals. Hygiene in the farrowing house and at service are issues of particular importance (Carr, 1992). The boar should not be forgotten as a potential source of infection.

- Group 2 — Infections resulting from certain common contagious microorganisms that are present on a high proportion of pig units.

A strong immunity to such infectious agents is usually developed during early postnatal life. Porcine enteroviruses and PPV are examples of group 2 organisms. Such viruses rarely cause clinical disease in adult sows and boars but they are highly contagious and can spread rapidly through a susceptible population.

PPV is endemic in most herds and may cause reproductive failure associated with embryonic death, mummifications, stillbirths and subsequent reduction in litter size. The virus has been recovered from aborted and stillborn piglets, piglets that died soon after birth, from vaginal mucus and semen (Cartwright and Huck, 1967). Infection must occur during the first half of pregnancy in order to result in disease. Transplacental infection has been demonstrated (Cartwright et al., 1969). Gilts are particularly susceptible at their first exposure, after which a life-long immunity will develop. Management of this disease requires exposure of all gilts to the virus before service by careful integration into the herd: an alternative is vaccination. Diagnosis is by serology, and serological testing also gives an indication of the immune status of the herd.

- Group 3 — Infections that occur relatively infrequently, but which tend to result in severe reproductive loss.

Leptospirosis

Reproductive losses from leptospirosis have been reported on a world-wide basis. The causative agents are a variety of spirochaetes belonging to the genus *Leptospira*. Serogroups of greatest importance to pig populations are *australis* (including the *bratislava* and *muenchen* serovars), *pomona* and *tarrasovi*. The last two groups have not yet been found in the UK (Ellis, 1992). Incidental infections in pigs may also result from *canicola*, *icterohaemorrhagiae*, *autumnalis*, *hardjo*, *mozdak* and *muenchen*. The epidemiology of the disease is complicated by the fact that some strains are specifically adapted to the pig, others to pigs, dogs, horses and hedgehogs and other wildlife.

The most important route of infection is thought to be via the mucous membranes of the eye, mouth, nose (Alston and Broom, 1958; Michna and Campbell, 1969) or vagina (Chaudhary et al., 1966). A bacteraemia occurs 1–2 days after infection, may last for a week and coincides with acute clinical disease. Leptospires then localize in the kidneys, multiply at this site and appear in the urine in varying degrees of intensity and for different lengths of time (Ellis, 1992). Leptospires also localize in the uterus of pregnant sows: when this happens in the last half of gestation abortions and stillbirths often result, occurring 1–4 weeks after infection (Hanson and Tripathy, 1986). Infection with the *bratislava* serovar has also resulted in persistence of leptospires in the uterine tube and uterus of non-pregnant sows (Ellis et al., 1986a) and in the genital tract of boars (Ellis et al., 1986b).

Symptoms of the acute phase of leptospirosis are relatively mild: anorexia, pyrexia and listlessness have resulted from experimental infection (Hanson and Tripathy, 1986). Primary signs of chronic leptospirosis are abortions, stillbirths and birth of weak piglets (Bohl et al., 1954; Fennestad and Borg-Petersen, 1966).

Diagnosis of leptospirosis usually is based on serology using the microscopic agglutination test (MAT) (Faine, 1982). Demonstration of leptospires in the fetus provides a definitive diagnosis of leptospiral abortion (Ellis, 1992).

Control of leptospirosis depends upon the combined use of antibiotic therapy and management. Systemic streptomycin at 25 mg/kg body weight (Dobson, 1974) or oral tetracyclines at levels of 800 g per tonne of feed (Stalheim, 1967) have been used to eliminate carriers, although this type of strategy is not always successful (Doherty and Baines, 1967; Hodges et al., 1979). The main management factor involves prevention of contact between pig populations and other domestic stock or wildlife. Vaccination is an option in some parts of the world, although vaccines are not available in many countries in Western Europe (Ellis, 1992).

Aujeszky's disease

The causative agent of Aujeszky's disease (or pseudorabies) is a herpesvirus. Aujeszky's infection usually gains access to the pig by inhalation or ingestion of the virus (Wrathall, 1975). It may also be transmitted by coitus although there is some argument as to whether true venereal transmission occurs.

Aujeszky's disease is characterized by nervous and respiratory signs associated with a rise in temperature and often death in young piglets. Infection in adults may result in stillbirths and abortion (Taylor, 1989). In adult boars and sows, the clinical signs of this disease are seldom severe and usually consist of pyrexia, depression and anorexia that lasts for up to a week. Of great significance to the breeding herd is that the virus causes embryonic death, fetal mummification and stillbirths.

Porcine reproductive respiratory syndrome (PRRS)

This disease was first recognized in the USA in 1987 (Dial and Parsons, 1989) and has since occurred in mainland Europe and Britain (Done et al., 1992). The effect on the reproductive performance of a herd may be described as devastating (Christianson et al., 1992). The clinical signs of PRRS are rather variable but include some or all of the following (de Jong et al., 1991; Loula, 1991; White, 1991; Done et al., 1992; Hopper et al., 1992):

- *In the sow*:
  - Inappetance (for 7–10 days), which may appear in waves in the herd.
  - Fever.
  - Listlessness.
  - Regular and irregular returns.
  - Vaginal discharge.
  - Anoestrus.
  - Abortions (not a major feature).
  - Early farrowings.
  - Stillbirths and mummifications.
  - Poor milking.
  - Secondary discharges due to cystitis or pyelonephritis.
  - Sudden death.
- *In the boar*:
  - Lethargy.
  - Inappetance.
  - Semen quality is affected for up to 13 weeks (personal communication).

- *In the piglets*:
  - Weakness.
  - Puffy eyes.
  - Lameness
  - High pre- and postweaning mortality.
  - Respiratory signs.

Gross pathological lesions tend to occur in the respiratory system with a confluent consolidation of the lungs affecting all lobes. Extensive broncho-pneumonia and occasionally fibrous pleuritis are also a feature of this disease (Loula, 1991).

The most likely method of spread of the disease is by the introduction of infected pigs on to the premises, although local airborne spread between herds has been suspected (Cromwijk, 1991; van Alstine, 1991) over distances of up to 3 km (Robertson, 1992).

The serious economic impact of this disease results from its devastating effect on herd productivity in terms of farrowing rate, number of live piglets born, pre- and postweaning mortality and performance of surviving piglets. De Jong et al. (1991) suggest that a herd may lose 10% of production.

Diagnosis of PRRS is made on the basis of clinical signs, changes in herd performance, serology and histopathology (Done et al., 1992).

Treatment involves the use of antibiotics for some of the secondary effects although they cannot prevent the reproductive losses (Wensvoort et al., 1991).

Brucellosis

Brucella suis is a widespread infection of pigs in the USA but has not appeared in Great Britain. In countries where it does occur it should always be considered as a cause of herd infertility or abortion. Pigs of both sexes are much more susceptible to infection after weaning. Once infection has been introduced into a susceptible herd (usually by pig movements) it spreads quite rapidly by ingestion or by venereal transmission (Wrathall, 1975). An infected animal suffers an initial generalized bacteraemia similar to undulant fever in humans, which may last for several weeks or months (Deyoe, 1967). Service by an infected boar results in uterine infection, although establishment and proliferation of the organism do not appear to interfere with fertilization. Abortion is the most significant effect of venereal infection and often occurs relatively early in pregnancy. The incidence of abortion is generally low and is most common during the third month. Sows usually abort only once. There is also a higher incidence of stillborn and weakly piglets. In sexually mature boars, infection can localize in the testis, resulting in clinical orchitis (Kernkamp et al., 1946) with consequent impairment of spermatogenesis, loss of libido and infertility. Poor reproductive performance of the boars exacerbates the overall fertility problem.

Herd diagnosis is made by means of a complement fixation test (CFT) or a serum agglutination test (SAT). *B. suis* may be isolated from aborted fetuses.

There is no treatment for swine brucellosis, nor is there any means of conferring artificial immunity. In infected commercial herds, all pigs should be slaughtered as they reach a suitable marketable weight and the unit left empty for 6 months before restocking. In the case of a valuable breeding herd, depopulation may be out of the question. In such situations all pigs are assumed infected, and a clean herd built up by isolating the piglets at birth and retaining those which pass the agglutination test at weaning age.

The public health issues should be borne in mind as this is an important zoonosis.

Other viruses

Other viruses that interfere with gestation include swine fever (hog cholera), foot and mouth disease, swine influenza, transmissible gastroenteritis, Japanese B encephalitis and Japanese haemagglutinating virus. Experimental infection with attenuated swine fever virus caused various effects that vary according to the stage of gestation at which sows were inoculated. In the USA, Dunne et al. (1965) have associated enteroviruses from two serologically distinct groups (A and B) with an epizootic disease of pigs characterized by stillbirths (S), mummification (M), embryonic death (ED) and infertility (I). The agents were termed SMEDI viruses.

VULVAL DISCHARGES

Pig producers often complain of a high incidence of vaginal discharge in the herd, and it is often worth considering the types and aetiology of these in some detail.

Vulval discharges are the most obvious clinical sign of bacterial genital infections although their detection varies according to a range of factors including the level of stockmanship and the type of sow accommodation. Discharges are also seen in a number of more generalized infectious forms of infertility (see above). The intermittent nature of most discharges confounds the problem (Meredith, 1991). The time of appearance of the discharge is also of significance to the investigation.

In most cases, uterine infections in non-pregnant sows do not appear to affect return intervals, although infection in early pregnancy can be associated with regular or irregular returns to service. In late pregnancy uterine infection can lead to abortion (Meredith, 1991).

Investigation of an outbreak of vulval discharge involves identification of the source of the discharge by speculum examination per vaginum. Discharges may originate from the vestibule, the vagina, the uterus or the bladder.

Cytological examination of the discharge differentiates between those composed of urinary sediments (which are rarely responsible for the disease) and those containing leucocytes and bacteria. The consistency of the discharge may vary from a thin pale yellow fluid without blood or mucus, to one with necrotic debris and mucus with or without blood (Muirhead, 1986). The latter type is closely correlated with cystitis that may be associated with *Corynebacterium suis* (Soltys, 1961). Microbiological sampling of the cervix generally yields a mixed flora of group 1 commensal organisms.

Differential diagnosis

Some discharges are quite normal, particularly those which are watery or slightly cloudy in appearance, and occur in pro-oestrus and oestrus. After mating, seminal fluids, including gel, may be expelled, and again these do not indicate a problem. A slight discharge may also be seen during pregnancy, and following parturition a lochia will be normally persist for up to 5 days (see Chapter 7).

Abnormal discharges can vary in quantity, consistency and colour (Table 27.5). Production of large volumes of creamy discharge (up to 500 ml)

Table 27.5 Differential diagnosis of vulval discharge (guidelines)

Type of discharge	Quantity	Consistency	Colour	Malodorous?
Normal				
Pro-oestrus/oestrus	Small	Watery, slightly tacky	Clear, cloudy or white (depending on cell content)	No
Seminal (during/shortly after mating or artificial insemination)	Varied	Mainly semen components, some fluid and cells from female	Clear, cloudy or white	No
Postmating (up to 2 days after service or artificial insemination)	Small	Thick, tenacious	White, grey or yellow	No
Pregnancy (probably from cervix)	Small	Thick, tenacious	White, grey or yellow	No
Postpartum lochia (up to 5 days postpartum)	Up to about 15 ml present at one time Decreasing by 3rd day	Usually thick	Varied	Slightly
Abnormal				
Vaginitis/cervicitis	Small	Thick, tenacious	White to yellow	Severe cases only
Endometritis	Varied	Varied	Varied	Severe cases
Endometritis (puerperal)	Often > 15 ml present at one time	Usually thin, may be lumps	Varied	Usually
Abortion (bacterial)	Varied	Varied	Varied (may be blood)	Occasionally
Urolithiasis (oxalates, phosphates)	Varied	Often gritty when rubbed between fingers	Cloudy, white or yellow	No
Cystitis/pyelonephritis	Varied	Varied	Often blood stained	Severe cases (ammoniacal)

Meredith (1991).

usually indicates endometritis. In the early stages, a tacky mucus can appear 15–21 days after service; these sows usually return to oestrus (Muirhead, 1986). Discharges immediately after farrowing have also been reported in association with the mastitis, metritis, agalactia syndrome (Leman et al., 1972). Muirhead (1986) did not recognize an association between postfarrowing discharges and those observed after service.

Treatment of discharges involves improved hygiene particularly in the service house, antibiotic injection of sows at weaning and a programme of in-feed medication. Boars can also be treated by a course of preputial infusion with a bovine intramammary antibiotic preparation (Muirhead, 1986).

ABNORMALITIES OF THE FEMALE REPRODUCTIVE TRACT

Anatomical defects of the female genitalia are relatively common in pigs and include intersexuality, gonadal hypoplasia and other miscellaneous abnormalities (Wrathall, 1975). That such anomalies are congenital rather than acquired is shown by their relatively higher incidence in gilts than sows. This aspect of pathological reproduction in swine has been studied by Wilson et al. (1949) and Nalbandov (1952), who found its incidence in sterile swine to be 21.5%. Despite the relative importance of a developmental abnormality in an individual, it should be remembered that on a herd scale such defects are not usually of great significance.

Inherited hypoplasia of the gonads

This is an important condition in farm livestock because it can lead to substantial reduction in fertility without being particularly obvious clinically (Wrathall, 1975). Both sexes may be affected but it is, of course, more readily apparent in the male. In pigs, gonad hypoplasia has not been studied extensively although it has been described in the boar (Holst, 1949).

Intersexuality

This abnormality is of far greater significance and prevalence in the pig, with up to 0.5% affected (Wrathall, 1975). It appears to be a hereditary condition determined by recessive genes. Most porcine intersexes are male pseudohermaphrodites; they have testes which may be subanal or intra-abdominal. The mammalian ovary has dual potentiality in the sense that initially it possesses two sets of tubular duct systems — the Wolffian ducts and the Müllerian ducts. If the embryo is male the Wolffian ducts are stimulated to develop, whereas the Müllerian ducts regress and are usually vestigial by the time of birth (Hunter, 1988b); in the case of the female, the reverse takes place, with the Müllerian duct system developing instead. In the intersex a combination of both duct systems are present, the animal possessing a mixed set of tubular organs (Figure 27.5) both Wolffian and Müllerian ducts developing side by side.

Externally, intersexes resemble the female and micturate through the vulva, although a phallus may be present. The animal may be considered a gilt until puberty, when it starts to demonstrate male behaviour.

Bilateral uterine tubal lesions

Structural sterility resulting from bilateral tubal lesions (e.g. hydrosalpinx, pyosalpinx and ovarobursal adhesions) has been shown to occur in 33.3% sows and gilts which failed to breed (Warnick et al., 1949). The incidence of such abnormalities appears to be lower in Europe (Perry, 1956; Teige, 1957). Apart from the uterine tubes, other parts of the tubular genital tract may show aplasia or duplication, but only when the whole tubular system is aplastic, or when the vagina, cervix or uterine body is imperforate, will sterility result. The condition of uterus unicornis (Figure 27.6) will lead only to lowered fecundity.

Absence of one or both ovaries

The absence of one or both ovaries and a generalized underdevelopment of the whole reproductive tract (infantilism) occurs occasionally. Other lesions include double vagina, septae or 'strings' in the vagina and hymenal residues; Teige (1957) suggested that this type of defect may cause problems at service. Meredith (1982) described incidents of pain and/or haemorrhage at mating associated with hymenal strictures and urethral intromission.

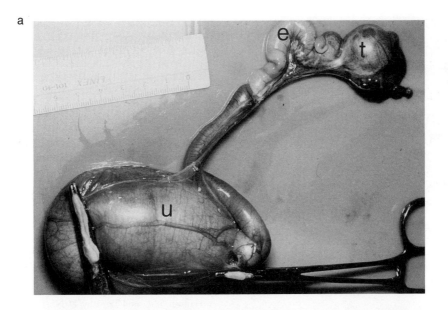

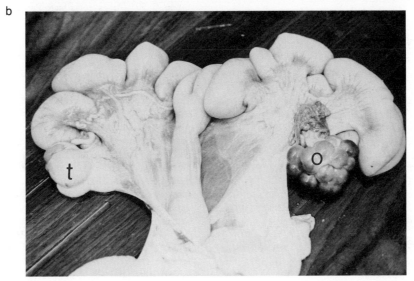

Fig. 27.5 Intersexuality. (a) Distended uterine horn (u), epididymis (e) and testis (t). (b) Genitalia of a porcine hermaphrodite showing testicle (t) and ovary (o). (Courtesy of R. G. A. Douglas and J. D. Mackinnon)

SEASONAL INFERTILITY

Reduction in fertility in pigs in the summer and early autumn has been reported in many countries and appears to manifest as a range of problems from delayed puberty in gilts, delayed postweaning oestrus in sows, regular and irregular returns to oestrus (Wrathall, 1987), delayed return to oestrus (Love, 1978, 1981), reduction in the farrowing rate, embryonic death, ovarian cysts and silent oestrus (Williamson et al., 1980). Autumn abortion syndrome may also be connected to seasonal infertility (Wrathall, 1987).

It has been suggested that heat stress is particularly damaging during the first 8 days postmating. Improvement of management of sows to avoid stressful and overheated conditions during the hot summer months can reduce the problem (Hennessy and Williamson, 1984; Hancock, 1988). More information is needed on the description and causes of this significant loss of production,

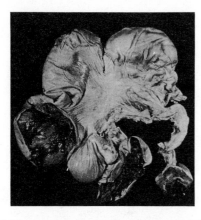

Fig. 27.6 Uterus unicornis: complete pregnant genital tract of a gilt showing uterus unicornis. Five piglets were present

particularly with the increasing trend to outdoor pig production in various parts of the world.

REFERENCES

Almond, G. W. and Dial, G. D. (1987) *J. Amer. Vet. Med. Assn*, **191**, 1987.

Alston, J. M. and Broom, J. C. (1958) *Leptospirosis in Man and Animals*, p. 65. Edinburgh: E. and S. Livingstone.

Bohl, E. H., Powers, T. E. and Ferguson, L. C. (1954) *J. Amer. Vet. Med. Assn*, **124**, 262.

Carr, J. (1992) *Pig Vet. J.*, **29**, 10.

Cartwright, S. F. and Huck, R. A. (1967) *Vet. Rec.*, **81**, 196.

Cartwright, S. F., Lucas, M. and Huck, R. A. (1969) *J. Comp. Pathol.*, **79**, 371.

Chaudhary, R. K., Fish, N. A. and Barnum, D. A. (1966) *Can. Vet. J.*, **7**, 106.

Christensen, R. K. (1981) *J. Anim. Sci.*, **52**, 821.

Christianson, W. T., Collins, J. E., Benfield, D. A., Harris, L., Molitor, T. W., Morrison, R. B. and Joo, H. S. (1992) *Proc. 12th IPVS Congr.*, p. 110.

Cromwijk, W. (1991) *EEC Seminar Report on the New Pig Disease*, p. 20. Brussels: PRRS.

de Jong, M. F., Cromwijk, W. and t'Veld, P. (1991) *EEC Seminar Report on the New Pig Disease*, p. 9. Brussels: PRRS.

Deyoe, B. L. (1967) *Amer. J. Vet. Res.*, **28**, 951.

Dial, G. D. and Parsons, T. (1989) *Proc. Amer. Assn Swine Practitioners 20th Annual Meeting*.

Dobson, K. J. (1974) *Aus. Vet. J.*, **50**, 471.

Doherty, P. C. and Baines, I. D. (1967) *Aust. Vet. J.*, **43**, 135.

Done, S. H., Paton, D. S., Edwards, S. Brown, I., White, M. E. C. and Robertson, I. B. (1992) *Pig Vet. J.*, **28**, 9.

Douglas, R. G. A. and Mackinnon, J. D. (1992) *Pig Vet. J.*, **29**, 26.

Dunne, H. W., Gobble, J. L., Hokanon, J. F., Kradel, D. C. and Bubash, G. R. (1965) *Amer. J. Vet. Res.*, **26**, 1284.

Einarsson, S., Larsson, K., Ersmar, M. and Edqvist, L. E. (1978) *Acta Vet. Scand.*, **19**, 156.

Ellis, W. A. (1992) *Pig Vet. J.*, **28**, 24.

Ellis, W. A., McParland, P. J., Bryson, D. G., Thierman, A. B. and Montgomery, J. (1986a) *Vet. Rec.*, **118**, 294.

Ellis, W. A., McParland, P. J., Bryson, D. G. and Cassells, J. A. (1986b) *Vet. Rec.*, **118**, 563.

English, P. R. (1991) *Pig Vet. J.*, **26**, 56.

Faine, S. (1982) *Guidelines for the Control of Leptospirosis.* Geneva: WHO.

Fennestad, K. L. and Borg-Petersen, C. (1966) *J. Infec. Dis.*, **116**, 57.

Fiennes, R. N. T. W. (1970) In: *Infection and Immunosuppression in Subhuman Primates*, ed. H. Balner, and W. I. B. Beveridge, pp. 149–154. Copenhagen: Munksgaard.

Glossop, C. E. (1991) *Pig Vet. J.*, **27**, 142.

Glossop, C. E. (1992) *Proc. Rencontres International de Production Porcine*, p. 97.

Glossop, C. E. and Foulkes, J. A. (1986) *Proc. 9th IPVS Congr.*, p. 15.

Glossop, C. E. and Foulkes, J. A. (1988) *Vet. Rec.*, **122**, 163.

Glossop, C. E. and Foulkes, J. A. (1990) *Proc. 11th IPVS Congr.*, p. 452.

Hancock, R. D. (1988) *Vet. Rec.*, **123**, 413.

Hanson, L. E. and Tripathy, D. N. (1986) *Diseases of Swine*, 6th edn, p. 591. Ames: Iowa State Press.

Hemsworth, P. (1988) Report, University of Minnesota Swine Health Clinic.

Hennessy, D. P. and Williamson, P. E. (1984) *Aust. Vet. J.*, **61**, 212.

Hodges, R. T., Thompson, J. and Townsend, K. G. (1979) *N. Z. Vet. J.*, **27**, 124.

Holst, S. J. (1949) *Nord. VetMed.*, **1**, 87.

Hopper, S. A., White, M. E. C. and Twiddy, N. (1992) *Vet. Rec.*, **131**, 140.

Hunter, R. H. F. (1988a) *P. V. S. Proc.*, **21**, 28.

Hunter, R. F. H. (1988b) *P. V. S. Proc.*, **21**, 135.

Hurtgen, J. P., Leman, A. D. and Crabo, B. (1980) *J. Amer. Vet. Med. Assn*, **176**, 119.

Kernkamp, H. C. H., Roepke, M. H. and Jasper, D. E. (1946) *J. Amer. Vet. Med. Assn*, **108**, 215.

Leman, A. D., Knudson, C., Rodeffer, H. E. and Mueller, A. G. (1972) *J. Amer. Vet. Med. Assn*, **161**, 1248.

Loula, T. (1991) *Agripractice*, **12**, 23.

Love, R. J. (1978) *Vet. Rec.*, **103**, 443.

Love, R. J. (1981) *Vet. Rec.*, **109**, 407.

Lynch, P. B. and O'Grady, J. F. (1984) *Pig News Info.*, **5**, 365.

Meredith, M. J. (1977) *Vet. Rec.*, **101**, 70.

Meredith, M. J. (1979) *Vet. Rec.*, **104**, 25.

Meredith, M. J. (1982) *Irish Vet. J.*, **36**, 17.

Meredith, M. J. (1983) *Pig News Info.*, **4**, 283.

Meredith, M. J. (1984) *Pig News Info.*, **5**, 213.

Meredith, M. J. (1991) *Pig Vet. J.*, **27**, 110.

Meulen van der, J., Helmond, F. A. and Oudenaarden, C. P. J. (1987) *Proc. Dutch Federation Meeting, Nijmegen, Holland*, p. 320.

Michna, S. W. and Campbell, R. S. F. (1969) *Vet. Rec.*, **84**, 135.

Muirhead, M. R. (1976) *Proc. Pig Vet. Soc.*, **1**, 49.

Muirhead, M. R. (1986) *Vet. Rec.*, **119**, 233.

Nalbandov, A. V. (1952) *Fertil. Steril.*, **3**, 100.

Perry, J. S. (1956) *J. Agr. Sci., Camb.*, **47**, 332.

PIC (1990–1991) *Pigtales Int. Rev.*

PIC (1993) *Pigtales Int. Rev.*

Robertson, I. B. (1992) *Pig Vet. J.*, **29**, 186.

Schilling, E. and Cerne, F. (1972) *Vet. Rec.*, **91**, 471.

Soltys, M. A. (1961) *J. Pathol.*, **81**, 441.

Stalheim, O. H. V. (1967) *Amer. J. Vet. Res.*, **28**, 161.

Taylor, D. J. (1989) *Pig Diseases*, 5th edn, p. 44.

Teige, J. (1957) *Nord. VetMed.*, **9**, 609.

van Alstine, W. G. (1991) *EEC Seminar Report on the New Pig Disease*, p. 65. Brussels: PRRS.

Walton, J. S. (1986) *J. Anim. Sci.*, **62**, 9.

Warnick, A. C., Grummer, R. H. and Casida, L. E. (1949) *J. Anim. Sci.*, **8**, 569.

Weitze, K. F., Rabeler, J., Willmen, T. and Waberski, D. (1990a) *Reprod. Domestic Anim.*, **25**, 191.

Weitze, K. F., Lotz, J. H., Everwand, A., Willmen, T. and Waberski, D. (1990b) *Reprod. Domestic Anim.*, **25**, 197.

Wensvoort, G., Terpstra, C. and Pol, J. M. A. (1991) *Vet. Rec.*, **128**, 574.

White, M. E. C. (1991) *Pig Vet. J.*, **28**, 62.

Williamson, P. E., Hennessy, D. P. and Cutler, C. (1980) *Aust. J. Agr. Res.*, **31**, 233.

Wilson, M. R. and Love, R. J. (1986) *Proc. 9th IPVS Congr.*, p. 21.

Wilson, R. F., Nalbandov, A. V. and Krider (1949) *J. Anim. Sci.*, **8**, 558.

Wrathall, A. E. (1971) *Vet. Rec.*, **89**, 61.

Wrathall, A. E. (1975) *Reproductive Disorders in the Pig, Review Series No. 11*. Commonwealth Bureau of Animal Health.

Wrathall, A. E. (1977) *Vet. Rec.*, **100**, 230.

Wrathall, A. E. (1987) *Proc. EC Seminar Definition of the Summer Infertility Problem in the Pig*, p. 45.

28

Infertility in the Bitch and Queen

In recent years there have been many physiological studies of reproduction in the bitch and queen. However, the number of investigations of infertility have been limited, indeed most attention has been paid to the prevention of conception because of the considerable problem world-wide of pet overpopulation (Olson and Moulton, 1993). However, there is no doubt that reproductive failure is common, and this may be attributed to the high degree of inbreeding (Wildt et al., 1983).

The extent of infertility in the bitch and queen is unknown. In the bitch, reduced fertility may not be fully appreciated because matings are relatively infrequent, when compared with other domestic species, and because the majority of breeding animals are housed singly or in small groups. The situation is further complicated because 'fertility' usually represents an owner's personal expectation of the reproductive performance of the bitch or queen; this expectation may differ between a commercial breeding establishment and the owner of an individual pet. In addition, there are wide breed variations, particularly in litter size, which make it difficult to compare animals of different breeds.

It is with increasing frequency that both individual breeders, and the managers of breeding colonies approach the veterinarian for help with breeding problems. This may be because of the value of an individual animal which fails to reproduce, or because of a concern for the decline in the productivity of a breeding colony. In the former case, continuation of a breeding line is the ultimate aim, whilst for the latter, greater productivity allows lower numbers of breeding animals to be maintained. The breeding of large numbers of dogs and cats is common for pharmaceutical and biological laboratories, and also for the production of working and assistance animals such as guide dogs for visually impaired people. For the latter, colony management requires not only a high output but a consistent production throughout the year.

The normal expectation of fertility in the bitch is a conception rate in the region of 70–80% (Hancock and Rowlands, 1949; Strasser and Schumacher, 1968; Andersen, 1970; England, 1992), whilst the queen may rear between one and three litters per year (Stabenfeldt and Shille, 1977; Cline et al., 1981; Concannon, 1991). There are considerable variations from this, depending upon age and breed. For the bitch, the peak in reproductive efficiency occurs at approximately 3 years of age, with a significant decline in the number of pups born in bitches aged 7 years and above (Blythe and England, 1993). Blythe and England (1993) also demonstrated a variation in the prolificacy between three breeds of dog. Similarly, in the cat an age-related reduction in the number of litters per year and average litter size has also been noted (Robinson and Cox, 1970; Schmidt, 1986), which is most marked after 6 years of age (Lawler and Bebiak, 1986). The decreased litter size in older bitches may be associated with an increased frequency of stillbirths. However, it should be remembered that there are marked breed variations for normal litter size in both the dog and cat (Lyngset and Lyngset, 1970; Robinson and Cox, 1970; Robinson, 1973); these should be considered when an animal is presented because of alleged subfertility.

The investigation of infertility in the bitch and queen is complicated by the fact that failure to conceive does not result in an immediate return to oestrus as occurs in polyoestrous species. However, the early diagnosis of pregnancy is now possible using real-time ultrasonography (Yeager and Concannon, 1990; England and Yeager, 1993) and the measurement of acute phase proteins in serum (Eckersall et al., 1993). These methods allow improved investigations into why an individual animal fails to produce live offspring.

As with other species, infertility in the bitch and queen may be categorized according to whether the cause is structural (including congenital, acquired and neoplastic diseases), functional (including endocrinological abnormalities), infectious or managemental. The influence of the male should always be investigated; collection and evaluation of a semen sample provides a basic assessment of the male's fertility (see Chapter 30). In addition, attention should also be given to the mating routine since owners, who are unfamiliar with normal mating behaviour, may inadvertently be hindering conception. Examples of this are: the belief that ovulation always occurs a set number of days after the onset of pro-oestrus in the bitch, and that only a single mating is necessary to induce ovulation in the queen.

THE BITCH

Structural abnormalities of the reproductive tract

Congenital abnormalities

Agenesis of an ovary is rare and does not cause infertility unless both ovaries are affected. In some cases there may also be agenesis of the ipsilateral uterine tube and/or uterine horn; although the latter may occur with a normal ovary. Ovarian dysplasia has also been reported in a bitch with an abnormal number of chromosomes (Johnston et al., 1985).

Bitches with uterine tube and/or uterine horn agenesis and normal ovaries usually exhibit typical oestrous behaviour, but either fail to become pregnant (bilateral lesion) or have low numbers of offspring (unilateral lesion). Diagnosis usually relies upon direct inspection of the reproductive tract via laparotomy or laparoscopy; the use of radiography following the injection of radiopaque contrast media into the uterus (Lagerstedt, 1993) is not as useful in the bitch as for other species.

Other congenital anomalies of the tubular genital tract include segmental aplasia of the Müllerian duct system. The aetiology of this condition remains uncertain; however, the inadvertent administration of exogenous hormones during pregnancy may result in the partial or complete absence of a connection between the Müllerian ducts and the urogenital sinus (Christiansen, 1984). Complete aplasia of the vagina results in infertility (Wadsworth et al., 1978; Hawe and Loeb, 1984) and allows the accumulation of

uterine fluid, producing similar signs to those of pyometra. In these cases the only treatment is ovariohysterectomy.

Strictures of the caudal reproductive tract are common in bitches. These may produce clinical signs associated with vulval pruritis or chronic vaginitis (Holt and Sayle, 1981; Soderberg, 1986); however, most commonly they are first recognized during a prebreeding examination or when there is pain associated with intromission. Circumferential strictures are most commonly found at the junction between the vestibule and the vagina; these may be stretched under general anaesthesia during pro-oestrus to allow mating during oestrus. Larger transverse fibrous bands may also be present; these require an episiotomy and extensive dissection to restore the vaginal lumen.

Congenital abnormalities of the external genitalia are rare. Vulval hypoplasia associated with perivulval dermatitis has been described (Christiansen, 1984); the relationship between this condition and early neutering has not fully been established. Masculinized female pups which have an abnormally shaped vulva may be produced following androgen or progestogen administration during pregnancy (see abnormalities of phenotypic sex below).

Intersex. Intersex animals have ambiguous genitalia. In the bitch this is usually recognized because of an abnormal phenotypic sex appearance; externally the animal appears as female but when it reaches puberty the clitoris enlarges and male-like behaviour is demonstrated. Intersex animals may be classified as those with abnormalities of chromosomal, gonadal or phenotypic sex. These conditions have recently been reviewed (Meyers-Wallen and Patterson, 1989; Meyers-Wallen, 1993).

Abnormalities of chromosomal number include phenotypic females (X0 or XXX) which have underdeveloped genitalia, and chimeras and mosaics which arise from two cell populations with different chromosome constituents. In chimeras and mosaics, there may be both ovarian and testicular tissue (true hermaphrodite); the phenotype of the animal depends upon the amount of functional testicular tissue (Meyers-Wallen and Patterson, 1989).

Animals with abnormalities of gonadal sex are those in which chromosomal and gonadal sex are dissimilar. Such individuals are called sex reversed. XX sex reversal is inherited as an autosomal recessive trait in the American cocker spaniel, and appears to be familial in other breeds (Meyers-Wallen and Patterson, 1988). Affected animals may conform to one of three categories: (1) true hermaphrodites with one ovotestis, bilateral uterine tubes, and normal external female genitalia, (2) true hermaphrodites with ovotestes and/or epididymides and masculinized external male genitalia and (3) XX males (Meyers-Wallen and Patterson, 1989). Animals with abnormalities of phenotypic sex are those in which chromosomal and gonadal sex are the same; however, the internal or external genitalia are ambiguous. Animals may be either female or male pseudohermaphrodites. Female pseudohermaphrodites generally occur as the result of androgen or progestogen administration during pregnancy; they have masculinization of the external or internal genitalia but with two ovaries. The clinical appearance may vary from simple clitoral enlargement to almost male-like external genitalia. Progestogens administered during pregnancy have been most frequently implicated since these agents are used by some veterinarians to prevent alleged luteal deficiency. Male pseudohermaphrodites have testes, but the internal or external genitalia are feminized. This may be the result of failure of Müllerian duct regression or the failure of androgen-dependent masculinization. In many cases, the exact aetiology remains unknown. However, removal of the reproductive tract including gonads is usually necessary. Following gonadectomy an enlarged clitoris may reduce in size although clitoridectomy may be necessary subsequently.

Acquired abnormalities

Acquired atrophy of the genitalia has been seen with neoplasia of the hypothalamus or pituitary (Arthur et al., 1989); this is termed Fröhlich's syndrome.

Other acquired abnormalities of the reproductive tract include endometrial hyperplasia and pyometra (which are discussed later) and vaginal hyperplasia (Figure 28.1). The latter condition, which is often wrongly called vaginal prolapse, may cause infertility by preventing mating. The aetiology is not clear; however, in some bitches the vaginal mucosa cranial to the urethral orifice becomes hyperplastic during pro-oestrus and oestrus and may protrude from the vulva and prevent mating. The hyperplasia appears to be an accentuated response to normal circulating oestrogen concentrations, which regresses at the beginning of metoestrus (dioestrus) but returns at the subsequent oestrus. In many cases, conservative therapy using emollient creams and topical antimicrobial

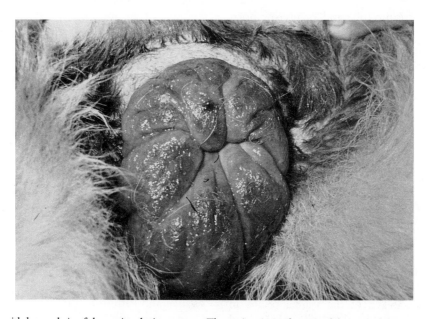

Fig. 28.1 Bitch with hyperplasia of the vagina during oestrus. The entire circumference of the vaginal mucosa is hyperplastic and protrudes from the vulva. Top is the dorsal commissure.

agents is sufficient. Recurrence may be prevented by performing an ovariohysterectomy during the subsequent anoestrus. However, if the bitch is required for breeding a submucosal resection may be performed during early oestrus. Breeding from these bitches should, however, be questioned since a familial tendency has been reported (Jones and Joshua, 1982).

True vaginal prolapse during oestrus has also been reported (Schuttle, 1967a), and recently chronic prolapse during pregnancy requiring hysteropexy has been described (Memon et al., 1993).

Neoplasia

Ovarian tumours are uncommon in the bitch, accounting for approximately 1% of all neoplasms (Cotchin, 1961; Hayes and Harvey, 1979). There is an increased incidence of ovarian neoplasia in older dogs (Jergins and Shaw, 1987); the mean age of occurrence is 8 years (Withrow and Susaneck, 1986). Ovarian tumours may be germ cell, epithelial or sex cord stromal in origin. The most important are granulosa cell tumours, which may become very large and produce clinical signs related to a mass effect or ascites. These tumours do not frequently metastasize and are usually endocrinologically inactive; however, they may secrete progesterone and produce cystic endometrial hyperplasia and pyometra, or oestrogen and pro-

duce signs of persistent oestrus or possibly bone marrow suppression. A less common tumour is the papillary cystadenocarcinoma which may occur bilaterally (Neilsen, 1963). These tumours commonly metastasize to the peritoneal lymphatics producing obstruction and ascites. This neoplasm has appeared after prolonged administration of stilboestrol.

The diagnosis of ovarian tumours is usually made on the basis of clinical signs, abdominal palpation, radiography and ultrasonography (Goodwin et al., 1990). Ovariectomy or ovariohysterectomy may be curative if performed early.

Uterine tumours are uncommon (Brodey and Roszel, 1967). The most frequently reported such lesions have been fibroleiomyomata. These are discrete and non-malignant, but haemorrhage may occur, resulting in a sanguineous vulval discharge. Uterine tumours may be diagnosed using real-time B-mode ultrasound (Figure 28.2).

Tumours of the cervix are rare, but benign tumours of the vagina and vestibule are more common and include fibromata, fibroleiomata and lipomata (Withrow and Susaneck, 1986) (Figure 28.3). These often originate from the ventral vaginal floor cranial to the urethral orifice and may cause a local vaginitis and haemorrhage. Usually they can be removed via an episiotomy; concurrent

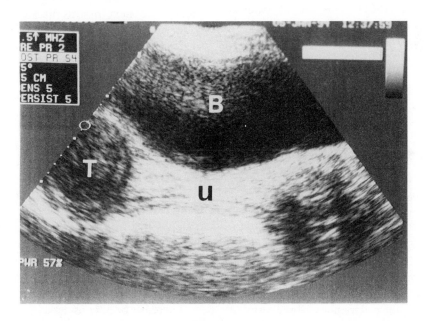

Fig. 28.2 Ultrasound image of the uterus of a bitch demonstrating a hypoechoic uterine tumour (T). The uterus (U) lies dorsal to the bladder (B).

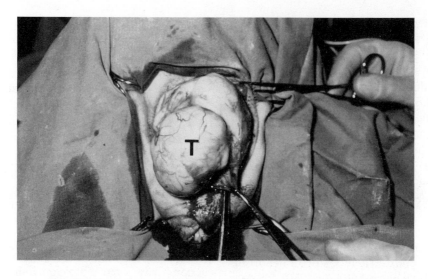

Fig. 28.3 Surgical removal of a large vaginal tumour (T) via an episiotomy.

ovariectomy/ovariohysterectomy reduces the risk of recurrence.

The transmissible veneral tumour (TVT) affects the vagina and external genitalia of the bitch and the penis of the dog (see Chapter 30). Transmission of the tumour occurs at coitus when infected cells 'seed' the genital mucosa of the recipient (Cohen, 1974). The lesions, which are often friable and multilobulated and may be single or multiple, generally reach their maximum size after 5–7 weeks and then regress spontaneously within 6 months (Moulton, 1961). The use of surgical debulking and various chemotherapeutic regimes have been described, including cyclophosphamide and vincristine, and radiation therapy (Calvert et al., 1982; Thrall, 1982). Such tumours are more common in tropical countries, and in the UK are generally only seen in imported animals (Booth, 1994).

Functional abnormalities of the reproductive tract

Delayed puberty and prolonged anoestrus

The age of puberty in the bitch ranges between 5 and 24 months (Andersen and Wooten, 1959; Rogers et al., 1970; Concannon, 1991), although this is influenced by the breed, body weight and environmental conditions (Christiansen, 1984; Feldman and Nelson, 1987a; Concannon, 1991). Bitches which do not reach puberty by 2 years of age are therefore considered to have delayed puberty. Since it is not uncommon for there to be few signs associated with the first oestrus, bitches which are thought to have delayed puberty may simply have had an unobserved oestrus. Failure to identify oestrus should also be considered in bitches which have prolonged interoestrus intervals. A high peripheral plasma progesterone concentration demonstrates that ovulation has occurred.

The normal interoestrus interval is between 26 and 36 weeks (Christie and Bell, 1971), and this is variable both within and between breeds (Linde-Forsberg and Wallen, 1992) and cannot be used to predict the next oestrus in an individual bitch (Bouchard et al., 1991). Therefore, it is difficult to define prolonged anoestrus, except that it is an interoestrus interval greater than that which was anticipated for a particular individual. The Basenji dog frequently exhibits its pubertal oestrus at approximately 300 days of age, and thereafter cycles only annually (Concannon, 1993).

To investigate both delayed puberty and prolonged anoestrus it is necessary to ensure that an oestrus has not been missed and that the animal's body weight and nutritional plane are normal. Debilitating disease may result in a failure to cycle, as may the use of certain drugs including progestogens, androgens and anabolic steroids. Progesterone-producing ovarian cysts have been described in the bitch (Burke, 1986), although these are very rare.

There has been considerable interest in the role of hypothyroidism as a cause of acyclicity in the bitch (Manning, 1979; Johnston, 1989). The mechanism of this is not fully understood although the administration of thyrotrophin-releasing hormone (TRH) causes the release of prolactin (Reimers et al., 1978); therefore, factors which affect TRH are likely to affect both thyroid function and prolactin secretion (Concannon, 1986). It is rare for only reproductive signs to be present in dogs with hypothyroidism. Recently, hypothyroidism was shown not to be related to poor reproductive performance in greyhounds (Beale et al., 1992).

Induction of Oestrus. It may be possible to induce cyclicity in bitches provided that there is no underlying disease. A variety of agents may be used for this purpose including oestrogens, luteinizing hormone (LH) and follicle-stimulating hormone (FSH), gonadotrophin-releasing hormone (GnRH) agonists and prolactin antagonists (England, 1994). Unlike other domestic species, it is not possible to induce oestrus in the bitch by shortening the luteal phase using prostaglandins since the luteal phase is followed by a variable period of anoestrus.

Exogenous oestrogens produce an increased responsiveness to basal concentrations of LH, which results in follicular growth and the production of endogenous oestrogen. Oestrogens have been used in a variety of regimens for oestrus induction; most have involved using low doses for 7–10 days with or without subsequent gonadotrophin administration. Results have been disappointing until recently, when Moses and Shille (1988) gave diethylstilboestrol (5 mg daily orally) until 2 days after the signs of pro-oestrus developed. If no response was elicited by day 7 the dose was increased to 10 mg daily for a maximum of a further 7 days. Subsequently, intramuscular injections of LH (5 mg) and FSH (10 mg) were given on days 5 (LH) and days 9 and 11 (FSH). All seven bitches in the study exhibited oestrous behaviour, were mated and whelped normally. However, subsequent studies by the same worker (Shille et al., 1989) were unsuccessful. Recently, diethylstilboestrol alone has been found to be very effective (Bouchard et al., 1993a). One concern over the use of oestrogens is the risk of toxicity, which may include dose-related bone marrow suppression, coat changes, mammary and vulval enlargement and potentiation of the stimulatory effects of progesterone on the uterus producing cystic endometrial hyperplasia and possibly pyometra.

Pharmacological doses of FSH and LH stimulate follicular growth and maturation, and therefore induce the release of endogenous oestrogens and stimulate ovulation. Many protocols using exogenous gonadotrophins for the induction of oestrus have been suggested. Equine chorionic gonadotrophin (eCG) and human chorionic gonadotrophin (hCG) were first used by Scorgie (1939). Other workers have subsequently used these preparations at different dosages and different regimens with varying success (Wright, 1972, 1980; Jones et al., 1973; Allen, 1982; Nakao et al., 1985). Recently, Arnold et al. (1989) showed that certain regimens could induce hyperoestrogenism and result in inhibition of implantation as well as bone marrow suppression and death. These workers found that low doses (20 IU/kg of eCG for 5 days) with a single administration of 500 IU of hCG on the fifth day produced more physiological changes in plasma hormones; six of six bitches exhibited oestrus and three became pregnant.

Exogenous pulsatile administration of GnRH may be used in an attempt to mimic natural profiles and induce physiological concentrations of FSH and LH. The pulsatile administration of GnRH to anoestrous bitches every 90 minutes for 6–12 days induced a fertile oestrus with pregnancy in three of eight bitches (Vanderlip et al., 1987). Pulsatile infusions are necessary because the constant infusion of GnRH produces initial stimulation followed by down-regulation of GnRH receptors. However, such techniques are not practical in the clinical situation. Concannon (1989) achieved some success in inducing oestrus using a GnRH superagonist administered via a subcutaneous osmotic pump. Concannon et al. (1993) recently showed that oestrus could be synchronized in a group of bitches by initially preventing oestrus using progesterone, and subsequently inducing oestrus using a GnRH agonist.

Prolactin appears to play a role in the regulation of interoestrous intervals possibly by affecting gonadotrophin secretion and/or ovarian responsiveness to gonadotrophins (Concannon, 1993). The use of prolactin antagonists, such as bromocriptine, cabergoline and metergoline, can result in shortening of the duration of anoestrus (Okkens et al., 1985; van Haaften et al., 1989) or induction of oestrus when anoestrus is prolonged (Arbeiter et al., 1988; Jochle et al., 1989; Handaja Kusuma and

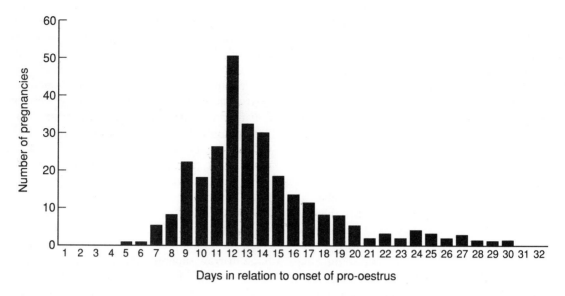

Fig. 28.4 The relationship between the calculated day of ovulation and the number of days from the onset of pro-oestrus in 278 bitches (England, unpublished observations).

Tainturier, 1993). The use of these drugs on a routine basis has not been entirely successful, and further investigations into their mode of action are warranted.

Silent oestrus

Normal cyclical endocrine changes may occur in some bitches without obvious external signs of pro-oestrus or oestrus. This may occur in up to 25% of greyhound bitches at the first cycle after puberty (Gannon, 1976). It is possible that oestrus events are not observed by the owner because there is only slight vulval swelling and minimal serosangineous discharge, or because the bitch is particularly fastidious. On some occasions overt pseudopregnancy occurs in the absence of a preceding oestrus. Ovulation can be confirmed by the measurement of peripheral plasma progesterone concentration, whilst weekly examination of exfoliative vaginal cytology will ensure that an oestrus is not missed.

Split oestrus (false oestrus)

Occasionally, at their first oestrus, bitches develop vulval swelling and a serosangineous vulval discharge of a short duration; however, ovulation does not occur; follicles presumably regress and the signs of pro-oestrus disappear. A normal oestrus follows several weeks later. The recognition of the split oestrus syndrome is important to ensure

that mating is achieved at the correct time in relation to ovulation.

Unpredictable ovulation time

Most bitches ovulate between 10 and 14 days after the onset of pro-oestrus (see Chapter 1). However, ovulation in normal bitches may occur as early as day 5 or as late as day 30 after the first signs of pro-oestrus (Figure 28.4). In addition to this large variation, bitches are not necessarily consistent between cycles (England et al., 1989a). Infertility may therefore result because of attempted matings at inappropriate times in relation to ovulation (see management factors affecting fertility, p. 534).

Prolonged pro-oestrus/oestrus

The normal interval between the onset of pro-oestrus and ovulation varies from 5 to 30 days (England et al., 1989a; England, unpublished observations). However, most bitches ovulate by day 14 after the onset of pro-oestrus, and those which ovulate later than this are often considered to have prolonged oestrus. These animals do not require treatment but careful assessment of the optimal mating time. Cases in which pro-oestrus or oestrus persists longer than 30 days (Wright, 1990) may require treatment. The induction of ovulation may be attempted by the administration of hCG (20 IU/kg).

Oestrogen-secreting follicular cysts are very rare

in the bitch, but these may produce persistent oestrus. Similar clinical signs may be seen with oestrogen-secreting ovarian tumours where high concentrations of oestrogen may lead to bone marrow suppression resulting in anaemia and thrombocytopenia. In such cases, treatment is by unilateral ovariectomy, although consideration should be given to the fact that the bitch may be normal or have a split oestrus syndrome. The administration of lithium carbonate may be useful in cases of oestrogen-induced bone marrow suppression (Hall, 1992).

Ovulation failure

Until recently, the diagnosis of ovulation failure was most commonly made on the basis of a shortened interoestrous interval (Johnston, 1988). However, following the introduction of routine monitoring of plasma progesterone concentrations bitches which fail to ovulate have been detected (Wright, 1990; Arbeiter, 1993). The incidence of ovulation failure has not been established; however, attempts at treatment may be made by the administration of hCG (Johnston, 1991).

Ovarian cysts

Cystic follicles (Figure 28.5) and corpora lutea are very rare; however, ovarian cystic structures are commonly observed at routine ovariohysterectomy. These are most frequently of parabursal origin (Figure 28.6) and of little clinical significance. Oestrogen-secreting follicular cysts may produce persistent oestrus with vulval discharge, flank alopecia and hyperkeratosis (Fayrer-Hosken et al., 1992); unilateral ovariectomy or ovariohysterectomy is necessary for the control of the clinical signs (Vaden, 1978; Burke, 1986). Attempts to cause luteinization of the cysts using hCG are usually disappointing (Arthur et al., 1989).

Luteal cysts have been identified in post-mortem studies (Dow, 1960); however, their significance is unknown. Burke (1986) suggested that they may secrete progesterone and produce prolonged anoestrus (sic) and cystic endometrial hyperplasia.

Andersen (1970) found that follicular and luteal cysts were most common in older bitches. Similar findings have been noted in the ovaries of aged bitches which have a mucohaemorrhagic vulval discharge, a condition referred to as metrorragie (Lesbouyries and Lagneau, 1950). These bitches are often attractive to male dogs but will not allow

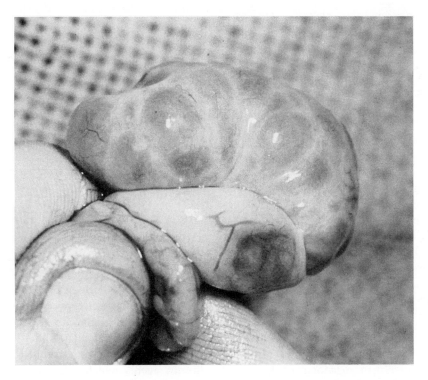

Fig. 28.5 An ovary of a labrador bitch demonstrating multiple follicular cysts.

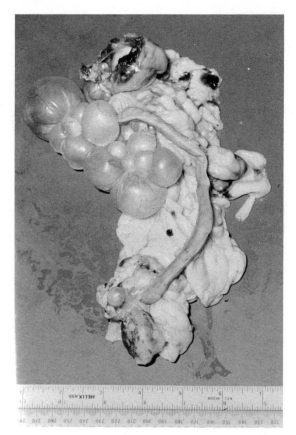

Fig. 28.6 The reproductive tract of a bitch demonstrating multiple parabursal cysts adjacent to the ovary and proximal uterine horn.

coitus; study of exfoliative vaginal cells demonstrates neutrophils, erythrocytes and parabasal epithelial cells.

Premature ovarian failure

Premature ovarian failure has been suggested as a cause of permanent anoestrus in previously normal bitches (Feldman and Nelson, 1987b). For an accurate diagnosis of these cases investigation of the karyotype and measurement of plasma concentrations of LH, FSH and thyroid hormone should be undertaken (Johnston, 1989). In valuable breeding animals, oestrus induction regimens may be contemplated; however, there is no information on the efficacy of these treatments in animals with premature ovarian failure.

Habitual abortion

There is little, other than anecdotal, evidence to suggest that habitual abortion is a clinical problem in the bitch. However, cases of abortion and resorption have been documented using real-time B-mode ultrasound (England, 1992; Muller and Arbeiter, 1993), although England (1992) suggested that there was no increased incidence in those bitches which had previously had reproductive disease. Cases of abortion are probably related to fetal defects and/or the result of infectious agents. However, progesterone deficiency due to poor luteal function is implicated by some workers (Feldman and Nelson, 1987a; Purswell, 1991). There is no doubt that the corpora lutea remain the principal source of progesterone production throughout gestation and that pregnancy may be terminated by ovariectomy (Andersen and Simpson, 1973) or the induction of luteolysis (Onclin et al., 1993) at any stage. However, the minimum concentration of progesterone required to support the pregnancy is only 2 ng/ml (Concannon and Hansel, 1977). Measurement of progesterone concentration at the time of an abortion often reveals that concentrations are low; however, this is likely to be the result of the abortion rather than the cause. Insufficient luteal function has been demonstrated following oestrus induction regimens (Barta et al., 1982) and in one case of oophoritis (Nickel et al., 1991). In the author's experience plasma progesterone concentrations of bitches with habitual abortion are not dissimilar to those of normal pregnant bitches. Progesterone or progestogen supplementation during pregnancy may produce masculinized female pups (Curtis and Grant, 1964) and cryptorchid male pups, and may possibly impair or delay parturition resulting in fetal death (see Chapter 6). Progestogen therapy should be restricted to those cases in which a true luteal insufficiency has been diagnosed.

Infectious agents

There are three categories of organisms which may exert an influence upon fertility. Firstly, those agents which are known to have a specific pathogenic effect upon the reproductive tract; secondly, those organisms which are present in the normal environment and which under certain circumstances can become opportunistic pathogens; and, thirdly, agents which cause systemic disease and exert their effect upon reproduction indirectly.

Normal vaginal bacterial flora

There is a widespread belief among breeders and veterinarians that infertility, vaginitis and fading puppy syndrome are caused by bacteria which inhabit the reproductive tract of the dog and bitch. This arose from the work of Stafseth et al. (1937) and Hare and Fry (1938), who concluded that streptococci, especially β-haemolytic types G and L, were responsible for infertility, abortion, anoestrus and weak pups. With the advent of virus isolation techniques, several specific viruses have been identified, and it seems likely that the earlier work over-emphasized the importance of the streptococci. Probably bacteria invade secondarily to viruses, or are contaminants.

Many aerobic and anaerobic bacteria normally inhabit the vestibule and vagina of the healthy bitch (Olson and Mathur, 1978), and the bacterial flora is normally mixed. The aerobic bacteria isolated from normal bitches include *Escherichia coli*, staphylococci and streptococci (Olson and Mathur, 1978; Allen and Dagnall, 1982) whilst the anaerobic bacteria include *Bacteroides* spp. and *Peptostreptococcus* spp. (Baba et al., 1983). Mycoplasmas have been isolated from between 30 and 88% of normal bitches (Bruchim et al., 1978; Doig, 1981; Baba et al., 1983). Greater numbers of bacteria are found within the vestibule compared with the vagina; the uterus is normally sterile (Olson et al., 1986). The stage of the oestrous cycle may influence the bacterial flora, because there is a significant increase in vaginal bacterial numbers when oestrogen concentrations are elevated (van Duijkeren, 1992). Several authors have examined the vaginal bacterial flora of normal bitches and compared them with those of infertile bitches. These studies were recently reviewed by van Duijkeren (1992), who showed that the bacterial species cultured from infertile bitches did not differ significantly from healthy bitches. Similarly, Hirsh and Wiger (1977) found that the organisms recovered from bitches with vaginal discharge were qualitatively the same as the normal bacterial flora, although the bacterial numbers were higher.

Therefore, the results of microbiological examination of the reproductive tract of the bitch must be treated with caution because the simple isolation of bacteria from the vagina does not constitute a diagnosis of reproductive disease.

Opportunist pathogens

The bacterial species found in bitches with reproductive disease do not differ significantly from those found in healthy bitches. However, disease may result if the uterine or vaginal defence mechanisms are depressed thereby allowing overgrowth of the normal commensals (Olson et al., 1986). Many of the normal vaginal inhabitants may become pathogens if a breakdown in local immunity occurs (van Duijkeren, 1992).

Bacteria may enter the uterus during oestrus when the cervix is relaxed, and could then cause infertility either directly by interfering with the zygote or by producing spermicidal factors (Jones and Joshua, 1982). Bacteria might persist within the uterus and be associated with the development of pyometra during the progesterone-dominant phase of the cycle.

If vaginal microbiological sampling reveal bacteria present in a pure growth or in very large numbers, then they may be considered significant; although pure growths of bacteria may also be isolated from normal dogs (Bjurstrom and Linde-Forsberg, 1992). Those bacteria most commonly thought to be significant include *Pseudomonas* spp., *Proteus* spp. and some streptococci. Repeated culture after one week should be performed to confirm the diagnosis before attempting treatment. Appropriate antimicrobial therapy, based upon sensitivity tests, should be administered parenterally and topically after investigation of possible predisposing causes such as anatomical, neoplastic or mechanical abnormalities of the vagina. It is prudent to refrain from breeding until the condition has been successfully treated, and preferably the bitch should be reswabbed at the beginning of pro-oestrus.

Mycoplasmas and ureaplasmas have been implicated in causing reproductive disease in the bitch (Lein, 1986). Mycoplasma colonization of the vagina has recently been demonstrated following treatment of bitches with oral ampicillin and potentiated sulfonamides (Strom and Linde-Forsberg, 1993), which suggests that the widespread use of antimicrobial agents in healthy bitches should be avoided.

Specific infections

Brucella canis. *B. canis* is a Gram-positive bacterium which can produce abortion and infertility. It is the only bacterium known to be a specific cause of infertility in the bitch. Brucella infertility was first reported in the USA (Moore and Bennet, 1967; Carmichael and Kenney, 1968) but has subsequently been found in several countries. Barton (1977) found that between 1.5 and 6.6% of dogs in the USA had antibodies diagnostic of infection; however, *B. canis* is not present in the UK, although Taylor et al. (1975) reported brucella abortion in one bitch. *B. canis* can be transmitted in several ways, including contact with aborted fetal or placental tissue, contact with the vaginal discharge of infected bitches, venereal transmission and congenital infection. The most common method of infection is venereal (Moore and Gupta, 1970). Abortion occurs most commonly between days 45 and 55 of pregnancy; however, there may be early fetal resorption, or the birth of stillborn or more rarely weak pups.

The isolation of the bacterium from blood or aborted tissue is diagnostic of the disease; however, there may be prolonged periods when the bitch is not bacteraemic, so that a negative blood culture does not rule out infection. Fortunately, diagnosis using the plate agglutination test for screening and tube agglutination for confirmation is not difficult, titres of 1:200 or greater being diagnostic of infection. Treatment of the condition with a combination of streptomycin and tetracycline is often effective in clinical cases; however, antimicrobial treatment does not remove the organism from tissues (Johnston et al., 1982). Since a carrier state can occur and these animals may be potential sources of infection, they are best neutered to remove them from the breeding programme.

Toxoplasma gondii. *T. gondii* infection causes abortion, premature birth, stillbirth and neonatal death (Cole et al., 1954; Siim et al., 1963). Surviving infected pups may carry the infection. The public health consequences of toxoplasma infection should be considered whenever it is diagnosed.

Canine herpesvirus. Canine herpesvirus in adult dogs generally produces a few mild signs limited to the respiratory or genital tract. However, the virus may cause genital lesions in the bitch that may be associated with infertility, abortion and stillbirths (Hashimoto and Hirai, 1986). It appears that infection of the pregnant bitch results in the production of placental lesions and the infection of the fetuses (Hashimoto et al., 1979). The infected placentae are macroscopically under-developed and possess small greyish-white foci which are characterized by focal degeneration, necrosis and the presence of eosinophilic intranuclear inclusion bodies. Experimental data suggests that infection during early pregnancy may result in fetal death and subsequent mummification, whilst infection during midpregnancy results in abortion, and infection during late pregnancy results in premature birth (Hashimoto et al., 1979). The virus has also been recovered from vesicular lesions on the genitalia of bitches (Post and King, 1971). Variable-sized vesicles are commonly observed in the vestibule (Hashimoto et al., 1983), and frequently these lesions are evident at the onset of pro-oestrus, suggesting that venereal transmission is probably important in adult dogs. Recrudescent canine herpes with virus shedding from the vesicular lesions may be stimulated by the stress of pregnancy and parturition. Pups may become infected at birth, during passage through the vagina, and subsequently die with characteristic widespread histological necrotizing lesions (Carmichael, 1970). Pups which survive the illness may show persistent neurological disorders (Percy et al., 1970). Pups are only at risk whilst *in utero* and during the first 3 weeks of life; attempts to produce the generalized disease in older pups have failed (Wright and Cornwell, 1970a). In the pups, the disease is rapidly fatal and treatment is often unrewarding; symptomatic therapy is all that is available since specific antiviral agents are not efficacious (Wright and Cornwell, 1970b).

Canine adenovirus. It is well established that infection with canine adenovirus during pregnancy can result in the birth of dead or weak pups which die within a few days of parturition (Spalding et al., 1964). In most cases, however, the virus is ingested and causes neonatal mortality (Cornwell, 1984). Carrier bitches may therefore act as a source of infection for pups.

Canine distemper virus. Experimental exposure of pregnant bitches to canine distemper virus was found to produce either clinical illness in the bitch with subsequent abortion, or subclinical infection of the bitch and the birth of clinically affected pups (Krakowka et al., 1977). This provides evidence for transplacental transmission, although the frequency of this under natural conditions is unknown.

Canine parvovirus. Canine parvovirus has

been implicted by some breeders as a cause of infertility in their kennels. However, Meunier et al. (1981) found that the conception rate, incidence of stillbirths, average litter size or average number of pups weaned per litter did not change after the introduction of canine parvovirus to a kennel of 2000 brood bitches. Canine parvovirus may cause an acute generalized infection in pups less than 2 weeks of age, which can occur as a consequence of uterine infection or as a result of exposure to the virus soon after birth (Guy, 1986).

Cystic endometrial hyperplasia and pyometra

Aetiology. Although the exact aetiology of cystic endometrial hyperplasia and pyometra is uncertain, this syndrome is probably best categorized as an infectious cause of infertility even though the role of the endocrine environment is significant. Pyometra may be lethal, but results in infertility if left untreated. It has been suggested that cystic endometrial hyperplasia, which precedes pyometra, may also result in infertility due to conception failure and embryonic resorption. The incidence of pyometra in the bitch is high; in fact, the disease is recognized as one of the common causes of illness and death in this species.

There has been considerable debate over the predisposing factors and the exact aetiology of pyometra. Most observers are of the opinion that the spontaneous disease is of middle-aged or old bitches. Dow (1958, 1959a) reported that the mean age of clinical cases was 8.2 years, with only 12% of the cases under 6 years of age. Several workers have suggested that the condition is more common in nulliparous bitches (Dow, 1958, 1959a; Frost, 1963) whilst others have suggested that it is more common in bitches with abnormal oestrous cycles and pseudopregnancy (Dow, 1959b; Whitney, 1967). Fidler et al. (1966), however, found no relationship to parity or oestrous characteristics; this opinion is now widely accepted. Pyometra is a disease of the luteal phase, with most bitches showing clinical signs between 5 and 80 days after the end of oestrus (Figure 28.7).

Early attempts to produce the condition by introducing bacteria into the uterus were unsuccessful (Benesch and Pommer, 1930; Teunissen, 1952); however, the latter worker managed to induce endometritis when bacteria were introduced into the oestrous uterus during laparotomy

when the uterine horn was also ligated. Although successful attempts to produce the disease following the administration of oestrogens have been reported (Bloom, 1944; von Schulze, 1955), it was the work of Teunissen (1952) which indicated the importance of progesterone in the aetiology of the condition, and also demonstrated the potentiation of the effects of progesterone by oestrogen. Teunissen's general conclusions were that progesterone was the main hormone concerned with inducing uterine glandular hyperplasia which preceded pyometra. Continuing glandular hyperplasia occurs under the influence of progesterone and regresses at the end of the luteal phase. However, during the animal's life there is progressive hyperplasia which ultimately results in the development of pathological lesions termed cystic endometrial hyperplasia. The mucosal epithelial cells are characteristically tortuous with a hypertrophic clear cytoplasm (Hardy and Osborne, 1974). It is not known whether all cases of spontaneous pyometra are preceded by cystic endometrial hyperplasia, but this seems likely.

Much attention has been paid to the work of Dow (1959b), who was able to produce pyometra experimentally in young ovariectomized bitches by the administration of cycles of oestrogen and progesterone. Cystic endometrial hyperplasia was induced following three such cycles of treatment but there were no inflammatory changes in the endometrium. If, however, in the fifth or sixth cycle the dose of progesterone was increased, typical acute endometritis became superimposed upon the cystic glandular hyperplasia. It is worth noting that the dose rates of the hormones used were very high. Successful induction of pyometra was achieved by Teunissen (1952) without the need for cycles of oestrogen and progesterone; this difference may have been due to the age of the bitches used in the study since Dow's bitches were between 1 and $1\frac{1}{2}$ years of age whereas Teunissen's bitches were up to 5 years old.

It was suggested that pyometra was the result of excessive and/or prolonged stimulation of the uterus by progesterone from 'retained' or 'cystic' corpora lutea (Hardy and Osborne, 1974). However, although corpora lutea are always present within the ovaries of bitches with clinical pyometra (the result of the long luteal phase), there is no evidence of excessive progesterone production (Christie et al., 1972). Progesterone

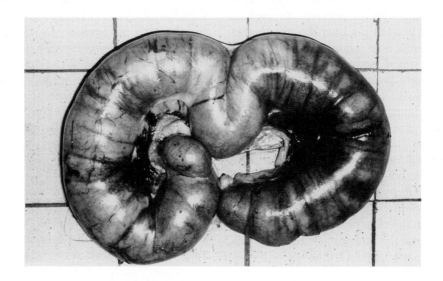

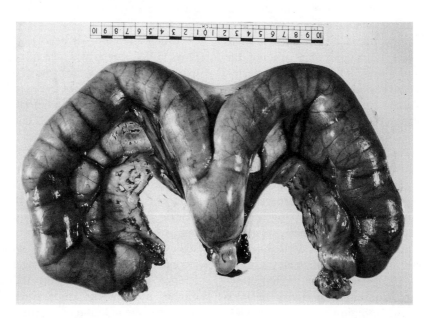

Fig. 28.7 The reproductive tracts from two bitches with pyometra. Note different degrees of distension.

concentrations in bitches with pyometra are similar to those in healthy bitches at the same stage of the luteal phase (Hadley, 1975a; Chaffaux and Thibier, 1978; De Coster et al., 1979) and the functioning capacity of the corpora lutea has been shown to be normal (Colombo et al., 1982).

Hadley (1975b) inadvertently produced a cystic endometrial hyperplasia in bitches which were subjected to repeated uterine biopsy during the early luteal phase of the cycle. These animals were much younger than those which normally develop the lesion and had not been subjected to any hormone therapy.

Organisms isolated from the uterine fluid in cases of pyometra are those found as part of the normal vaginal and vulval microflora. It is generally agreed that the predominant bacterium isolated is *E. coli* (Dow, 1960; Grindlay et al., 1973). Sandholm et al. (1975) found that the progesterone-sensitized endometrium and myometrium had an affinity for *E. coli*. These workers postulated that urinary tract infection was associated with pyometra; the uterus becoming infected during early metoestrus when receptors for *E. coli* develop within the endometrium, thus enhancing the colonization of the uterus with bacteria. It is likely that the long luteal phase of the bitch is an important contributory factor in the development of the condition since it has been shown that in the cow, progesterone increases the susceptibility of the genital tract to infection (Rowson et al., 1953). Brodey (1968) hypothesized that ano-genital bacteria entered the uterus during oestrus and were able to proliferate during metoestrus. This suggestion offers a plausible explanation of the aetiology, since the condition is more likely to develop when there is cystic endometrial hyperplasia; however, it has also been suggested that bacteria may enter the uterus either haematogenously or via lymphatic spread (Teunissen, 1952). A further factor that must be considered in the aetiology of pyometra is the use of exogenous reproductive hormones. Anderson et al. (1965) reported the occurrence of pyometra following the use of medroxyprogesterone acetate for the prevention of oestrus. Similar findings have been observed with several other progestogens. The experimental use of oestrogens in the bitch does not usually result in the development of pyometra. However, oestrogens enhance the stimulatory effects of progesterone on the uterus. For this reason when oestrogens are administered post-mating to prevent conception, pyometra may be induced (Durr, 1975; Nelson and Feldman, 1986); this probably relates to the increasing concentrations of progesterone seen during oestrus.

Clinical Signs. There are a wide range of clinical signs associated with pyometra in the bitch. When a complete history is available it is usually found that the bitch was in oestrus a few weeks prior to the illness. In some cases, when there is a vulval discharge, the owner may consider this to be a continuation of oestrus (Table 28.1).

If presented early, the general history is that the animal has been lethargic with a reduced appetite. Increased thirst and vomiting are variable findings.

Some bitches may be presented later when there is a vulval discharge, which in some cases is associated with improvement in the general health. In other cases, the bitch remains unwell and there is no discharge of pus. The bitch's abdomen may become distended and she may be thought to be pregnant although systemic illness is common. These cases generally end fatally often within 14–21 days from the onset of clinical signs; the cervix remains closed throughout. Death may be due to toxaemia alone or it may be associated with peritonitis due to rupture of the uterus. Occasionally, the cervix relaxes and there is an outpouring of pus just before death.

In a further category, there may be intermittent opening of the cervix, with relative good health following the discharge of pus, and malaise during the intervening periods. Such cases generally succumb from toxaemia in the course of a month or two.

Some cases of open-cervix pyometra may persist for years with a more or less continuous vulval discharge. Body temperature may be normal or slightly elevated in cases of open-cervix pyometra, whilst there is commonly an elevated body temperature in cases of closed-cervix pyometra. In toxaemic patients the temperature may be subnormal.

The character of the vulval discharge may vary considerably. Most often it is of thin consistency, light chocolate brown in colour and has a characteristic odour. In other cases it is yellow in colour, often blood tinged, and varying from a watery to a creamy consistency. The vulva is generally enlarged and there may be discoloration or scalding of the perivulval tissues and perineum.

An increased thirst is commonly observed in advanced cases and is due to reduced permeability for water in the distal convoluted tubule of the kidney (Asheim, 1964). Renal dysfunction is probably caused by the formation of immune complexes (Sandholm et al., 1975).

Diagnostic Features.

Abdominal palpation. Before examination the animal should be given the opportunity to urinate and defecate. In cases of open-cervix pyometra the uterine horns may be detected as thickened, often irregular and slightly turgid structures from 1 to 3 cm in diameter. Their location within the abdomen is not generally altered from normal. Occasionally, some areas of the uterine horns are turgid

Table 28.1 Differential diagnosis of vulval discharge in the bitch

Nature of the discharge	Condition	History	Condition of the vulva	Cytological findings[a]	Comments
Clear or straw coloured	Oestrus	Expected in 'heat'	Swollen or slightly soft	LIEC, AEC, RBC, no WBC	Attractive to male
Mucoid	Metoestrus	Recent oestrus	Large but soft	PBC, SIEC, VSIEC, WBC	No malaise
Mucoid	Normal pregnancy	Pregnant/recent oestrus	Large but soft	PBC, SIEC, WBC	No malaise, does not threaten pregnancy
Purulent	Juvenile vaginitis	Before first 'heat'	Normal	PBC, SIEC, WBC	May respond to antibiotics but recurs. Recovery after puberty
Purulent	Vaginitis	Variable but often excessive licking, attractive to male	Depends on the stage of the cycle	Depends on the stage of the cycle	Specific causes include: certain bacterial or viral infections, chemical irritation (urine), mechanical irritation (foreign body), neoplasia and anatomical abnormalities
Purulent/ haemorrhagic	Pyometra	Oestrus 2–8 weeks previously	Slightly swollen	WBC, SIEC, LIEC, RBC, bacteria, cell debris	Diagnosis using ultrasonography or radiography. Often malaise
Purulent/ haemorrhagic	Metritis	Recent parturition	Large	Multinucleated cells, LIEC, uterine cells	Severe malaise
Haemorrhagic	Pro-oestrus	Expected in 'heat'	Swollen	SIEC, LIEC, RBC, WBC	Attractive to male
Haemorrhagic	Oestrus	Expected in 'heat'	Swollen or slightly soft	LIEC, AEC, RBC, no WBC	Attractive to male
Haemorrhagic	Follicular cysts	Persistent discharge	Swollen	LIEC, RBC, ± WBC	No malaise, attractive to male, may develop bone marrow suppression
Haemorrhagic	Vaginal ulceration	Recent trauma or mating	Depends on the stage of the cycle	RBC, depends on the stage of the cycle	Rare, may start up to 2 weeks after mating
Haemorrhagic	Placental separation	Pregnant	Normal or slightly swollen	RBC, mucus	Ultrasound, radiography, etc., will confirm pregnancy
Haemorrhagic	Subinvolution of placental sites	Persistent discharge after whelping	Normal or slightly swollen	RBC, large polynucleated vacuolated cells	No malaise, refractory to treatment

Haemorrhagic	Transmissible venereal tumour	Not all countries of the world	Depends on the stage of the cycle	RBC, tumour cells?	Identification of tumour on vulva or in vagina confirms diagnosis
Haemorrhagic	Cystitis	Frequent urination	Depends on the stage of the cycle	RBC, mucus	Small volumes of urine, dysuria
Haemorrhagic	Urinary tract neoplasia	Dysuria	Depends on the stage of the cycle	RBC, tumour cells?	Endoscopy may show origin of haemorrhage, positive contrast cystourethrography may be diagnostic
Haemorrhagic/brown coloured	Abortion	Pregnant	Slightly enlarged	RBC, mucus	Ultrasound shows uterus with similar appearance to postpartum
Green/brown coloured	Parturition	Pregnant	Slightly swollen	RBC, SIEC, uterine cells	Panting, nest making, milk production
Green/brown coloured	Dystocia, placental separation	Non-productive straining	Slightly swollen	RBC, SIEC, uterine cells	Ultrasound will confirm pregnancy and fetal viability

[a] PBC, parabasal cells; SIEC, small intermediate epithelial cells; LIEC, large intermediate epithelial cells; AEC, anuclear epithelial cells; RBC, erythrocytes; WBC, polymorphonuclear leucocytes; VSIEC, vacuolated small intermediate epithelial cells ('metoestrus cells').
Adapted from Allen and Renton (1982).

and solid to palpate whilst others, which are distended by pus, may be indistinguishable from the surrounding bowel. Care must be taken not to confuse the colon with thickened uterine horns. In cases of closed-cervix pyometra the degree of uterine distension may be greater, and there may be visible abdominal enlargement. In large or obese patients, abdominal palpation may not be possible.

Ultrasonography. Ultrasound is particularly valuable for detecting the uterus which is filled with fluid. The uterus has an increased diameter and may be folded upon itself so that several sections of each horn may be imaged in a single plane (Figure 28.8). The diameter of the uterus may vary depending upon whether the cervix is open or closed. The uterine wall is usually relatively hypoechoic and is increased in thickness. The uterine lumen is usually grossly dilated with anechoic fluid, although small echogenic particles and mass lesions may be identified. The diagnosis is most simple when the diameter of the uterus increases above that of the small intestine. In cases where there are large volumes of uterine fluid there is usually a far enhancement effect (Feeney and Johnston, 1986). Poffenbarger and Feeney (1986) noted that when the uterus was imaged at its proximal end the transverse image had a target configuration. Recently, Renton et al. (1993) sug-

gested that ultrasonography could be used to monitor cases of pyometra during treatment.

Radiography. The detection of a soft tissue opacity mass lesion within the caudal abdomen causing cranial displacement of the small intestine and dorsal displacement of the colon has been used for some time to indicate enlargement of the uterus (Engle, 1940; Schnelle, 1940; Walker, 1965). It should be remembered, however, that these findings are not specific for pyometra since early pregnancy has a similar radiographic appearance. Pneumoperitoneography may be a useful aid which allows clearer radiographic differentiation of the uterus in cases of pyometra (Glenney, 1954) but this is not routinely performed.

Haematology. The total number of leucocytes is frequently elevated in cases of pyometra (Khuen et al., 1940), although the degree is much less marked in cases of open-cervix pyometra compared with closed-cervix pyometra (Morris et al., 1942). However, an elevated white cell count is not always present (Sheridan, 1979).

Rectal examination. It may be possible to palpate the distended uterus per rectum especially if slight backward pressure is applied to the abdominal wall.

Treatment. Ovariohysterectomy is the treatment of choice for pyometra. Bitches that are presented early in the course of the disease are usually a low surgical risk, and success rates up to

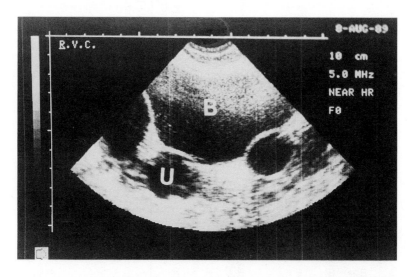

Fig. 28.8 Ultrasound image of the reproductive tract of a bitch with pyometra. The uterine horns (U) are distended with anechoic fluid and can be seen in three cross-sectional planes dorsal to the bladder (B).

92% have been reported (Austad, 1952). Lower success rates may be obtained with bitches that are toxaemic. Intravenous fluid therapy is essential in all cases to ensure minimum renal toxic effects (Ewald, 1961). Attention should also be paid to plasma electrolytes and acid–base status since complications associated with septicaemia, bacteraemia and uraemia are common (Feldman and Nelson, 1987a). Whilst the ideal situation is to administer intravenous broad-spectrum antimicrobial agents and fluid therapy, it is not always possible to stabilize the patient before surgery.

If the condition is not life threatening and the animal is particularly valuable, the question of restoration of fertility may be considered. Attempts have been made to drain the uterine fluid using a catheter placed via the cervix (Stephenson and Milks, 1934; Funkquist et al., 1983). However, this technique is difficult to perform, and surgically introduced drains have been advocated by some workers (Mara, 1971; Gourley, 1975). These are inserted transcervically via a hysterotomy and are used to flush the uterus after surgery. High success rates have been reported using this method (Mara, 1971).

In those cases where it is essential to retain reproductive function, or where surgery is not possible because of intercurrent disease, medical therapy may be considered. There have been several reports of successful medical management using oestrogens (presumably to induce cervical relaxation) (Watson, 1942; Fethers, 1943), drugs to induce uterine contraction including ergometrine (Hornby, 1943), quinine (Cowie and Muir, 1957), etamiphylline (Thomas, 1980) and several other agents (Spalding, 1923; Linde, 1966). However, since pyometra is a disease of the luteal phase and ovariectomy has been shown to produce resolution of the clinical signs (Watson, 1957), there has been considerable interest in the use of prostaglandins to cause lysis of the corpora lutea as well as for their uterine spasmogenic action (Swift et al., 1979; Sokolowski, 1980; Henderson, 1984; Wheaton and Barbee, 1993). Recently, prostaglandins have been used successfully in the treatment of cases of open-cervix pyometra (Nelson et al., 1982; Gilbert et al., 1989), even in those cases in which progesterone concentrations were low (Renton et al., 1993).

A protocol of 0.25 mg/kg of dinoprost administered daily by subcutaneous injection has been recommended (Feldman and Nelson, 1987b), although the twice daily administration of 0.125 mg/kg may result in fewer adverse effects. These, which include restlessnes, pacing, hypersalivation, tachypnoea, vomiting, diarrhoea, pyrexia and abdominal pain, may be severe and can persist for up to 60 minutes. Hospitalization and careful observation of the patient is necessary during such treatment. Prostaglandin therapy should be combined with appropriate broad-spectrum antimicrobial agents and intravenous fluid administration. Whilst prostaglandins have been used in cases of closed-cervix pyometra (Feldman and Nelson, 1987b), this is not recommended because of the risk of uterine rupture (Jackson, 1979; Renton et al., 1993). Reported success rates have varied: one bitch of three treated by uterine drainage subsequently became pregnant (Lagerstedt et al., 1987), whilst Feldman and Nelson (1987b) found that 37 of 42 bitches subsequently whelped after treatment of open-cervix pyometra with prostaglandin. Gilbert et al. (1989) achieved a clinical cure in 33 of 40 bitches, and of these, nine eventually produced litters. The long-term complications were anoestrus, recurrence of metritis, failure to conceive and abortion.

Management factors affecting fertility

It is generally accepted that the majority of bitches presented for fertility investigation are normal healthy fertile animals whose apparent infertility is related to a misunderstanding of the proper breeding management (Feldman and Nelson, 1987a). In modern breeding protocols, the dog and bitch are often not allowed to display normal courtship behaviour since they are introduced when the owner considers that the time for mating is correct. This is usually based simply upon the number of days from the onset of vulval swelling and the appearance of a serosanguineous vulval discharge.

Whilst the majority of bitches ovulate between 10 and 14 days after the onset of pro-oestrus this event may occur as early as day 5 or as late as day 30. In addition, bitches are not necessarily consistent between cycles (England et al., 1989a). Therefore, should a bitch be mated on days 12–16 after the onset of pro-oestrus (which is common breeding

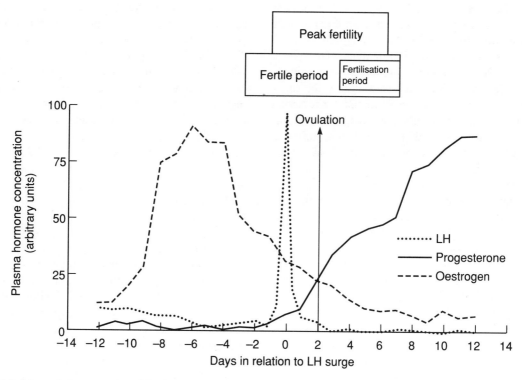

Fig. 28.9 Schematic representation of the changes in peripheral plasma hormones during pro-oestrus, oestrus and early metoestrus (dioestrus) and the relationship to the fertile period and the fertilization period in the bitch.

practice) this may be inappropriate and result in a failure of conception.

The fertilization period and fertile period

A surge in plasma LH concentration is the trigger for ovulation, which occurs 40–50 hours later (Phemister et al., 1973). Ovulation is spontaneous and eggs are ovulated as primary oocytes (Evans and Cole, 1931; Doak et al., 1967). The oocytes are immature at ovulation and must reach the metaphase of the second meiotic division after extrusion of the first polar body before fertilization (Baker, 1982); this further stage of maturation lasts 48–60 hours (Tsutsui, 1989). Eggs remain fertilizable for a further 2–3 days (Holst and Phemister, 1974; Concannon et al., 1989a), therefore the time-span over which fertilization may occur, termed the 'fertilization period' (Jeffcoate and Lindsay, 1989), is between 4 and 7 days after the LH surge (Figure 28.9).

Dog sperm can remain viable and fertile within the uterus and uterine tubes for at least 6 days or more (Doak et al., 1967). Therefore, it is possible for matings, which take place before the fertiliza-

tion period, to result in conception. A second term may therefore be used, the 'fertile period', which differs from the 'fertilization period' in that it encompasses the period of sperm survival within the female reproductive tract before ovulation and oocyte maturation. The fertile period extends from 3 days before until 7 days after the preovulatory LH surge, and may be even longer for dogs with exceptional semen quality. Determination of the time to mate can therefore be assessed on the basis of the time of the LH surge, or methods that may reliably indicate the 'fertilization period' or the 'fertile period'.

Whilst it was initially thought that the LH surge occurred synchronously with the onset of standing oestrus (Concannon et al., 1975), it was subsequently shown that this may occur between 3 days before, to 9 days after, the onset of oestrus (Mellin et al., 1976; Wildt et al., 1978a; Concannon and Rendano, 1983). Therefore, teasing the bitch has little value in determining the fertile period. Clinical assessment of the volume and colour of the vaginal discharge is similarly unreliable for determining the fertile period (Rowlands, 1950; Bell and Christie, 1971).

The optimal mating time

The optimal time for mating is likely to be during or immediately preceding the fertilization period, and the period of peak fertility for natural matings ranges from 1 day before to 5 or 6 days after the LH surge (Holst and Phemister, 1974; Concannon et al., 1989a; England et al., 1989a) (Figure 28.9). Determination of the time to breed could therefore be based upon methods for estimating the time of the LH surge.

Hormone Measurement. Measurement of peripheral plasma concentrations of LH is a reliable and accurate method of determining the optimum time to mate. However, there is no readily available commercial assay for canine LH, and at present measurement requires radioimmunoassay, a technique which is time-consuming and expensive. An enzyme-linked immunosorbent assay has recently been described for the measurement of LH concentration in fox plasma (Maurel et al., 1993), but has yet to be evaluated in the dog.

Plasma progesterone concentrations begin to increase towards the end of pro-oestrus at the time of the LH surge (Concannon et al., 1975; Hadley, 1975a). The progesterone is produced by luteinizing follicles, and, therefore, serial monitoring of plasma progesterone concentrations allows anticipation of ovulation. Recently, commercial test kits designed to measure the concentration of plasma progesterone by enzyme-linked immunosorbent assay (ELISA) have become available. These kits have been shown to be useful for predicting the optimum mating time in the bitch (Eckersall and Harvey, 1987; England and Allen, 1989b; Dietrich and Moller, 1993; Fieni et al., 1993). Progesterone concentration may also be measured using this method on whole blood (England, 1991; Bouchard et al., 1993b) and vaginal fluid (England and Anderton, 1992).

Vaginal Cytology. The examination of exfoliative vaginal cells is now commonly used to monitor the oestrous cycle. During pro-oestrus,

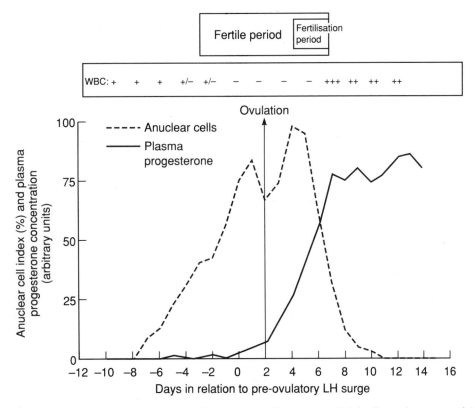

Fig. 28.10 Schematic representation of the changes in the percentage of anuclear epithelial cells in relation to ovulation and the fertile period in the bitch.

increased plasma oestrogen concentrations cause thickening of the vaginal mucosa, which becomes a keratinized squamous epithelium. Vaginal epithelial cells may be collected using either a moistened swab or by aspiration. The relative proportions of different types of epithelial cells can be used as a marker of the endocrine environment (Plate 7). Several methods for staining of cells and various indices of cornification and keratinization have been suggested as markers for the stage of the cycle (Schutte, 1967b; Klotzer, 1974). In general, the fertile period can be predicted by calculating the percentage of epithelial cells which appear cornified using a modified Wright–Giemsa stain (van der Holst and Best, 1976), although staining with a modified trichrome stain, allowing an assessment of the percentage of keratinized cells, has been suggested as being most useful (Schutte, 1967a). A schematic representation of the changes of exfoliative vaginal cells is given in Figures 1.31 and 28.10.

Polymorphonuclear leucocytes are absent from the vaginal smear during oestrus because the keratinized epithelium is impervious to these cells. Their reappearance during late oestrus reflects the breakdown of this epithelium (Evans and Cole, 1931). The return of polymorphonuclear leucocytes to the vaginal smear has been used by some workers as an indicator of the time of optimum fertility (Andersen, 1980).

Feldman and Nelson (1987a) suggested that breeding should be attempted throughout the period when more than 80% of epithelial cells are cornified in nature. Whilst this is a good guide, some bitches reach peak values of only 60% cornification, whilst in others there may be two peaks of cornification (van der Holst and Best, 1976). Some bitches demonstrate poor cellular changes in the vaginal smear (Tsutsui, 1975) and typical metoestrus cells may be found during pro-oestrus (Fowler et al., 1971). Allen (1985) noted that polymorphonuclear leucocytes may be found throughout the entire oestrous period; the extent of these variations has not been quantified. Recently, the aspiration of cells from the cranial vagina and the assessment of the anuclear cell index was found to increase the pregnancy rate and litter size of a group of bitches compared with a similar group mated only on the basis of the onset of pro-oestrus (England, 1992). The technique is particularly useful for bitches with irregular oestrous cycles and those with prolonged pro-oestrus or prolonged oestrus.

Vaginal Endoscopy. Vaginoscopy is the technique of examination of the vaginal mucosa using either a rigid endoscope or a paediatric proctoscope. Vaginoscopic assessment is based upon observation of the mucosal fold contours and profiles, the mucosal colour and on the characteristic colour of any fluid present (Lindsay, 1983a). Enlarged oedematous pink or pink/white mucosal folds are present during pro-oestrus and oestrus. Progressive shrinking of these folds is accompanied by pallor, effects which are probably the result of an abrupt withdrawal of the water-retaining effect of oestrogen during its preovulatory decline (Concannon, 1986). Subsequently, mucosal shrinkage is accompanied by wrinkling of the mucosal folds which become distinctly angulated and dense cream to white in colour. These gross changes have been used to assess the fertile period (Lindsay, 1983a,b). Jeffcoate and Lindsay (1989) proposed a scoring scheme to allow description and recording of the vaginoscopic changes. These workers also suggested that vaginoscopy could be used to indicate the end of the fertilization period.

Ultrasound Examination. Real-time B-mode ultrasound imaging has been used in several species to monitor follicular growth and to identify the time of ovulation. Imaging of the bitch's ovaries and the detection of ovulation was achieved by Inaba et al. (1984). Subsequent work suggested that a dramatic decrease in the size or number of follicles occurred at ovulation (Wallace et al., 1989), although no details of ovarian morphology were published. England and Allen (1989a) suggested that ovulation was difficult to detect since follicles did not collapse and because corpora lutea had central fluid-filled cavities unoccupied by luteal tissue (Figure 28.11). The central anechoic appearance of the corpora lutea was confirmed in a combined ultrasonographic and histological study (England and Allen, 1989b).

Recent work showed that ovulation could be detected by a decrease in follicle number, and a subjective decrease in follicle size (Wallace et al., 1992), whilst England and Yeager (1993) found that ovulation was characterized by a decrease in the number of fluid-filled follicles and their replacement by similar sized hypoechoic structures; these structures declined in number after ovulation and were replaced by fluid filled corpora lutea.

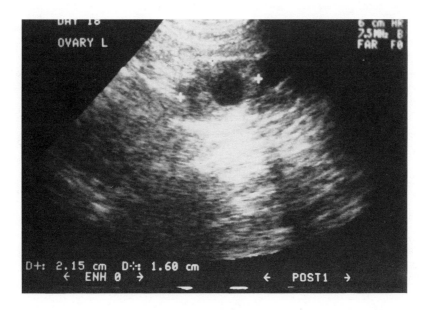

Fig. 28.11 Ultrasound image of an ovary of a bitch during metoestrus (dioestrus). A single large cavitated anechoic corpus luteum can be seen within the ovary (crosses).

Study of the Cervicovaginal Secretion. Variations in the electrical resistance of the vaginal secretion during the oestrous cycle have been described and Klotzer (1974) reported that the resistance decreased during the last part of oestrus in all bitches. These results were confirmed by Gunzel et al. (1986), and although the technique has been poorly investigated in the dog, it is used commercially for the detection of insemination time of the fox (Fougner, 1989).

Van der Holst and Best (1976) suggested that the amount of glucose within the vaginal discharge was a useful indicator of the optimum time of breeding. The principle of this technique is related to a change in the pH of vaginal secretion, since glucose is liberated from carboglutelin, which is then converted into lactic acid (Vogel and van der Holst, 1973). Although initial results were promising, this technique has not found clinical acceptance, presumably due to individual bitch variations.

Crystallization of mucus collected from the anterior vagina has been described in the bitch (Figure 28.12), occurring after the peak in plasma oestrogen concentrations (England and Allen, 1989c). Assessment of the mucus, which originates from cervical glandular tissue (England, 1993), may be useful when combined with vagi-

nal cytology for determining the optimal mating time (England and Allen, 1989c).

Vulval Softening. During pro-oestrus the vulva becomes enlarged and turgid. There is often a distinct softening and decrease in swelling following the preovulatory LH surge (Concannon, 1986). This method is imprecise but is probably the single clinical event that has proven to be useful for assessing the optimal mating time.

THE CAT

Structural abnormalities of the reproductive tract

Congenital abnormalities

The range of congenital abnormalities of the reproductive tract of the queen are similar to those of the bitch. Ovarian agenesis is rare and results in permanent anoestrus and infertility. Small ovarian remnants containing fibrous tissue may be identified at laparotomy or laparoscopy (Schmidt, 1986).

Ovarian hypoplasia is also rare (Herron, 1986) although phenotypically normal queens may have non-functional ovaries secondary to chromosomal abnormalities (Centerwall and Benirschke, 1975; Johnston et al., 1983).

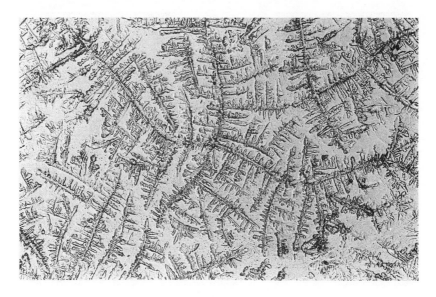

Fig. 28.12 Photomicrograph of the cervicovaginal fluid collected from a bitch during oestrus. Crystallization of the mucus has resulted in the formation of a fern-like pattern.

There are few reports of aplasia of the tubular genital tract although unilateral and/or bilateral agenesis of the uterine tube and uterine horn have been identified (Herron, 1986). It is not uncommon for these lesions to be associated with absence of the ipsilateral kidney and ureter. The queen may be fertile when the abnormality is unilateral, although litter size is often reduced. Vaginal aplasia may result in the retention of uterine fluid and cause endometrial changes and infertility. Vulval and vaginal atresia may occur separately or simultaneously. Small labia with or without stenosis of the vestibule are observed in the former, whilst stenosis of the vagina is observed in the latter (Saperstein et al., 1976).

Intersex. Several female cats with ambiguous genitalia have been described (Herron and Boehringer, 1972; Felts, 1982). In many cases the external genitalia are underdeveloped until puberty, when the animal may demonstrate male-like behaviour. Clitoral enlargement has not been reported (Herron, 1986). An exact diagnosis may not always be reached; however, removal of the reproductive tract including gonads is necessary in most cases. Animals may be classified as having abnormalities of either chromosomal, gonadal or phenotypic sex; a full description is given for the bitch (see p. 517).

Acquired abnormalities

Acquired abnormalities of the reproductive tract of the queen are rare. Occasionally ovarobursal adhesions of unknown aetiology are seen, but these are usually unilateral and cause reduced fertility rather than infertility. The most common acquired abnormality is pyometra (see later), although hydrometra has also been reported.

Neoplasia

Ovarian tumours are uncommon in the queen. They generally reach a large size before diagnosis and are not frequently metastatic, often being granulosa–theca cell tumours (Herron, 1986). These may be endocrinologically active and result in clinical signs of persistent oestrus, cystic endometrial hyperplasia and bilaterally symmetrical alopecia (Barrett and Theilen, 1977). The treatment of choice is ovariectomy. Malignant endometrial adenocarcinoma is the most common uterine neoplasm, although benign tumours have also been reported (Herron, 1986). These tumours may be associated with a persistent haemorrhagic vulval discharge and straining. In all cases, ovariohysterectomy is curative provided that metastases have not developed. Tumours of the vagina include pedunculated leiomyomata and fibromata. These are rare and generally produce clinical signs of vaginitis and straining to defecate, since they may impinge upon the colon and rectum. Local excision is usually curative, and ovariohysterectomy may reduce the risk of recurrence.

Functional abnormalities of the reproductive tract

Delayed puberty and prolonged anoestrus
The onset of puberty in the queen is influenced both by body weight and the season of birth. In most cases puberty occurs in the spring, therefore those animals born in autumn may exhibit their first oestrus at 6 months of age. However, queens born in winter or spring time may not exhibit puberty until 12 months of age (Goodrowe et al., 1989).

Queens that do not reach puberty by their second spring are considered to have delayed puberty. In the northern hemisphere, queens generally commence oestrous behaviour in January or February; an event which is dependent upon photoperiod (Herron, 1986). Prolonged anoestrus may be associated with systemic disease, poor nutrition or a high parasite burden (Mosier, 1975). If these factors are eliminated, 14 hours of daylight should abolish anoestrus in the healthy normal queen (Gruffydd-Jones, 1990). Attention should also be given to whether progestogens have been used for the control of dermatological or behavioural problems, since their use will prevent oestrus.

Induction of Oestrus. When it is necessary to breed the queen it may be possible to induce cyclicity providing that there is no underlying disease. Crude extracts of FSH and LH have been used to induce oestrous behaviour and ovulation (Foster and Hisaw, 1935). More recent work has utilized pregnant mare serum gonadotrophin administered daily for 8 days with reasonable success (Colby, 1970). The queen appears to be sensitive to the effects of exogenous gonadotrophins, and high doses may result in large numbers of cystic unovulated follicles (Wildt et al., 1978a). When anoestrous queens were given a single bolus of 100 IU of eCG, followed 5–7 days later by 50 IU of hCG, ovulation and pregnancy rates were similar to those at natural cycles (Cline et al., 1980). Similarly, the administration of FSH for 5–7 days resulted in a high pregnancy rate (Wildt et al., 1978a). More recently, a decreasing dose regime of

FSH-P combined with a single dose of hCG was shown to be successful (Pope et al., 1993).

Silent oestrus
Cases of silent oestrus are usually identified in queens which are low in the hierarchy of a cat colony. The incidence of silent oestrus is unknown, and the diagnosis is made upon the absence of behavioural oestrus whilst endocrinological events are normal. Cases are best evaluated by the study of vaginal cytology to demonstrate oestrus (see later), removal of the queen to a new environment or the induction of oestrus.

Prolonged oestrus
Some queens appear to have a behavioural oestrus which persists for the duration of two follicular cycles, even though the endocrinological events are normal. In these cases, oestrogen concentrations return to basal values between the follicular waves, although in some cases persistently elevated oestrogen concentrations have been identified (Feldman and Nelson, 1987b). The fertility of these cycles is uncertain, although it is likely that fertility may be reduced because of inappropriate mating time; however, treatment is not warranted since prolonged oestrus is generally a sporadic occurrence.

Ovulatory failure
Cats are induced ovulators with eggs being fertilizable at ovulation following mating or artificial stimulation of the genitalia (Greulich, 1934). Copulation produces a rapid pituitary-mediated release of LH (Robinson and Sawyer, 1987), and usually multiple copulations are required to ensure that ovulation occurs (Concannon et al., 1980). Failure of ovulation may occur if the queen is not mated a sufficient number of times. However, approximately 90% of queens ovulate if mated three times at 4 hour intervals for the first 3 days of oestrus (Schmidt, 1986). Ovulatory failure may be diagnosed by a return to oestrus after 3 weeks, and by measurement of plasma progesterone concentrations which remain basal following cessation of behavioural oestrus. Ovulation may be facilitated by ensuring that sufficient matings occur, or by the administration of a single dose of hCG (500 IU) on the first day of oestrus (Wildt and Seager, 1978).

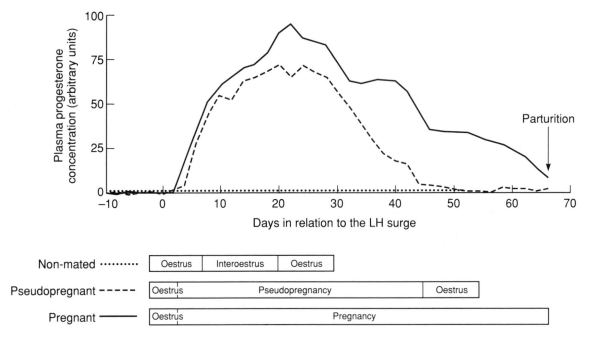

Fig. 28.13 Schematic representation of the changes in peripheral plasma progesterone concentrations in the non-mated, pseudopregnant and pregnant queen. The hormone profiles are plotted in relation to the time of the LH surge for the mated animals and the onset of oestrus in the unmated animals.

Pseudopregnancy

Whilst in the bitch pseudopregnancy is not a cause of infertility, in the queen the absence of cyclical activity may be explained by this condition.

Non-fertile matings, or occasional spontaneous ovulations (Lawler et al., 1993), result in the formation of corpora lutea which secrete progesterone. During the life-span of the corpora lutea the queen does not demonstrate oestrous activity, and this results in interoestrus intervals of between 35 and 70 days, with an average of 45 days (Verhage et al., 1976; Wildt et al., 1981). Diagnosis of the condition is based upon the demonstration of elevated concentrations of plasma progesterone (Figure 28.13). Late in the breeding season, however, pseudopregnancy may be followed by anoestrus.

Ovarian cysts

In the queen, cystic structures can be associated with the ovaries. However, the majority of these are not of ovarian origin, being remnants of mesonephric and rete tubules. These cysts are endocrinologically inactive and do not produce clinical signs. True follicular cysts, associated with hyperoestrogenism, have been reported (Herron, 1986), and

may be associated with exaggerated sexual behaviour and prolonged oestrus. Diagnosis may be made on the basis of clinical signs, measurement of plasma oestrogen concentrations or by the demonstration of persistent cornification of vaginal epithelial cells. hCG may be administered in an attempt to induce ovulation; however, in most cases, either ovariectomy or the use of progestogens to suppress the clinical signs is necessary.

Premature ovarian failure

Premature ovarian failure has been suggested as a cause of permanent anoestrus in previously fertile queens which results in a shortening of their reproductive life (Feldman and Nelson, 1987b). The condition is difficult to confirm, and diagnosis relies upon elimination of other causes of anoestrus. In valuable breeding animals oestrus induction regimens may be contemplated; however, there is no information on the efficacy of these treatments.

Habitual abortion

There is little non-anecdotal evidence to show that habitual abortion occurs in the queen; however, the condition is commonly diagnosed and treated. In many cases it is suggested that habitual abortion is the result of progesterone deficiency (Christiansen, 1984), although evidence for this is lacking. As in the bitch, the minimum plasma concentration of progesterone required to maintain pregnancy is approximately 1–2 ng/ml, with ovarian-derived progesterone being the major source throughout pregnancy (Verstegen et al., 1993a). The administration of progesterone or progestogens has been advocated to prevent habitual abortion (Christiansen, 1984); however, this therapy is empirical and suffers the risk of prolonging gestation and producing masculinized female kittens and cryptorchid male kittens. Progestogen administration should be limited to those cases in which a true luteal insufficiency has been diagnosed.

Infectious agents

There are no reported venereally transmitted infections nor specific genital infections that are recognized as causes of infertility in cats. However, there are several opportunistic pathogens and specific infectious agents which may have a direct effect upon fertility.

Opportunist pathogens

The vestibule and vagina of the queen is normally inhabited by many aerobic and anaerobic bacteria. It has been suggested that a variety of these bacteria may enter the uterus at mating and subsequently cause abortion because the progesterone-dominant uterine environment allows them to proliferate (Christiansen, 1984; Troy and Herron, 1986a). It is not clear, however, whether bacteria isolated from aborted fetuses have caused the abortion, or whether they have invaded the uterus after dilation of the cervix at the time of the abortion. Bacteria commonly isolated include *E. coli*, staphylococci, streptococci, salmonellae and mycobacteria (Troy and Herron, 1986b). Immediately prior to an abortion, the queen may become pyrexic and lethargic. Treatment includes the administration of broad-spectrum antimicrobial agents, fluid therapy and drugs to stimulate uterine evacuation. Hysterotomy to remove fetal tissue is rarely necessary, although ovariohysterectomy may be required should a severe metritis develop.

Specific infections

Feline Leukaemia Virus (FeLV). FeLV has been implicated in a variety of clinical syndromes including infertility, embryonic resorption and abortion (Hardy, 1981). FeLV is believed to be the single most common cause of infertility in the queen (Jarrett, 1985). Fetal resorption is seen frequently, although abortion and the birth of permanently infected kittens also occurs. The aetiology of the reproductive disease is uncertain, and whilst it is known that the virus may cross the placenta, one possibility is that secondary bacterial infections occur because of FeLV-induced immunosuppression (Jarrett, 1985). Diagnosis of FeLV may be achieved either by virus isolation, immunofluorescence or an ELISA method. Owners should be discouraged from breeding from FeLV-positive queens since all offspring are born persistently infected. These kittens usually develop an FeLV-related disease soon after birth. Vaccines are now available which provide protection against FeLV and its related diseases.

Feline Herpesvirus. Feline herpesvirus 1 may result in abortion during the fifth or sixth week of gestation. Lesions may be found within the uterus; however, placental lesions have only been demonstrated following experimental infection (Hoover and Griesemer, 1971). In the naturally occurring disease, abortions are thought to be the result of a non-specific reaction to the infection (Troy and Herron, 1986a). Transmission of virus occurs via the respiratory tract, with up to 80% of cats remaining as chronic carriers. The diagnosis of herpesvirus infection is based upon the clinical signs and the isolation of virus. Vaccination of queens provides good immunity and should be recommended for all breeding animals.

Feline Panleucopenia Virus. Feline panleucopenia virus is transmitted by direct contact with saliva, faeces and urine. Infection of pregnant queens may result in abortion, stillbirths, neonatal deaths and fetal cerebellar hypoplasia (Troy and Herron, 1986a). These effects are the result of transplacental infection leading to fetal death and resorption in early pregnancy (Gillespie and Scott, 1973), and cerebellar hypoplasia when infection occurs from the middle third of pregnancy onwards (Gaskell, 1985). Diagnosis may be made on the basis of the clinical signs, histopathological findings, virus isolation and paired serum samples which demonstrate a rising antibody titre. There is no treatment for kittens with cerebellar hypoplasia.

Feline Infectious Peritonitis Virus. Feline infectious peritonitis virus has been implicated as a cause of infertility, stillbirths, endometritis, resorption and abortion, chronic upper respiratory tract disease and fading kitten syndrome (Scott et al., 1979; Troy and Herron, 1986b). Queens are not always ill and may suffer resorption or abortion which is unnoticed. Abortion generally occurs during the last 2 weeks of pregnancy (Norsworthy, 1974, 1979). Diagnosis is made by serological and pathological investigation.

Toxoplasmosis. Toxoplasmosis (*T. gondii* infection) has been incriminated as a rare cause of abortion and congenital infection of cats (Troy and Herron, 1986b). Serological screening is necessary to demonstrate the role of this protozoan in cases of abortion.

Chlamydiae. There is evidence that the feline strain of *Chlamydia psitacci* causes abortion in the queen. The mode of transmission has not been elucidated, although the organism has been isolated from the genital tract of infected cats and there is circumstantial evidence associating infection with reproductive disease (Willis et al., 1984). As well as direct isolation of the organism, diagnosis is possible by demonstrating high antibody titres. It is difficult to confirm whether the isolation of this organism indicates its role in an abortion since it may simply be an opportunistic bacterium.

Cystic endometrial hyperplasia and pyometra

Aetiology. Both natural and experimentally induced cystic endometrial hyperplasia and pyometra have been described in the queen (Dow, 1962a,b). The syndrome is more common in older animals (Lein and Concannon, 1983) and is uncommon during winter, when queens are acyclic. In naturally occurring cases, corpora lutea are present within the ovaries, suggesting that progesterone is involved in the pathogenesis, in a similar manner to the bitch (see p. 527). Interestingly, approximately half of the cases are seen in unmated queens, in which there should be no luteal phase. This may be explained by the observation of Dow (1962b) and Lawler et al. (1991) that a proportion of queens ovulate without mating. Recently, Lawler et al. (1993) showed that 35% of queens ovulated spontaneously without copulation or mechanical stimulation of the cervix. Reports of the relationship between the incidence of pyometra with parity (Colby, 1980) have been disputed (Feldman and Nelson, 1987b).

The bacteria isolated from cases of pyometra are similar to those found in the bitch, frequently being opportunistic organisms which are normal inhabitants of the genital tract of cats including *E. coli* (Joshua, 1971; Choi and Kawata, 1975; Lawler et al., 1991). Culture of vaginal swabs is therefore of limited value.

Clinical Signs and Diagnostic Features. The severity and clinical signs of the cystic endometrial hyperplasia–pyometra complex vary considerably. In early cases there may simply be mild endometrial hyperplasia with glandular dilation. This leads to a hostile uterine environment which may lead to fetal resorption. Queens with endometrial hyperplasia are often clinically normal, although occasionally the uterus may be enlarged and can be palpated. Ultrasound examination of these cases can reveal the presence of anechoic regions within the uterine mucosa, representing cystic glandular tissue; occasionally free uterine fluid may be detected. In breeding queens, it may be necessary to confirm the diagnosis using histological examination of a uterine biopsy. At laparotomy, a transverse wedge of uterus of full thickness to include endometrium is removed. In some cases, a presumptive macroscopic diagnosis can be made on gross examination of the uterus.

Cases of pyometra are not often difficult to diagnose since many queens have a malodorous vulval discharge, although the queen may be particularly fastidious and regularly clean her perineum. Often oestrus will have been observed within 2 months of the onset of the discharge. The range of diagnostic methods described in the bitch (see p. 527) may be helpful to confirm the diagnosis. The use of real-time diagnostic ultrasound provides the most accurate method, although radiography, haematology and clinical examination are also rewarding. Care must be exercised in palpating the abdomen because of the risk of causing rupture of the uterus.

Treatment. As in the bitch, ovariohysterectomy is the treatment of choice for cases of pyometra. Attention should always be paid to the electrolyte and acid–base status of the animal prior to surgery; intravenous fluid therapy is always warranted. The complete reproductive tract from a queen following ovarohysterectomy is shown in Figure 28.14.

A variety of methods have been investigated for promoting uterine drainage, although cervical

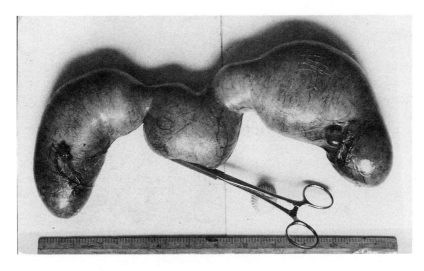

Fig. 28.14 Reproductive tract of a queen with pyometra.

catheterization has not been reported in the queen. Surgical drainage and lavage of the uterus via a laparotomy and uterotomy have been described (Gourley, 1975; Vasseur and Feldman, 1982). Following lavage, an indwelling drainage tube is placed in each uterine horn and passed through the cervix and vagina to allow postsurgical lavage.

Medical therapy may be useful and has been shown to have a good success rate (Feldman and Nelson, 1987b; Davidson et al., 1992). The former authors only treated queens that were less than 6 years of age which had open-cervix pyometra using 0.1 or 0.25 mg/kg of dinoprost daily for 5 days, and found that 12 of 14 queens subsequently produced litters. The adverse effects of prostaglandin administration in the queen are similar in duration and effect to those noted in the bitch and include tachycardia, salivation, vocalization, defecation and altered behaviour. Prostaglandin therapy should be combined with appropriate broad-spectrum antimicrobial agents and fluid therapy. Prostaglandins are known to have a direct luteolytic effect in the cat (Verstegen et al., 1993b) which, combined with their uterine spasmogenic action, explains why this regimen appears to be very successful. However, recently the luteotrophic action of prolactin and the luteolytic effects of prolactin antagonists such as cabergoline have been demonstrated (Verstegen et al., 1993b); it is possible that these agents may be used in the treatment of pyometra in the future.

Management factors affecting fertility

In the queen, modern breeding protocols may hamper reproductive performance because of a misunderstanding of the normal reproductive physiology.

Ovulation is considered to be induced by an adequate surge of plasma LH, released following coitus. In one study single copulations induced an LH surge sufficient to cause ovulations in only 50% of queens (Concannon et al., 1980). When four to 12 unrestricted matings were allowed in a 4 hour period the mean concentrations of LH were three to six times higher than for single matings and all queens ovulated (Concannon et al., 1980). Matings at limited, predetermined intervals on single or sequential days of oestrus can result in LH release of variable incidence, magnitude and duration (Wildt et al., 1978b, 1980; Banks and Stabenfeldt, 1982). It can be seen, therefore, that restricted mating regimens, which are common breeding practice, may result in failure of ovulation in a high proportion of queens. Multiple matings should result in ovulation although Glover et al. (1985) suggested that repeated matings very early in oestrus may not result in adequate LH release, whilst similar matings later in oestrus are likely to be successful at inducing ovulation. Therefore, not only is it important that multiple matings are allowed, but also normal courtship to ensure that matings occur throughout oestrus and not simply at the time the breeder considers to be correct.

It is difficult to accurately identify the stages of pro-oestrus or oestrus in the queen; however, unlike the bitch the behavioural events are more repeatable. During the 1–2 days of pro-oestrus the queen refuses copulation but is more active and may show interest in the male; this period can only truly be identified in the presence of a male. Oestrus may last between 3 and 20 days, with an average of 8 days. During this time the queen displays a crouching and lordotic stance which facilitates mounting by the male. This response can be elicited by firmly grasping the queen by the skin on the back of the neck. Mating should be attempted commencing at midoestrus, 3–4 days after the initial signs of pro-oestrus.

Vulval swelling during oestrus does not occur; therefore, clinical assessments of the queen are of little value for determining the optimum breeding time. A small amount of white vulvar discharge may occasionally be noticed during oestrus (Tsutsui and Stabenfeldt, 1993). The examination of exfoliative vaginal cytology is useful in the queen for determining the stage of the cycle; however, the technique does not enable the prediction of the onset of oestrus; up to one-third of queens may show signs of oestrus before the vaginal smear contains evidence of cornified cells (Shille et al., 1979). The technique is therefore most useful for verifying oestrus (Banks, 1986). The smear may be collected using either a moistened cotton swab or by irrigation with an eye-dropper containing sterile saline. Staining of the epithelial cells can be achieved using a variety of stains including a modified Wright–Giemsa stain. Erythrocytes are not found within the vaginal smear, because uterine diapedesis is not a feature of oestrus in the queen. The changes in the vaginal smear are therefore limited to changes in morphology of epithelial cells, because polymorphonuclear leucocytes are also usually absent except during early metoestrus and pregnancy. The percentage of epithelial cells which are cornified changes in a similar manner to that seen in the bitch (see p. 535). During oestrus more than 80% of cells are cornified. If the queen does not ovulate, the exfoliative cells return to a state similar to that observed during anoestrus or early pro-oestrus. Early metoestrus is characterized by increasing numbers of parabasal and small intermediate epithelial cells, whilst debris, mucus and

polymorphonuclear leucocytes also become evident.

Care should always be used when collecting vaginal epithelial cells since the technique may induce ovulation.

REFERENCES

Allen, W. E. (1982) *J. Small Anim. Pract.*, **23**, 223.

Allen, W. E. (1985) *J. Small Anim. Pract.*, **26**, 343.

Allen, W. E. and Dagnall, G. R. J. (1982) *J. Small Anim. Pract.*, **23**, 325.

Allen, W. E. and Renton, J. P. (1982) *Brit. Vet. J.*, **138**, 188.

Andersen, A. C. (1970) *The Beagle as an Experimental Dog*, p. 31. Ames: Iowa State University Press.

Andersen, A. C. and Simpson, M. E. (1973) *The Ovary and Reproductive Cycle of the Dog (Beagle)*. California: Geron-X.

Andersen, A. C. and Wooten, E. (1959) *Reproduction in Domestic Animals I.*, p. 359. New York: Academic Press.

Andersen, K. (1980) *Current Therapy in Theriogenology*, p. 661. Philadelphia: Saunders.

Anderson, R. K., Gilmore, C. E. and Schnelle, G. B. (1965) *J. Amer. Vet. Med. Assn*, **146**, 1311.

Arbeiter, K. (1993) *J. Reprod. Fertil. Suppl.*, **47**, 453.

Arbeiter, K., Brass, W., Ballabio, R. and Jochle, W. (1988) *J. Small Anim. Pract.*, **29**, 781.

Arnold, S., Arnold, P., Concannon, P. W., Weilenmann, R., Hubler, M., Casal, M., Dobeli, M., Fairburn, A., Eggenberger, E. and Rusch, P. (1989) *J. Reprod. Fertil. Suppl.*, **39**, 115.

Arthur, G. H., Noakes, D. E. and Pearson, H. (1989) *Veterinary Reproduction and Obstetrics*, 6th edn, p. 488. London: Baillière Tindall.

Asheim, A. (1964) *Acta Vet. Scand.*, **5**, 88.

Austad, R. (1952) *Nord. VetMed.*, **14**, 67.

Baba, E., Hata, H. and Fukata, T. (1983) *Amer. J. Vet. Res.*, **44**, 606.

Baker, T. G. (1982) *Reproduction in Mammals I. Germ Cells and Fertilization*, p. 17. Cambridge: Cambridge University Press.

Banks, D. H. and Stabenfeldt, G. H. (1982) *Biol. Reprod.*, **16**, 603.

Banks, D. R. (1986) *Current Therapy in Theriogenology*, p. 795. Philadelphia: Saunders.

Barrett, R. E. and Theilen, G. H. (1977) *Current Veterinary Therapy*, p. 1179. Philadelphia: Saunders.

Barta, M., Archibald, L. F. and Godke, R. A. (1982) *Theriogenology*, **18**, 541.

Barton, C. L. (1977) *Vet. Clin. N. Amer. Small Anim.*, **7**, 705.

Beale, K. M., Bloomberg, M. S., Gilder, J. V., Wolfson, B. B. and Keisling, K. (1992) *J. Amer. Anim. Hosp. Assn*, **28**, 263.

Bell, E. T. and Christie, D. W. (1971) *Vet. Rec.*, **88**, 536.

Benesch, F. and Pommer, A. (1930) *Wien. Tierartzl. Monatsschr.*, **17**, 1.

Bjurstrom, L. and Linde-Forsberg, C. (1992) *Amer. J. Vet. Res.*, **53**, 665.

Bloom, F. (1944) *N. Amer. Vet.*, **25**, 483.

Blythe, S. A. and England, G. C. W. (1993) *J. Reprod. Fertil. Suppl.*, **47**, 549.

Booth, M. J. (1994) *J. Small Anim. Pract.*, **35**, 39.

Bouchard, G., Youngquist, R. S., Vaillancourt, D., Krause, G. F., Guay, P. and Paradis, M. (1991) *Theriogenology*, **36**, 41.

Bouchard, G., Gross, G., Ganjam, V. K., Youngquist, R. S., Concannon, P. W., Krause, G. F. and Reddy, C. S. (1993a) *J. Reprod. Fertil. Suppl.*, **47**, 515.

Bouchard, G., Malugani, N., Youngquist, R. S., Krause, G. F., Concannon, P. W., Ganjam, V. K., Plata-Madrid, H., Tamassia, M. A. and Reddy, C. S. (1993b) *J. Reprod. Fertil. Suppl.*, **47**, 517.

Brodey, R. S. (1968) *Current Veterinary Therapy*, p. 652. Philadelphia: Saunders.

Brodey, R. S. and Roszel, J. F. (1967) *J. Amer. Vet. Med. Assn*, **149**, 1047.

Bruchim, A., Lutsky, I. and Rosendal, S. (1978) *Res. Vet. Sci.*, **25**, 243.

Burke, T. J. (1986) *Small Animal Reproduction and Infertility*. Philadelphia: Lea and Febiger.

Calvert, C., Leifer, C. E. and MacEwen, E. G. (1982) *J. Amer. Vet. Med. Assn*, **183**, 987.

Carmichael, L. E. (1970) *J. Amer. Vet. Med. Assn*, **156**, 1714.

Carmichael, L. E. and Kenny, R. M. (1968) *J. Amer. Vet. Med. Assn*, **152**, 605.

Centerwall, W. R. and Benirschke, K. (1975) *Amer. J. Vet. Res.*, **26**, 1275.

Chaffaux, S. and Thibier, M. (1978) *Ann. Rech. Vet.*, **9**, 587.

Choi, W. and Kawata, K. (1975) *Jpn. J. Vet. Res.*, **23**, 141.

Christansen, Ib. J. (1984) *Reproduction in the Dog and Cat*. London: Baillière Tindall.

Christie, D. W. and Bell, E. T. (1971) *J. Small Anim. Pract.*, **12**, 159.

Christie, D. W., Bell, E. T., Parkes, M. F., Pearson, H., Frankland, A. L. and Renton, J. P. (1972) *Vet. Rec.*, **90**, 704.

Cline, E. M., Jennings, L. L. and Sojka, N. J. (1980) *Lab. Anim. Sci.*, **30**, 1003.

Cline, E. M., Jennings, L. L. and Sojka, N. J. (1981) *Feline Pract.*, **11**, 10.

Cohen, D. (1974) *Transplant*, **17**, 8.

Colby, E. D. (1970) *Lab. Anim. Care*, **20**, 1075.

Colby, E. D. (1980) *Current Therapy in Theriogenology*, p. 869. Philadelphia: Saunders.

Cole, C. R., Sanger, V. L., Farrell, R. L. and Kornder, J. D. (1954) *N. Amer. Vet.*, **35**, 265.

Colombo, G., Baccani, D., Masi, I., Mattioli, M., Pannelli, I., Straini, R. and Cairoli, F. (1982) *Clin. Vet. (Milano)*, **105**, 196.

Concannon, P. W. (1986) In: *Small Animal Reproduction and Infertility*, p. 23. Philadelphia: Lea and Febiger.

Concannon, P. W. (1989) *J. Reprod. Fertil. Suppl.*, **39**, 149.

Concannon, P. W. (1991) *Reproduction in Domestic Animals*, 4th edn, p. 517. New York: Academic Press.

Concannon, P. W. (1993) *J. Reprod. Fertil. Suppl.*, **47**, 3.

Concannon, P. W. and Hansel, W. (1977) *Prostaglandins*, **13**, 533.

Concannon, P. W. and Rendano, V. (1983) *Amer. J. Vet. Res.*, **44**, 1506.

Concannon, P. W., Hansel, W. and Visek, W. J. (1975) *Biol. Reprod.*, **13**, 112.

Concannon, P. W. Hodson, B. and Lein, D. (1980) *Biol. Reprod.*, **23**, 111.

Concannon, P. W., McCann, J. P. and Temple, M. (1989a) *J. Reprod. Fertil. Suppl.*, **39**, 3.

Concannon, P. W., Lein, D. and Hodson, B. (1989b) *Biol. Reprod.*, **40**, 1179.

Concannon, P. W., Temple, M., Montanez, A. and Frank, D. (1993) *J. Reprod. Fertil. Suppl.*, **47**, 522.

Cornwell, H. J. C. (1984) *Canine Medicine and Therapeutics*, p. 340. Oxford: Blackwell Scientific.

Cotchin, E. (1961) *Res. Vet. Sci.*, **2**, 133.

Cowie, R. S. and Muir, R. W. (1957) *Vet. Rec.*, **69**, 772.

Curtis, E. M. and Grant, R. P. (1964) *J. Amer. Vet. Med. Assn*, **144**, 395.

Davidson, A. P., Feldman, E. C. and Nelson, R. W. (1992) *J. Amer. Vet. Med. Assn*, **200**, 825.

De Coster, R., D'ieteren, G., Josse, M., Jacovljevic, S., Ectors, F. and Derivaux, J. (1979) *Ann. Med. Vet.*, **123**, 233.

Dietrich, E. and Moller, R. (1993) *J. Reprod. Fertil. Suppl.*, **47**, 524.

Doak, R. L., Hall, A. and Dale, H. E. (1967) *J. Reprod. Fertil.*, **13**, 51.

Doig, P. A. (1981) *Can. J. Comp. Med.*, **45**, 233.

Dow, C. (1958) *Vet. Rec.*, **70**, 1102.

Dow, C. (1959a) *J. Comp. Path.*, **69**, 237.

Dow, C. (1959b) *J. Path. Bact.*, **78**, 267.

Dow, C. (1960) *J. Comp. Path.*, **70**, 59.

Dow, C. (1962a) *J. Comp. Path.*, **72**, 303.

Dow, C. (1962b) *Vet. Rec.*, **74**, 141.

Eckersall, P. D. and Harvey, M. J. A. (1987) *Vet. Rec.*, **120**, 5.

Eckersall, P. D., Harvey, M. J. A., Ferguson, J. M., Renton, J. P., Nickson, D. A. and Boyd, J. S. (1993) *J. Reprod. Fertil. Suppl.*, **47**, 159.

England, G. C. W. (1991) *Vet. Rec.*, **129**, 221.

England, G. C. W. (1992) *J. Small Anim. Pract.*, **33**, 577.

England, G. C. W. (1993) *J. Reprod. Fertil. Suppl.*, **47**, 551.

England, G. C. W. (1994) *Vet. Annu.*, **34**, 189.

England, G. C. W. and Anderton, D. J. (1992) *Vet. Rec.*, **130**, 143.

England, G. C. W. and Yeager, A. E. (1993) *J. Reprod. Fertil. Suppl.*, **47**, 107.

England, G. C. W. and Allen, W. E. (1989a) *J. Reprod. Fertil. Suppl.*, **39**, 91.

England, G. C. W. and Allen, W. E. (1989b) *Vet. Rec.*, **125**, 555.

England, G. C. W. and Allen, W. E. (1989c) *J. Reprod. Fertil.*, **86**, 335.

England, G. C. W., Allen, W. E. and Blythe, S. A. (1989a) *Vet. Rec.*, **125**, 624.

England, G. C. W., Allen, W. E. and Porter, D. J. (1989b) *Vet. Rec.*, **125**, 107.

Engle, J. B. (1940) *N. Amer. Vet.*, **21**, 358.

Evans, H. M. and Cole, H. H. (1931) *Mem. Univ. Calif.*, **9**, 65.

Ewald, B. H. (1961) *Small Anim. Clinic*, **4**, 383.

Fayrer-Hosken, R. A., Durham, D. H., Allen, S., Miller-Liebl, D. M. and Caudle, A. B. (1992) *J. Amer. Vet. Med. Assn*, **201**, 107.

Feeney, D. A. and Johnston, G. J. (1986) *Textbook of Veterinary Diagnostic Radiology*, p. 467. Philadelphia: Saunders.

Feldman, E. C. and Nelson, R. W. (1987a) *Canine and Feline Endocrinology and Reproduction*, p. 399. Philadelphia: Saunders.

Feldman, E. C. and Nelson, R. W. (1987b) *Canine and Feline*

Endocrinology and Reproduction, p. 525. Philadelphia: Saunders.

Felts, J. (1982) *J. Amer. Vet. Med. Assn*, **181**, 925.

Fethers, G. (1943) *Aust. Vet. J.*, **19**, 30.

Fieni, F., Decouvelaere, E., Bruyas, J. F. and Tainturier, D. (1993) *J. Reprod. Fertil. Suppl.*, **47**, 529.

Fidler, I. J., Brodey, R. S., Howson, A. E. and Cohen, D. (1966) *J. Amer. Vet. Med. Assn*, **149**, 1043.

Foster, M. A. and Hisaw, F. L. (1935) *Anat. Rec.*, **62**, 75.

Fougner, J. A. (1989) *J. Reprod. Fertil. Suppl.*, **39**, 317.

Fowler, E. H., Feldman, M. K. and Loeb, W. F. (1971) *Amer. J. Vet. Res.*, **32**, 327.

Frost, R. C. (1963) *Vet. Rec.*, **75**, 653.

Funkquist, B., Lagerstedt, A. S., Linde, C. and Obel, N. (1983) *Zbl. Vet Med.*, **30**, 72.

Gannon, J. (1976) *Racing Greyhound*, **1**, 12.

Gaskell, R. M. (1985) *Feline Medicine and Therapeutics*, p. 251. Oxford: Blackwell Scientific.

Gilbert, R. O., Nothling, J. O. and Oettle, E. E. (1989) *J. Reprod. Fertil. Suppl.*, **39**, 225.

Gillespie, J. H. and Scott, F. W. (1973) *Adv. Vet. Sci. Comp. Med.*, **17**, 164.

Glenney, W. C. (1954) *Vet. Med.*, **49**, 535.

Glover, T. E., Watson, P. F. and Bonney, R. C. (1985) *J. Reprod. Fertil.*, **75**, 145.

Goodrowe, K. L., Howard, J. G., Schmidt, P. M. and Wildt, D. E. (1989) *J. Reprod. Fertil. Suppl.*, **39**, 73.

Goodwin, J.-K., Hager, D., Phillips, L. and Lyman, R. (1990) *Vet. Radiol.*, **31**, 265.

Gourley, I. M. (1975) *Current Techniques in Small Animal Surgery*, p. 244. Philadelphia: Lea and Febiger.

Greulich, W. W. (1934) *Anat. Rec.*, **58**, 217.

Grindlay, M., Renton, J. P. and Ramsay, D. H. (1973) *Res. Vet. Sci.*, **14**, 75.

Gunzel, A., Koivisto, P. and Fougner, J. A. (1986) *Theriogenology*, **25**, 559.

Gruffydd-Jones, T. J. (1990) *Manual of Small Animal Endocrinology*, p. 143. Cheltenham: British Small Animal Veterinary Association.

Guy, J. S. (1986) *Vet. Clin. N. Amer. Small Anim.*, **16**, 1145.

Hadley, J. C. (1975a) *Vet. Rec.*, **96**, 545.

Hadley, J. C. (1975b) *J. Small Anim. Pract.*, **16**, 249.

Hall, E. J. (1992) *J. Amer. Vet. Med. Assn*, **200**, 814.

Hancock, J. L. and Rowlands, I. W. (1949) *Vet. Rec.*, **61**, 771.

Handaja Kusuma, P. S. and Tainturier, D. (1993) *J. Reprod. Fertil. Suppl.*, **47**, 363.

Hardy, R. M. and Osborne, C. A. (1974) *J. Amer. Anim. Hosp. Assn*, **10**, 245.

Hardy, W. D. (1981) *J. Amer. Anim. Hosp. Assn*, **17**, 941.

Hare, T. and Fry, R. M. (1938) *Vet. Rec.*, **50**, 1540.

Hashimoto, A. and Hirai, K. (1986) *Current Therapy in Theriogenology*, p. 516. Philadelphia: Saunders.

Hashimoto, A., Hirai, K., Okada, K. and Fujimoto, Y. (1979) *Amer. J. Vet. Res.*, **40**, 1236.

Hashimoto, A., Hirai, K., Fukushi, H. and Fujimoto, Y. (1983) *Jpn. J. Vet. Sci.*, **45**, 123.

Hawe, R. S. and Loeb, W. F. (1984) *J. Amer. Anim. Hosp. Assn*, **20**, 123.

Hayes, A. and Harvey, H. J. (1979) *J. Amer. Vet. Med. Assn*, **174**, 1304.

Henderson, R. T. (1984) *Aust. Vet. J.*, **61**, 317.

Herron, M. A. (1986) *Current Therapy in Theriogenology*, p. 829. Philadelphia: Saunders.

Herron, M. A. and Boehringer, B. T. (1972) *Feline Pract.*, **5**, 30.

Hirsch, D. C. and Wiger, N. (1977) *J. Small Anim. Pract.*, **18**, 25.

Holst, P. A. and Phemister, R. D. (1974) *Amer. J. Vet. Res.*, **35**, 401.

Holt, P. E. and Sayle, B. (1981) *J. Small Anim. Pract.*, **22**, 67.

Hoover, E. A. and Griesemer, R. A. (1971) *Amer. J. Pathol.*, **65**, 173.

Hornby, R. B. (1943) *Vet. Rec.*, **55**, 6.

Inaba, T., Matsui, N., Shimizu, R. and Imori, T. (1984) *Vet. Rec.*, **115**, 267.

Jackson, P. G. G. (1979) *Vet. Rec.*, **131**, 105.

Jarrett, J. O. (1985) *Feline Medicine and Therapeutics*, p. 271. Oxford: Blackwell Scientific.

Jeffcoate, I. A. and Lindsay, F. E. F. (1989) *J. Reprod. Fertil. Suppl.*, **39**, 277.

Jergins, A. E. and Shaw, D. P. (1987) *Comp. Cont. Ed.*, **9**, 489.

Jochle, W., Arbeiter, K., Post K., Ballabio, R. and D'ver, A. S. (1989) *J. Reprod. Fertil. Suppl.*, **39**, 199.

Johnston, C. A., Bennett, M., Jensen, R. K. and Schirmer, R. (1982) *J. Amer. Vet. Med. Assn*, **180**, 1330.

Johnston, S. D. (1988) *Fertility and Infertility in Veterinary Practice*, p. 160. London: Baillière Tindall.

Johnston, S. D. (1989) *J. Reprod. Fertil. Suppl.*, **39**, 65.

Johnston, S. D. (1991) *Vet. Clin. N. Amer. Small Anim.*, **21**, 421.

Johnston, S. D., Buoen, L. C. and Madl, J. E. (1983) *J. Amer. Vet. Med. Assn*, **182**, 986.

Johnston, S. D., Buon, L. C., Weber, A. F. and Madl, J. E. (1985) *Theriogenology*, **24**, 597.

Jones, D. E. and Joshua, J. O. (1982) *Reproductive Clinical Problems in the Dog*. London: Wright.

Jones, G. E., Boyns, A. R., Bell, E. T., Christie, D. W. and Parkes, M. F. (1973) *Acta Endocrinol.*, **72**, 573.

Joshua, J. O. (1971) *Vet. Rec.*, **88**, 511.

Khuen, E. C., Park, S. E. and Adler, A. E. (1940) *N. Amer. Vet.*, **21**, 666.

Klotzer, I. (1974) *Kleintierprax*, **19**, 125.

Krakowka, S., Hoover, E. A. and Koestner, A. (1977) *Amer. J. Vet. Res.*, **38**, 919.

Lagerstedt, A.-S. (1993) Thesis, Veterinarmedicinska faculteten, Uppsala, Sweden.

Lagerstedt, A.-S., Obel, N. and Stavenborn, M. (1987) *J. Small Anim. Pract.*, **28**, 215.

Lawler, D. F. and Bebiak, D. M. (1986) *Vet. Clin. N. Amer. Small Anim.*, **16**, 495.

Lawler, D. F., Evans, R. H., Reimers, T. J., Colby, E. D. and Monti, K. L. (1991) *Amer. J. Vet. Res.*, **52**, 1747.

Lawler, D. F., Johnston, S. D., Hegstad, R. L., Keltner, D. G. and Owens, S. F. (1993) *J. Reprod. Fertil. Suppl.*, **47**, 57.

Lein, D. H. (1986) *Current Veterinary Therapy IX*, p. 1240. Philadelphia: Saunders.

Lein, D. H. and Concannon, P. W. (1983) *Current Veterinary Therapy. Small Animal Practice*, p. 936. Philadelphia: Saunders.

Lesbouyries, G. and Lagneau, F. (1950) *Rec. Med. Vet.*, **126**, 19.

Linde, N. N. (1966) *Mod. Vet. Pract.*, **47**, 79.

Linde-Forsberg, C. and Wallen, A. (1992) *J. Small Anim. Pract.*, **33**, 67.

Lindsay, F. E. F. (1983a) *J. Small Anim. Pract.*, **24**, 1.

Lindsay, F. E. F. (1983b) *Current Veterinary Therapy. Small Animal Practice*, p. 912. Philadelphia: Saunders.

Lyngset, A. and Lyngset, O. (1970) *Nord. VetMed.*, **22**, 186.

Manning, P. J. (1979) *Amer. J. Vet. Res.*, 40, 820.

Mara, J. L. (1971) *Current Veterinary Therapy. Small Animal Practice*, p. 762. Philadelphia: Saunders.

Maurel, M. C., Mondain-Monval, M., Farstad, W. and Smith, A. J. (1993) *J. Reprod. Fertil. Suppl.*, **47**, 121.

Mellin, T. N., Orczyk, G. P., Hichens, M. and Behrman, H. R. (1976) *Theriogenology*, **5**, 175.

Memon, M. A., Pavletic, M. M. and Kumar, M. S. A. (1993) *J. Amer. Vet. Med. Assn*, **202**, 295.

Meunier, P. C., Glickman, L. T. and Appel, M. J. G. (1981) *Cornell Vet.*, **71**, 96.

Meyers-Wallen, V. N. (1993) *J. Reprod. Fertil. Suppl.*, **47**, 441.

Meyers-Wallen, V. N. and Patterson, D. F. (1988) *Hum. Genet.*, **80**, 23.

Meyers-Wallen, V. N. and Patterson, D. F. (1989) *J. Reprod. Fertil. Suppl.*, **39**, 57.

Moore, J. A. and Bennet, M. (1967) *Vet. Rec.*, **80**, 604.

Moore, J. A. and Gupta, B. N. (1970) *J. Amer. Vet. Med. Assn*, **156**, 1737.

Morris, M. L., Allison, J. B. and White, J. I. (1942) *Amer. J. Vet. Res.*, **3**, 100.

Moulton, J. E. (1961) *Tumours of Domestic Animals*. University of California Press.

Moses, D. L. and Shille, V. M. (1988) *J. Amer. Vet. Med. Assn*, **192**, 1541.

Mosier, J. E. (1975) *Mod. Vet. Pract.*, **56**, 699.

Muller, K. and Arbeiter, K. (1993) *J. Reprod. Fertil. Suppl.*, **47**, 558.

Nakao, T., Aoto, Y., Fukushima, S., Moriyoshi, M. and Kawata, K. (1985) *Jpn. J. Vet. Sci.*, **47**, 17.

Neilsen, S. W. (1963) *J. Amer. Vet. Anim. Hosp. Assn*, **19**, 13.

Nelson, R. W. and Feldman, E. C. (1986) *Vet. Clin. N. Amer. Small Anim.*, **16**, 561.

Nelson, R. W., Feldman, E. C. and Stabenfeldt, G. H. (1982) *J. Amer. Vet. Med. Assn*, **181**, 889.

Nickel, R. F., Okkens, A. C., van der Gaag, I. and van Haaften, B. (1991) *Vet. Rec.*, **128**, 333.

Norsworthy, G. D. (1974) *Feline Pract.*, **4**, 34.

Norsworthy, G. D. (1979) *Feline Pract.*, **9**, 57.

Okkens, A. C., Bevers, M., Dieleman, S. and Willemse, S. (1985) *Vet. Quart.*, **7**, 173.

Olson, P. N. S. and Mather, E. C. (1978) *J. Amer. Vet. Med. Assn*, **172**, 708.

Olson, P. N. and Moulton, C. (1993) *J. Reprod. Fertil. Suppl.*, **47**, 433.

Olson, P. N. S., Jones, R. L. and Mather, E. C. (1986) *Current Therapy in Theriogenology*, p. 469. Philadelphia: Saunders.

Onclin, K., Silva, L. D. M., Donnay, I. and Verstegen, J. P. (1993) *J. Reprod. Fertil. Suppl.*, **47**, 403.

Percy, D. H., Carmichael, L. E. and Albert, D. M. (1970) *Vet. Pathol.*, **8**, 37.

Phemister, R. D., Holst, P. A., Spano, I. S. and Hopwood, M. L. (1973) *Biol. Reprod.*, **8**, 74.

Poffenbarger, E. M. and Feeney, D. A. (1986) *J. Amer. Vet. Med. Assn*, **189**, 90.

Pope, C. E., Keller, G. L. and Dresser, B. L. (1993) *J. Reprod. Fertil. Suppl.*, **47**, 189.

Post, G. and King, N. (1971) *Vet. Rec.*, **88**, 229.

Purswell, B. J. (1991) *J. Amer. Vet. Med. Assn*, **199**, 902.

Reimers, T. J., Phemister, R. D. and Niswender, G. D. (1978) *Biol. Reprod.*, **19**, 673.

Renton, J. P., Boyd, J. S. and Harvey, M. J. A. (1993) *J. Reprod. Fertil. Suppl.*, **47**, 465.

Robinson, B. L. and Sawyer, C. H. (1987) *Brain Res.*, **418**, 41.

Robinson, R. (1973) *Vet. Rec.*, **92**, 221.

Robinson, R. and Cox, H. W. (1970) *Lab. Anim.*, **4**, 99.

Rogers, A. L., Templeton, J. W. and Stewart, A. P. (1970) *Lab. Anim. Care*, **20**, 1133.

Rowlands, I. W. (1950) *Proc. Conf. Soc. Study Fertil., London*, **2**, 40.

Rowson, L. E. A., Lamming, G. E. and Fry, R. M. (1953) *Vet. Rec.*, **65**, 335.

Sandholm, M., Vaseius, H. and Kvisto, A.-K. (1975) *J. Amer. Vet. Med. Assn*, **167**, 1006.

Saperstein, G., Harris, S. and Leipold, H. W. (1976) *Feline Pract.*, **6**, 18.

Schmidt, P. M. (1986) *Vet. Clin. N. Amer. Small Anim.*, **16**, 435.

Schnelle, G. B. (1940) *N. Amer. Vet.*, **21**, 349.

Schutte, A. P. (1967a) *J. S. Afr. Vet. Med. Assn*, **38**, 197.

Schutte, A. P. (1967a) *J. Small Anim. Pract.*, **8**, 313.

Schutte, A. P. (1967b) *J. Small Anim. Pract.*, **8**, 301.

Scorgie, N. J. (1939) *Vet. Rec.*, **51**, 265.

Scott, F. W., Weiss, R. C. and Post. J. E. (1979) *Feline Pract.*, **9**, 44.

Sheridan, V. (1979) *Vet. Rec.*, **104**, 417.

Shille, V. M., Lundstrom, K. E. and Stabenfeldt, G. H. (1979) *Biol. Reprod.*, **21**, 953.

Shille, V. M., Thatcher, M. J., Lloyd, M. L., Miller, D. D., Seyfert, D. F. and Sherrod, J. D. (1989) *J. Reprod. Fertil. Suppl.*, **39**, 103.

Siim, J. C., Biering-Sorenson, U. and Moller, T. (1963) *Advances in Veterinary Science*, p. 335. New York: Academic Press.

Soderberg, S. F. (1986) *Vet. Clin. N. Amer. Small Anim.*, **16**, 543.

Sokolowski, J. H. (1980) *J. Amer. Anim. Hosp. Assn*, **16**, 119.

Spalding, R. H. (1923) *J. Amer. Vet. Med. Assn*, **64**, 338.

Spalding, V. T., Rudd, H. K., Langman, B. A. and Rogers, S. E. (1964) *Vet. Rec.*, **76**, 1402.

Stabenfeldt, G. H. and Shille, V. M. (1977) *Reproduction in Domestic Animals*, p. 499. New York: Academic Press.

Stafseth, H. J., Thompson, N. W. and Neu, L. (1937) *J. Amer. Vet. Med. Assn*, **90**, 769.

Stephenson, H. C. and Milks, H. J. (1934) *Cornell Vet.*, **24**, 132.

Strasser, H. and Schumacher, W. (1968) *J. Small Anim. Pract.*, **9**, 603.

Strom, B. and Linde-Forsberg, C. (1993) *Amer. J. Vet. Res.*, **54**, 891.

Swift, G. A., Brown, R. H. and Nuttall, J. E. (1979) *Vet. Rec.*, **105**, 64.

Taylor, D., Renton, J. P. and McGregor, A. (1975) *Vet. Rec.*, **96**, 428.

Teunissen, G. H. B. (1952) *Acta Endocrinol.*, **9**, 407.

Thrall, D. E. (1982) *Vet. Radiol.*, **23**, 217.

Thomas, K. W. (1980) *Vet. Rec.*, **107**, 452.

Troy, G. C. and Herron, M. A. (1986a) *Small Animal Reproduction and Infertility*, p. 258. Philadelphia: Lea and Febiger.

Troy, G. C. and Herron, M. A. (1986b) *Current Therapy in Theriogenology*, p. 834. Philadelphia: Saunders.

Tsutsui, T. (1975) *Jpn. J. Anim. Reprod.*, **21**, 37.

Tsutsui, T. (1989) *J. Reprod. Fertil. Suppl.*, **39**, 269.

Tsutsui, T. and Stabenfeldt, G. H. (1993) *J. Reprod. Fertil. Suppl.*, **47**, 29.

Vaden, P. (1978) *Vet. Med. Small Anim. Clin.*, **73**, 1160.

van der Holst, W. and Best, A. P. (1976) *Tijdschr. Diergeneesk.*, **19**, 125.

Vanderlip, S. L., Wing, A. E., Felt, P., Linke, D., Rivier, J., Concannon, P. W. and Lasley, B. L. (1987) *Lab. Anim. Sci.*, **37**, 459.

van Duijkeren, E. (1992) *Vet. Rec.*, **131**, 367.

van Haaften, B., Dieleman, S. J., Okkens, A. C., Bevers, M. M. and Willemse, A. H. (1989) *J. Reprod. Fertil. Suppl.*, **39**, 330.

Vasseur, P. B. and Feldman, E. C. (1982) *J. Amer. Anim. Hosp. Assn*, **18**, 870.

Verhage, H. G., Beamer, N. B. and Brenner, R. M. (1976) *Biol. Reprod.*, **14**, 579.

Verstegen, J. P., Onclin, K., Silva, L. D. M., Wouters-Ballman, P., Delahaut, P. and Ectors, F. (1993a) *J. Reprod. Fertil. Suppl.*, **47**, 165.

Verstegen, J. P., Onclin, K., Silva, L. D. M. and Donnay, I. (1993b) *J. Reprod. Fertil. Suppl.*, **47**, 411.

Vogel, F. and van der Holst, W. (1973) *Tijdschr. Diergeneesk.*, **98**, 75.

von Durr, A. (1975) *Schweiz. Arch Tierheilkd.*, **117**, 349.

von Schulze, W. (1955) *Dtsch. Tierarztl. Wochenschr.*, **62**, 504.

Wadsworth, P. F., Hall, J. C. and Prentice, D. E. (1978) *Lab. Anim.*, **12**, 165.

Walker, R. G. (1965) *J. Small Anim. Pract.*, **6**, 437.

Wallace, S. S., Mahaffey, M. B., Miller, D. M. and Thompson, F. N. (1989) *J. Reprod. Fertil. Suppl.*, **39**, 331.

Wallace, S. S., Mahaffey, M. B., Miller, D. M., Thompson, F. N. and Chakraborty, P. K. (1992) *Amer. J. Vet. Res.*, **53**, 209.

Watson, M. (1942) *Vet. Rec.*, **54**, 489.

Watson, M. (1957) *Vet. Rec.*, **69**, 774.

Wheaton, L. G. and Barbee, D. D. (1993) *Theriogenology*, **40**, 111.

Whitney, J. C. (1967) *J. Small Anim. Pract.*, **8**, 247.

Wildt, D. E. and Seager, S. W. J. (1978) *Horm. Res.*, **9**, 144.

Wildt, D. E., Chakraborty, P. K., Panko, W. B. and Seager, S. W. J. (1978a) *Biol. Reprod.*, **18**, 561.

Wildt, D. E., Kinney, G. M. and Seager, S. W. J. (1978b) *Lab. Anim. Sci.*, **28**, 301.

Wildt, D. E., Guthrie, S. C. and Seager, S. W. J. (1978c) *Horm. Behav.*, **10**, 251.

Wildt, D. E., Seager, S. W. J. and Chakraborty, P. K. (1980) *Endocrinology*, **107**, 1212.

Wildt, D. E., Chan, S., Seager, S. W. J. and Chakraborty, P. K. (1981) *Biol. Reprod.*, **25**, 15.

Wildt, D. E., Bush, M., Howard, J. G., O'Brien, S. J., Meltzer, D., Vadn-Dyk, A., Ebedes, H. and Brand, D. J. (1983) *Biol. Reprod.*, **29**, 1019.

Willis, J. M., Gruffydd-Jones, T. J., Richmond, S. J. and Paul, I. D. (1984) *Vet. Rec.*, **114**, 344.

Withrow, S. J. and Susaneck, S. J. (1986) *Current Therapy in Theriogenology*, p. 521. Philadelphia: Saunders.

Wright, N. G. and Cornwell, H. J. C. (1970a) *J. Small Anim. Pract.*, **10**, 669.

Wright, N. G. and Cornwell, H. J. C. (1970b) *Res. Vet. Sci.*, **11**, 221.

Wright, P. J. (1972) *Proc. 7th Int. Cong. Anim. Reprod. AI*, **2**, 1075.

Wright, P. J. (1980) *Aust. Vet. J.*, **56**, 137.

Wright, P. J. (1990) *J. Small Anim. Pract.*, **31**, 335.

Yeager, A. E. and Concannon, P. W. (1990) *Theriogenology*, **34**, 655.

6

Part Six

The Male Animal

ANATOMY AND PHYSIOLOGY

The reproductive organs (Figure 29.1) of the male animal may be considered to fulfil three major functions. These are, firstly, the production of spermatozoa in the testis; secondly the maturation, storage and transport of spermatozoa within the duct system and, finally, the deposition of semen within the female genital tract via the penis. Likewise, the functions of the male hormones may be considered to be three-fold: the maintenance of spermatogenesis, the production of masculine behaviour (libido and aggression) and the development of the masculine body form.

Anatomy of the testis, spermatic cord and scrotum

The testes of all domestic male animals are located at the inguinal region within a scrotum. In the bull and the ram this structure is pendulous and has an elongated neck, but in most other domestic species the scrotum is closely applied to the inguinal region. The scrotum consists of a skin pouch overlying various fibroelastic and muscular layers, of which the most prominent is the tunica dartos (see Figure 29.2). The dartos layers are confluent between the testes, where they form the intertesticular septum. In the boar, the external spermatic fascia is also prominent. The testis itself is surrounded by two layers of peritoneum, which are formed during the descent of the testis as a single outpouching of the parietal peritoneum, through the inguinal canal. The outer layer of peritoneum, the processus vaginalis (tunica vaginalis reflexa), is reflected onto the testis to form the serous outer layer of that organ, the tunica vaginalis propria. Accompanying this outpouching of peritoneum through the inguinal canal is a diverticulum of the internal abdominal oblique muscle, which inserts on to the cremasteric fascia and the vaginal tunics. This muscle, the cremaster, raises or lowers the testis in response to temperature or noxious stimuli.

The capsule, or tunica albuginea, of the testis is composed principally of fibrous tissue, but has a smooth muscle component whose function is largely unknown. Overlying the capsule is the tunica vaginalis propria. The main blood vessels of the testis are distributed over the surface of the tunica albuginea before penetrating the capsule to supply the testicular parenchyma; while the innervation of the testis is mainly confined to the periphery and little nervous tissue is found in its substance. The substance of the testis (Figure 29.3) is composed of two main tissues: seminiferous tubules and interstitial tissue. Each seminiferous tubule is a highly convoluted, unbranched tube, which opens at both ends into collecting tubules and which, in turn, open into the single epididymal duct. The seminiferous tubules are limited by a basement membrane which is partially surrounded by contractile myoid cells. Within the tubule, the seminiferous epithelium is composed of two main cell lines, somatic Sertoli cells and the sperm-producing germinal cell lines. Interstitial tissue, which consists of steroid-producing Leydig cells, blood vessels and lymphatics, exhibits much variation in its quantity and morphology between species. For example, there is prolific interstitial tissue in the boar and the stallion, but relatively little in ruminants.

The epididymis is a single, highly convoluted tube, into which the vasa efferentia drain the seminiferous tubules. Grossly, the epididymis appears as an approximately cylindrical organ, which is divided into a prominent head, situated close to the suspension of the testis from the spermatic cord, a smaller, medially situated body and a distended tail, which is continuous with the vas deferens. The muscular wall of the epididymal duct moves sperm through its lumen by peristalsis, so that during passage of the epididymis, sperm, which are immature on release from the testis,

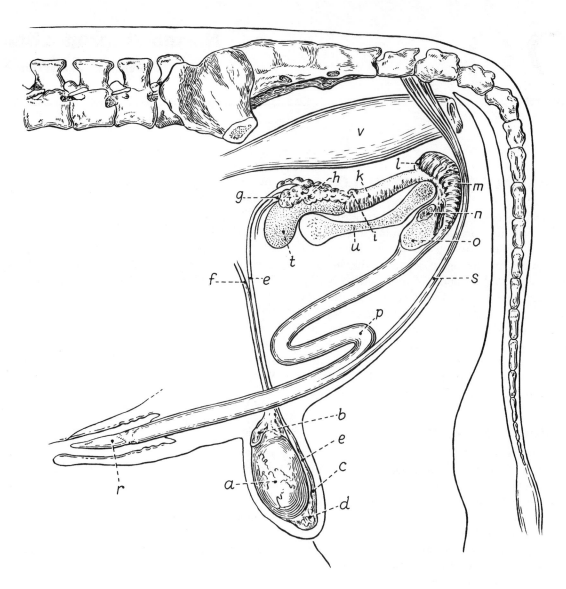

Fig. 29.1 The genital organs of the bull. a, testis; b, head of epididymis; c, body of epididymis; d, tail of epididymis; e, vas deferens; f, vascular part of spermatic cord; g, ampulla of vas deferens; h, seminal vesicle; i, body of prostate; k, pelvic urethra surrounded by urethralis muscle; l, bulbourethral gland; m, bulbocavernosus muscle; n, crus penis; o, ischiocavernosus muscle; p, distal sigmoid flexure of penis; r, glans penis; s, retractor penis muscle; t, urinary bladder; u, pubic symphysis; v, rectum. (From Blom and Christensen (1947).)

undergo final maturation. The tail of the epididymis also acts as a reservoir for fully mature sperm, and becomes turgid with stored sperm in sexually active animals.

The vas deferens is a relatively thick-walled, muscular tube, which acts both as a reservoir for sperm and the means of their conduction between the epididymis and the penis. It is situated mediocaudally within the spermatic cord, in a small diverticulum of peritoneum. In addition to the

vas deferens, the spermatic cord also contains the arteries, veins and nerves supplying the testis, all of which are contained within the peritoneal vaginal tunics. Together, these structures form the spermatic cord. The spermatic sac includes the spermatic cord, the internal spermatic fascia, cremaster muscle and cremasteric fascia. The cremaster muscle is situated on the opposite side of the sac to the vas deferens, i.e. on the anterolateral surface. The vasa deferentia enter the abdomen through the

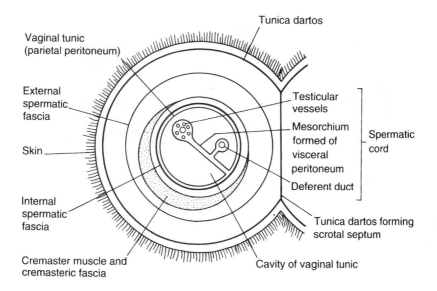

Fig. 29.2 Diagram of the anatomy of the fascial, muscular and peritoneal tissues of the neck of the scrotum. The vaginal tunic is strongly reinforced by the closely adherent and much thicker internal spermatic fascia. All of the layers are closely apposed to their adjacent structures so that the only (potential) space is the cavity of the vaginal tunic. (Redrawn from Cox (1982), with permission.)

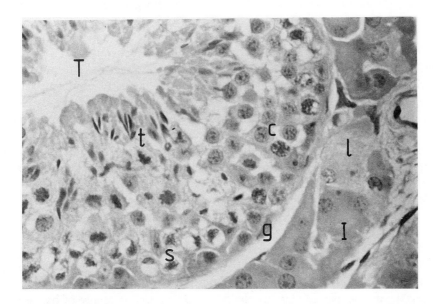

Fig. 29.3 Histology of the testis. Interstitial tissue (I) containing Leydig cells (l), blood, nervous tissue and lymphatic tissue is interspersed between seminiferous tubules (T), whose lumen is lined, in some sections, by formed spermatozoa. The periphery of the tubules is composed of spermatogonia (g) and Sertoli cells (s), with spermatocytes (c) and spermatids (t) occurring deeper in the tubules.

inguinal canals, whence they run in a caudal direction to join the pelvic urethra where the latter organ joins the neck of the bladder.

A number of short ligaments exist between the various structures within the scrotum, as shown in Figure 29.4. The proper ligament of the testis joins the ventral pole of the testis to the tail of epididymis, which is also joined to the vaginal tunic by the caudal ligament of the epididymis. These ligaments are derived from the gubernaculum. Finally, on the external surface of the vaginal tunic, the scrotal ligament joins the tunic to the scrotal fascia.

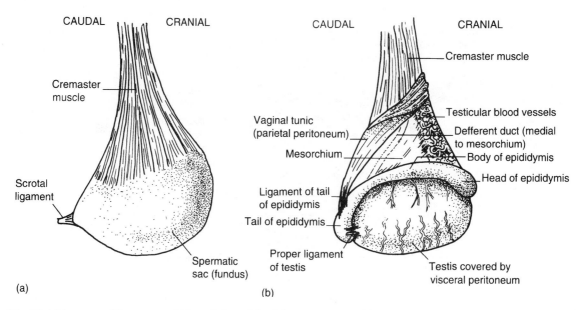

Fig. 29.4 Ligaments of the scrotum. (a) Lateral view of the right spermatic sac of the horse. (b) Lateral aspect of the contents of the right spermatic sac of the horse. The most ventral part of the spermatic sac shown in Figure 29.2 has been incised so as to enter the lumen of the vaginal tunic. (Redrawn from Cox (1982), with permission.)

Blood and nervous supply to the testis

The testes are supplied with blood through the spermatic arteries, which arise from the caudal aorta, close to the renal arteries. In the domestic species, these arteries pass through the inguinal canal, enclosed in peritoneum, forming a major component of the spermatic cord. In animals with scrotal testes, the spermatic artery becomes highly convoluted from the point at which it passes through the inguinal canal, although the degree of convolution is less if the scrotum is inguinal than if pendulous. The testis is drained by an anastomosing plexus of veins (the pampiniform plexus) which arise in the tunica albuginea and return to the spermatic cord through the inguinal canal and, thence, to the inferior vena cava. Initially, many veins are identifiable in the plexus, but as the plexus ascends the spermatic cord, fewer and fewer collateral branches are apparent, until a few main veins penetrate the inguinal canal. These finally join, as a single vein, into the caudal vena cava or renal vein (Setchell, 1970). The spermatic artery surrounds, and is in very intimate contact with, the pampiniform plexus, such that artery and vein frequently share a common tunica intima. This complex vascular anatomy fulfils several functions. The length of the spermatic artery is greatly extended by its convolutions, such that the arterial

pulse is almost completely eliminated by the time the artery reaches the testis (Waites and Moule, 1970), as it appears that a pulsatile arterial blood supply to the testis is incompatible with normal spermatogenesis. Secondly, spermatogenesis is more efficient at temperatures below the mammalian core body temperature. The close apposition of artery and veins allows heat exchange to occur between spermatic artery and vein, such that the temperature in the testis is several degrees lower than the core body temperature. Thirdly, it is possible that some counter-current exchange of small molecules, such as testosterone, may occur between spermatic vein and artery, although the importance of such transfers remains to be established.

The nervous supply of the testis (see Hodson, 1970) is derived from the thoracolumbar sympathetic outflow, whose visceral motor fibres innervate the smooth muscle of the testicular arterioles and of the testicular and epididymal capsules. These fibres and their accompanying visceral sensory fibres run in the spermatic cord. The scrotum has both visceral and somatic innervation, derived from nerves that pass through the inguinal canal and which arise as branches of the pudendal nerve. A further prominent feature of the innervation of the scrotum is the motor supply to the cremaster muscle and dartos. However, as might be expected from the interspecies variation in anatomy of the scrotum, there is also considerable variation in the detail of its nervous supply.

Development of the testis

Early in embryonic development, primordial germ cells migrate from the yolk sac into the meso-

nephros, where they induce formation of the gonadal ridge. In male embryos, the presence of testis-determining genes on the Y chromosome induces development of undifferentiated gonad into a testis. Recent evidence suggests that the critical stage in the formation of the testis is in the differentiation of the somatic component of the primitive gonad. Sertoli cells are not only crucial for the formation

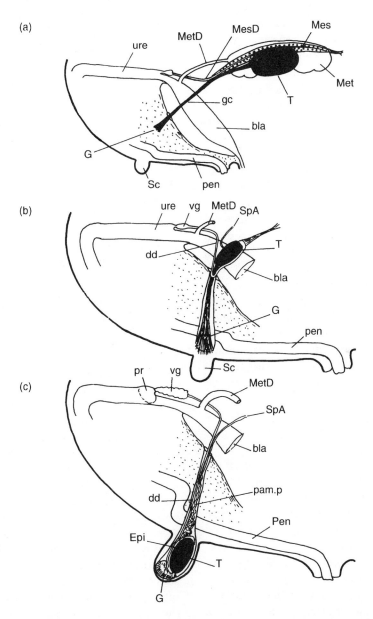

Fig. 29.5 Descent of the testis in the bull. (a) 65 day fetus, (b) 96 day fetus and (c) 140 day fetus. The changing relationships between the gubernaculum (G), testis (T) and vaginal tunics will be noted. bla, bladder; dd, ductus deferens; Epi, epididymis; gc, gubernacular cord; Mes, mesonephros; Met, metanephros; MetD, metanephric duct; pam.P; pampiniform plexus; pen, shaft of penis; pr, prostate; Sc, scrotum; SpA, spermatic artery; ure, urethra; vg, vesicular gland. (Redrawn from Gier and Marion (1970), with permission.)

of the testis, but are also responsible for producing müllerian duct inhibiting factor, which prevents development of the female genital tubular genitalia, and a meiotic inhibiting factor, which maintains meiotic arrest until puberty. Leydig cells produce testosterone, which stimulates development of the mesonephric (wolffian) ducts to form the tubular parts of the male genital tract. The only critical effector of the XY germ cell is its spermatogenesis gene, which lies on the Y chromosome, and is responsible for the onset of spermatogenesis (Burgoyne, 1988; McLaren, 1988).

As the testis develops in the mesonephros, differentiation of the definitive kidney (the metanephros) begins and, as it grows, the metanephros replaces the mesonephros as the organ of osmoregulation. The testis then migrates from its position within the abdomen towards its definitive position in the scrotum, in a process referred to as the descent of the testis. The testis traverses the abdomen (see Gier and Marion, 1970; Figure 29.5(a) and (b)) partly as a result of differential growth between the pelvis, abdomen, kidney and testis, and partly due to the tension exerted upon the testis by the gubernaculum. Before the testis itself passes through the inguinal canal, the canal is distended by a thickening of the gubernaculum and by the passage of the tail of the epididymis. Thus, the gubernaculum, tail of epididymis and tip of the vaginal process precede the testis through the inguinal canal. Final passage of the testis is achieved by tension from the gubernaculum and pressure from the abdominal viscera (Figure 29.5(c)). The times at which the testis is first present within the scrotum are given for the main domestic species in Table 29.1.

Spermatogenesis does not commence until the time of puberty. Thus, the seminiferous tubules of the prepubertal animal consist of immature Sertoli cells and relatively undifferentiated spermatogonial stem cells. As puberty approaches, the number and complexity of Sertoli cells increase, to reach maximal numbers at the onset of spermatogenesis. Mitoses in the spermatogenic cells occur at an increasing rate as puberty approaches, with puberty itself being characterized by the onset of meiosis and sperm production. Maximum spermatogenic rate is not reached until some time after the occurrence of puberty, for both the rate of cell divisions and the size of the testis continue to

Table 29.1 Age at which testes descend into the scrotum

Species	Time of testicular descent
Cat	2–5 days after birth
Dog	Between the last few days of gestation and the first few after birth
Horse	Between 9 months of gestation and a few days after birth
Cattle	3.5–4 months of gestation
Sheep	Midgestation (80 days)
Pig	After 85 days of gestation

increase into adulthood (see Hochereau-de-Reviers et al., 1987).

Physiology of the testis

Endocrinology

All aspects of male reproductive physiology are under the endocrine control of the two major gonadotrophins, luteinizing hormone (LH) and follicle-stimulating hormone (FSH). The secretion of LH is pulsatile, with irregular episodes of secretion occurring every 2–4 hours. The actions of LH are primarily upon the Leydig cell, where, acting through adenylate cyclase, it promotes steroidogenesis by regulating the rate-limiting step of steroidogenesis; namely, conversion of cholesterol into the testosterone precursor, pregnenolone. Peak testosterone concentrations follow those of LH by about 40 minutes and decline back to prestimulation values over a further 40–80 minutes (D'Occhio et al., 1982a; Figure 29.6). Testosterone is required for the production of sperm in the testis and their subsequent maturation in the epididymis, for the function of the accessory sex glands and for the development of masculine secondary sexual characteristics. After aromatization into oestrogen within the brain, testosterone is also responsible for negative-feedback regulation of LH secretion and for male behaviour. Curiously, in long-term castrated animals, neither negative feedback nor libido can be restored by testosterone administration, for brain aromatase activity is eventually lost and oestrogen itself has to be given for the restoration of these effects. (D'Occhio et al., 1982b). Within the lumen of the seminiferous tubule testosterone is converted by 5-reduction into 5-dihydrotestosterone (DHT), which is not susceptible to aromatization and is a more potent

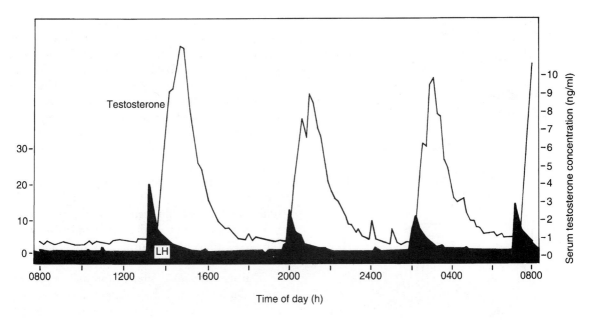

Fig. 29.6 Typical profile of the patterns of LH and testosterone secretion in the ram. (Redrawn from D'Occhio et al. (1982a).)

androgen than testosterone itself. Both testosterone and DHT are bound within the tubule lumen by the secretory product of the Sertoli cells, androgen-binding protein (ABP). The role of ABP therefore appears to be to maintain high androgen concentrations in the lumina of the seminiferous tubule and epididymis.

The main target of FSH is the Sertoli cell, where it also acts through adenylate cyclase-linked enzyme systems. Under the influence of FSH, Sertoli cells secrete ABP (Gunsalus et al., 1981) and aromatize testosterone into oestrogens (Setchell et al., 1983). Adeqate FSH stimulation is also required to permit Sertoli cells to support spermatogenesis. Some evidence suggests that the production of pyruvate and lactate, which act as energy substrates for germ cells, may be a key role of the FSH-stimulated activity of the Sertoli cell in maintaining spermatogenesis. Debate remains over the pattern of secretion of FSH; some consider it to be pulsatile, a manner analogous to LH, while others consider its secretion only to exhibit longer-term fluctuations. FSH secretion is regulated by both gonadal steroids and inhibin, the regulatory protein secreted by Sertoli cells (Baird et al., 1991).

The actions of the gonadotrophins are, however, not limited to the somatic cells of the testis, as both LH and FSH regulate aspects of germ cell activity. For example, experiments upon hypophy-

sectomized rams indicated that the rate of division of stem spermatogonia is controlled by LH, while the rate of subsequent divisions and the ability of cells to undergo meiosis is regulated by FSH (Courot and Ortavant, 1981). Whilst these actions upon germ cells are, in part, mediated through the stimulation of activity in the somatic component of the testis by the gonadotrophins, circumstantial evidence indicates direct actions upon germ cells themselves. A schematic summary of the endocrine relationships of the testis is given in Figure 29.7 (Amann and Schanbacher, 1983).

Spermatogenesis

Spermatogenesis is the basic process of male reproduction, resulting in the production of spermatozoa. It is carried out in the seminiferous tubule of the adult testis and comprises three main processes. Initially, the relatively undifferentiated spermatogonia undergo a period of mitotic, multiplication, divisions, which is followed by the meiotic reduction of the diploid to haploid genome. Finally, the postmeiotic cells undergo the morphological transformation of spermiogenesis, resulting in the release of formed spermatozoa into the lumen of the tubule.

These processes of spermatogenesis are reflected in the functional morphology of the seminiferous tubule (see Courot et al., 1970).

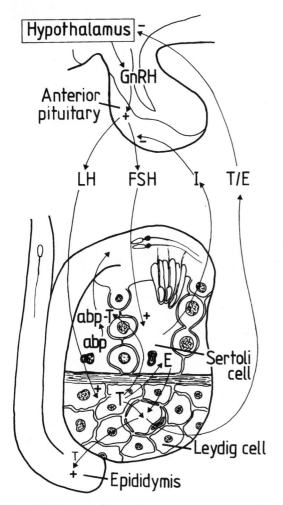

Fig. 29.7 Diagram of the endocrine relationships controlling the testis. abp, androgen-binding protein; E, oestrogen; GnRH, gonadotrophin-releasing hormone; I, inhibin; T, testosterone. (Redrawn and adapted from Amann and Schanbacher (1983).)

The basement membrane of the seminiferous tubule is surrounded externally by fibroblasts and myoid cells. The blood supply is limited by the basement membrane and does not pass into the tubule itself. Within the tubule there are somatic Sertoli cells and the various stages of the seminiferous cell line, which together form the seminiferous epithelium. Sertoli cells rest upon the basement membrane, but extend through the entire thickness of the seminiferous epithelium, so that the germinal cells in all stages of spermatogenesis are in contact with the plasmalemma of Sertoli cells. Sertoli cells are irregularly cylindrical in shape, with large, variably shaped nuclei situated close to the basement membrane. They multiply during fetal and prepubertal life, with the full complement being present at the time of puberty. Until recently it was considered that Sertoli cell numbers were fixed at the time of puberty, but it is now evident that there is an annual cycle of loss and regeneration in at least some seasonally breeding species (Johnson and Thompson, 1983; Hochereau-de-Reviers et al., 1987). Sertoli cells secrete oestrogens, inhibin, a gonadotrophin-releasing hormone (GnRH)-like peptide, proteins (including ABP), lactate, pyruvate and tubule fluid. The cells are joined by specialized tight-cell-like junctions, so that the seminiferous epithelium is separated into apical and basal compartments by the blood–testis barrier formed by these junctions (see Hochereau-de-Reviers et al., 1990).

During early fetal life, primordial germ cells enter the body from the yolk sac. In the gonadal ridge these cells differentiate into gonocytes, which undergo mitosis throughout fetal and prepubertal life. Gonocytes in turn differentiate into spermatogonia, at which stage development in the seminiferous cells is arrested until the onset of puberty. In the mature animal, spermatogonia are divided into A, intermediate and B classes, with each class further subdivided according to morphology and degree of differentiation. Thus, in the bull and ram, A_0, A_1, A_2, A_3, intermediate, B_1 and B_2 spermatogonia occur (Hochereau-de-Reviers, 1976). A-series spermatogonia are the least differentiated and form the reservoir of stem cells within the seminiferous tubule. It is likely that stem cells are regenerated by asymmetrical divisions of early A-series spermatogonia; with one daughter cell remaining as an uncommitted stem cell, the other being committed to undergo further mitotic and meiotic divisions. All spermatogonia remain in contact with the basement membrane, but, as the final meiotic division of spermatogonia give rise to the primary spermatocytes, the cytoplasm of the Sertoli cells starts to intervene between the basement membrane and the primary spermatocytes. DNA synthesis occurs during mitotic divisions and then, to its greatest extent, during the formation of tetraploid nuclei during meiosis (for a review, see Hochereau-de-Reviers et al., 1990). RNA synthesis occurs during preleptotene and late pachytene (Kierszenbaum and Tres, 1974). The first meiotic division then proceeds through the highly sensitive zygotene and pachytene stages. The pachytene stage is

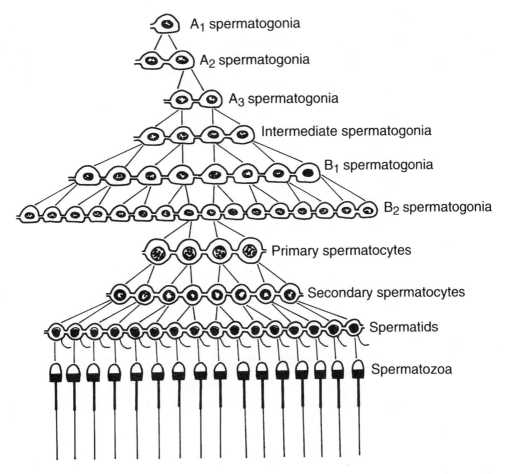

A_1 spermatogonia

A_2 spermatogonia

A_3 spermatogonia

Intermediate spermatogonia

B_1 spermatogonia

B_2 spermatogonia

Primary spermatocytes

Secondary spermatocytes

Spermatids

Spermatozoa

Fig. 29.8 Multiplication of cells during spermatogenesis in the bull. A_1 spermatogonia undergo a series of mitotic divisions, to produce A_2, A_3, intermediate, B_1 and B_2 spermatogonia. The final mitotic division produces primary spermatogonia, which enter meiosis, producing secondary spermatocytes after the first meiotic division and spermatids after the second. Spermatids then differentiate into spermatozoa without further cellular division.

particularly sensitive to noxious damage, such as by high testicular temperature and inadequate maintenance of spermatogenesis by inappropriate gonadotrophin levels. During the first meiotic division, the cells move deeper into the seminiferous epithelium and the tight cell junctions of the Sertoli cells form beneath the spermatocytes and degenerate above them (Russell, 1977, 1978), so that the cells effectively pass through the blood–testis barrier. Thus, the progeny of the first meiotic division, the secondary spermatocytes, move from the basal to the apical compartment of the seminiferous epithelium and are thereafter separated from the general tissue fluid compartment. The second meiotic division produces spermatids, which do not divide further. The spermatids thereafter differentiate into spermatozoa (Figures 29.8 and 29.9).

At the end of meiosis, spermatids are round cells with round nuclei, which have to then undergo the very marked changes in cell function and morphology that occur during spermiogenesis. Immediately after completion of meiosis, the spermatids undergo a period of RNA synthesis, which is then followed by the beginnings of nuclear chromatin condensation (Monesi, 1971). Simultaneously, acrosomal contents are synthesized in the Golgi, whose vesicles progressively fuse to form the acrosome. As the nucleus condenses and elongates, the acrosome forms over the basal pole of the nucleus (Courtens, 1979), while at the opposite pole the flagellum starts to form from one of the centrioles. A transient microtubular structure, the manchette, appears during the formation of the flagellum in the postnuclear cytoplasm of the elongating spermatid. The function of the

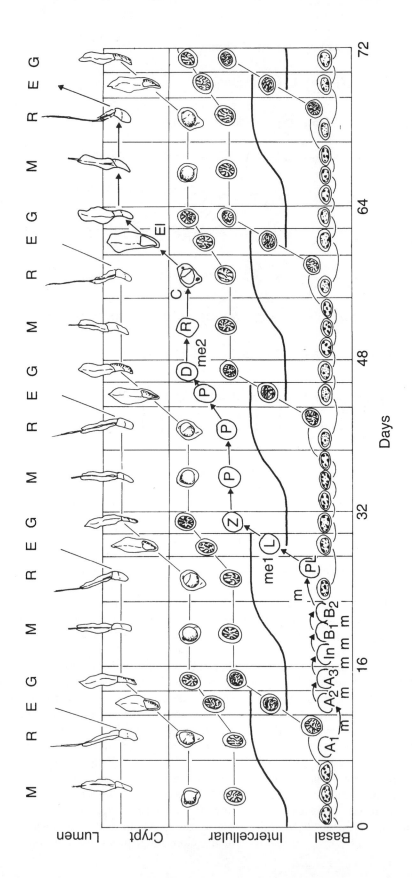

Fig. 29.9 Spermatogenesis in the bovine testis. Stem cells undergo mitotic (m) divisions producing successive generations of diploid spermatogonia (A_1, A_2, A_3, intermediate (In), B_1 and B_2), before entering the first meiotic division (me1). Preleptotene primary spermatocytes (PL) pass through the successive stages of the long first meiotic prophase (L, leptotene; Z, zygotene; P, pachytene; D, diakinesis), becoming short-lived secondary spermatocytes. These proceed through the second meiotic division (me2), producing early round spermatids (R). These differentiate into spermatozoa without further division, after nuclear condensation (C) and elongation (El). The solid horizontal line indicates the position of tight junctions between Sertoli cells: the site of the blood–testis barrier. Four major groupings of cells can be determined, based upon the morphology of the spermatids/spermatozoa: E, elongation; G, grouping; M, maturation; R, release. These recur every 16 days. (Adapted from an original drawing by Brian Setchell.)

manchette is unknown and it disappears after the flagellum is formed (Fawcett, 1970; Zirkin, 1971). The last stage of flagellum formation is the development of the midpiece, when a helix of mitochondria condense around the proximal part of the flagellum. During formation of the acrosome and flagellum, the cytoplasm of the spermatid is deeply invaded by a process of the Sertoli cell which extends between the forming flagellum and the residual cytoplasm. It is suggested that this process is responsible for the reduction in cytoplasmic volume of the spermatid which occurs during spermiogenesis. Finally, most remaining cytoplasm is engulfed by the Sertoli cell as the formed spermatozoon, with its remnant cytoplasmic droplet, is expelled from the crypt of the Sertoli cell into the lumen of the seminiferous tubule (see Fouquet, 1974).

The duration of spermatogenesis, i.e. the time between spermatogonial divisions and the release of the spermatozoan, is approximately 60 days in most domestic animals. Epididymal transit takes a further 8–14 days. Thus, the interval between the most sensitive stage of spermatogenesis, meiotic prophase, and ejaculation, is approximately 30 days (see Amann and Schanbacher, 1983). Hence, the interval between damage to the testis and the appearance of abnormal spermatozoa in the ejaculate is generally between 30 and 60 days, depending upon the site of damage.

The seminiferous epithelium appears as concentric layers of spermatogonia, spermatocytes and spermatids, with characteristic associations between generations of cells throughout the depth of the seminiferous epithelium. Each generation of seminiferous cells is linked by cytoplasmic bridges, so that developmental stages are synchronous within each generation, and substantial areas of seminiferous epithelium exhibit cells at a similar stage of development. Cellular associations are generally classified into type I, where two generations of primary spermatocytes and one of spermatids are present, and type II, where there is only one generation of primary spermatocytes but two of spermatids (see Hochereau-de-Reviers et al., 1990). Transition between type I and type II occurs after the maturation divisions, while type II changes into type I with the release of spermatozoa and the arrival of a new generation of spermatocytes from the last spermatogonial division.

Physiology of the epididymis

Considerable changes occur to spermatozoa as they pass through the epididymis (for reviews, see Amann, 1987; Hammerstedt and Parkes, 1987). The epididymis is highly androgen-dependent; thus, if androgen levels are suppressed, epididymal function is immediately impaired. The protoplasmic remnant, which is initially sited close behind the sperm head, migrates distally to the end of the midpiece, before being finally shed in the tail of the epididymis. Sperm are immotile in the head of the epididymis, but they acquire the capacity for motility as they pass through its body. Similarly, in the head of epididymis, sperm do not have the ability to fertilize, but this is acquired during passage of the epididymal body. Less obvious, but of equal or greater importance to the morphological changes exhibited by sperm during their passage of the epididymis, are the changes in their plasma membrane, to which surface glycoproteins are added or modified by epididymal secretions and luminal cells. It is likely that these act to stabilize the acrosome while the sperm is within the female genital tract, to reduce the surface immunogenicity of the sperm and to enhance the ability of the sperm membrane to bind to the zona pellucida.

Spermatozoa take between 8 and 14 days to traverse the epididymis, according to species. In the bull, sperm take 5 days to pass through the head and body of the epididymis and a further 5–9 days to traverse the epididymal tail. The transit times of the head and body are fixed, but the tail of the epididymis has dual functions of both a site of maturation and storage, so that, in periods of high ejaculation frequency, the passage time of the tail may be reduced and relatively immature sperm ejaculated. Although sperm held in the tail of the epididymis have the capacity for motility, motility is not itself acquired until the time of ejaculation. Thus, sperm within the epididymis exhibit little motility, but are rapidly activated upon mixing with seminal plasma during ejaculation.

Structure and function of spermatozoa

Spermatozoa are divided into three main segments: the head, midpiece and tail (Figure 29.10). The head consists of little other than the condensed nucleus and the overlaying acrosome. Of the

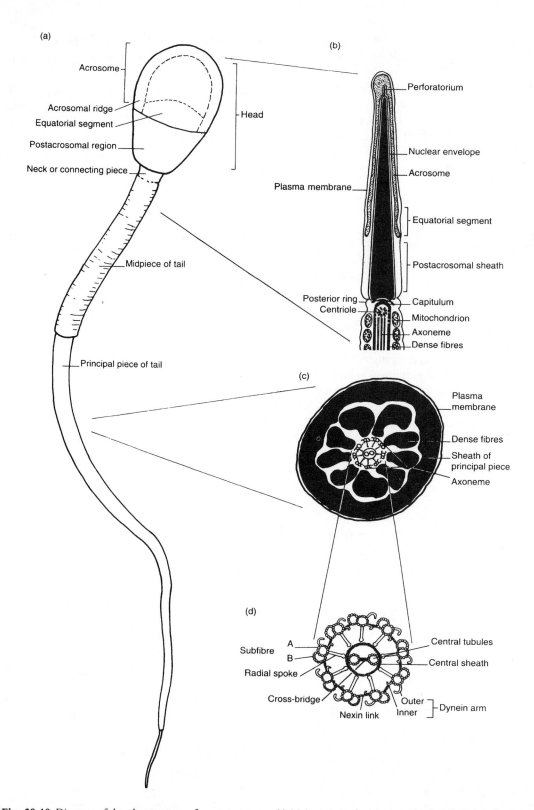

Fig. 29.10 Diagram of the ultrastructure of a spermatozoan. (a) Main structural regions as revealed by light microscopy. (b) Generalized ultrastructural features of the head and connecting piece. (c) Ultrastructure of the proximal principal piece of the tail. (d) Generalized detail of the ultrastructure of the axoneme of the tail. (Redrawn and adapted from Bedford and Hoskins (1990).)

other enzymes contained within the acrosome, the main two are acrosin and hyaluronidase (Morton, 1977). During the acrosome reaction, the outer acrosomal membrane fuses with the plasmalemma, under the control of intra- and extracellular calcium, whereupon exocytosis of the contents of the acrosome occurs (see Harrison and Roldan, 1990). The main functions ascribed to the acrosomal enzymes are dispersal of the cumulus oophorus and local lysis of the zona pellucida; although it has been questioned recently whether the latter function is indeed a function of the released acrosomal enzymes *per se*. The inner membrane of the acrosome is relatively stable and remains intact after the acrosome reaction has occurred, and some of the acrosomal enzymes are probably bound to the inner acrosomal membrane. Penetration of the zona pellucida and fusion with the oolemma are both receptor-mediated events, with specific areas of the sperm head binding to target components of the oocyte (see Wassarman, 1990).

The midpiece and tail of the sperm may be considered to form a single functional entity. The tail itself consists of a central axoneme, which, in the region of the midpiece, is sheathed in a helix of mitochondria (reviewed by Bedford and Hoskins, 1990). Sperm metabolize simple molecules, principally sugars and their derivatives (e.g. fructose, glucose, mannose and pyruvate), by both aerobic and anaerobic pathways, to provide energy for motility and the maintenance of ionic gradients across membranes (see Harrison, 1977). Forward motility of sperm results from coordinated waves of flagellar bending progressing from neck along the length of the tail. Bending of the tail occurs as the result of forces generated between adjacent peripheral doublets of the axoneme (Satir et al., 1981). The dynein arms of the doublet, which in the resting state are bound to the adjacent doublet, unbind, elongate and then bind to a new site further along the filament. The unbinding process, which is the ATP-using step, is then repeated, resulting in a progressive bending of the flagellum. The doublets on one side of the axoneme work in opposition to each other, providing the alternating beat of the tail. After capacitation, the rate and amplitude of the flagellar beat greatly increases, and the rate of energy usage by the sperm is correspondingly elevated (Yanagimachi, 1981). The motility of the cell itself probably

Table 29.2 Accessory sex glands of the main domestic species

Species	Ampulla	Prostate	Vesicular gland	Bulbourethral gland
Cat		++		++
Dog	(+)	+++		
Horse	++	++	++	+
Cattle	(+)	++	+++	+
Sheep	(+)	++	+++	+
Pig		+	++	+++

The relative size and importance is indicated by the number of + symbols. Ampullary glands are present in species marked (+) but are not anatomically prominent.

has little role in the movement of spermatozoa through the cervix and uterus, for this is accomplished mainly through contractions of the female genital tract (Hunter, 1980). However, passage through the uterotubal junction and within the oviduct does require sperm motility, while the enhanced, whiplash motility of the capacitated sperm is necessary for penetration of the cumulus and zona pellucida.

Accessory glands

The accessory glands include the ampullae, prostate, vesicular glands and bulbourethral (or Cowper's) glands. There is much variation between the anatomy of the accessory glands between species, which is summarized in Table 29.2.

Ampullae are present as dilations of the terminal portion of the vasa deferentia, just before they enter the pelvic urethra, where their main function is to act as reservoirs of sperm. In the bull, ram and dog, the ampullary glands which are present, contribute slightly to the seminal plasma, whereas their contribution to the ejaculate is relatively important in the stallion. The main constituent of ampullary secretion in the stallion is ergothionine (Mann et al., 1956).

Vesicular glands are prominent in ruminants, the stallion and the boar. They are sac-like in the stallion and boar, and are firm, lobulated structures in the ram and bull. The glands are adjacent to the neck of the bladder and lateral to the ampullae. They open into the urethra just distally to the vasa deferentia. Their secretion, which is generally watery, contributes substantially to the volume of the semen. In all species its secretion contains large quantities of citrate, while in the ruminants it also contains fructose and, in the boar, inositol (Mann et al., 1949, 1956; Mann, 1954; Marley et al., 1977).

The *prostate* is intimately related to the pelvic urethra and, in most species, is in two parts; its body surrounds the neck of the bladder and its disseminated part spreads around the pelvic urethra into which it has several openings. In the dog, the prostate is the main accessory gland and is relatively large, forming a discrete organ around the urethra. The prostatic secretion is watery and, in the dog, contains large quantities of chloride ions, but neither citrate, fructose nor inositol is present in high concentration (see Huggins, 1945).

In the stallion, bull and ram, the *bulbourethral* (or Cowper's) *glands* are small, rounded structures lying between the anus and urethra. Their watery secretion is discharged prior to coitus and is considered to cleanse the urethra of urine. In the boar, the bulbourethral glands are large, cylindrical structures lying along each side of the intrapelvic urethra. In this species, their secretion is very viscid, due to its high sialomucin concentration (Boursnell et al., 1970) and combines with the secretion of the vesicular glands to produce a gelatinous phase of the seminal plasma (Boursnell and Butler, 1973).

The physiological functions of the various constituents of seminal plasma remains a matter of debate (for a review, see Brooks, 1990). There is much interspecies variation in the composition of seminal plasma, so it has been difficult to ascribe absolute functions to many of its constituents. Provision of energy, maintenance of osmotic pressure, chelation of free calcium ions and buffering are some of the suggested functions; while other possibilities include immunosuppression in the female genital tract and regulation of spermatozoan motility. Seminal plasma is also responsible for the coagulation of semen which occurs shortly after ejaculation in many species. On the other hand, it has been argued that the wide variety in constitution of seminal plasma between species indicates that it has no critical role; an argument which is emphasized by the ability of sperm to survive in relatively simple media, which bear little resemblance to seminal plasma. Paradoxically, the seminal plasma of many species appears to contain spermicidal factors, especially in the post-sperm-rich fraction of the species which produce a fractionated ejaculate.

The penis

The penis comprises three tracts of erectile tissue and the penile urethra. The urethra is surrounded by the corpus spongiosum penis (CSP), which arises at the bulb of the penis and terminates in the glans penis. The dorsum of the penis is made up of the paired corpora cavernosa penis (CCP; Figure 29.11), which arise in the two crura (roots) of the penis and terminate behind the glans. The blood supply of all three tracts is via branches of the pudendal artery, but the venous drainage of the CCP is markedly different from that of the CSP. The CCP is drained via the root of the penis, into the pudendal vein, whereas the CSP drains into the dorsal vein of the penis from its distal extremity (Ashdown and Gilanpour, 1974). Thus, both the supply and drainage of blood to the CCP is via the root of the penis, whereas the supply of the CSP is through the bulb and its drainage from its distal part. The roots of the penis are surrounded by the ischiocavernosus muscles, which, on contraction, occlude the veins draining the CCP against the ischium of the pelvis, so that the cavernous spaces of the erectile tissue in the blind-ending CCP become engorged with blood, causing stiffening and lengthening of the penis (Beckett et al., 1974). However, the detailed anatomy of the penis varies greatly between species (Figure 29.12) and, as a result, details of the functional anatomy of erection are similarly variable.

In Artiodactylae, the penis has a thick, fibrous tunica albuginea overlying the CCP and surrounding the urethra, and the individual cavernous spaces within the CCP are relatively small. The penis also has a sigmoid flexure, which is either caudal (postscrotal), as in the ruminants, or cranial (prescrotal) to the scrotum, as in the boar. In these species, relatively little blood enters the penis during erection, although the blood pressures achieved are considerable, exceeding 40 000 mmHg during ejaculation. In order that the increased pressure induced by ischiocavernosus muscle activity can be transmitted throughout the length of the penis, specialized artery-like vascular canals, the longitudinal canals, run the length of the penis. Paired canals arise in the crura of the penis, which fuse shortly afterwards to produce a single dorsal canal. Either side of the dorsal canal thereafter gives rise to a series of branches, which join together to form paired ventral canals. The dorsal

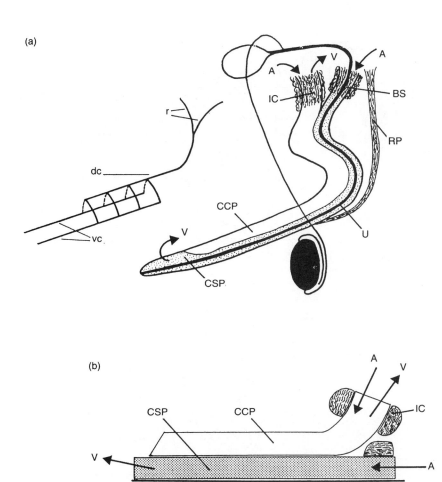

Fig. 29.11 Functional vascular anatomy of the bovine penis: (a) representational and (b) diagrammatic. Blood enters and leaves the corpus cavernosum (CCP) via the arteries (A) and veins (V) of the crura (roots) of the penis, so that contraction of the overlying ischiocavernosus (IC) muscles occludes the venous drainage and forces blood into the penis under pressure. The blood passes through the penis in longitudinal canals (inset). Two canals arise in the roots (r) of the penis and unite to form a single dorsal longitudinal canal (dc). This gives of a series of lateral branches in the region of the sigmoid flexure, which unite to form paired ventral canals (vc). The corpus spongiosum (CSP) is drained from its distal end, so contraction of the bulbospongiosus (BS) muscle only produces a transient increase in hydrostatic pressure. This is of sufficient magnitude to temporarily occlude the urethra, so that a bolus of semen can be propelled along its length. During detumescence, vascular pressure is lost and the penis is returned to the preputial cavity by the retractor penis (RP) muscle. (Redrawn and adapted from Laing et al. (1988), with permission.)

canal runs for the proximal third of the penis, the ventral canals for the remaining distance, with a short distance of overlap with the dorsal canal. Lengthening of the penis is achieved partly by longitudinal expansion of the cavernous spaces between the trebeculae of the CCP, but mainly by straightening of the sigmoid flexure of the penis (Ashdown, 1970). As a result, the penis, which is normally carried high in the preputial cavity, is fully exteriorized from the narrow

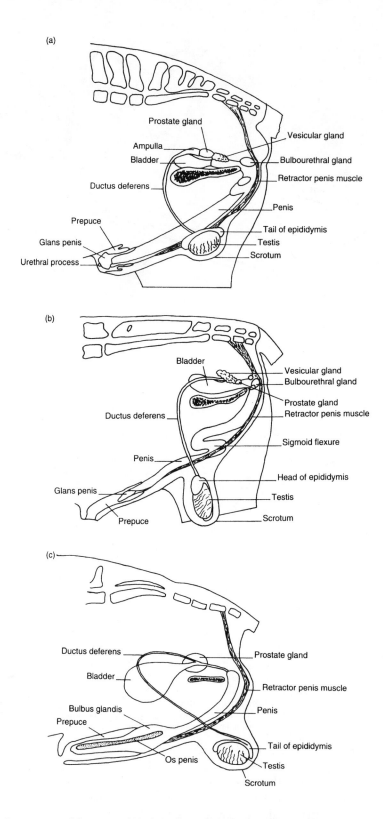

Fig. 29.12 Comparative anatomy of the penes of (a) the stallion, (b) bull and (c) dog. (Redrawn and adapted from Laing et al. (1988), with permission.)

preputial orifice. Obliteration of the sigmoid flexure and forward movement of the penis is made possible by the very loose arrangement of the connective tissue that surrounds the penis and prepuce. In the ruminants, full erection is only briefly attained during the single ejaculatory thrust, but copulation is more prolonged in the boar. Erection is terminated by cessation of ischiocavernosus muscular contraction, and the penis is returned to the preputial cavity by contraction of the retractor penis muscles, which restores the sigmoid flexure.

The other domestic species have a musculocavernous penis, in which the tunica albuginea is less pronounced and the cavernous spaces of the erectile tissue larger than in the artiodactyls. In the stallion (see Nickel et al., 1973; Amann, 1993), tracts of longitudinally oriented smooth muscle fibres are associated with the trabeculae of the CCP. These are normally in a state of tonic contraction, holding the penis in the prepuce. The tone in these muscles falls during erection and micturition, leading to prolapse of the penis from the prepuce. In the stallion and dog (Evans and deLahunta, 1988), erection produces increases in both length and girth of the penis and, as there is no sigmoid flexure, the lengthening of the penis is caused entirely by vascular engorgement.

The ejaculation reflex is stimulated by sensory nerves within the glans penis which transmit to the spinal cord through the dorsal nerve of the penis, a branch of the pudendal nerve. Thereafter, erection and ejaculation are primarily coordinated as spinal reflexes in the lower lumbar and sacral segments of the spinal cord. The integrity of this nerve is essential for the ejaculation reflex to take place and, if it becomes damaged, ejaculation, though not erection, becomes impossible (Beckett et al., 1978). Pressure, tactile sensation and, in the bull, temperature are the main stimulants to ejaculation. During ejaculation, the glans of the penis of the bull and goat become coiled (Ashdown and Smith, 1969), while the vermiform appendage of the penis of the ram shows a vigorous flicking movement. It is probable that these conformational changes are to assist with deposition of semen in and around the external os of the cervix. The glans penis of the stallion and boar engage in the cervical canal, with ejaculation occurring through the cervix into the uterine lumen. Thus, the penis of the boar adopts a spiral conformation during copulation which mirrors that of the cervix of the sow, but the stallion shows only a very pronounced enlargement of the glans penis during ejaculation. The penis of the dog is unique amongst the domestic animals in having an os penis, in whose grooved ventral floor lies the urethra. During copulation, the penis of the dog is gripped by the levator vestibuli of the vagina of the bitch, whereupon engorgement of the bulbus glandis occurs. Ejaculation occurs over a prolonged period of time, with the brief production of the pre-ejaculatory and sperm-rich fractions being followed by a very protracted deposition of prostatic fluid during the copulatory tie.

Propulsion of semen along the urethra is achieved by contraction of the bulbospongiosus muscle that overlies the CSP in the bulb of the penis. Because the CSP drains from its distal end, the high pressures achieved in the CCP cannot be attained. Thus, each contraction of the bulbospongiosus muscle causes a transient wave of increased pressure in the CSP which progresses from the bulb to the glans, where it dissipates by dorsal venous drainage of the blood. Because the CCP is turgid, the increased pressure within the CSP causes a wave of occlusion of the urethra. This progessive wave of urethral occlusion, assisted by the contraction of the muscle which surrounds the extrapelvic urethra, causes conduction of boluses of semen along the urethra.

Development of the penis

Initial development of the phallus from the genital tubercle is similar in both male and female fetuses, but, in the male fetus, rapid enlargement occurs early in development. At birth, the penis is fused with the prepuce throughout its length, with small lateral veins draining the erectile tissue. During prepubertal development, the connective tissue joining penis and prepuce breaks down and the veins become occluded. The frenulum is the most substantial of the connections between the penis and prepuce, frequently containing quite large blood vessels. It is often the last part to break down and may not infrequently persist into post-pubertal life.

Libido and mating behaviour

Libido is primarily dependent upon androgenic steroid hormones, which allow mating and aggressive behaviour to occur, as well as maintaining the function of all parts of the male reproductive system. Libido seldom is expressed in animals that are castrated before puberty although, if a mature animal which has learnt to copulate is castrated, erection and copulation may persist for long periods or, occasionally, indefinitely. Despite the dependency of male behaviour upon androgen, there has been much debate over the relationship between absolute concentrations of androgen and libido (Foote et al., 1976; Wodzicka-Tomaszewska et al., 1981). Some have argued a permissive role of androgen, while others have demonstrated positive correlations between testosterone concentrations and measures of libido. Breeds of bull which are aggressive and respond quickly to the presence of an oestrous female tend to have higher testosterone concentrations than the more phlegmatic breeds, but whether this is a causal relationship remains unclear.

The males of those domestic species which are naturally herd animals spend a great deal of time detecting oestrus (see Chenoweth, 1981). Oestrous females of many species secrete pheromones to attract males, while others, notably the cow and some breeds of pig, exhibit homosexual behaviour as a signal to the male of the presence of oestrus. All males smell the perineal region of the female,

and the odour of the oestrous female induces the so-called 'flehmen' reaction in the bull, ram and stallion: a characteristic raised posture of the head an an elevation of the upper lip. Females which are not in oestrus signal their objection to the advances of the male and, at the least, will respond by moving away or, perhaps, by attacking the male in the offensive manner peculiar to the species. During pro-oestrus, the interest of the male in the female is increased but, whereas she associates with the male, she will not permit mounting. Oestrous females signal receptivity by squatting, urinating, moving the tail to one side and remaining stationary (Figure 29.13). During this foreplay the male becomes progressively aroused; there are frequent erections of the penis, with emission of accessory fluid and many unsuccessful attempts to mount the female. Finally, mounting and copulation occur.

Stallion

Following intromission, the stallion performs a succession of copulatory movements of the hindquarters which, within a minute, culminate in ejaculation. During ejaculation, successive waves of urethral peristalsis can be palpated on the lower surface of the penis, while the stallion exhibits a characteristic 'flagging' movement of the tail (Figure 29.14). The stallion then dismounts.

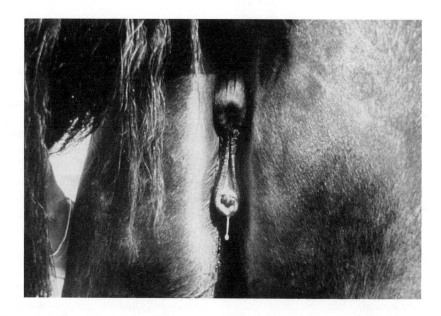

Fig. 29.13 Signs of oestrus in the mare include squatting, urination and moving the tail to one side.

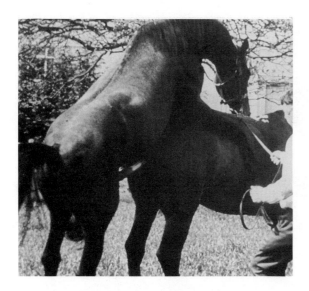

Fig. 29.14 The main external sign of ejaculation in the stallion is tail flagging. Peristaltic waves can also be palpated in the penile urethra.

Ruminants

Copulation in all of the domestic species of ruminants is brief. After detecting an oestrous female, mounting is followed quickly by the single ejaculatory thrust. The male then immediately dismounts, but frequent subsequent matings occur. Farm management of rams and bulls should take this high mating frequency into account. Thus, whereas individual sires can service quite large groups of spontaneously cyclic females, the groups of females have to be much reduced if these have undergone oestrus synchronization. Furthermore, care has to be exercised in the use of young sires. The testis does not reach its full size and sperm-producing capacity until 1–2 years after puberty, nor does the epididymis reach its full length until the same time (reviewed by Salisbury et al., 1978). Until maturity has been reached, groups of females should be smaller than for adult animals. If overused, both the numbers of sperm produced are too few for adequate conception rates to be achieved and sperm from the tail of the epididymis are ejaculated before their functional maturation is complete. Thus, sperm numbers and sperm maturity are both adversely affected, causing severe limitation upon the chance of conception.

Boar

Copulation is relatively prolonged in pigs, lasting for between 5 and 15 minutes. Following intro-

mission, the first phase is occupied by a series of vigorous thrusting movements of the hindquarters of the boar. During this phase, the first part of the fractionated ejaculate is produced, which comprises only accessory fluid. The second phase is quieter and accompanied by production of the sperm-rich fraction of the ejaculate. This is followed by a final, more vigorous phase, in which the third jelly-like accessory secretion is discharged. Ejaculation occurs directly into the uterus, which is distended with semen immediately after copulation, while the cervix is often sealed with a gelatinous plug. The large volume of semen produced by the boar is necessary to convey its spermatozoa through the extensive length of the uterus of the sow.

Dog

The dog achieves intromission by vigorous thrusting of the hindquarters. Once intromission has been achieved, the bulbus glandis swells considerably, while the constrictor vulvae muscles of the bitch contract behind it, thus forming the 'copulatory tie'. The sperm-rich fraction of canine semen is ejaculated within as little as 80 seconds of intromission, so that conception may occur even if copulation does not proceed through to its second stage. In this second stage, the dog dismounts but remains connected and faces away from the bitch (Figure 29.15). This change of position causes the penis to become bent through an angle of 180°; the efferent veins of the penis are thereby occluded and the penis remains turgid. The function of the tie may be to prevent penile detumescence during the prolonged second stage of copulation, during which some 30 ml of sperm-free accessory fluid is pumped into the vagina and thence to the uterus, where it flushes the sperm-rich fraction through the uterus. The sexes remain locked until the vulval muscles relax and penile erection wanes.

Cat

During mating, the tom mounts the queen and grasps her neck with his teeth. As the tom adjusts his position the queen paddles her hindlegs, continuing to do so at an increasing frequency during the 10 seconds or so for which coitus lasts. The queen cries out during copulation and, as the tom dismounts, she may strike out at him, displaying the typical 'rage' reaction. This is followed by a

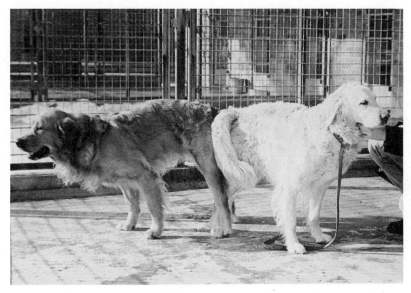

Fig. 29.15 The copulatory tie in the dog.

period of frantic rolling and licking at the vulva. As soon as the postcoital reaction has ceased, the tom will attempt to mount again. Several matings may therefore occur within the first 30–60 minutes. The cat is an induced ovulator (Shille et al., 1983), so the number and frequency of matings are important in ensuring that the LH surge is of sufficient magnitude to cause ovulation (Tsutsui and Stabenfeldt, 1993).

REFERENCES

Amann, R. P. (1987) *J. Reprod. Fertil. Suppl.*, **34**, 115.

Amann, R. P. (1993) In: *Equine Reproduction*, ed. A. O. McKinnon and J. L. Voss, pp. 645–657. Philadelphia: Lea and Febiger.

Amann, R. P. and Schanbacher, B. D. (1983) *J. Anim. Sci.*, **57**(Suppl. 2), 380.

Ashdown, R. R. (1970) *J. Anat.*, **106**, 403.

Ashdown, R. R. and Gilanpour, H. (1974) *J. Anat.*, **117**, 159.

Ashdown, R. R. and Smith, J. A. (1969) *J. Anat.*, **104**, 153.

Baird, D. T., Campbell, B. K., Mann, G. E. and McNeilly, A. S. (1991) *J. Reprod. Fertil. Suppl.*, **43**, 125.

Beckett, S. D., Walker, D. F., Hudson, R. S., Reynolds, T. M. and Vachou, R. I. (1974) *Amer. J. Vet. Res.*, **35**, 761.

Beckett, S. D., Hudson, R. S., Walker, D. F. and Purhoit, R. C. (1978) *J. Amer. Vet. Med. Assn*, **173**, 838.

Bedford, J. M. and Hoskins, D. D. (1990) In: *Marshall's Physiology of Reproduction*, ed. G. E. Lamming, Vol. 2, pp. 379–568. Edinburgh: Churchill Livingstone.

Blom, E. and Christensen, N. O. (1947) *Skand. Vet.*, **37**, 1.

Boursnell, J. C. and Butler, E. J. (1973) *J. Reprod. Fertil.*, **34**, 457.

Boursnell, J. C., Hartree, E. F. and Briggs, P. A. (1970) *Biochem. J.*, **117**, 981.

Brooks, D. E. (1990) In: *Marshall's Physiology of Reproduction*, ed. G. E. Lamming, Vol. 2, pp. 569–690. Edinburgh: Churchill Livingstone.

Burgoyne, P. S. (1988) *Phil. Trans. R. Soc. Lond. B.*, **322**, 63.

Chenoweth, P. J. (1981) *Theriogenology*, **16**, 155.

Courot, M. and Ortavant, R. (1981) *J. Reprod. Fertil. Suppl.*, **30**, 47.

Courot, M., Hochereau de Reviers, M. T. and Ortavant, R. (1970) In: *The Testis*, ed. A. D. Johnson, W. R. Gomes and N. L. VanDemark, Vol. 1, pp. 339–432. New York: Academic Press.

Courtens, J. L. (1979) *Ann. Biol. Anim. Biochim. Biophys.*, **19**, 989.

Cox, J. E. (1982) *Surgery of the Reproductive Tract in Large Animals*, 2nd edn. Liverpool: Liverpool University Press.

D'Occhio, M. J., Schanbacher, B. D. and Kinder, J. E. (1982a) *Endocrinology*, **110**, 1547.

D'Occhio, M. J., Kinder, J. E. and Schanbacher, B. D. (1982b) *Biol. Reprod.*, **26**, 249.

Evans, H. E. and deLahunta, A. (1988) *Guide to the Dissection of the Dog*. Philadelphia: Saunders.

Fawcett, D. W. (1970) *Biol. Reprod. Suppl.*, **2**, 90.

Foote, R. H., Munkenbeck, N. and Green, W. A. (1976) *J. Dairy Sci.*, **59**, 2011.

Fouquet, J. P. (1974) *J. Microscopie*, **19**, 161.

Gier, H. T. and Marion, G. B. (1970) In: *The Testis*, ed. A. D. Johnson, W. R. Gomes and N. L. VanDemark, Vol. 1, pp. 1–46. New York: Academic Press.

Gunsalus, G. L., Larrea, F., Musto, N. A., Becker, R. R., Mather, J. P. and Bardin, C. W. (1981) *J. Steroid Biochem.*, **15**, 291.

Hammerstedt, R. H. and Parkes, J. E. (1987) *J. Reprod. Fertil. Suppl.*, **34**, 133.

Harrison, R. A. P. (1977) In: *Frontiers in Reproduction and*

Fertility Control, ed. R. O. Greep and M. A. Koblinsky, pp. 379–401. Cambridge, Mass.: MIT Press.

Harrison, R. A. P. and Roldan, E. R. S. (1990) *J. Reprod. Fertil. Suppl.*, **42**, 51.

Hochereau-de-Reviers, M. T. (1976) *Andrologia*, **8**, 137.

Hochereau-de-Reviers, M. T., Monet-Kuntz, C. and Courot, M. (1987) *J. Reprod. Fertil. Suppl.*, **34**, 101.

Hochereau-de-Reviers, M. T., Coutens, J. L., Courot, M. and de Reviers, M. (1990) In: *Marshall's Physiology of Reproduction*, ed. G. E. Lamming, Vol. 2, pp. 106–182. Edinburgh: Churchill Livingstone.

Hodson, H. (1970) In: *The Testis*, ed. A. D. Johnson, W. R. Gomes and N. L. VanDemark, Vol. 1, pp. 47–100. New York: Academic Press.

Huggins, C. (1945) *Phys. Rev.*, **25**, 281.

Hunter, R. F. H. (1980) *Physiology and Technology of Reproduction in Female Domestic Animals*, pp. 104–144. London: Academic Press.

Johnson, L. and Thompson, D. L. (1983) *Biol. Reprod.*, **29**, 777.

Kierszenbaum, A. L. and Tres, L. L. (1974) *J. Cell Biol.*, **63**, 923.

Laing, J. A., Morgan, W. J. B. and Wagner, W. C. (1988) *Fertility and Infertility in Veterinary Practice*. London: Baillière Tindall.

Mann, T. (1954) *Proc. R. Soc. London B.*, **142**, 21.

McLaren, A. (1988) *Trends Genetics*, **4**, 153.

Mann, T., Davies, D. V. and Humphrey, G. F. (1949) *J. Endocrinol.*, **6**, 75.

Mann, T., Leone, E. and Polge, C. (1956) *J. Endocrinol.*, **13**, 279.

Marley, P. B., Morris, S. R. and White, I. G. (1977) *Theriogenology*, **8**, 33.

Monsei, V. (1971) *J. Reprod. Fertil. Suppl.*, **13**, 1.

Morton, D. B. (1977) In: *Immunobiology of Gametes*, ed. M. Edidin and M. H. Johnson, pp. 115–155. Cambridge: Cambridge University Press.

Nickel, R., Schummer, A. and Sieferle, E. (1973) *The Viscera of the Domestic Animals*. Berlin: Paul Parey.

Russell, L. D. (1977) *Amer. J. Anat.*, **148**, 313.

Russell, L. D. (1978) *Anat. Rec.*, **90**, 99.

Salisbury, G. W., VanDemark, N. L. and Lodge, J. R. (1978) *Physiology of Reproduction and Artificial Insemination of Cattle*, Chapt. 23. San Francisco: Freeman.

Satir, P., Wais-Steder, J., Lebduska, S., Nasr, A. and Avolio, J. (1981) *Cell Motil.*, **1**, 303.

Setchell, B. P. (1970) In: *The Testis*, ed. A. D. Johnson, W. R. Gomes and N. L. VanDemark, Vol. 1, pp. 101–240. New York: Academic Press.

Setchell, B. P. (1982) In: *Reproduction in Mammals*, ed. C. R. Austin and R. V. Short, Vol. I. Cambridge: Cambridge University Press.

Setchell, B. P., Laurie, M. S., Flint, A. P. F. and Heap, R. B. (1983) *J. Endocrinol.*, **96**, 127.

Shille, V. M., Munro, C., Farmer, S. W. and Papkoff, H. (1983) *J. Reprod. Fertil.*, **69**, 29.

Tsutsui, T. and Stabenfeldt, G. H. (1993) *J. Reprod. Fertil. Suppl.*, **47**, 29.

Waites, G. M. H. and Moule, G. R. (1960) *J. Reprod. Fertil.*, **1**, 223.

Wassarman, P. M. (1990) *J. Reprod. Fertil. Suppl.*, **42**, 79.

Wodzicka-Tomaszewska, M., Kilgour, R. and Ryan, M. (1981) *Appl. Anim. Ethology*, **7**, 203.

Yanagimachi, R. (1981) In: In Vitro *Fertilization and Embryo Transfer*, ed. J. D. Biggers and L. Mastroianni, pp. 65–100. New York: Academic Press.

Zirkin, B. R. (1971) *Mikroskopie*, **27**, 10.

30

EXAMINATION FOR BREEDING SOUNDNESS

Examinations of male animals are made for two main purposes: either to ascertain whether normal fertility can be expected from the animal, or for the diagnosis of infertility. In either situation the requirements are a history of the animal, a general examination, a detailed examination of the genital tract, observation of copulation and collection and evaluation of semen.

History-taking is an important part of the examination of a suspected infertile male animal. Many of the causes of infertility do not manifest themselves until a considerable period of time has elapsed from the original insult, so that careful questioning of the owner, often over matters he or she may have considered as trivial at the time of their occurrence, may be needed to elucidate such causes. History-taking is also a useful way of assessing owners' expectations of their animals, for many cases of so-called 'infertility' result from no more than an unrealistic expectation of a sire's capabilities.

The history must establish whether or not the sire is likely to be the cause of the infertility, the duration of infertility and the circumstances of its onset. The number of females with which the sire's infertility has been manifest must be determined, as must the conditions under which mating has occurred. For example, it is not uncommon for dogs to be presented for infertility examination after failure to achieve pregnancy on no more than one or two occasions, with bitches that were scarcely in oestrus. Clearly, under such circumstances, the probability of a pathological cause of infertility is minimal. Amongst agricultural animals, the sizes of groups of females and the system under which mating was taking place must be determined. A common cause of apparent infertility in rams derives from no more than using

groups of too many ewes, especially if these have undergone synchronization of oestrus or are being used in out-of-season breeding regimens. Table 30.1 gives suggested ratios of females to males for the main agricultural species, under various mating systems. The time of year when the infertility was noticed may give helpful clues as to its cause, and may help to determine whether female factors are likely to have been of importance. Similarly, information regarding the previous achievements of the animal are of great importance in differentiating between congenital and acquired conditions, or between managemental and pathological causes. Any available records of the management and reproductive performance of the herd are invaluable in ascertaining the overall level of the fertility of the herd; while they may provide also useful comparative information for other contemporary sires and may help to pinpoint the onset and duration of the period of low fertility. Similarly, observation of the normal environment of the sire is usually advisable. Seeing how the animal is handled, how it is housed, fed and cleaned, observing the area in which it is required to serve, how it is moved there and how it is handled during service, all may assist with one's assessment of the infertility of the animal.

The general examination of the sire must take into consideration its age and likely sexual experience, body condition, the possibility of intercurrent illness and its temperament. Considerable importance can be attached to the body condition and general degree of maturity of young animals; for, on one hand, puberty can be delayed in poorly grown animals, while, on the other, animals which have achieved very high growth rates during rearing may have a body conformation which belies their sexual immaturity. It is also noticeable that young bulls of some later maturing breeds, notably the Charolais and Holstein, may remain relatively subfertile for longer than their earlier-maturing counterparts (Figure 30.1; Coulter, 1980). Thus,

Table 30.1 Numbers of females per male of agricultural animals in various mating systems

Species	Mating system			Overall ratio (females in herd per male)
Bull	Spontaneously cyclic groups	Oestrus synchronized	In hand[a]	
Immature	10–20	NA	2–4	20–60
Mature	20–40	10	4–12	80–120
Ram	Spontaneously cyclic groups	Oestrus synchronized (in breeding season)	Oestrus synchronized (out of season)	
Immature	20–30	NA	NA	20–30
Mature	40–80	10–20	5–10	40–80
Boar	Group synchronized by weaning[b]	In hand[a]		
Immature	1–2	1–2		20
Mature	2	1–4		20–30

Derived from Roberts (1986) and Levis (1992).
[a] In hand: number of supervised double services per week.
[b] Overall ratio of boars:sows. Boars would be rotated with larger groups of sows, with periods of sexual rest to give an overall service frequency of 1–4 per week.

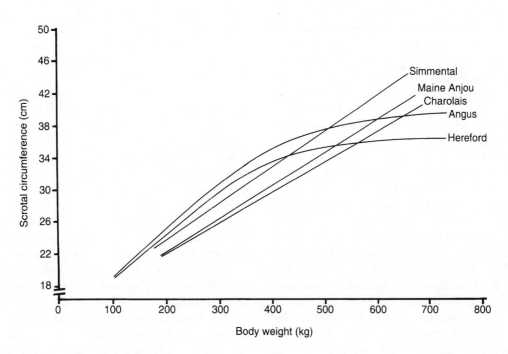

Fig. 30.1 Relationship between body weight and scrotal circumference of beef bulls. British beef breeds initially exhibit faster testicular growth than their Continental counterparts, but, as the former reach mature body weights, testicular growth ceases. The later-maturing Continental sires therefore have a longer period of testicular growth, related to their greater mature body weight. (Redrawn from Coulter (1980), with permission.)

the assessment of young sires can present some difficulty, for allowance has to be made for the maturity characteristics of the beed, yet the use of young bulls in which puberty is excessively delayed is best avoided in view of the evidence that the age of puberty in a sire is highly correlated with the age of puberty in his daughters. This problem is further compounded by the pressure of time imposed by the requirements of progeny testing. In a seasonally calving national herd, such as that of the UK, semen from young bulls has to be available roughly 12 months after their birth, if progeny testing is to be carried out successfully. For Friesians, this target presented little difficulty, but a significant proportion of young Holstein bulls do not produce consistently usable semen until 15 or even 18 months of age. By the time they reach this age, the majority of cows in the national herd will already be pregnant, so progeny testing is delayed until the following season. Young sires used in natural-mating regimens present further difficulties. Firstly, it must be ascertained that they have learnt to mount and successfully copulate. Indeed, where young sires are running with fully mature females, copulation may not by physically achievable. Furthermore, it is not uncommon for those young boars or rams which are run with large, mature females to be bullied by these females, to achieve no pregnancies and to lose a great deal of body condition. Secondly, young sires are most unlikely to achieve high pregnancy rates amongst large groups of females and are generally unsuitable for use in groups of oestrus-synchronized females.

Body condition is also important in adult males. Spermatogenesis tends to be limited when body condition is poor, and can also be limited by specific micronutrient deficiencies. In general, chronic and continuing deficiencies of protein and energy are likely to be of greater overall importance than micronutrient deficiencies, although the effects upon fertility can be severe when these occur simultaneously (see Salisbury et al., 1978). For most agricultural species, sires should be maintained in moderate condition, although rams should start the breeding season in a high condition score, due to the considerable weight loss they experience during the season. Conversely, ruminants which are fed on very poor-quality roughage can develop such great rumen fill that normal copulation can be physically difficult to achieve. Moreover, as excess weight can lead to damage to females during mounting, it is important to determine that the size of sire and females is compatible.

Whereas any systemic illness can affect reproductive performance, three groups of conditions can be noted as of particular importance; namely, diseases of the locomotor system, conditions causing pain in the caudal abdomen and conditions which have resulted in prolonged pyrexia. Specific conditions will be considered under the first two headings later in the chapter but, in principle, it is important to note that hindleg, hindfoot or back pain are incompatible with normal mating behaviour. Furthermore, not only does locomotor pain limit mating directly, but also the stress of prolonged, unresolved pain may cause corticosteroid-mediated impairment of spermatogenesis. Systemic illness causing prolonged pyrexia can result in increased temperatures in the testis, thereby causing temperature-limited impairment of spermatogenesis.

Reproductive examination

A complete examination of the reproductive system requires physical examination of the genital system, observation of the response of the animal to an oestrous female, observation of mating and the collection of semen. In practice, which of these procedures are actually carried out and the order in which they are undertaken depends upon the species and the nature of the owner's complaint. For example, it is frequently desirable to observe mating or to collect semen before the animal has undergone the stress of a physical examination. Thus, for a bull, collection of semen by an artificial vagina (AV) is often better undertaken before palpation of the genitalia (especially before examination of the internal genitalia per rectum). Also, observing mating (or collecting semen by an AV) is the easiest way of observing the penis of a bull. Conversely, in the ram, it is generally best to examine the external genitalia first, as this frequently obviates the need for causing the animal stress by collecting of semen by electroejaculation.

Choosing the conditions for the observation of mating behaviour is important. Where the inherent libido of the animal is high, such as in boars and dairy bulls, it will often be willing to mount females that are not in oestrus, or even to mount other males, castrates or dummy animals. Indeed, the willingness of a cow to be haltered and tied is often a more important criterion for her use than whether or not she is in oestrus: few bulls are willing even to attempt to mount a fractious cow that is fighting against unfamiliar restraint! Rams and beef bulls, although usually of high inherent libido, commonly refuse to mount an oestrous female in the presence of a human observer, and considerable tenacity and patience are often required before mounting occurs. Animals which are stressed by recent transport are also often unwilling to mount straight away. Taken together, these many caveats mean that, although the results of observations of mating are valuable and often provide diagnostic information in infertility examinations, one should be most cautious about condemning an animal that does not perform under observation.

Conversely, high libido is generally associated with good reproductive performance, such that direct testing of libido is widely used as a method of evaluating bulls. Such tests may utilize either females in oestrogen-induced oestrus or non-oestrous females; and score the number and vigour of matings or mating attempts. While such tests are subject to many of the caveats described above, libido testing of young bulls is a useful means of either selecting animals of genetically high libido or of screening out older bulls whose libido is limited either by pathological causes or a waning of sexual interest (see Chenowith, 1986). Libido is highly heritable in cattle, so early selection of animals for high libido is likely to result in an overall increase in this aspect of reproductive performance.

During examination of the genital tract, all parts of the genitalia that are accessible externally should be palpated. When examining the contents of the scrotum, the temperature, size, texture, resilience and evenness of the testes and epididymes should be determined. The testes should be freely movable within the scrotum. It is generally possible to palpate the head and tail of the epididymis, but the body is often difficult to feel, due to its medial site. The vasa deferentia should be palpated throughout the scrotal neck and (particularly in rams) the presence or absence of vasectomy scars confirmed. The spermatic cord should be palpated up to the level of the inguinal ring for the presence of abdominal contents (scrotal hernia) or abnormalities of spermatic vasculature.

Measurement of scrotal circumference is useful in animals with a pendulous scrotum (see Figure 30.2), while, in the stallion, measurement of their width by calipers or ultrasonography is similarly valuable. Likewise, ultrasonography of the testes of stallions and dogs to visualize fluid-filled structures within their substance is proving to be a valuable additional examination (Figure 30.3). Scrotal circumference of yearling bulls should exceed 30 cm, while mature bulls should be over 36 cm for British beef breeds and over 38 cm for most other breeds. Scrotal circumference of mature rams depends upon body weight: values over 28 cm are acceptable for smaller breeds, and over 34 cm for larger breeds.

After palpation of the preputial part of the penis, exteriorization of its free part where possible, palpation of the sigmoid flexures and palpation of the prepuce and preputial orifice, such of the internal genitalia as are within reach should be

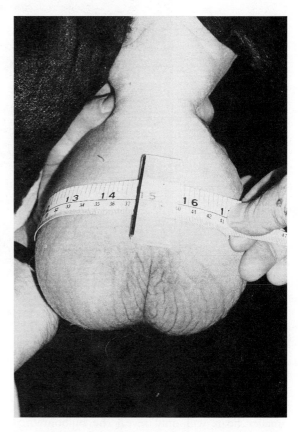

Fig. 30.2 Measurement of the scrotal circumference of the bull. The tape should be placed around the fullest part of the scrotum while the testes are held in their base by grasping the scrotal neck.

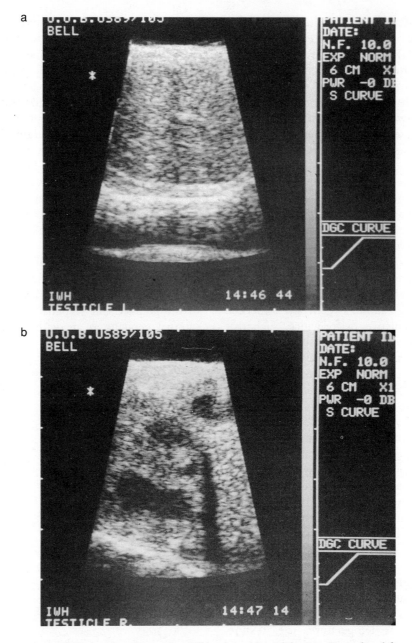

Fig. 30.3 Ultrasonograms of (a) normal canine testes and (b) a dog with epididymitis. (Reproduced from Barr (1990), with permission.)

palpated per rectum. In the bull and stallion, all accessory glands can be palpated thus, but they are generally out of reach to a digital examination of the ram. In large boars, rectal examination is potentially feasible, but digital examination of smaller boars will only reveal the bulbourethral glands. In smaller dogs, digital examination of the prostate is possible, but radiography, which is essential when prostatic disease is suspected, is required in any case for examination of the prostate in larger dogs.

Collection and assessment of semen

Collection from the bull

Representative samples of semen can be obtained from most bulls by means of the AV (Figure 30.4),

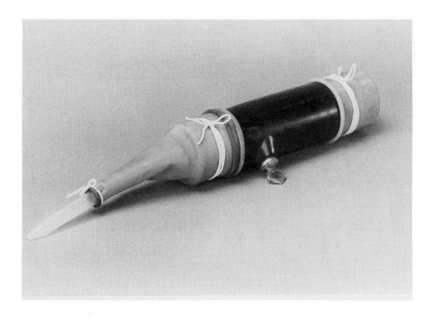

Fig. 30.4 Artificial vagina for use in the bull.

which consists of a strong outer rubber cylinder, containing a latex liner. At one end of the AV, a latex extension cone carrying a graduated collecting tube is attached. The length of the AV should be adjusted so that the bull ejaculates into the extension cone, thereby producing semen which is largely devoid of particulate or bacterial contamination. The space between the rubber cone and latex liner is filled with warm water, so that the temperature in the lumen of the AV is between 45 and 48°C. If this temperature falls below about 43°C, ejaculation is unlikely. The main stimulus to ejaculation is the temperature of the AV, but its pressure upon the bull's penis is relatively less important. Clearly, however, the larger the bull's penis, the less water is required. A little inert lubricant (liquid paraffin, soft paraffin or gynaecological jelly) is placed in the lumen of the AV just prior to use.

Control of the bull and the safety of all personnel are of paramount importance during semen collection. A halter-trained, oestrous cow is the ideal object for a bull to mount, although such an animal is often difficult to provide on most farms. Where a service crate is available, the cow should be restrained in this, otherwise she should be tied to a post. The bull is led to the cow, but not allowed to mount at once. Rather, he should be allowed to see and smell the cow, but then be led away before mounting takes place. This usually causes complete or partial erection, with production of pre-ejaculatory accessory gland secretions, and is considered to cause a better ejaculation of semen when the bull is finally allowed to mount. The bull is led up to the cow with the collector standing to the right of the shoulder of the bull. Before mounting, the bull usually nuzzles the perineum of the cow, then a pumping action of the tail head can be seen as the ischiocavernosus muscles start to pump blood in to the erecting penis. As the bull mounts, full erection is achieved and the bull usually makes a single ejaculatory thrust after achieving intromission. Small, preliminary thrusts occur as the bull locates the vulva and, during these, the collector grasps the prepuce (not penis) with the left hand and deflects the penis to the right of the hindquarters of the cow, allowing it to find the entrance to the AV. The bull will then normally make the ejaculatory thrust into the AV (Figure 30.5). The entire procedure must be carried out quietly and methodically, keeping the bull under continual careful observation before, during and after collection: many bulls are at their most aggressive immediately after ejaculation.

Where older bulls have been used for natural service for a number of years, they may be unwilling to ejaculate into an AV. Providing the libido of

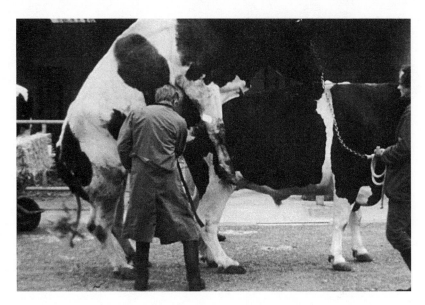

Fig. 30.5 Semen collection from the bull by means of an AV.

the bull is sufficient, repeated teasing or allowing the bull to mount, but deflecting his penis so he does not ejaculate, will usually provide enough stimulation for ejaculation to occur when presented with the AV. More difficulty is experienced with bulls that are unwilling to mount in the presence of humans, or which are no longer halter trained. Some such bulls can sometimes be stimulated by allowing the cow to mount the bull, but, for many, plentiful supplies of both patience and freshly heated AVs are the only route to success.

The main alternative to collection by an AV is collection of semen by electroejaculation. Early bull electroejaculators were undoubtedly unpleasant devices, but modern, variable voltage models are much more acceptable. Electrodes are worn on two fingers over a gloved hand, which are placed over the ampullae per rectum. Gently increasing voltages first produce accessory gland secretion, after which semen may be dribbled through the prepuce or ejaculated from the erect penis. Electroejaculation is not as widely used in the UK as it is in North America, where it is frequently used on bulls of low libido or which are otherwise unwilling to mount. If carefully and properly carried out, electroejaculation appears to be well tolerated by most bulls, although if performed by unskilled operators or with poor equipment, considerable distress can be caused.

Semen can also be collected by rectal massage of the internal genitalia. This technique involves the location of the vesicular glands per rectum and stroking them against the pubis, which causes accessory fluid to drip from the prepuce. The ampullae are then located and 'milked' between the finger and thumb. Success is indicated by the dripping of semen from the prepuce. It should finally be noted that, in some animals, semen can only be obtained by aspiration of the ejaculate from the vagina of a freshly served cow. Both of these last two methods have many disadvantages, and really only allow assessment of motility and morphology of sperm and do not provide accurate information over sperm numbers. Even so, the information yielded by such imprecise methods can still be diagnostic.

The stallion

Semen can be obtained from stallions by the use of an AV, a large condom or by examining the residual drips of semen left in the urethra after dismounting. Collection from the vagina of a mare is not normally possible, due to the intrauterine site of ejaculation. The AV for a stallion is larger than that used for a bull and, for large stallions, may be exceedingly heavy. The stallion is presented with a mare in full oestrus, which is often restrained with a twitch or service hobbles. After mounting, the penis is deflected into the AV and its lower surface palpated for the presence of peristaltic ejaculatory

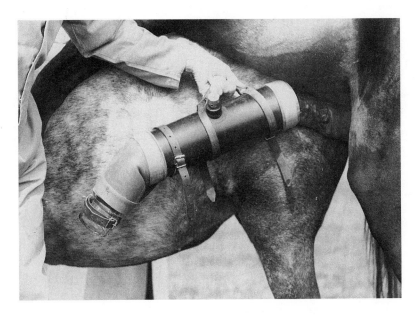

Fig. 30.6 Semen collection from the stallion. The urethra is palpated for the peristaltic waves that characterize ejaculation.

waves (Figure 30.6). Stallions can be quite fastidious about the temperature and pressure in the AV before they will ejaculate, and some stallions object so vehemently to even the sight of an AV that collection is impossible. Care must be exercised by the collector to avoid getting trapped between the forelegs of the stallion and the body of the mare, as the force of the clasping movements of the legs of the stallion are quite sufficient to break an arm.

The ram

Semen can be collected from rams by electro-ejaculation or by the use of an AV which is, essentially, a smaller version of that used for the bull. Some workers consider that the spermatozoa of the ram are more susceptible to temperature shock than are those of the bull, so a warmed ejaculation cone should be provided. Most rams will not use an AV until trained to do so, and virtually all require a ewe in oestrus to mount. In consequence, most semen examinations of farm rams are undertaken by electroejaculation. A probe, containing two electrodes (Figure 30.7), is placed into the rectum of the ram and located on to the brim of the pelvis (Figure 30.8). Rhythmic stimulations of the ampullae and sacral nerve plexus should cause erection and ejaculation within a few moments. Electroejaculation is generally well tolerated but, as the electrical stimula-tion also causes relatively widespread muscle contraction, attempts to collect by this method should be discontinued for several minutes if the ram has not ejaculated within the first 4–6 stimulations. Where rams are taken directly from pasture, housing them on straw for 1–2 days before attempting collection produces drier faeces in the rectum and appears to cause less widespread dissemination of current. Semen collected by electro-ejaculation is usually of lower volume and density than that collected by an AV, and occasionally is completely immotile or completely aspermic. For these reasons, some Breed Societies' rules of sale require that infertility can only be diagnosed on semen collected by an AV. In all circumstances, further collections should be made after an immotile or aspermic sample, to ensure that the initial findings should not rightly be attributed to operator error.

Although sheep are seasonal breeders, semen can be collected from most domestic rams throughout the year. Semen quality can be maintained to a considerable extent by regular ejaculation; a phenomenon that is used to maintain production of (frozen) semen in ovine artificial insemination (AI) centres. Farm rams exhibit a more profound decline in semen quality in the non-breeding season but, even so, epididymal reserves are sufficient for evaluation.

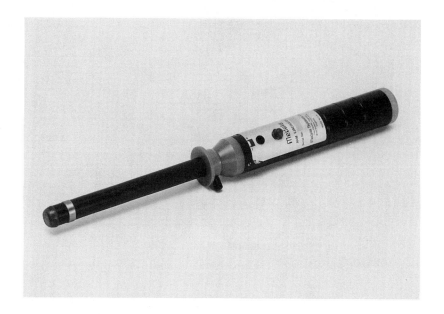

Fig. 30.7 Electroejaculator for the ram.

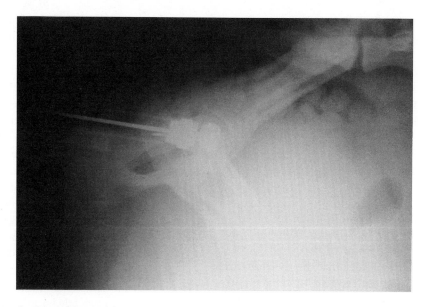

Fig. 30.8 Radiograph of the hindquarters of a ram indicating the position of the electroejaculator relative to the brim of the pelvis.

The boar

The main prerequisite for ejaculation in the boar seems to be the locking of the corkscrew-shaped penis in the spirally disposed cervix of the sow. This can quite easily be simulated by firmly encircling the protruded penis with the hand and fingers which are covered by a warm, lubricated, latex glove. The boar is much less sensitive to temperature than is the bull, but firm pressure is essential.

The use of an AV has been advocated in the past, as an alternative to this simple method of manual collection. The AV was based upon the bovine pattern but included an air pump to vary the internal pressure. One such AV, that designed by Melrose and O'Hagen (1959) also had a tapering latex extension, intended to simulate the cervical canal of the sow. In general, the use of such AVs was less satisfactory than the manual collection method; the latter being the more widely used.

At AI centres, a dummy, which does not necessarily resemble the sow, is used for the boar to mount. As the boar mounts and makes thrusting movements, the penis is directed into the AV or gloved hand. Thrusting becomes less vigorous as ejaculation begins. The ejaculate is allowed to pass through a funnel containing cotton gauze, which retains the gel fraction, but allows the fluid to pass down to an insulated bottle that is kept at 30°C. After ejaculation of the sperm-rich fraction, the boar begins to thrust again as the postsperm gel fraction is produced.

The dog

Semen can be taken fairly readily from most dogs by digital manipulation or, less commonly, by the use of an AV. In either case, the presence of a teaser bitch, preferably in oestrus, facilitates procedures. It is generally considered that semen collected by digital manipulation is of better quality and quantity, probably due to deleterious effects of the latex of the AV upon canine sperm. Erection can be induced by applying encircling pressure with the thumb and forefinger behind the bulbus glandis. When erection is obtained, the penis can be deflected into an AV, or digital collection continued. Where an AV is used, rhythmic changes in pressure are applied until the dog attempts to tie. The AV is then repositioned to allow the penis to be directed backwards, as in the tie, while ejaculation continues. In small dogs, the AV is cumbersome to use, and it does not allow for collection of the separate fractions of the ejaculate.

In order to induce ejaculation by digital manipulation, the bulbus glandis may be rhythmically compressed (Figure 30.9), although many dogs will induce ejaculation by their own thrusting. Before production of the presperm accessory fluids quite vigorous thrusting occurs, but the dog is relatively quiet during the initial phase of ejaculation. Firstly, during this quiescent phase, between 0.5 and 5.0 ml of watery, pre-ejaculatory fluid is produced, over a period of up to 50 seconds. Ejaculation of the sperm-rich fraction then follows immediately, when 0.5–2.0 ml of thick, creamy fluid is produced within a few seconds. The dog then attempts to turn and tie, whereupon the postsperm, prostatic fluid fraction of the ejaculate is produced. This third component is again watery, comprising up to 30 ml of fluid, which is ejaculated over 3–30 minutes.

Semen examination

The purpose of semen examination is to ascertain whether the numbers of functionally normal spermatozoa present in an ejaculate are sufficient to cause pregnancy and whether the sire has an adequate capacity to produce enough spermatozoa to achieve pregnancies amongst all the females he is required to service. Details of the methodologies and interpretation of semen examination are given later in this chapter.

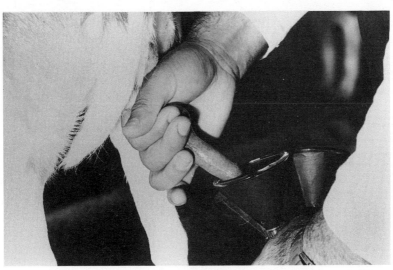

Fig. 30.9 Digital collection of semen from the dog.

REPRODUCTIVE ABNORMALITIES OF MALE ANIMALS

Reproductive abnormalities causing absolute or relative infertility in male animals have classically been divided into two main classes, namely conditions causing failure of normal service (*impotentia coeundi*) and conditions causing failure of conception after normal service (*impotentia generandi*). The first group can be further divided into, firstly, conditions causing an unwillingness to mount and, secondly, conditions which prevent normal copulation from occurring, despite normal libido. Superimposed upon both groups are considerations of whether the infertility represents a pathological condition of the genital (or other) system, or whether infertility is primarily managemental in origin and could simply be alleviated by modifying aspects of the husbandry of the animal. Much of the differentiation between these major groups of conditions can be achieved by careful history-taking. A scheme of diagnosis for some of the major causes of infertility in the bull is given in Figure 30.10.

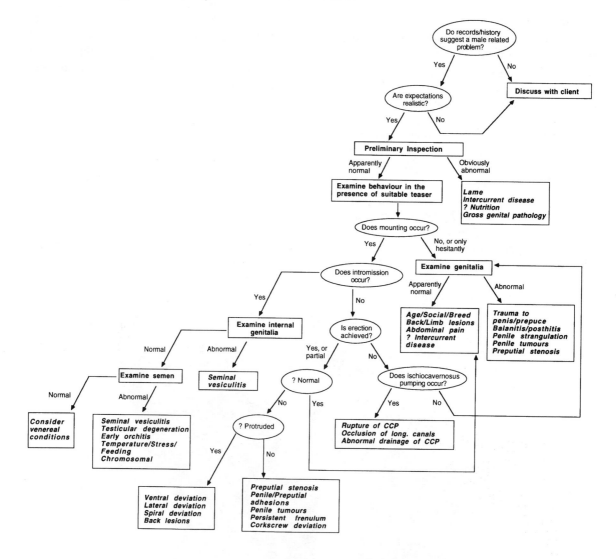

Fig. 30.10 Scheme for the diagnosis of the major conditions causing infertility in the bull. (Reproduced from Parkinson (1991), with permission.)

Conditions causing a lack of libido

Inability and unwillingness to copulate are relatively frequent presenting signs that accompany many disorders of the male reproductive system. The syndrome of lack of libido is, however, one of the most difficult for the clinician to unravel, for it is not only caused by genital pathology, but also can result from intercurrent disease, management, age, maturity or season. Furthermore, many diseases which would normally be expected to show other presenting signs can, if neglected, frequently result in a sexually disinterested animal. Finally, the difficulties of achieving a diagnosis in cases of low libido are further compounded by the unwillingness of some, quite normal, sires to copulate in human company.

Maturity, age and experience

Many animals which are presented for lack of libido are either young or of advanced age. The age of the sire must be considered in relation to the normal time at which its species (and breed) exhibits puberty. The conditions under which a young male has been reared can also affect its behaviour. For example, where bull calves are reared in small groups, they continuously exhibit mounting behaviour as puberty approaches and usually learn to copulate quite quickly. However, where reared in isolation, such mounting behaviour does not occur and can seem to take an age to learn, especially in those AI stations where steers are the sole objects available for the young bull to mount. Similarly, young colts in racing yards may be violently dissuaded from exhibiting male behaviour by their grooms. When such animals then go to become stud stallions, much behavioural reinforcement has to be unlearnt, before successful mating can occur.

Where immaturity is suspected as the cause of low libido, little can be achieved other than by the exercise of much patience and the provision of a plentiful supply of appropriately sized, oestrous females. Hormone therapy has been suggested, giving large doses of human chorionic gonadotrophin (hCG) (5000–10 000 IU) or gonadotrophin-releasing hormone (GnRH), in an attempt to stimulate libido through the production of elevated testosterone concentrations. Considerable caution should be exercised in the use of such hormones, however, for the high levels of testosterone they produce exert as great an effect upon aggression as on libido. Moreover, hCG, although having luteinizing hormone (LH)-like properties, is not the same substance as LH, and may damage spermatogenesis through the testicular oedema that it produces. In general, the efficacy of such treatments is low. Most animals fail to respond at all, a few exhibit a short period of enhanced libido, while only in very few can success be attributed to the treatment. More seriously, the correlation between the age of onset of reproductive activity of sires and their offspring means that it is positively undesirable to attempt to breed from animals which exhibit a gross delay in the onset of sexual activity.

Unwillingness to copulate can also result from poor service management. Slippery floors, roofs that are too low, females that are too big and stockmen that are insensitive in their handling of their charges can all contribute to unwillingness to copulate. Similar problems pertain amongst companion animals. Tom cats frequently become conditioned to mating in one particular environment and, if that environment should later be changed, an unwillingness to mate ensues. Dogs, which are frequently travelled before mating, can also have stress-induced impairment of libido. Finally, young males of many species, notably the pig, are frequently unwilling to mate if in the sight or sound of an older, more dominant, male.

Locomotor dysfunction

Most lesions affecting locomotion impair ability and willingness to copulate. Lesions of the back and hindlegs are clearly the most important of such incapacities, but, for example, in the boar, where the forelegs are used to clasp the female, painful lesions of the carpus can also preclude mating. In dogs and in aged animals of all species, lesions of the joints of the hindlimbs are important locomotor causes of impaired libido.

Amongst the large herbivores, foot lesions are probably of greatest significance. Gross pathology of the foot, such as penetrations of the sole, separations of the white line, foot rot, foul in the foot, etc., produce pain, so that the sire is unwilling to take his weight on the foot during copulation. Less obvious lesions of the foot, such as the interdigital growths of Hereford bulls, can also be important. However, it is the author's opinion that the most common locomotor-related cause of impaired libido is poor conformation of the foot. Animals

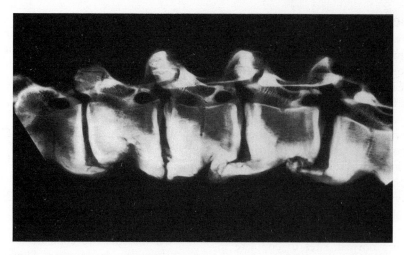

Fig. 30.11 Radiograph of the lumbar spine of an aged bull. Several of the vertebrae have substantial amounts of new bone deposition.

with overgrown hooves, where the distribution of weight has been adversely affected, are frequently unwilling to mount or, if they do mount, are unwilling to remain mounted for long enough for successful copulation to occur. For this reason, valuable sires in AI studs receive considerable attention to the conformation of their feet. By contrast, many farm sires, especially bulls, receive little such attention until overt lameness has developed.

Similarly, any lesion of the trunk affects ability to mate. In young bulls which are overzealous in their early attempts to mate, the lumbodorsal fascia may rupture, producing the so-called condition of 'honeymoon back'. In this condition, the pain caused by the rupture of the fascia is such that the forelimb cannot be raised in preparation for mounting. This condition can be diagnosed by palpation of crepitus in the lumbodorsal region or by the presence of swollen muscle masses protruding through the fascia, and is most common in bulls that are 15–21 months old. As bulls age, progressive deposition of new bone occurs around the intervertebral joints (Figure 30.11), causing several related syndromes of incapacity. These conditions, which are most common in housed bulls receiving diets that are relatively high in calcium (Krook et al., 1969), rarely present under 7 years of age (Bane and Hansen, 1962). Firstly, progressive growth of exostoses can merely make the bull appear 'stiff', so that mounting requires increasing effort. Animals with back pain may mount, but frequently dismount again quite quickly. Affected bulls are unwilling to make the ejaculatory thrust and, if AV collection of semen is attempted, may spend a long time in the AV without thrusting (Almquist and Thomson, 1977). More seriously, spondyles of bone can fracture, usually during mounting, causing immediate, acute, back pain which is accompanied by a complete, but usually temporary, unwillingness to mount. However, where complete bridges of bone form between several adjacent vertebrae, flexing forces upon the spine can cause fractures within the spinal column, typically straight across a vertebral body. Such fractures typically occur at the moment of ejaculation, whereupon the bull becomes immediately paraplegic by spinal cord severance. The bull therefore collapses off the teaser into a dog-sitting position and exhibits complete loss of sensation of its hindlimbs.

Abnormalities of gait are a further cause of inability to mate. Details of such are beyond the scope of this chapter (for a review see Greenhough et al., 1972) other than to mention four conditions of the bull: spastic paresis, crampy syndrome, straddle gaits and the congenital ataxia of the Charolais breed. Attention is drawn to these conditions because of the importance of their recognition during examinations of bulls on behalf of prospective purchasers. However, similar conditions occur in many other domestic species.

Failure to copulate

Inability to copulate is a relatively frequent cause of infertility in domestic animals. Conditions which cause failure of copulation include failure of the penis to become turgid (i.e. failure of erection), abnormalities of erection which prevent intromission, and lesions of the penis and prepuce which prevent protrusion of the penis. Most of the conditions can be differentiated relatively easily and a prognosis can usually be given at an early stage of investigation.

Failure of erection

Erection is achieved by the action of the ischio-cavernosus muscles pumping blood into the corpus cavernosum penis (CCP). Because the CCP is, essentially, a blind-ending chamber, whose venous drainage is close to its arterial supply in the crura of the penis, the effect of the activity of the ischiocavernosus muscles is to occlude the veins

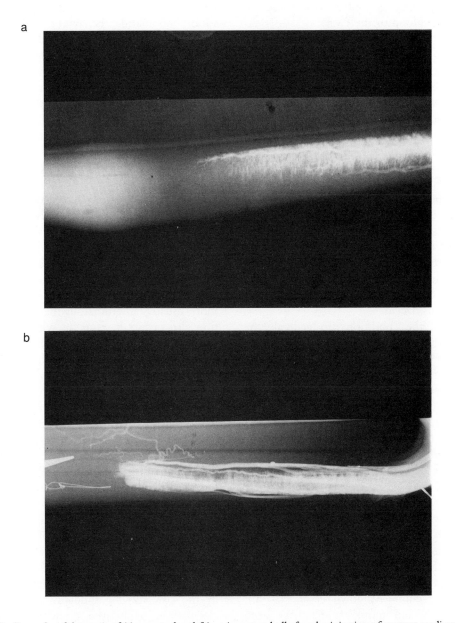

Fig. 30.12 Radiographs of the penis of (a) a normal and (b) an impotent bull after the injection of contrast medium into the CCP near the root of the penis. In the normal animal, the contrast medium is contained within the CCP, but in the impotent animal, contrast medium is leaking into the dorsal vein of the penis, indicating the presence of ectopic veins draining the CCP. The CCP was therefore not blind-ending and could not become turgid.

and force blood into the arteries, thereby raising the hydrostatic pressure within the CCP. The hydrostatic pressures thus generated produces the lengthening and stiffening of the penis that characterizes erection (Watson, 1964; Beckett et al., 1975). Thus, if any aspect of the vascular system of the CCP is perturbed, failure of erection ensues. Two main classes of abnormalities occur: those which allow blood to leak from the CCP so that it is not blind-ending, and those which prevent normal access of blood to the CCP.

Abnormal Venous Drainage of the CCP. This condition (Young et al., 1977; Ashdown et al., 1979a) is most commonly seen in young bulls, which are presented with normal libido, eager to mount, but never achieving erection or intromission. Observation of the mating behaviour of such bulls reveals that considerable activity is present in the ischiocavernosus muscles before and during mounting, to such an extent that the tail head appears to be 'pumping' up and down. However, the penis remains flaccid throughout its length. The cause of this condition is almost invariably failure of occlusion of the veins which drain the CCP during fetal life. Thus, because of the presence of veins draining the CCP, it is not a closed vessel, the high blood pressures required to produce erection cannot be achieved and the penis therefore remains flaccid.

Diagnosis of the condition can generally be made on clinical signs and history alone. However, if further confirmation of the cause of the condition is required, the presence of ectopic veins can be diagnosed by injecting radiographic contrast media into the CCP of the anaesthetized bull, then observing drainage of contrast into the dorsal veins of the penis (Figure 30.12). Because there are nearly always many small veins along both lateral edges of the CCP, surgical correction is rarely possible.

Occlusion of the Longitudinal Canals of the Penis. During erection, the changes in blood pressure which are initiated by ischiocavernosus activity are transmitted throughout the length of the CCP by the longitudinal canals. Congenital absence or acquired blockage of these canals therefore prevents erection (Ashdown et al., 1979b). Both young bulls and animals which have been successfully used as sires over a number of years can be afflicted with this condition. Young bulls present in a very similar way to animals with

abnormal venous drainage of the CCP and, in many ways, differentiation of the two conditions is rather academic, the prognosis for both being hopeless. In young bulls, the condition is typically caused by a congenital failure of cannulation of the short segment of the single, dorsal longitudinal canal (between the point of fusion of the two crural canals and the origin of the first of the lateral branches that form the ventral canal). In young bulls, the condition is diagnosed by observation of mating behaviour, when the penis remains flaccid despite considerable ischiocavernosus activity. It can be differentiated from abnormal drainage of the CCP by palpation of base of the penis. Although the great majority of the penis is flaccid, a short length of turgid tissue is present, in the part of the penis proximal to the occlusion. This can be appreciated by palpating the root of the penis just beneath the tail head, where the penis may become so turgid that the animal may resent it being touched.

Older bulls can be afflicted with a very similar condition. Such animals generally have a history of a long period of normal service behaviour, which has latterly changed into failure of erection. Libido remains normal. The other clinical signs are similar to those exhibited by a young bull. In such animals the longitudinal canals are blocked by fibrinous or, more usually, atheromatous material. This condition also occurs in rams, in which the CCP can rupture proximal to the site of obstruction, causing a peripenile haematoma in the region of the escutcheon. Similar ruptures occur infrequently in affected bulls.

Rupture of the Corpus Cavernosum Penis. This is a relatively common and potentially serious condition of bulls. It also occurs sporadically in boars and rams. The condition has many names, including rupture of the CCP, ruptured penis, fractured penis and broken penis. Rupture of the tunica albuginea occurs spontaneously if pressures within the CCP rises substantially above the pressures achieved during normal copulation (Noordsy et al., 1970; Beckett et al., 1974). Such abnormal increases in pressure can occur if the penis is suddenly subjected to shearing forces, for example by the cow moving suddenly at the moment of ejaculation, or by the ejaculatory thrust being directed against the escutcheon of the cow rather than the vagina. Rupture (Figure 30.13) occurs most commonly either in the region of the

a

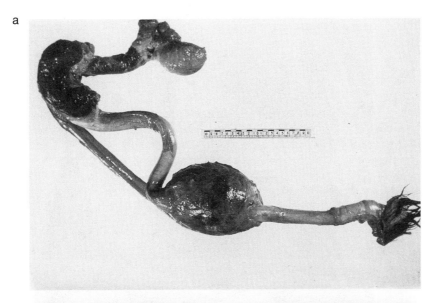

b

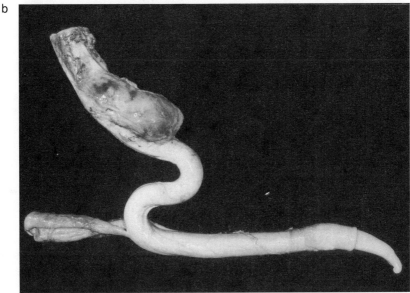

Fig. 30.13 (a) Peripenile haematoma from the rupture of the CCP, close to the insertion of the retractor penis muscles in a 3-year-old Jersey bull. (b) Organized haematoma following rupture of the CCP above the proximal sigmoid flexure.

insertion of the retractor penis muscle, or on the dorsal aspect of the distal sigmoid flexure where the trabeculae of the CCP are relatively weak. In rams, it is more common to see rupture of the CCP near to the root of the penis, above the proximal sigmoid flexure, presumably as a result of being butted from behind at the time of ejaculation.

The aetiology of the condition makes it more common in young than older bulls, probably due to the enthusiasm and inexperience of the former.

Immediately after rupture, the animal may be noticeably subdued and, in most cases, will immediately refuse to make further attempts to copulate. However, a few bulls continue to attempt to mate for short periods. Other clinical signs include shortness of gait and general indications of mild discomfort. Haemorrhage occurs from the site of rupture, with haematomata collecting in the surrounding tissues: cranial to the scrotum in ruptures of the distal sigmoid flexure (Figure 30.14(a)), behind the scrotum with proximal ruptures.

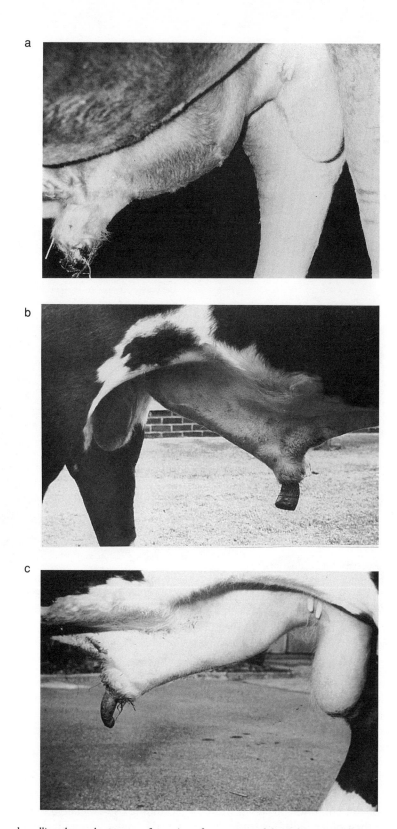

Fig. 30.14 (a) Prescrotal swelling due to haematoma formation after rupture of the CCP in a bull. (b) Prolapse of the preputial mucosa after rupture of the penis in a Hereford bull. (c) Prolapse of the penis secondary to rupture of the penis.

These haematomata can become very large, especially if mating behaviour is not immediately inhibited. Distal ruptures are also characterized by preputial oedema, which is often sufficiently severe to cause eversion of the preputial mucosa (Figure 30.14(b)). Occasionally, the penis itself may be prolapsed (Figure 30.14(c)). In light-coloured bulls, the rupture of the CCP may be of sufficiently explosive nature to cause blood staining of the overlying skin. Urination is not affected.

The haematoma is initially soft and fluctuant, but later, as the clot becomes organized, it becomes firm and hard. It is not possible to determine the extent of the haematoma during the initial phase, when the prepuce is oedematous, so assessment must take place after the oedema has subsided. If untreated, a substantial proportion of haematomata become infected and produce abscesses (Figure 30.15(a)), while others develop fibrous adhesions between the penis and prepuce and within the

a

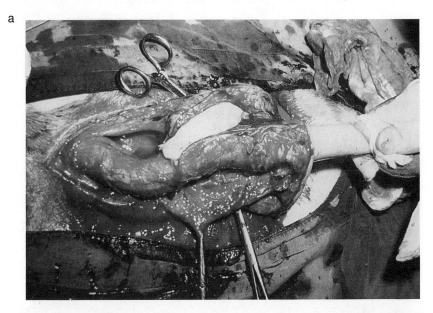

b

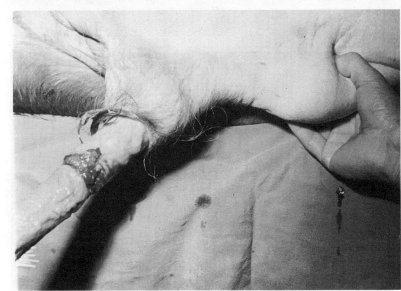

Fig. 30.15 (a) Secondary abscess formation in a peripenile haematoma in a bull. (b) Preputial fibrosis in a yearling bull with a small penile haematoma. The fibrotic lesion prevented protrusion and required resection.

fascial planes of the prepuce (Figure 30.15(b)). Diagnosis is relatively straightforward in recent cases, but neglected cases must be differentiated from preputial trauma and abscessation, tumours and urinary infiltration of the prepuce after urethral rupture. Peripenile haematomata may also be caused by trauma to the ventral abdomen or from peripenile vessels (Noordsy et al., 1970).

The time taken for recovery is such that treatment is inappropriate for all but the most valuable bulls, so that, in many cases, slaughter for salvage of the carcass price should be recommended. Where treatment is considered, several alternatives need to be considered, whose relative merits and demerits are still the subject of debate (see Pattridge, 1953;

Vandeplassche et al., 1963; Metcalfe, 1965; Pearson, 1972; Walker and Vaughan, 1980; Cox, 1982). Conservative treatment, consisting of sexual rest for 90 days, with initial antibiotic therapy to prevent abscess formation in the haematoma, and daily massage of the affected area to limit formation of peripenile adhesions, has been reported in some surveys to allow as many as 50% of bulls to regain service ability. However, other surveys have indicated that a successful response to conservative therapy occurs in as few as 10% of animals. Selection of cases to which conservative treatment is applied may account for some of the variation between surveys, for bulls with relatively small, freely movable, circumscribed, haematomata that

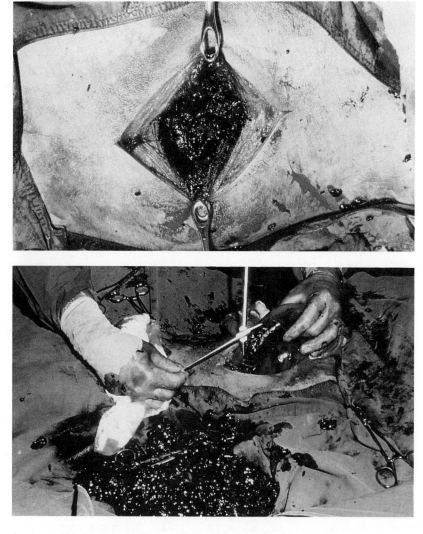

Fig. 30.16 Surgical evacuation of a peripenile haematoma in a bull.

are little bigger than the diameter of the normal penis respond best to conservative treatment. Larger haematomata carry a greater risk of abscess formation and of resulting in peripenile adhesions. Surgical treatment of such cases is best confined to evacuation of the haematoma, with strict attention to asepsis (Figure 30.16). More radical surgery, in which the site of rupture of the tunica albuginea is isolated, resected and sutured closed, has been suggested, but appears to result in a high proportion of animals developing peripenile adhesions and consequential inability to protrude the penis. In either case, surgery should not be delayed for more than 7 days after injury, as adhesions can become extensive thereafter. Sexual rest after surgery should only last for a few days, for a long period of inactivity also promotes peripenile adhesions. Affected bulls should therefore be teased regularly in order to induce penile movement and counteract the effect of contracting scar tissue. Mounting should, however, be prevented. Initially, protrusion of the penis is limited, but during ensuing weeks, a progressively greater length of penis is protruded.

Sequelae of rupture of the CCP include abscessation of the blood clot, if this is not evacuated. Peripenile adhesions are likely to be more severe if the clot is not removed, but even quite small areas of fibrosis can prevent penile protrusion. A proportion of animals develop ectopic veins that drain the CCP through the site of rupture. Such veins prevent vascular engorgement of the CCP. In such cases, surgical location of the site of the venous drainage and closure of the vein is often feasible, for, unlike congenital venous drainage of the CCP, such acquired cases usually only possess a single abnormal vein.

Abnormalities of erection

Persistence of the Penile Frenulum. Persistence of the penile frenulum is most frequently encountered in young bulls (Ashdown, 1962; Carrol et al., 1964), in which it either limits the amount of penis that can be protruded or causes the protruded penis to be deviated ventrally (Figure 30.17). Transecting the frenulum after ligating the frenular blood vessels if they are sufficiently prominent gives a good prognosis for the recovery of breeding ability (see Elmore, 1981; Cox, 1982). A familial predisposition has been suggested for the Angus and Beef Shorthorn breeds (Carrol et al., 1964), although the lesion occurs in all breeds. Persistence of the penile frenulum has also been occasionally reported in boars and dogs (e.g. Joshua, 1962).

Congenital Abnormalities of the Penis Preventing Protrusion. Considerable growth of the penis and changes in the relationships between the penis and the peripenile tissues occurs during the pre-pubertal period. Failure of these developmental changes can result in failure of normal erection.

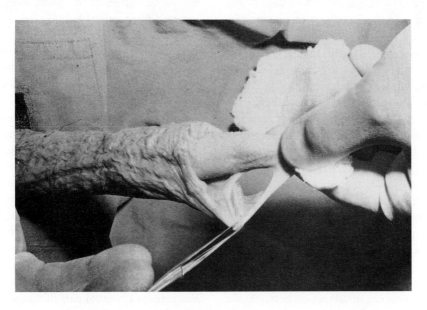

Fig. 30.17 Persistent penile frenula in an 18-month-old Friesian bull.

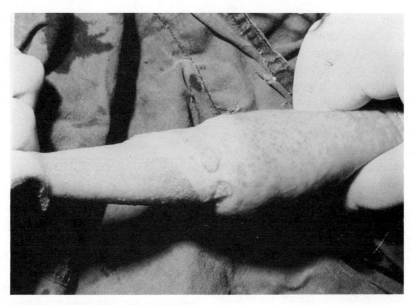

Fig. 30.18 Localized fibrosis responsible for ventral deviation of the penis. The animal was treated by excision of the lesion.

For example, failure of the penis to undergo normal growth causes a congenital shortness of the organ, such that normal intromission cannot be achieved. Alternatively, if such failure of growth is confined to the sigmoid flexure, it may be impossible to exteriorize the penis (see Roberts, 1986). Similarly, the retractor penis muscles can fail to develop, causing inability to protrude the penis. Although treatable by myectomy, this condition, like so many others affecting the bovine penis, is probably inherited (DeGroot and Numans, 1946), so correction should, perhaps, not be undertaken.

At birth, the integument of the penis and the penile part of the prepuce are fused but, during the prepubertal period, the bridging connective tissue normally breaks down (Ashdown, 1962). Where the connective tissue remains substantially intact, the penis cannot properly be protruded, such that only a few centimetres appear through the preputial orifice. This condition is most frequently encountered in bulls that were reared in isolation, which have never had the opportunity to indulge in the calf-hood riding behaviour which normally causes stretching and dislocation of the connective tissue between penis and prepuce (see Cox, 1982). The condition is frequently self-limiting once sexual activity begins, although it may result in persistence of the frenulum. It must be differentiated from other causes of adhesions between penis and prepuce.

Deviation of the Penis. Ventral deviation of the penis, often referred to as 'rainbow' deviation, can arise through a number of underlying conditions, of which the most common is persistence of the penile frenulum. In the absence of a persistent frenulum, the condition usually arises from defects in the fibrous architecture of the tunica albuginea. Such defects can be congenital, but can also arise from injuries to the penis which result in scar formation within the tunica (Figure 30.18). True ventral deviation of the penis must also be differentiated from partial failure of erection, when the penis appears deviated ventrally due to its flaccidity. Lateral deviation of the penis is also often attributed to injuries to the tunica, but may arise from inadequate development of the dorsal apical ligament of the penis or congenital defects of the tunica albuginea. Treatment is occasionally successful but is generally unrewarding (Milne, 1954; Walker, 1970; Boyd and Henskelka, 1972; Walker and Vaughan, 1980), due to the difficulty in identifying the site of the causal lesion. For bulls of moderate value, attempting treatment is therefore rarely worthwhile, while for valuable sires, collection of semen for cryopreservation and artificial insemination is often the most viable option.

The most spectacular deviation of the bovine penis is the spiral deviation. Spiralling of the tip of the penis is a normal part of the process of ejaculation in the bull, occurring after intromission,

a

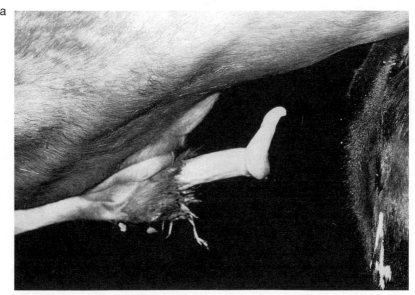

b

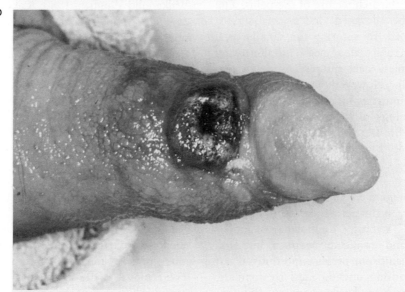

Fig. 30.19 (a) Spiral deviation of the penis manifested after protrusion. (b) Traumatic ulceration of the glans penis, secondary to spiral deviation of the penis.

during the ejaculatory thrust (Ashdown and Coombs, 1967, 1968; Seidel and Foote, 1967, 1969; Ashdown et al., 1968). If spiralling occurs prior to intromission, the latter cannot be achieved and the bull is described as suffering from a spiral deviation. Premature spiralling occurs in most afflicted bulls as the tip of the penis touches the hindquarters of the cow (Figure 30.19(a)), but may occur while the penis is still contained within the prepuce. In such cases, the spiralled penis can be clearly seen just behind the preputial orifice, through which it cannot pass. An affected bull

may escape the farmer's attention for quite long periods of time, for bulls generally mount keenly enough but, unless they are observed carefully, the characteristic absence of the ejaculatory thrust may be missed. Moreover, bulls do not invariably display premature spiralling, such that some cows may be successfully served. Persuading affected bulls to undergo premature spiralling during clinical examination can also require some patience: the author's experience is that it may take a long time of quite intense teasing before the abnormality is displayed. The onset of the condition may be at any age, although it is least common in yearlings and most common in animals in their second or third season of use (Pearson and Ashdown, 1976). Continual premature spiralling can result in the penile integument becoming traumatized as it comes into contact with the perineum of the cow. The pain caused by the consequent ulcer on the glans penis (Figure 30.19(b)) may, in time, impair the libido of the bull to the extent that it will not mount.

The cause of premature spiralling of the penis is not clear. Originally, it was suggested to be due to deficiency of the dorsal apical ligament of the penis (Walker, 1970), but later investigations indicated that this was unlikely (Ashdown et al., 1968; Ashdown and Pearson, 1971). Given that spiralling is a normal part of copulation, it appears more probable that the cause is neural or behavioural rather than a defect of the architecture of the penis. The condition can be alleviated, and normal service behaviour allowed, by suturing the dorsal apical ligament to the tunica albuginea with alternating catgut and stainless steel sutures (Ashdown and Pearson, 1973a). However, increasingly strong evidence is accumulating for an inherited component in the aetiology of the condition (Ashdown and Pearson, 1981; Blockey and Taylor, 1984), so it is questionable whether surgical correction is justifiable.

Lesions of the prepuce preventing penile protrusion
Adhesions between the peripenile tissues can arise from localized trauma, haemorrhage and/or abscessation in and around the prepuce. Infection of the penis (balanitis) or prepuce (posthitis) is not only painful, causing unwillingness to copulate, but also can result in development of adhesions between the two organs, preventing protrusion of the penis.

Preputial Injuries. In cattle, intermittent protrusion of varying lengths of preputial mucosa is a normal occurrence, which normally coincides with non-erectile movement of the penis within the sheath (Long and Hignett, 1970; Long et al., 1970; Ashdown and Pearson, 1973b). Pathological eversion of the prepuce is associated with aplasia or hypoplasia of the retractor muscles of the prepuce, which normally stabilize the preputial mucosa during penile movement. It is most commonly observed in naturally polled members of breeds with a pendulous prepuce (Long, 1969; Lagos and Fitzhugh, 1970; Bellenger, 1971). The result-

ing damage to the prepuce occurs most commonly in the segment of preputial mucosa that is closest to the preputial orifice and therefore most likely to be everted. In such cases, eversion of the preputial mucosa is followd by acute inflammatory changes which cause local hyperaemia and oedema. Unless replaced soon after eversion, the mucosa may become permanently prolapsed, with severe and diffuse fibrosis and thickening, often with chronic fissure formation and granulation tissue. Penile protrusion is substantially impaired by such lesions, usually to the extent that, at most, only the tip of the glans protrudes at full erection.

Acutely affected animals may be treated by the application of emollient dressings and replacement of the everted preputial tissue (Wheat, 1951; Hattangady et al., 1968; Larsen and Bellenger, 1971; Walker and Vaughan, 1980; Roberts, 1986). However, chronically inflamed tissue generally requires surgical removal, with the objective of restoring free movement of the preputial mucosa during penile erection. Many variations of surgical procedure have been described to remove the effete and fibrosed preputial tissue (Wheat, 1951; Milne, 1954; Walker, 1966; Larsen and Bellenger, 1971; Pearson, 1972; Walker and Vaughan, 1980), which is generally achieved by either submucosal resection (Figure 30.20), or amputation of the prolapse if the fibrotic change extends deeply into the submucosal tissues. In principle, a circumferential incision is made in the outer layer of preputial mucosa, after which the dissection is then deepened so as to excise all the fibrotic tissue before the inner mucous membrane of the prepuce is cut. The removal of the submucous lesions may cause considerable venous bleeding, such that careful haemostatis is essential. The inner layer of the mucosa is then sectioned in quadrants, so that suturing of mucosal frills can be performed without risk of retraction of the inner membrane into the preputial cavity. Interrupted sutures of catgut or polyglycolic acid are suitable. Resection of lesions around the preputial orifice inevitably reduces the effective length of the penis at erection, so the amount of tissue removed should therefore be limited to the minimum necessary to restore penile movement. Postoperative oedema may cause temporary protrusion of the sutured tissues, but this soon subsides. After 2 weeks sexual rest, the bull should be teased as frequently as possible until penile protrusion is

a

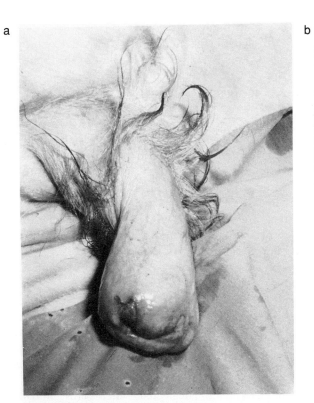

b

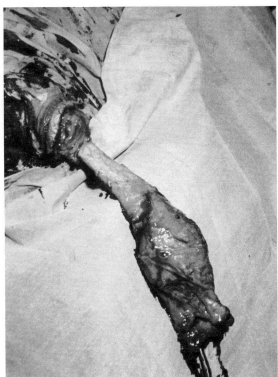

c

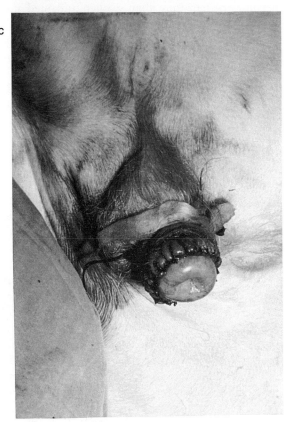

Fig. 30.20 (a) Chronic fibrosis in a prolapse of the distal prepuce in a Hereford bull. (b) Submucosal resection. (c) Final repair of the lesion.

adequate for intromission. Such teasing should persist for at least 3 months after surgery before an animal is condemned.

Alternatively, preputial lesions may occur at the site of the reflection of the preputial mucosa onto the penile integument (Figure 30.21). This site is less common than at the preputial orifice, but presents greater difficulty in treatment. The cause of such lesions is not always clear, but may result from partial or complete avulsion of the prepuce from the penis during copulation or AV collection of semen. Alternatively, lesions may occur when the prepuce becomes lacerated deep within the preputial cavity: usually as a result of the ventral prepuce bursting during the ejaculatory thrust. The site of such lesions is not always clear on clinical examination, for the changing relationships between penis and prepuce make it difficult to correlate the apparent site of a lesion with its position when the penis is protruded under anaesthesia. Intrapreputial lesions present difficulties of exposure for surgery. Even under general anaesthesia it may be difficult to expose the penis fully without tearing the tissues at the site of fibrotic change. After the penis is extruded, forcibly if necessary, all fibrotic tissue masses are excised, down to the tunica albuginea, between two circumferential mucosal incisions at the proximal and distal extremities of the lesion. The mucosal edges are repaired as for distal resections and the animals are managed similarly in the postoperative period. Such surgery is surprisingly effective, although somewhat unpredictable. Much depends upon the length of mucosa that requires resection.

Phimosis. Phimosis indicates a stricture of the preputial orifice which prevents the penis from being protruded. It has been recorded in most of the domestic species, and may arise from the injuries described above. It may also be a congenital defect, particularly in dogs of the German shepherd and golden retriever breeds. Severely congenitally affected puppies may be unable to urinate adequately, with the consequential balanoposthitis leading to septicaemia and death (see Johnston, 1986). Where dogs are affected by congenital lesions or a simple stricture of the preputial orifice, they may be treated by removing a wedge of preputial skin, fascia and mucosa, from just behind the ventral aspect of the preputial orifice. Mucosa and skin are then sutured together. Mild urine scalding may occur after surgery, as urine

does not run away freely (see Burke, 1986; Allen, 1992). In afflicted bulls and rams, a wedge of tissue should similarly be removed from the ventral aspect of the prepuce.

Paraphimosis. Inability to withdraw the penis into the prepuce results from congenital or acquired strictures of the prepuce, paralysis of the penis and, occasionally, from balanoposthitis. Although not strictly constituting paraphimosis, some coital injuries to the penis also prevent its return to the prepuce and thus, giving similar clinical signs, are considered under the same heading. The condition is most common in the dog and the stallion, but is also reported occasionally in most domestic species.

Paraphimosis following copulation or spontaneous erection is relatively common in the dog. It may also occur when the preputial opening becomes constricted by a band of hair, thereby preventing return of the penis to the prepuce (Johnston, 1986). In cases that have occurred recently, the penis can often be returned to the prepuce with careful manipulation and plentiful lubrication. If neglected, the penis initially becomes oedematous, then swollen, inflamed and suffers damage to its increasingly friable integument. In such cases, the preputial orifice may need to be surgically enlarged before the penis can be replaced (Chaffee and Knecht, 1975; Walker and Vaughan, 1980; Johnston, 1986). If the condition is left untreated, the penis can become strangulated within a relatively short space of time. The prognosis for cases that have not been treated promptly is therefore guarded, depending upon the severity of trauma and the degree of necrosis the penis has sustained. Unfortunately, the dorsal nerves of the penis are highly susceptible to ischaemic damage and, as these are required for the ejaculation reflex to be operative, inability to ejaculate is a relatively common sequel of relatively minor penile damage.

In stallions, prolapse of the penis is the sequel to many conditions. For example, it generally occurs transiently after the administration of phenothiazide tranquillizers (Pearson and Weaver, 1978; Lucke and Sansom, 1979). On occasions, this prolapse is irreversible (Figure 30.22(a)). Penile prolapse can also follow exhaustion, severe systemic illness and in the terminal stages of disorders of the central nervous system. It may be seen secondary to the preputial oedema that follows

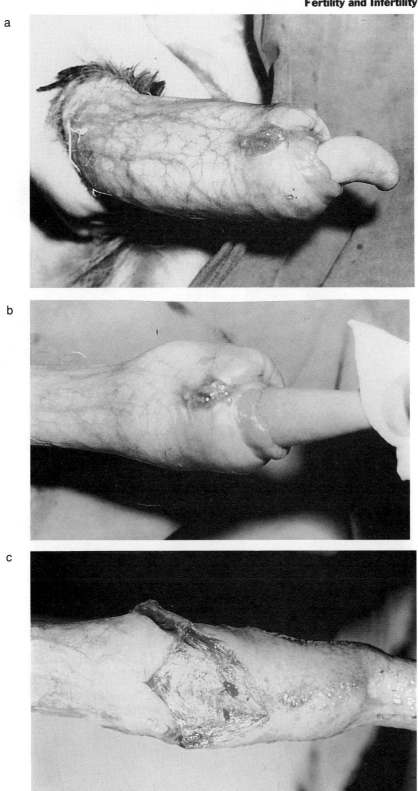

Fig. 30.21 (a) Severe preputial adhesion in a bull. (b) Preputial avulsion and fibrosis at the attachment of the preputial mucosa to the penis. (c) Mucosal tearing as the penis is forcibly withdrawn for the resection of the fibrotic tissues.

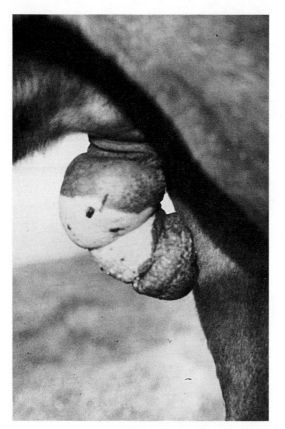

a

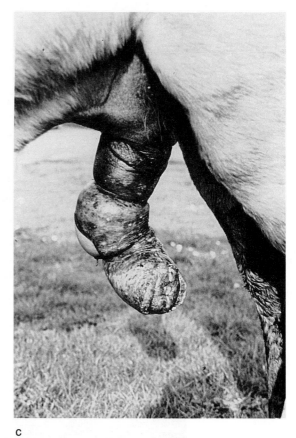

c

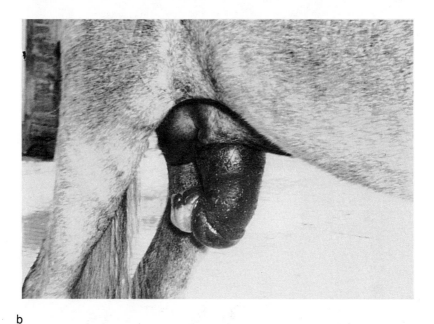

b

Fig. 30.22 (a) Priapism, 9 days after administration of neuroleptanalgesia for castration. (b) Penile prolapse in a horse after a kick at service. (c) Penile prolapse in a horse after an inguinal stake wound.

castration or other inguinal surgery (see Vaughan, 1993). However, it most commonly occurs after injury to the penis, such as occurs during copulation (Figure 30.22(b)), due to the use of ill-fitting stallion rings, malicious damage to the penis, accidents (Figure 30.22(c)), or injuries sustained during fighting. The pathology of the condition is similar to that of the dog, namely development of swelling, oedema, inflammation, followed by trauma, ischaemia and necrosis.

The earlier treatment is instigated, the greater the chance of obtaining a satisfactory outcome. Treatment (Walker and Vaughan, 1980; Cox, 1982; Vaughan, 1993) must aim to reduce oedema, prevent trauma to the penile integument and provide support for the penis until it can be returned to the prepuce. In the early stages, oedema may be dissipated by the use of cold water hosing, cold packs and exercise, whereas in the later stages the use of anti-inflammatory drugs and diuretics may also be helpful. The surface of the penis must be protected by the use of ointments which prevent drying, or by antiseptic ointments if open wounds are present. Finally, the penis must be supported. Arguably, providing adequate support for the penis is the most important aspect of treatment of this condition; for the drainage of fluid from the penis is greatly facilitated by reducing the tension on the lymphatics that is caused by the weight of the swollen, pendulous

penis. Effective supports have been made out of nylon stocking material or U-section plastic guttering, appropriately slung around the horse's hind quarters.

Strangulation and Necrosis of the Penis. Strangulation may occur as a consequence of paraphimosis or as a result of constriction of the penis by hair or maliciously placed objects. It is most common in long-haired breeds of dog and long-woolled breeds of sheep (Figure 30.23). As with paraphimosis, the prognosis depends upon the duration of the vascular constriction and the degree of necrosis that has ensued. Restoration of penile anatomy is relatively easy to achieve, for, providing gross necrosis has not occurred, the ability of the organ to heal is relatively good. However, loss of function, particularly impairment of the ejaculation reflex, occurs after relatively short periods of ischaemia. The prognosis should therefore always be guarded in the first instance. Where gross necrosis has occurred, amputation of the penis may be indicated. However, recourse to this option should not be taken at too early a stage, for, in the stallion at least, resolution of even a severe case of paraphimosis may take several weeks.

Necrosis of the penis, which does require immediate action, occurs in the ram following obstruction of the urethra by urethral calculi. This condition is seen most commonly in ram or

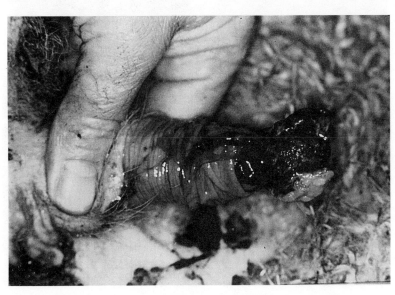

Fig. 30.23 Strangulation of the penis of a ram after long strands of fleece became wrapped around the glans during successive copulations.

a

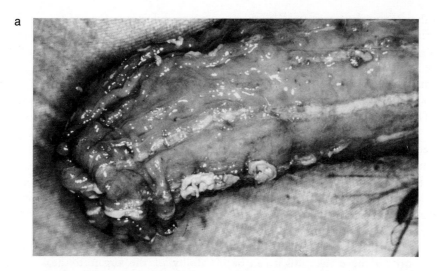

b

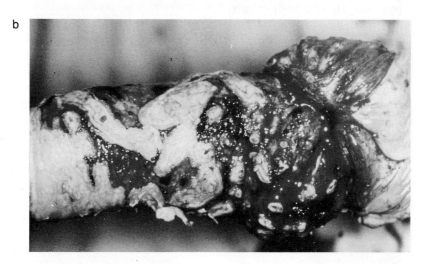

c

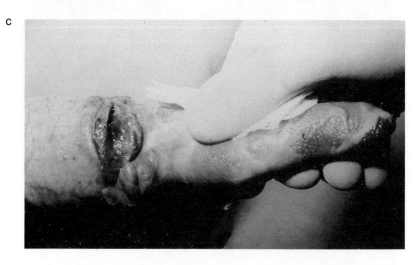

Fig. 30.24 Balanoposthitis in the bull. (a) Acute balanoposthitis, which prevented penile protrusion. (b) Acute balanoposthitis caused by IBR infection. (c) Diffuse fibrosis, following balanoposthitis.

wether lambs that have been growing very rapidly on diets that contain a high proportion of concentrate feeds, but may occur in any male sheep. At first, the calculi may lodge in the vermiform appendage and, if caught at this stage, the condition can easily be resolved, without impairing the fertility of the animal, by amputation of the appendage. However, calculi rapidly build up thereafter in the urethra, with penile necrosis rapidly ensuing. In such cases, amputation of the necrotic tissue, often accompanied by perineal urethrostomy, is often the only recourse. In animals that have been neglected for the regrettably long periods that frequently characterize the history of such cases, urethral rupture may occur, leading to infiltration of urine into perineal tissues, the prepuce and the scrotum. Alternatively, rupture of the bladder may occur. In both situations, extreme uraemia occurs and, where urine has infiltrated into tissue, necrosis and sloughing of the tissue invariably follows. The best that can be hoped for is the recovery of the carcass value of the animal, but even this is rarely achievable in neglected cases.

Balanoposthitis. Infections of the penis and prepuce are common in the dog, bull and ram, occasionally in the stallion, and rare in the boar and cat. Low-grade infection of the preputial cavity is very common, and rarely causes clinical disease. Severe balanoposthitis can cause pain, unwillingness to mate, preputial stenosis, adhesions between penis and prepuce, and peripenile adhesions.

Mild balanoposthitis is particularly common in the dog, in which the prepuce almost always contains a mild seropurulent exudate which is rarely indicative of clinical disease. It does cause a great deal of anxiety to some dog owners, however, who find both the discharge of such material from the preputial orifice and their dogs' efforts to cleanse themselves of the material, offensive. Prophylactic treatment of these mild infections is also frequently requested by owners of stud dogs. Such requests should be received with some caution for, whereas the use of mild antiseptic douches or bland antibiotic or antiseptic ointments rapidly clears any infection, the loss of the normal bacteriological flora from the preputial cavity can predispose to the establishment of opportunist infections by organisms of clinical significance. Occasionally, a canine herpesvirus causes a more severe balano-

posthitis (see Roberts, 1986), which is characterized by ulceration of the penis and unwillingness to copulate. However, it is more common to find that a traumatic aetiology underlies the relatively infrequent cases of the condition that are of clinical significance.

Similarly, many organisms are able to colonize the preputial cavity or penile integument of the bull. Most of these do not cause any clinical problems, although there are also a number which produce venereally transmitted diseases. Most of these diseases do not cause any gross lesions of the penis, and the bull is a symptomless carrier. A spectacular exception to this generality is the condition caused by the infectious bovine rhinotracheitis–infectious pustular vulvovaginitis (IBR–IPV) virus (Studdert et al., 1964; and see Roberts, 1986; McEntee, 1990). IBR–IPV causes an acute, ulcerative inflammation of the penis and prepuce (Figure 30.24), accompanied by an initial period of pyrexia. Secondary bacterial infection of the ulcers results in a severe, purulent balanoposthitis, causing very considerable discomfort to the bull. Affected bulls may exhibit swelling and pain in the region of the penis and may appear dysuric. Treatment is symptomatic, and consists of sexual rest and infusion of oily suspensions of antibiotics into the prepuce. Healing occurs over 2–8 weeks. In neglected cases, fibrinous adhesions may develop between adjacent ulcers on the penis and prepuce, eventually resulting in an impaired protrusion of the penis. Pustular vulvovaginitis usually occurs in cows served by bulls in the early stages of the disease. A few cases have been recorded in which the bull was relatively asymptomatic, despite characteristic lesions of pustular vulvovaginitis in the cows. The virus is transmissible in semen, which presents considerable risk if bulls which either have active infection or are seropositive are used in AI programmes. For this reason, many regulatory authorities preclude the use of seropositive bulls in AI studs.

Bulls are also susceptible to granulomata formation on the penis, which is a non-transmissible and usually asymptomatic condition (see Cox, 1982; Roberts, 1986). Occasionally it causes pain, producing the clinical sign of unwillingness to mate. The condition is characterized by hypertrophy of the lymphoid nodules of the penis, in the absence of an obvious, purulent balanoposthitis. Sexual rest and prophylactic infusions of oily suspensions of

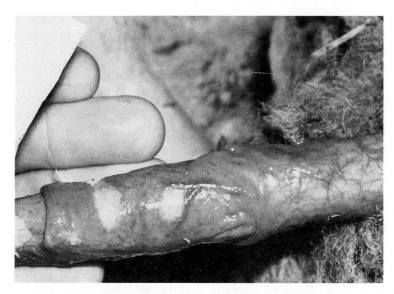

Fig. 30.25 Scars left on the ovine penis by healed orf lesions.

antibiotic into the prepuce usually produces a resolution of clinical signs. Tuberculous balanoposthitis has been described in areas where the disease is epizootic (Williams, 1943). Its signs include enlarged, granulomatous lesions of the penis, which may bleed, peripenile adhesions and secondary phimosis. This condition must be differentiated from actinomycosis of the prepuce, which causes a similar syndrome.

Balanoposthitis of the ram, colloquially known as 'pizzle-rot', is most commonly caused by the orf virus. Lesions may be present upon the preputial orifice, prepuce and glans penis, where the shallow ulcers are generally covered by a scab. Lesions may also be present in the other sites characteristic of orf, namely the lips, nostril and feet and, in females of the same flock, the vulva and teats. The disease is spread by contact, including venereal contact. Affected rams are generally unwilling to achieve intromission, but their libido is often maintained sufficiently to allow mounting to continue. Thus, the condition may escape notice for quite long periods of time, until it is realized that there is a very high incidence of returns to oestrus amongst the ewes. In consequence, the primary lesions are often healed by the time animals are presented for clinical examination, with little evidence, other than the scars left on the glans penis by the healing ulcers (Figure 30.25), that infection has occurred.

The most serious cause of balanoposthitis in the

stallion is the notifiable disease of dourine (Bowen, 1987; De Vries, 1993). Dourine is caused by the protozoan parasite *Trypanosoma equiperdum*, and occurs in the Middle East, North Africa and South America. Pockets of infection also occur in the Balkans, and South Africa. Infection is predominantly venereal, but can also be transmitted through infected AI equipment and can be passed to foals through vaginal discharges from the mare. The initial sign is oedema of the prepuce, penis, scrotum and surrounding skin, which may be sufficiently severe to cause paraphimosis. Inguinal lymph nodes are often enlarged, and a mucopurulent urethral discharge may also be present. Death may occur rapidly, but a chronic condition is more common outside Europe. Death occurs as the consequence of vascular degeneration causing peripheral nerve degeneration, muscle wasting, emaciation and paralysis. The condition can be treated in its early stages by trypanocidal drugs, although affected animals are slaughtered in many countries, such as those of Northern and Western Europe, the USA, Canada and Australasia, where eradication policies are in force.

In parts of the world where *Habronema muscae* occurs, larval infection produces granulomata in the equine penile and preputial integument. These fungoid growths are infiltrated with eosinophils, bleed easily, cause pruritus and may interfere with urination. In cool climates, lesions may temporarily regress during the winter. Treatment, by administration of systemic insecticide and corticosteroids, generally causes resolution of the disease (Wheat, 1961; Vaughan, 1993). Occasionally, surgery is required to relieve urethral obstruction or to remove the scar tissue that may form during healing (Stick, 1981).

A more common condition of stallions is equine coital exanthema, or 'horse pox' (see Cox, 1982; Couto and Hughes, 1993; De Vries, 1993). The herpesvirus (equine herpesvirus 3) that causes the disease is dissimilar to both the equine rhinopneumonitis and equine cytomegaloviruses and, while its mode of transmission is predominantly venereal, it may also be transmitted by vectors or vomites. Lesions occur mainly on the free part of the penis, consisting of papules that are surrounded by an area of hyperaemia and oedema, and whch progress to form ulcers. Where the density of lesions is sufficiently great, large ulcerated areas may appear. Mild infections do not impair libido, although lesions with severe secondary infection may do so. Control is achieved by preventing affected animals from mating, while individual animals may need affected areas to be washed weekly with antiseptic solution to limit the establishment of secondary infection.

Penile Neoplasia. Virally induced fibropapillomata of the skin, genitalia and alimentary tract are common in young cattle. The penile integument, particularly its terminal 5 cm, is a common site for such tumours, which may be single or multiple, sessile or pedunculated (Figure 30.26). Tumours can be found in intact and castrated animals, but rarely persist beyond 3 years of age. Clinical effects vary according to the size and the morphology of the lesions. Haemorrhage and ulceration are the most common sequelae; the pain caused by the latter sometimes being sufficiently severe to impair libido. Large lesions can prevent retraction of the protruded penis back into the sheath, resulting in the tumour-bearing segment remaining outside the preputial orifice and becoming traumatized and infected. Multiple or large lesions can cause complete irreducible prolapse of the penis, which then undergoes secondary changes of venous congestion and oedema. Rapid growth of penile tumours within the preputial cavity can result in compression of the urethra, which may even rupture, allowing extensive infiltration of urine into peripenile tissues.

Fibropapillomata sometimes undergo necrosis and sloughing, others become detached during coitus, while yet other lesions regress spontaneously. However, such resolutions cannot be assumed, so recourse to surgery is frequently indicated (Pearson, 1972). Single, pedunculated lesions can sometimes be removed during coitus, but most tumours require careful removal with the bull very heavily sedated or under general anaesthesia. Pedunculated lesions can be ligated relatively easily, but excision of sessile lesions often leads to profuse haemorrhage, which may be difficult to control if a large area of mucosa has had to be removed. However, although such haemorrhage may persist for some time, it is rarely dangerous and, provided the tumour does not recur, the wounds generally heal quickly. Care should be exercised to avoid incising the urethra, for its highly vascular mucosa may continue to bleed at ejaculation for long periods afterwards. Penile fibropapillomata do not metastasize, but a small proportion of tumours exhibit a remarkably aggressive recurrence after surgical removal. There is debate of the incidence of such recurrences, but possibly 10% of lesions recur with sufficient rapidity to be obvious again within 3–4 weeks of surgery (Pearson, 1977). Cryotherapy of the affected area usually prevents further recurrences (Pearson and Lane, unpublished findings), while administration of an autogenous tissue vaccine markedly reduces the incidence of recurrences (Desmet et al., 1974). The prognosis for use as breeding animals is generally good, although libido may take some time to recover in animals that have had long-standing, painful, ulcerated lesions.

Penile tumours are also common in the horse. Squamous cell carcinomata of the glans penis (Figure 30.27(a)) or preputial ring occur in aged geldings, in which they develop as large, fungating tissue masses which may cause bloody preputial discharge or penile prolapse. The tumour develops in response to the carcinogenic properties of the smegma that accumulates around the penis of geldings (Plaut and Kohn-Speyer, 1947). Its growth is relatively slow and it is slow to metastasize, although it does spread within the preputial cavity and, eventually, metastasizes to local lymph nodes. However, local lymphadenitis may also occur due to the secondary infection which invariably occurs with these tumours, so care must be exercised in giving a prognosis. Occasionally,

a

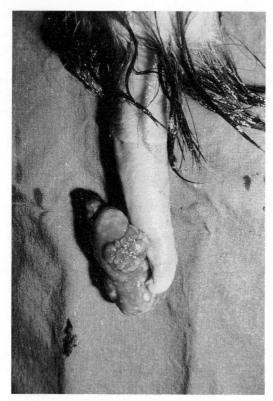

b

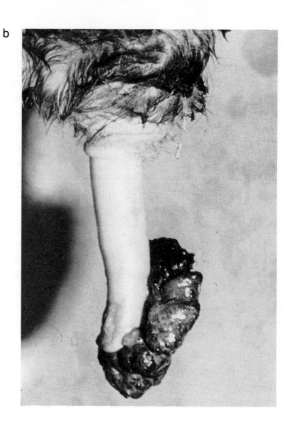

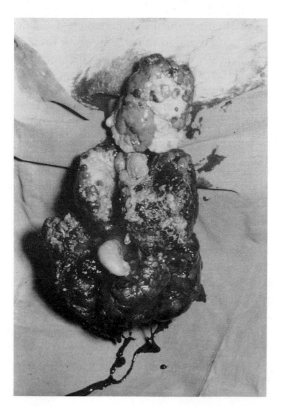

Fig. 30.26 Penile fibropapillomata in the bull. (a) Lesions exposed in conscious bull by means of pudendal nerve block. (b) Lesion covering an extensive area of the tip of the penis. (c) Massive tumour causing penile prolapse, urethral rupture and localized cellulitis in a 10-month-old castrate.

c

penile carcinomata behave in a malignant, invasive manner and rapidly destroy the body of the penis (Figure 30.27(b)). Penile carcinomata are best treated by radical amputation of the penis, with a urethrostomy on the penile stump within the sheath or directly to the preputial skin (see Walker and Vaughan, 1980). Some lesions of the more loosely attached preputial mucous membrane can be dealt with by simple or reefing excision.

Sarcoids also frequently develop on the preputial skin and mucosa in both castrated and entire horses, donkeys and othe Equidae. Sarcoids also occur on the scrotal integument. In most circumstances, such lesions can be extirpated without difficulty, using a variety of surgical methods (see Vaughan, 1993). However, the presence of multiple, recurrent sarcoids on the inner or external surfaces of the prepuce (Figure 30.27(c)) may necessitate its complete ablation and amputation of the penis (Cox, 1992). Grey horses may develop melanomata of the penis or prepuce (Figure 30.27(d)). Their progress is generally slow and only produce local invasion of tissue, but aggressive lesions which metastasize also occur from time to time.

In the dog, the most common penile tumour is the transmissible venereal tumour (see Jones and Joshua, 1982; Roberts, 1986). This tumour, which is mostly commonly found in the tropics, is spread by coitus and has an incubation period of 5–6 weeks. A fetid, bloody preputial discharge may be present and, on exteriorization of the penis, characteristic fleshy, greyish-red, nodular masses are observed (Bloom et al., 1951). The tumours ulcerate easily and are friable (Figure 30.28), so bleed when handled. In neglected cases, spread to local lymph nodes occurs. Treatment, where this is possible, is by removal of the penis and prepuce. The recurrence rate is relatively high. The use of chemotherapy has also been advocated (Wittrow and Susaneck, 1986).

Penile papillomata (Figure 30.29) also occur in the dog but, unlike those of the bull, are generally ulcerative, locally keratinized and poorly circumscribed (Arthur et al., 1989). They may also be completely sessile, with a sharply demarcated, ulcer-like border. Such lesions bleed profusely with sexual or other excitement, but their development may be remarkably slow, even over a number of years.

Miscellaneous Conditions of the Penis Complete avulsion of the preputial mucosa from its attachment to the glans penis is an occasional injury of bulls which usually results from careless use of an AV (Roberts, 1986). Diaphallus, or duplication of the penis, is a rare condition of the bull. Hypospadias and epispadias are congenital abnormalities of the penis, in which the urethra opens in the perineum or on the ventral or dorsal surface of the penis. The consequences of such lesions depend upon the site of the urethral opening. Where this is close to the distal end of the penis, the condition may be undetected and have no effect upon fertility. However, more proximal lesions adversely affect fertility.

The retractor penis muscle may undergo disuse atrophy after the penis has been unable to achieve erection for a long period. However, calcification of the retractor penis muscle, which occurs in aged bulls, does not affect erection. Finally, some bulls exhibit profuse arterial haemorrhage at the time of ejaculation. This condition, which is difficult both to investigate and to treat, may be due to unhealed traumatic lesions of the penile integument but, more commonly, is due to leakage of blood from the corpus spongiosum penis into the urethral lumen (Ashdown and Majeed, 1978).

Conditions causing failure of ejaculation

There are a few conditions in which ejaculation does not occur, despite normal mounting. Such conditions can be broadly divided into those where the ejaculation reflex is impaired and those in which localized pain makes the animal unwilling to ejaculate. The former conditions generally occur when some damage has occurred to the neural pathways between the glans penis and the spinal cord. Strangulation of the penis, with ensuing damage to the sensory dorsal nerve of the penis, causes ejaculation failure, while in older bulls, compression of the spinal nerve roots by age-related exostoses can also preclude ejaculation.

Localized pain is similarly effective in preventing ejaculation. Localized peritonitis in the caudal abdomen of ruminants causes pain during the ejaculatory thrust, so affected animals are often willing to mount but less willing to ejaculate. Animals with back pain behave similarly, although they may be less willing to mount. Finally, some painful conditions of the penis, notably orf in rams, make the animal unwilling to achieve intromission and ejaculate, despite their willingness to mount.

a

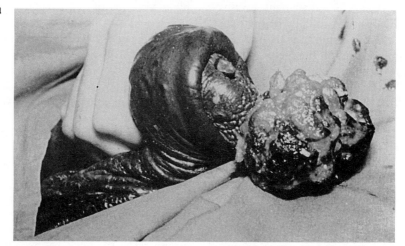

b

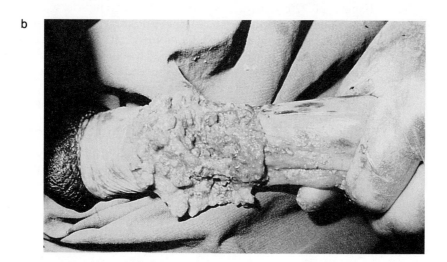

c

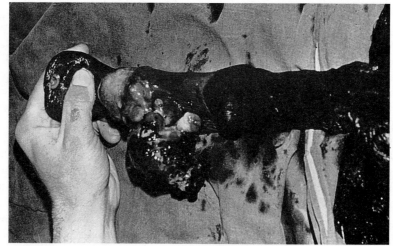

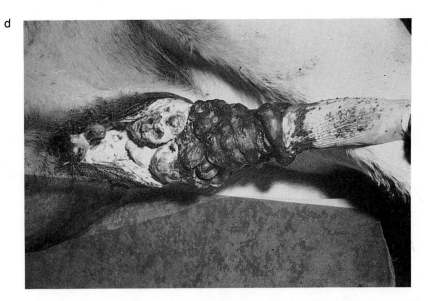

Fig. 30.27 Penile and preputial tumours in the stallion. (a) Squamous cell carcinoma of the penis in an aged gelding. (b) Squamous cell carcinoma of the penis associated with tissue infiltration and destruction. (c) Multiple sarcoids of the penis and prepuce. (d) Multiple melanomata formation in the prepuce of an aged grey gelding.

Conditions causing failure of fertilization

Fertilization failure, despite normal copulation, generally characterizes diseases of the testis (including abnormalities of spermatogenesis), epididymis and accessory glands. Many of the conditions causing failure of fertilization can be diagnosed by an examination of the external genitalia of the sire, but many more can only be diagnosed by semen evaluation, which is therefore an essential component of one's clinical examination. However, a diagnosis of failure of fertilization on the part of the male animal always requires careful differentiation from the many female factors which can present with apparently identical signs. For this reason, it is generally advisable to undertake an evaluation of the group of females with which the apparent infertility of a sire has been manifest, before examining the sire.

Furthermore, it is important to separate causes of fertilization failure which represent pathologies of the reproductive tract from causes which are non-pathological. In the latter category are two important factors. Firstly, the time of year when the sire was used must be considered in relation to the endogenous breeding season of the species. Secondly, the number of females the sire was required to impregnate and the system of mating under which he was being used must also be considered, in relation to the normal reproductive expectations of the species and breed.

Conditions affecting the testis and epididymis

Cryptorchidism. Cryptorchidism occurs when the normal process of testicular descent is perturbed, such that one or both testes fail to complete their descent into the scrotum. Spermatogenesis is generally markedly impaired or absent in testes that are not scrotal, due to high intratesticular temperature. Animals which have a single cryptorchid testis are usually fertile, although the inhibition of spermatogenesis in retained testes means that the sperm density is often below expectation for the species. Where both testes are cryptorchid, the ejaculate is either aspermic or very severely oligospermic. Testosterone secretion is unaffected by a cryptorchid position, so the libido of affected animals is normal. Indeed, it is far more common for cryptorchidism to be detected in supposedly castrated animals which continue to exhibit masculine behaviour than as a cause of subfertility in intact males.

Cryptorchidism occurs most commonly in the stallion (Hayes, 1986) and the boar (Huston et al., 1978), and in some breeds of dog (see Patterson, 1977). It is uncommon in other species, except as an iatrogenic condition of bulls and rams. In these species, unskilled use of rubber rings for castration can result in one testis being either forced back

a

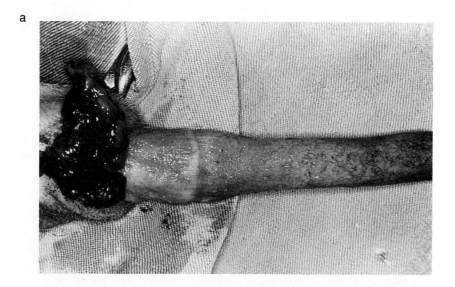

b

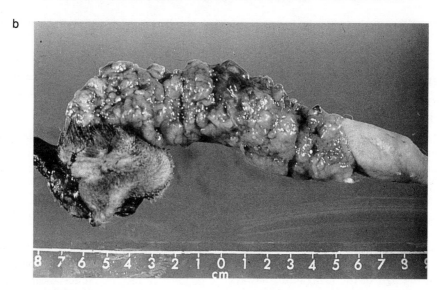

Fig. 30.28 Transmissible venereal tumour of the dog. (a) Tumour formation over most of the penile integument. The characteristic fleshy, greyish-red, nodular masses of the tumour are readily apparent. (b) Tumour developing in the preputial fornix.

into the inguinal canal or, more commonly, into a subcutaneous position cranial to the scrotum. Occasionally, a high incidence of cryptorchidism has been recorded in individual flocks of sheep. Such flocks, together with the clear breed incidences of the condition in other species (e.g. Red Danish cattle — Blom and Christensen, 1947; Angora goat — Warwick, 1961), indicate the probability of an inherited basis for the disease. For this reason, the use of cryptorchid animals as sires should be avoided, and their castration recommended. In the dog and the stallion,

retained testes exhibit a similarly high incidence of neoplasia to that reported in humans: a further reason for the castration of such animals (Willis and Rudduck, 1943; Pendergass and Hayes, 1975).

Testes may be retained in the abdomen or inguinal canal. The incidence of different sites of retention in the horse is shown in Table 30.2. In supposedly castrated animals, diagnosis of the presence of a testis in the inguinal canal may be achieved by careful palpation of that region, but many cases require demonstration of the presence of male hormones for confirmation. All affected

a

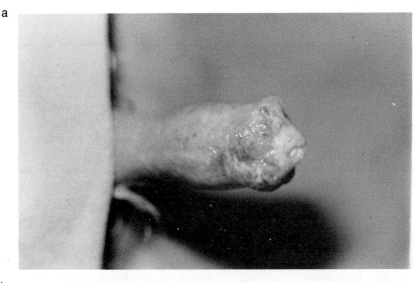

b

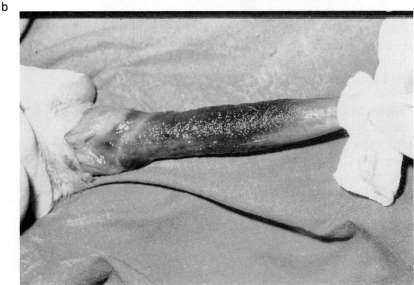

Fig. 30.29 Penile papillomata of the dog. (a) Localized lesion and (b) diffuse 'florid' lesion.

stallions exhibit testosterone concentrations that are not only higher than in castrated animals, but also are responsive to LH stimulation (Cox et al., 1973; Cox, 1975). Thus, after collection of an initial blood sample, 3000 IU of hCG are given intravenously, then a further blood sample collected 40 minutes later. Both are assayed for testosterone concentrations. In older animals (4 years and over), the presence of oestrone sulfate in the blood also confirms the presence of testicular tissue. Removal of retained testes from the horse may be effected by initial surgical exploration of the inguinal canal. Many testes will be found in this site, while others can be withdrawn from an

abdominal position through the inguinal ring without much difficulty. Other abdominal testes can be withdrawn through a parapenile abdominal incision (Arthur, 1961; Walker and Vaughan, 1980; Cox, 1982). Providing the gubernacular attachments of the testis are left intact during surgery, it is very uncommon to find an abdominal testis at a site other than near the internal inguinal ring.

Testicular Degeneration. The seminiferous epithelium of the tesis is highly susceptible to damage, with a wide variety of agents causing reversible or irreversible degeneration. Testicular degeneration occurs in response to raised intra-testicular

Table 30.2 Sites of testes in the cryptorchid stallion

Position of left testis	Position of right testis			Total
	Abdominal	Inguinal	Scrotal	
Abdominal	125 (7.0)	12 (0.7)	545 (30.7)	682
Inguinal	2 (0.001)	69 (3.9)	254 (14.3)	325
Scrotal	291 (16.4)	446 (25.1)	—	
Total	418	527		1744

Compiled from Hobday (1914), Silbersiepe (1937), Stanic (1960), Arthur (1961), Wright (1963), Bishop *et al.* (1966), Stickle and Fessler (1978) and Cox *et al.* (1979).

temperature, toxins, endocrine disturbances and infection (see Humphrey and Ladds, 1975; McEntee, 1990). Many of the causes of testicular degeneration do not manifest themselves in infertility immediately, due to the protracted time taken for spermatogenesis. There is therefore normally a lag interval, which may be of several weeks, between the time at which the testis is damaged and the time at which effects upon semen quality are first noted.

Raised temperature in the testis can itself emanate from many causes. Many animals exhibit a period of relative infertility during and after high summer temperatures. This phenomenon is well recognized in the boar (see Crabo, 1986), even in Northern European conditions, and is sufficiently important in the bull for some AI studs to provide air-conditioned accommodation for the sires to limit summer maxima of temperature (Roberts, 1986). Temperature-induced summer infertility of males is a very important cause of infertility in European breeds of domestic animals that are imported into tropical and subtropical climates. In rams, raised scrotal temperature can result from excessive amounts of wool over the scrotum, or from leaving animals unshorn during the summer (Hulet et al., 1956). Thus, the practice of showing rams in full fleece in mid-summer accounts for the very high proportion of such animals which become infertile during the subsequent autumn breeding season. Excessive deposition of fat in the scrotum, such as occurs in rapidly grown bulls and rams, can prevent heat loss from the scrotum and result in infertility (Jubb and Kennedy, 1970). Local inflammation to the scrotal skin or other structures in the scrotum can also raise the testicular temperature sufficiently to impair spermatogenesis (Rhodes, 1976; Burke, 1986; Roberts, 1986), and inflammation of one

testis or epididymis almost invariably causes a temperature-dependent degeneration in the opposite testis. Abnormalities of the testicular circulation, such as occurs in varicocoele (Figure 30.30), perturbs the heat exchange mechanism responsible for maintaining the testis at a temperature below that of the body, again resulting in temperature-dependent testicular degeneration

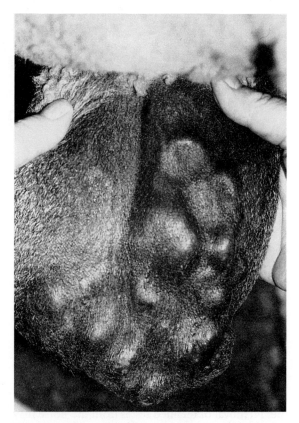

Fig. 30.30 Varicocoele of the scrotum of a ram. The distended arterial masses which extend over the surface of the scrotum impaired thermal regulation of the scrotum, thereby causing infertility.

(Ott et al., 1982). Degeneration results from inguinal or scrotal hernias, for the same reason. Finally, prolonged pyrexia, such as occurs with systemic infections, can cause testicular damage, although short periods of illness are unlikely to be detrimental. Conversely, scrotal frostbite also can result in testicular degeneration (Faulkner et al., 1967).

Toxic causes of testicular degeneration are, likewise, many (see Humphrey and Ladds, 1975). Heavy metal or radiation contamination are well-recognized causes of testicular damage, but many other materials have been implicated at various times. Establishing causal relationships between such substances and infertility is particularly difficult, given the time interval between their ingestion and appearance of infertility. Stress-related degeneration occurs largely due to the inhibition of LH secretion by the corticosteroids that are released during stress (Welsh et al., 1981). Stress-related degeneration has been described in beef bulls after movement (Knudsen, 1954; Jackowski, et al., 1961) and in other animals due to chronically unsuitable housing and management (see Clarke and Tilbrook, 1992). Hormonal degeneration is described in dogs whose gonadotrophin

secretion is impaired either by a primary lesion of the anterior pituitary or due to the presence of oestrogenic tumours, such as Sertoli cell or adrenal tumours (see Roberts, 1986). Aged animals undergo a progressive, irreversible degeneration, initially characterized by increased percentages of sperm with primary abnormalities, with later oligospermia and testicular fibrosis (Bishop, 1970; McEntee, 1990).

Many infectious causes of degeneration have also been described. The most severe of such infectious causes, orchitis, is considered under a separate heading, but many other, more mild conditions affect the efficiency of spermatogenesis. Ascending infection by enterocytopathic bovine orphan (ECBO) viruses and infection by IBR or, where it occurs, Epivag virus have been specifically associated with testicular degeneration, although viral causes are frequently implicated even when a causal organism cannot be conclusively demonstrated (Humphrey and Ladds, 1975; Roberts, 1986). Bacterial contamination of such testes frequently leads an inherently mild bout of degeneration to progress to purulent or necrotic orchitis.

Clinical signs of infertility and oligospermia usually supervene 4–8 weeks after the onset of

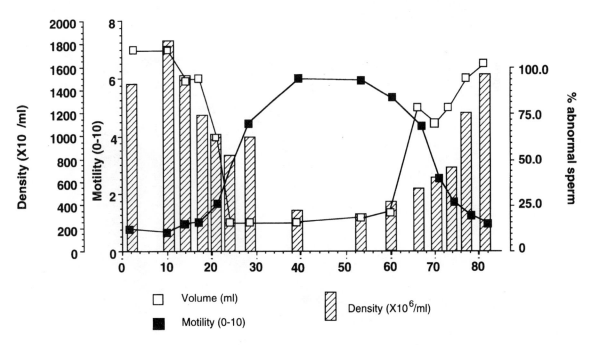

Fig. 30.31 Changes in semen quality of a bull during a period of testicular degeneration and the subsequent restoration of normal spermatogenesis. The cause of the degeneration was presumed to be high summer temperatures. (Redrawn from Parkinson (1991) with permission.)

the cause of the degeneration. Ejaculate volume is usually unaffected, but the number and motility of spermatozoa fall, while the proportion of sperm exhibiting abnormal morphology rises (Figure 30.31). In severe cases, the ejaculate may become virtually aspermic, with such sperm as are present having such bizarre morphology as to be scarcely recognizable. After such an acute phase, the condition may resolve in one of two main ways. In many animals, resolution of the degeneration occurs over a period of weeks or months, with an eventual recovery of semen parameters back to, or close to, normality. Some residual oligospermia or increased proportion of morphologically abnormal sperm may be present. In more severe cases, permanent loss of seminiferous tubules occurs, with fibrosis and calcification (Figure 30.32) of the testis following. Such animals never regain normality, but present with shrunken, firm, irregular testes and virtually aspermic semen. It is

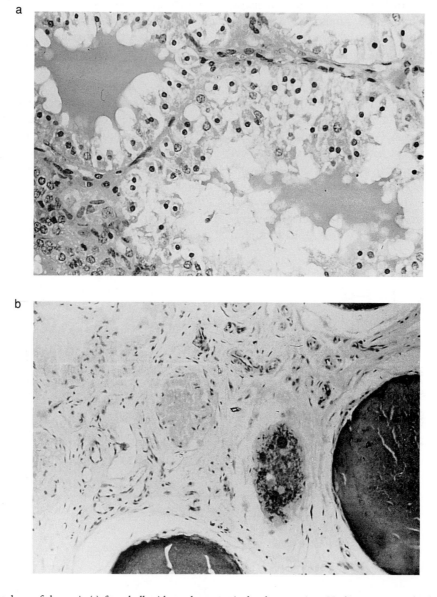

a

b

Fig. 30.32 Histology of the testis (a) from bull with moderate testicular degeneration. Healing may completely restore normal testicular architecture, or may result (b) in loss of seminiferous tubules, together with fibrosis and calcification of interstitial tissue. (Reproduced from Parkinson (1991), with permission.)

important to note that the severity of the initial changes in semen quality is of very little prognostic value: the author has seen animals which have very severe changes in semen quality that have returned to normal fertility in a matter of months, whereas other animals, with quite mild initial seminal changes have never again produced acceptable semen. Testicular biopsy can be a valuable aid to prognosis, although very great care is needed if such samples are to be collected from ruminant species, due to the very considerable risk of severe haemorrhage into the testis or betwen the vagina tunics (Gassner and Hill, 1955). However, biopsies can be collected from the dog (Soderberg, 1986) and stallion (Threlfall and Lopate, 1993) although, even in these species, considerable damage to testicular parenchyma can result in individual animals. Intact basement membranes of the seminiferous tubules, the presence of spermatogonia within the tubules and the patency of the lumina of the tubules all indicate a good prognosis for restoration of fertility (Kenney, 1970). Where collection of biopsies is not undertaken, the progress of the animal must be monitored by regular collection of semen until signs of resolution of the condition are observed. An early sign of resolution which occurs in some animals is that the grossly abnormal morphology of the spermatozoa is replaced by relatively high percentages of cells with cytoplasmic droplets at the distal end of the midpiece.

Orchitis and Epididymitis. *Orchitis* ranges from a mild infection of the testis, scarcely distinguishable from testicular degeneration, through to gross suppurative or necrotic destruction of the organ. Orchitis can arise from a primary infection or by haematogenous spread of bacteria into the testis superinfecting pre-existing traumatic, viral or parasitic damage. Primary testicular damage can arise from ECBO infection in bulls (Humphrey and Ladds, 1975), but, in rams, it is likely that many infections become established after fighting injury to the testis. *Brucella* species cause orchitis in many domestic animals: *B. abortus*, *B. canis*, *B. melatensis* and *B. suis* affecting bulls, dogs, goats and boars, respectively (reviewed by Plant et al., 1976; Jones and Joshua, 1982; Roberts, 1986; Smith, 1986). In cattle, a further important primary bacterial pathogen is *Mycobacterium tuberculosis*. However, the majority of isolates from cases of orchitis are either non-specific bacteria and mycoplasma, or are the particular pyogenic organ-

ism for the animal species (e.g. *Actimomyces pyogenes* in cattle). Ascending infection from the urinary tract is postulated, but haematogenous spread seems more probable.

Orchitis is more commonly unilateral than bilateral and may involve the epididymis. During the acute phase of the disease, the affected testis is inflamed, with consequent hyperaemia, heat and swelling (Figures 30.33 and 30.34). The testis may become grossly enlarged; up to two or three times its normal size. The testis is often very painful, so that the animal resents it being touched. The pain may be sufficiently severe to produce an altered gait. A systemic pyrexia may occur. The localized inflammation usually causes temperature-dependent degeneration in the unaffected testis. If the condition progresses to the chronic phase, the testis becomes shrunken, fibrotic and adherent to the tunic and scrotum. Abscesses may break through the scrotal skin.

Orchitis invariably causes a great deal of destruction of the affected testis. The infection may be purulent, with large, coalescent abscesses occupying much of the testicular parenchyma, or it may be necrotic, when the substance of the testis is almost entirely destroyed. Because of the degree of destruction that occurs, the prognosis for saving the affected testis is hopeless. If it is hoped to salvage an affected animal for breeding, removal of a unilaterally affected testis should therefore be advocated at the earliest possible stage of the disease, to limit degeneration of the unaffected testis. If bilateral orchitis occurs, the prognosis for future breeding is hopeless, and castration should be performed as soon as it is safe to do so.

Epididymitis can also occur as a primary infection or by spread from an infected testis (Humphrey and Ladds, 1975). Orchitis in the associated testis can also occur following a primary epididymitis. In Australia, North and South America and central Europe, *Brucella ovis* causes an epididymitis, which causes epididymal obstruction and granuloma formation (Bruere, 1986). The general signs of epididymitis are similar to those of orchitis, namely heat, swelling and pain of the affected organ. Any inflammation of the epididymis causes obstruction of the single, highly convoluted tube of which the organ is composed, so a loss of function normally ensues. Unilateral epididymitis therefore results in reduced fertility, whereas bilateral obstruction results in sterility. Furthermore,

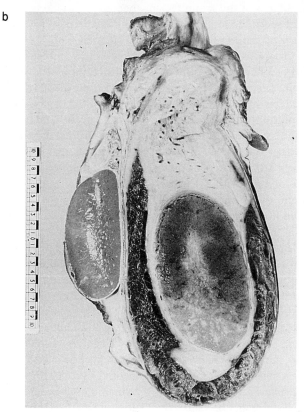

Fig. 30.33 Orchitis in the bull. (a) Simmental bull with acute orchitis. (b) Longitudinal section of the scrotum, showing inflammation within the substance of the testis and in the vaginal tunics. Degeneration of the contralateral testis has caused a reduction in its size. (Reproduced from Parkinson (1991), with permission.)

as with orchitis, unilateral epididymitis causes temperature-induced degeneration in the contralateral testis, so early removal of the affected epididymis and its associated testis shold be recommended.

Obstruction of the epididymis can occur fol-

a
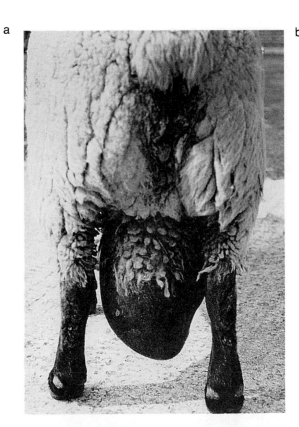

b
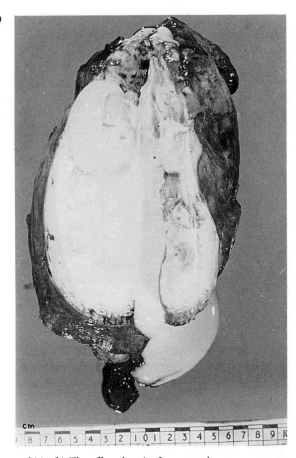

Fig. 30.34 Orchitis in the ram. (a) Ram with acute orchitis. (b) The affected testis after removal.

lowing localized rupture of the duct and leakage of sperm into the surrounding stromal tissue. The granulomata formed in response to the presence of foreign (sperm) antigen in the tissue cause an obstruction of the epididymes (Parkinson et al., 1993; Figure 30.35). Leakage of sperm into the tail of the epididymis also occurs in animals that have been vasectomized. In vasectomized rams, the epididymal tail can be nearly as large as the testis (Figure 30.36), where innumerable small sperm granulomata have formed. Surprisingly, this condition does not appear to be painful, and the libido of such vasectomized rams is normal.

Testicular Hypoplasia. Testicular hypoplasia implies an incomplete development of the germinal epithelium of the seminiferous tubules, due to inadequate numbers of germinal cells within the testis. Lack of germinal cells may arise through partial or complete failure of the germinal cells to develop in the yolk sac, failure to migrate to the genital ridge, failure to multiply in the devel-

oping gonad, or widespread degeneration of embryonic germinal cells within the primitive gonad (see Roberts, 1986). Mild cases may exhibit moderate oligospermia or poor sperm morphology, but severe cases may be aspermic. A hereditary form of hypoplasia exists in Swedish Highland cattle (Lagerlof, 1936, 1951; Eriksson, 1950), affecting the left testis more commonly than the right. Formerly, in the UK, many cases were detected when bulls were licensed at 10 months of age; however, the abandoning of such licensing means that the frequency of animals with relative hypoplasia is likely to increase. A high incidence of hypoplasia occurs in the Welsh Mountain pony (Arthur et al., 1989), in which the right testis is most commonly affected, and in which an inherited aetiology is probable. Sporadic cases of hypoplasia occur in all species, occasionally, but not often, with a clear familial predisposition (e.g. Holst, 1949; Gunn et al., 1942; Soderberg, 1986; Siliart et al., 1993). The condition (Figure 30.37) is

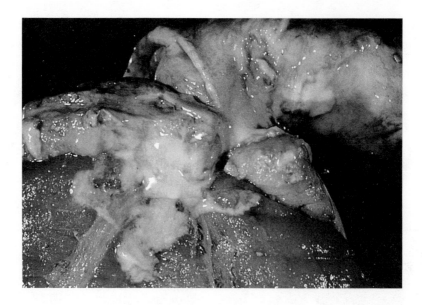

Fig. 30.35 Abscess-like sperm granuloma formation in the epididymal head of a Devon bull after rupture of the epididymal duct. (Reproduced from Parkinson et al. (1993), with permission.)

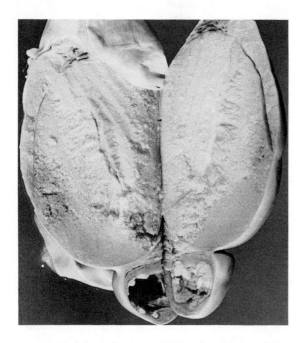

Fig. 30.36 Multiple sperm granuloma formation in the epididymal tail of a vasectomized ram.

relatively common in rams (see Bruere, 1986).

Klinefelter's syndrome (karyotype XXY) is a sporadic cause of testicular hypoplasia in bulls (Logue et al., 1979), and has been reported in rams, boars and dogs (Breeuwsma, 1968; Bruere et al., 1969; Clough et al., 1970). It is also par-

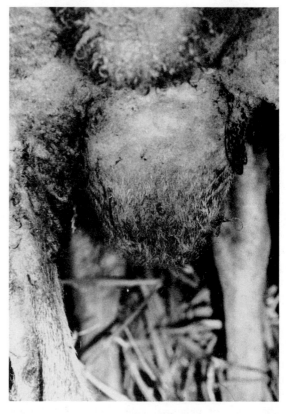

Fig. 30.37 Testicular hypoplasia in a ram. The scrotal circumference of 22 cm was well below the 30–35 cm expected for a ram during the breeding season.

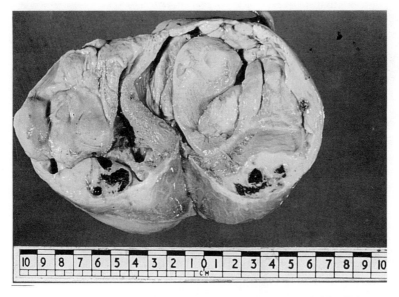

Fig. 30.38 Testicular teratoma in the undescended testis of a shire colt.

ticularly associated with male tortoiseshell and calico cats (Smith and Jones, 1966; Centerwall and Benirschke, 1975; Long et al., 1981). The spermatogonia of such animals fail to develop, so the seminiferous tubules are virtually devoid of spermatogenic cells. The semen of such animals is therefore aspermic although, the Leydig cells being unaffected, libido is normal.

Diagnosis of the condition is by measurement of scrotal circumference, which is below acceptable limits for the species and breed. Palpation of the testes reveals one or both to be small and flabby, but regular in outline and freely movable in the scrotum. Semen analysis may reveal aspermic or oligospermic ejaculates, sometimes with markedly abnormal morphology or motility characteristics of such sperm as are present. By contrast, libido is generally normal and, for this reason, the condition may escape the owner's attention until the failure to achieve satisfactory pregnancy rates is noticed.

Because of the probable inherited basis of testicular hypoplasia, attempting to breed from an affected animal should be avoided. Attempts at treatment with exogenous hormones are invariably unsuccessful, so castration and (for meat animals) slaughter for recovery of the carcass value should be recommended.

Testicular Neoplasia Testicular neoplasia (reviewed by Humphrey and Ladds, 1974; Roberts, 1986; McEntee, 1990; Schumacher and Varner, 1993) is rare in the bull, ram and boar and, although common in dogs, rarely presents as a cause of infertility. Interstitial cell tumours are the most common tumour of the dog, and are recorded occasionally as incidental findings in aged bulls. They are very rare in stallions. Seminomata, the next most common canine testicular tumour, are also occasionally found in bulls (and stallions) while Sertoli cell tumours rarely occur in species other than the dog. In cryptorchid stallions, a further testicular tumour is found relatively commonly: the teratoma, a benign growth that contains many different tissue types, including hair, bone, teeth and cartilage (Figure 30.38). Overall, testicular tumours account for over 10% of tumours in male dogs, with a considerably increased incidence in animals with cryptorchid testes.

Interstitial cell tumours usually occur in scrotal testes of aged dogs, but are usually too small to be palpated. They may result in increased circulating concentrations of androgen and, thereby, predispose to androgen-related disease, such as prostatic hyperplasia and circumanal gland adenoma. In bulls, interstitial cell tumours may cause irregular texture of the testis and, sometimes, enlargement. They cause no clinical signs in bulls and no impairment to fertility.

The incidence of seminomata in cryptorchid dogs is about 20 times that of dogs with scrotal

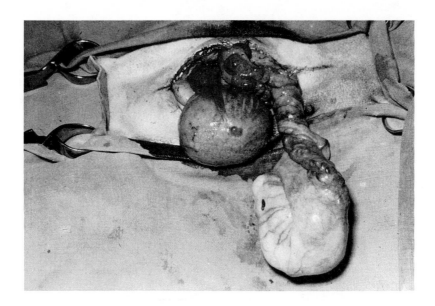

Fig. 30.39 Torsion of the spermatic cord of an undescended testis.

testes. Seminomas may become large but are generally innocuous in scrotal testes. They often grow slowly for long periods, but may undergo a sudden increase in the rate of growth, for no apparent reason. The tumours may become necrotic or haemorrhagic, whereupon affected dogs may exhibit lameness, pain, crouching or hunching. Occasionally they metastasize to local lymph nodes.

Sertoli cell tumours are usually characterized by feminization, in response to the tumour's oestrogen-secreting properties. Feminization is typified by gynaecomastia, symmetrical alopecia, penile atrophy, a pendulous prepuce and attraction to male dogs, and occurs more often and to a greater extent if the neoplastic testis is inguinal or intraabdominal than scrotal. If the tumour is unilateral, the contralateral testis is generally markedly atrophied. The oestrogenic secretion of the Sertoli cell tumour causes squamous metaplasia of the prostate gland, which may be of sufficient magnitude to cause obstructive uropathy. Metastases are uncommon but, when they occur, retain the oestrogen-secreting properties of the parent tumour.

Teratomata (Figure 30.38) occur most frequently in the stallion and very occasionally in other species. The tumour is most commonly found in cryptorchid testes, particularly of draught horses. They are either solid or cystic

and may have many tissue types identifiable within their substance. Hair, bone, teeth, fat, cartilage and nerve tissue appear most frequently. The tumours can become very large, so that their removal may be quite difficult to achieve. However, they rarely metastasize.

In addition to their hormonal and malignant effects, tumours of undescended testes predispose the spermatic cord to undergo torsion, which results in gradual testicular infarction. In exceptional cases, both spermatic cords may be tightly twisted through several rotations (Figure 30.39). Torsion of normal scrotal testes occurs occasionally (Young, 1979), but the condition is most frequently associated with neoplastic changes in undescended gonads (Pearson and Kelly, 1975). The susceptibility of such testes to tumour formation is therefore a strong justification for their removal.

Aplasia of the Mesonephric Ducts. Segmental aplasia of the mesonephric ducts (Blom and Christensen, 1951) is most commonly manifested as an absence of parts of the epididymis (Figure 30.40). In the bull, the condition is probably inherited (Konig et al., 1972). Absence of the head or tail of epididymis can be determined relatively easily by careful palpation of the scrotum, but the medially sited epididymal body is rarely palpable. Only in thin-skinned bulls and rams can it occasionally be felt; even then the scrotum must have little fat

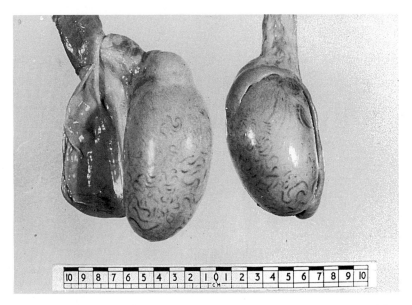

Fig. 30.40 Aplasia of the mesonephric ducts in the bull. Absence of the entire epididymis.

within it. Epididymal aplasia also occurs sporadically in other species (see McEntee, 1990). Oligospermia occurs if one epididymis is aplastic; aspermia if both are affected. Parts of the epididymis distal to the site of obstruction are often enlarged and tense, but the testis undergoes degenerative atrophy. Stasis of secretory material within the epididymis and the possibility of sperm leakage into the surrounding tissue predisposes to secondary pyogenic infection.

Aplasia of the vas deferens is less common. In bulls (Blom and Christensen, 1951), the condition may, sometimes, be diagnosed by rectal palpation, when strictures, or dilations distal to the site of stricture, may be discerned. As with epididymal aplasia, unilateral aplasia usually does not affect fertility, whereas sterility is the consequence of bilateral lesions.

Lesions of the accessory glands

Vesicular Glands. Infection of the vesicular glands (seminal vesicles) is relatively common in bulls. Incidences range between 0.2 (Blom, 1979) and 9% (Bagshaw and Ladds, 1974), depending upon the country and class of bull in which the survey has been undertaken. Bacteriological examination of infected glands usually reveals the presence of *A. pyogenes*, although a wide variety of organisms, including *Corynebacterium renale*, *Actinobacillus actinoides*, *Escherichia coli*, *Pseudomonas aeruginosa*, streptococci and staphylococci can be recovered. It is, however, unlikely that these are the causative organisms, for these are more commonly regarded as secondary infections of a previously damaged organ. Primary causative organisms may include *B. abortus*, *Chlamydia* spp., and the Epivag, ECBO and IBR–IPV viruses. Seminal vesiculitis occurs most commonly in young bulls of less than 2 years old and in aged bulls. Curiously, it is not a common disease of younger mature animals. Infection of the vesicular glands also occurs in the stallion (Varner et al., 1993), from whch a similarly mixed series of organisms have been isolated (*B. abortus*, *Klebsiella pneumoniae*, *P. aeruginosa*, streptococci and staphylococci). The disease is rare in rams.

In bulls, during the acute phase of the disease, localized peritonitis may occur in the caudal abdomen, producing the signs associated with that syndrome. One sign of localized peritonitis that itself affects reproductive performance is the unwillingness of affected animals to undertake movements that cause stretching of the area of inflammation. Foremost amongst such actions are mounting and, more particularly, the ejaculatory thrust. Hence, in the early stages of vesiculitis, animals may present with these signs. Later, animals generally present as infertile despite normal service behaviour. Occasionally, abscesses form in infected glands, which can burst, causing

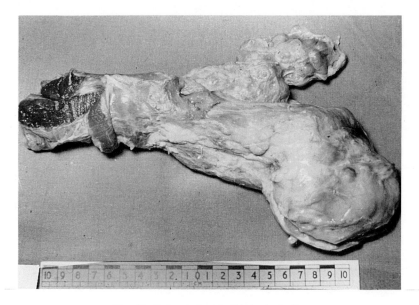

Fig. 30.41 Seminal vesiculitis in the bull.

generalized peritonitis, or fistulate, generally into the rectum. Infection is more commonly unilateral, but may be bilateral.

The main consequence of infection of the vesicular gland is a decline in semen quality, which exhibits a decrease in motility, accompanied by elevated pH, low fructose concentrations and the presence of polymorphonuclear leucocytes. In moderate or severe cases, the semen may appear overtly purulent and may be tinged brownish, due to the presence of degenerating blood from the damaged gland. In most cases these changes in semen quality lead to a decrease in fertility, although cases have been reported in which affected bulls have produced normal conception rates. Diagnosis of the condition can be confirmed by rectal palpation of the vesicular glands (Figure 30.41), which are characteristically enlarged, tense and painful during the acute phase, or lobular and fibrous, and sometimes shrunken, in the chronic phase.

Treatment is sometimes possible if the disease is noticed in its earliest stage, by the administration of very large doses of intravenous bacteriocidal antibiotics (Roberts, 1986; Arthur et al., 1989; Varner et al., 1993). However, in many cases antibiotic treatment is ineffective and, in such animals, amputation of a unilaterally infected gland is the only means of restoration of fertility (McEntee, 1962; King and McPherson, 1969). In bilaterally infected animals, the prognosis is hopeless. No treatment should be attempted in animals infected with *Brucella*, instead the bull should be slaughtered.

It would be natural to assume that a sire with an infection of the vesicular glands would transmit the infection venereally to females. Cases of such transmission have been reported in bulls infected with streptococci (e.g. Webster, 1932), associated with herd infertility, a yellowish–white postcoital discharge and pronounced cervicitis. However, other cases of streptococcal infection have had no associated signs in cows. Nevertheless, it would be prudent to advise that a bull with vesiculitis should not be used for service and a very cautious prognosis given in the first instance.

Prostate. Prostatic disease is rare in species other than the dog, in which prostatic infection and hyperplasia are common (see Barsanti and Finco, 1986). Tumours and senile atrophy of the canine prostate are also rare. The route of infection is generally ascending, with *B. canis*, *E. coli*, *Proteus* spp. and *Streptococcus* spp. commonly being recovered. Prostatitis and prostatic hyperplasia often occur together; the prostate undergoing a diffuse or local suppurative reaction, with a tendency to abscess formation. Polymorphonuclear lucocytes, bacteria and blood are often found in the urine of affected animals. During the acute phase of the diseases, affected animals may show systemic signs of infection, constipation and abdominal pain, especially on digital examination per rectum. Prostatic hyperplasia is a common age-related change, with the gland forming numerous small, or a few large, cysts. Constipation, but not pain or signs of systemic illness, characterize this condition. Neither condition is commonly characterized by changes in fertility. Prostatitis may be treatable with broad-spectrum antibiotics, whereas hyperplasia, being androgen-dependent, is best treated by the administration of oestrogens or by castration.

Abnormalities of semen

Semen examination

Semen can be collected by the methods described earlier in this chapter, and assessed so as to provide information about the fertilizing potential of the ejaculate. Classically, assessment of the numbers of sperm, their motility and morphology, and the presence of extraneous material in the ejaculate, has been used to give an approximate indication of the quality of the ejaculate. However, while such assessments are adequate to identify ejaculates of low fertilizing potential, correlations between the parameters of classic semen evaluation and conception rates of individual sires has been only mediocre. Hence, such assessments are a valuable part of the evaluation of potentially infertile sires but, if accurate predictions of fertility are required, more sophisticated examinations are needed.

Much care is needed in the handling of semen, if the results of its examination are to be meaningful. Spermatozoa are very sensitive to cooling, therefore the semen must be maintained at temperatures close to that of the body (above 30°C), prior to and during assessment, which should be undertaken as promptly as possible after collection. Futhermore, any microscope slides or material in which the semen is to be diluted must also be maintained at around 30°C. Semen is initially inspected for the presence of urine, fresh or changed blood, pus and extraneous material. The colour and consistency are noted, for watery samples are usually oligospermic, and samples that are not homogeneous often contain pus. Some normal bulls have semen which is bright yellow in colour, due to excretion of grass pigments in the seminal plasma.

Motility. Sperm motility is markedly influenced by temperature, so temperature control during this stage of semen examination is, clearly,

most critical. Ideally, this is achieved by using prewarmed slides on a heated microscope stage, but in the field, improvised methods are needed. The use of a small burner to warm the slides, or placing a small, flat-sided, clear glass bottle full of warm water on the microscope stage beneath the slide, have proved effective methods. Temperatures must be kept below 50°C, above which sperm rapidly die. For the bull and ram, a drop of semen is placed on the slide and examined under low power. At low magnification, individual sperm cannot be seen, but mass sperm movement can be observed in the form of recurrent swirling waves. It is important to differentiate between true movement and the apparent movement exhibited by dead sperm that are being moved passively by living sperm beneath them. For other species, it is essential, and for the bull and ram desirable, that a small drop of semen, either neat or diluted (in warm 0.9% saline or 2.9% sodium citrate solution) is placed on a slide, covered and observed at higher power for assessment of individual sperm motility. Progressive, forward motility, with a characteristic swing of the head and tail is the ideal, but other forms of motility are seen. Moderately damaged sperm may swim around in circles or backwards, while more severely damaged and dying sperm roll from side to side, alternately presenting the broad and narrow edges of their heads.

Sperm Count. Ranges of sperm density and ejaculate volume are given in Table 30.3. For field use, sperm density can most readily be estimated using a haemocytometer. Ram and bull semen should be diluted 1:100 in 0.9 saline/0.02% formalin solution; other species, whose semen is less dense, may require lower dilution factors. The total sperm count is then derived as the product of volume and density. Where a large number of semen samples require evaluation, such as occurs in AI studs, estimation of sperm density can be facilitated by the use of spectrophotometry, in which the optical density of the sample is compared with a calibration curve (Salisbury et al., 1943). Alternatively electronic particle counters can be used, although the small size and flattened shape of the sperm head make it a relatively difficult cell to count.

Live:Dead Ratio and Sperm Morphology. A further estimate of the proportion of dead sperm in an ejaculate can be obtained by the use of a vital

Table 30.3 Semen characteristics of domestic animals

Characteristic	Species				
	Bull	*Ram*	*Stallion*	*Boar*	*Dog*
Volume (ml)	4 (2–10)	1.0 (0.5–2.0)	60 (30–250)	250 (125–500)	10 (2–19)
Fractionated	N	N	Y	Y	Y
Density ($\times 10^6$/ml)	1250 (600–2800)	2000 (1250–3000)	120 (30–600)	100 (25–1000)	125 (20–540)
Motility (motile sperm, %)	>70	>90	>60	>60	>85
Normal spermatozoa (%)	>75	>85	>60	>60	>90

Figures in parentheses indicate the normal range. Compiled from Arthur et al. (1989), Roberts (1986) and Morrow (1986).

stain, such as eosin B (Lasley et al., 1942). This stain is most commonly used as part of a combined stain, eosin–nigrosin, which is used to evaluate both the proportion of dead sperm and sperm morphology (Swanson and Bearden, 1951). For vital staining to be effective, great care has to be taken of temperature control and conditions must be standardized. Semen which has been frozen is difficult to assess with eosin, as cryoprotectants, such as glycerol (Mixner and Saroff, 1954), enhance penetration of the vital stain into the cells, thereby giving artificially high percentages of dead cells. Also, until considerable experience has been obtained, repeatability of live:dead ratio counts is low.

Assessment of sperm morphology is, by contrast, a useful and important aspect of semen examination. Nigrosin, a simple background stain, is adequate for most purposes, but specialist sperm stains, such as aniline blue plus eosin B (Casarett, 1953) are also widely used. Defects of the acrosome are often difficult to see in stained preparations, although specialized stains such as that of Wells and Awa (1970) are used to visualize acrosomal vacuoles. More commonly, phase contrast or differential interference contrast microscopy of wet preparations are used to examine acrosomal defects (Aalseth and Saacke, 1985).

Sperm Function Tests. Semen analysis provides enough information to recognize sires of very low fertility, but has been increasingly considered to be a poor discriminator between moderate and high fertility levels (see Watson, 1990). In order to attempt to improve the accuracy of semen assessments, a number of tests of sperm function have been employed, with varying success. The simplest of such tests incubate semen at various temperatures (typically 4 or 40°C) and, by relating the duration of sperm survival under these conditions to survival in female genital tract, produce reasonable correlations with fertility (see Roberts, 1956). Other tests utilize additional measurements upon the semen, such as pH, ATP content or asparate transaminase concentration (see Salisbury et al., 1978). These have been moderately successful, but have not been of sufficiently greater value than conventional semen assessment to justify their use. In medical practice, much value is placed upon the ability of sperm to penetrate cervical mucus and the behaviour of the sperm at the interface between semen and the mucus (Linford, 1974; Blasco, 1984). Failure of mucous penetration is frequently a sign of failure of sperm function and occurs in sperm that have been damaged by cryopreservation and in the presence of anti-sperm antibodies.

Of more widespread use in veterinary practice is computer-assisted analysis of sperm swimming characteristics. In medical practice, such analyses are regarded as a useful prognostic tool in assessment of fertility because high correlations have been demonstrated between such measurements and fertility. The most important swimming characteristics are rate of forward progress, lateral movement of the sperm head and characteristics of the flagellar beat. Although the use of sperm motility analysis in veterinary practice at present is largely confined to Thoroughbred stallions (Amann, 1988) and AI stud bulls (Budworth et al., 1988) it is probable that the use of such systems will rapidly increase as cost of analysis programs decreases.

Assessments of sperm viability have also been improved in recent years. Fluorescent markers which stain live, but not dead, sperm have been used, and high correlations with fertility demon-

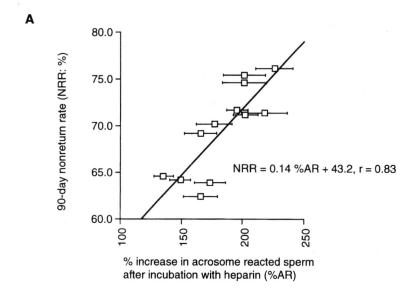

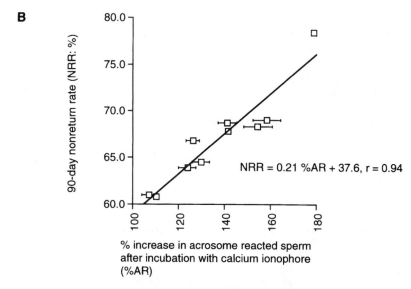

Fig. 30.42 Relationship between acrosome reactions induced in bovine semen in vitro by (A) heparin and (B) A23187 and fertility, as expressed by the proportion of cows not represented for service 90 days after AI (90 day NRR).

strated (Garner et al., 1986). Assessment of the proportion of sperm with intact acrosomes has been highly correlated with fertility (Saacke, 1972). The most recent innovation in assessment of sperm function has derived from the development of *in vitro* fertilization (IVF) procedures, in which sperm from different sires were observed to have widely differing fertilization success rates. Subsequently, the ability of sperm to undergo acrosome reaction *in vitro* was identified as a critical stage in the IVF procedure and, in the

bull, tests of sperm function based upon *in vitro* induction of acrosome reactions have been found to have very high correlation with fertility in the field (Ax and Lenz, 1987; Whitfield and Parkinson, 1994; Whitfield and Parkinson, unpublished data; Figure 30.42).

Abnormalities of spermatozoa

Three main classifications of sperm morphology have been proposed. Firstly, defects can be classified according to their site on the sperm. By this

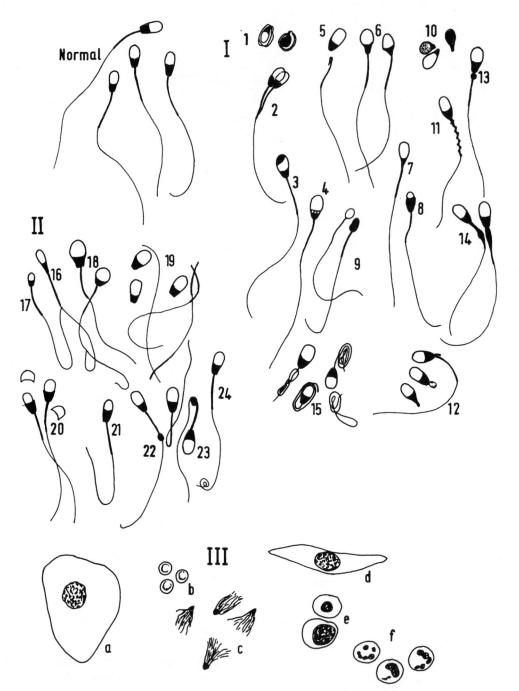

Fig. 30.43 Classification of spermatozoal abnormalities into major and minor defects according to their effect upon fertility. Major defects (I) include: 1, underdeveloped cells; 2, double forms; 3, acrosome ('knobbed sperm') defect; 4, diadem defect; 5, decapitated sperm defect (the tails appear active); 6, pear-shaped heads; 7, heads which are narrow at the base; 8, heads with an abnormal contour; 9, small abnormal heads; 10, free (detached) abnormal heads; 11, the 'corkscrew defect' of the midpiece; 12, other midpiece defects; including the 'tail-stump' defect and accessory tails; 13, proximal cytoplasmic droplet; 14, pseudodroplet and other thickened midpieces; 15, coiled or strongly folded tails (including 'Dag defect').

Minor defects (II) include: 16, narrow heads; 17, small, normal heads; 18, giant and short, broad heads; 19, detached normal heads; 20, detached acrosomal membranes; 21, abaxial implantation of the tail; 22, distal droplet; 23, simple bent tail; 24, terminally coiled tail.

Other cellular elements which may also be present (III) include: a, epithelial cells; b, erythrocytes; c, medusa formations; d, boat cells; e, mononuclear cells; f, neutrophils. (Redrawn and adapted from Blom (1983), with permission.)

classification, sperm are classified into head, mid-piece and tail defects and sperm bearing protoplasmic droplets. A rather more useful classification is that based upon the site within the genital tract where the sperm defect has arisen (Blom, 1950). By this classification, defects are divided into primary abnormalities, which arise during spermatogenesis, secondary defects, which arise within the epididymis, and tertiary defects, which arise after ejaculation, for example, from inadequate temperature, pH or osmotic control during handling of the semen. Thus, defects of the head and midpiece are mostly primary, protoplasmic droplets secondary and looped tails tertiary. The final classification (Blom, 1983; Figure 30.43) categorizes defects, according to empirical observations upon their effects on fertility in the bull, into major and minor abnormalities. Major abnormalities include most defects of the head, proximal protoplasmic droplets and congenital acrosomal defects, while most other defects, including, somewhat surprisingly, detached heads, are classified as minor abnormalities.

Using the principles of the effect of specific abnormalities upon fertility, criteria have been established for maximal percentages of each class of sperm abnormality in an ejaculate. In the UK, a maximum of 20% total sperm abnormalities, with not more than 5% of any individual class, is allowed in bovine semen for use in AI. In bull studs in the USA, a maximum of 10% major abnormalities or 20% minor abnormalities is allowed. However, in bulls destined for use in natural service, different criteria would be applied, which may need to take into account the frequency of use of the sire and the use to which its progeny (i.e. slaughter or breeding) are to be put. In other species, the criteria for acceptance of semen are also different. For example, equine, porcine and canine semen can exhibit quite high percentages of abnormal sperm without materially affecting fertility, whereas in the ram only a very low percentage of abnormalities is acceptable.

Abnormalities of the Sperm Head. Two aspects of the morphology of the sperm head appear to be essential for normal fertility. Firstly, the shape of the sperm head is critical, as small changes in the overall size, acrosomal area and width at the base of the head markedly reduce the ability of sperm to fertilize (reviewed by Barth

and Oko, 1989). Secondly, the morphology and stability of the acrosome are also important. Therefore, most abnormalities of the sperm head are major defects, i.e. having relatively serious effects upon fertility (Blom, 1950, 1980; Wilmington, 1981). The majority of such defects arise within the testis as abnormalities of spermatogenesis (primary abnormalities). Such defects include heads which are narrow at the base, pear shaped, small and mis-shaped, and grossly abnormal and bizarre (Figure 30.44). Less serious defects of the head include giant heads (which have a diploid chromosome complement), double heads, narrow heads and small, normally shaped heads. The diadem defect (figure 30.44(c)) represents pouches in the nuclear material. This defect is common at low percentages, may be present at high percentages for short periods of time after testicular damage, or may be continuously present as an inherited defect (see Barth and Oko, 1989).

Acrosomal defects are also of serious consequence for fertility. Many acrosomal defects arise as primary abnormalities of spermatogenesis, although acrosomal damage may also arise during epididymal transit and storage, or even after ejaculation. Many of the acrosomal defects that arise during spermatogenesis are present at high percentage in the ejaculate, in which case they are usually inherited, but identical abnormalities can be found at low percentages in most ejaculates, indicating that they can also arise spontaneously. Furthermore, the significance of these defects depends upon the species. For example, the fertility of bulls is impaired by single-figure percentages of the knobbed acrosome defect, but percentages have to be much higher before the fertility of stallions or boars is affected. However, in general, all defects of the acrosome should be regarded as serious, and careful consideration given to the likelihood to the inheritance of the condition before use of the sire is sanctioned. Defects of the acrosome can be difficult to see in stained preparations, so the use of phase contrast or differential interference microscopy upon wet smears is often needed. Some acrosomal defects can be seen if smears are stained with nigrosin alone, while others can be readily observed when the stain of Wells and Awa (1970) is used. Acrosomal defects with a suspected or known heritable basis include the knobbed sperm defect and the presence of vacuoles in the acrosome, whereas simple ridges

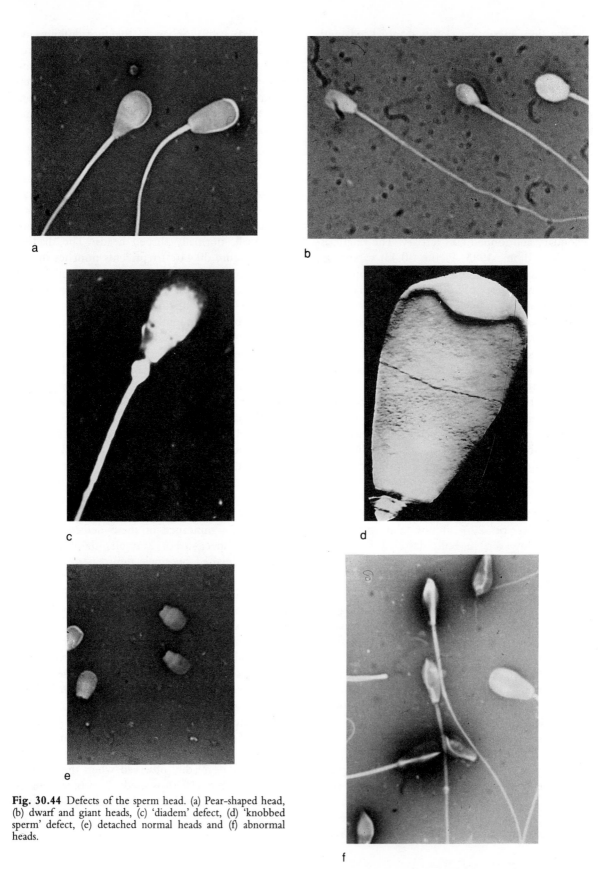

Fig. 30.44 Defects of the sperm head. (a) Pear-shaped head, (b) dwarf and giant heads, (c) 'diadem' defect, (d) 'knobbed sperm' defect, (e) detached normal heads and (f) abnormal heads.

on the acrosome may be inherited or acquired. Acrosomal morphology may deteriorate preceding the appearance of major head abnormalities in cases of testicular degeneration, orchitis or epididymitis, so repeated evaluations of the semen may need to be undertaken.

Detached acrosomes may be observed in wet or nigrosin-stained smears, although observation under phase contrast or differential interference contrast microscopy offers the best means of evaluating the acrosome. The site of origin of such defects is not always clear, for this abnormality may arise at any time between spermatogenesis and insemination. In particular, it may be seen in frozen–thawed semen of animals whose sperm do not survive cryopreservation well. At low percentages, detachment of the acrosome has been regarded as a minor defect, with fertility only being impaired with higher levels of the abnormality. However, recent data from the bull indicate that the percentage of detached acrosomes may be related in a linear fashion with fertility and, therefore, the significance of this abnormality is being reassessed.

Abnormalities of the Midpiece and the Tail and of Attachment of the Head. Abnormalities of attachment of the sperm head are, generally, primary defects of spermatogenesis. Some are inherited defects of the centriole or axoneme, occurring at high percentages, while others are sporadic or occur as acquired defects. Surprisingly, many such defects have minor effects upon fertility, unless present at high percentages. Detached heads are generally an acquired defect, occurring particularly during testicular degeneration. The separated tails are usually immotile. However, an inherited condition of Guernsey and Hereford bulls (Blom and Birch-Anderson, 1970; Blom, 1977) occurs, in which most sperm are decapitated and the detached tails are motile. The semen of such bulls exhibits apparently normal wave motion. Detached heads may be present in the semen of animals which have not ejaculated for a considerable period of time, as a senescent change in the sperm. It is also relatively common in the semen of aged bulls. Sperm with fractures of the attachment between head and tail ('fractured neck') may arise from senescent changes, or due to congenital weakness of the attachment.

Abaxial implantation of the tail is generally of minor significance (Bishop and Hancock, 1955)

and some degree of abaxial implantation may be regarded as normal in the stallion. Some bulls with abaxially implanted tails exhibit a curious, additional, vestigial tail (Figure 30.45(d)) beside the main flagellum, which causes a serious impairment of fertility if the abnormality is present in a high percentage (e.g. Williams and Savage, 1925). Most other defects of development of the midpiece and tail are of serious consequences for fertility: deformity of the tail precluding motility. The coiled tail defect (Figure 30.45(a)) is a primary abnormality that is commonly found during testicular degeneration. The somewhat similar 'Dag' defect (Blom, 1966) is usually of inherited origin, especially in Jersey bulls, in which it is relatively common. It has also been seen sporadically in most other domestic animals, either as a permanent defect—in which case it is probably inherited—or transiently, as a response of the testis to some insult. The apparently loose coils of the sperm tail in the Dag defect represent a serious perturbation of the genesis of the flagellum (Figure 30.45(b)), resulting in immotile sperm. This condition is common in Jersey bulls, in whch it is inherited. The 'tail-stump' defect occurs as an inherited condition of several breeds of bull (see Blom and Birch-Anderson, 1980), in which morphologically normal heads are attached to a vestigial structure which appears like a protoplasmic droplet (Figure 30.45(f)). On electron microscopy, this droplet-like structure can be seen to consist of small segments of flagellar material and represents a vestigial tail. Affected bulls are sterile.

Other, less spectacular, but nevertheless serious, defects of the midpiece occur. These include the corkscrew defect, so-called because the loose arrangement of the helix of mitochondria gives the appearance of a corkscrew to the midpiece of the sperm, which may be inherited when present at high percentages, and various thickenings of the midpiece which arise from other malformations of the mitochondrial helix.

Tail defects are, by contrast, generally minor defects. These include looped tails and terminally coiled tails. Care should be exercised in the interpretation of the presence of looped tails, for looping of the tail is a common response of sperm to noxious stimuli. Thus, while looped tails can arise as defects of spermatogenesis or epididymal function, they more commonly occur in response to poor temperature control of the semen, or in

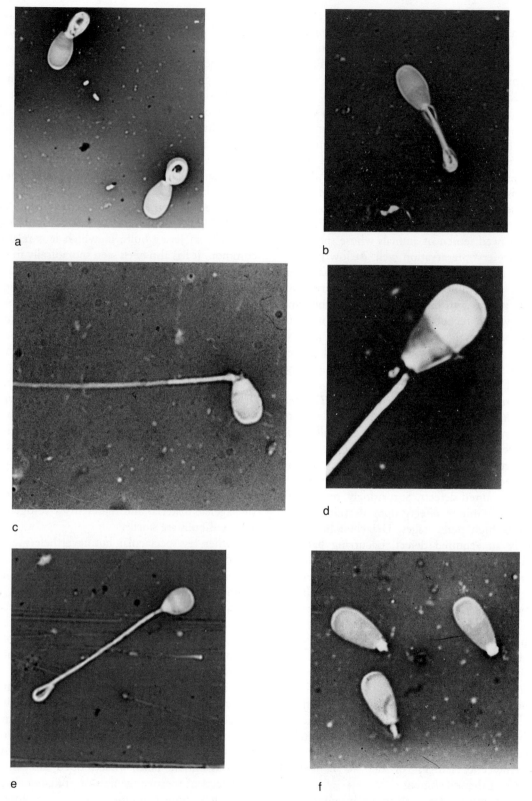

a

b

c

d

e

f

Fig. 30.45 Defects of the sperm midpiece and tail (1). (a) 'Coiled-tail' — a defect of formation of the midpiece — (b) 'Dag' defect, (c) fractured neck, (d) accessory tail, (e) terminally coiled tail and (f) the tail-stump defect.

response to hypotonic stress such as may occur if the semen becomes contaminated by water. Departure of seminal pH from its normal range can also cause looped tails and, as such, may be an early indicator of the increase in pH that occurs during infection of the accessory glands.

Protoplasmic Droplets. The residual cytoplasm that remains at the end of spermiation is removed during the passage of sperm through the epididymis, as a maturational change. The presence of sperm with protoplasmic droplets (Figure 30.46(a) and (b)) therefore indicates that epididymal maturation is incomplete by the time of ejaculation. Sperm with droplets close to the head (proximal droplets) are more immature than those with droplets at the distal end of the midpiece (distal droplets), although it has recently been argued that proximal droplets also arise as defects of spermiation (i.e. as a primary abnormality).

Protoplasmic droplets are often observed in

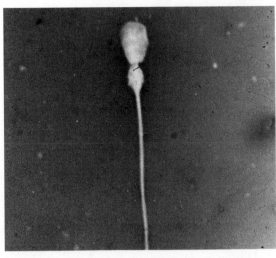

a

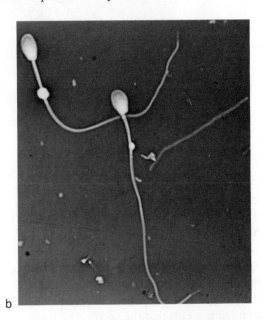

b

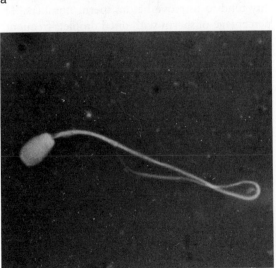

c

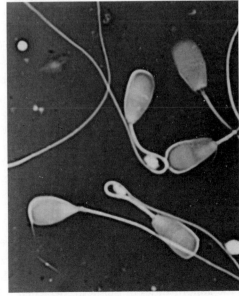

d

Fig. 30.46 Defects of the sperm midpiece and tail (2). (a) Proximal cytoplasmic droplet, (b) distal cytoplasmic droplet, (c) looped tail and (d) looped tail with a cytoplasmic remnant enclosed in the loop.

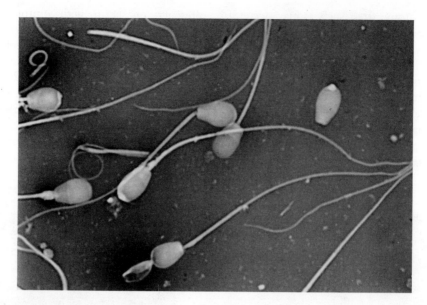

Fig. 30.47 Sperm morphology from a bull with severe testicular degeneration. Many abnormal cells are present, including sperm with abnormal heads, detached heads and various defects of the midpiece, and sperm with proximal droplets. The ejaculate was also characterized by oligospermia and low sperm motility.

young sires that are being overused. In such animals, daily sperm production rates are lower than in fully mature animals and, in addition, the epididymis has not fully developed to its final length. Hence, if a young sire is overused, not only does the number of sperm in the ejaculate decline, but also the withdrawal of sperm from the tail of the epididymis means that the sperm which are ejaculated are often functionally immature. The fertility of such animals therefore can decline spectacularly. Where young sires are heavily used, such as in AI programmes, careful monitoring of the percentages of sperm with protoplasmic droplets is therefore advisable.

Semen Changes During Testicular Degeneration. The initial changes in semen quality during testicular degeneration are a decrease in motility and an increase in the percentage of abnormal sperm (see Figure 30.31), particularly sperm with proximal droplets. If the semen is being cryopreserved, a precipitous decline in post-thaw motility may occur at this stage. Subsequently, sperm numbers generally start to decline, although ejaculate volume is usually unaffected. As sperm numbers decrease, the proportion of abnormal sperm increase, with high percentages of primary defects occurring (Figure 30.47). These include abnormalities of the head, detached heads

and coiled tails. Bizarre abnormalities occur, including small, abnormal heads, acrosomal defects and the presence of premeiotic cells and stellate forms in the ejaculate. Sperm numbers may decline to the extent that the ejaculate becomes virtually aspermic.

During recovery, sperm morphology and motility tend to improve before sperm numbers. The percentage of sperm with distal droplets frequently increases during the recovery phase. Recovery may occur almost immediately after the nadir of semen quality, but may be protracted. The extent and severity of semen changes cannot be correlated with either the duration of illness or the likelihood of recovery.

REFERENCES

Aalseth, E. P. and Saacke, R. G. (1985) *J. Reprod. Fertil.*, **74**, 473.

Allen, W. E. (1992) *Fertility and Obstetrics in the Dog.* Oxford: Blackwell Scientific.

Almquist, J. O. and Thomson, R. G. (1977) *J. Amer. Vet. Med. Assn*, **163**, 163.

Amann, R. P. (1988) *Proc. Am. Assoc. Eq. Pract.*, 453.

Arthur, G. H. (1961) *Vet. Rec.*, **73**, 385.

Arthur, G. H., Noakes, D. E. and Pearson, H. (1989) *Veterinary Reproduction and Obstetrics*, 6th edn. London: Baillière Tindall.

Ashdown, R. R. (1962) *Vet. Rec.*, **74**, 1464.

Ashdown, R. R. and Coombs, M. A. (1967) *Vet. Rec.*, **80**, 737.

Ashdown, R. R. and Coombs, M. A. (1968) *Vet. Rec.*, **81**, 126.

Ashdown, R. R. and Majeed, Z. Z. (1978) *Vet. Rec.*, **103**, 12.

Ashdown, R. R. and Pearson, H. (1971) *Res. Vet. Sci.*, **12**, 183.

Ashdown, R. R. and Pearson, H. (1973a) *Vet. Rec.*, **93**, 30.

Ashdown, R. R. and Pearson, H. (1973b) *Res. Vet. Sci.*, **15**, 13.

Ashdown, R. R. and Pearson, H. (1981) Unpublished observations.

Ashdown, R. R., Ricketts, S. W. and Wardley, R. C. (1968) *J. Anat.*, **103**, 567.

Ashdown, R. R., David, J. S. E. and Gibbs, C. (1979a) *Vet. Rec.*, **104**, 423.

Ashdown, R. R., David, J. S. E. and Gibbs, C. (1979b) *Vet. Rec.*, **104**, 589.

Ax, R. L. and Lenz, R. W. (1987) *J. Dairy Sci.*, **70**, 1477.

Bagshaw, P. A. and Ladds, P. W. (1974) *Vet. Bull.*, **44**, 343.

Bane, A. and Hansen, H. J. (1962) *Cornell Vet.*, **52**, 362.

Barsanti, J. A. and Finco, D. R. (1986) In: *Current Therapy in Theriogenology*, 2nd edn, ed. D. A. Morrow, pp. 553–560. Philadelphia: Saunders.

Barr, F. J. (1990) *Diagnostic Ultrasound in the Dog and Cat.* Oxford: Blackwell Scientific.

Barth, A. D. and Oko, R. J. (1989) *Abnormal Morphology of Bovine Spermatozoa.* Ames: Iowa State University.

Beckett, S. D., Reynolds, T. M., Walker, D. F., Hudson, R. S. and Purhoit, R. C. (1974) *Amer. J. Vet. Res.*, **35**, 761.

Beckett, S. D., Purhoit, R. C. and Reynolds, T. M. (1975) *Biol. Reprod.*, **12**, 289.

Beckett, S. D., Hudson, R. S., Walker, D. F. and Purhoit, R. C. (1978) *J. Amer. Vet. Med. Assn*, **173**, 838.

Bellenger, C. R. (1971) *Res. Vet. Sci.*, **12**, 299.

Bishop, M. H. W. (1970) *J. Reprod. Fertil. Suppl.*, **15**, 65.

Bishop, M. H. W., David, J. S. E. and Messervey, A. (1966) *Proc. R. Soc. Med.*, **59**, 769.

Bishop, M. H. W. (1955) *Vet. Rec.* **67**, 363.

Blasco, L. (1984) *Fert. Steril.*, **41**, 177.

Blockey, M. A. de B. and Taylor, E. G. (1984) *Aust. Vet. J.*, **61**, 141.

Blom, E. (1950) *Fert. Steril.*, **1**, 223.

Blom, E. (1966) *Nature*, **209**, 739.

Blom, E. (1977) *Nord. VetMed.*, **29**, 119.

Blom, E. (1979) *Nord. VetMed.*, **31**, 241.

Blom, E. (1983) *Nord. VetMed.*, **35**, 105.

Blom, E. and Birch-Anderson, A. (1970) *J. Reprod. Fertil.*, **23**, 67.

Blom, E. and Birch-Anderson, A. (1980) *Acta Path. Microbiol. Scand., Sec. A*, **88**, 397.

Blom, E. and Christensen, N. O. (1947) *Skand. Vet. Tidskr.*, **37**, 1.

Blom, E. and Christensen, N. O. (1951) *K. Vet. Hojsk, Arsskr.*, 1.

Bloom, F., Paff, G. H. and Noback, C. R. (1951) *Amer. J. Pathol.*, **27**, 119.

Bowen, J. M. (1987) In: *Current Therapy in Equine Medicine*, 2nd edn, ed. N. E. Robinson, pp. 567–570. Philadelphia: Saunders.

Boyd, C. L. and Henskelka, D. V. (1972) *J. Amer. Vet. Med. Assn*, **161**, 275.

Breeuwsma, A. J. (1968) *J. Reprod. Fertil.*, **16**, 119.

Bruere, A. N. (1969) *N. Z. Vet. J.*, **18**, 189.

Bruere, A. N., Marshall, R. B. and Ward, D. J. P. (1969) *J. Reprod. Fertil.*, **19**, 103–108.

Bruere, A. N. (1986) In: *Current Therapy in Theriogenology*, 2nd edn, ed. D. A. Morrow, pp. 874–880. Philadelphia: Saunders.

Budworth, P. R., Amann, R. P. and Chapman, P. L. (1988) *J. Androl.*, **9**, 41.

Burke, T. J. (1986) *Small Animal Reproduction and Infertility.* Philadelphia: Lea and Febiger.

Carrol, E. J., Aanes, W. A. and Ball, L. (1964) *J. Amer. Vet. Med. Assn*, **144**, 747.

Casarett, G. W. (1953) *Stain Tech.*, **28**, 125.

Centerwall, W. R. and Benirschke, K. (1975) *Amer. J. Vet. Res.*, **36**, 1275.

Chaffee, V. W. and Knecht, C. D. (1975) *Vet. Med. Small Anim. Clin.*, **70**, 1418.

Chenowith, P. J. (1986) In: *Current Therapy in Theriogenology*, ed. D. A. Morrow, pp. 136–142. Philadelphia: Saunders.

Clarke, I. J. and Tilbrook, A. J. (1992) *Anim. Reprod. Sci.*, **28**, 219.

Clough, E., Pyle, R. L., Hare, W. C. D., Kelly, D. F. and Patterson, D. E. (1970) *Cytogenetics*, **9**, 71.

Coulter, G. H. (1980) *8th Tech. Conf. AI Reprod.*, p. 160 (Abstr.).

Couto, M. A. and Hughes, J. P. (1993) In: *Equine Reproduction*, ed. A. O. McKinnon and J. L. Voss, pp. 845–854. Philadelphia: Lea and Febiger.

Cox, J. E. (1975) *Equine Vet. J.*, **7**, 179.

Cox, J. E. (1982) *Surgery of the Reproductive Tract in Large Animals.* Liverpool: Liverpool University Press.

Cox, J. E., Williams, J. H., Rowe, P. H. and Smith, J. A. (1973) *Equine Vet. J.*, **5**, 85.

Cox, J. E., Edwards, G. B. and Neal, P. A. (1979) *Equine Vet. J.*, **11**, 113.

Crabo, B. G. (1986) In: *Current Therapy in Theriogenology*, 2nd edn, ed. D. A. Morrow, pp 975–978. Philadelphia: Saunders.

DeGroot, R. and Numans, S. R. (1946) *Tijdschr. Diergeneesk.*, **71**, 732.

Desmet, P., De Moor, A., Bouters, R. and Meurichy, W. (1974) *Vlaams Diergeneesk. Tijdschr.*, **43**, 357.

De Vries, P. J. (1993) In: *Equine Reproduction*, ed. A. O. McKinnon and J. L. Voss, pp. 878–884. Philadelphia: Lea and Febiger.

Elmore, R. G. (1981) *Vet. Med. Small Anim. Clin.*, **76**, 701.

Eriksson, K. (1950) *Nord. VetMed.*, **2**, 943.

Faulkner, L. C., Hopwood, M. L., Masken, J. F., Kingman, H. E. and Stoddard, H. L. (1967) *J. Amer. Vet. Med. Assn*, **151**, 602.

Garner, D. L., Pinkel, D., Johnson, L. A. and Pace, M. M. (1986) *Biol. Reprod.*, **34**, 127.

Gassner, F. X. and Hill, H. J. (1955) *Fert. Steril.*, **6**, 290.

Greenhough, P. R., MacCallum, F. J. and Weaver, A. D. (1972) *Lameness in Cattle*, 2nd edn. Edinburgh: Oliver and Boyd.

Gunn, R. M. C., Sanders, R. N. and Granger, W. (1942) *Bull. CISRO*, **148**.

Hattangady, S. R., Wadia, D. S. and George, P. O. (1968) *Vet. Rec.*, **82**, 666.

Hayes, H. M. (1986) *Equine Vet. J.*, **18**, 467.

Hobday, F. T. G. (1914) *Castration Including Cryptorchids and Caponing) and Ovariectomy.* Edinburgh: Johnson.

Holst, S. J. (1949) *Nord. VetMed.*, **1**, 87.

Hulet, C. V., El-Sheikh, A. S., Pope, A. L. and Casida, L. E. (1956) *J. Anim. Sci.*, **15**, 617.

Humphrey, J. D. and Ladds, P. W. (1974) *Vet. Bull.*, **45**, 787.

Huston, R., Saperstein, G., Schoneweis, D. and Leipold, H. W. (1978) *Vet. Bull.*, **48**, 645.

Jaskowski, L., Walkowski, L. and Korycki, S. (1961) *Proc. 4th Int. Congr. Reprod., The Hague*, **2**, 801.

Johnston, S. D. (1986) In: *Current Therapy in Theriogenology*, 2nd edn, ed. D. A. Morrow, pp. 549–551. Philadelphia: Saunders.

Jones, D. E. and Joshua, J. O. (1982) *Reproductive Clinical Problems in the Dog*. Bristol: Wright.

Joshua, J. O. (1962); *Vet. Rec.*, **74**, 1550.

Jubb, K. V. F. and Kennedy, P. C. (1970) *Pathology of the Domestic Animals*, 2nd edn, Vol. 1. New York: Academic Press.

Kenney, R. M. (1970) *Proc. VI Ann. Conf. Cattle Dis., Oklahoma*, p. 295.

King, G. J. and McPherson, J. W. (1969) *J. Dairy Sci.*, **52**, 1837.

Knudsen, O. (1954) *Acta Path. Microbiol. Scand. Suppl.*, **101**, 12.

Konig, H., Weber, W. and Kupferschmeid, H. (1972) *Schweizer Arch. Tierheilk.*, **114**, 73.

Krook, L., Lutwak, L. and McEntee, K. (1969) *Amer. J. Clin. Nutr.*, **22**, 115.

Lagerlof, N. (1936) *Vet. Rec.*, **48**, 1159.

Lagerlof, N. (1951) *Fert. Steril.*, **2**, 230.

Lagos, F. and Fitzhugh, H. A. (1970) *J. Anim. Sci.*, **30**, 949.

Larsen, L. H. and Bellenger, C. R. (1971) *Aust. Vet. J.*, **47**, 349.

Lasley, J. F., Easley, G. I. and McKenzie, F. F. (1942) *Anat. Rec.*, **82**, 167.

Levis, D. G. (1992) *Vet. Clin. N. Amer. Food Anim. Pract.*, **8**, 517.

Linford, E. (1974) *J. Reprod. Fertil.*, **37**, 239.

Logue, D. N., Harvey, M. J. A., Munro, C. D. and Lennox, B. (1979) *Vet. Rec.*, **104**, 500.

Long, S. E. (1969) *Vet. Rec.*, **84**, 495.

Long, S. E. and Hignett, P. G. (1970) *Vet. Rec.*, **86**, 165.

Long, S. E., Hignett, P. G. and Lee, R. (1970) *Vet. Rec.*, **86**, 192.

Long, S. E., Gruffydd-Jones, T. J. and David, M. (1981) *Res. Vet. Sci.*, **30**, 274.

Lucke, J. N. and Sansom, J. (1979) *Vet. Rec.*, **105**, 21.

McEntee, K. (1962) *Proc. 66th US Livestock Sanit. Assoc., Washington*, p. 160.

McEntee, K. (1990) *Reproductive Pathology of Domestic Animals*. San Diego: Academic Press.

Melrose and O'Hagen (1959) *Proc. 6th Int. Cong. Anim. Reprod., The Hague*, **4**, 855.

Metcalfe, F. L. (1965) *J. Amer. Vet. Med. Assn*, **147**, 1319.

Milne, F. J. (1954) *J. Amer. Vet. Med. Assn*, **124**, 6.

Mixner, J. P. and Saroff, J. (1954) *J. Dairy Sci.*, **37**, 1094.

Morrow, D. A. (1986) *Current Therapy: Theriogenology*, 2nd edn, p. 1084. Philadelphia: Saunders.

Noordsy, J. L., Trotter, D. M., Carnham, D. L. and VestWeber, J. G. (1970) *Proc. Ann. Conf. Cattle Dis., Oklahoma*, p. 333.

Ott, R. S., Heath, E. H. and Bane, A. (1982) *Amer. J. Vet. Res.*, **43**, 241.

Parkinson, T. J. (1991) *In Practice*, **13**, 3.

Parkinson, T. J., Brown, P. J. and Crea, P. R. (1993) *Vet. Rec.*, **132**, 509.

Patterson, D. F. (1977) In: *Current Veterinary Therapy*, ed. R. W. Kirk, Vol. 6, pp. 73–89. Philadelphia: Saunders.

Pattridge, P. D. (1953) *South-western Vet.*, **7**, 31.

Pearson, H. (1972) *Vet. Rec.*, **91**, 498.

Pearson, H. (1977) *Vet. Annu.*, **17**, 40.

Pearson, H. and Ashdown, R. R. (1976) *9th Int. Cong. Dis. Cattle, Paris*, **1**, 89.

Pearson, H. and Kelly, D. F. (1975) *Vet. Rec.*, **97**, 200.

Pearson, H. and Weaver, B. M. Q. (1978) *Equine Vet. J.*, **10**, 85.

Pendergass, T. W. and Hayes, H. M. (1975) *Teratology*, **12**, 51.

Plant, J. W., Claxton, D., Jakovljevic, D. and deSaram, W. (1976) *Aust. Vet. J.*, **52**, 17.

Plaut, A. and Kohn-Speyer, A. C. (1947) *Science*, **105**, 391.

Rhodes, A. P. (1976) *Aust. Vet. J.*, **52**, 250.

Roberts, S. J. (1956) *Veterinary Obstetrics and Genital Diseases*. Ithaca, New York: self-published.

Roberts, S. J. (1986) *Veterinary Obstetrics and Genital Diseases*, 3rd edn. Ithaca, New York: self-published.

Saacke, R. G. and White, J. M. (1972) *Proc. 4th Tech. Conf. AI, Reprod., Chicago*, 22.

Salisbury, G. W., Beck, G. H., Elliott, I. and Willett, E. L. (1943) *J. Dairy Sci.*, **26**, 69.

Salisbury, G. W., VanDemark, N. L. and Lodge, J. R. (1978) *Physiology of Reproduction and Artificial Insemination of Cattle*, 2nd edn. San Francisco: Freeman.

Schumacher, J. and Varner, D. D. (1993) In: *Equine Reproduction*, ed. A. O. McKinnon and J. L. Voss, p. 871–877. Philadelphia: Lea and Febiger.

Seidel, G. E. and Foote, R. H. (1967) *J. Dairy Sci.*, **50**, 970.

Seidel, G. E. and Foote, R. H. (1969) *J. Reprod. Fertil.*, **20**, 313.

Silbersiepe, E. (1937) *Berl. Mun. Tierarztl. Wochenschr.*, **53**, 432.

Siliart, B,. Fontbonne, A. and Badinand, F. (1993) *J. Reprod. Fertil. Suppl.*, **47**, 560 (Abstr.).

Smith, H. A. and Jones, T. C. (1966) *Veterinary Pathology*, 3rd edn. Philadelphia: Lea and Febiger.

Smith, M. C. (1986) In: *Current Therapy in Theriogenology*, 2nd edn, ed. D. A. Morrow, pp. 544–550. Philadelphia: Saunders.

Soderberg, S. F. (1986) In: *Current Therapy in Theriogenology*, 2nd edn, ed. D. A. Morrow, pp. 544–550. Philadelphia: Saunders.

Stanic, M. N. (1960) *Mod. Vet. Pract.*, **41**, 30.

Stick, J. A. (1981) *Vet. Med. Small Anim. Clin.*, **76**, 410.

Stickle, R. L. and Fessler, J. F. (1978) *J. Amer. Vet. Med. Assn*, **172**, 343.

Studdert, M. H., Barker, C. A. V. and Savan, M. (1964) *Amer. J. Vet. Res.*, **25**, 303.

Swanson, E. W. and Bearden, H. J. (1951) *J. Anim. Sci.*, **10**, 981.

Threlfall, W. R. and Lopate, C. (1993) In: *Equine Reproduction*, ed. A. O. McKinnon and J. L. Voss, pp. 943–949. Philadelphia: Lea and Febiger.

Vandeplassche, M., Bouckaert, J. H., Oyaert, W. and Bouters, R. (1963) *Proc. XVII World Vet. Cong., Hannover*, **2**, 1135.

Varner, D. D., Taylor, T. S. and Blanchard, T. L. (1993) In: *Equine Reproduction*, ed. A. O. McKinnon and J. L. Voss, pp. 861–863. Philadelphia: Lea and Febiger.

Vaughn, J. T. (1993) In: *Equine Reproduction*, ed. A. O. McKinnon and J. L. Voss, pp. 885–894. Philadelphia: Lea and Febiger.

Walker, D. F. (1964) *J. Amer. Vet. Med. Assn*, **145**, 677.

Walker, D. F. (1966) *Arburn. Vet.*, **22**, 56.

Walker, D. F. (1970) *Proc. VI Ann. Conf. Cattle Dis., Oklahoma*, p. 322.

Walker, D. F. and Vaughn, J. T. (1980) *Bovine and Equine Urogenital Surgery*. Philadelphia: Lea and Febiger.

Warwick, B. L. (1961) *J. Anim. Sci.*, **20**, 10.

Watson, J. W. (1964) *Nature*, **204**, 95.

Watson, P. F. (1990) In: *Marshall's Physiology of Reproduction*, ed. G. E. Lamming, Vol. 2, pp. 747–869. Edinburgh: Churchill Livingstone.

Webster, W. M. (1932) *Aust. Vet. J.*, **8**, 199.

Wells, M. E. and Awa, O. A. (1970) *J. Dairy Sci.*, **53**, 227.

Welsh, T. H., Randell, R. D. and Johnson, B. H. (1981) *Archiv. Androl.*, **6**, 141.

Wheat, J. D. (1951) *J. Amer. Vet. Med. Assn*, **118**, 295.

Wheat, J. D. (1961) *Vet. Med.*, **56**, 477.

Whitfield, C. H. and Parkinson, T. J. (1994) *Theriogenology*, **38**, 11.

Williams, W. L. (1943) *Diseases of the Genital Organs of Domestic Animals*, 3rd edn. Ithaca, New York: self-published.

Williams, W. W. and Savage, A. (1925) *Cornell Vet.*, **15**, 353.

Willis, R. A. and Rudduck, H. B. (1943) *J. Pathol. Bact.*, **55**, 165.

Willmington, J. A. (1981) *Proc. AVTRW, Scarborough*, 1.

Wittrow, S. J. and Susaneck, S. J. (1986) In: *Current Therapy: Theriogenology*, 2nd edn, ed. D. A. Morrow, pp. 521–528. Philadelphia: Saunders.

Wright, J. G. (1963) *Vet. Rec.*, **75**, 1352.

Young, A. C. B. (1979) *J. Small Anim. Pract.*, **20**, 229.

Young, S. A., Hudson, R. S. and Walker, D. F. (1977) *J. Amer. Vet. Med. Assn*, **171**, 643.

The successful use of artificial insemination (AI) as a means of animal breeding relies upon three major premises: firstly, that spermatozoa can survive outside the body; secondly, that they can be reintroduced into the female genital tract in a way which results in an acceptable conception rate; and, thirdly, that the fertile period of the female can be identified. The degree to which these underlying premises can be fulfilled dictates, to a large degree, the success with which AI can be applied to an animal species. For example, in cattle, spermatozoa can be preserved outside the body almost indefinitely after cryopreservation. A technically straightforward intrauterine insemination means that the number of spermatozoa for each insemination dose is low; hence, each ejaculate can be used for serving many females. Conception rates achieved thus are identical to those of natural service, while the oestrous behaviour of cows means that detection of the fertile period is not difficult. Hence, in this species, in which all three premises are fulfilled, the use of AI is widespread. However, in many other species, where one or more of the premises are less adequately fulfilled, AI is less successful and therefore less widely used.

AI regimes have been developed for most domestic and many semidomestic species. It is routinely practised in cattle, sheep, pigs, goats, fowl, turkeys, salmon and trout, and is used in dogs, domestic foxes, buffalo, horses and even bees. Of these, cattle and sheep/goats account for the vast majority of mammalian inseminations. The use of AI in turkey breeding is essential, as natural mating is not possible in this species, so that very large numbers of inseminations are performed. AI in salmonid farming is also very widespread. The use of AI in pigs has been surprisingly low, with estimates of around 9% of the national herd being typical for Western Europe and the USA (Iritani, 1980), although its use is increasing (Reed, 1985). However, it is much more widely practised in Eastern Europe, with perhaps as much as 30% of national herds bred thus (Reed, 1982). The discussion of AI in this chapter will be limited to the major domestic mammals.

ADVANTAGES AND DISADVANTAGES OF AI OVER NATURAL BREEDING

Artificial insemination offers several potential advantages over natural service. Of these, the reason most commonly advocated for AI is as a means of genetic improvement. In most food-producing animals, each ejaculate can be divided into many insemination doses, such that each AI sire can potentially be used to breed a very large number of females. Hence, the total number of sires needed is reduced. In consequence, the selection intensity that can be applied to male-side selection becomes very much more intense than for natural service. In dairy cattle, only the best 1% of cows are selected as potential bull mothers, and only about the best 1–3% of their male progeny eventually become sires of the next generation. In beef cattle and pigs the selection intensity is not quite so great, but nevertheless very much more intense than can be achieved in natural breeding.

Direct genetic selection of sires is not, however, the most widely used application of AI for achieving genetic improvement. More common is the use of AI to allow rapid dissemination of new breeds. In the UK, AI was one of the main means whereby the Friesian breed of cattle displaced the indigenous British dairy breeds. Subsequently, AI has also been the means by which the Friesian has been displaced by the Holstein. In such breed substitution programmes, AI can be used to rapidly change the gene pool of a national herd; a commonly used technique for upgrading unimproved cattle in remote areas. In this process, AI has the advantage of being both cheap and simple, for local distribution of extended and chilled semen from small numbers of imported sires is within the economic capabilities of even the poorest countries.

International trade in livestock is also facilitated by AI. Improved stock can be imported in the form of semen for AI, rather than having to move animals themselves. Thus, many problems of acclimatization, lack of resistance to local diseases, etc., can be eliminated. Importing semen also allows the importing country to exert far greater control over the health status of the donor sires than if the livestock itself were imported.

The second major advantage of AI is in the reduction of the numbers of sires that individual farmers need to maintain. The males of agricultural species generally require accommodation in which they can be segregated from the breeding females, so that breeding can be controlled, in buildings which preclude, as far as possible, injury to farm staff. The significant housing and labour costs involved with keeping such animals can therefore be obviated by the use of AI; moreover, the farmer generally has access to genetic material through AI centres which would be far beyond his pocket if the sire was bought outright.

The third major advantage to AI is in the control of venereal disease. In the UK in the 1940s a major impetus to the development of cattle AI was the need to control the epizootic venereal pathogens *Tritrichomonas fetus* and *Campylobacter fetus*, which were virtually eliminated by the use of AI (see Chapter 23). However, the converse is also true, namely that uncontrolled use of sires in AI can disseminate disease. Many diseases are transmissible through semen, including not only the classic venereal diseases, but also other conditions which would not generally be regarded as primarily venereal (see Roberts, 1986). Rigorous monitoring of the health of AI donor sires is therefore regarded in many countries as an integral part of national disease control programmes.

However, although AI carries many advantages over natural breeding, the technique is not without drawbacks. Detection of the fertile period in the female oestrous cycle is potentially the most problematic aspect of AI programmes. In cattle, the prominent homosexual behaviour of oestrous females allows relatively accurate human identification of the fertile period, but in most other species its detection is less easy. In such species, detection

of oestrus therefore requires the presence of infertile (e.g. vasectomized) males, or the timing of oestrus must be controlled by pharmacological (e.g. oestrus synchronization/induction regimens) or mangemental (e.g. timing of weaning in sows) procedures. Thus, for ewes, which do not normally display any signs of oestrus in the absence of a male, AI requires either the presence of vasectomized rams to detect oestrus, or the use of pharmacological means of oestrus manipulation, to ensure that the fertile period occurs at a predetermined time. Hence, detection of the fertile period of the ewe is, to a greater or lesser extent, a costly procedure, thereby detracting from the attraction of AI in that species. It may therefore be considered that an economic 'trade-off' exists in such species, between the genetic advantages conferred by the use of superior AI sires on one hand and the costs of maintaining teaser males or pharmacological manipulation on the other.

Once oestrus has been identified, the female animal has to be restrained for insemination, which generally requires separation from the herd and holding in specialized pens. The process of insemination also requires trained personnel, which may require a limited degree of technical proficiency, as is the case in insemination of sows, or may be very demanding, as in the case of laparoscopic intrauterine insemination of ewes.

A consequence of the need to detect oestrus is the necessity of maintaining an adequate recording system so that not only are insemination dates recorded but also expected dates of return to oestrus need to be known, so that appropriate observations can be made. Similarly, where males are not present in the herd, some form of positive pregnancy diagnosis is also advantageous. It is also imperative that the identities of the sires are recorded and their pedigrees known, so that inbreeding is avoided.

The ability of AI as a rapid means of transmission of the genes of superior sires has already been identified. However, a corresponding disadvantage exists: namely, that genetic faults can also be widely disseminated if they are present in an AI sire. Dominant traits should rarely be transmitted in this way, but recessive traits may be very widely transmitted, especially if the recessive gene is present in the general population at such a low incidence that many breedings may have to be performed before the condition is expressed in a homozygous progeny. Hence, AI programmes must be underpinned by an efficient reporting system for monitoring abnormalities in the progeny, with clearly defined criteria for the withdrawal of sires for use if they proved to be carrying deleterious genes. In cattle, achondroplasia is transmitted as a simple recessive gene (Marlowe, 1964) which, when present in the homozygous condition, causes failure of long bone development, resulting in the birth of so-called 'bulldog' (achondroplastic) calves (see Chapter 4). The incidence of this gene in the general cattle population is so low that the birth of one or two calves with this deformity is regarded as sufficient reason to slaughter the bull and withdraw all stocks of semen. Spastic paresis is similarly transmitted and dealt with in a similar manner (Keith, 1981). However, other defects may be less readily appreciated as such and may even result from breeding programmes. For example, the high incidence of dystocia in Friesian cattle has resulted from the selection of sires producing progeny with a level pelvis, which has also caused a lengthening of the pelvic canal (see Chapter 11). Likewise, a Canadian Holstein bull that was popular in the UK in recent years produced progeny with very straight hindlegs, considered desirable at the time, but many of which later proved to have severe hock malconformation. A further concern, which has been frequently expressed but has yet to prove of major impact, is the reduction in the gene pool of highly selected breeds. For example, in Holstein cattle, concern has been expressed that the number of blood lines from which sires are drawn is becoming progressively reduced, yet no unequivocal evidence of inbreeding depression has been identified in the breed so far.

PREPARATION OF SEMEN FOR USE IN AI

The methods for collection of semen from domestic mammals are described in Chapter 30. In most AI regimes, semen evaluation is limited to measuring sperm numbers, motility and, usually, morphology. More sophisticated analyses may be used in determining whether an individual sire produces semen of acceptable quality for acceptance into an

AI programme, but such evaluations are rarely carried out on the day-to-day collections of semen. Unless the semen is to be directly inseminated without delay into a single female, it is usually then diluted and either cooled or frozen. Direct inseminations are performed most commonly in the bitch, usually in response to some incapacity of the sire which precludes normal mating (Roberts, 1986) or in the mare with chronic endometritis (Asbury, 1986).

Dilution
The ejaculates of most domestic animals contain more sperm than are needed for achieving pregnancies. Hence, by diluting the semen, it can potentially be used for seveal inseminations. In species such as the dog and the horse, the whole sperm-rich fraction of the ejaculate is diluted and chilled, then either used for sequential inseminations of the same female over her extended oestrus period or after various determinations of the fertile period (see Jeffcoate and Lindsay, 1989; Brinsko and Varner, 1993). In food animal species, the ejaculate is generally diluted so that it can be used to inseminate many females. In either case, the maximum degree of dilution is determined from the minimum number of spermatozoa and the volume of inseminate that is required to achieve acceptable pregnancy rates. These are themselves determined by the site of insemination, the survival of sperm in diluent and the idiosyncrasies of individual species and sires. In general, where an intrauterine insemination can be achieved, the minimum numbers of sperm are one or two orders of magnitude lower than for an intracervical insemination; which is itself one or two orders of magnitude lower than for an intravaginal insemination. Hence, where widespread use of sires is required, great advantage exists in devising methods of achieving intrauterine insemination, even where, as in the ewe, this requires such a complex procedure as a laparoscopic insemination.

The major properties of a semen diluent (see Watson, 1979) are:

1. *Addition of volume.* Insemination doses must be prepared in a volume which is a compromise between ease of handling and an appropriate volume for the site of insemination. Thus, for ovine intracervical inseminations, minimizing

volume is important to reduce retrograde loss from the cervix (Evans and Maxwell, 1987), while for porcine intrauterine inseminations, a minimum volume of 50 ml is required to spread the semen through that capacious organ (Reed, 1982).

Dilution of semen is not entirely straightforward, for mammalian sperm placed in simple diluents exhibit an initial increase in motility, which is then rapidly followed by loss of motility and increase in vital staining (Mann, 1964). This phenomenon, known as the 'dilution effect', represents a loss of cell viability, probably through leaching of structural components of the cell membrane. Although it was of great concern amongst the early practitioners of AI, the use of diluents containing macromolecules such as proteins or polyvinyl alcohol was found to abrogate the dilution effect (Suter et al., 1979; Clay et al., 1984).

2. *Buffers.* Spermatozoa generally have a narrow range of tolerance to changes in pH, so provision of buffering capacity is necessary. Buffering is especially important where the semen is only to be chilled and not cryopreserved, as the metabolic activity of cooled semen remains appreciable (Salisbury et al., 1978). In many diluents, the major volume component is also the major buffering solution, although buffers may be a minor addition to the diluent. Simple buffers are effective, with citrate being widely used (Willett and Salisbury, 1942). Phosphate-buffered saline is rather less suitable, as it predisposes to head-to-head agglutination of sperm. More recently, organic buffers have been used: Tris (tris(hydroxymethyl)aminomethane) is probably the most widely employed of such buffers (Davis et al., 1963), but the successful use of many similar materials (e.g. TES, HEPES Tricene) is described. The proteins contained in skimmed milk products also provide considerable buffering capacity to diluents.

3. *Maintenance of osmotic pressure.* Seminal plasma has an osmotic pressure of 285 mOsm, although sperm can tolerate a moderate range of tonicity (Foote, 1969). Some debate has centred on whether sperm respond better to a slightly hyperosmotic (Foote, 1970) or isosmotic diluent, with the former being generally favoured. Apart from the osmotic activity of the ionic component of diluents, a substantial contribution is made by proteins and, particularly, by sugars, which are added to provide nutrition for the sperm or to

contribute to the cryoprotective properties (see Watson, 1990) of the diluent.

4. *Energy substrate.* Most diluents make some provision of energy substrates for sperm. In general, simple sugars, such as glucose, fructose, mannose and arabinose are suitable substrates, although the rate at which these sugars are metabolized varies substantially between species (reviewed by Bedford and Hoskins, 1990). Lactose, which is present in milk-based diluents, is not metabolizable to any appreciable extent. However, egg yolk, also a component of many diluents, provides many substrates for sperm metabolism (Salisbury et al., 1978). The provision of energy is relatively less important where sperm are to be frozen, for they will only remain active for a few hours at most before freezing suspends metabolic activity. However, if semen is to be used chilled, when sperm metabolism has to be sustained for several days, provision of energy is important.

5. *Antimicrobial activity.* Antibiotics are added to most semen diluents as a prophylactic measure against the transmission of pathogenic bacteria and to reduce the load of non-pathogenic organisms that contaminate the semen. In cattle AI, benzylpenicillin and streptomycin (Melrose, 1962) are the most widely used antibiotics, for these are efficacious against *C. fetus.* Most other antibiotics either fail to control this organism or are directly detrimental to sperm. Recently, concern over the potential transmission of *Mycoplasma* and *Ureaplasma* species in bovine semen has led to the incorporation of lincomycin and spectimomycin (Almquist and Zaugg, 1974) into semen diluents in an effort to control these organisms. There is evidence that the efficiency of antibiotics may be reduced in the presence of some components of diluents, notably egg yolk (Morgan et al., 1959). Hence, in some bovine AI centres it is common to preincubate the raw semen with antibiotic cocktails before the main dilution occurs.

The lifespan of spermatozoa at ambient temperatures is generally short, but can be extended by inhibiting their metabolism and motility with carbon dioxide (VanDemark et al., 1965; Foote, 1967). For most species, the alternative method of inhibiting sperm activity, namely cooling, has been the method of choice. However, the spermatozoa of some species, notably the boar, do not tolerate cooling well, so ambient temperature dilutions have been needed. The earliest of such diluents, the Illinois variable temperature (IVT) diluent, used glucose, citrate, bicarbonate and egg yolk and was gassed with carbon dioxide (see Salisbury and VanDemark, 1961). Variations of this diluent formed the basis of diluents used in early pig AI programmes, although more modern diluents, such as the Guelph (Haeger and Mackle, 1971) or Zorlesco (Gottardi et al., 1980) diluents, have largely supplanted these now. Such diluents allow boar semen to remain viable for over 3 days at ambient temperature.

The lifespan of spermatozoa of most other species can more conveniently be prolonged by either cooling or freezing. Cooling sperm, however, results in considerable damage to the cells, with the leakage of intracellular potassium, enzymes, lipoprotein and ATP occurring (Salisbury et al., 1978). This phenomenon of cold shock is exacerbated by rapid cooling rates, but cannot be prevented even by slow cooling. The most effective way of protecting sperm against the detrimental effects of cooling is by the inclusion of lecithins, proteins, lipoproteins and similar complexes of large molecules that are found in egg yolk and milk (Blackshaw, 1954; Melrose, 1956; Blackshaw and Salisbury, 1957). Of these, lipoprotein appears to be the most critical, although its mode of action is poorly understood (Watson, 1990). Possibly it prevents the leaching of similar materials from the sperm plasmalemma, or possibly it mitigates and limits the consequences of such leaching when it occurs. Unfortunately, neither egg yolk nor milk adequately protects boar spermatozoa against cooling, nor does any other readily available or fully synthetic compound (Watson and Plummer, 1985). Furthermore, some of the constituents of egg are toxic to the sperm of some species, notably the goat, in which a toxic interaction occurs between yolk and components of the seminal plasma, causing sperm death (Corteel and Paquignon, 1984). Moreover, whole milk is also toxic to sperm, for it contains a protein, 'lactenin', which is spermicidal. Thus, milk for use as a semen diluent must be heat treated (e.g. in the skimming process) to inactivate this toxic factor (Flipse et al., 1954).

The fertility of bovine semen stored at 5°C in such a diluent remains acceptable for 2–4 days (Foote et al., 1960), although that of ram semen only persists for 12–24 hours (Salamon and Robinson, 1962; Evans and Maxwell, 1987). The decline in fertility that occurs after this time is initially due to decreased motility and survival in the female genital tract rather than to sperm death per se. Short-term storage of semen by chilling to 5°C is, however, a very cheap and effective way of establishing an AI programme for cattle and is of value for on-farm collection and insemination of sheep, while the use of liquid boar semen at ambient temperatures remains, effectively, the basis of the technique in that species. Short-term 5°C storage is also widely used in the horse and the dog, for it avoids the unpredictable response to freezing that characterizes the semen of those species.

Cryopreservation

Longer-term storage of semen is achieved through cryopreservation. Cryopreservation maintains the fertile life of semen virtually indefinitely, although a large proportion of individual spermatozoa fail to survive the considerable stresses of freezing and thawing. For sperm to survive freezing, they need to be extended in a diluent that not only contains substances that protect them against cold shock, but also cryoprotectants, such as glycerol, which protect them from the deleterious consequences of freezing.

The general responses of cells to freezing (reviewed by Farrant, 1980; Watson, 1990) were not understood until long after empirical methods of cryopreservation had become widely adopted. Initially, as the temperature of the external medium falls below its freezing point, crystals of pure water start to form. The concentration of solutes in the unfrozen part of the medium therefore rises as, in consequence, does its osmotic pressure. Ice crystals do not extend into the cell at this stage, as they are excluded by the cell membrane. Thus, the intracellular contents undergo a period of supercooling, during which the cell loses water to the unfrozen part of the extracellular medium by osmosis (Figure 31.1). A variable degree of cell dehydration follows, which is terminated by the formation of intracellular ice crystals. Thus, damage can occur to cells in one of two ways. Where a substantial degree of cellular dehydration occurs, the high concentrations of solutes in the residual intracellular water can be damaging, whereas, if only slight dehydration occurs, large ice crystals can form within the cell, which cause physical damage to its internal and bounding membranes. The degree to which each affects the cell is determined by the rate of cooling — the slower the rate the more dehydration, the faster the rate the greater the damage by ice formation — and the size of the cell, such that the larger the cell the slower its inherent rate of dehydration.

Cryoprotective agents may either penetrate or remain outside the cell, but both act by binding water and therefore alter the availability of water either for dehydrative loss or for ice crystal formation. Penetrating cryoprotectants, such as glycerol or dimethyl sulfoxide (DMSO) appear to not only reduce the loss of water from the cell, thereby reducing solute damage, but also bind it in a form that renders it unavailable for crystal formation, thereby reducing the effects of intracellular ice. Non-penetrating cryoprotectants, such as disaccharides or proteins, may hasten dehydration during very rapid cooling, thereby minimizing intracellular ice formation. Notwithstanding the aforegoing, precise understanding of the mode of action of cyroprotectants remains elusive, and much information relating to their practical use remains empirical.

Glycerol (Polge et al., 1949) is the main primary cryoprotectant used in preparing mammalian semen for freezing (see Watson, 1990), despite the fact that it has some directly toxic effects upon sperm (Watson, 1979). The concentrations used depend upon species and the other components of the diluent. For example, diluents for bovine semen that contain disaccharides can utilize lower percentages (3–4%) of glycerol than diluents that lack such disaccharides, which have a final glycerol concentration of at least 7% (Unal et al., 1978). Whether the toxic effects of glycerol are exacerbated at high temperatures has been a matter of debate. Certainly Polge (1953) considered that the addition of glycerol was more damaging to bovine sperm at 28°C than at 4°C, although Salisbury et al. (1978), reviewing the (by then) copious literature concluded that the effects of temperature of glycerolization were equivocal. Nevertheless, the practice in commercial bovine AI centres is, in general, that where the final concentration of glycerol contrations is required to be high, a primary dilution of the semen is made with a diluent containing little or no glycerol, with glycerolization being carried out after reducing the temperature to 4°C, whereas diluents which utilize lower final concentrations are added in one step, at 30°C. With boar semen, by contrast, the toxicity of glycerol at high temperatures is much less equivocal, and low-temperature glycerolization is desirable (see Paquignon, 1985).

Originally, diluted semen was placed in glass ampoules for freezing in a mixture of alcohol and solid carbon dioxide at −79°C, or drops of diluted semen were placed directly onto the

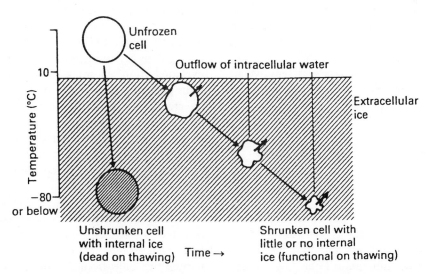

Fig. 31.1 Shrinkage of cells during cryopreservation. Extracellular freezing induces conditions that allow osmotically induced loss of water from cells during slow freezing. This correlates with survival on thawing. Rapidly cooled cells do not have time to shrink, form intracellular ice and are dead on thawing. (Reproduced from Farrant (1980), with permission.)

surface of a block of solid carbon dioxide where they froze in pellet form (see Salisbury et al., 1978). Long-term storage at −79°C was not satisfactory, however, as deterioration occurred at that temperature (Pickett et al., 1961; Stewart, 1964). Storage in liquid nitrogen at −196°C has subsequently become established as the standard medium for long-term preservation of semen and, over the 40 years for which it has been practised, has maintained sperm fertility unscathed. At the present time, semen is frozen in one of two main ways. Diluted semen is packed into thin, plastic tubes of 0.25 or 0.5 ml capacity, then, in the simpler techniques, these tubes ('straws' or 'paillettes') are suspended in the vapour from liquid nitrogen, which is at about −120°C, for about 10 minutes (Cassou, 1964; Jondet, 1964). The straws are then plunged into the liquid nitrogen (Figure 31.2(a)). More recently, a greater degree of control of freezing rate has been exercised by the use of microprocessor-controlled freezers, with improved sperm survival justifying the increased cost of the processing (e.g. Landa and Almquist, 1979; Parkinson and Whitfield, 1987).

Thawing of the semen needs to be rapid; slow thawing allows recrystallization of ice within the cells, causing membrane damage (see Salisbury et al., 1978). In practice, the rate of thawing is rarely critical: the surface area-to-volume ratio of the 0.25 ml tubes being so great that any temperature of the thawing water between 0 and 40°C will thaw adequately (Figure 31.2(b)). Of greater importance is the temperature control of the thawed semen. This should not be allowed to cool below the final temperature achieved during thawing, otherwise substantial sperm losses can occur. Rethawed spermatozoa are as sensitive to fluctuations in temperature as are their unfrozen counterparts (Roberts, 1986).

Diseases transmissible in semen

Many infectious agents can be transmitted through semen. Foot and mouth virus can be transmitted in the semen of all species which are susceptible to its infection (see Callis and McKercher, 1980; Radostits et al., 1994). Indeed, control of foot and mouth transmission has, until recently, underpinned the UK legislation controlling AI of cattle, with broadly similar regulations in force throughout much of the

developed world. Most of the other serious viral diseases of cattle can also potentially be transmitted thus, as can the somewhat less serious viral diseases such as infectious bovine rhinotracheitis–infectious pustular vulvovaginitis (IBR–IPV) (Chapman et al., 1979; Kahrs et al., 1980). Recently, it has become apparent that the bovine viral diarrhoea (BVD) virus can be present in the semen of bulls (Barlow et al., 1986), potentially causing early embryonic death and abortions in inseminated cows (Grahn et al., 1984).

A number of bacterial diseases are transmissible in semen, including tuberculosis, brucellosis, leptospirosis and, possibly, Johne's disease (see Roberts, 1986). *Haemophilus somnus*, to which the possibility of causing reproductive failure has been attributed, may also be present in semen (Humphrey et al., 1982). Many species of *Mycoplasma* and *Ureaplasma* are present as commensals of the prepuce of the bull, and are harmless when inseminated into cows, but some species are responsible for a granulomatous vaginitis in cows, which causes infertility and unwillingness to mate (Ashfar et al., 1966; Radostits et al., 1994). Most importantly, the classic venereal pathogens of cattle, *T. fetus* and *C. fetus* (Garlick, 1939; Rasbech, 1951; Willett et al., 1955), are transmissible by AI; control of these two organisms remains the second major precept upon which legislation governing cattle AI is based.

Two other conditions warrant specific mention. Firstly, EBL (enzootic bovine leucosis) virus, which is generally considered not to be transmissible in semen (Radostis, 1979), rightly causes such anxiety to regulating authorities that infected bulls are excluded from AI studs. Secondly, blue tongue virus generally causes little or no clinical signs in infected cattle (Radostits et al., 1994). However, the disease it causes in sheep is so severe that semen from potentially infected bulls (Bowen and Howard, 1984) is carefully excluded from most countries in which sheep production is of economic importance.

In cattle, control of these diseases rests upon three major strategies. Diseases which can be detected by serology, such as brucellosis, IBR, EBL, Q fever, etc., are controlled by exclusion of seropositive bulls from AI studs. Likewise, tuberculosis is controlled by exclusion of bulls which react to tuberculin testing. *Leptospira* spp. may be

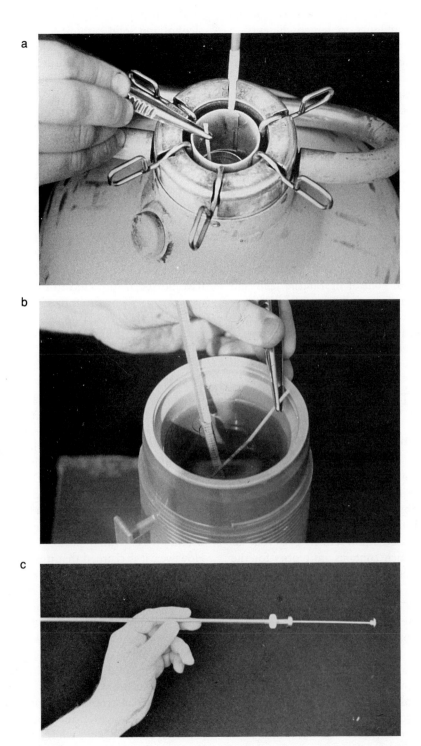

Fig. 31.2 Semen handling for bovine artificial insemination. (a) Withdrawing a straw of frozen semen from the liquid nitrogen flask. The canister containing the semen should not be lifted above the level of the top of the neck of the flask. (b) Thawing. After checking the identity of the sire, the straw is thawed. Water temperature is not really critical, but placing the straw in water at 37°C for 10 seconds is a typical thawing regime. (c) The straw is placed in an insemination catheter, which is then covered with a plastic sheath. The catheter is then ready for use, but care must be exercised not to allow the semen to become chilled again before it is inseminated.

killed by freezing and thawing, but it is also routine practice to add antibiotics to semen diluents to destroy not only such organisms, but also contaminant organisms derived from the penis and prepuce during semen collection and, most importantly, *C. fetus*. Antibiotics are also used to control *Mycoplasma* and *Ureaplasma* species. The final, and most potent means of control of disease, is the quarantine of semen after its collection. After semen has been frozen, it is placed in a container where it remains untouched for 28 days. If during that period, the donor bull develops any disease, the semen is destroyed. If not, it is released for use.

Control of diseases in other species is generally much less stringent than in cattle, although a progressive trend towards increased disease security exists. For dogs, control of *Brucella canis* and leptospira infection is generally required for international shipments of semen, and pigs are generally screened for diseases such as Aujeszky's disease before entry to studs.

AI OF CATTLE

Collection, handling and storage of semen

Semen is usually collected by an artificial vagina, although electroejaculation is occasionally used. After assessment for motility, density and morphology, the semen is diluted into insemination doses, with a diluent based upon either egg yolk or skimmed milk, which contains antibiotics for the control of contaminating bacteria. The semen is then cooled to 4°C. If it is destined for use in this form, the motility of the sperm will be reassessed, then the semen released for use. If the semen is destined for cryopreservation, glycerol will be added, then the semen packed into 0.25 or 0.5 ml paillettes, or 0.5 or 1.0 ml glass ampoules. The semen is then equilibrated for 1–4 hours. It was originally considered that this was the period over which glycerol penetrated the sperm, although more recent observations indicate that the penetration of glycerol is very rapid and that most of the equilibration period is concerned with membrane stabilization during exposure to low temperatures (see Watson, 1979). The semen is then frozen in the vapour of liquid nitrogen, or

in a microprocessor-controlled freezer. Freezing in alcohol and solid carbon dioxide or in pellets on blocks of solid carbon dioxide, although formerly used widely, has now virtually ceased. The semen thereafter remains in liquid nitrogen until thawed for use.

The ability to perform an intrauterine insemination in cattle means that a relatively low dose of sperm is required to achieve acceptable pregnancy rates. Typically, of the 20–30 million sperm that are required in each insemination dose, 6–7 million survive freezing; a figure which is generally regarded as the minimum dose compatible with acceptable fertility (Milk Marketing Board, 1967; Sullivan and Elliott, 1968). Lower numbers of sperm can be used where unfrozen semen is used (Salisbury and VanDemark, 1961) — for these cells have not been subjected to the stress and damage of freezing — with studies from New Zealand indicating that as few as 2.5 million live sperm can be used (Shannon, 1968; Moller et al., 1972).

Insemination

Cows ovulate at about 12 hours after the end of the oestrus period. The ideal time for insemination is therefore 6–24 hours prior to ovulation (see Roberts, 1986). Where the technician service provided by an AI centre is used, the optimum insemination times achieved in practice are on the same day (morning or afternoon) where oestrus is first observed in the morning, or on the morning of the next day, where oestrus is first observed in the afternoon (Olds and Seath, 1954; Foote, 1979). However, it is claimed that it is possible to achieve a better timing of insemination in relation to the most fertile period of oestrus by farmers inseminating their own cattle at appropriate intervals after the first observation of oestrus. For this reason, and because of the cost of using AI centre technicians, technician services have fallen somewhat into disfavour, compared to farmers' own ('do-it-yourself') inseminations.

Cows are inseminated just into the short uterine body. Insemination into the cervix produces a lower fertilization rate, while insemination deeper into the uterus runs the risks of either inseminating into the uterine horn contralateral to the ovulation site, or of scoring the endometrium with the tip of the insemination catheter. Reduced fertility is the consequence of both of the latter two errors. The standard technique of insemination is to grasp the cervix through the rectum with the left hand. A catheter, into the tip of which a paillette of semen has been inserted (Figures 31.2(c) and 31.3(a)), is then passed into the vagina and manipulated into and through the cervix by the right hand. This technique, the rectovaginal method of insemination, requires considerable practice for success. The vulval lips are opened by downwards pressure from the arm in the rectum, while the circular folds of vaginal mucosa are obliterated by pushing the cervix forward. The catheter is initially inserted pointing upwards at an angle of about 30°, to avoid entering the urethral meatus or fossa, and is then moved horizontally until it engages in the external os of the cervix. The left hand squeezes the anterior vagina onto the caudally projecting external os of the cervix, thereby obliterating the fornix of the vagina (Figure 31.3(b)) and facilitating entry of the catheter into the cervix. Entry into the external os is accompanied by a characteristic 'gritty' sensation. The catheter is then introduced through the convoluted cervical canal by manipulation of the cervix through the rectal wall. One finger is placed over the internal os of the cervix, so that the tip of the catheter can be palpated as it emerges from the cervical canal (Figure 31.3(c)). As soon as the catheter has emerged, deposition of semen in to the uterus begins: the catheter is advanced no deeper into the uterus. In this way, semen should be equally distributed between the two uterine horns (Figures 31.3(d) and 31.4).

No forwards pressure should be exerted on the catheter with the right hand, for the uterine wall is friable and easily penetrated if the catheter moves suddenly. The most common faults of insemination (Figure 31.5) are twisting the cervix in the left hand, so that one uterine horn is partly occluded. Alternatively, the catheter may be partly withdrawn during the deposition of semen, resulting in a partially intracervical insemination. The cervix of maiden cattle is difficult to penetrate at oestrus, and impossible at other stages of the oestrous cycle: such animals are therefore often beyond the capabilities of inexperienced inseminators. However, the cervix of parous cattle can, with greater or lesser difficulty, be traversed at most stages of the oestrous cycle and early pregnancy. It is therefore imperative that it is known whether an animal is likely to be pregnant before insemination is attempted, for abortion can be induced if an insemination catheter penetrates the fetal membranes or if infection is introduced into a pregnant uterus by poor insemination hygiene.

Management of insemination

Insemination can be performed at an observed or induced oestrus. The former is more common in dairy cattle, for considerable opportunity exists for the observation of oestrus, but in beef cattle and dairy or beef heifers the time required for observation makes the use of induced oestrus relatively more attractive. Oestrus can be induced and synchronized by the use of prostaglandin $F_{2\alpha}$ ($PGF_{2\alpha}$) or its analogues, progesterone-like hormones, or combinations of progesterone and a luteolytic agent. Most such regimens require the use of fixed-time insemination, although, particularly in the case of $PGF_{2\alpha}$, the accuracy with which the timing of oestrus can be predicted is sufficiently imprecise for some observation to be advisable, and re-insemination performed if animals exhibit signs of oestrus after fixed-time insemination has occurred.

Fertility to AI is generally very similar to that achieved to natural service, with a calving rate to a single insemination of around 50% (e.g. Barrett et al., 1948). The true fertilization rate is much higher than this, at around 90%, but subsequent embryonic losses bring the apparent figure to the lower value (Ayalon et al., 1968). In practice, AI companies are generally unable to obtain complete data on the calving rates, so they estimate fertility from the proportion of cows which are re-presented for insemination by either 49 or 60–90 days after the initial service. The proportion of cows which are not re-presented is closely related to the proportion which actually have become and remained pregnant. The figure thereby obtained, the non-return rate, is an overestimate of calving rate, but is generally in fixed ratio to the calving rate, so is usable for monitoring fertility (reviewed by Salisbury et al., 1978). AI centres therefore use the 'non-return rate' to monitor both the fertility of their bulls and the results obtained by their technicians. Bulls or technicians which produce consistently low figures are generally slaughtered, or dismissed, respectively. No such control exists over the technical proficiency of farmers who inseminate their own cattle, nor, necessarily, over the fertility of the bulls they use.

a

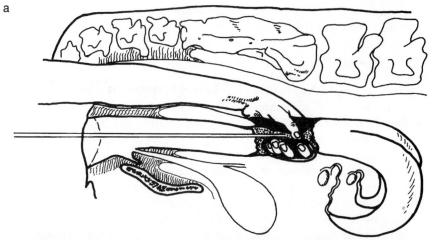

b

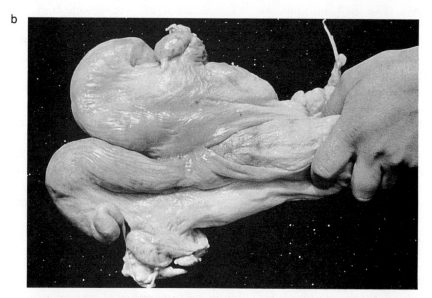

c

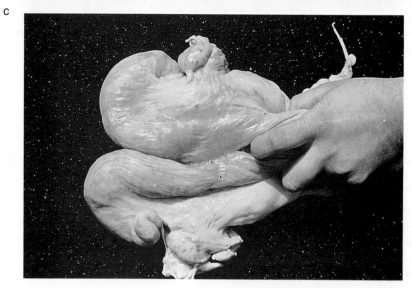

d

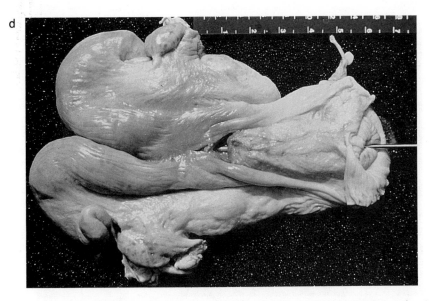

Fig. 31.3 Rectovaginal method of insemination. (a) General method. Partially dissected bovine uterus showing; (b) grip on the cervix for the obliteration of the vaginal fornix, to facilitate entry of the catheter into the external os of the cervix; (c) second grip on the cervix to allow passage of the catheter through the tortuous cervical canal — the index finger is gently pressed over the internal os in order to feel the tip of the catheter as it emerges from the cervical canal; (d) site of deposition of semen in the uterine body — the recommended site is no more than 0.5 cm deep to the internal cervical os. (Redrawn from Salisbury et al. (1978) with permission.)

Regulation of cattle AI varies from country to country, but is generally under some form of state control. In the UK, AI centres are licensed by the Ministry of Agriculture, with the right to distribute semen, or to employ technicians to inseminate cattle, also granted by ministry licence. Further licenses grant individual farmers the right to inseminate their own cattle and to store frozen semen on their farms. The greatest degree of control is exercised over the health status of donor bulls and the hygiene of technicians who, by travelling between farms, offer considerable risk as disease vectors. Surprisingly, although cattle AI is generally closely regulated, AI of most other species, including those of agricultural importance, has generally received scant attention from regulating authorities.

AI OF SHEEP AND GOATS

Artificial insemination of sheep and goats has recently been comprehensively reviewed by Evans and Maxwell (1987). The sheep is, in many ways, less amenable to artificial insemination than is the cow. Oestrus cannot readily be detected without the presence of rams, insemination is less straightforward and the semen of rams less easy to freeze. However, Eastern Europe, South America and Australasia use AI a great deal in their sheep-breeding programmes, although its use is of much less significance in Western Europe and North America, mainly due to the high costs of handling and inseminating sheep compared with the costs of natural service in the latter countries.

Insemination of sheep

Ewes normally only display oestrous behaviour in the presence of a ram. Thus, in order to determine the time at which AI should be performed, it is necessary either to use raddled, vasectomized rams to detect oestrus, or to use pharmacological methods to induce and synchronize oestrus, so that the time of the fertile period is defined. Much of the cost benefit that exists for AI in the bovine species is therefore negated in the sheep, for substantial costs, either of maintaining rams, or of the drugs plus their administration, have to be set against the financial benefits gained from the superior carcass or wool characteristics of the progeny born to AI.

Furthermore, insemination is more difficult for sheep than cattle. It is seldom possible to pass a catheter right through the ovine cervix, so insemination has, until recently, been limited to an intracervical site. This has had two consequences. Firstly, the number of sperm is much higher than is required if an intrauterine site can be achieved

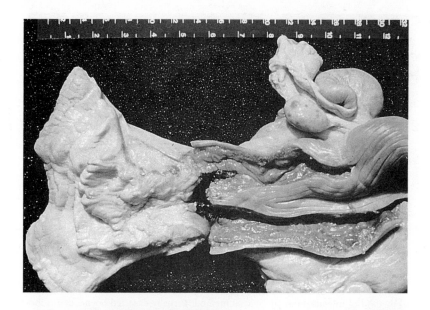

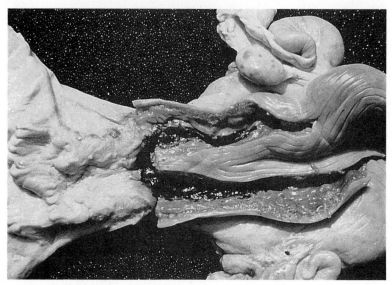

Fig. 31.4 Distribution of semen in the cow after artificial insemination. A dark-coloured dye has been placed into the uterine body and runs equally into both uterine horns. As inseminators are trained not to palpate the uterus or ovaries, they should be unaware of the side on which ovulation will occur, so semen must have access to both uterine horns.

(150–200 million total sperm: Salamon and Robinson, 1962; Langford and Marcus, 1982). Secondly, the permissible volume of inseminate is limited by the anatomy of the cervical canal to below about 0.25 ml (Evans and Maxwell, 1987). Such a high number of sperm in such a low volume of diluent means that dilution rates of ram semen are low (1:1 to 1:3), resulting in mediocre postfreezing survival of sperm; for insufficient protection can be afforded by the diluent to the sperm against cold shock and freezing damage (see Miller, 1986). A method of direct intrauterine, laparoscopic insemination has been developed which overcomes many of these difficulties. In this method, ewes are restrained in a cradle, and laparoscopy performed close to the udder, whereupon the uterus is located and semen injected into the uterine lumen (Killeen and Caffery, 1982). Conception rates to frozen semen inseminated by this method are higher than for intracervical insemination (Maxwell et al., 1984), probably because, as lower sperm numbers are required for the intrauterine insemination, more appropriate dilution levels can be used, resulting in more successful cryopreservation of semen. Conversely, the laparoscopy is technically demanding and there are far greater implications for the welfare of the ewes than with intracervical insemination. Use of laparoscopic AI is already widespread throughout Australasia, but the method has had only a limited uptake in Western Europe, mainly due to concerns for the welfare of its subjects and, as with sheep AI in general, the lack of a clear cost benefit.

Collection, handling and storage of semen
Most of the inseminations of sheep are performed using semen on the day of collection, after the addition of simple diluents. This practice remains common in Eastern Europe, where the semen is collected from farm rams and inseminated directly into the ewes of the same flock. Semen is collected by an artificial vagina or electroejaculation. The semen may be directly inseminated or diluted in buffers containing glucose, or heat-treated cows' milk, egg yolk–citrate or egg yolk–phosphate solutions and stored at 4°C until needed. Such semen has to be used within 12 hours of collection. Between 50 million and 150 million motile sperm are inseminated, in a volume of less than 0.25 ml, into the cervix. Conception rates of 65–80% are typical when this method is used in the ewes' breeding season, with a somewhat lower figure when used in out of season breeding regimes.

Freezing of semen for intracervical insemination suffers from the difficulties outlined earlier, principally the low dilution rates that can be achieved. Furthermore, the semen of many individual rams does not respond well to cryopreservation. However, the semen of rams has been relatively successfully frozen in pellet form on the surface of blocks of solid carbon dioxide (Salamon, 1971), or in paillettes in the vapour of liquid nitrogen (Fiser and Fairfull, 1984), using diluents based upon egg yolk, skimmed milk, citrate and/or lactose. Higher numbers of sperm are needed for intracervical insemination than when using fresh semen, but, despite this, conception rates are below those of natural service or fresh semen insemination (Colas, 1979). Embryonic mortality

is generally considered to be similar with frozen and fresh semen (Evans and Maxwell, 1987), although some reports exist of higher embryonic losses after the use of frozen semen.

Laparoscopic, intrauterine insemination of ewes is undoubtedly the most significant development in sheep AI, for it circumvents many of the problems of the traditional methods. The numbers of sperm required for insemination are lower and the volume of inseminate greater, allowing more appropriate dilution rates, and therefore better preservation of sperm. Hence, conception rates are closer to those of natural service and embryonic mortality is reduced to an acceptable level. The method also allows for the possibility of genuine progeny testing of rams, as semen from an individual sire can be used in many flocks, over prolonged periods of time. Laparoscopic AI is therefore already the basis of several sire referencing schemes world-wide.

Insemination of goats

As with the ewe, an intrauterine insemination is difficult to achieve in the female goat, although a higher proportion can be so inseminated than for ewes. Hence, many of the limitations of AI that apply to the sheep also pertain to this species. Nevertheless, both in the substantial flocks of goats that are maintained for milk production and in the small flocks of goats maintained by many amateur farmers, AI has been making an increasing contribution to breeding. In the Western world, AI of goats is based predominantly upon frozen semen, inseminated by an intracervical route (see Haibel, 1986).

Cryopreservation of goat semen differs from that of the ram in one important aspect; namely that the seminal plasma must be removed before dilution in, for example, yolk-containing media. A bulbourethral phospholipase coagulates egg yolk media and hydrolyses lecithin to fatty acids and spermicidal lysolecithins. Therefore, either diluents for goat semen have been based upon skimmed milk, in which goat semen survives adequately, or the seminal plasma has been removed before using egg yolk-based diluents (Corteel, 1974). Although much variation exists between individual animals, overall results with doses of 50 million motile frozen-thawed sperm,

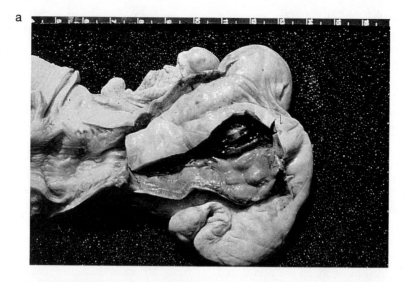

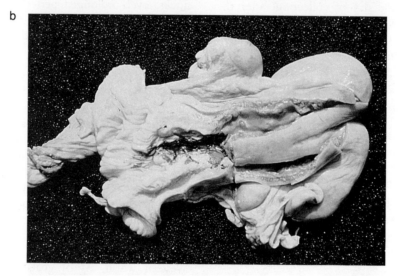

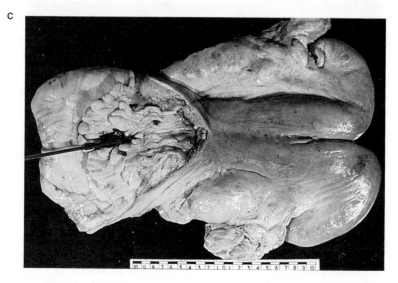

d

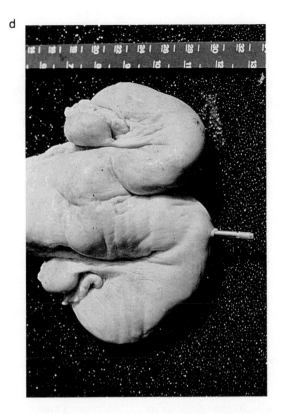

Fig. 31.5 Distribution of dye in the reproductive tract of the cow after faulty insemination. (a) Uterus twisted during insemination, occluding one uterine horn. The dye is present throughout one horn; typically the right. (b) Catheter withdrawn into the cervix during semen deposition. Some dye is present in the uterine body, but most is within the cervical canal. (c) Failure to penetrate the cervix: semen deposited in the caudal cervical canal. (d) Penetration of the uterine horn following excessively deep insemination. Such penetrations are usually associated with the use of undue force on the catheter during passage of the cervical canal.

inseminated into the uterus, are comparable with those of natural service (Ritar and Salamon, 1983).

AI OF PIGS

One of the main impetus to the use of AI in pig breeding is the possibility it confers of maintaining a closed herd, by obviating the necessity of introducing purchased boars to the herd. Furthermore, because the traits of economic importance in the pig — carcass conformation, growth rate and feed conversion efficiency — have high heritabilities and can be evaluated in the sires themselves, genetic selection can be intense, so that the potential value of AI boars in enhancing the genetic base of a breeding herd is considerable.

The use of AI in pig breeding has been greatest in the large farms of Eastern Europe and in the countries of Western Europe with high densities of pigs, such as Holland and Denmark. In the UK, uptake of AI has traditionally been at quite a low level, but in recent years a modest but sustained increase has occurred. Most inseminations are performed by farm staff, for the costs of a technician service are too great to be economically viable, other than in areas of very high pig density (see Reed, 1982, 1985).

Two main difficulties exist in pig AI. Firstly, the fertile period is not particularly easy to detect in sows (see Evans and McKenna, 1986) and, secondly, the semen of boars has a short storage life, due to its inability to adequately survive cryopreservation. Hence, for optimum conception rate and litter size, multiple inseminations are required during the oestrus period, using semen that has been extended, but not chilled (Reed, 1982). Moreover, only about 30 inseminations can be obtained from each ejaculate, due to the high number of sperm (1000–2000 million) required for each dose and the fact that double insemination is generally practised.

Collection, handling and distribution of semen

Semen is manually collected from boars every 5–7 days in the presence of a dummy sow. The pre-ejaculatory fluid is generally discarded, while the postsperm rich fraction is filtered to separate the gel fraction. Between 100 and 150 ml of sperm-rich semen is produced which, after evaluation for density, motility and sperm morphology, is diluted to between 1000 million and 2000 million sperm per insemination dose in a volume of 50–100 ml. In the UK, a volume of 70 ml is most widely used. It is necessary to use a sufficiently great volume to stimulate uterine motility in the sow, thereby ensuring that adequate numbers of sperm reach the site of fertilization. Diluents, which are designed to be used at ambient temperature, were based upon the Illinois variable temperature (IVT) diluent throughout the 1960s and 1970s (see Paquignon, 1984), but have more recently been superseded by diluents such as the Kiev (also called Guelph or EDTA diluent) and Zorlesco diluents (Haeger and Mackle, 1971; Gottardi et al., 1980). The Kiev diluent is simpler than the IVT diluent to prepare, but maintains the fertility of semen for a similar length of time. The more complicated Zorlesco diluent was claimed to maintain semen fertility for up to 12 days, although field trials have indicated that it is no greater value than the Kiev diluent. In general, diluents maintain fertility for 3 days, with fertility declining over the next 2 days.

The semen of boars does not generally respond well to cryopreservation. Recovery after thawing is poor and highly variable between individual sires, and fertility of semen is invariably substantially below that of extended semen. Typical results for frozen semen are 40–50% sows conceiving to a double insemination, with 6–8 piglets born per litter. This compares with 65–75% conception rate and 9–11 piglets per litter following double insemination with extended semen (Reed, 1982). A great deal of research into the factors affecting survival of boar semen during cryopreservation has failed to substantially improve matters (e.g. Johnson and Larson, 1987), for there appear to be two major limitations to success. Firstly,

neither egg yolk nor skimmed milk provide anything like the degree of protection against cold shock that they provide to the sperm of most other species (see Watson, 1979). Nor, indeed, do any other cheaply available or natural sources of phospholipids. Secondly, while glycerol is probably the best cryoprotectant for the sperm of boars, its toxic effects upon sperm are more pronounced in this species than in most others (Wilmut and Polge, 1974). In consequence, the numbers of sperm that are required to obtain even the mediocre conception rates that follow the use of cryopreserved semen are very high indeed: typically 5000–6000 million sperm per insemination dose (Paquignon, 1984). Hence, only about five animals can be inseminated per ejaculate, when frozen semen is used. This low dilution rate effectively limits the use of frozen semen to international traffic in pig genetics and to the preservation of gene stocks for future use.

Insemination services

1. *Inseminator service.* Technicians employed by AI centres take the semen from the centre to the farm, where they inseminate the sows. This was the main form of insemination service in Western Europe when pig AI first started, but has become progressively disfavoured, except in regions of exceptionally high pig density. Inseminator services generally provide only a single insemination of the sow in a given oestrus period, resulting in significantly lower conception rates and lower numbers of piglets per litter than are achieved by natural service. Also, the cost of a technician service is expensive in relation to the value of the progeny, especially as litter sizes are lower than with natural service. Furthermore, itinerant inseminators are significant vectors for disease transmission between farms. The trends towards closed herds and 'minimal disease' precautions on most pig farms has therefore mitigated against the use of such technicans.

2. *Semen delivery service.* This system was devised in the UK in the mid-1960s (Melrose et al., 1968), since when it has undergone a steady expansion. Processed semen is either collected from the AI centre, or is despatched by rail or post to farms, where the sows are inseminated by the farm staff. This system overcomes most of the disadvantages of technician services, in that double

inseminations can be performed, the risk of disease transmission is minimal and the cost is much reduced. It does require some technical proficiency on the part of the farm staff.

The use of AI with delivered semen has also received considerable impetus from increased use of batch management of pig herds. Thus, large groups of sows are weaned simultaneously, in the knowledge that most of them will be in oestrus at a predictable interval after weaning. Standing or advance orders are placed for the semen to inseminate these sows, with small numbers of boars kept to mate the small proportion of sows that return to oestrus outside the predicted time period, and to detect and mate animals that fail to conceive.

3. *On-farm collection and insemination programmes.* This method has been widely used on the state farms and combines of Eastern Europe and has been used in other countries to a lesser extent. In most cases, inseminations are performed with raw semen immediately after collection. However, in Spain and the USA, AI centres have provided producers with semen diluent for on-farm insemination programmes (see Crabo and Dial, 1992). This method minimizes the risk of disease transmission, but limits each farm to using the boars it has available. Access to performance/progeny-tested sires is therefore limited.

Insemination of sows

The optimum time for AI is during a 24 hour period in the middle of the 50–60 hours of oestrus. A positive reaction to the 'back-pressure' test is the best indication of the correct time for AI (Madden, 1959), although up to 30% of gilts might pass through oestrus without giving a positive reaction. Oestrous behaviour is manifested most strongly in the presence of a boar, but if a boar is not available, oestrous behaviour can be elicited by spraying an aerosol containing the androgenic steroid that is contained in the saliva of boars which is responsible for boar odour (Reed et al., 1974). Oestrous detection can be difficult where sows are tethered in stalls, and the management of AI is also difficult in herds of pigs that are kept out of doors.

Insemination is achieved (Rowson, 1962; Melrose and O'Hagen, 1969) by passing a spiral rubber catheter into the cervix of the sow. The catheter is rotated into the cervix, until its spiral groove becomes locked into the cervical canal. The cervical lock prevents the catheter from becoming dislodged if the sow moves during insemination, and prevents loss of the large volume of fluid that has to be inseminated. The patience, gentleness and quietness of the inseminator greatly affects the success of insemination.

AI OF HORSES

AI of horses has been practised for many years; indeed, legend holds that, in medieval times, semen would be stolen from the freshly served mares of one's neighbours, in order to inseminate one's own mare! Today, AI of horses is practised widely in the former USSR and in China, while, in the West, it is used in most classes of horse other than the Thoroughbred. The lack of use of AI in this breed is due to the refusal of the Thoroughbred Breeders' Association to allow registration of foals conceived by AI. Some other breed societies follow similarly restrictive practices, with the result that AI has failed to generally achieve its potential in Western horse breeding. Even in the face of venereal disease, such as the outbreak of contagious equine metritis, the restriction on the use of AI in Thoroughbreds was not relaxed, thereby precluding the substantial benefits offered by the technique in the control of such diseases. Certainly, in other breeds, AI after appropriate treatment of the semen with antibiotics has proved a most useful method of achieving pregnancies in mares that regularly have postcovering endometritis.

AI of horses is more technically demanding than it is for cattle. Firstly, collection of semen from stallions is, arguably, more difficult than from bulls, for coitus is both more prolonged and more violent in horses than cattle. Secondly, the stallion produces a fractionated ejaculate, from which the viscous, post-sperm-rich fraction requires separation and discarding (see Brinsko and Varner, 1993). Thirdly, stallion semen has proved more difficult to store than has that of the bulls, with cryopreservation proving difficult to achieve with any reliability (see Amann, 1984). Finally, the peculiarities of the oestrus period of the mare makes pinpointing the moment of peak fertility more difficult than in the cow. Thus, mares do not adequately display visible signs of oestrus in the absence of a stallion and, furthermore, the oestrous period is prolonged, so that unless the ovaries of the mare are palpated to determine the time of ovulation, repeated insemination is likely to be required to ensure that the fertile period is covered.

Handling, dilution and storage of semen

After collection, the semen of stallions requires careful temperature control to prevent damage to the sperm by cold shock (Brinsko and Varner, 1993). If the mares that are to be inseminated are close by, insemination can be performed directly, using raw semen. Alternatively, the semen can be diluted (1:3) in a simple diluent (e.g. skimmed milk plus antibiotics) and stored at 4°C for 12–48 hours before insemination. More complex diluents, together with the removal of seminal plasma by centrifugation, may extend the storage life of semen for up to 72 hours (Martin et al., 1979). However, the length of time for which semen remains fertile depends primarily upon the quality of the initial sample and upon the idiosyncrasies of individual stallions. Most equine AI is performed using direct insemination of chilled semen that has been stored for a short period (Klug, 1992; Brinsko and Varner, 1993).

Stallion semen has been successfully cryopreserved (see Pickett and Amann, 1993), using low concentrations (4%) of glycerol, in diluents containing either glucose, skimmed milk and egg yolk (Rajamannan, 1968), or lactose, EDTA and egg yolk (Nishikawa et al. 1972; Cochran et al., 1984). In all cases, the seminal plasma was removed before freezing. Freezing (see Amann and Pickett, 1987) may be undertaken in controlled-rate freezers, using moderate (-10°C/min between $+20$ and -15°C, -25°C/min between -15 and -120°C) freezing rates, or, using less accurately controlled conditions, in the vapour of liquid nitrogen or as pellets on the surface of blocks of solid carbon dioxide. The timing of insemination in relation to ovulation is critical when cryopreserved semen is used, with even less tolerance than for unfrozen semen.

Insemination of mares

Unless palpation of the ovaries of the mare is undertaken to determine the timing of ovulation, AI needs to be performed every other day throughout oestrus when chilled, extended semen is used, or daily if the semen has been cryopreserved. However, if the presence of an ovulable follicle is determined, and insemination of frozen–thawed semen performed within 6 hours of ovulation (Kloppe et al., 1988) acceptable success rates can be achieved. Rather more latitude exists for chilled semen: inseminations with semen from stallions of high fertility produce acceptable pregnancy rates within 48 hours of ovulation, although less inseminations of fertile stallions need to be within 12–24 hours. Thus, at best, similar success rates are achievable when natural service, chilled, or cryopreserved (with adequate postfreezing motility) semen is used. In most field studies, however, pregnancy rates achieved with frozen–thawed semen are significantly lower than with other methods (see Pickett and Amann, 1993).

Insemination is best performed with the mare restrained in stocks. After applying a tail bandage and cleaning the perineal area, a hand is inserted into the vagina and the cervix located. The index finger is inserted into the cervix and an insemination catheter passed through the vagina, then alongside the index finger and, so, into the uterus. Debate exists over the numbers of sperm and volume of semen required for adequate fertility. Initially, inseminations with chilled, extended semen used 1000–2000 million sperm in a volume of 10–50 ml (Arthur et al., 1989). Insemination doses have thereafter been progressively reduced to a minimum of around 100 million motile sperm, although it is possible that the semen of fertile stallions could be further diluted (Pace and Sullivan, 1975; Pickett, 1980). However, there is very considerable variation between stallions, even in the survival of diluted and chilled semen. For routine insemination with chilled semen, around 250–500 million total sperm are used (Klug, 1992; Brinsko and Varner, 1993). Sperm numbers required for acceptable fertility with frozen–thawed semen are of the order of 100–200 million motile sperm.

AI OF DOGS

It was upon the dog that the earliest recorded studies of AI were undertaken, by the Italian natural philosopher Spallanzani. Despite such an impeccable pedigree, relatively little demand exists for AI of dogs, with a significant degree of resistance to it by many breed societies. Thus, AI of dogs is limited to two main circumstances. Firstly, it is used where copulation is not possible. Secondly AI is employed as a means of using sires that are geographically remote from the bitch, particularly where these reside in a different country. For many breed societies, this latter circumstance is the only one under which they will allow registration of puppies conceived by AI.

Handling and storage of dog semen

Semen is collected from the dog by digital manipulation or an artificial vagina. The pre-ejaculatory fluid, sperm-rich fraction and a little of the post-ejaculatory (prostatic) fluid is collected. If the reason for AI is inability to copulate, the whole ejaculate may then be immediately inseminated into the bitch's vagina. However, it is more common, even in this circumstance, to dilute the semen, if only so that multiple inseminations can be performed.

Dog semen can be stored in a chilled condition at 4°C, after dilution in simple diluents (e.g. skimmed milk), for 24–72 hours (Harrop, 1962). This is generally long enough for at least two inseminations to be performed on the bitch, or for air freight transport to most international destinations. Hence, this method is very widely used in dog AI.

Insemination of bitches

The bitch has a prolonged period of receptivity to the male, but a relatively short fertile period. When natural service is used, many breeders allow bitches only a single mating, which typically occurs 12 days after the onset of pre-oestrous bleeding. For successful AI, much closer attention to the time of the fertile period is needed, with the timing of ovulation predicted from vaginal cytology or the preovulatory rise in circulating progesterone concentrations. Timing of insemination in relation to ovulation is particularly crucial when cryopreserved semen is used, although more latitude exists where chilled semen is used (Jeffcoate and Lindsay, 1989; Linde-Forsberg and Forsberg, 1989, 1993; Morton and Bruce, 1989).

Where the reason for AI is failure of copulation, semen is collected from the dog by digital manipulation, and the whole ejaculate may be inseminated into the vagina of the bitch immediately after collection. It may, however, be preferable to dilute the semen, inseminating one portion immediately and the remainder 48 hours later. Similarly, where chilled semen has been transported from the sire to the bitch, insemination may be performed upon receipt of the semen and 48 hours later. It is therefore imperative to ensure that the recipient bitch is approaching the fertile period of oestrus before semen is collected.

When fresh or chilled semen is used, intravaginal insemination is undertaken, with the semen deposited as close as possible to the external os of the cervix (see Burke, 1986). The semen may be deposited through a shortened bovine insemination catheter, which may require the use of a speculum to be guided into the correct site. Once inseminated, the hindquarters of the bitch should be raised for a few minutes, to prevent retrograde loss of semen. Some authors recommend inserting one or two fingers into the vulva after insemination, in order to promote the motility of the female genital tract that normally occurs during the copulatory tie. Intrauterine insemination has been described (Andersen, 1975) and is sometimes recommended for use with cryopreserved semen.

The fertility achieved in canine AI primarily depends upon achieving a correct insemination timing in relation to that of ovulation in the bitch. The inherent fertility of the dog is also of importance, with the longevity of his sperm in the female tract being a critical determinant of fertility. Dogs with long-lived sperm can achieve pregnancies even if the timing of insemination is not optimal, whereas with dogs whose sperm have poor survival, sperm death is more likely to have occurred prior to ovulation under such circumstances. Where frozen semen is used, timing of insemination is critical and, as with most species, there is very considerable sire-to-sire variation in the ability of sperm to survive cryopreservation.

REFERENCES

Almquist, J. O. and Zaugg, N. L. (1974) *J. Dairy Sci.*, **57**, 1211.

Amann, R. P. (1984) *Proc. 10th Int. Cong. Anim. Reprod. AI, Urbana*, **4**, II 28.

Amann, R. P. and Pickett, B. W. (1987) *Equine Vet. Sci.*, **7**, 145.

Andersen, K. (1975) *Zuchthygiene*, **10**, 1.

Arthur, G. H., Noakes, D. E. and Pearson, H. (1989) *Veterinary Reproduction and Obstetrics*, 6th edn. London: Baillière Tindall.

Asbury, A. C. (1986) In: *Current Therapy in Theriogenology*, 2nd edn, ed. D. A. Morrow, pp. 718–722. Philadelphia: Saunders.

Ashfar, A., Stuart, P. and Huck, R. A. (1966) *Vet. Rec.*, **78**, 512.

Ayalon, N., Weiss, Y. and Lewis, I. (1968) *Proc. 6th Int. Cong. Anim. Reprod. AI, Paris*, **1**, 393.

Barlow, R. M., Nettleton, P. F., Gardiner, A., Greig, A., Campbell, J. R. and Bonn, J. M. (1986) *Vet. Rec.*, **118**, 321.

Barrett, G. R., Casida, L. E. and Lloyd, C. A. (1948) *J. Dairy Sci.*, **31**, 682.

Bedford, J. M. and Hoskins, D. D. (1990) In: *Marshall's Physiology of Reproduction*, ed. G. E. Lamming, Vol. 2, pp. 379–568. Edinburgh: Churchill Livingstone.

Blackshaw, A. W. (1954) *Aust. J. Biol. Sci.*, **7**, 573.

Blackshaw, A. W. and Salisbury, G. W. (1957) *J. Dairy Sci.*, **40**, 1099.

Bowen, R. A. and Howard, T. H. (1984) *Amer. J. Vet. Res.*, **45**, 1386.

Brinsko, S. P. and Varner, D. D. (1993) In: *Equine Reproduction*, ed. A. O. McKinnon and J. L. Voss, pp. 790–797. Philadelphia: Lea and Febiger.

Burke, T. J. (1986) *Small Animal Reproduction and Infertility*. Philadelphia: Lea and Febiger.

Callis, J. J. and McKercher, P. D. (1980) *Bov. Pract.*, **15**, 170.

Cassou, R. (1964) *Proc. 5th Int. Cong. Anim. Reprod. AI, Trento*, p. 540.

Chapman, Lucas, M. H., Herbert, C. N. and Goodey, R. G. (1979) *Vet. Sci. Commun.*, **3**, 137.

Clay, C. M., Squires, E. L. Amman, R. P. and Pickett, B. W. (1984) *Proc. 10th Int. Cong. Anim. Reprod. AI, Urbana*, **2**, 187 (Abstr.).

Cochran, J. D., Amann, R. P., Froman, D. P. and Pickett, B. W. (1984) *Theriogenology*, **22**, 25.

Colas, G. (1979) *Livestock Prod. Sci.*, **6**, 153.

Corteel, J. M. (1974) *Ann. Biol. Anim. Biochim. Biophys.*, **14**, 741.

Corteel, J. M. and Paquignon, M. (1984) *Proc. 10th Int. Cong. Anim. Reprod. AI, Urbana*, **4**, II 20.

Crabo, B. G. and Dial, G. D. (1992) *Vet. Clin. N. Amer. Food Anim. Pr.*, **8**, 533.

Davis, I. S., Bratton, R. W. and Foote, R. H. (1963) *J. Dairy Sci.*, **46**, 333.

Evans, L. E. and McKenna, D. J. (1986) In: *Current Therapy in Theriogenology*, 2nd edn, ed. D. A. Morrow, pp. 946–949. Philadelphia: Saunders.

Evans, G. and Maxwell, W. M. C. (1987) *Salamon's Artificial Insemination of Sheep and Goats*. Sydney: Butterworth.

Farrant, J. (1980) In: *Low Temperature Preservation in Medicine and Biology*, ed. M. J. Ashwood-Smith and J. Farrant, pp. 1–17. Tunbridge Wells: Pitman Medical.

Fiser, P. S. and Fairfull, R. W. (1984) *Cryobiology*, **21**, 542.

Flipsse, R. J., Patton, S. and Almquist, J. O. (1954) *J. Dairy Sci.*, **37**, 1205.

Foote, R. H. (1967) *J. Dairy Sci.*, **50**, 1338.

Foote, R. H. (1969) In: *Reproduction in Domestic Animals*, 2nd edn, ed. H. H. Cole and P. T. Crupps, pp. 313–353. New York: Academic Press.

Foote, R. H. (1970) *J. Dairy Sci.*, **53**, 1478.

Foote, R. H. (1979) *J. Dairy Sci.*, **62**, 355.

Foote, R. H., Gray, L. C., Young, D. C. and Dunn, H. O. (1960) *J. Dairy Sci.*, **43**, 1330.

Garlick, G. (1939) *Vet. Med.*, **34**, 43.

Gottardi, L., Brunel, L. and Zanelli, L. (1980) *Proc. 9th Int. Cong. Anim. Reprod. AI, Madrid*, **5**, 49.

Grahn, T. C., Fahning, M. L. and Zemjanis, R. (1984) *J. Amer. Vet. Med. Assn*, **185**, 429.

Haeger, O. and Mackle, N. (1971) *Dtsche Tierarztl. Wochensch.*, **78**, 395.

Haibel, G. K. (1986) In: *Current Therapy in Theriogenology*, 2nd edn, ed. D. A. Morrow, pp. 624–626. Philadelphia: Saunders.

Harrop, A. E. (1962) In: *The Semen of Animals and Artificial Insemination*, ed. J. P. Maule, pp. 304–315. Farnham Royal: Commonwealth Agricultural Bureau.

Iritani, A. (1980) *Proc. 9th Int. Cong. Reprod. AI, Madrid*, **1**, 115.

Jeffcoate, I. A. and Lindsay, F. E. F. (1989) *J. Reprod. Fertil. Suppl.*, **39**, 277.

Johnson, L. A. and Larson, K. (1987) *Deep Freezing of Boar Semen*. Uppsala: Swedish University of Agricultural Sciences.

Jondet, R. (1964) *Proc. 5th Int. Cong. Anim. Reprod. AI, Trento*, p. 463.

Keith, J. R. (1981) *Vet. Med. Small Anim. Clin.*, **76**, 1043.

Kahrs, R. F., Gibbs, E. P. J. and Larsen, R. J. (1980) *Theriogenology*, **14**, 151.

Killeen, I. D. and Caffery, G. J. (1982) *Aust. Vet. J.*, **59**, 95.

Kloppe, L. H., Varner, D. D., Elmore, R. G., Bretzlaff, K. N. and Shull, J. W. (1988) *Theriogenology*, **29**, 429.

Klug, E. (1992) *Anim. Reprod. Sci.*, **28**, 39.

Landa, C. A. and Almquist, J. O. (1979) *J. Anim. Sci.*, **49**, 1190.

Linde-Forsberg, C. and Forsberg, M. (1989) *J. Reprod. Fertil. Suppl.*, **39**, 299.

Linde-Forsberg, C. and Forsberg, M. (1993) *J. Reprod. Fertil. Suppl.*, **47**, 313.

Madden, D. H. L. (1959) *Vet. Rec.*, **72**, 227.

Mann, T. (1964) *The Biochemistry of Semen and the Male Reproductive Tract*, 2nd edn. London: Methuen.

Marlowe, T. J. (1964) *J. Anim. Sci.*, **23**, 454.

Martin, J. C., Klug, E. and Gunzel, A. R. (1979) *J. Reprod. Fertil. Suppl.*, **27**, 47.

Maxwell, W. M. C., Butler, L. C. and Wilson, H. R. (1984) *J. Agr. Sci. (Cambridge)*, **102**, 233.

Melrose, D. R. (1956) *Proc. 3rd Int. Cong. Anim. Reprod. AI, Cambridge*, **3**, 68.

Melrose, D. R. (1962) In: *The Semen of Animals and Artificial Insemination*, ed. J. P. Maule, pp. 1–181. Farnham Royal: Commonwealth Agricultural Bureau.

Melrose, D. R. and O'Hagen, C. (1959) *Proc. 6th Int. Cong. Anim. Reprod., The Hague*, **4**, 855.

Melrose, D. R., Reed, H. C. B. and Pratt, J. H. (1968) *Proc. 6th Int. Cong. Anim. Reprod. AI, Paris*, p. 181 (Abstr.).

Milk Marketing Board (1967) *Report of Breeding and Production Organisation, 1966–1967*, No. 17, p. 123.

Miller, S. J. (1986) In: *Current Therapy in Theriogenology*, 2nd edn, ed. D. A. Morrow, pp. 884–887. Philadelphia: Saunders.

Moller, K., Macmillan, K. L. and Shannon, P. (1972) *N. Z. J. Agr. Res.*, **15**, 252.

Morgan, W. J. B., Melrose, D. R. and Stewart, D. L. (1959) *J. Comp. Pathol.*, **69**, 257.

Morton, D. B. and Bruce, S. G. (1989) *J. Reprod. Fertil. Suppl.*, **39**, 311.

Nishikawa, Y., Iritani, A. and Shinomiya, S. (1972) *Proc. 7th Int. Cong. Anim. Reprod. AI, Munich*, **2**, 306 (Abstr.).

Olds, D. and Sheath, D. M. (1954) *Kentucky Agric. Expt. Sta. Bull.*, 605.

Pace, M. M. and Sullivan, J. J. (1975) *J. Reprod. Fertil. Suppl.*, **23**, 115.

Paquignon, M. (1984) In: *The Male in Farm Animal Reproduction*, ed. M. Courot, pp. 202–218. Dordrecht: Martinus Nijhoff.

Paquignon, M. (1985) In: *Deep Freezing of Boar Semen*, ed. L. A. Johnson and K. Larson, pp. 129–145. Uppsala: Swedish University of Agricultural Sciences.

Parkinson, T. J. and Whitfield, C. H. (1987) *Theriogenology*, **27**, 781.

Pickett, B. W. (1980) In: *Current Veterinary Therapy*, ed. D. A. Morrow, p. 692. Philadelphia: Saunders.

Pickett, B. W. and Amann, R. P. (1993) In: *Equine Reproduction*, ed. A. O. McKinnon and J. L. Voss, pp. 769–789. Philadelphia: Lea and Febiger.

Pickett, B. W., Fowler, A. K. and Cowen, W. A. (1961) *J. Dairy Sci.*, **43**, 281.

Polge, C. (1953) *Vet. Rec.*, **65**, 557.

Polge, C., Smith, A. U. and Parkes, A. S. (1949) *Nature*, **164**, 666.

Radostits, O. M., Blood, D. C. and Gay, C. C. (1994) *Veterinary Medicine*, 8th edn. London: Baillière Tindall.

Rajamannan, A. H. J. (1968) *Proc. 6th Int. Cong. Anim. Reprod. AI, Paris*.

Rasbech, N. O. (1951) Cited by *Vet. Rec.*, **63**, 657.

Reed, H. C. B. (1982) In: *Control of Pig Reproduction*, ed. D. J. A. Cole and G. R. Foxcroft, pp. 65–90. London: Butterworth.

Reed, H. C. B. (1985) In: *Deep Freezing of Boar Semen*, ed. L. A. Johnson and K. Larson, pp. 225–238. Uppsala: Swedish University of Agricultural Sciences.

Reed, H. C. B., Melrose, D. R. and Patterson, R. L. S. (1974) *Brit. Vet. J.*, **130**, 61.

Ritar, A. J. and Salamon, S. (1983) *Aust. J. Biol. Sci.*, **36**, 49.

Roberts, S. J. (1986) *Veterinary Obstetrics and Genital Diseases*, 3rd edn. Ithaca, New York: self-published.

Rowson, L. E. A. (1962) In: *The Semen of Animals and Artificial Insemination*, ed. J. P. Maule, pp. 263–280. Farnham Royal: Commonwealth Agricultural Bureau.

Salamon, S. (1971) *Aust. J. Biol. Sci.*, **24**, 183.

Salamon, S. and Robinson, T. J. (1962) *Aust. J. Agr. Res.*, **13**, 271.

Salisbury, G. W. and VanDemark, N. L. (1961) *Physiology of Reproduction and Artificial Insemination*. San Francisco: Freeman.

Salisbury, G. W., VanDemark, N. L. and Lodge, J. R. (1978) *Physiology of Reproduction and Artificial Insemination of Cattle*, 2nd edn. San Francisco: Freeman.

Shannon, P. (1968) *Proc. N. Z. Soc. Anim. Prod.*, **28**, 23.

Stewart, D. L. (1964) *Proc. 5th Int. Int. Cong. Anim. Reprod. AI, Trento*, p. 617.

Sullivan, J. J. and Elliott, F. I. (1968) *Proc. 6th Int. Cong. Anim. Reprod. AI, Paris*, **2**, 1307.

Suter, D., Chow, P. Y. W. and Martin, I. C. A. (1979) *Biol. Reprod.*, **20**, 505.

Unal, M. B., Berndtson, W. E. and Picketts, B. W. (1978) *J. Dairy Sci.*, **61**, 83.

VanDemark, N. L., Koyama, K. and Lodge, J. R. (1965) *J. Dairy Sci.*, **48**, 586.

Watson, P. F. (1979) *Oxford Rev. Reprod. Biol.*, **1**, 283.

Watson, P. F. (1990) In: *Marshall's Physiology of Reproduction*, ed. G. E. Lamming, Vol. 2, pp. 747–869. Edinburgh: Churchill Livingstone.

Watson, P. F. and Plummer, J. M. (1985) In: *Deep Freezing of Boar Semen*, ed. L. A. Johnson and K. Larson, pp. 113–127. Uppsala: Swedish University of Agricultural Sciences.

Willett, E. L. and Salisbury, G. W. (1942) *Mem. Cornell Univ. Agric. Exp. Stn*, 249.

Willett, E. L., Ohms, J. I., Frank, A. H., Bryner, J. H. and Bartlett, D. E. (1955) *J. Dairy Sci.*, **38**, 1369.

Wilmut, I. and Polge, C. (1974) *J. Reprod. Fertil.*, **38**, 105.

7

Part Seven

Exotic Species

The one-humped (dromedary) camel is economically important in northern Africa, particularly Sudan and Somalia, as well as in the Arabian states and in the Indian subcontinent; the two-humped (Bactrian) camel is bred mainly in Russia and Central Asia. Many camels are exported from the Sudan and Somalia to Egypt and Sauda Arabia.

She-camels reach puberty at 2 years but are not usually mated until 3 years. Male camels are sexually active at 3 years but are not usually used as stud animals until 5 years. Both sexes breed throughout their lives but it is customary to breed from the female in alternate years, the gestation period being 370–375 days.

MALE REPRODUCTION

When sexually mature, male camels show an annual rut, roughly from November to July, after which they are sexually quiescent. During the rut, the temperament changes towards an aggressive, less tractable nature, including a predisposition to fight other males and an inclination to bite other animals, as well as human beings. Rutting males are notoriously unpredictable and should be approached with due regard to their potential aggression. When urinating they stand with hindlegs spread apart and spray the urine around their hindquarters by vigorous movements of the tail. A prominent feature of rutting behaviour is frothing at the mouth and loud vocal gurgling, accompanied by the protrusion of the markedly oedematous and mobile soft palate. An additional peculiarity is a profuse secretion of fetid fluid from the poll glands. The rutting peculiarities of male camels are especially marked in the presence of an oestrous female, and when the male smells her urine he displays the characteristic flehmen response.

The testicles are relatively small. They are descended at birth. The non-erect penis is directed backwards and its extremity ends in a hook; otherwise it resembles that of the bull, and extension of it at coitus depends mainly on the straightening of the sigmoid flexure of the organ.

FEMALE REPRODUCTION

The structure and function of the genitalia of the she-camel show several noteworthy features. The uterus is bicornuate, with a well-developed uterine body, from which the two horns diverge and taper anteriorly to give a combined uterine shape intermediate between that of the letters Y and T. The left horn is longer than the right, even in the fetus. The endometrium shows irregularly raised mainly longitudinal folds, which are more conspicuous in the right horn. The cervix resembles that of the cow but has five annular mucosal folds. A few centimetres behind the cervix is a concentric fringe-like fold of the anterior vaginal mucosa, which tends to obscure the os uteri externum, and behind it are several progressively less prominent circular folds.

The uterine tubes are 22–24 cm long. Their width increases towards the ovarian end where the tubes are obviously funnel-shaped.

The mesosalpinx and the mesovarium together form a very well developed bursa which closely invests the ovary.

The size and shape of the ovaries vary with their content of follicles and corpora lutea. The anoestrous ovary is roughly oval and thin, measuring about 4 × 2.5 × 0.5 cm. Its surface is uneven and shows many small follicles and, in mature animals, projections of old corpora lutea. The latter, corpora albicantia, are cream-coloured and up to 0.6 cm in diameter.

Mature follicles and current corpora of the breeding season project from the main contour of the ovary and give the latter an exaggerated, lobular form. Graafian follicles may grow to a size of 10 cm in diameter, but a commoner ovulating size is 1.5–3.0 cm. The mature follicle can easily be detached from the ovary as a discrete sphere by gentle pressure at its attachment. Follicles also develop, but do not ovulate, at the beginning and end of pregnancy. The wall of the mature follicle is vascular; the follicular fluid is at first yellowish and later red.

Because ovulation is a sequel to coitus, corpora lutea are to be expected only in pregnant camels; however, smaller apparently functional corpora lutea occur and probably they are a legacy of early pregnancy failures. The young corpus luteum is soft and spherical, brownish on section, with a central blood clot. It can be detached from the ovary by digital pressure exerted at its base. The mature corpus luteum is a compact sphere of 2.6 cm diameter and flesh-coloured, with a central area of grey connective tissue. Older corpora lutea have a greenish or bluish-grey external appearance. Corpora lutea persist throughout pregnancy and the established corpus luteum cannot be detached from the ovary by finger pressure.

Corpora lutea presumably from previous pregnancies (corpora albicantia) appear as creamy bodies of up to 0.6 cm diameter in the substance of, or projecting from, the flat main body of the ovary.

By repeated rectal palpation of the genital organs of she-camels during the breeding season Musa (1975) found that a period of about 6 days is required for a developing follicle to reach its full size (of 1.5–3 cm, but occasionally up to 10 cm); full size is maintained for an average of 13 days and then follicular regression occurs during the following 8 days. Another follicle then begins to develop in the other ovary. During the breeding season, from December to June in the Sudan, there are six or seven of these follicular cycles in unmated animals. This breeding season is followed by an anoestrous period of 6 months duration. However, camel breeders in Saudi Arabia say that well-fed camels will cycle and breed throughout the year, but in natural conditions food shortage probably decreases breeding activity. The author's experience in that country was that new-born camels could be seen throughout the whole period from September to May and that there was a concentration of births in December, January and February.

The left and right ovaries function equally and ovulate alternately. Because ovulation is induced by coitus the length of oestrus depends on whether and when mating occurs. In the absence of a male, oestrus may last about 2 weeks, whereas if copulation occurs on the first day of oestrus, receptivity may disappear after 3 days. Twin ovulation occurs in 14% of matings (Musa, 1975).

During the last decade, studies in China on the ovulation mechanism of the Bactrian camel (Chen et al., 1985) revealed that ovulation is induced by a factor or factors in seminal plasma. Furthermore, ovulation could be stimulated by either intrauterine or intramuscular injection of seminal plasma, while bovine seminal plasma had the same effect. The intervals from the intramuscular injection to the subsequent luteinizing hormone (LH) peak in peripheral blood, and to ovulation, were the same as those that follow natural mating. The authors concluded that there is a gonadotrophin-releasing (GnRH)-like hormone in seminal plasma.

The signs of oestrus are restlessness, bleating, vulval swelling and mucous vaginal discharge. The she-camel urinates and moves its tail up and down in rapid succession on the approach of the male or when hearing the gurgling voice of the rutting male. At range, the rutting male pursues the oestrous female and, on catching up with her, presses his head on her neck and induces her to sit down. The male then mounts in a squatting posture. Copulation lasts from 8 to 15 minutes; it is accompanied by much male oral frothing and gurgling, with intermittent protrusion of the soft palate, and by female bleating. During these mating activities, which are interspersed with several bouts of male pelvic thrusting and correspondingly louder vocal responses from the female, the rest of the herd becomes alerted and assembles in a circle round the copulating pair. During the phase of follicular growth the uterus develops an increasing tone, and when the follicle is ripe the cervix will admit two fingers.

Pregnancy

Despite the equal function of the right and left ovaries, 99% of pregnancies are in the left horn (and uterine body) and although the incidence of twin ovulation is 14%, twin births occur to an extent of only 0.4% (Musa, 1975). Embryonic migration from the right horn to left is frequent and seems always to occur when the right ovary ovulates and the left ovary does not. When both ovaries ovulate at the same oestrus embryos develop initially in both horns but the one in the right horn dies when it reaches a size of 2–3 cm. This embryonic death occurs despite the coalescence of the chorions of two embryos. Presumably, allantoic vascular anastomosis does not take place, as in the bovine, and there is no record of a free-martin among the small number of twins born. It is a unique biological curiosity that successful placentation of a right-horn embryo does not develop in the corresponding horn, whereas the placenta of a left-horn embryo regularly intrudes into the right horn and develops extensively throughout the right horn.

As in the cow, the allantois of the camel elongates quickly and soon protrudes from the left horn into the uterine body and the right horn. Because the uterine body is relatively large, the shape of the whole placenta resembles more closely that of the mare than the cow. Moreover, the camel placenta is diffuse, like the mare's, not cotyledonary.

The amount of allantoic fluid increases from about 1.5 litres at a fetal body length 0–10 cm to approximately 5–6 litres at a body length 11–20 cm. This volume is maintained fairly constantly until 90–100 cm, when it rises to 6 litres; finally, at a fetal body length of 101–107 cm, the allantoic volume is about 8 litres. The allantoic fluid is like pale urine and sometimes contains yellow-brown hippomanes. From the gestation stage when the fetal body length is 41 cm, Musa (1975) noticed an inner amnion which very closely invests all the fetus except its orifices.

The volume of amniotic fluid rises from 13 ml at a fetal body length of 0–10 cm to a final volume of nearly 1 litre, i.e. its amount is always small relative to the allantoic fluid. The amniotic fluid is usually watery but sometimes cloudy and brown with bits of meconium and hippomanes.

Fetal growth is of a linear pattern. Posterior presentations predominate (54–60%) from early pregnancy to a fetal body length 41–50 cm, at which point the situation changes to an anterior presentation of 51%. Thenceforward anterior presentations increase sharply to 93% at a fetal body length of 61–70 cm and then to the final gestation

presentation of nearly 100% anterior. By post-mortem manipulation, Musa and Abusineina (1976) found they could not alter the presentation beyond the stage of 61–70 cm fetal body length. There is no tendency in late pregnancy for the amnion to separate from the allantochorion as it may do in the cow.

Pregnancy diagnosis

An intriguing and commonly held belief among camel owners is that a she-camel, when pregnant, will curl its tail dorsally on being approached by a rutting male. Until recently, veterinarians have regarded this sign as unreliable. However, Abdel Rahim and Al-Nazeer (1992), in a well-conducted study of housed camels, have stated that from 2 weeks after mating this is a constant reaction of pregnant camels to a male-camel approach.

Clinical methods

Rectal palpation. Barmintsev (1951), working with the Bactrian camel, and Musa and Abusineina (1978), using the dromedary, have given accounts of the rectal method of diagnosis. The technique of palpation of the genital organs is the same as for the cow but the she-camel needs to be restrained in the sitting position. In connection with early diagnosis it is important to remember four features of camel reproduction:

1. Large corpora lutea are only present in pregnancy.
2. 99% of pregnancies are in the left horn.
3. The empty (or early pregnant) right horn is congenitally shorter than the left.
4. The amount of fetal fluid at all stages of camel pregnancy is less than in the cow.

From the foregoing it is clear that the presence of a palpable corpus luteum in one or both ovaries is a very strong indication of pregnancy. However, a corpus luteum would form after a sterile mating and would be present initially in the cases where embryonic death occurs; but in both these instances the corpus luteum would not persist.

The earliest palpable swelling of the pregnant (left) uterine horn is at 1 month in the Bactrian camel according to Barmintsev. In the dromedary, however, Musa and Abusineina are emphatic that no swelling is palpable until the eighth week, when the whole of the left horn is uniformly enlarged. At this time both ovaries (one or both with corpora lutea), together with the uterus, are within the pelvis. It should be noted that because the camel placenta is non-cotyledonary it is not possible to 'slip the fetal membrane' as in the cow. By the eighth week, vaginal palpation or inspection reveals a plug of adhesive mucus in the os uteri externum.

At the end of the third month the pregnant left horn is clearly larger and softer and in front of the non-pregnant right horn. It is at the pelvic brim and its corresponding ovary is in the abdomen. At the fourth month the uterus is just in front of the pelvic brim but most of it is palpable. A month later the limits of the uterus cannot be defined, although its dorsal surface is still palpable. During the sixth month, and for the remainder of pregnancy, the fetus can be palpated and the ovary on the non-pregnant (right) side can be felt until the tenth or eleventh month. From the seventh month individual parts of the fetus, namely head and legs, can be identified. External observation of the right flank reveals spontaneous fetal movements from the ninth month and the fetus can be ballotted from the tenth month.

In the eleventh month the vulva is slightly swollen and hypertrophy of the udder is first noticed. In the following month there is abdominal enlargement and the camel is lethargic. The caudal part of the uterus now projects backwards and occupies the anterior two-thirds of the pelvis. The sacrosciatic ligaments begin to relax.

In the thirteenth month relaxation of the pelvic ligaments is pronounced, tumefaction of the vulva is marked and hypertrophy of the udder is more evident. The fetus can be ballotted from both flanks.

Incidentally, regarding the length of gestation in the camel, almost incredible variations of from 308 to 440 days have been given. The mean duration is probably around 375 days.

Ultrasonography. Diagnosis of pregnancy by transrectal ultrasound scanning can be made consistently at 17–18 days after mating (Tinson and MacKinnon, 1992). The conceptus then appears as a discrete, non-echogenic, fluid-filled structure in the left horn, of about 4–6 mm diameter and 10–15 mm length. The embryo is first visible at about 20 days, when its heart beat is also detectable, and the amnion can be recognized as a slightly echogenic band around the embryo at about day 35.

Electronic Pulse Detector. It is expected that this technique could be successfully used from mid-pregnancy, applying the probe to the right flank or above the uterus per rectum.

Laboratory methods

Progesterone Test. Because persistent corpora lutea are said to be present only in pregnancy, a progesterone assay carried out after a suitable interval from copulation should be effective in distinguishing pregnancy from non-pregnancy. This has been confirmed by Elias et al. and by Xu et al. in 1985, and later by other investigators, as follows: unmated and anovulatory camels have basal progesterone levels; those which ovulate but do not conceive show a peak value at 6–10 days after mating which declines to the baseline by day 12; pregnant camels show raised progesterone levels throughout gestation. Obviously, embryonic death could occur after a positive test result, and it remains to be determined in what percentage of instances this would negate the result. Presumably milk, in lactating animals, or blood could be used for this test.

Gonadotrophin Test. El Azab and Musa (1976) have demonstrated the presence of follicle-stimulating hormone (FSH) in the blood of pregnant camels using immature female mice as in the method devised by Cole and Saunders (1935) in the mare. The mouse ovaries showed marked follicular activity when injected with the blood of camels pregnant with fetuses of fetal body lengths between 11 and 58 cm. However, the authors did not mention any spate of follicular activity in the maternal camel ovaries as occurs in the mare when pregnant mare serum gonadotrophin is present. The present author has seen no such activity in his study of the pregnant camel, neither has he found endometrial cups which are the source of equine gonadotrophin. The source of the gonadotrophic factor in the camel is therefore unknown but it is presumably of placental origin.

Oestrogen Test. El Ghannam et al. (1974) found that the Cuboni test for the demonstration of oestrogenic substances in urine can be successfully applied for pregnancy diagnosis in camels. The technique is the same as that described for the mare. In this connection no inordinate growth of fetal gonads during the second half of pregnancy like that of the mare has been seen in the camel. In the mare the fetal gonads are believed to be the source of the large amount of oestrogen present in the blood and urine of the mare.

Parturition

The premonitory signs of parturition are abdominal distension, mammary hypertrophy, with presence of colostrum, and oedema of the vulva. Most camels calve in winter and spring. Almost 100% of presentations are anterior.

First-stage labour lasts 24–48 hours and the period of expulsion is half an hour. If the placenta is retained for more than a day the mother is said to become ill due to the development of endometritis.

During the second stage the she-camel adopts a sitting posture. The allantochorion ruptures before reaching the vulva. There are bouts of straining at intervals of 30–60 seconds and the fetal nose, covered by the amnion, appears first. Later one front foot and then the other are protruded alongside the head and with further straining they are both extended well beyond the head. Maximum straining effort then leads to complete emergence of the head and the rest of the body quickly follows. One's comparative obstetric impression of second-stage labour in the camel is of a rather elegant, untrammelled expulsion of a well-lubricated and beautifully streamlined fetal body. The umbilical cord ruptures as the offspring wriggles away from its mother or when the mother gets up, as she does immediately after the birth. She noses and nibbles at the offspring but does not lick it as do other animals.

During the third stage the she-camel shows intermittent restlessness and may get up and down several times. The afterbirth progressively emerges and includes large retention sacs of allantochorion, containing up to 5 litres of allantoic fluid which presumably exert a gravitational pull on that part of the afterbirth still attached. The fetal membranes may be completely expelled soon after the fetus or, more commonly, within about 30 minutes of birth. They are not eaten by the mother. The young camel can stand, after many unsuccessful attempts, within half an hour.

Dystocia

There is a scarcity of published information. However, conversations with Bedouin camel owners indicate their familiarity with the recognition and treatment of dispositional dystocias such as carpal flexion, lateral deviation of the head and hock and hip flexion, although posterior presentation is uncommon. Fetopelvic disproportion, monstrosities and transverse presentations are rare and the frequency of twin births is of the order of 0.1–0.4%. Uterine inertia occurs to a small extent; Petris (1956) recorded two cases of torsion of the uterus. In these respects the camel resembles the mare rather than the cow and the overall impression is that the incidence of camel dystocia is very low.

In the correction of limb and neck flexions, where substantial fetal retropulsion is required because of the length of the neck and the limbs, the she-camel is placed, front-end first, into a deep pit, excavated in the sand. Head and limb extension seems much more difficult to achieve than in the cow. Limited experience indicates that the camel fetus survives dystocia better than the equine fetus and that the camel is a good subject for caesarean operation in cases of irreducible malpresentation with a living fetus. When a malpositioned fetus is dead, fetotomy using Thygesen's embryotome seems feasible. For caesarean operations the camel is cast on its right side under xylazine sedation and the operation is performed under regional infiltration anaesthesia, along a vertical incision in the posterior aspect of left sublumbar area. The writer and his colleagues have delivered by caesarean operation a live fetus, with irreducible hock flexion, 17 hours after rupture of the allantochorion.

Infertility

The fertility of camels is good. According to Bedouin breeders, of every 100 she-camels mated 80–90 bring calves. About 1% are sterile. Poor nutrition in seasons of low rainfall and resultant poor grazing is a cause of reduced sexual activity in both sexes. Abortion is rarely seen. Unthriftiness due to disease leads to infertility and pleuropneumonia is a cause of abortion.

Fertility of she-camels is maintained throughout life; breeding in alternate years, which is the usual practice, a female can yield a total of 12 offspring, although an average of something less than eight seems more likely. One mating per oestrus is usually allowed and it is possible for a male to serve five or six females in a day. It is said that one male can suffice for 200 females, with controlled breeding, but a much smaller number is customary.

In abattoir genital tracts, endometritis, associated with a partially involuted uterus and a regressing corpus luteum, is sometimes seen. These are presumably postparturient or postabortion cases. The author has seen no cases of ovarobursal adhesions or of cystic ovaries and has not read of any in the literature. As mentioned in the discussion of the observed incidence of corpora albicantia, embryonic death after twin conception and fetal death after single or twin conception are probably common.

Wernery and Wernery (1992) studied the uterine bacterial flora of 80 barren camels in two herds bred for racing in Dubai — some with and some without endometritis. Their main findings were as follows:

1. The range of organisms isolated was very similar to those obtained from equine and bovine uteri except that *Streptococcus zooepidemicus*, which is the commonest pathogen recovered from equine uteri, and the organism of contagious equine metritis (*Taylorella equigenitalis*), were not found.

2. *Campylobacter fetus* and *Tritrichomonas fetus* were both isolated from infertile camels.

According to Bedouins, unsuccessful copulation due to incomplete intromission is not uncommon. In the belief that intromission is intracervical they treat this condition by gentle and gradual digital dilatation of the cervix, using butter as a lubricant. After this treatment complete intromission is said to be possible and pregnancy ensues.

Prolapse of vagina

Several cases of vaginal prolapse have been seen in pregnant camels whose exercise was restricted and which were fed ad libitum on lucerne and barley. Bedouins control the condition by the application of a body truss of bandages which exerts constant pressure on the perineum. One case, for which veterinary attention was requested, was successfully treated by the Bühner technique of vulval circumferential, subcutaneous suture (see p. 138).

ARTIFICIAL INSEMINATION

Progress in the application of artificial insemination (AI) to camel breeding had been slow because of two main factors: firstly, the nomadic, pastoral nature of typical camel husbandry in arid regions militates against frequent herding, enclosure and restraint of animals and, secondly, she-camels in natural circumstances ovulate only in response to mating. However, despite these two constraints it has been shown that AI is possible in camels kept intensively and by using (1) service by a vasectomized male, or (2) an injection of seminal plasma, or (3) an injection of human chorionic gonadotrophin (hCG) or a GnRH analogue.

Chen et al. (1990), working with Bactrian camels in China, and Sieme et al. (1990), using dromedaries in Sudan, have reported pioneering studies on the collection, dilution and storage, including freezing, of camel semen and its use for insemination.

Semen collection

An artificial vagina (AV), as used for bulls, is prepared as usual and the final internal temperature brought to 40–50°C (camels are not as sensitive to this requirement as bulls). An oestrous she-camel is restrained in the natural sitting posture and the well-controlled male is brought up to her side and allowed to nuzzle her head and then to sniff her perineum before mounting. The operators kneel on each side of the squatting male; one holds the AV and the other directs the penis into it by holding the sheath. Copulation lasts from 5 to 15 minutes; it is characterized by several bouts of male pelvic thrusting at intervals of a few minutes, and these coincide with ejaculatory squirts of semen into the collecting cup.

The semen sample is greyish-white in colour and quite gelatinous, but it soon liquefies on standing at room temperature; volumes vary from 2 to 10 ml and average 3 ml. Normal sperm counts are from 200×10^6 to 400×10^6 / ml. The fresh semen can be diluted three or four times with an egg yolk lactose extender, for use with inseminating doses of 2 ml. For freezing, Musa et al. (1992) recommended the technique used for boar semen, while Chen et al. (1990) used a diluent containing sucrose, egg yolk and glycerol, with the addition of penicillin and streptomycin for their frozen semen studies.

Insemination

The oestrous she-camel must have a palpable follicle of at least 1.2 cm. Of the methods available for promoting ovulation, Anouassi et al. (1992) obtained best results after preliminary service by a vasectomized male 24 hours before the insemination. However, for general use this was considered an impracticable method. The Chinese workers prefer two inseminations, 24 hours apart; the first with 0.8 ml of whole undiluted semen, and the second with 2 ml of the diluted semen. The experience of workers experimenting with embryo transfer in camels indicates that the most convenient method of inducing ovulation is the injection of 20 µg of a GnRH analogue (buserelin) or 3000 IU of hCG (McKinnon and Tinson 1992). Remarkable fertility from frozen semen inseminations was reported by Chen et al. (1990); for 31 animals inseminated the conception rate was 93.54%.

EMBRYO TRANSFER

The preliminary trials of embryo transfer in camels are quite recent and have been performed in Israel and in racing camel breeding studs in the United Arab Emirates (Anouassi et al. 1992; Yagil and van Creveld 1990; McKinnon and Tinson 1992; Skidmore et al., 1992). Compared with cattle, the technique is more difficult in camels because the non-pregnant camel does not have a cyclical corpus luteum and does not ovulate spontaneously; these factors make superovulation of the donors and preparation of the recipients less reliable. A substantial and meticulously conducted trial of embryo transfer was carried out in the United Arab Emirates and reported in 1992 by McKinnon and Tinson.

Donors were given daily injections of 100 mg of progesterone for 10–15 days. From the last day of that series, twice-daily injections of 1–3 mg of ovine FSH were given for 5 days. Then the ovaries were examined to assess follicular development for mating: those follicles of 1.6–1.8 cm were considered optimum and they were most commonly found 8–12 days after the gonadotrophic treat-

ment was begun. Ovulation was then induced by one or two natural matings, 12 hours apart. Alternatively, ovulation could be induced by injection of 3000 IU of hCG or by 20 µg of GnRH (buserelin), and followed by AI.

Recipients were prepared like donors by daily injection for 10–15 days of 100 mg of progesterone. This schedule was designed to terminate on the day that gonadotrophin was first given to the donor. Five days after these progesterone injections ceased, the ovaries of potential recipients were examined and grouped according to follicular size. On the day the donor was expected to ovulate, the recipient was injected with either 2000–5000 IU of hCG or 20 µg of GnRH (75% of the recipients prepared in this way ovulated at the correct time). Immediately before embryo transfer all recipients were scanned to ensure ovulation had occurred and that the genital tract was normal.

The day of mating was 'day 0', and embryo recovery was attempted on days 6.5 or 7.5, when the donor was tranquillized and given epidural anaesthesia. One litre of flushing fluid was injected and recovered in 30–70 ml aliquots, which were filtered and scanned for embryos; the latter were assessed to estimate age and normality. The embryos were placed in straws and introduced by means of a special injection gun into the left uterine horn of the recipient.

Commenting on their experimental study in which an overall pregnancy rate of 22% was achieved from these non-surgical transfers of 121 embryos, the authors concluded that: (1) best responses to the hormonal treatments were obtained during the natural breeding season, (2) more embryos were recovered from donors over 11 years old, on day 7 or 7.5 after mating, and from matings by particular bulls, and (3) more favourable pregnancy rates occurred in recipients under 11 years old and which had ovulated 0.5–1.5 days after the donor.

REFERENCES

Abdel Rahim, S. E. A. and Al-Nazeer, A. E. (1992) *Proc. 1st Int. Camel Conf., Dubai*, p. 115.

Anouassi, A., Adnani, M. and El Raed (1992) *Proc. 1st Int. Camel Conf., Dubai*, p. 175.

Barmintsev, Y. N. (1951) *Konevodsevo*, **1**, 138.

Chen, B. X. Yuen, Z. X. and Pan, G. W. (1985) *J. Reprod. Fertil.*, **74**, 335.

Chen, B. X. Zhao, X. X. and Huang, Y. M. (1990) *Proc. UCDEC Workshop, Paris.*

Cole, H. H. and Saunders, F. J. (1935) *Endocrinology,* **19**, 199.

El Azab, E. A. and Musa, B. (1976) *Zuchthygiene,* **11**, 166.

El Ghannam, F., El Azab, E. A. and El Sawaf (1974) *Zuchthygiene,* **9**, 46.

Elias, E., Bedrak, E. and Cohen, D. (1985) *J. Reprod. Fertil.,* **75**, 519.

McKinnon, A. C. and Tinson, A. H. (1992) *Proc. 1st Int. Camel Conf., Dubai,* p. 203.

Musa, B. (1975) Personal communication.

Musa, B. and Abusineina, M. E. A. (1976) *Acta Vet. Beograd.,* **26**, 107.

Musa, B. and Abusineina, M. E. A. (1978) *Vet. Rec.,* **102**, 7.

Musa, B., Siema, H., Merkt, H. and Hago, B. E. D. (1992) *Proc. 1st Int. Camel Conf., Dubai,* p. 179.

Petris, M. A. (1956) *Vet. Rec.,* **68**, 274.

Sieme, H., Merkt, H., Musa, B., Badreldin, H. and Willmen, T. (1990) *Proc. Unité de Coordination pour l'Elevage Camelin,* pp. 273–284.

Skidmore, J., Allen, W. R., Cooper, M. J., Ali Chaudhry, M., Billah, M. and Billah, A. M. (1992) *Proc. 1st Int. Camel Conf., Dubai,* p. 137.

Tinson, A. H. and McKinnon, A. O. (1992) *Proc. 1st Int. Camel Conf., Dubai,* p. 129.

Wernery, H. and Wernery, R. (1992) *Proc. 1st Int. Camel Conf., Dubai,* p. 155.

Xu, Y. S., Jian, L. G., Wang, H. Y., Zing, G. Q., Jiang, G. T. and Gao, Y. H. (1985) *J. Reprod. Fertil.,* **74**, 341.

Yagil, R. and van Creveld, C. (1990) *Proc. UCDEC Workshop,* pp. 293–311. *Paris.*

The world population of domestic buffaloes (*Bubalus bubalis*) is about 150 million. There are two distinct types of domestic buffalo which have been named according to whether they wallow in stagnant pools (swamp buffalo), or in running water (river buffalo). These types also differ in conformation, chromosome number, geographical distribution and uses. The swamp buffalo, found in the eastern half of Asia from Assam to China, has 48 chromosomes and is mainly used for draught purposes and for meat. The river buffalo, distributed in the western half of Asia, mainly in India and Pakistan, has 50 chromosomes and provides milk for human consumption.

Buffaloes and cattle are in the family Bovidae but belong to different genera. Both species were domesticated for draught, milk and meat around the same period in history. Despite several similarities in their reproductive process, and the recent progress made in understanding the hormonal control of many reproductive events in the buffalo, there has been no significant improvement in the reproductive efficiency of the buffalo at the farm level.

PUBERTY

The buffalo attains puberty later than cattle. On recommended levels of nutrition, the average age at puberty in the female (first oestrus) is about 15–18 months for the river buffalo and 21–24 months for the swamp buffalo. However, most conceptions occur when the buffalo weighs about 250–275 kg. Spermatogenesis commences at 12–15 months in both buffalo types but viable spermatozoa appear in the ejaculate only at about 24 months. The faster growing F_1 river × swamp cross-breed reaches puberty earlier than the slower-growing swamp buffalo.

FEMALE REPRODUCTION

Anatomy of the reproductive organs

The structure and location of the internal reproductive organs of the buffalo are similar to those of cattle. However, the cervix is less conspicuous and the uterine horns are smaller and more coiled than in cattle. The ovaries are ovoid and measure 2–3 cm in length, 1–2 cm from surface to surface and 1–2 cm from the attached to the free border. They are located within the pelvic cavity, caudal and lateral to the uterine horns. The genital tract and ovaries, including the cyclic corpus luteum and mature follicles (>10 mm), may be palpated per rectum.

The oestrous cycle

Breeding season

The buffalo is polyoestrous, breeding throughout the year, but rainfall, feed supply, ambient temperature and photoperiod may influence the annual calving pattern. Decreasing day-length and cooler ambient temperatures favour cyclicity whereas long day-length and the high summer temperatures depress cyclicity. In the Indian subcontinent, most buffaloes calve between November and March.

Cyclic periodicity

The oestrous cycle is about 21 days, and 'standing' oestrus is usually less than 24 hours. Oestrus commences towards late evening, with peak sexual activity during the night and the early morning hours. Matings are noted less frequently during daylight hours, particularly in the swamp buffalo. Ovulation is spontaneous and usually occurs 15–18 hours after the end of oestrus.

Signs of oestrus

Overt signs of oestrus in buffalo are not as pronounced as in cattle. Heterosexual behaviour or standing to be mounted by a male is the most reliable sign of oestrus in the buffalo because homosexual behaviour or standing to be mounted by other females is observed only occasionally. Signs such as swelling of the vulva, a clear mucoid vulval discharge, reduction in milk production, vocalization, restlessness and frequent urination are not dependable signs of oestrus because their occurrence varies from animal to animal and in relation to standing oestrus.

Mating behaviour

Mating behaviour in many respects resembles that of cattle. On contacting a female, the male sniffs her urine, then displays the 'flehmen' reaction and proceeds to nuzzle and lick the perineum and vulva. An oestrous female responds by standing immobile for the male to mount and ejaculate; mating lasts 20–30 seconds. Rhythmic pelvic thrusts during intromission and the forward leap at ejaculation are less marked in buffalo than cattle. The male dismounts and gradually retracts the penis into the sheath while the female remains with her back arched and tail elevated for a few minutes.

Methods of oestrus detection

A male buffalo fitted with a chinball mating device may be used for routine oestrus detection. The male is either kept in a corral with females from late evening until the next morning or is led behind them if they are in stanchions, twice daily. If no male is available, a female buffalo can be androgenized for oestrus detection.

Oestrus detection aids such as pressure-sensitive indicators placed on the sacrum or painting the tailhead (tail painting) are unsatisfactory because wallowing interferes with their efficiency. Where routine oestrus detection is not practised, as in the villages of India and Pakistan, buffaloes are submitted for insemination on the basis of a vulval discharge of clear mucus, a drop in milk yield or a change in temperament. In these situations, inseminators often palpate the uterus for the presence of tone before inseminating an animal.

Cyclic changes in the internal genitalia

Ovaries. The rising level of oestrogens, particularly oestradiol-17β secreted by the Graafian follicle, combined with the declining level of pro-gesterone secreted by the regressing corpus luteum, triggers a surge of luteinizing hormone (LH). The LH surge induces a mature follicle, if present in the ovary, to ovulate about 24 hours later (Kaker et al., 1980).

During oestrus, a mature ovarian follicle, 10–20 mm in diameter, is rectally palpable as a turgid area bulging slightly from the surface of the ovary. On the day of ovulation (days 1–2), the follicle softens and the site of ovulation is felt as a pit or depression. Only one egg is shed per cycle.

The growth, maintenance and regression of the corpus luteum are closely correlated with progesterone levels in blood plasma (Jainudeen et al., 1983a,b). The developing corpus luteum (days 2–8) is soft and difficult to palpate per rectum but the mature corpus luteum (days 8–16) is palpable as a firm projection on the surface of the ovary. The mature corpus luteum secretes up to about 3.5 ng/ml progesterone into the bloodstream. With the regression of the corpus luteum (day 17), progesterone secretion rapidly declines to reach levels below 0.2 ng/ml at the next oestrus. Old corpora lutea appear as white scars on the surface of the ovary.

Uterus, Cervix and Vagina. The uterine horns are turgid and coiled with maximum tone during oestrus, then lose their turgidity and tonicity after ovulation to become flaccid during the luteal phase of the cycle. The cervix dilates sufficiently during oestrus to enable the passage of an insemination catheter into the uterus. The clear, copious mucus that is secreted during oestrus changes to an opaque, thick, scanty discharge after ovulation. Hyperaemia of the vaginal mucous membrane and some swelling of the vulva occur during oestrus. Blood in the vulval discharge or metoestrus bleeding, usually seen in cattle, rarely occurs in the buffalo.

Pregnancy and its diagnosis

Gestation length

The buffalo has a longer gestation than cattle, being 305–320 days for the river buffalo and 320–340 days for the swamp buffalo. Male calves are carried 1–2 days longer than female calves. River × swamp hybrids have an intermediate gestation length of 315 days.

Physiology of pregnancy

Placentation. The epitheliochorial placenta of the buffalo is of the cotyledonary type. The fetal membranes and fetus mostly develop in one uterine horn. Most of the 60 to 90 placentomes are distributed throughout the gravid uterine horn. As pregnancy advances the placentomes enlarge to mushroom-like structures measuring 5–7 cm in diameter.

Endocrinology. Oestrus is generally suspended during pregnancy but a few animals may experience one or more periods of anovulatory oestrus. The corpus luteum is maintained throughout gestation but its role in the maintenance of pregnancy is yet not known. As in cattle, plasma progesterone levels remain elevated throughout pregnancy.

Methods of pregnancy diagnosis

Rectal Palpation. Pregnancy can be accurately diagnosed per rectum from about 45 days of pregnancy. Manual slipping of the allantochorion is possible from about 42 to 56 days of gestation. The uterus is suspended at the level of the pelvic floor up to the fourth month of gestation, then descends to the abdominal floor. In most buffaloes, placentomes and the fetus may be palpated beyond the third month of pregnancy. However, in some deep-bellied river buffalo breeds, the fetus may be difficult to palpate, particularly between the sixth and eighth months of pregnancy. In such cases, palpation of the hypertrophy and fremitus in the uterine arteries as well as recognition of the placentomes should aid in the diagnosis.

Hormone Assays. As in cattle, pregnancy can be diagnosed on progesterone concentrations in milk or blood plasma at 22–24 days after breeding. This test is accurate for non-pregnancy but not for pregnancy for the same reasons as stated for cattle (see p. 84).

PARTURITION AND PUERPERIUM

Parturition

Signs of approaching parturition

About 1–2 weeks before parturition, the female exhibits marked abdominal enlargement, udder development, hypertrophy and oedema of the vulval lips. As parturition approaches, the animal isolates herself from the rest of the herd. The relaxation of the pelvic ligament leads to an elevation of the tail head while liquefaction of the cervical seal of pregnancy results in a string of clear mucus hanging from the vulva, particularly when the animal lies down.

Initiation of parturition

Little is yet known of the mechanism initiating parturition in the buffalo. Plasma concentrations of progesterone remain elevated throughout gestation but about 15 days before parturition, plasma levels of both oestrone and prostaglandin $F_{2\alpha}$ metabolite (PGFM) increase and reach peak values, 3–5 days prepartum (Perera et al., 1981; Arora and Pandey, 1982; Batra and Pandey, 1982). At parturition, the sharp decline in plasma concentrations of progesterone is associated with a significant increase in plasma concentrations of cortisol (Prakash and Madan, 1984); whether the cortisol originates in the mother or the fetus remains to be established.

Stages of labour

About 12–24 hours before parturition, uterine contractions increase both in frequency and amplitude, causing the animal some abdominal discomfort. The cervix takes about 1–2 hours to fully dilate (stage I labour).

As the fetus enters the birth canal, the dam lies down in sternal or lateral recumbency and starts straining (stage II labour) (Figure 33.1). The allantochorion ruptures before it reaches the vulva. Next, the fetus, within the amnion, appears at the vulva. Strong abdominal contractions lead to the rupture of the amniotic sac and the delivery of the fetus, usually in anterior presentation and dorsal position, with extended limbs; posterior presentation is uncommon. This stage of labour lasts 30–60 minutes but may extend up to 6 hours, particularly in primipara. After delivery, abdominal straining ceases and the fetal membranes are expelled within 4–5 hours (stage III labour). Twinning is rare in the buffalo, and the incidence is less than 1 per 1000 births.

Dystocia

Dystocia is less common in buffalo than cattle and is more often due to fetal rather than maternal

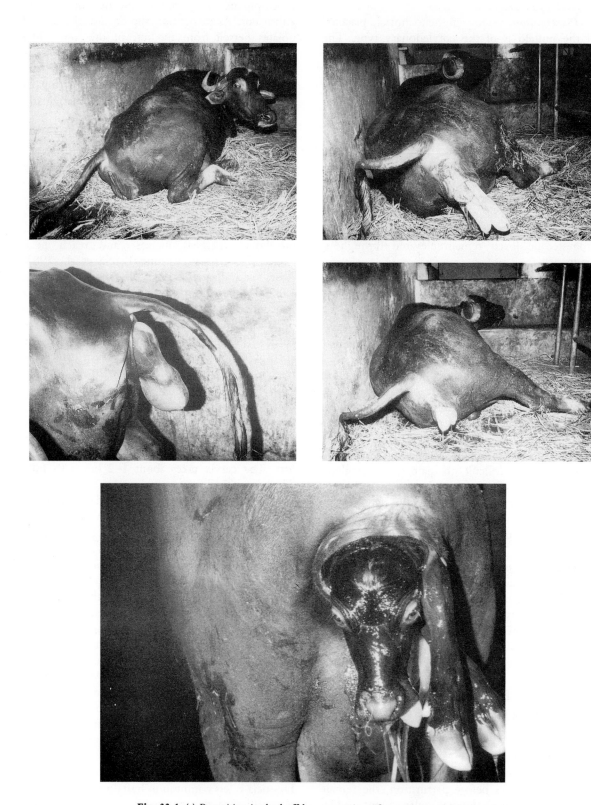

Fig. 33.1 (a) Parturition in the buffalo: progression of second-stage labour.

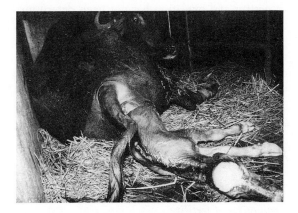

Fig. 33.1 (b) Parturition in the buffalo: end of second-stage labour.

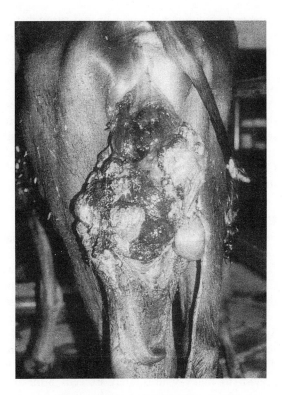

Fig. 33.2 Prolapse of the uterus.

causes. Stabled river buffaloes are more prone than the free-ranging swamp type to dystocia. The common forms of fetal dystocia are disproportion between the size of the fetus and the maternal birth canal and abnormal presentation, position and posture. Maternal forms of dystocia include uterine inertia, uterine torsion and failure of the cervix to dilate. The same obstetrical procedures used for cattle are applicable for the relief of dystocia in the buffalo.

Other conditions related to parturition
Retention of the fetal membranes and prolapse of the uterus (Figure 33.2) occur particularly in the river type buffalo. Infections, uterine inertia, dystocia and poor management practices have been implicated in the pathogenesis of retention of the fetal membranes. Prolapse of the uterus occurs within the first 6 hours after expulsion of the fetus and involves a complete inversion of the gravid uterine horn. Treatment for both conditions is the same as previously described for cattle.

Puerperium
Involution of the uterus
The uterus is rectally palpable by the second week postpartum as a well-defined structure, the size of a football, anterior and slightly ventral to the pelvic brim. Involution, based on the time when both uterine horns reach normal non-gravid size and position, is completed by about 30 days in the suckled swamp buffalo and about 45 days in the hand-milked river buffalo. Uterine involution is

delayed in cases of dystocia and retention of the fetal membranes (Jainudeen, 1984). Although the relationship between uterine involution and fertility has not been established, buffaloes are usually bred at about 60 days postpartum.

Resumption of ovarian activity
The corpus luteum of the previous pregnancy (corpus albicans) completely regresses by day 30 postpartum. Follicular activity commences between days 30–60 postpartum, but only a few animals ovulate. The first postpartum oestrus and ovulation occur at about 60 and 90 days, respectively, in well-managed buffalo herds.

MALE REPRODUCTION

Normal sexual apparatus
Anatomy
The reproductive organs are like those of the bull but the testes and scrotum are smaller and the penile sheath is less pendulous. As in cattle, the

testis and epididymis can be palpated through the scrotal wall whereas the prostate, seminal vesicles and ampullae can be felt per rectum.

Spermatogenesis

Among farm animals, the buffalo has one of the shortest spermatogenic cycles. The durations of the seminiferous epithelial cycle and spermatogenesis are 8.6 days and 38 days respectively (Sharma and Gupta, 1980). In general, the frequency of the cell stages in buffalo and cattle are comparable.

Examination of semen

Semen is collected either with a bovine artificial vagina (AV) or by electroejaculation. Either a female or a castrated male buffalo can be used as the teaser. The temperature of the water jacket of the AV should be about 40–42°C and the pressure within the AV adjusted to suit individual males. Sperm concentration is increased by allowing two to three false mounts before the actual collection. The normal ejaculate collected with an AV is greyish to milky-white, rarely exceeds 5 ml and has a sperm concentration of between 500 and 1500 million cells/ml. Motility of spermatozoa is lower than in cattle semen. Semen can also be collected with cattle electroejaculators provided suitable restraining facilities are available.

ARTIFICIAL INSEMINATION

Artificial insemination (AI) has been practised in the river buffalo for over 30 years in the Indian subcontinent but has lagged behind cattle largely because of the difficulty of detecting oestrus. Chilled semen (5°C), diluted in a variety of extenders is still widely used in buffalo AI.

Buffalo semen can be frozen in extenders used for bovine semen. One such extender is a Tris buffer containing 7% glycerol and 20% egg yolk. Extended semen is packed in 0.25 or 0.5 ml French straws to contain 30 million motile spermatozoa per dose. Straws are exposed to nitrogen vapour at −120 to −140°C for 7–10 minutes before being stored in liquid nitrogen. Semen should be thawed at 37–40°C. The post-thaw progressive motility of buffalo semen varies from 35 to 60%.

The optimum time of insemination in relation to oestrus and ovulation has not been determined for the buffalo. Most inseminations are usually performed between 12 and 24 hours from the onset of oestrus. At this time, the cervix is sufficiently dilated for the deposition of semen in the uterine body by the rectovaginal technique of AI.

FERTILITY AND INFERTILITY

Fertility

Evaluation of fertility

Most buffaloes are reared under low input–low output management systems where there is little economic necessity to maintain breeding records. Female fertility in the buffalo is commonly expressed in terms of the calving interval. A buffalo produces, on average, two calves every 3 years. Caution should be exercised in interpreting conception rates based on non-return rates in the buffalo because of the inherent difficulty of detecting oestrus. Pregnancy rates based on rectal palpation in swamp buffaloes usually range from 20 to 75% during a 3–4 month breeding season, depending upon the nutritional and lactational status of the females at joining. The first service: pregnancy rate for the river buffalo varies between 50 and 75% for hand matings and 30–50% for inseminations with chilled or frozen semen.

Female infertility

The reproductive efficiency of the female is lower for buffalo than in cattle. The seasonal pattern of the reproductive cycle and long calving intervals under traditional management systems provide few opportunities for a buffalo to calve during the most favourable months of two successive years. Both infectious and non-infectious factors contribute to the long calving interval through anoestrus, repeat-breeding and abortion.

Anoestrus

As in cattle, two forms of anoestrus occur in the buffalo. In the first form, the animal possesses a palpable corpus luteum in one ovary but is not detected in oestrus ('apparent' anoestrus or 'silent oestrus'), whereas in the second form, the animal lacks a palpable corpus luteum and does not exhibit oestrus ('true' anoestrus). In the past, silent oestrus was commonly believed to be a major problem in buffalo breeding but recent evidence suggests that it may be related to the poor oestrus detection techniques adopted in these herds. The incidence has been drastically reduced in herds where routine oestrus detection practices stated previously have been adopted (Jainudeen, 1984). Factors that contribute to postpartum anoestrus include poor body condition, lactation and suckling. Hand-milked river buffaloes have a lower incidence of postpartum anoestrus than suckled swamp buffaloes. Affected animals have smaller than normal ovaries which are devoid of follicles or a corpus luteum.

Cystic ovaries

Cystic ovaries are more common in the high producing river buffalo than the suckled swamp buffalo. In a survey, cystic ovaries accounted for 6% of the reproductive failure in over 12 000 river buffaloes in India; most cases occurred before day 45 postpartum (Rao and Sreemannarayanan, 1982). The clinical findings and treatment are similar to those in cattle.

Repeat breeding and abortion

The incidence and causes of early embryonic deaths are not known. Diseases that cause repeat breeding and abortion in cattle such as brucellosis, leptospirosis, vibriosis, trichomoniasis and infectious bovine rhinotracheitis (IBR) occur in the buffalo, but their contribution to female infertility, except for brucellosis, has not been clearly defined. Abortion caused by *Brucella abortus* occurs during the latter half of gestation.

Endometritis and acquired abnormalities

A high incidence of endometritis has been reported in infertile river buffaloes (Samad et al., 1984). The common organisms isolated include *Escherichia coli*, *Actinomyces (Corynebacterium) pyogenes* and *Staphylococcus aureus*. This high incidence has been attributed to the practice of stimulating milk let-down by the introduction of instruments or the hand into the vagina and to the unhygienic facilities at parturition. Pathology of the ovarian bursa and oviducts were the common findings observed in infertile river buffaloes in several abattoir surveys.

Male infertility

Less is known concerning male infertility in buffalo than cattle. Several sperm defects have been reported but their relationship to fertility has not been ascertained. Common pathological conditions that cause infertility in the buffalo include testicular degeneration and hypoplasia, orchitis, epididymitis and seminal vesiculitis (Rao, 1984). High environmental temperatures during the summer months exert a deleterious effect on libido as well as semen quality. This effect has partly been overcome by providing water sprinklers to cool the animals during the hotter part of the day.

Several South-East Asian countries have embarked upon cross-breeding the indigenous swamp to the river buffalo. The chromosome complement of 49 for the F_1 river × swamp hybrid buffalo (Bongso and Jainudeen, 1979) is intermediate to that of its parents. Doubts have been cast on the fertility of the hybrid buffalo because interspecies hybrids with chromosome complements different to their parents are mostly sterile, while some may be partially fertile (female), e.g. cattalo (bison × cattle), mule (horse × donkey) or hinny (donkey × horse). However, both male and female hybrid buffaloes are fertile. The hybrid female buffalo produces viable calves and the male hybrid, despite the presence of a high percentage of degenerating spermatocytes and abnormal spermatids in the testes (Bongso et al., 1983), is capable of achieving calf crops comparable to male swamp buffaloes.

Improving fertility

In the past, attention was given mainly to the control of infectious diseases and pathological conditions affecting infertility. However, with the recent development of sensitive methods for measuring reproductive hormones such as LH and progesterone, veterinarians are now giving more attention to the non-infectious factors contributing to infertility in the buffalo.

Improvements in nutrition could increase growth rates and advance the onset of puberty. Similarly, management practices such as early weaning and high plane of feeding during the early postpartum period have advanced the restoration of postpartum ovarian activity and reduced the incidence of anoestrus.

Higher conception rates to AI could be

achieved by inseminating only those buffaloes which are in 'standing' oestrus, depositing the semen in the body of the uterus rather than in either the vagina or the cervix and adopting hygienic measures at insemination.

The difficulty of detecting oestrus, a major limitation to the widespread use of AI, could be overcome by two methods of oestrus induction: (1) premature regression of the corpus luteum by injection of $PGF_{2\alpha}$ or its synthetic analogues; and (2) prolongation of the lifespan of the corpus luteum by a progesterone-releasing intravaginal device (PRID). Buffaloes are usually inseminated at fixed times following oestrus induction and conception rates vary between 20 and 40%. These techniques depend on the presence of a corpus luteum and are of limited value in lactating or suckled buffaloes because of the high incidence of true anoestrus. Since $PGF_{2\alpha}$ causes abortion, buffaloes should be examined for pregnancy before treatment.

There are no special management programmes for reproduction in the buffalo. Most reproductive management programmes adopted for cattle (see Chapter 24) can be effectively applied for the buffalo.

REFERENCES

Arora, R. C. and Pandey, R. S. (1982) *Gen. Comp. Endocrinol.*, **48,** 43.

Batra, S. K. and Pandey, R. S. (1982) *Biol. Reprod.*, **27,** 1055.

Bongso, T. A. and Jainudeen, M. R. (1979) *Kajian Vet.*, **11,** 6.

Bongso, T. A., Hilmi, A. and Basrur, P. K. (1983) *Res. Vet. Sci.*, **35,** 253.

Jainudeen, M. R. (1984) *Proc. Xth Int. Congr. Anim. Reprod. Artif. Insem.*, **4,** xiv.

Jainudeen, M. R., Bongso, T. A. and Tan, H. S. (1983a) *Anim. Reprod. Sci.*, **5,** 181.

Jainudeen, M. R., Sharifuddin, W. and Bashir Ahmad, F. (1983b) *Vet. Rec.*, **113** 369.

Kaker, M. L., Razdan, M. N. and Galhotra, M. M. (1980) *J. Reprod. Fertil.*, **60,** 419.

Perera, B. M. O. A., Abeygunawardena, H., Thamotheram, A., Kindahl, H. and Edqvist, L. E. (1981) *Theriogenology*, **15,** 463.

Prakash, B. S. and Madan, M. L. (1984) *Theriogenology*, **22,** 241.

Rao, A. R. (1984) *Proc. Xth Int. Congr. Anim. Reprod. Artif. Insem.*, **4,** xiv.

Rao, A. V. and Sreemannarayanan, O. (1982) *Theriogenology*, **18,** 403.

Samad, H. A., Ali, C. S. and Ahmad, K. M. (1984) *Proc. Xth Int. Congr. Anim. Reprod. Artif. Insem.*

Sharma, A. K. and Gupta, R. C. (1980) *Anim. Reprod. Sci.*, **3,** 217.

8

Part Eight

Embryo Transfer

The term 'embryo transfer', taken literally, refers solely to the collection of an embryo from a donor animal and its placement into the uterine tube or uterus of a recipient. However, by common usage, it has become accepted to cover a whole range of allied techniques, including superovulation of the donor, and storage and manipulation of embryos *in vitro*.

The first successful embryo transfer was carried out nearly 100 years ago in rabbits (Heape, 1891) but it was some time before the technique was successfully applied to farm animals. Warwick and Berry (1949) produced the first lamb by embryo transfer, but despite intense research effort, the first calf was not born until 1951 (Willett et al., 1951). Even then it was not until much later that the technique had advanced sufficiently to be of practical use in cattle breeding (Rowson et al., 1969). Since then embryo transfer has been used successfully to increase the reproductive rate of cattle, horses, sheep, goats and pigs.

Embryo transfer has been applied most extensively in the cow, consequently the technology has advanced most rapidly in this species. In the early 1970s general anaesthesia and laparotomy were necessary both for recovery and transfer of bovine embryos, and embryo transfer was used in the UK and North America mainly for the rapid multiplication of imported exotic beef breeds. With the advent of efficient non-surgical techniques for recovery of embryos and effective methods for preserving embryos in liquid nitrogen in the latter part of the decade, demand for embryo transfer services increased dramatically in both the beef and dairy industries.

According to figures collected by the European Embryo Transfer Association, the number of transfers per annum peaked in 1990 in the EU, and the trend is now downwards. Nevertheless, in 1992 around 88 000 transfers were carried out in the EU, of which around 8000 were in the UK.

International trade in frozen embryos now contributes significantly to these figures. The commercial application of embryo transfer has been much more restricted in the other domestic species. A reluctance on the part of the breed associations to register progeny produced by embryo transfer has partly been responsible in the horse, and economic factors, together with the need for surgery, have militated against widespread use in pigs, sheep and goats.

APPLICATIONS OF EMBRYO TRANSFER

Over the years embryo transfer has been, and continues to be, a valuable research tool (review — Sreenan, 1983). It has been used exclusively in studies of uterine capacity, uterine environment, maternal recognition of pregnancy, embryo–uterine relations and endocrinology of pregnancy. Embryo transfer has also been used in disease transmission studies and to investigate the genetics of reproduction; for instance, litter size, gestation length, birth weight and postnatal production. The rapid development of new technologies is now expanding the scope of embryo transfer in research.

The production of identical twins and clones will accelerate progress in many fields of research and the ability to manipulate fertilization and modify the genome of the early embryo will advance the frontiers of knowledge in a hitherto undreamed of manner. However, the most practical application of embryo transfer today depends on its capacity to increase the reproductive rate of female animals. The rapid uptake of embryo transfer by cattle breeders in particular, has depended on the ability to increase the number of progeny from valuable brood cows, either as a means of rapid herd improvement or to produce surplus embryos, pregnancies or stock for sale.

Genetic improvement

The rate of genetic improvement within a breed depends on four variables: the amount of genetic variation for the traits under question, the accuracy with which the parents of the next generation can be selected, the selection intensity and the generation interval. Embryo transfer can be used to influence all four variables and improve rates of progress.

Genetic variation

This can be increased by introduction of a breed genetically superior for the desired traits. Embryo transfer can be used both to introduce the breed in question through the medium of frozen embryos, and to increase the reproductive rate of resulting females to facilitate its distribution.

Selection of dams

The breeding value of females can be calculated from their own performance and conformation data, together with that of close relatives. The accuracy of the calculation depends on the numbers of relatives available for recording, and embryo transfer can be used to increase numbers in species with a low reproductive rate, allowing, for instance, sibling or progeny testing of cows (Nicholas and Smith, 1983).

Selection intensity

In dairy cattle, the majority of female offspring in a herd are needed as replacements to produce the next generation. Using embryo transfer to increase the reproductive rate of the best cows, selection can be restricted to the top 5–10% of females. Similarly, in a national bull selection programme the use of embryo transfer would allow the proportion of bull dams selected to be reduced from say, 2 to 1%, by ensuring that a bull calf was produced from virtually every mating (Cunningham, 1976).

Generation interval

A method for dairy cattle improvement using embryo transfer intensively on selected individuals within one nucleus herd has been proposed by Nicholas and Smith (1983). Sets of full and half siblings within this type of scheme can be recorded for traits in question in a uniform environment, and the selection of males and females to produce the next generation can then be made on the basis of sibling testing rather than progeny testing, as in conventional improvement schemes. Breeding programmes based on this system have become known as MOET (multiple ovulation and embryo transfer) schemes and have been applied in practice in dairy and beef cattle and sheep. The practical application of MOET in dairy cattle has been described by Christie et al. (1992).

This approach allows a dramatic cut in generation interval, and consequently allows the opportunity for more rapid genetic improvement than can be achieved with the application of a traditional progeny-testing system.

Genetic screening

Embryo transfer has also been used to expedite the screening of both dams and sires for genetic defects such as syndactyly in cattle (Baker et al., 1980).

Disease control

There is increasing evidence to suggest that embryos are unlikely to spread viral and bacterial diseases when transferred into recipients. The zona pellucida would appear to be an effective barrier to infection of the embryonic cells from the uterine environment, and washing of embryos, or treating with trypsin, has been shown to remove viral contamination from the zona pellucida *in vitro* (Singh, 1984). Singh (1984) cites data from several authors: for instance 407 embryos transferred from enzootic bovine leucosis-seropositive donors have resulted in no seropositive recipients or calves. Similarly, 67 embryos transferred from blue tongue virus-infected donors and 62 embryos (trypsin treated) transferred from infectious bovine rhinotracheitis virus infected donors resulted in seronegative recipients and calves. Embryo transfer has also been effectively used for the introduction of new blood lines into specific pathogen-free pig herds (Wrathall, 1984). Sufficient transfers have been conducted with embryos from bovine leucosis, infectious bovine rhinotracheitis, and foot and mouth disease infected donors to determine that these viruses will not be transmitted via embryos, provided they are washed properly (Stringfellow and Seidel, 1990). As the

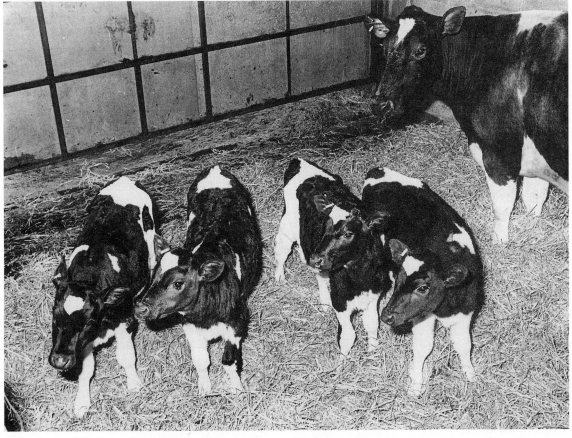

Fig. 34.1 Embryo transfer can be used to circumvent certain types of infertility. This cow had ceased to breed because of senility but four young surrogates were able to carry her calves to term.

results of current and future experimental work become available, it is likely that similar conclusions will be drawn for additional pathogens. However, more field trials will be necessary before the risk of disease transmission by embryos can be fully assessed.

Import and export

The development of efficient methods for cryopreservation of embryos of the cow, sheep and goat have stimulated a growing international trade in genetic material. Economy and convenience have been major considerations, but many governments are now making import regulations for embryos less stringent than those for live animals or semen, in recognition of the relatively lower risk of introduction of disease by embryo transfer. An additional advantage of embryo transfer in this situation lies in the fact that a calf resulting from an imported embryo transferred into an indigenous

recipient acquires colostral immunity to local diseases and consequently may thrive better than an animal imported on the hoof.

Circumvention of infertility

Embryo transfer techniques have proved valuable in diagnosis, treatment and circumvention of certain types of infertility in cows (Elsden et al., 1979; Mapletoft et al., 1980; Figure 34.1). Careful screening of donors is necessary to ensure that the infertility is due to injury, disease or senility, and is not of genetic origin, otherwise reproductive problems could be propagated.

Twinning in cattle

Studies have shown that the efficiency of beef production from suckler herds could be increased by twinning in intensively managed units (Sreenan, 1977).

Genetic selection for twinning has largely been

unsuccessful (Sreenan, 1979) and gonadotrophin treatments to increase ovulation rates are not reliable (Gordon et al., 1962). Twinning by embryo transfer, either by transfer of two embryos or one embryo to a previously inseminated recipient, is a practical alternative (Sreenan and Diskin, 1982). The relatively high cost of embryo transfer has precluded practical application in the past. However, the technology of *in vitro* fertilization applied to oocytes aspirated from abattoir ovaries has now dramatically reduced unit costs per embryo, opening up possibilities for commercial application of twinning to improve beef production (Lu and Polge, 1992).

Conservation

Embryo transfer can be used to increase the population of rare or endangered breeds or species, provided there are recipients of a more plentiful breed or species that will accept the embryo.

EMBRYO TRANSFER IN THE COW

Superovulation

Single embryos can be recovered and transferred to other cows 6–8 days after service at natural oestrus, but because of the high costs involved, this is not usually an economic procedure in the practical situation. Consequently, a critical aspect of embryo transfer technology is the use of gonadotrophins to induce multiple ovulations in the ovaries of the donor cow (superovulation). For optimum response, gonadotrophin treatment is initiated on days 9–14 (oestrus = day 0) of a normal oestrous cycle. Prostaglandin is administered 48–72 hours later to cause regression of the mid-cycle corpus luteum and induce oestrus,

which usually occurs 40–56 hours later. Manifestation of oestrus is usually normal and it is common practice to inseminate donors on at least two occasions 12–18 hours apart when using frozen semen as ovulations may occur over a prolonged period of time (Maxwell et al., 1978). The superovulated donor would appear to be a sensitive indicator of the fertility of semen (Newcomb et al., 1978a) and only bulls of high fertility should be used.

Several different gonadotrophins have been used to superovulate cattle and these include pregnant mare serum gonadotrophin (eCG) (Betteridge, 1977), pituitary follicle-stimulating hormone (FSH) of porcine (Elsden et al., 1978), equine (Christie and Green, 1984) or ovine (Jordt and Lorenzini, 1990) origin, and human menopausal gonadotrophin (hMG) (Newcomb, 1980).

eCG has a longer biological half-life in the cow than either FSH or hMG, consequently a single injection of 2000–3000 IU will induce superovulation. FSH and hMG require a multiple injection treatment regimen for optimum effect; for instance, porcine FSH is usually administered twice daily for 4–5 days. The long half-life of eCG can be a disadvantage, as its effect persists even after induced oestrus, and in some cows embryo transport is adversely affected. This is manifest, over large numbers, by a poorer recovery rate of embryos after superovulation with eCG, compared with other gonadotrophins (Table 34.1). There is evidence that an eCG antiserum administered at oestrus will improve results (Saumande et al., 1984). The presence of substantial luteinizing hormone activity in eCG and in the crude FSH preparations commonly available for superovulation can adversely affect the viability of some ovulated oocytes by causing premature maturation (Moor et al., 1984). Fertilization failure has also been attributed to abnormalities of oocyte

Table 34.1 A survey of superovulatory response and egg recovery after treatment with each of three gonadotrophins in cows

Gonadotrophin	No. of cows	Mean ovulation rate	Mean No. of eggs recovered	Recovery rate (%)	Mean No. of viable eggs (%)
eCG (2500–3500 IU)	149	10.6	7.54	71.1	6.4 (84.7)
Equine FSH (20–24 mg)	52	11.83	9.62	81.3	7.13 (74.2)
Porcine FSH (40–50 mg)	54	11.52	9.48	82.3	7.41 (78.1)

From Christie and Green (1984).

maturation (Moor et al., 1985) and to asynchrony between maturation of the oocyte and the follicle (Loos et al., 1991). The problems are compounded by deficiencies in sperm transport in superovulated animals, resulting in reduced numbers of sperm in the uterine tube at the time of fertilization (Hawk, 1988). There is some evidence that the use of purified FSH preparations will improve fertilization rates and embryo quality (Donaldson and Ward, 1986).

Donor cows can be superovulated repeatedly at approximately 6–8 week intervals with no adverse effect on subsequent fertility (Christie et al., 1979a), but ovarian response to superovulation treatment is very variable, both between animals and between treatments of the same animal (Newcomb et al., 1979). With experience, variability can be reduced by adjusting dose rates but this still remains one of the problem areas of embryo transfer, with some donors yielding no embryos and occasionally 30 or more being recovered.

Embryos are located under a stereoscopic microscope after settling and siphoning or aspiration of the flushing medium (Newcomb et al., 1978b), or after filtering through a plankton filter (Pugh et al., 1980). A modified phosphate buffered saline (PBS) (Whittingham, 1971) is commonly used both for flushing the uterus and for storage. Embryos can be kept in PBS on the bench for at least 8 hours with no loss of viability and can be cultured for up to 48 hours with acceptable results on transfer (Trounson et al., 1976a). It is also possible to cool embryos to +4° C and maintain them in a state of suspended development for up to 3 days (Lindner et al., 1983), or store them long-term by deep freezing (see later).

Collection of embryos

In the cow the egg usually enters the uterus on day 4 after oestrus, at which time non-surgical embryo recovery becomes feasible by flushing the uterus through the cervix. Collection attempts are usually made on day 7 or 8 after oestrus but recovery and successful transfer is possible up to day 16 (Betteridge et al., 1976).

There are several methods of non-surgical embryo recovery in use but the commonest fall broadly into the types depicted in Figures 34.2 and 34.3. The earliest reported method was the variable-distance three-way (Sugie et al., 1972) but

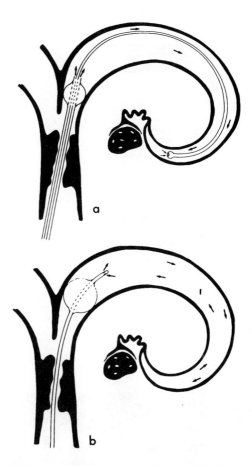

Fig. 34.2 Techniques for recovering bovine embryos non-surgically: (a) variable-distance three-way (continuous flow); (b) two-way (ebb and flow). (From Newcomb et al. (1978b).)

the fixed-distance three-way (Newcomb et al., 1978b) is the most common technique in use in the UK. This method has the advantage of a continuous flow of medium within the distal third of the uterine horn and a consequent efficient flush of the region of the horn where the majority of early-stage embryos are situated (Newcomb et al., 1976) (see also Figure 34.4). The ebb and flow two-way technique (Elsden et al., 1976; Greve et al., 1977) is simpler but requires larger volumes of flushing medium and is more time-consuming. In non-superovulated cattle, a skilled operator using these techniques can recover an egg in six or seven out of 10 attempts. The results which can be expected from superovulated donors are summarized in Table 34.1.

Day 7 bovine embryos are about 150–190 μm in diameter, are still within the zona pellucida and at the late morula or blastocyst stage of development

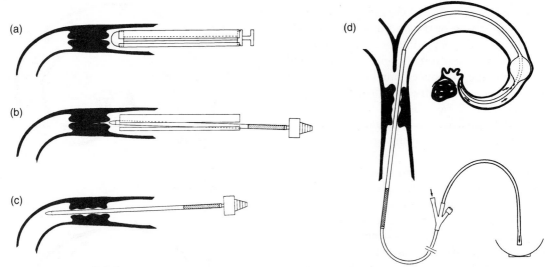

Fig. 34.3 A fixed-distance three-way technique for recovering bovine embryos non-surgically: (a) speculum in the vagina; (b) introducer passed through the speculum to the cervix; (c) introducer passed through the cervix into one uterine horn; (d) PVC catheter passed through the introducer to the tip of the horn and the cuff inflated. (From Newcomb et al. (1978b).)

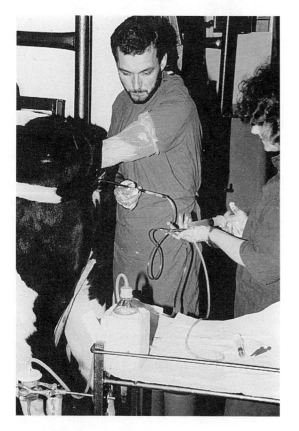

Fig. 34.4 A fixed-distance three-way uterine flush in progress.

(Figure 34.5). They can be handled easily using fine glass pipettes and are evaluated under the microscope at 50–100 × magnification. An assessment of viability can then be made by taking into account stage of development relative to age, and the appearance of the cells. Embryos are usually classified good, moderate or poor in quality, and this can be related to pregnancy rate on transfer (Table 34.2).

Transfer

Many factors will affect the suitability of a recipient for embryo transfer. The animals used should be healthy, fertile heifers or young cows which are in good body condition and can be reasonably expected to deliver the transferred calf, trouble-free, at term. Nutritional status should be good and ideally the recipient should be on a rising plane for at least 6 weeks before and after transfer to achieve optimum results.

It has been shown conclusively that the oestrous cycle of the donor and recipient should be closely synchronized if transferred embryos are to survive (Rowson et al., 1972). An asynchrony of more than 24 hours results in a marked fall in pregnancy rate, and it is more economic to freeze and transfer later, when suitable recipients are available, than to step outside these limits. Of great importance too is the side of the transfer. Pregnancy rates are greatly reduced unless the

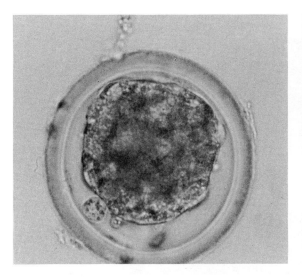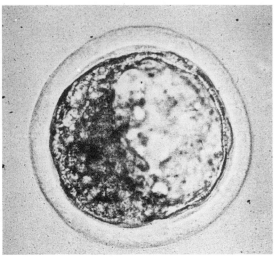

Fig. 34.5 Day 7 bovine embryos: Left, morula; right, blastocyst.

Table 34.2 The quality of eggs/embryos recovered from superovulated cows and pregnancy rate achieved on transfer — a survey of 1437 eggs

	Quality of egg/embryo			
	Good	*Moderate*	*Poor*	*Unfertilized/degenerate*
Percentage in each category	50.4	13.2	10.7	25.7
Pregnancy rate (%)	79.0	63.8	38.6	Discarded

From Christie (1982).

embryo is placed in the lumen of the uterine horn on the same side as the corpus luteum (Christie et al., 1979b).

Embryos can be transferred either surgically or non-surgically. For surgical transfer, the uterus is exposed through a flank incision under local anaesthesia (Newcomb, 1979). A puncture is made with a blunt needle and the embryo transferred to the lumen using a fine pipette or catheter (Rowson et al., 1969) (see Figure 34.6). Under controlled conditions a pregnancy rate of approximately 70% can be consistently achieved with embryos transferred on the same day as recovery.

Similar equipment to that used for artificial insemination can be used for non-surgical transfer but stricter asepsis must be observed and the embryo is usually placed some distance into the appropriate uterine horn. Success appears to be skill-related, suggesting that trauma to the endometrium may be a limiting factor with this technique. However, experienced and dextrous individuals can achieve a pregnancy rate approaching that of surgical transfer, and as a consequence welfare considerations must mitigate against continued use of the surgical technique.

EMBRYO TRANSFER IN SHEEP AND GOATS

Embryo transfer techniques are well established in sheep, mainly because the ewe has been used extensively in research as a low-cost model for the cow. Commercial use of the technique in sheep has not been widespread, with rapid multiplication of recently imported breeds and MOET schemes for breed improvement being the commonest applications. The use of embryo transfer in the goat mushroomed in the late 1980s, in line with the increased demand for valuable

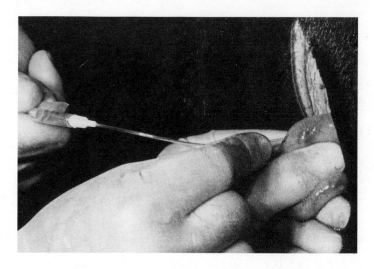

Fig. 34.6 Surgical transfer. A fine catheter is passed through a puncture into the uterine lumen to deliver the embryo.

pure-bred Angora and Cashmere stock in the UK and Australasia, but has subsequently decreased to a low level.

Techniques for superovulation, embryo recovery and transfer are very similar for both species (Armstrong and Evans, 1983). The gonadotrophin preparations used are the same as those used in the cow, and they are administered in similar treatment regimens. Gonadotrophin treatment is usually initiated mid- to late cycle and prostaglandin is administered 24–72 hours later, inducing oestrus within 24–36 hours. Oestrus and ovulation can also be controlled by progesterone or progestogen administration in the form of injections, implants or vaginal sponges. Sheep are treated for 12–14 days and goats for 14–18 days; using this method, superovulation can be induced outside the breeding season.

Insemination is commonly achieved by natural service or artificially, using freshly collected semen. However, fertilization failure can occur commonly in the ewe, particularly when the ovarian response to gonadotrophin is high. This can be overcome by surgical insemination directly into the uterus, either by laparotomy (Trounson and Moore, 1974) or by a laparoscopic technique (Maxwell, 1984).

Surgical techniques for the recovery of embryos from the ewe and the doe have changed very little since the first reports (Hunter et al., 1955) and involve general anaesthesia, midline laparotomy

and flushing of the catheterized uterus and uterine tube. Non-surgical recovery in the ewe has been reported (Coonrod et al., 1986) although the tortuous nature of the cervix makes catheter passage very difficult. Laparoscopy has been shown to be as effective as laparotomy (McKelvey et al., 1986) and is now widely used. The transcervical passage of catheters is much easier in the doe and non-surgical techniques could be more successful in this species.

Collections are normally carried out 3–7 days after oestrus and embryos can be evaluated and handled in the laboratory in a similar manner to the cow.

Most transfers are performed using general anaesthesia and midline laparotomy or laparoscopy. Embryos earlier than the eight-cell stage of development are best transferred to the uterine tube, and later-stage embryos to the uterus. Uterine transfer of day 6 and 7 embryos by laparoscope is as effective as laparotomy in the ewe (McKelvey et al., 1985) and has the advantage of not requiring exteriorization of the tract. Recipients are synchronized using prostaglandin treatments or intravaginal progestogens and oestrus is detected by the use of a harnessed, vasectomized ram or buck.

The requirements for synchrony of oestrus between donor and recipient are similar to the cow.

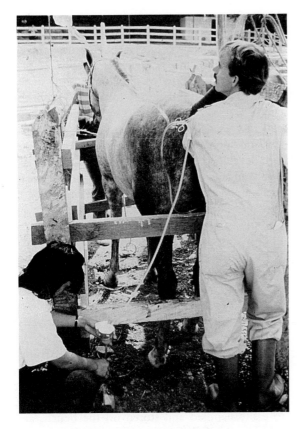

Fig. 34.7 A uterine flush in progress in a mare.

EMBRYO TRANSFER IN THE MARE

Embryo transfer in the mare is a relatively new procedure compared to the cow and many breed societies have been reluctant to register progeny (Figure 34.7). This, coupled with the difficulty in inducing superovulation, has limited commercial application. The major uses, apart from the production of multiple offspring, are for the production of foals from subfertile mares, for the removal of the risks of gestation and parturition from older valuable brood mares and for the production of foals from mares while they are in competition.

Limited success has been achieved with superovulation in mares using large doses of equine pituitary extract injected daily during dioestrus (Squires and McKinnon, 1986). In this study, two embryos were collected per mare compared with 0.65 embryos per untreated control. Porcine FSH was even less effective and eCG has been shown to

have no effect at all on follicular development in the mare (Douglas, 1979). Consequently, it is routine for most groups involved in equine embryo transfer to collect single embryos.

Embryos are recovered non-surgically 6–8 days postovulation using a Foley-type catheter and an ebb and flow flush of the uterus with modified PBS. Day 9 embryos have been found to be less viable on transfer, possibly due to their relatively large size and consequent predisposition to handling damage (Squires et al., 1982). The use of prostaglandin on the day of recovery allows repeat collections to be made at approximately 17–18 day intervals without compromising embryo recovery.

The early equine embryo grows very rapidly and can usually be seen with the naked eye in flushing media, ranging from 0.1 to 4.5 mm in diameter from 6–9 days postovulation.

The degree of synchrony between donor and recipient is not so critical in the mare as in other large domestic species. Squires et al. (1985) found no difference in pregnancy rate between recipients ovulating 1 day before, or up to 3 days after the donor, although those ovulating after tended to be best. Ovulation can be synchronized using progesterone and human chorionic gonadotrophin (hCG) treatments.

Transfer can be performed either non-surgically through the cervix or surgically through a flank incision. As with the cow, the results with non-surgical transfer are more variable than with surgery, and are dependent on operator skill. Pregnancy rates of 50–70% can, however, be achieved by an experienced technician.

EMBRYO TRANSFER IN THE PIG

Embryo transfer has not been widely used in the pig, except as a research procedure. Potentially the major applications in the pig are international movement of genetic material and disease control, either to establish disease free herds from infected donors (James et al., 1983) or for the introduction of new bloodlines into specific pathogen-free herds.

The basic procedures in pigs are well established (review — Polge, 1982). When superovulation is required, gonadotrophins such as eCG are best administered during the early follicular phase of the cycle, 15 or 16 days after the onset of oestrus (Hunter, 1964). Oestrus then occurs $3\frac{1}{2}$–4 days later, and an average of 25–30 ovulations may be expected following a dose of 1000–1500 IU eCG. Synchronization of oestrus of donors and recipients can be easily achieved by use of the oral progestogen altrenogest (Polge, 1982).

Embryo recovery in the pig is generally very successful and involves general anaesthesia and mid-ventral laparotomy 3–7 days after oestrus. Ovulation in pigs occurs 36–40 hours after the onset of oestrus and embryos remain in the uterine tubes for less than 48 hours after ovulation. Consequently, embryo recovery from the uterine horns is the general practice. Modified PBS is flushed into the uterus from the fimbrial end of the uterine tube and is collected through a cannula in the uterine horn (Hancock and Hovell, 1962). Donors can be used for collection two or three times if care is taken with the surgery.

Average recovery rates of over 90% can be achieved and embryos can be stored for short periods in modified PBS before transfer. Embryos must be maintained at a temperature above 15°C in the laboratory, as they are extremely sensitive to cooling (Polge, 1977). Embryo survival after culture periods of more than 24 hours are low (Pope and Day, 1977).

Transfers are also performed using midline surgery, the usual method being to use a fine pipette which is passed through a puncture in the isthmus of the uterine tube and into the uterus. Embryos need only be transferred to one uterine horn, from which they will migrate throughout the uterus (Dzuik et al., 1964). About 14 embryos are routinely transferred to each recipient but a minimum of four are required to establish pregnancy (Polge et al., 1966). Optimum pregnancy rates of 70% and embryo survival rates of 60–65% is achieved when day 3–7 embryos are transferred to recipients that were in oestrus on the same day or 1–2 days after the donor (Polge, 1982).

CRYOPRESERVATION OF EMBRYOS

The earliest report of successful cryopreservation of mammalian embryos was by Whittingham et al.

(1972). This group used the mouse as an experimental animal and demonstrated the importance of cooling rate, thawing rate and cryoprotectant on embryo survival. Initial attempts to apply the best method for the mouse to the cow resulted in the birth of a calf (Wilmut and Rowson, 1973) but the success rate was very low. The sheep was subsequently used experimentally as a model for the cow and soon practical methods for both species were developed (Willadsen, 1977; Willadsen et al., 1978) and later extended to the goat and the horse. There are variations between species, however, in the stages of embryonic development that tolerate exposure to low temperatures.

The early experiments with mouse embryos (Whittingham et al., 1972, Wilmut, 1972) had demonstrated that embryos from one cell to blastocyst stage could survive deep freezing. However, Trounson et al. (1976b) showed that early bovine embryos were sensitive to cooling, but an increased tolerance developed once they had reached the compacted morula or blastocyst stage. Consequently, interest centred on day 6, 7 or 8 embryos in this species, particularly in view of the fact that these stages are readily recovered non-surgically, are easily handled and stored on the bench, and can be successfully transferred surgically or non-surgically into recipients. In the mare, embryos do not enter the uterus from the uterine tube until day 6, at which stage they can be successfully recovered non-surgically.

Day 6 embryos have been successfully frozen in the mare (Slade et al., 1985), but later-stage embryos do not withstand freezing so well. In contrast, pig embryos at any stage of development appear to be extremely intolerant of cooling (Polge, 1977). There has, however, been a report of the birth of piglets after transfer of frozen/thawed expanded blastocysts (Hayashi et al., 1989), although with a low rate of success.

The principles of cryopreservation in the larger domestic animals are best discussed by referring to the cow, as techniques are well documented in this species (review — Lehn-Jensen, 1984). The important features of successful bovine programmes are applicable to sheep, goats and mares, including the use of a modified PBS (Whittingham, 1971) as a freezing medium and glycerol as a cryoprotectant.

The cryoprotective effect of compounds such as glycerol depends on their presence intracellularly

(Willadsen, 1980); consequently a period of equilibration is necessary. Early reports suggested addition of glycerol in four to six steps of 5 minutes each in gradually increasing concentration. More recent evidence, however, suggests that embryos can be placed directly into 1.5 M glycerol in PBS at room temperature and that equilibration will occur in 10–15 minutes without deleterious effect (Schneider and Mazur, 1984). In contrast, it is important that glycerol is removed slowly from the embryo after thawing, in order to avoid osmotic lysis of cells.

This can be achieved by serial dilution in four to six steps of 10 minutes each and gradually decreasing concentration of glycerol in PBS. Alternatively, a sucrose gradient can be used (Nieman et al., 1982). Sucrose does not permeate the embryonic cell membrane and when added to the medium during cryoprotectant removal, the resulting high extracellular osmotic pressure prevents the intermittent swelling of blastomeres that would otherwise occur during stepwise cryoprotectant removal. Several authors have reported an improvement in embryo survival after thawing in a sucrose gradient compared with the stepwise method (Nieman et al., 1982, Bielanski et al., 1986).

Glycerol can be removed in one step by transferring the thawed embryo directly into 0.25–1.0 M sucrose in PBS for 10–20 minutes before placing in PBS. The latter is the basis of a 'one-step' procedure for direct transfer of embryos after thawing. This technique requires that the embryo is placed in a plastic straw in a column of medium containing glycerol. The remainder of the straw is then filled with a column of 0.25–1.0 M sucrose in a medium separated from the embryo by air bubbles. The fluid columns are mixed after thawing, by shaking the straw and the embryo is transferred non-surgically after an equilibration period (Renard et al., 1982; Leibo, 1983). More recently, ethylene glycol has been shown to be an effective cryoprotectant for bovine embryos. Ethylene glycol diffuses across the cell membrane much more rapidly than glycerol, allowing direct transfer of frozen–thawed embryos without cryoprotectant removal (Voelkel and Hu, 1992).

Plastic straws (0.25 or 0.5 ml) are commonly used as containers for freezing, although glass ampoules are used by some. There appears to be no effect of either container type on embryo survival after thaw (Bielanski et al., 1986).

The 6–8 day bovine embryo does not appear to be adversely affected by rapid temperature change above $-7°C$, and embryos can be placed directly into the freezing machine at this temperature and left to equilibrate rapidly. Induction of ice formation, or 'seeding', in the freezing medium is necessary once the temperature has reached the true freezing point of the medium, otherwise supercooling, spontaneous freezing, and intracellular ice formation will occur, with a consequent adverse effect on embryo viability (Bilton and Moore, 1976). Seeding is usually accomplished by pinching the container gently with a pair of forceps cooled in liquid nitrogen, but some modern freezing machines include automatic seeding in the programme. Most laboratories are using programmable freezing machines to obtain the precise cooling rates necessary for optimal embryo survival but it is possible to use a relatively simple device with good success (Lehn-Jensen, 1984).

The damage incurred by cells during freezing and thawing is thought to be mainly caused by the formation of intracellular ice and the dehydration of the embryo. The cells dehydrate during cooling, as the water in the medium crystallizes to form extracellular ice and the solute portion becomes increasingly hypertonic. The cryoprotectant helps protect the cells from the damaging effects of hypertonicity, and the intracellular ice formation is minimized if the cells are allowed sufficient time to dehydrate before they reach the temperature at which they would freeze internally (Whittingham, 1980). It is evident, therefore, that the cooling rate, plunge temperature and thawing rate will be critical in balancing these effects for optimal survival.

Slow cooling from the seeding temperature ($0.3–0.5°C$/min, plunging between -30 and $-40°C$) and a rapid thaw (approximately $360°$ C/minute) is favoured by most laboratories, with some slowing the rate of cooling to $-0.1°C$/min for the final 30 minutes prior to plunge (Willadsen et al., 1978; Elsden et al., 1982). Using this type of technique, very acceptable results can be achieved in commercial embryo transfer programmes in the cow (Table 34.3).

A further cause of damage to the embryo during freezing is the formation of random fracture planes in the extracellular ice during rapid cooling to the storage temperature (Lehn-Jensen

Table 34.3 The effect of quality of bovine embryos on pregnancy rate after transfer (direct or frozen/thawed) to recipients synchronized for oestrus within ±12 hours of the donor

Quality of embryos	Frozen transfers: No. pregnant/No. of embryos frozen (%)	Direct transfers: No. pregnant/No. transferred (%)
Good	747/1224 (61.0)	338/545 (74.4)
Moderate	73/169 (43.2)	69/124 (55.6)
Poor	9/34 (26.5)	34/86 (39.5)
Total	829/1427 (58.1)	441/664 (66.4)

From Christie (1986).

and Rall, 1983) and possibly also during rapid thaw. Fracture planes involving the embryo itself will cause varying degrees of cell damage and consequently affect viability. Damage restricted to the zona, in the form of cracks or holes, does not appear to be of any significance (Lehn-Jensen, 1984) although the presence of a zona, intact or otherwise, may well be beneficial in that it acts as a physical barrier to the growth of extracellular ice (Lehn-Jensen and Rall, 1983).

The optimum thawing rate depends on the method used for freezing. When embryos are frozen slowly and plunged into liquid nitrogen between −30 and −40°C, rapid thawing is essential to prevent residual water in the cells crystallizing during warming (Willadsen, 1977). When using ampoules, Elsden et al. (1982) found that thawing in a water bath at 37°C was superior to one at 25°C, and this is now the method of choice.

Although there are probably as many different techniques for freezing embryos as there are groups involved in bovine embryo transfer, the majority differ only in minor detail. Good results are more dependent on fastidious attention to detail in the laboratory and on good management and critical selection of suitable recipients, than to minor changes in equilibration times or cooling rates. Future research is needed to simplify techniques without prejudicing embryo survival. Field transfer of frozen/thawed embryos can now be carried out without the use of a laboratory set-up (Renard et al., 1982; Leibo, 1983; Massip and van der Zwalmen, 1984; Voelkel and Hu, 1992), but the protocols for freezing embryos are time-consuming and still require the use of sophisticated, programmable freezing machines.

Rall and Fahy (1985), however, showed that mouse embryos could be successfully cryopreserved by a simple, rapid vitrification technique requiring minimal equipment. This is a new approach dependent on the fact that concentrated solutions of cryoprotectants in PBS do not crystallize when cooled to low temperatures but become increasingly viscous and form a glass-like solid. Rall and Fahy used a mixture of four cryoprotectants in the mouse, but Massip et al. (1986) have reported successful vitrification of bovine embryos using a simplified technique which resulted in seven pregnancies from 13 transfers (53.8%). The embryos were equilibrated in two steps with 25% glycerol and 25% 1,2-propanediol, and then immediately plunged into liquid nitrogen. A rapid thaw technique and one-step dilution of cryoprotectant in 1 M sucrose in PBS was used, and this suggests that a 'one-step' transfer procedure could be applied successfully, making available an effective field technique, both for freezing and thawing, which requires minimal laboratory equipment.

There is no doubt that simple field methods for freezing and thawing bovine embryos are becoming more widely used. Whether they are generally applied will depend on the comparative results. Bovine embryos are still expensive to recover and most embryos collected commercially are potentially valuable. Consequently, even a few per cent advantage in pregnancy rate would mean continuous use of programmable freezing machines and laboratory thawing for a few years yet.

MANIPULATION OF EMBRYOS

The technologies associated with manipulation of oocytes and embryos are advancing at a very rapid rate. In vitro maturation and fertilization of oocytes has been achieved in the sheep (Staigmiller and Moor, 1984), and preovulatory oocytes collected from ovaries and fertilized *in vitro* have resulted in live calves (Brackett et al., 1982; Sirard and Lambert, 1986; Lu et al., 1987, 1988a) and piglets (Cheng, 1985). Successful cloning of 16-cell embryos has been reported in the ewe (Willadsen, 1986; Wilmut and Smith, 1988) and foreign genes have been injected into the nucleus and incorporated into the genome of single-cell, fertilized eggs of pig (Hammer et al., 1985) and sheep

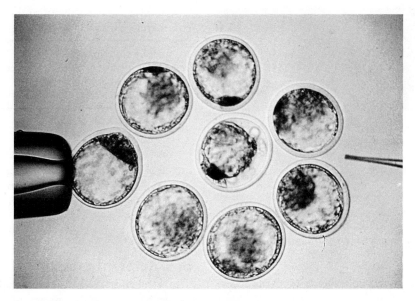

Fig. 34.8 A group of bovine embryos at the expanded blastocyst stage of development produced by in vitro maturation, fertilization and culture.

(Simons et al., 1988). Many other manipulations of the fertilization process, such as androgenesis, gynogenesis and parthenogenesis may also be possible in future (Seidel, 1982).

In vitro maturation and fertilization of oocytes

These techniques have recently become highly developed in cattle, with banks of cheap embryos now available for commercial transfer on a limited scale in the UK (Lu and Polge, 1992) (Figure 34.8).

The vast number of oocytes normally wasted in the abattoir are tapped by recovering the ovaries and releasing the oocytes from 2–5 mm follicles by aspiration. Maturation is achieved by culturing the oocytes for 24–26 hours in medium containing serum from a cow in oestrus (Lu et al., 1987). Most oocytes will reach the second metaphase stage of meiosis during culture but not all have the full potential for development.

Matured oocytes are then cultured with sperm capacitated *in vitro* (Parrish et al., 1986), and up to 90% fertilization can be achieved with some bulls.

Embryos must be at the morula or blastocyst stage of development before they can be transferred to the uterus of a recipient. This can be achieved either by culture of the newly fertilized embryo or by transfer to a temporary host. The sheep is the host of choice for the latter approach.

Several hundred one- or two-cell embryos can be transferred to the uterine tube of a ewe and recovered 6 days later for evaluation, transfer or freezing.

Culture of early embryos in chemically-defined media has not been very successful. In contrast, however, co-culture with bovine uterine tube epithelial cells (Lu et al., 1988b) produces acceptable results and is the method of choice in the practical situation.

Commercial exploitation of these techniques has already begun, with the ultimate aim of increasing the quality and size of the calf crop by twinning or transfer into the genetically inferior dairy herds using embryos of cross-bred beef breed derivation.

Recently, a technique for aspiration of oocytes from the ovaries of live cows has been described (Pieterse et al., 1991). This has opened up the prospect of a dramatic increase in embryo production from valuable, pedigree cattle where slaughter is not an option. Van der Schans et al. (1991) were able to collect an average of 9.4 oocytes per aspiration from cows aspirated twice weekly over a 3 month period. Follicle aspiration was achieved using a transvaginal, ultrasound-guided puncture technique, and there appeared to be no significant detrimental effect of repeat sampling on the ovary or genital tract.

Follicle aspiration and *in vitro* fertilization in

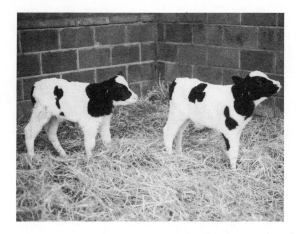

Fig. 34.9 Identical twin calves produced by micromanipulation of a day 7 embryo.

Table 34.4 The results of embryo bisection in a commercial embryo transfer programme

Number of embryos bisected	43
Number of demi-embryos transferred	86
Number of recipients pregnant (%)	52 (60.5)
Number of genetically identical pairs	16

From Christie and Green (1984).

Embryo division is being used commercially to increase the number of progeny produced in bovine embryo transfer programmes and could also be a valuable method for producing identical twins for research.

practice is particularly applicable to repeat breeders which are unsuitable for conventional embryo transfer, or normal cows which do not respond to superovulation treatments.

Micromanipulation

Division of embryos using microsurgical instruments is a practical method for creating identical siblings. Identical quadruplet sheep (Willadsen, 1981), triplet calves (Willadsen and Polge, 1981), and twin horses (Willadsen et al., 1980) and pigs (Polge, 1985) have been produced by separation of blastomeres of two-, four- and eight-cell embryos. Success rates are high when embryos are divided into two but drop off considerably when they are quartered. Identical quintuplets have been produced in sheep by mixing cells of four- and eight-cell embryos, when the more advanced cells apparently developed into the fetus and the less advanced contributed to the placenta (Willadsen and Fehilly, 1983).

A simpler and more practical method of producing identical twins (Figure 34.9) from morulae and early blastocysts involves microsurgical division of the embryo into two groups of cells and immediate transfer into recipients (Willadsen and Godke, 1984; Williams et al., 1984). The half embryos can be replaced in surrogate zonae pellucidae before transfer or transferred naked. Pregnancy rates of 50% or more per half embryo have been reported, resulting in a net pregnancy rate of over 100% per original embryo (Table 34.4).

Sex determination

The efficiency of livestock breeding enterprises would be considerably increased if it was possible to predetermine the sex of offspring. The vast majority of claims to alter the sex ratio significantly by the separation of X and Y chromosome-bearing spermatozoa have not been substantiated in practice. Recently, however, a method has been described for separation of spermatozoa on the basis of their DNA content, by fluorescent labelling and cell sorting (Cran, 1992). The method has significant production limitations and is therefore more compatible with *in vitro* fertilization systems, where low sperm numbers per oocyte are required, than with artificial insemination, where sperm numbers per insemination are high.

Embryos have been sexed by cytological methods (review — King, 1984). These involve chromosome analysis of cells in metaphase which have been sampled from the embryo using an embryo division technique. However, biopsy and karyotyping procedures are tedious, time-consuming and relatively inaccurate, making them impractical for routine commercial use.

An alternative approach is to use an antibody to the HY antigen, a protein present on the surface of male mammalian cells. The HY antibody binds to male embryos and can be detected by adding a fluorescently labelled antibody directed against the first, such that male embryos fluoresce in appropriate light. This procedure sexes mouse embryos with 80% accuracy (White et al., 1982) but has not been successfully applied to large domestic species.

A more accurate method for determination of sex has become available with the development of DNA probes which are specific for the Y chromosome. Only a few cells need to be sampled for testing, with a consequent minimal effect on embryo viability. Effective probes have been developed for several species including the cow (Jones et al., 1987; Leonard et al., 1987; Ellis et al., 1988; Herr and Reed, 1991). Several probes have been developed for commerical use in combination with polymerase chain reaction (PCR) technology, but the relatively high cost of the test has prevented widespread application.

The manipulation of eggs and embryos of the large domestic species will have a major impact on the efficiency of animal production in the future. Although much of the research involved is in its infancy, it is growing fast and there are exciting prospects ahead for the geneticist and the animal breeder. It should be remembered, however, that it is through embryo transfer that new developments may be exploited and that the use of this breeding technique will expand accordingly over the next decade.

REFERENCES

Armstrong, D. T. and Evans, G. L. (1983) *Theriogenology*, **19**, 31.

Baker, R. D., Snider, G. W., Leipold, H. W. and Johnson, T. L. (1980) *Theriogenology*, **13**, 87.

Betteridge, K. J. (ed.) (1977) In: *Embryo Transfer in Farm Animals*, p. 1. Ottawa: Agriculture Canada.

Betteridge, K. J., Mitchell, D., Eaglesome, M. D. and Randall, G. C. B. (1976) *Proc. 8th Int. Cong. Anim. Reprod. AI, Krakow*, **3**, 237.

Bielanski, A., Schneider, U., Pawlyshyn, V. P. and Mapletoft, R. J. (1986) *Theriogenology*, **25**, 429.

Bilton, J. R. and Moore, N. W. (1976) *Theriogenology*, **6**, 635.

Brackett, B. G., Bousquet, D., Boice, M. L., Donawick, W. J., Evans, J. F. and Dressel, M. A. (1982) *Biol. Reprod.*, **27**, 147.

Cheng, W. T.-K. (1985) Ph.D. Thesis, Council for National Academic Awards.

Christie, W. B. (1982) In: *The Veterinary Annual*, ed. C. S. G. Grunsell and F. W. G. Hill, p. 113. Bristol: Scientechnica.

Christie, W. B. (1986) *Proc. 5th Ann. Conv. American E. T. Assn*, p. 33.

Christie, W. B. and Green, D. (1984) Unpublished observations.

Christie, W. B., Newcomb, R. and Rowson, L. E. A. (1979b) *J. Reprod. Fertil.*, **56**, 701.

Christie, W. B., McGuirk, B. J., Strathie, R. J. and Mullan, J. S. (1992) *Ann. Zootech.*, **41**, 347.

Coonrod, S. A., Coren, B. R., McBride, B. L., Bowen, M. J. and Kraemer, D. C. (1986) *Theriogenology*, **25**, 149 (Abstr.).

Cran, D. G. (1992) In: *Embryonic Development and Manipulation in Animal Production*, ed. A. Lauria and F. Gandolfi, p. 125. London: Portland Press.

Cunningham, E. P. (1976) In: *Egg Transfer in Cattle*, ed. L. E. A. Rowson, EUR 5491, p. 345. Luxembourg: Commission of the European Communities.

Donaldson, L. E. and Ward, D. N. (1986) *Vet. Rec.*, **119**, 625.

Douglas, R. H. (1979) *Theriogenology*, **11**, 33.

Dzuik, P. J., Polge, C. and Rowson, L. E. A. (1964) *J. Anim. Sci.*, **23**, 37.

Ellis, S. B., Bondioli, K. R., Williams, M. E., Pryor, J. H. and Harpold, M. M. (1988) *Theriogenology*, **29**, 242 (Abstr.).

Elsden, R. P., Hasler, J. F. and Seidel, G. E. Jr (1976) *Theriogenology*, **6**, 523.

Elsden, R. P., Nelson, L. D. and Seidel, G. E. Jr (1978) *Theriogenology*, **9**, 17.

Elsden, R. P., Nelson, L. D. and Seidel, G. E. Jr (1979) *Theriogenology*, **11**, 170.

Elsden, R. P., Seidel, G. E. Jr, Takeda, T. and Farrand, G. D. (1982) *Theriogenology*, **17**, 1.

Gordon, I., Williams, G. and Edward, J. (1962) *J. Agric. Sci.*, **59**, 143.

Greve, T., Lehn-Jensen, H. and Rasbech, N. O. (1977) *Theriogenology*, **7**, 239.

Hammer, R. E., Pursel, V. G., Rexroad, C. E. Jr, Wall, R. J., Bolt, D. J., Ebert, K. M., Palmiter, R. D. and Brinster, R. L. (1985) *Nature, Lond.*, **315**, 680.

Hancock, J. L. and Hovell, G. J. R. (1962) *J. Reprod. Fertil.*, **2**, 295.

Hawk, H. W. (1988) *Theriogenology*, **29**, 125.

Hayashi, S., Kobayashi, K., Mizuno, J., Saitho, K. and Hirano, S. (1989) *Vet. Rec.*, **125**, 43.

Heape, W. (1891) *Proc. R. Soc. Lond.*, **48**, 457.

Herr, C. M. and Reed, K. C. (1991) *Theriogenology*, **35**, 45.

Hunter, G. L., Adams, C. E. and Rowson, L. E. A. (1955) *J. Agric. Sci.*, **46**, 143.

Hunter, R. H. F. (1964) *Anim. Prod.*, **6**, 189.

James, J. E., James, D. M., Martin, P. A., Reed, D. E. and Davis, D. L. (1983) *J. Amer. Vet. Med. Assn*, **183**, 525.

Jones, K. W., Singh, L. and Edwards, R. G. (1987) *Human Reprod.*, **2**, 439.

Jordt, T. and Lorenzini, E. (1990) *Proc. 6e Renunion AETE, Lyon*, p. 158.

Lehn-Jensen, H. (1984) *Proc. 10th Int. Cong. Anim. Reprod. and AI, Urbana-Champaign*, **4**, II–1–11.

Lehn-Jensen, H. and Rall, W. F. (1983) *Theriogenology*, **19**, 263.

Leibo, S. P. (1983) *Cryo-Letters*, **4**, 387.

Leonard, M., Kirszenbaum, M., Cotinot, C., Chesne, P., Heyman, Y., Stinnakre, M. G., Bishop, C., Delouis, C., Vaiman, M. and Fellous (1987) *Theriogenology*, **27**, 248 (Abstr.).

Lindner, G. M., Anderson, G. B., Bon Durant, R. H. and Cupps, P. T. (1983) *Theriogenology*, **20**, 311.

Loos, F. de Bevers, M. M., Dieleman, S. J. and Kruip, Th. A. M. (1991) *Theriogenology*, **35**, 537.

Lu, K. H., Gordon, I., Gallagher, M. and McGovern, H. (1987) *Vet. Rec.*, **121**, 259.

Lu, K. K., Gordon, I., Gallagher, M. and McGovern, H. (1988a) *Theriogenology*, **29**, 272 (Abstr.).

Lu, K. H., Gordon, I., Chen, H. B., Gallagher, M. and McGovern, H. (1988b) *Vet. Rec.*, **122**, 539.

Lu, K. H. and Polge, C. (1992) *Proc. 12th Int. Cong. Anim. Reprod., The Hague*, **3**, 1315.

McKelvey, W. A. C., Robinson, J. J. and Aitken, R. P. (1985) *Vet. Rec.*, **117**, 492.

McKelvey, W. A. C., Robinson, J. J., Aitken, R. P. and Robertson, I. S. (1986) *Theriogenology*, **25**, 855.

Massip, A. and van der Zwalmen, P. (1984) *Vet. Rec.*, **115**, 327.

Massip, A. and van der Zwalmen, P., Scheffen, B. and Ectors, F. (1986) *Cryo-Letters*, **7**, 270.

Maxwell, D. P., Massey, J. M. and Kraemer, D. C. (1978) *Theriogenology*, **9**, 97 (Abstr.).

Maxwell, W. M. C. (1984) In: *Reproduction in the Sheep*, ed. D. R. Lindsay and D. T. Pierce, p. 291. Canberra: Australian Academy of Science.

Moor, R. M., Kruip, Th. A. M. and Green, D. (1984) *Theriogenology*, **21**, 103.

Moor, R. M., Osborne, J. C. and Crosby, I. M. (1985) *J. Reprod. Fertil.*, **74**, 167.

Newcomb, R. (1979) *Vet. Rec.*, **105**, 432.

Newcomb, R. (1980) *Vet. Rec.*, **106**, 48.

Newcomb, R., Rowson, L. E. A. and Trounson, A. O. (1976) In: *Egg Transfer in Cattle*, ed. L. E. A. Rowson, EUR 5491, p. 1. Luxembourg: Commission of the European Communities.

Newcomb, R., Christie, W. B. and Rowson, L. E. A. (1978a) *Vet. Rec.*, **102**, 414.

Newcomb, R., Rowson, L. E. A. and Trounson, A. O. (1978b) *Vet. Rec.*, **103**, 415.

Newcomb, R., Christie, W. B., Rowson, L. E. A., Walters, D. E. and Bousfield, W. E. D. (1979) *J. Reprod. Fertil.*, **56**, 113.

Nicholas, F. W. and Smith, C. (1983) *Anim. Prod.*, **36**, 341.

Nieman, H., Sacher, B., Schilling, E. and Schmit, D. (1982) *Theriogenology*, **17**, 102 (Abstr.).

Parrish, J. J., Susko-Parrish, J. L., Liebfried-Rutledge, M. L., Critser, E. S., Eyestone, W. H. and First, N. L. (1986) *Theriogenology*, **25**, 591.

Pieterse, M. C., Vos, Plam, Kruip, Th. A. M., Warth, Y. A., Van Bereden, Th. H., Willemse, A. H. and Taverne, M. A. M. (1991) *Theriogenology*, **35**, 19.

Polge, C. (1977) In: *The Freezing of Mammalian Embryos*, G. B. A. Found. Symp. No. 52, p. 3. Amsterdam: Elsevier.

Polge, C. (1982) In: *Control of Pig Reproduction*, ed. D. J. A. Cole and G. R. Foxcroft, p. 277. London: Butterworth.

Polge, C. (1985) *J. Reprod. Fertil. Suppl.*, **33**, 93.

Polge, C., Rowson, L. E. A. and Chang, M. C. (1966) *J. Reprod. Fertil.*, **12**, 395.

Pope, C. E. and Day, B. N. (1977) *J. Anim. Sci.*, **44**, 1036.

Pugh, A., Trounson, A. D., Aarts, M. H. J. and McPhee, S. (1980) *Theriogenology*, **13**, 281.

Rall, W. F. and Fahy, G. M. (1985) *Theriogenology*, **23**, 220 (Abstr.).

Renard, J. P., Heyman, Y. and Ozil, J. P. (1982) *Vet. Med. — US*, **126**, 23.

Rowson, L. E. A., Moor, R. M. and Lawson, R. A. S. (1969) *J. Reprod. Fertil.*, **18**, 517.

Rowson, L. E. A., Lawson, R. A. S. and Moor, R. M. (1972) *J. Reprod. Fertil.*, **28**, 427.

Saumande, J., Procureur, R. and Chupin, D. (1984) *Theriogenology*, **21**, 727.

Schneider, V. and Mazur, P. (1984) *Theriogenology*, **21**, 68.

Seidel, G. E. Jr (1982) *Theriogenology*, **17**, 23.

Simons, J. P., Wilmut, I., Clark, A. J., Archibald, A. L., Bishop, J. O. and Lathe, R. (1988) *Biotechnology*, **6**, 179.

Singh, E. L. (1984) *Proc. 10th Int. Cong. Anim. Reprod. AI, Urbana-Champaign*, **IV**, IX–17.

Sirard, M. A. and Lambert, R. D. (1986) *Vet. Rec.*, **119**, 167.

Slade, N. P., Takeda, T., Squires, E. L. and Elsden, R. P. (1985) *Theriogenology*, **24**, 45.

Squires, E. L. and McKinnon, A. O. (1986) *Proc. 5th Ann. Conv. Am. E. T. Assn*, p. 73.

Squires, E. L., Iuliano, M. F. and Shideler, R. K. (1982) *Theriogenology*, **17**, 35.

Squires, E. L., Garcia, R. H. and Ginther, O. J. (1985) *Equine Vet. J.*, **3**, 92.

Sreenan, J. M. (1977) In: *Embryo Transfer in Farm Animals*, ed. K. J. Betteridge, p. 62. Ottawa: Agriculture Canada.

Sreenan, J. M. (1983) *Vet. Rec.*, **112**, 494.

Sreenan, J. M. and Diskin, M. G. (1982) *Ir. Vet. J.*, **36**, 138.

Staigmiller, R. B. and Moor, R. M. (1984) *Gamete Research*, **9**, 221.

Stringfellow, D. A. and Seidel, S. M. (eds) (1990) *Manual of the International Embryo Transfer Society*, p. 12. Champaign, Ill.: IETS.

Sugie, T., Soma, T., Fukumitsu, S. and Otsuiki, K. (1972) *Bull. Nat. Inst. Anim. Ind.*, **25**, 27.

Trounson, A. O. and Moore, N. W. (1974) *Aust. J. Biol. Sci.*, **27**, 301.

Trounson, A. O., Willadsen, S. M. and Rowson, L. E. A. (1976a) *J. Reprod. Fertil.*, **47**, 367.

Trounson, A. O., Willadsen, S. M., Rowson, L. E. A. and Newcomb, R. (1976b) *J. Reprod. Fertil.*, **46**, 173.

Van der Schans, A., Van der Westerlaken, L. A. J., De Wit, A. A. C., Eyestone, W. H. and De Boer, H. A. (1991) *Theriogenology*, **35**, 288.

Voelkel, S. A. and Hu, Y. X. (1992) *Theriogenology*, **37**, 23.

Warwick, B. L. and Berry, R. O. (1949) *J. Hered.*, **40**, 297.

Wite, K. L., Lindner, G. M., Anderson, G. B. and Durant, R. H. (1982) *Theriogenology*, **18**, 655.

Whittingham, D. G. (1971) *Nature*, **233**, 125.

Whittingham, D. G. (1980) *Proc. 9th Int. Cong. Anim. Reprod. AI, Madrid*, **2**, 237.

Whittingham, D. G., Leibo, S. and Mazur, P. (1972) *Science*, **178**, 411.

Willadsen, S. M. (1977) In: *The Freezing of Mammalian Embryos*, G. B. A. Found. Symp. No. 52, p. 175. Amsterdam: Elsevier.

Willadsen, S. M. (1980) *Proc. 9th Int. Cong. Anim. Reprod. AI, Madrid*, **2**, 255.

Willadsen, S. M. (1981) *J. Embryol. Exp. Morph.*, **65**, 165.

Willadsen, S. M. (1986) *Nature*, **320**, 63.

Willadsen, S. M. and Fehilly, D. B. (1983) In: *Fertilisation of the Human Egg In Vitro: Biological Bases and Clinical Applications*, ed. H. M. Beier and H. R. Lindner, p. 353. Berlin: Springer-Verlag.

Willadsen, S. M. and Godke, R. A. (1984) *Vet. Rec.*, **114**, 240.

Willadsen, S. M. and Polge, C. (1981) *Vet. Rec.*, **108**, 211.

Willadsen, S. M., Polge, C. and Rowson, L. E. A. (1978) In: *Control of Reproduction in the Cow*, ed. J. M. Sreenan, p. 427. Luxembourg: Commission of the European Communities.

Willadsen, S. M., Polge, C. and Rowson, L. E. A. (1978) *J. Reprod. Fertil.*, **52**, 391.

Willadsen, S. M., Pashen, R. L. and Allen, W. R. (1980) *Proc. Ann. Conf. Soc. Study Fert.*, p. 28 (Abstr.).

Williams, T. J., Elsden, R. P. and Seidel, G. E. Jr (1984) *Theriogenology*, **21**, 276.

Wilmut, I. (1972) *Life Science*, **II**(Part 2), 1071.

Wilmut, I. and Rowson, L. E. A. (1973) *Vet. Rec.*, **92**, 686.

Wilmut, I. and Smith, L. C. (1988) *Proc. 4th Cong. Europ. E. T. Assn, Lyons*, p. 19.

Wrathall, A. E. (1984) *Proc. 10th Int. Cong. Anim. Reprod. AI, Urbana-Champaign*, **IX**, IX–10.

The preparations listed in this appendix are those that are available in the UK at the time of publication. The recommendations are not necessarily those of the manufacturers, since some have been modified by the authors in the light of their experience. Readers are warned of the importance of checking the current recommendations in case changes have been made.

Gonadotrophin (luteinizing)-releasing hormone and analogues (GnRH or LHRH)

Naturally occurring hormone, produced by the hypothalamus and transferred to the anterior pituitary gland in the hypophyseal portal circulation. It is a peptide and stimulates the release of follicle-stimulating hormone (FSH) and luteinizing hormone (LH).

Commercially available products

Fertirelin, synthetic GnRH peptide ('Ovalyse', Upjohn Ltd, Crawley).

Gonadorelin, synthetic GnRH peptide ('Fertagyl', Intervet Animal Health UK Ltd, Cambridge).

Buserelin, synthetic GnRH peptide analogue ('Receptal', Hoechst Animal Health UK, Milton Keynes).

Pharmacological action

Stimulates a short surge of FSH and LH following a single bolus injection.

Indications

Cattle: follicular cysts;
  delayed ovulation or anovulation;
  acyclicity (doubtful if a single bolus is very effective);
  improved pregnancy rates following use of

buserelin when injected as a single bolus 12 days after insemination.

Horse: induce ovulation (preovulatory gonadotrophin surge lasts several days in mare); single bolus may not be effective, requires frequent repeated doses.

Dose rate

Buserelin: cow, 10–20 g; horse 40 g preferably i.m. but can be given i.v. or s.c.
Gonadorelin: cow, 0.5 mg i.m., s.c. or i.v.
Fertirelin: cow, 100 μg i.m.

Gonadotrophins

1. FSH and LH. FSH and LH can be obtained in a semi-purified form but both are expensive. Porcine FSH and recombinant-derived FSH are used to induce superovulation in donor cows for embryo transfer.

2. Equine chorionic gonadotrophin (eCG). Originally called pregnant mare's serum gonadotrophin (PMSG) but in order to use consistent nomenclature it is now called eCG. A protein hormone produced by the endometrial cups of the mare from about 40–120 days of pregnancy.

Commercially available products

eCG or serum gonadotrophin ('Folligon', Intervet UK Ltd, Cambridge; 'Fostim', Paines and Byrne Ltd, West Byfleet).

Pharmacological action

Mainly FSH-like in its action but has some LH activity.

Indications

Cattle: Superovulation of donor cows for embryo transfer; over-stimulation can be a problem;

impaired spermatogenesis in bulls (doubtful value).

Sheep and goats: in association with intravaginal progestogen sponges to advance the onset of breeding season.

Pig: in association with hCG to stimulate onset of cyclical activity after farrowing.

Dog: induce oestrus during physiological anoestrus.

Dose rate
Cattle, 1500–3000 IU s.c. or i.m.
Sheep and goats, 500–800 IU s.c. or i.m.
Pig, 1000 IU s.c. or i.m.
Dog, 50–200 IU.

3. Human menopausal gonadotrophin (hMG). Extracted from the urine of menopausal women, this has primarily an FSH-like action. Used to a limited extent in superovulating donor cows for embryo transfer. It has a shorter biological half-life than eCG.

4. Human chorionic gonadotrophin (hCG). A protein hormone extracted from the urine of pregnant women, this hormone has primarily an LH-like effect and hence is used as a substitute for the more expensive LH; it also has a longer half-life than LH.

Commercially available products
'Chorulon' injection (Intervet UK Ltd, Cambridge).

'LH 1500' (Paines and Bryne Ltd, West Byfleet).

Pharmacological action
Stimulates androgen production by the thecal cells of the ovary and Leydig cells of the testis, stimulates follicular maturation and ovulation, corpus luteum formation and maintenance.

Indications
Cattle: delayed ovulation or anovulation;
  ovarian cysts (especially follicular);
  luteal deficiency;
  improve chances of pregnancy in cyclic non-breeders (repeat-breeder cows), rationale is not always apparent;
  improve libido in bull (may make temperament more aggressive).

Horse: induce or hasten ovulation;
  'rig test', stimulates rise in testosterone in peripheral blood of suspected cryptorchid.

Pig: with eCG to stimulates onset of cyclical activity after farrowing;
  improve libido in boar.

Sheep and goat: improve libido in ram and male goat;
  cystic ovaries in female goat.

Dog: curtail pro-oestrus/oestrus in bitches with prolongation of these phases;
  cystic ovaries;
  improve libido in male dog.

Cat: induce ovulation.

Dose rate
Cattle, 1500–3000 IU i.v. or i.m.
Horse, 1500–3000 IU i.v. or i.m.
Pig, 500–1000 IU i.m. or s.c.
Sheep and goat, 100–500 IU i.v. or i.m.
Dog, 100–500 IU i.m.
Cat, 100–200 IU i.m.

Gonadotrophins with other hormones
A number of commercial preparations are available in which gonadotrophins are combined with other hormones as a single injectable substance. The rationale for their use is frequently doubtful since they are attempting to overcome complex hormone deficiencies somewhat simplistically.

Commercially available preparations and manufacturers' indications for usage
hCG with progesterone ('Nymfalon', Intervet UK Ltd, Cambridge). Indications are essentially those listed above for hCG in the cow and mare.

eCG and hCG ('PG 600', Intervet UK Ltd, Cambridge). Indicated for the induction of oestrus in sows and gilts after weaning. There is evidence that this can be a useful method of overcoming postpartum anoestrus.

Oxytocin and posterior pituitary extracts
Oxytocin is a peptide hormone produced by the neurones of the supraoptic nucleus and is trans-

ported to, and stored in, the posterior pituitary gland. Synthetic oxytocin is available commercially and is thus highly purified; however, aqueous extracts of mammalian pituitary glands are also available. These latter products will also contain other posterior pituitary hormones such as vasopressin and antidiuretic hormone (ADH).

Commercially available products

Oxytocin (Leo Laboratories Ltd, Aylesbury).

Oxytocin (Intervet UK Ltd, Cambridge).

'Hyposton', posterior pituitary extract (Paines and Bryne Ltd, West Byfleet).

Pharmacological action

Causes milk let-down, myometrial contractions to facilitate gamete transport, myometrial contractions during parturition and postpartum.

Indications

Cattle: induce milk let-down;
    hasten uterine involution following dystocia, caesarean operation, replacement of uterine prolapse, uterine trauma or haemorrhage.

Horse: induce foaling;
    cause expulsion of retained placenta;
    induce milk let-down.

Sheep: as for cow.

Pig: induce milk let-down;
    hasten second stage of parturition;
    treatment of uterine inertia;
    cause expulsion of retained placentas;
    hasten uterine involution.

Dog: treat uterine inertia;
    cause expulsion of retained placentas;
    hasten uterine involution after caesarean operation (perhaps treat sub-involution of placental sites);
    induce milk let-down.

Where there is trauma to the uterus, especially with haemorrhage, pituitary extracts should *not* be used.

Dose rate

Many recommended dose rates are too high. The myometrium is very sensitive to the effects of oxytocin and high dose rates can cause spasm rather than synchronized contractions. The myometrium will also become refractory to its effect, hence increasing incremental dose rates should be used. Most effective when used in an intravenous drip in saline.

Cattle, 10 IU i.m. or i.v.
Horse, 10 IU i.m. or i.v.
Pig, 5 IU i.m. or i.v.
Sheep and goat, 2–5 IU i.m. or i.v.
Dog and cat, 1–5 IU i.m. or i.v.

Spasmolytics

These substances have a wide range of effects; some are specific for the myometrium, whilst others exert their action upon all smooth muscles. Assessment of their efficacy is frequently rather subjective during their clinical application.

Commercially available preparations

Hyoscine *N*-butylbromide and dipyrone ('Buscopan Compositum', Boehringer Ingelheim Ltd, Bracknell).

Phenylbutane HCl ('Monzaldon', Boehringer Ingelheim Ltd, Bracknell).

Clenbuterol HCl ('Planipart', Boehringer Ingelheim Ltd, Bracknell). Clenbuterol HCl is a β-adrenergic stimulant.

Pharmacological action

Abolish or reduce myometrial contractions and tone, thus causing relaxation of the uterus at caesarean operations and during embryo transfer and enabling easier repulsion of the fetus in obstetrical manipulations. Clenbuterol HCl can be used specifically to postpone parturition in cattle as a management aid, or to allow adequate softening and relaxation of the birth canal to occur.

Indications

Cattle: relaxation of myometrium to facilitate obstetrical manipulation to treat dystocia and during caesarean operations;
    aid relaxation and softening of the birth canal;
    in embryo transfer to facilitate manipulation of the uterus;
    postpone parturition (clenbuterol HCl only).

Horse, sheep, pig and dog: as for cattle except it cannot be used to postpone parturition.

Cat: some spasmolytics are contraindicated in this species and should be checked before use.

Dose rate

These should be checked for each product and species before use.

Clenbuterol HCl, when used to postpone calving during the night, should be given at a dose rate of 0.3 mg (10 ml) i.m. at about 1800 hours followed by a second injection of 0.21 mg (7 ml) 4 hours later. This should postpone calving for 8 hours after the second injection. It must not be used if the cervix is fully dilated and second stage has commenced.

Oestrogens

Oestrogens, which are steroids, play a wide role in the reproductive process. However, there are relatively few rational indications for oestrogen therapy in the treatment of reproductive disorders in domestic species. In recent years, several of the synthetic oestrogens have been withdrawn from use in the EC because of concern about residues in human food products.

Commercially available products

Oestradiol benzoate (Intervet UK Ltd, Cambridge). This contains 5 mg/ml of hormone in a sterile oily solution.

Pharmacological actions

Oestrogens are primarily responsible for oestrous behaviour in the female; they stimulate changes in the tubular genital tract which control gamete transport and, with progestogens, cause development of the mammary gland. They potentiate the ecbolic action of oxytocin and prostaglandins on the myometrium. They stimulate the preovulatory surge of gonadotrophins.

Indications

Horse: ripening of the cervix before oxytocin-induced foaling.

Cattle: treatment of endometritis (contraindicated in acute toxic metritis).

Dog: treatment of misalliance in the bitch within 4 days of mating;
urinary incontinence in the spayed bitch;
prostatic hyperplasia in the male dog;
to depress hypersexuality in the male dog.

Dose rate

Horse, 3–6 mg i.m.
Cattle, 3–5 mg i.m.
Dog, for misalliance 0.1 mg/kg up to a maximum of 3 mg i.m.; for urinary incontinence 1 mg daily for 3 days then 1 mg every third day; for prostatic hyperplasia 1 mg/day.

Progestogens

These include the naturally occurring steroid progesterone and a number of synthetic progestogens which are much more potent and have a longer half-life. Progestogens are used widely in all domestic species, mainly to control cyclical activity; this is because, as a group, they exert a powerful negative feedback effect upon the hypothalamus and anterior pituitary gland, thus inhibiting gonadotrophin release. The consequence of this effect is to suppress cyclical activity so that, following cessation of treatment in polyoestrous species, there is ovarian rebound within a few days.

1. Progesterone

Commercially available products

Progesterone-releasing intravaginal device ('PRID', Sanofi Animal Health, Watford). Each device contains 1.55 g progesterone (in addition to a 10 mg capsule of oestradiol ester). Used for synchronization of oestrus in cows and heifers, preferably in conjunction with prostaglandin $F_{2\alpha}$ ($PGF_{2\alpha}$); treatment of acyclicity (true anoestrus) in cows and heifers; treatment of non-observed oestrus in cows. The oestradiol ester is a weak luteolysin. One device should be inserted into the vagina and left *in situ* for up to 12 days, with $PGF_{2\alpha}$ administered 24 hours before removal. Oestrus occurs 2–5 days after withdrawal.

Intravaginal progesterone release device (EASI-BREED 'CIDR' Animal Reproductive Technologies Ltd, Leominster). Each device contains 1.9 g progesterone, which should be left in place for 7–12 days with $PGF_{2\alpha}$ treatment at the time of removal. Same indications as for PRID.

Progesterone in oil ('progesterone injection', Intervet UK Ltd, Cambridge). Used to suppress cyclical activity but requires injection i.m. daily, and to prevent pregnancy failure due to endogenous progesterone deficiency; the latter is of doubtful value.

Dose rate: cow, 100 mg per day; bitch, 2–3 mg/kg per day; cat, 2.5–5 mg every 3 days.

2. Synthetic progestogens

Commercially available products

Allyltrenbolone ('Regumate Equine', Hoechst Animal Health, Milton Keynes). A liquid in-feed substance containing 2.2 mg of allyltrenbolone per 1 ml. Used to suppress cyclical activity where this may cause managemental or behavioural problems, to control timing of oestrus to meet the availability of the stallion, to induce cyclical activity in the breeding season. Dose rate of 27.5 or 33 mg in the feed as a single dose per day for 10 or 15 consecutive days. Oestrus occurs within 8 days of last dose and ovulation after 7–13 days.

Altrenogest ('Regumate Porcine', Hoechst Animal Health, Milton Keynes). A liquid in-feed suspension which is placed on the food as a top dressing when gilts are eating, so that it is immediately consumed. It is used to synchronize oestrus in sexually mature, and therefore cyclical gilts, by administering the suspension for 18 consecutive days. Oestrus occurs 2–3 days after cessation of treatment. Dose rate of 20 mg (5 ml) per day.

Norgestamet ('Crestar', Intervet UK Ltd, Cambridge). An implant, containing 3 mg of the synthetic progestogen norgestamet, which is inserted beneath the outer surface of the ear using a special applicator. In addition, for oestrous synchronization, there is a fluid containing 3 mg of norgestamet and 5 mg of oestradiol benzoate per 2 ml for intramuscular injection. The implant can be removed either by withdrawing it along the injection tract or preferably, by making a very small incision with a stylus over the distal end of the implant and expressing it by gentle squeezing with thumb and forefinger. The product must only be used in beef animals in which milk is not used for human consumption or dairy heifers. For the synchronization of oestrus, the implant is inserted on day 0 and followed immediately with the intramuscular injection. On day 9, the implant is removed and, if the animals were acyclical at the time of the implant insertion, an injection of eCG should be given. The dose rate will vary from 400 to 700 IU. Animals can be inseminated at observed oestrus or at a fixed time. Beef heifers should be inseminated at 48 hours and nursing cows at 56

hours after implant removal; alternatively the latter group can be inseminated twice at 48 and 72 hours.

Fluorogestone acetate intravaginal sponges ('Chronogest', Intervet UK Ltd, Cambridge). Medroxyprogesterone acetate intravaginal sponges ('Veramix' and 'Veramix Plus', Upjohn Ltd, Crawley). Used to synchronize ewes and female goats or, in conjunction with eCG (PMSG) injections, to advance the time of onset of the breeding season by up to 6 weeks. Dose rate: each ewe receives a single sponge inserted into the anterior vagina where it should remain 12–14 days before withdrawal, oestrus occurs 48–72 hours later. When the breeding season is being advanced, eCG is normally given at the time of sponge removal or just before. At least one ram per 10 ewes should be available.

Medroxyprogesterone acetate tablets ('Perlutex tablets', Leo Laboratories Ltd, Aylesbury). Used to interrupt oestrus in bitches and queen cats when pro-oestrus is observed and to postpone oestrus for a long period following treatment during anoestrus. Dose rate: bitch (interruption of oestrus), 10–20 mg daily for 4 days from the first sign of pro-oestral bleeding followed by 5–10 mg daily for 12 days; bitch (postponement of oestrus), 5–10 mg daily for as long as postponement is required; queen cat (interruption of oestrus), 2.5 mg per day for as long as is required; the same regime and dose rate are recommended for postponement.

Medroxyprogesterone acetate injection ('Perlutex for Injection', Leo Laboratories Ltd, Aylesbury; 'Promone-E', Upjohn Ltd, Crawley). Used for prevention of oestrus in bitches and prostatic hyperplasia in dogs. Dose rate: bitches (prevention of oestrus), 50–150 mg s.c. in anoestrus; dog (prostatic hyperplasia), 50–100 mg s.c. every 3–6 months.

Megoestrol acetate tablets ('Ovarid', Mallinckrodt Veterinary, Harefield). Used for the interruption of oestrus in bitches and queen cats when given at the first signs of pro-oestrus or the postponement of oestrus when given during anoestrus. Dose rates: bitch (interruption of oestrus), 2 mg/kg daily for 8 days; postponement of oestrus, 0.5 mg/kg daily for up to 40 days and then, if required, at a dose of 0.1 to 0.2 mg/kg twice weekly for not more than 4 months; queen cats (interruption of oestrus), 5 mg per day for 3 days commencing at the first signs of pro-oestrus/oestrus; postponement of oestrus, 2.5 mg per day.

Proligestone injection ('Covinan', Intervet UK Ltd, Cambridge; 'Delvosteron', Mycofarm UK Ltd, Cambridge). Used to interrupt and postpone oestrus in the bitch and queen cat. Dose rate: bitch (interruption of oestrus), 100–600 mg by s.c. injection at the first signs of pro-oestrus. The same dose rate can be given when the bitch is anoestrus to temporarily postpone oestrus, or at 3, 4 and then 5-monthly intervals to postpone oestrus for a longer period of time. Queen cat, 100 mg by s.c. injection at the first signs of pro-oestrus or oestrus; postponement involves a similar injection regimen to that described for the bitch.

Progestogens in bitches and queen cats are not without dangers, since they predispose to pyometra and should be used with utmost caution in those individuals that are subsequently intended for breeding.

Androgens
Testosterone is the principal circulating androgen in the male being produced by the interstitial cells of the testis. As well as being responsible for the secondary sex characteristics, it is also involved in spermatogenesis. Androgens, either naturally occurring or synthetic analogues, have limited application in animal reproduction or disease.

Commercially available preparations
Methyltestosterone tablets ('Orandrone', Intervet UK Ltd, Cambridge).

Testosterone phenylpropionate injection ('Andro-ject', Intervet UK Ltd, Cambridge).

Testosterone esters injection ('Durateston', Intervet UK Ltd, Cambridge).

Pharmacological actions
Since testosterone is involved in controlling libido in the male it is used to improve any deficiency that might be present, although it must be stressed that libido and sexual behaviour are complex and not just a reflection of endogenous androgens; therefore, the results of such therapy will usually be disappointing. Androgens have anabolic effects and can be used to treat debilitated animals. They

have been used to postpone oestrus in bitches and overcome some of the behavioural problems associated with pseudopregnancy in bitches.

Dose rate
These should be checked for each product and each species.

Combined androgens and oestrogens
Commercially available preparations
Ethinyloestradiol and methyltestosterone tablets ('Sesoral', Intervet UK Ltd, Cambridge). Used to control overt pseudopregnancy in bitches.

Prostaglandins and prostaglandin analogues
Only $PGF_{2\alpha}$ and synthetic analogues are available commercially for use in domestic species.

Commercially available products
Dinoprost ('Lutalyse', Upjohn Ltd, Crawley). For use in cattle, sheep, pigs, horses, goats and dogs.

Cloprostenol ('Estrumate' and 'Planate', Mallinckrodt Veterinary, Harefield). For use in cattle, sheep, pigs, horses and goats.

Luprostiol ('Prosolvin', Intervet UK Ltd, Cambridge). For use in cattle, sheep, pigs, horses and goats.

Tiaprost ('Iliren', Hoechst Animal Health, Milton Keynes). For use in pigs.

Pharmacological activity
$PGF_{2\alpha}$ and analogues are potent luteolytic agents except in the bitch and cat. They play a role in ovulation, parturition and gamete transport, in the latter two by virtue of their effect on the smooth muscle of the genital tract. They have a short biological half-life because 90% of prostaglandins are metabolized at one passage through the pulmonary circulation.

Indications
Cattle: synchronization of oestrus in cow and heifers;
    treatment of non-visible oestrus;
    induction of calving;

inducing abortion and expulsion of mummified calves;
treatment of pyometra;
treatment of endometritis;
treatment of luteal (luteinized) cysts.

Horse: inducing abortion before 35 days;
treatment of prolonged dioestrus;
induction of foaling;
hasten return to oestrus if service is missed;
hasten return to oestrus after the foal heat;
planning the time of oestrus for efficient use of stallion.

Sheep: synchronization of oestrus;
inducing abortion.

Pig: induction of farrowing.

Dog: treatment of open pyometra in the bitch (only dinoprost, use with care).

Dose rates

Dinoprost. Cattle, 25–35 mg; horse, 5 mg; pig, 10 mg; sheep, 6–8 mg; dog, 0.25–0.5 mg/kg. All i.m.
Cloprostenol. Cattle, 500 g; horse, 12.5–500 g; sheep and goats, 125–250 g; pig, 350 g. All i.m.
Tiaprost. Pig, 300–600 mg.
Luprostiol. Cattle, 15 mg; horse, 7.5 mg; sheep and goats, 7.5 mg; pigs, 7.5 mg.

Anti-androgens

These are substances which counteract the behavioural actions of androgens.

Commercially available products

Delmadinone acetate ('Tardak', Pfizer Animal Health Ltd, Tadworth).

Indications

Dog: hypersexuality in the male dog; prostatic hyperplasia and prostatitis.

Dose rate

1.0–2.0 mg/kg body weight, s.c. or i.m.

Melatonin

Melatonin, an indoleamine, is produced by the pineal gland. Its level of secretion is influenced by the photoperiod, with reducing day-length stimulating, and increasing day-length inhibiting, its secretion. Melatonin modulates, either directly or indirectly, the frequency of GnRH secretion from the hypothalamus, thus influencing the secretion of gonadotrophins and cyclical ovarian activity.

Commercially available product

Melatonin implant ('Regulin', Hoechst Animal Health, Milton Keynes).

Indications

Advancing the onset of normal cyclical ovarian activity in pure and cross-bred lowland breeds of sheep so that early lambing occurs.

Dose rate and treatment regimen

One implant (18 mg of melatonin) per ewe inserted subcutaneously on the outer aspect of the base of the ear. The earliest time of use of implants is determined by the breed of the ewe; details should be checked against the manufacturer's instructions. It can also be used in goats. It is critical to ensure that ewes (and does) are out of sight, sound and smell of rams (and bucks) for at least 7 days before and at least 30 days after the implant is inserted.

Vaccines

Equine herpesvirus 1

'Pneumabort-K' (Willows Francis Veterinary, Crawley). Killed virus vaccine of equine herpesvirus 1 for use in healthy pregnant mares to prevent infection which might result in abortion, or in contact mares. Pregnant mares should be injected with a 2 ml dose i.m. during the fifth, seventh and ninth month of gestation together with in-contact maiden and barren mares.

Leptospira hardjo

'Leptavoid-H' (Mallinckrodt Veterinary, Harefield). Formol-killed cultures of *L. hardjo* for vaccination against this organism. Primary course of immunization involves two subcutaneous injections with an interval of at least 4 weeks before and not more than 6 weeks after the main season of the year for transmission of the disease. Thereafter, an annual booster can be given at about the same time of the year.

'Vaxall' (Webster Animal Health, Ickenham). An

adjuvanted vaccine containing inactivated cells of *L. hardjo*.

Bovine para-influenza virus (PI3)

'Imuresp' (Pfizer Animal Health Ltd, Tadworth). Freeze dried live virus strain of PI3 virus administered intranasally.

Infectious bovine rhinotracheitis (IBR)

'Tracherine', (Pfizer Animal Health Ltd, Tadworth). Freeze-dried live virus strains for intranasal administration.

'Inbovac' IBR (Intervet UK Ltd, Cambridge). A living avirulent strain given by intranasal or intramuscular injection.

Infectious bovine rhinotracheitis (IBR) and bovine para-influenza virus (PI3)

'Imuresp' (Pfizer Animal Health Ltd, Tadworth.) Combined virus vaccine.

Ovine enzootic abortion

Ovine enzootic abortion vaccine (Mallinckrodt Veterinary, Harefield). A 20% suspension of formalin-inactivated yolk-sac membranes infected with ovine *Chlamydia* strains A22 and S26/3 as a 50/50 mixture. 1 ml of the suspension s.c. before tupping and repeated after 3 years. May not prevent abortion in infected ewes.

Equine viral arteritis (EVA)

'Artervac' (Willows Francis Veterinary, Crawley). A killed vaccine is available in the UK, although in some other countries a modified live virus vaccine is available.

Index